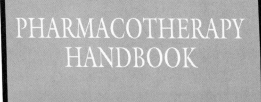

PHARMACOTHERAPY HANDBOOK

Sixth Edition

Barbara G. Wells, PharmD, FASHP, FCCP, BCPP
Dean and Professor
Executive Director, Research Institute of Pharmaceutical Sciences
School of Pharmacy, The University of Mississippi
Oxford, Mississippi

Joseph T. DiPiro, PharmD, FCCP
Professor and Executive Dean
South Carolina College of Pharmacy
Medical University of South Carolina, Charleston,
and University of South Carolina, Columbia

Terry L. Schwinghammer, PharmD, FCCP, FASHP, BCPS
Professor and Chair, Dept of Clinical Pharmacy
School of Pharmacy, West Virginia University
Morgantown, West Virginia

Cindy W. Hamilton, PharmD
Principal, Hamilton House
Virginia Beach, Virginia
Assistant Clinical Professor
Virginia Commonwealth University School of Pharmacy
Richmond, Virginia

McGraw-Hill
Medical Publishing Division

New York Chicago San Francisco Lisbon London Madrid
Mexico City Milan New Delhi San Juan Seoul
Singapore Sydney Toronto

Pharmacotherapy Handbook, Sixth Edition

Copyright © 2006 by The McGraw-Hill Companies, Inc. All rights reserved. Printed in the United States of America. Except as permitted under the United States Copyright Act of 1976, no part of this publication may be reproduced or distributed in any form or by any means, or stored in a data base or retrieval system, without the prior written permission of the publisher.

Previous edition copyright © 2003, 2000, by The McGraw-Hill Companies, Inc.; copyright © 1998 by Appleton & Lange.

1 2 3 4 5 6 7 8 9 0   DOC/DOC   0 9 8 7 6 5

ISBN 0-07-143322-8

This book was set in Times Roman by TechBooks, Inc.
The editors were Michael Brown and Christie Naglieri.
The Production Supervisor was Sherri Souffrance.
Project management was provided by TechBooks, Inc.
The cover designer was Elizabeth Pisacreta.
The index was prepared by Ron Prottsman.
RR Donnelley was the printer and binder.

Please tell the authors and publisher what you think of this book by sending your comments to *pharmacotherapy@mcgraw-hill.com*. Please put the author and title of the book in the subject line.

Cataloging-in-Publication Data for this book is on file at the Library of Congress.

International Edition ISBN 0-07-110503-4
Copyright © 2006. Exclusive rights by The McGraw-Hill Companies, Inc., for manufacture and export. This book cannot be re-exported from the country to which it is consigned by McGraw-Hill. The International Edition is not available in North America.

CONTENTS

BONE AND JOINT DISORDERS
Edited by Terry L. Schwinghammer

CARDIOVASCULAR DISORDERS
Edited by Terry L. Schwinghammer

DERMATOLOGIC DISORDERS
Edited by Terry L. Schwinghammer

ENDOCRINOLOGIC DISORDERS
Edited by Terry L. Schwinghammer

GASTROINTESTINAL DISORDERS
Edited by Joseph T. DiPiro

Contents

GYNECOLOGIC AND OBSTETRIC DISORDERS
Edited by Barbara G. Wells

HEMATOLOGIC DISORDERS
Edited by Cindy W. Hamilton

INFECTIOUS DISEASES
Edited by Joseph T. DiPiro

Contents

Contents

RENAL DISORDERS
Edited by Cindy W. Hamilton

RESPIRATORY DISORDERS
Edited by Terry L. Schwinghammer

UROLOGIC DISORDERS
Edited by Cindy W. Hamilton

APPENDICES
Edited by Barbara G. Wells

PREFACE

This sixth edition of the pocket companion to *Pharmacotherapy: A Pathophysiologic Approach,* sixth edition, is designed to provide practitioners and students with critical information that can be easily used to guide drug therapy decision making in the clinical setting. To ensure brevity and portability, the bulleted format provides the user with essential textual information, key tables and figures, and treatment algorithms. For the first time, the sixth edition is available in both print and PDA.

Corresponding to the major sections in the main text, disorders are alphabetized within the following sections, which appear as a tabbing guide on the back of the book: Bone and Joint Disorders; Cardiovascular Disorders; Dermatologic Disorders; Endocrinologic Disorders; Gastrointestinal Disorders; Gynecologic and Obstetric Disorders; Hematologic Disorders; Infectious Diseases; Neurologic Disorders; Nutritional Disorders; Oncologic Disorders; Ophthalmic Disorders; Psychiatric Disorders; Renal Disorders; Respiratory Disorders; and Urologic Disorders. Drug-induced conditions associated with allergic and pseudoallergic reactions, hematologic disorders, liver disease, pulmonary disorders, and renal disease appear in six tabular appendices. In the sixth edition, a chapter has been added on skin disorders and cutaneous drug eruptions.

Carrying over a popular feature from *Pharmacotherapy,* each chapter is organized in a consistent format:

- Disease state definition
- Concise review of relevant pathophysiology
- Clinical presentation
- Diagnosis
- Desired outcome
- Treatment
- Monitoring

The treatment section may include nonpharmacologic therapy, drug selection guidelines, dosing recommendations, adverse effects, pharmacokinetic considerations, and important drug-drug interactions. When more in-depth information is required, the reader is encouraged to refer to the primary text, *Pharmacotherapy: A Pathophysiologic Approach,* sixth edition.

It is our sincere hope that students and practitioners find this book helpful as they continuously strive to deliver the highest quality care to patients. We invite your comments on how we may improve subsequent editions of this work.

Barbara G. Wells
Joseph T. DiPiro
Terry L. Schwinghammer
Cindy W. Hamilton

Please provide your comments about this book, Wells et al., *Pharmacotherapy Handbook,* sixth edition, to its Authors and Publisher by writing to pharmacotherapy@mcgraw-hill.com. Please indicate the author and title of this handbook in the subject line of your e-mail.

ACKNOWLEDGMENTS

The editors wish to express their sincere appreciation to the authors whose chapters in the sixth edition of *Pharmacotherapy: A Pathophysiologic Approach* served as the basis for this book. The dedication and professionalism of these outstanding practitioners, teachers, and clinical scientists are evident on every page of this work. The authors of the chapters from the sixth edition are acknowledged at the end of each respective *Handbook* chapter. We also wish to thank our spouses, Richard Wells, Cecily DiPiro, Donna Schwinghammer, and Raleigh Hamilton, for their love, encouragement, and patience.

Basic and clinical research provides a continuous flow of biomedical information that enables practitioners to use medications more effectively and safely. The editors, authors, and publisher of this book have made every effort to ensure accuracy of information provided. However, it is the responsibility of all practitioners to assess the appropriateness of published drug therapy information, especially in light of the specific clinical situation and new developments in the field. The editors and authors have taken care to recommend dosages that are consistent with current published guidelines and other responsible literature. However, when dealing with new and unfamiliar drug therapies, students and practitioners should consult several appropriate information sources.

Bone and Joint Disorders
Edited by Terry L. Schwinghammer

Chapter 1

▶ GOUT AND HYPERURICEMIA

▶ DEFINITIONS

- The term *gout* describes a disease spectrum including hyperuricemia, recurrent attacks of acute arthritis associated with monosodium urate crystals in leukocytes found in synovial fluid, deposits of monosodium urate crystals in tissues (tophi), interstitial renal disease, and uric acid nephrolithiasis.
- Hyperuricemia may be an asymptomatic condition, with an increased serum uric acid concentration as the only apparent abnormality. A urate concentration greater than 7.0 mg/dL is abnormal and associated with an increased risk for gout.

▶ PATHOPHYSIOLOGY

- In humans, uric acid is the end product of the degradation of purines. It serves no known physiologic purpose and therefore is regarded as a waste product. The size of the urate pool is increased severalfold in individuals with gout. This excess accumulation may result from either overproduction or underexcretion.
- The purines from which uric acid is produced originate from three sources: dietary purine, conversion of tissue nucleic acid to purine nucleotides, and de novo synthesis of purine bases.
- Abnormalities in the enzyme systems that regulate purine metabolism may result in overproduction of uric acid. An increase in the activity of phosphoribosyl pyrophosphate (PRPP) synthetase leads to an increased concentration of PRPP, a key determinant of purine synthesis and thus uric acid production. A deficiency of hypoxanthine–guanine phosphoribosyl transferase (HGPRT) may also result in overproduction of uric acid. HGPRT is responsible for the conversion of guanine to guanylic acid and hypoxanthine to inosinic acid. These two conversions require PRPP as the cosubstrate and are important re-utilization reactions involved in the synthesis of nucleic acids. A deficiency in the HGPRT enzyme leads to increased metabolism of guanine and hypoxanthine to uric acid and more PRPP to interact with glutamine in the first step of the purine pathway. Complete absence of HGPRT results in the childhood Lesch–Nyhan syndrome, characterized by choreoathetosis, spasticity, mental retardation, and markedly excessive production of uric acid.
- Uric acid may also be overproduced as a consequence of increased breakdown of tissue nucleic acids, as with myeloproliferative and lymphoproliferative disorders.
- Dietary purines play an unimportant role in the generation of hyperuricemia in the absence of some derangement in purine metabolism or elimination.
- About two thirds of the uric acid produced each day is excreted in the urine. The remainder is eliminated through the gastrointestinal tract after enzymatic degradation by colonic bacteria. A decline in the urinary excretion of uric acid to a level below the rate of production leads to hyperuricemia and an increased miscible pool of sodium urate.
- Drugs that decrease renal clearance of uric acid through modification of filtered load or one of the tubular transport processes include diuretics, salicylates (less

than 2 g/day), pyrazinamide, ethambutol, nicotinic acid, ethanol, levodopa, cyclosporine, and cytotoxic drugs.

- Normal individuals produce 600 to 800 mg of uric acid daily and excrete less than 600 mg in urine. Individuals who excrete more than 600 mg after being on a purine-free diet for 3 to 5 days are considered overproducers. Hyperuricemic individuals who excrete less than 600 mg of uric acid per 24 hours on a purine-free diet are defined as underexcretors of uric acid. On a regular diet, excretion of more than 1000 mg per 24 hours reflects overproduction; less than this is probably normal.

- Deposition of urate crystals in synovial fluid results in an inflammatory process involving chemical mediators that cause vasodilation, increased vascular permeability, and chemotactic activity for polymorphonuclear leukocytes. Phagocytosis of urate crystals by the leukocytes results in rapid lysis of cells and a discharge of proteolytic enzymes into the cytoplasm. The inflammatory reaction that ensues is associated with intense joint pain, erythema, warmth, and swelling.

- Uric acid nephrolithiasis occurs in 10% to 25% of patients with gout. Factors that predispose individuals to uric acid nephrolithiasis include excessive urinary excretion of uric acid, acidic urine, and highly concentrated urine.

- In acute uric acid nephropathy, acute renal failure occurs as a result of blockage of urine flow secondary to massive precipitation of uric acid crystals in the collecting ducts and ureters. This syndrome is a well-recognized complication in patients with myeloproliferative or lymphoproliferative disorders and results from massive malignant cell turnover, particularly after initiation of chemotherapy. Chronic urate nephropathy is caused by the long-term deposition of urate crystals in the renal parenchyma.

- Tophi (urate deposits) are uncommon in gouty subjects and are a late complication of hyperuricemia. The most common sites of tophaceous deposits in patients with recurrent acute gouty arthritis are the base of the great toe, the helix of the ear, olecranon bursae, Achilles tendon, knees, wrists, and hands.

▶ CLINICAL PRESENTATION

- Acute attacks of gouty arthritis are characterized by rapid onset of excruciating pain, swelling, and inflammation. The attack is typically monoarticular at first, most often affecting the first metatarsophalangeal joint (podagra), and then, in order of frequency, the insteps, ankles, heels, knees, wrists, fingers, and elbows. Attacks commonly begin at night, with the patient awakening from sleep with excruciating pain. The affected joints are erythematous, warm, and swollen. Fever and leukocytosis are common. Untreated attacks may last from 3 to 14 days before spontaneous recovery.

- Although acute attacks of gouty arthritis may occur without apparent provocation, attacks may be precipitated by stress, trauma, alcohol ingestion, infection, surgery, rapid lowering of serum uric acid by ingestion of uric acid–lowering agents, and ingestion of certain drugs known to elevate serum uric acid concentrations.

▶ DIAGNOSIS

- The definitive diagnosis is accomplished by aspiration of synovial fluid from the affected joint and identification of intracellular crystals of monosodium urate monohydrate in synovial fluid leukocytes.

- When joint aspiration is not a viable option, a presumptive diagnosis of acute gouty arthritis may be made on the basis of the presence of the characteristic signs and symptoms, as well as the response to treatment.

▶ DESIRED OUTCOME

The goals in the treatment of gout are to terminate the acute attack, prevent recurrent attacks of gouty arthritis, and prevent complications associated with chronic deposition of urate crystals in tissues.

▶ TREATMENT

ACUTE GOUTY ARTHRITIS

Nonpharmacologic Therapy
- Patients may be advised to reduce their intake of foods high in purines (e.g., organ meats), avoid alcohol, and lose weight if obese.

Indomethacin
- **Indomethacin** is as effective as colchicine in the treatment of acute gouty arthritis and is preferred because acute gastrointestinal toxicity occurs far less frequently than with colchicine (Figure 1–1). Begin treatment with a relatively large dose for the first 24 to 48 hours and then taper the dose over 3 to 4 days to minimize the risk of recurrent attacks. For example, 75 mg of indomethacin may be given initially, followed by 50 mg every 6 hours for 2 days, then 50 mg every 8 hours for 1 or 2 days.
- Side effects unique to indomethacin include headache and dizziness. All non-steroidal anti-inflammatory drugs (NSAIDs) have been implicated in causing gastric ulceration and bleeding, but this is unlikely with short-term therapy.

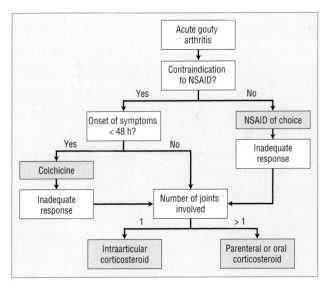

Figure 1–1. Treatment algorithm for acute gouty arthritis.

TABLE 1–1. Dosage Regimens of Nonsteroidal Anti-inflammatory Drugs (NSAIDs) for Treatment of Acute Gouty Arthritis

Generic (Brand) Name	Dosage and Frequency
Fenoprofen (Nalfon)	800 mg q 6 h
Flurbiprofen (Ansaid)	100 mg q.i.d for 1 day, then 50 mg q.i.d
Ibuprofen (Motrin)	600–800 mg q.i.d
Ketoprofen (Orudis)	50 mg q.i.d or 75 mg t.i.d
Meclofenamate (Meclomen)	100 mg t.i.d–q.i.d
Naproxen (Naprosyn)	750 mg initially, then 250 mg q 8 h
Piroxicam (Feldene)	40 mg/day
Sulindac (Clinoril)	200 mg b.i.d
Tolmetin (Tolectin)	400 mg t.i.d–q.i.d

Other NSAIDs
- Other NSAIDs are also effective in relieving the inflammation of acute gout (Table 1–1). NSAIDs should be used with caution in individuals with a history of peptic ulcer disease, heart failure, chronic kidney disease, or coronary artery disease.

Colchicine
- **Colchicine** is usually given in an oral dose of 1 mg initially, followed by 0.5 mg every 2 hours until the joint symptoms subside, the patient develops abdominal discomfort or diarrhea, or a total dose of 8 mg has been given. About 75% to 90% of patients with acute gouty arthritis respond favorably to colchicine when treatment is begun within 24 to 48 hours of the onset of joint symptoms. The major problem associated with oral colchicine is that gastrointestinal (GI) toxicity occurs in 50% to 80% of patients before relief of the attack.
- This high incidence of GI toxicity may be circumvented by administering colchicine intravenously. The initial intravenous (IV) dose is 2 mg (if renal function is normal). If relief is not obtained, an additional 1-mg dose may be given at 6 and 12 hours to a total dose of 4 mg for a specific attack. Colchicine should be diluted with 20 mL of normal saline before administration to minimize sclerosis of the vein. Local extravasation of IV colchicine can cause inflammation and necrosis of surrounding tissue. Very small, difficult-to-inject veins and renal impairment are relative contraindications to IV colchicine therapy. IV colchicine should not be used in individuals who are neutropenic, have severe renal impairment (creatinine clearance less than 10 mL/min), or have combined renal and hepatic insufficiency.
- Colchicine should be discontinued within 7 days after either IV or oral therapy to reduce the risk of bone marrow toxicity. The dose should be reduced by 50% in patients with creatinine clearances between 10 and 50 mL/min and limited to a total dose of 2 mg in those receiving oral maintenance colchicine.

Corticosteroids
- Corticosteroids may be used to treat acute attacks of gouty arthritis, but they are reserved primarily for resistant cases or for patients with contraindications to colchicine and NSAID therapy.
- **Prednisone,** 30 to 60 mg orally once daily for 3 to 5 days, may be used in patients with multiple-joint involvement. Because rebound attacks may occur

upon steroid withdrawal, the dose should be gradually tapered in 5-mg increments over 10 to 14 days and discontinued.
- **Adrenocorticotropic hormone (ACTH)** gel, 40 to 80 USP units, may be given intramuscularly every 6 to 8 hours for 2 to 3 days and then reduced in stepwise fashion and discontinued.
- **Triamcinolone hexacetonide,** 20 to 40 mg given intra-articularly, may be useful for acute gout limited to one or two joints.

PROPHYLACTIC THERAPY
General Approach
- If the first episode of acute gouty arthritis was mild and responded promptly to treatment, the patient's serum urate concentration was only minimally elevated, and the 24-hour urinary uric acid excretion was not excessive (less than 1000 mg/24 h on a regular diet), then prophylactic treatment can be withheld.
- If the patient had a severe attack of gouty arthritis, a complicated course of uric acid lithiasis, a substantially elevated serum uric acid (greater than 10 mg/dL), or a 24-hour urinary excretion of uric acid of more than 1000 mg, then prophylactic treatment should be instituted immediately after resolution of the acute episode.
- Prophylactic therapy is also appropriate for patients with frequent attacks of gouty arthritis (i.e., more than two or three per year) even if the serum uric acid concentration is normal or only minimally elevated.

Colchicine
- **Colchicine** given in low oral doses (0.5 to 0.6 mg twice daily) may be effective in preventing recurrent arthritis in patients with no evidence of visible tophi and a normal or slightly elevated serum urate concentration. Treated patients who sense the onset of an acute attack should increase the dose to 1 mg every 2 hours; in most instances, the attack aborts after 1 or 2 mg.

Uric Acid Lowering Therapy
- Patients with a history of recurrent acute gouty arthritis and a significantly elevated serum uric acid concentration are probably best managed with uric acid lowering therapy.
- **Colchicine,** 0.5 mg twice daily, should be administered during the first 6 to 12 months of antihyperuricemic therapy to minimize the risk of acute attacks that may occur during initiation of uric acid lowering therapy.
- The therapeutic objective of antihyperuricemic therapy is to reduce the serum urate concentration below 6 mg/dL, well below the saturation point.

Uricosuric Drugs
- **Probenecid** and **sulfinpyrazone** increase the renal clearance of uric acid by inhibiting the renal tubular reabsorption of uric acid. Therapy with uricosuric drugs should be started at a low dose to avoid marked uricosuria and possible stone formation. Maintenance of adequate urine flow and alkalinization of the urine with sodium bicarbonate or Shohl's solution during the first several days of uricosuric therapy further diminish the possibility of uric acid stone formation.
- Probenecid is given initially at a dose of 250 mg twice daily for 1 to 2 weeks, then 500 mg twice daily for 2 weeks. Thereafter, the daily dose is increased by 500-mg increments every 1 to 2 weeks until satisfactory control is achieved or a maximum dose of 2 g/day is reached.

- The initial dose of sulfinpyrazone is 50 mg twice daily for 3 to 4 days, then 100 mg twice daily, increasing the daily dose by 100-mg increments each week up to 800 mg/day.
- The major side effects associated with uricosuric therapy are GI irritation, rash and hypersensitivity, precipitation of acute gouty arthritis, and stone formation. These drugs are contraindicated in patients who are allergic to them and in patients with impaired renal function (creatinine clearance less than 50 mL/min) or a history of renal calculi, and in patients who are overproducers of uric acid.

Xanthine Oxidase Inhibitor

- **Allopurinol** and its major metabolite, oxypurinol, are xanthine oxidase inhibitors and impair the conversion of hypoxanthine to xanthine and xanthine to uric acid. Allopurinol also lowers the intracellular concentration of PRPP. Because of the long half-life of its metabolite, allopurinol can be given once daily. An oral daily dose of 300 mg is usually sufficient. Occasionally, as much as 600 to 800 mg/day may be necessary.
- Allopurinol is the antihyperuricemic drug of choice in patients with a history of urinary stones or impaired renal function, in patients who have lymphoproliferative or myeloproliferative disorders and need pretreatment with a xanthine oxidase inhibitor before initiation of cytotoxic therapy to protect against acute uric acid nephropathy, and in patients with gout who are overproducers of uric acid.
- The major side effects of allopurinol are skin rash, leukopenia, occasional GI toxicity, and increased frequency of acute gouty attacks with the initiation of therapy. An allopurinol hypersensitivity syndrome characterized by fever, eosinophilia, dermatitis, vasculitis, and renal and hepatic dysfunction occurs rarely but is associated with a 20% mortality rate.

▶ EVALUATION OF THERAPEUTIC OUTCOMES

- Patients should be monitored for symptomatic relief of joint pain as well as potential adverse effects and drug interactions related to drug therapy. The acute pain of an initial attack of gouty arthritis should begin to ease within about 8 hours of treatment initiation. Complete resolution of pain, erythema, and inflammation usually occurs within 48 to 72 hours.

See Chapter 13, Gout and Hyperuricemia, authored by David W. Hawkins and Daniel W. Rahn, for a more detailed discussion of this topic.

Chapter 2

▶ OSTEOARTHRITIS

▶ DEFINITION

Osteoarthritis (OA) is a common, slowly progressive disorder affecting primarily the weight-bearing diarthrodial joints of the peripheral and axial skeleton. It is characterized by progressive deterioration and loss of articular cartilage resulting in osteophyte formation, pain, limitation of motion, deformity, and progressive disability. Inflammation may or may not be present in the affected joints.

▶ PATHOPHYSIOLOGY

- Early in OA, cartilage water content increases, possibly as a result of a damaged collagen network that is unable to constrain proteoglycans, which subsequently gain water. As OA progresses, cartilage proteoglycan content decreases, possibly through the action of metalloproteinases.
- Changes in glycosaminoglycan composition also occur, with decreased keratan sulfate and an increased ratio of chondroitin 4-sulfate to chondroitin 6-sulfate. These changes may interfere with proper collagen-proteoglycan interaction in cartilage. The collagen content does not appear to change until severe disease is present. Increases in collagen synthesis and altered distribution and diameter of the fibers are seen.
- Enhanced metabolic activity characterized by increased matrix synthesis controlled by chondrocytes suggests a reparative response to damage. However, there continues to be a loss of proteoglycan, reflecting a net loss as degradation proceeds faster than synthesis.
- The subchondral bone adjacent to articular cartilage also undergoes more rapid bone turnover, with increases in both osteoclast and osteoblast activity. There is associated release of vasoactive peptides and matrix metalloproteinases, neovascularization, and subsequent increased permeability of the adjacent cartilage. This sequence of events leads to continued cartilage degradation and eventually cartilage loss, resulting in painful, deformed joints.
- Fibrillation, a splitting of the noncalcified cartilage, exposes the underlying bone, which may ultimately lead to microfractures of the subchondral bone. With continued progression, cartilage is eroded completely, leaving denuded subchondral bone that becomes dense, smooth, and glistening (eburnation).
- Microfractures result in the production of callus and osteoid. New bone (osteophytes) forms at the joint margins, away from the area of cartilage destruction. Osteophytes may be an attempt to stabilize joints rather than a destructive aspect of OA.
- Inflammation, noted clinically as synovitis, occurs and may result from release of inflammatory mediators such as prostaglandins from chondrocytes.

▶ CLINICAL PRESENTATION

- The prevalence and severity of OA increase with age. Potential risk factors include obesity, repetitive use through work or leisure activities, joint trauma, and heredity.
- The clinical presentation depends on duration and severity of disease and the number of joints affected. The predominant symptom is a localized deep, aching pain associated with the affected joint. Early in OA, pain accompanies

joint activity and decreases with rest. With progression, pain occurs with minimal activity or at rest.

- Joints most commonly affected are the distal and proximal interphalangeal (DIP and PIP) joints of the hand, the first carpometacarpal (CMC) joint, knees, hips, cervical and lumbar spine, and the first metatarsophalangeal (MTP) joint of the toe.
- In addition to pain, limitation of motion, stiffness, crepitus, and deformities may occur. Patients with lower extremity involvement may report a sense of weakness or instability.
- Upon arising, joint stiffness typically lasts less than 30 minutes and resolves with motion. Joint enlargement is related to bony proliferation or to thickening of the synovium and joint capsule. The presence of a warm, red, and tender joint may suggest an inflammatory synovitis.
- Joint deformity may be present in the later stages as a result of subluxation, collapse of subchondral bone, formation of bone cysts, or bony overgrowths.
- Physical examination of the affected joints reveals tenderness, crepitus, and possible joint enlargement. Heberden's and Bouchard's nodes are bony enlargements (osteophytes) of the DIP and PIP joints, respectively.

▶ DIAGNOSIS

- The diagnosis of OA is dependent on patient history, clinical examination of the affected joint(s), and radiologic findings.
- *Primary (idiopathic) OA*, the most common type, has no known cause. Subclasses of primary OA are *localized OA* (involving one or two sites) and *generalized OA* (affecting three or more sites. The term *erosive OA* indicates the presence of erosion and marked proliferation in the proximal and distal interphalangeal hand joints.
- *Secondary OA* is associated with a known cause such as rheumatoid arthritis or another inflammatory arthritis, trauma, metabolic or endocrine disorders, and congenital factors.
- Criteria for the classification of OA of the hips, knees, and hands were developed by the American College of Rheumatology (ACR). The criteria include the presence of pain, bony changes on examination, a normal erythrocyte sedimentation rate (ESR), and characteristic radiographs.
  - For hip OA, a patient must have hip pain and two of the following: (1) an ESR less than 20 mm/h, (2) radiographic femoral or acetabular osteophytes, or (3) radiographic joint space narrowing.
  - For knee OA, a patient must have knee pain and radiographic osteophytes in addition to one of the following: (1) age greater than 50 years, (2) morning stiffness of 30 minutes' or less duration, or (3) crepitus on motion.
- Radiologic evaluation is necessary for the accurate diagnosis of OA. Radiographic changes are often absent in early, mild OA. With disease progression and loss of cartilage, there may be joint space narrowing, subchondral bony sclerosis, and development of marginal osteophyte and cysts. In late OA, subluxation and deformity may be apparent. Osteopenia and joint erosions are uncommon except in erosive OA.
- Joint arthroscopic examination can confirm the diagnosis or establish the extent of OA present in a particular joint but is rarely needed.
- No specific clinical laboratory abnormalities occur in primary OA. The ESR may be slightly elevated in patients with generalized or erosive inflammatory OA. The rheumatoid factor test is negative. Analysis of the synovial fluid

reveals fluid with high viscosity. This fluid demonstrates a mild leukocytosis (less than 2000 WBC/mm^3) with predominantly mononuclear cells.

▶ DESIRED OUTCOME

The major goals for the management of OA are to (1) educate the patient, care-givers, and relatives; (2) relieve pain and stiffness; (3) maintain or improve joint mobility; (4) limit functional impairment; and (5) maintain or improve quality of life.

▶ TREATMENT

NONPHARMACOLOGIC THERAPY

- The first step is to educate the patient about the extent of the disease, prognosis, and management approach. Dietary counseling for overweight OA patients is warranted.
- Physical therapy—with heat or cold treatments and an exercise program—helps to maintain and restore joint range of motion and reduce pain and muscle spasms. Exercise programs using isometric techniques are designed to strengthen muscles, improve joint function and motion, and decrease disability, pain, and the need for analgesic use.
- Assistive and orthotic devices such as canes, walkers, braces, heel cups, and insoles can be used during exercise or daily activities.
- Surgical procedures (e.g., osteotomy, joint debridement, osteophyte removal, partial or total arthroplasty, joint fusion) are indicated for patients with severe pain unresponsive to conservative therapy or pain that causes substantial functional disability and interference with lifestyle.

PHARMACOLOGIC THERAPY

General Approach

- Drug therapy in OA is targeted at relief of pain. Because OA often occurs in older individuals who have other medical conditions, a conservative approach to drug treatment is warranted.
- An individualized approach to treatment is necessary (Figure 2–1). For mild or moderate pain, topical analgesics or acetaminophen can be used. If these measures fail or if there is inflammation, nonsteroidal anti-inflammatory drugs (NSAIDs) may be useful. Appropriate nondrug therapies should be continued when drug therapy is initiated.

Acetaminophen

- **Acetaminophen** is recommended by the ACR as first-line drug therapy for pain management of OA. The dose is 325 to 650 mg four times daily (maximum dose 4 g/day). Comparable relief of mild to moderate OA pain has been demonstrated for acetaminophen (2.6 to 4 g/day) compared with aspirin (650 mg four times daily), ibuprofen (1200 or 2400 mg daily), naproxen (750 mg daily), and other NSAIDs. However, some patients respond better to NSAIDs.
- Acetaminophen is usually well tolerated, but potentially fatal hepatotoxicity with overdose is well documented. It should be used with caution in patients with liver disease and those who chronically abuse alcohol. Chronic alcohol users (three or more drinks daily) should be warned about an increased risk of liver damage or GI bleeding with acetaminophen. Other individuals do not appear to be at increased risk for GI bleeding. Renal toxicity occurs less frequently than with NSAIDs.

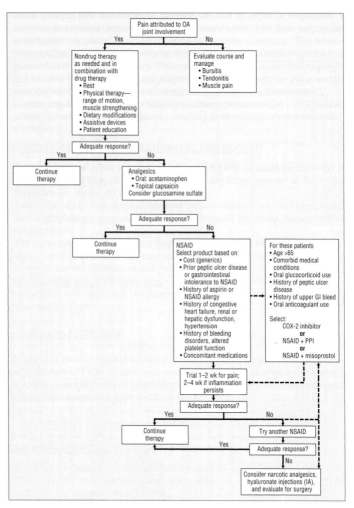

Figure 2–1. Treatment for osteoarthritis. NSAID, nonsteroidal anti-inflammatory drug; COX, cyclooxygenase; PPI, proton pump inhibitor; IA, intra-articular.

Nonsteroidal Anti-Inflammatory Drugs

- NSAIDs at prescription strength are often prescribed for OA patients after treatment with acetaminophen proves ineffective, or for patients with inflammatory OA. Analgesic effects begin within 1 to 2 hours, whereas anti-inflammatory benefits may require 2 to 3 weeks of continuous therapy.
- All NSAIDs have similar efficacy in reducing pain and inflammation in OA (Table 2–1), although individual patient response differs among NSAIDs.

TABLE 2–1. Medications Commonly Used in the Treatment of Osteoarthritis

Medication	Dosage and Frequency	Maximum Dosage (mg/day)
Oral analgesics		
Acetaminophen	325–650 mg every 4–6 h or 1 g 3–4 times/day	4000
Tramadol	50–100 mg every 4–6 h	400
Topical analgesics		
Capsaicin 0.025% or 0.075%	Apply to affected joint 3–4 times/day	—
Nutritional supplements		
Glucosamine sulfate	500 mg 3 times/day or 1500 mg once daily	1500
Nonsteroidal anti-inflammatory drugs (NSAIDs)		
Carboxylic acids		
Acetylated salicylates		
Aspirin, plain, buffered, or enteric-coated	325–650 mg every 4–6 h for pain; anti-inflammatory doses start at 3600 mg/day in divided doses	3600[a]
Nonacetylated salicylates		
Salsalate	500–1000 mg 2–3 times/day	3000[a]
Diflunisal	500–1000 mg 2 times/day	1500
Choline salicylate[b]	500–1000 mg 2–3 times/day	3000[a]
Choline magnesium salicylate	500–1000 mg 2–3 times/day	3000[a]
Acetic acids		
Etodolac	800–1200 mg/day in divided doses	1200
Diclofenac	100–150 mg/day in divided doses	200
Indomethacin	25 mg 2–3 times/day; 75 mg SR once daily	200; 150
Ketorolac[c]	10 mg every 4–6 h	40
Nabumetone[d]	500–1000 mg 1–2 times/day	2000
Propionic acids		
Fenoprofen	300–600 mg 3–4 times/day	3200
Flurbiprofen	200–300 mg/day in 2–4 divided doses	300
Ibuprofen	1200-3200 mg/day in 3–4 divided doses	3200
Ketoprofen	150–300 mg/day in 3–4 divided doses	300
Naproxen	250–500 mg twice a day	1500
Naproxen sodium	275–550 mg twice a day	1375
Oxaprozin	600–1200 mg daily	1800
Fenamates		
Meclofenamate	200–400 mg/day in 3–4 divided doses	400
Mefenamic acid[e]	250 mg every 6 h	1000
Oxicams		
Piroxicam	10–20 mg daily	20
Meloxicam	7.5 mg daily	15
Coxibs		
Celecoxib	100 mg twice daily or 200 mg daily	200 (400 for RA)
Valdecoxib	10 mg daily	10 (40 for dysmenorrheic pain)

[a]Monitor serum salicylate levels over 3–3.6 g/day.
[b]Only available as a liquid; 870 mg salicylate/5 mL.
[c]Not approved for treatment of OA for more than 5 days.
[d]Nonorganic acid but metabolite is an acetic acid.
[e]Not approved for treatment of OA.
RA, rheumatoid arthritis; SR, sustained-release.

- Selection of an NSAID depends on prescriber experience, medication cost, patient preference, toxicities, and adherence issues. An individual patient should be given a trial of one drug that is adequate in time (2 to 3 weeks) and dose. If the first NSAID fails, another agent in the same or another chemical class can be tried; this process may be repeated until an effective drug is found. Combining two NSAIDs increases adverse effects without providing additional benefit.
- COX-2 selective inhibitors (e.g., celecoxib, valdecoxib) demonstrate analgesic benefits that are similar to traditional nonselective NSAIDs. Although COX-2 selective inhibition was designed to reduce NSAID-induced gastropathy (e.g., ulcers, bleeding, perforation), concerns about adverse cardiovascular events (e.g., myocardial infarction, stroke) have led authorities to recommend their use only in selected patients who are at high risk for NSAID-related gastrointestinal effects and low risk for cardiovascular toxicity.
- Gastrointestinal complaints are the most common adverse effects of NSAIDs. Minor complaints such as nausea, dyspepsia, anorexia, abdominal pain, flatulence, and diarrhea occur in 10% to 60% of patients. NSAIDs should be taken with food or milk, except for enteric-coated products (milk or antacids may destroy the enteric coating and cause increased GI symptoms in some patients).
- All NSAIDs have the potential to cause gastric and duodenal ulcers and bleeding through direct (topical) or indirect (systemic) mechanisms. Risk factors for NSAID-associated ulcers and ulcer complications (perforation, gastric outlet obstruction, GI bleeding) include age more than 65 years, comorbid medical conditions (e.g., cardiovascular disease), concomitant corticosteroid or anticoagulant therapy, and history of peptic ulcer disease or upper GI bleeding.
- For OA patients who need an NSAID but are at high risk for GI complications, the ACR recommendations include either a COX-2 selective inhibitor or a nonselective NSAID in combination with either a proton pump inhibitor or misoprostol.
- NSAIDs may also cause renal complications, hepatitis, hypersensitivity reactions, rash, and central nervous system complaints of drowsiness, dizziness, headaches, depression, confusion, and tinnitus. All nonselective NSAIDs inhibit COX-1-dependent thromboxane production in platelets, thereby increasing bleeding risk. NSAIDs should be avoided in late pregnancy because of the risk of premature closure of the ductus arteriosus.
- The most potentially serious drug interactions include the concomitant use of NSAIDs with lithium, warfarin, oral hypoglycemics, high-dose methotrexate, antihypertensives, angiotensin-converting enzyme (ACE) inhibitors, β blockers, and diuretics.

Capsaicin
- **Capsaicin,** an extract of red peppers that causes release and ultimately depletion of substance P from nerve fibers, has been beneficial in providing pain relief in OA when applied topically over affected joints. It may be used alone or in combination with oral analgesics or NSAIDs.
- To be effective, capsaicin must be used regularly, and it may take up to 2 weeks to work. It is well tolerated, but some patients experience temporary burning or stinging at the site of application. Patients should be warned not to get the cream in their eyes or mouth and to wash their hands after application.
- Use is recommended 4 times daily, but tapering to twice-daily application may enhance long-term adherence with adequate pain relief.

Glucosamine and Chondroitin

- **Glucosamine** and **chondroitin** are dietary supplements that have been shown to be superior to placebo in alleviating pain from knee or hip OA in 17 double-blind, placebo-controlled studies. Use of the drugs has also been associated with slower loss of cartilage than placebo in knees affected by OA. A meta-analysis found that glucosamine reduced joint space narrowing.
- A follow-up survey completed 5 years after a 3-year study comparing glucosamine and placebo found that rates of lower limb joint replacement were twofold higher in subjects given placebo compared with subjects given glucosamine. Subjects treated with glucosamine also had lower rates of pain, joint space narrowing, and limitations of physical function. An ongoing study sponsored by the NIH should help to define the role of these supplements in the treatment of OA.

Corticosteroids

- Systemic corticosteroid therapy is not recommended in OA, given the lack of proven benefit and the well-known adverse effects with long-term use.
- Intra-articular corticosteroid injections can provide relief when local inflammation or joint effusion exists, but their long-term benefit remains controversial. Therapy is generally limited to 3 or 4 injections per year because of the potential systemic effects of the drugs and because the need for more frequent injections indicates poor response to therapy. After injection, the patient should minimize joint activity and stress on the joint for several days.

Hyaluronate Injections

- High-molecular-weight hyaluronic acid is a constituent of normal cartilage that provides lubrication with motion and shock absorbency during rapid movements. Because the concentration and molecular size of endogenous hyaluronic acid decreases in OA, exogenous administration has been studied in an attempt to reconstitute synovial fluid and reduce symptoms.
- Hyaluronic acid injections temporarily and modestly increase synovial fluid viscosity and were reported to decrease pain, but many studies were short term and poorly controlled with high placebo response rates.
- Two intra-articular agents containing hyaluronic acid are available for the treatment of pain associated with OA of the knee: **sodium hyaluronate** (Hyalgan) and **hylan G-F 20** (Synvisc). A treatment cycle consists of a 2-mL intra-articular injection into the affected knee once weekly for 3 (hylan G-F 20) or 5 (sodium hyaluronate) consecutive weeks.
- Injections are well tolerated, but acute joint swelling and local skin reactions (e.g., rash, ecchymoses, or pruritus) have been reported.
- These products may be beneficial for OA patients unresponsive to other therapy, but they are expensive because treatment includes both drug and administration costs.

Narcotic Analgesics

- Low-dose narcotic analgesics may be very useful in patients who experience no relief with acetaminophen, NSAIDs, intra-articular injections, or topical therapy.
- They are particularly useful in patients who cannot take NSAIDs because of renal failure, or for patients in whom all other treatment options have failed and who are at high surgical risk, precluding joint arthroplasty.
- Low-dose narcotics should be used initially, usually in combination with acetaminophen. Sustained-release compounds usually offer better pain control throughout the day and are used when simple narcotics are ineffective.

▶ EVALUATION OF THERAPEUTIC OUTCOMES

- To monitor efficacy, the patient's baseline pain can be assessed with a visual analog scale (VAS), and range of motion for affected joints can be assessed with flexion, extension, abduction, or adduction.
- Depending on the joint affected, measurement of grip strength and 50-feet walking time can help assess hand and hip/knee OA, respectively.
- Baseline radiographs can document the extent of joint involvement and follow disease progression with therapy.
- Other measures include the clinician's global assessment based on the patient's history of activities and limitations caused by OA, as well as documentation of analgesic or NSAID use.
- Disease-specific quality of life (QOL) questionnaires for arthritis are valuable for assessing clinical response to interventions.
- Patients should be asked if they are having adverse effects from their medications. They should also be monitored for any signs of drug-related effects, such as skin rash, headaches, drowsiness, weight gain, or hypertension from NSAIDs.
- Baseline serum creatinine, hematology profiles, and serum transaminases with repeat levels at 6- to 12-month intervals are useful in identifying specific toxicities to the kidney, liver, GI tract, or bone marrow.

See Chapter 90, Osteoarthritis, authored by Karen E. Hansen and Mary Elizabeth Elliott, for a more detailed discussion of this topic.

Chapter 3

▶ OSTEOPOROSIS

▶ DEFINITION

- Osteoporosis is characterized by low bone mass and deterioration of bone tissue leading to bone fragility and an increased fracture risk. The World Health Organization classifies bone mass on the basis of T scores. A T score is the number of standard deviations from the mean bone mineral density (BMD) for the young normal population. Normal bone mass is a T score greater than -1, osteopenia is a T score of -1 to -2.5, and osteoporosis is a T score less than -2.5.
- Three categories of osteoporosis have been described: (1) postmenopausal osteoporosis affects primarily trabecular bone in the decade after menopause, (2) age-related osteoporosis results from bone loss that begins shortly after peak bone mass is obtained and affects both cortical and trabecular bone, and (3) secondary osteoporosis is caused by certain medications and diseases and affects both types of bone.

▶ PATHOPHYSIOLOGY

- Estrogen deficiency increases bone resorption more than formation. Tumor necrosis factor and other cytokines stimulate osteoclastic activity. Reduced transforming growth factor β associated with estrogen loss also enhances osteoclast action.
- Age-related bone loss results from increased bone resorption. Increased osteocyte apoptosis may decrease responses to mechanical strain and hinder bone repair. Aging also increases fracture risk because of comorbid conditions, cognitive impairment, medications, deconditioning, inadequate calcium intake, and inadequate intake and absorption of vitamin D.
- The lower osteoporosis incidence in men may result from higher peak BMD, slower rate of bone loss after the peak, shorter life expectancy, fewer falls, and a more gradual cessation of hormone production.
- Drug-induced osteoporosis may result from systemic corticosteroids (prednisone doses greater than 7.5 mg/day), thyroid hormone replacement, some antiepileptic drugs (e.g., phenytoin, phenobarbital), and long-term heparin use (greater than 15,000 to 30,000 units daily for more than 3 to 6 months).

▶ CLINICAL PRESENTATION

- The usual presentation of osteoporosis is shortened stature, kyphosis, lordosis, bone pain, or a fracture, most commonly of a vertebra, hip, or forearm. Fractures can occur after bending, lifting, or falling or independent of any activity. Vertebral fractures are the most common, and multiple fractures may lead to dorsal kyphosis and exaggerated lordosis (referred to as *dowager's* or *widow's hump*). Collapsed vertebrae rarely lead to spinal cord compression. Chest wall changes can lead to pulmonary and cardiovascular complications.
- Acute fracture pain usually resolves in 2 to 3 months. Chronic fracture pain may be manifested as a deep, dull, nagging pain near the fracture site.

▶ DIAGNOSIS

- A patient history should be obtained to identify history of adult fractures, comorbidities, surgery, falls, and the presence of risk factors for osteoporosis.

- Genetic risk factors include Caucasian or Asian ethnicity, family history of osteoporosis or fractures, and small body frame (tall, thin, low body mass index).
- Lifestyle and dietary factors include sedentary lifestyle with minimal exercise, smoking, excessive alcohol ingestion, minimal sun exposure, low calcium intake at any time in life, lactose intolerance, high caffeine intake, high phosphorus intake, high animal protein intake, weight loss greater than 10% after age 50, and anorexia nervosa.
- Gynecologic factors include late menarche, surgical or early natural menopause, oophorectomy without estrogen replacement therapy, nulliparity, and amenorrhea.
- Chronic illnesses that may increase risk include hyperthyroidism, Cushing's syndrome, bone cancer, and type 1 diabetes mellitus.
- Medications increasing risk include corticosteroids, thyroid supplements, long-term high-dose heparin therapy, and anticonvulsants.
- A complete physical examination and laboratory analysis are needed to rule out secondary causes and to assess kyphosis and back pain. A complete blood count, chemistry panel (with calcium corrected for serum albumin level), erythrocyte sedimentation rate, parathyroid hormone (PTH) concentration, thyroid function tests, 25(OH) vitamin D, and 24-hour urine for calcium and creatinine may be obtained.
- Lateral spine radiographs may be done with new or severe back pain to detect vertebral fractures.
- Measurement of central (hip and spine) BMD with dual-energy x-ray absorptiometry (DXA) is the gold standard for osteoporosis diagnosis. For every 1 standard deviation (SD) below mean young adult BMD, the fracture risk increases about twofold. Measurement at peripheral sites (forearm, heel, and phalanges) with ultrasound or DXA is used only for screening purposes and to determine the need for further testing.
- Bone biopsy is rarely useful for osteoporosis but can rule out suspected secondary causes, such as osteomalacia.
- Biochemical markers of bone turnover are currently used only in clinical trials. Markers for bone resorption include C-terminal or N-terminal telopeptides and deoxypyridinoline. Bone formation markers include bone-specific alkaline phosphatase and osteocalcin.

▶ DESIRED OUTCOME

- The goal from birth to ages 20 to 30 years is to achieve the highest peak bone mass possible. Beyond this age, the goals are to maintain BMD and minimize age-related and postmenopausal bone loss.
- Prevention of osteoporosis is the goal in individuals with osteopenia.
- For patients with osteoporosis who are at risk of fractures, the aims are to increase BMD, prevent further bone loss, and prevent falls, fractures, and their complications.
- For those who experience an osteoporosis-related fracture, the goals are to achieve adequate pain control, maximize rehabilitation to restore independence and quality of life, and prevent subsequent fractures or death.

▶ PREVENTION AND TREATMENT

Figure 3–1 provides a management algorithm that incorporates both nonpharmacologic and pharmacologic approaches.

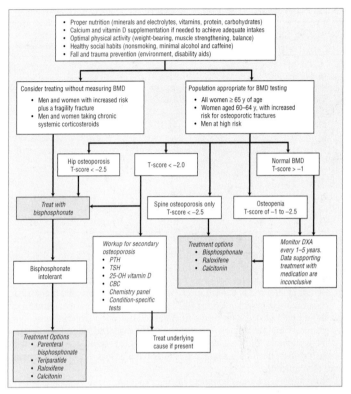

Figure 3–1. Bone Health Therapeutic Algorithm. BMD, bone mineral density; CBC, complete blood count; DXA, dual-energy x-ray absorptiometry; PTH, parathyroid hormone; TSH, thyroid-stimulating hormone.

NONPHARMACOLOGIC PREVENTION AND TREATMENT

- All individuals should have a balanced diet with adequate intake of **calcium** and **vitamin D** (Table 3–1). Table 3–2 lists dietary sources of calcium and vitamin D. If adequate dietary intake cannot be achieved, calcium supplements are necessary.
- Although 2 to 5 cups of coffee produce small increases in calcium excretion, this effect can be offset by increased calcium intake.
- Smoking cessation increases BMD, whereas continued smoking decreases BMD and increases fracture risk.
- Weight-bearing aerobic and strengthening exercises may prevent bone loss and decrease falls and fractures.

PHARMACOLOGIC PREVENTION AND TREATMENT

Antiresorptive Therapy
Calcium
- **Calcium** should be ingested in adequate amounts to prevent secondary hyperparathyroidism and bone destruction. Higher calcium intake has been shown to

TABLE 3–1. Daily Calcium and Vitamin D Requirements

	Adequate Calcium Intake (mg)	Adequate Vitamin D Intake (units)
Infant		
Birth to 6 months	210	200
6 months–1 yr	270	200
Children		
1–3 yr	500	200
4–8 yr	800	200
9–13 yr	1300	200
Adolescents		
14–18 yr	1300	200
Adults		
19–50 yr	1000	200
51–70 yr	1200	400
≥ 71 yr	1200	600

prevent or reduce bone loss in adults. Its effects are enhanced when combined with other antiresorptive therapies or exercise. The combination of calcium and vitamin D decreases nonvertebral, vertebral, and hip fractures.

- **Calcium carbonate** is the salt of choice because it contains the highest concentration of elemental calcium (40%) and is the least expensive (Table 3–3). It should be ingested with meals to enhance absorption from increased acid secretion. **Calcium citrate** absorption is acid independent and need not be taken with meals. Because the fraction of calcium absorbed decreases with increasing dose, maximum single doses of 600 mg or less of elemental calcium are recommended.
- Constipation is the most common adverse reaction; it can be treated with increased water intake, dietary fiber (given separately from calcium), and exercise. Calcium carbonate can create gas, sometimes causing flatulence or upset stomach.

Vitamin D and Metabolites
- **Vitamin D** deficiency results from insufficient intake, decreased sun exposure, decreased skin production, decreased liver and renal metabolism, and winter residence in northern climates.
- Supplemental vitamin D has been shown to increase BMD, and it may reduce fractures.
- Although the vitamin D intakes included in Table 3–1 are usually recommended, many experts feel that adult intake should be 800 to 1000 units daily.

Bisphosphonates
See Table 3–4.

- Bisphosphonates bind to hydroxyapatite in bone and decrease resorption by inhibiting osteoclast adherence to bone surfaces. The estimated terminal half-lives of bisphosphonates reflect the slow rates of bone turnover (many years).
- Of the antiresorptive agents available, bisphosphonates provide the greatest BMD increases and fracture risk reductions. The BMD increases range from 5% to 8% at the lumbar spine and 2% to 4% at the femoral neck. The risk of fracture is reduced by 45% to 55% at all skeletal sites: vertebral, nonvertebral, and hip.

TABLE 3–2. Dietary Sources of Calcium and Vitamin D[a]

Food	Serving Size	Calcium content (mg)	Vitamin D content (units)
Milk	1 cup	300	100
Powdered nonfat milk	1 teaspoon	50	
Ice cream	1 cup	200	
Yogurt, fortified	1 cup	240–415	60
American cheese	1 oz	150	
Cheddar cheese	1 oz	211	
Cottage cheese	1/2 cup	100	
Swiss cheese	1 oz	250	
Parmesan cheese	1 tablespoonful	70	
Cheese pizza	1 slice	150	
Macaroni and cheese	1 cup	360	
Slim Fast	11 oz	400	140
Orange juice, fortified	1 cup	350	100
Soymilk, fortified	1 cup	80–300	100
Bread, fortified	1 slice	100	
Cereals, fortified	1 cup	100–250	60
Sardines with bones	3 oz	370	230
Salmon with bones	3 oz	170–210	310
Catfish	3 oz		570
Halibut	3 oz		680
Tuna	4 oz		260
Almonds	1 oz	80	
Bok choy	1/2 cup	125	
Broccoli	1 cup	130–160	
Collards	1/2 cup	180	
Cornbread	1 slice	85	
Egg, medium	1	55	25
Figs, dried	5 medium	125	
Kale	1/2 cup	95	
Orange	1	52	
Soybeans	1 cup	130	
Spinach	1/2 cup	110	
Tofu	4 oz	140	
Turnip greens	1/2 cup	125	

[a]To calculate calcium content, multiply percentage on package by 1000. To calculate vitamin D content, multiply percentage on package by 400.

- BMD increases are greatest in the first year of therapy, continue for at least 2 to 3 years, and then plateau for the duration of therapy. After discontinuation, the increased BMD is sustained for at least 1 year and remains higher than that of nonusers.
- Combination therapy with either estrogen therapy or raloxifene produces greater BMD increases than either agent alone; however, alendronate appears to blunt the effects of teriparatide.
- **Alendronate**, **risedronate**, and **ibandronate** are FDA approved for prevention and treatment of postmenopausal osteoporosis. Alendronate is also approved for osteoporosis in men. Alendronate and risedronate are indicated for corticosteroid-induced osteoporosis.
- Bisphosphonates must be administered carefully to optimize the clinical benefit and minimize the risk of adverse GI effects. All bisphosphonates are poorly

TABLE 3–3. Calcium and Vitamin D Product Selection[a]

Product[b]	Calcium (mg)	Vitamin D (units)
Calcium carbonate (40%)		
Trade and generic products	200–600	
Generic suspension	500/5 mL	
Titralac Liquid	400/5 mL	
Titralac Chewable	168	
Titralac Extra Strength	300	
Tums Chewable	200	
Tums E-X	300	
Tums Ultra	500	
Other chewable brands	168–500	
Mylanta Soothing Lozenges	240	
Cal Carb-HD powder	2.4 g/7-g packet	
Calcium carbonate with vitamin D		
Generic + vitamin D	600	125
Calcilyte + vitamin D[c]	500	200
Calel-D + vitamin D	500	200
Caltrate + vitamin D	600	200
Os-Cal + vitamin D	500	125
Viactiv chews[d]	500	100
Caltrate 600 plus[e]	600	200
Olay vitamins		
Essential Bone		
Health Formulation[f]	600	200
Calcium citrate (24%)		
Generic	240	
Citracal	200	
Citracal Liquitab[d]	500	
Citracal + vitamin D	316	200
Calcium phosphate tribasic (39%)		
Posture	600	
Posture-D	600	125
Dical-D chewable wafers + vitamin D	232	200
Multivitamin (D_3)		
Vitamin A (5000 units)	40	400
Cod liver oil (D_3)		
5 mL: vitamin A (4000 units)		500
Gel caps: vitamin A (1250–2500 units)		130–270
Ergocalciferol (D_2)		
Drops (per mL)		8000
Tablets		50,000

[a]Only calcium products with 500–600 mg per tablet or with an alternative dosage form (i.e., chewable, liquid, or dissolvable tablet) are listed.

[b]Many products beginning to add magnesium, boron, zinc, copper, and manganese, and adding "Plus" or "Ultra" to name.

[c]Tablet for solution.

[d]Also contains vitamin K.

[e]Also contains magnesium, zinc, copper, boron, and manganese.

[f]Also contains phosphorus and magnesium.

TABLE 3–4. Medications Used to Prevent and Treat Osteoporosis

Drug	Dosage	Pharmacokinetics	Adverse Effects	Drug Interactions
Calcium	200–1500 mg/day; see Table 3–3; divided doses	Absorption: predominantly active transport; fractional absorption 10–60%; fecal elimination for the unabsorbed and renal elimination for the absorbed calcium	Constipation, gas, upset stomach, rare kidney stones	• Absorption is decreased with proton pump inhibitors • Decreases absorption of iron, tetracycline, quinolones, alendronate, risedronate, etidronate, phenytoin, and fluoride when given concomitantly • Fiber decreases calcium absorption if given concomitantly
Vitamin D_2 or D_3	200–1000 units/day	Hepatic and renal metabolism to active compound 1.25 (OH) vitamin D; active and inactive metabolites	Hypercalcemia, (weakness, headache, somnolence, nausea, cardiac rhythm disturbance); hypercalciuria	• Phenytoin, barbiturates, carbamazepine, rifampin increase vitamin D metabolism • Cholestyramine, colestipol, orlistat, or mineral oil decrease vitamin D absorption
Bisphosphonates Alendronate (Fosamax) Risedronate (Actonel) Ibandronate (Boniva)	5 mg daily (prevention); 10 mg daily; 70-mg tablet or 75-mL single-use oral dose weekly (treatment) 5 mg daily, 35 mg weekly 2.5 mg daily,[a] 100–150 mg monthly,[b] 3 mg IV every 3 months[c]	Poorly absorbed, decreasing to zero with food or beverage intake; long half-lives (2–10 yr); renal elimination (of absorbed) and fecal elimination (of unabsorbed)	Nausea; GI irritation, perforation, ulceration, and/or bleeding	• Do not coadminister with any other medication, including calcium

continued

TABLE 3-4. (Continued)

Drug	Dosage	Pharmacokinetics	Adverse Effects	Drug Interactions
Selective estrogen receptor modulators				
Raloxifene (Evista)	60 mg daily	Hepatic metabolism	Hot flushes, leg cramps; venous thromboembolism	None
Calcitonin (Miacalcin)	200 units daily, intranasally (alternating nares every other day)	3% nasal availability; renal elimination	Rhinitis, epistaxis	None
Teriparatide (Forteo)	20 mcg subcutaneously daily for up to 2 yr	95% bioavailability; T_{max}: ~30 min; half-life ~60 min; hepatic metabolism	Pain at injection site, dizziness, leg cramps	None
Testosterone (used in men)		Hepatic metabolism; highly protein bound to SHBG	Weight gain, acne, dyslipidemia, hepatotoxicity, gynecomastia, priapism, prostate disorders, testicular atrophy, sleep apnea, aggressive behavior, erythrocytosis, skin reaction to patches, drug absorption by sex partner	• Potentiation of oral anticoagulants • Can increase or decrease glucose, necessitating monitoring of antidiabetic medications at start of therapy
Androderm	2.5–5 mg daily			
Testoderm TTS	5-mg patch/day			
Androgel	5 mg/day			
Testim gel	5 mg/day			
Injectable products	10–400 mg 1 M every 2–4 wk			
Pellets	150–450 mg/implant every 3–6 months			

T_{max}, time to maximum concentration; SHBG, sex hormone-binding globulin; IV, intravenous; IM, intramuscular; FDA, Food and Drug Administration.
[a] FDA approved at time chapter was prepared.
[b] Filed for FDA review, May 2004.
[c] Filed for FDA review, December 2004.

absorbed (bioavailability 1% to 5%) even under optimal conditions. Each oral tablet should be taken in the morning with at least 4 oz of plain tap water (not coffee, juice, mineral water, or milk) at least 30 minutes before consuming any food or any other supplement or medication. The patient should remain upright (sitting or standing) for at least 30 minutes after administration to prevent esophageal irritation and ulceration.

- Once-weekly bisphosphonate administration is preferred by most patients. This dosing schedule also lowers GI tract drug exposure. Once-weekly alendronate achieved similar BMD results, had similar GI adverse effects, and did not impair bone mineralization when compared with daily doses of 10 mg.
- The most common bisphosphonate adverse effects are nausea, abdominal pain, and dyspepsia. Esophageal, gastric, or duodenal irritation, perforation, ulceration, or bleeding may occur when administration directions are not followed or when bisphosphonates are prescribed for patients with contraindications.

Selective Estrogen Receptor Modulators (SERMs)
- **Raloxifene** is an estrogen agonist in bone tissue but an antagonist in the breast and uterus. It is approved for prevention and treatment of postmenopausal osteoporosis. It increases spine and hip BMD by 2% to 3% and decreases vertebral fractures. Nonvertebral fractures are not prevented by raloxifene.
- In contrast to bisphosphonates, raloxifene discontinuation results in the BMD decreasing immediately at a rate similar to that of placebo.
- Raloxifene (like tamoxifen) is associated with decreased breast cancer risk. Raloxifene is associated with decreases in total and low-density lipoprotein (LDL) cholesterol, neutral effects on high-density lipoprotein (HDL) cholesterol, but slight increases in triglycerides; no beneficial cardiovascular effects have yet been demonstrated.
- Raloxifene is well tolerated overall, but hot flushes occasionally cause women to discontinue therapy. Raloxifene is associated with a threefold increased risk of venous thromboembolism, similar to the risk with estrogen. Raloxifene is contraindicated in women with active thromboembolic disease. Therapy should be stopped if a significant period (several hours or more) of immobility is anticipated.
- On the basis of current evidence, a bisphosphonate is probably a better choice than raloxifene for women with severe osteoporosis, particularly when hip fracture risk reduction is desired.

Calcitonin
- **Calcitonin** is released from the thyroid gland when serum calcium is elevated. Salmon calcitonin is used clinically because it is more potent and longer lasting than the mammalian form. Pharmacologic doses decrease bone resorption.
- Calcitonin is indicated for osteoporosis treatment for women at least 5 years past menopause. Although it is also used in men, it is not FDA approved for this indication.
- A 200-unit regimen of nasal calcitonin increased spine BMD and reduced new vertebral fractures by 36%. Calcitonin does not consistently affect hip BMD and does not decrease hip fracture risk.
- Because calcitonin reduces fracture risk to a lesser extent than other osteoporosis medications, it is reserved for second-line treatment. It may provide pain relief to some patients with acute vertebral fractures, but this effect is minimal.
- The intranasal dose is 200 units daily, alternating nares every other day. Subcutaneous administration of 100 units daily is available but rarely used.

Estrogen and Hormonal Therapy

- Estrogens decrease osteoclast recruitment and activity, inhibit PTH peripherally, increase calcitriol concentrations and intestinal calcium absorption, and decrease renal calcium excretion.
- The enhanced BMD effects from estrogen therapy (ET) and combined estrogen-progestin hormonal therapy (HT) are less than those from bisphosphonates or teriparatide but greater than those from raloxifene. Pooled results from prevention studies showed that ET or HT increased lumbar spine BMD by 4.9% and 7%, femoral neck BMD by 2.3% and 4.1%, and forearm BMD by 3% and 4.5% in the first and second years, respectively. Oral and transdermal estrogens at equivalent doses and continuous or cyclic HT regimens have similar BMD effects. Most gains in BMD were seen within the first few years of treatment, with slight increases or a plateau thereafter. Effects on BMD are increased when ET or HT is combined with bisphosphonates or parathyroid hormone. When ET or HT was discontinued, bone loss was accelerated for a short time compared with placebo in most studies.
- HT was shown to decrease vertebral, hip, and all fractures by 34%, 34%, and 24%, respectively. The estrogen-only arm of the Women's Health Initiative (WHI) trial also found decreased hip fractures in ET users.
- However, the beneficial bone benefits of ET and HT do not outweigh their negative effects. They do not prevent primary or secondary cardiovascular disease and may even increase events within the first years of use. In the WHI, for every 10,000 woman-years of HT, 5 hip fractures and 6 colorectal cancers were prevented, but 7 coronary heart disease events, 8 strokes, 8 breast cancer cases, and 8 pulmonary emboli were caused. Also, overall mortality was not changed with either HT or ET.
- Thus, ET and HT are not advocated for prevention of osteoporosis and fractures, because other better and safer medications exist. The lowest dose of ET and HT necessary should still be used for preventing and controlling menopausal symptoms, with use discontinued upon symptom abatement.
- Many contraindications to ET and HT exist and must be identified before starting therapy. For women with an intact uterus, a progestin (e.g., medroxyprogesterone 2.5 to 5 mg daily) should also be used to decrease the risk of endometrial cancer.

Phytoestrogens

- The isoflavonoids (soy proteins) and lignans (flaxseed) are the most common forms of phytoestrogens. Beneficial bone effects may be related to bone estrogen receptor agonist activity or effects on osteoblasts and osteoclasts.
- Bone density results are difficult to interpret because of different phytoestrogen products, quantities, and preparations; differing age and race of the study populations; small sample sizes; and suboptimal study designs.
- Some isoflavone studies using larger doses have reported decreased bone resorption markers and small increases in bone density. However, inconsistencies and negative results have also been reported. Thus, these products can be used for preventive bone-sparing effects but are probably not sufficient when used alone for treatment.
- Ipriflavone is a synthetic isoflavone available in health food stores. Although short studies showed either increases or no change in BMD, a 4-year study in 474 postmenopausal women showed no effect of ipriflavone 200 mg three times daily on either BMD or vertebral fractures. Subclinical lymphocytopenia occurred in 13% of subjects. For these reasons, use of this agent should be discouraged.

Testosterone and Anabolic Steroids

- In a few studies, women receiving oral **methyltestosterone** 1.25 or 2.5 mg daily or **testosterone** implants 50 mg every 3 months had increased BMD. Various salt forms of testosterone were associated with increased BMD in some studies of hypogonadal men or senior men with normal hormone levels or mild hormonal deficiency. Transdermal gel, oral, intramuscular, and pellet testosterone products are available.
- Anabolic steroids (nandrolone decanoate) have shown minimal to no effect on BMD but do increase muscle strength.
- The virilizing and estrogenic adverse effects of these products are listed in Table 3–4. Patients using them should be evaluated within 1 to 2 months of onset and then every 3 to 6 months thereafter.

Bone Formation Therapy
Teriparatide (Parathyroid Hormone)

- **Teriparatide** contains the first 34 amino acids in human PTH. Although hyperparathyroidism leads to bone loss, therapeutic doses for shorter periods improve BMD and reduce fracture risk. Anabolic activity may result from decreased osteoblast apoptosis and increased bone formation from the longer-lived osteoblasts.
- In postmenopausal women with osteoporosis and preexisting fractures, teriparatide reduced the risk of new vertebral fractures by 65% compared with placebo. New nonvertebral fracture risk was reduced by 53% with the 20-mcg/day dosage. In men with osteoporosis, teriparatide increased BMD, but its impact on fracture rate remains undetermined.
- The dose is 20 mcg administered subcutaneously in the thigh or abdominal area (see Table 3–4). The initial dose should be given with the patient either lying or sitting in case orthostatic hypotension occurs. Each prefilled 3-mL pen device delivers a 20-mcg dose each day for up to 28 days; the pen device should be kept refrigerated.
- Teriparatide is contraindicated in patients with Paget's disease of the bone, unexplained alkaline phosphatase elevations, or a history of previous skeletal radiation therapy.
- Teriparatide should not be used in combination with alendronate because the bisphosphonate may blunt teriparatide's beneficial effects.
- Because of adverse effects and cost concerns, teriparatide is reserved for patients at high risk of osteoporosis-related fracture who cannot or will not take or have failed bisphosphonate therapy.

► CORTICOSTEROID-INDUCED OSTEOPOROSIS

- Corticosteroids decrease muscle strength and bone formation and increase bone resorption. They also decrease calcium absorption, increase renal calcium excretion, and result in secondary hyperparathyroidism.
- Although bone loss is continuous throughout corticosteroid therapy, the greatest loss occurs during the first 6 to 12 months. Trabecular bone (ribs, vertebrae, and pelvis) is affected more than cortical bone. Oral daily doses greater than 7.5 mg of prednisone or equivalent and inhaled doses greater than 800 to 1200 mcg of beclomethasone, 800 to 1000 mcg of budesonide, 750 mcg of fluticasone, and 1000 mcg of flunisolide generally are required for significant bone loss to occur. Men, women, and children are all susceptible.
- Guidelines for managing corticosteroid-induced osteoporosis recommend measuring BMD at the beginning of chronic therapy (prednisone 5 mg or

more daily or equivalent for 3 months) and follow-up monitoring with DXA in 6 to 12 months. BMD should be measured in patients taking chronic therapy whose baseline values were not obtained.

- If drug discontinuation is not possible, corticosteroids should be used in the lowest possible dose and for the shortest duration. Alternate-day therapy and pulse (intermittent) therapy may also have negative effects on bone density.
- All patients receiving chronic corticosteroid therapy should adopt bone-healthy lifestyle changes and ingest adequate amounts of calcium and vitamin D. Calcium intake should be higher than normal: 800 mg for children between 1 and 5 years, 1200 mg for children between 6 and 10 years, and 1500 mg for other patients. All children should receive 400 units and adults 800 units of vitamin D per day.
- Bisphosphonates are the best choice for treating corticosteroid-induced osteoporosis. Data do not support routine use of calcitonin for this purpose.

▶ EVALUATION OF THERAPEUTIC OUTCOMES

- Patients receiving pharmacotherapy for low bone mass should be examined at least annually.
- Patients should be asked about possible fracture symptoms (e.g., bone pain, disability) at each visit.
- Medication adherence and tolerance should be evaluated at each visit.
- Some clinicians measure BMD every 1 to 2 years after beginning therapy with the goal of identifying medication nonadherence or secondary osteoporosis. Others advocate no subsequent BMD measurement because of expense and lack of correlation to fracture risk reduction.

See Chapter 90, Osteoporosis and Osteomalacia, authored by Mary Beth O'Connell and Mary E. Elliott, for a more detailed discussion of this topic.

Chapter 4

▶ RHEUMATOID ARTHRITIS

▶ DEFINITION

Rheumatoid arthritis (RA) is a chronic and usually progressive inflammatory disorder of unknown etiology characterized by polyarticular symmetric joint involvement and systemic manifestations.

▶ PATHOPHYSIOLOGY

- RA results from a dysregulation of the humoral and cell-mediated components of the immune system. Most patients produce antibodies called rheumatoid factors; these seropositive patients tend to have a more aggressive course than patients who are seronegative.
- Immunoglobulins can activate the complement system, which amplifies the immune response by enhancing chemotaxis, phagocytosis, and release of lymphokines by mononuclear cells that are then presented to T lymphocytes. The processed antigen is recognized by the major histocompatibility complex (MHC) proteins on the lymphocyte surface, resulting in activation of T and B cells.
- Tumor necrosis factor (TNF), interleukin-1 (IL-1), and interleukin-6 (IL-6) are proinflammatory cytokines important in the initiation and continuance of inflammation.
- Activated T cells produce cytotoxins, which are directly toxic to tissues, and cytokines, which stimulate further activation of inflammatory processes and attract cells to areas of inflammation. Macrophages are stimulated to release prostaglandins and cytotoxins.
- Activated B cells produce plasma cells, which form antibodies that, in combination with complement, result in accumulation of polymorphonuclear leukocytes (PMNs). PMNs release cytotoxins, oxygen free radicals, and hydroxyl radicals that promote cellular damage to synovium and bone.
- Vasoactive substances (histamine, kinins, prostaglandins) are released at sites of inflammation, increasing blood flow and vascular permeability. This causes edema, warmth, erythema, and pain and makes it easier for granulocytes to pass from blood vessels to sites of inflammation.
- Chronic inflammation of the synovial tissue lining the joint capsule results in tissue proliferation (pannus formation). Pannus invades cartilage and eventually the bone surface, producing erosions of bone and cartilage and leading to joint destruction. The end results may be loss of joint space, loss of joint motion, bony fusion (ankylosis), joint subluxation, tendon contractures, and chronic deformity.

▶ CLINICAL PRESENTATION

- Nonspecific prodromal symptoms that develop insidiously over weeks to months may include fatigue, weakness, low-grade fever, loss of appetite, and joint pain. Stiffness and myalgias may precede development of synovitis.
- Joint involvement tends to be symmetric and affect the small joints of the hands, wrists, and feet; the elbows, shoulders, hips, knees, and ankles may also be affected.
- Joint stiffness typically is worse in the morning, usually exceeds 30 minutes, and may persist all day.

- On examination, joint swelling may be visible or may be apparent only by palpation. The tissue feels soft and spongy and may appear erythematous and warm, especially early in the course of the disease.
- Chronic joint deformities commonly involve subluxations of the wrists, metacarpophalangeal (MCP) joints, and proximal interphalangeal (PIP) joints (swan-neck deformity, boutonniere deformity, ulnar deviation).
- Extra-articular involvement may include rheumatoid nodules, vasculitis, pleural effusions, pulmonary fibrosis, ocular manifestations, pericarditis, cardiac conduction abnormalities, bone marrow suppression, and lymphadenopathy.

▶ DIAGNOSIS

- The American Rheumatism Association criteria for classification of RA are included in Table 4–1.
- Laboratory abnormalities that may be seen include normocytic, normochromic anemia; thrombocytosis or thrombocytopenia; leukopenia; elevated erythrocyte sedimentation rate (ESR); positive rheumatoid factor (60% to 70% of patients); and positive antinuclear antibodies (ANA) (25% of patients).
- Examination of aspirated synovial fluid may reveal turbidity, leukocytosis, reduced viscosity, and normal or low glucose relative to serum concentrations.
- Radiologic findings include soft tissue swelling and osteoporosis near the joint (periarticular osteoporosis). Erosions occurring later in the disease course are usually seen first in the MCP and PIP joints of the hands and metatarsophalangeal (MTP) joints of the feet.

TABLE 4–1. American Rheumatism Association Criteria for Classification of Rheumatoid Arthritis—1987 Revision

Criteria[a]	Definition
1. Morning stiffness	Morning stiffness in and around the joints lasting at least 1 h before maximal improvement.
2. Arthritis of three or more joint areas	At least three joint areas simultaneously have soft tissue swelling or fluid (not bony overgrowth alone) observed by a physician. The 14 possible joint areas are (right or left): PIP, MCP, wrist, elbow, knee, ankle, and MTP joints.[b]
3. Arthritis of hand joints	At least one joint area swollen as above in wrist, MCP, or PIP joint.
4. Symmetric arthritis	Simultaneous involvement of the same joint areas (as in 2) on both sides of the body (bilateral involvement of PIP, MCP, or MTP joints is acceptable without absolute symmetry).
5. Rheumatoid nodules	Subcutaneous nodules, over bony prominences, or extensor surfaces, or in juxta-articular regions, observed by a physician.
6. Serum rheumatoid factor	Demonstration of abnormal amounts of serum rheumatoid factor by any method that has been positive in less than 5% of normal control subjects.
7. Radiographic changes	Radiographic changes typical of rheumatoid arthritis on posteroanterior hand and wrist x-rays, which must include erosions or unequivocal bony decalcification localized to or most marked adjacent to the involved joints (osteoarthritis changes alone do not qualify).

[a] For classification purposes, a patient is said to have rheumatoid arthritis if he or she has satisfied at least four of these seven criteria. Criteria 1 through 4 must be present for at least 6 weeks. Patients with two clinical diagnoses are not excluded. Designation as classic, definite, or probable rheumatoid arthritis is not to be made.

[b] PIP, proximal interphalangeal; MCP, metacarpophalangeal; MTP, metatarsophalangeal.

▶ DESIRED OUTCOME

- The ultimate goal of RA treatment is to induce a complete remission, although this is seldom achieved.
- The primary objectives are to reduce joint swelling, stiffness, and pain; preserve range of motion and joint function; improve quality of life; prevent systemic complications; and slow destructive joint changes.

▶ TREATMENT

NONPHARMACOLOGIC THERAPY

- Adequate rest, weight reduction if obese, occupational therapy, physical therapy, and use of assistive devices may improve symptoms and help maintain joint function.
- Patients with severe disease may benefit from surgical procedures such as tenosynovectomy, tendon repair, and joint replacements.
- Patient education about the disease and the benefits and limitations of drug therapy is important.

PHARMACOLOGIC THERAPY

General Approach

- A disease-modifying antirheumatic drug (DMARD) should generally be started within the first 3 months of symptom onset (Figure 4–1). DMARDs should be used in all patients except those with limited disease or those with class IV disease in whom little reversibility is expected. Early use of DMARDs results in a more favorable outcome and can reduce mortality.
- First-line DMARDs include **methotrexate, hydroxychloroquine, sulfasalazine**, and **leflunomide**. The order of agent selection is not clearly defined. Hydroxychloroquine or sulfasalazine may be used initially in mild disease, but

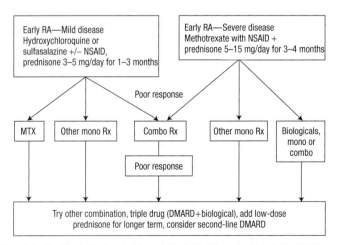

Figure 4–1. Algorithm for treatment of rheumatoid arthritis. RA, rheumatoid arthritis; NSAID, non-steroidal anti-inflammatory drugs; Rx, therapy; DMARD, disease-modifying antirheumatic drug.

methotrexate is often chosen initially in more severe cases because of long-term data suggesting superior outcomes than other DMARDs and lower cost than biologic agents. Leflunomide appears to have long-term efficacy similar to methotrexate.

- Biologic agents with disease-modifying activity include the anti-TNF agents (**etanercept, infliximab, adalimumab**) and the interleukin-1 receptor antagonist **anakinra**. Biologic agents are effective for patients who fail treatment with other DMARDs.
- DMARDs that are less frequently used include **azathioprine, penicillamine, gold salts** (including **auranofin**), **minocycline, cyclosporine**, and **cyclophosphamide**. These agents have either less efficacy or high toxicity, or both.
- Combination therapy with two or more DMARDs may be effective when single-DMARD treatment is unsuccessful. Combinations that are particularly effective include (1) methotrexate plus cyclosporine, and (2) methotrexate plus sulfasalazine and hydroxychloroquine.
- Nonsteroidal anti-inflammatory drugs (NSAIDs) and/or corticosteroids may be used for symptomatic relief if needed. They provide relatively rapid improvement compared with DMARDs, which may take weeks to months before benefit is seen. However, NSAIDs have no impact on disease progression, and corticosteroids have the potential for long-term complications.
- See Tables 4–2 and 4–3 for usual dosages and monitoring parameters for DMARDs and NSAIDs used in rheumatoid arthritis.

Nonsteroidal Anti-inflammatory Drugs (NSAIDs)

- NSAIDs act primarily by inhibiting prostaglandin synthesis, which is only a small portion of the inflammatory cascade. They possess both analgesic and anti-inflammatory properties and reduce stiffness but do not slow disease progression or prevent bony erosions or joint deformity. They should seldom be used as monotherapy for rheumatoid arthritis.
- Cyclooxygenase-2 (COX-2) selective NSAIDs have a better gastrointestinal (GI) safety profile and similar efficacy as conventional NSAIDs. However, concerns about adverse cardiovascular events (e.g., myocardial infarction, stroke) have led authorities to recommend their use only in selected patients who are at high risk for NSAID-related GI effects and low risk for cardiovascular toxicity.
- Common NSAID dosage regimens are shown in Table 4–4.

Methotrexate

- **Methotrexate** (MTX) inhibits cytokine production and purine biosynthesis, which may be responsible for its anti-inflammatory properties. Its onset is relatively rapid (as early as 2 to 3 weeks), and 45% to 67% of patients remained on it in studies ranging from 5 to 7 years.
- Toxicities are GI (stomatitis, diarrhea, nausea, vomiting), hematologic (thrombocytopenia, leukopenia), pulmonary (fibrosis, pneumonitis), and hepatic (elevated enzymes, rare cirrhosis). Concomitant folic acid may reduce some adverse effects without loss of efficacy. Liver injury tests (aspartate aminotransferase [AST] or alanine aminotransferase [ALT]) should be monitored periodically, but a liver biopsy is recommended only in patients with persistently elevated hepatic enzymes. MTX is teratogenic, and patients should use contraception and discontinue the drug if conception is planned.
- Methotrexate is contraindicated in pregnant and nursing women, chronic liver disease, immunodeficiency, pleural or peritoneal effusions, leukopenia, thrombocytopenia, preexisting blood disorders, and creatinine clearance less than 40 mL/min.

TABLE 4–2. Usual Doses and Monitoring Parameters for Antirheumatic Drugs

Drug	Usual Dose	Initial Monitoring Tests	Maintenance Monitoring Tests
NSAIDs	See Table 4–4	S_{cr} or BUN, CBC every 2–4 wk after starting therapy for 1–2 months; *salicylates:* serum salicylate levels if therapeutic dose and no response	Same as initial plus stool guaiac every 6–12 months
Methotrexate	Oral or IM: 7.5–15 mg/wk	Baseline: AST, ALT, ALK-P, albumin, total bilirubin, hepatitis B and C studies, CBC with platelets, S_{cr}	CBC with platelets, AST, albumin every 1–2 months
Leflunomide	Oral: 100 mg daily for 3 days, then 10–20 mg daily	Baseline: ALT	ALT monthly initially, and then periodically when stable
Hydroxychloroquine	Oral: 200–300 mg twice daily; after 1–2 months may decrease to 200 mg once or twice daily	Baseline: color fundus photography and automated central perimetric analysis	Ophthalmoscopy every 9–12 months and Amsler grid at home every 2 wk
Sulfasalazine	Oral: 500 mg twice daily, then increase to 1 g twice daily max	Baseline: CBC with platelets, then every week for 1 month	Same as initial every 1–2 months
Etanercept	25 mg SC twice weekly or 50 mg every 7 days	None	None
Infliximab	3 mg/kg IV at 0, 2, and 6 wk, then every 8 wk	None	None
Adalimumab	40 mg SC every 2 wk	None	None
Anakinra	100 mg SC daily	None	None
Auranofin	Oral: 3 mg once or twice daily	Baseline: UA, CBC with platelets	Same as initial every 1–2 months
Gold thiomalate	IM: 10-mg test dose, then weekly dosing 25–50 mg; after response may increase dosing interval	Baseline and until stable: UA, CBC with platelets preinjection	Same as initial every other dose
Azathioprine	Oral: 50–150 mg daily	CBC with platelets, AST every 2 wk for 1–2 months	Same as initial every 1–2 months
Penicillamine	Oral: 125–250 mg daily, may increase by 125–250 mg every 1–2 months; max 750 mg/day	Baseline: UA, CBC with platelets, then every week for 1 month	Same as initial every 1–2 months, but every 2 wk if dose changes
Cyclophosphamide	Oral: 1–2 mg/kg/day	UA, CBC with platelets every week for 1 month	Same tests as initial but every 2–4 wk
Cyclosporine	Oral: 2.5 mg/kg/day	S_{cr}, blood pressure every month	Same as initial
Corticosteroids	Oral, IV, IM, IA, and soft-tissue injections: variable	Glucose; blood pressure every 3–6 months	Same as initial

ALK-P, alkaline phosphatase; ALT, alanine aminotransferase; AST, aspartate aminotransferase; BUN, blood urea nitrogen; CBC, complete blood cell count; IA, intra-articular; IM, intramuscular; IV, intravenous; SC, subcutaneously; S_{cr}, serum creatinine; UA, urinalysis.

TABLE 4–3. Clinical Monitoring of Drug Therapy in Rheumatoid Arthritis

Drug	Toxicities Requiring Monitoring	Symptoms to Inquire About[a]
NSAIDs and salicylates	GI ulceration and bleeding, renal damage	Blood in stool, black stool, dyspepsia, nausea/vomiting, weakness, dizziness, abdominal pain, edema, weight gain, shortness of breath
Corticosteroids	Hypertension, hyperglycemia, osteoporosis[b]	Blood pressure if available, polyuria, polydipsia, edema, shortness of breath, visual changes, weight gain, headaches, broken bones or bone pain
Azathioprine	Myelosuppression, hepatotoxicity, lymphoproliferative disorders	Symptoms of myelosuppression (extreme fatigue, easy bleeding or bruising, infection), jaundice
Gold (intramuscular or oral)	Myelosuppression, proteinuria, rash, stomatitis	Symptoms of myelosuppression, edema, rash, oral ulcers, diarrhea
Hydroxychloroquine	Macular damage, rash, diarrhea	Visual changes including a decrease in night or peripheral vision, rash, diarrhea
Methotrexate	Myelosuppression, hepatic fibrosis, cirrhosis, pulmonary infiltrates or fibrosis, stomatitis, rash	Symptoms of myelosuppression, shortness of breath, nausea/vomiting lymph node swelling, coughing, mouth sores, diarrhea, jaundice
Leflunomide	Hepatitis, GI distress, alopecia	Nausea/vomiting, gastritis, diarrhea, hair loss, jaundice
Penicillamine	Myelosuppression, proteinuria, stomatitis, rash, dysgeusia	Symptoms of myelosuppression, edema, rash, diarrhea, altered taste perception, oral ulcers
Sulfasalazine	Myelosuppression, rash	Symptoms of myelosuppression, photosensitivity, rash, nausea/vomiting
Etanercept, adalimumab, anakinra	Local injection-site reactions, infection	Symptoms of infection
Infliximab	Immune reactions, infection	Postinfusion reactions, symptoms of infection

[a] Altered immune function increases infection, which should be considered, particularly in patients taking azathioprine, methotrexate, corticosteroids, or other drugs that may produce myelosuppression.
[b] Osteoporosis is not likely to manifest early in treatment, but all patients should be taking appropriate steps to prevent bone loss.

Leflunomide

- **Leflunomide** (Arava) inhibits pyrimidine synthesis, which reduces lympho-cyte proliferation and modulation of inflammation. Its efficacy for RA is similar to that of MTX.
- A loading dose of 100 mg/day for the first 3 days may result in a therapeutic response within the first month. The usual maintenance dose of 20 mg/day may be lowered to 10 mg/day in cases of GI intolerance, complaints of hair loss, or other dose-related toxicity.
- The drug may cause liver toxicity and is contraindicated in patients with pre-existing liver disease. The ALT should be monitored monthly initially and pe-riodically thereafter. It is teratogenic and should be avoided during pregnancy. Leflunomide causes bone marrow toxicity so rarely that hematologic monitor-ing is not required.

TABLE 4–4. Dosage Regimens for Nonsteroidal Anti-Inflammatory Drugs

| | Recommended Total Daily Anti-inflammatory Dosage | | |
Drug	Adult	Children	Dosing Schedule
Aspirin	2.6–5.2 g	60–100 mg/kg	4 times daily
Celecoxib	200–400 mg	–	Once or twice daily
Diclofenac	150–200 mg	–	3–4 times daily Extended release: twice daily
Diflunisal	0.5–1.5 g	–	Twice daily
Etodolac	0.2–1.2 g (max, 20 mg/kg)	–	3–4 times daily
Fenoprofen	0.9–3.0 g	–	4 times daily
Flurbiprofen	200–300 mg	–	2–4 times daily
Ibuprofen	1.2–3.2 g	20–40 mg/kg	3–4 times daily
Indomethacin	50–200 mg	2–4 mg/kg (max, 200 mg)	2–4 times daily Extended release: once daily
Ketoprofen	150–300 mg	–	3–4 times daily Extended release: once daily
Meclofenamate	200–400 mg	–	3–4 times daily
Meloxicam	7.5–15 mg	–	Once daily
Nabumetone	1–2 g	–	Once or twice daily
Naproxen	0.5–1.0 g	10 mg/kg	twice daily Extended release: once daily
Naproxen sodium	0.55–1.1 g	–	Twice daily
Nonacetylated salicylates	1.2–4.8 g		2–6 times daily
Oxaprozin	0.6–1.8 g (max, 26 mg/kg)		1–3 times daily
Piroxicam	10–20 mg		Once daily
Sulindac	300–400 mg	–	Twice daily
Tolmetin	0.6–1.8 g	15–30 mg/kg	3–4 times daily
Valdecoxib	10 mg	–	Once daily

Hydroxychloroquine

- **Hydroxychloroquine** lacks the myelosuppressive, hepatic, and renal toxicities seen with some other DMARDs, which simplifies monitoring. Its onset may be delayed for up to 6 weeks, but the drug should not be considered a therapeutic failure until after 6 months of therapy with no response.
- Short-term toxicities include GI (nausea, vomiting, diarrhea), ocular (accommodation defects, benign corneal deposits, blurred vision, scotomas, night blindness, rare retinopathy), dermatologic (rash, alopecia, skin pigmentation), and neurologic (headache, vertigo, insomnia) effects. Periodic ophthalmologic examinations are necessary for early detection of reversible retinal toxicity.

Sulfasalazine

- **Sulfasalazine** use is often limited by adverse effects. Antirheumatic effects should be seen in 1 to 2 months.
- Adverse effects include GI (anorexia, nausea, vomiting, diarrhea), dermatologic (rash, urticaria), hematologic (leukopenia, rare agranulocytosis), and

hepatic (elevated enzymes) effects. GI symptoms may be minimized by starting with low doses, dividing the dose more evenly throughout the day, and taking the drug with food.

Gold Preparations

- **Aurothioglucose** (Solganol) (suspension in oil) and **gold sodium thiomalate** (Myochrysine, Aurolate) (aqueous solution) are intramuscular (IM) preparations with an onset that may be delayed for 3 to 6 months. They require weekly injections for about 22 weeks before a less frequent maintenance regimen may be initiated.
- **Auranofin** (Ridaura) is an oral gold preparation that is more convenient but less effective than IM gold.
- Adverse effects are GI (nausea, vomiting, diarrhea), dermatologic (rash, stomatitis), renal (proteinuria, hematuria), and hematologic (anemia, leukopenia, thrombocytopenia). Gold sodium thiomalate is associated with nitritoid reactions (flushing, palpitations, hypotension, tachycardia, headache, blurred vision). Patients receiving IM gold may experience a postinjection disease flare for 1 to 2 days after an injection.

Azathioprine

- **Azathioprine** is a purine analog that is converted to 6-mercaptopurine and is thought to interfere with DNA and RNA synthesis.
- Antirheumatic effects may be seen in 3 to 4 weeks. It should be discontinued if no response is observed after 12 weeks at maximal doses.
- Its major adverse effects are bone marrow suppression (leukopenia, macrocytic anemia, thrombocytopenia, pancytopenia), stomatitis, GI intolerance, infections, drug fever, hepatotoxicity, and oncogenic potential.

Penicillamine

- **Penicillamine** onset may be seen in 1 to 3 months, and most responses occur within 6 months.
- Early adverse effects include skin rash, metallic taste, hypogeusia, stomatitis, anorexia, nausea, vomiting, and dyspepsia. Glomerulonephritis may occur, which manifests as proteinuria and hematuria.
- Penicillamine is usually reserved for patients who are resistant to other therapies because of the rare but potentially serious induction of autoimmune diseases (e.g., Goodpasture's syndrome, myasthenia gravis).

Cyclosporine

- **Cyclosporine** reduces production of cytokines involved in T-cell activation and has direct effects on B cells, macrophages, bone, and cartilage cells.
- Its onset appears to be 1 to 3 months. Important toxicities at doses of 1 to 10 mg/kg/day include hypertension, hyperglycemia, nephrotoxicity, tremor, GI intolerance, hirsutism, and gingival hyperplasia.
- Cyclosporine should be reserved for patients refractory to or intolerant of other DMARDs. It should be avoided in patients with current or past malignancy, uncontrolled hypertension, renal dysfunction, immunodeficiency, low white blood cell or platelet counts, or elevated liver function tests.

Biologic Agents

Etanercept

- **Etanercept** (Enbrel) is a fusion protein consisting of two p75-soluble TNF receptors linked to an Fc fragment of human IgG_1. It binds to and inactivates TNF, preventing it from interacting with the cell-surface TNF receptors and thereby activating cells.

- Most clinical trials used etanercept in patients who failed DMARDs, and responses were seen in 60% to 75% of patients. It has been shown to slow erosive disease progression to a greater degree than oral MTX in patients with inadequate response to methotrexate monotherapy.
- Adverse effects include local injection-site reactions, and there have been case reports of pancytopenia and neurologic demyelinating syndromes. No laboratory monitoring is required.
- The drug should be avoided in patients with preexisting infection and in those at high risk for developing infection. Treatment should be discontinued temporarily if infections develop during therapy.

Infliximab

- **Infliximab** (Remicade) is a chimeric anti-TNF antibody fused to a human constant-region IgG$_1$. It binds to TNF and prevents its interaction with TNF receptors on inflammatory cells.
- To prevent formation of antibodies to this foreign protein, MTX should be given orally in doses used to treat RA for as long as the patient continues on infliximab.
- In clinical trials, the combination of infliximab and MTX halted progression of joint damage and was superior to MTX monotherapy.
- Infliximab may increase the risk of infection, especially upper respiratory infections. An acute infusion reaction with fever, chills, pruritus, and rash may occur within 1 to 2 hours after administration. Autoantibodies and lupus-like syndrome have also been reported.

Adalimumab

- **Adalimumab** (Humira) is a human IgG$_1$ antibody to TNF that is less antigenic than infliximab. It has response rates similar to other TNF inhibitors.
- Local injection site reactions were the most common adverse event reported in clinical trials. It has the same precautions regarding infections as the other biologics.

Anakinra

- **Anakinra** (Kineret) is an IL-1 receptor antagonist (IL-1ra) that binds to IL-1 receptors on target cells, preventing the interaction between IL-1 and the cells. IL-1 normally stimulates release of chemotactic factors and adhesion molecules that promote migration of inflammatory leukocytes to tissues.
- The drug is approved for moderately to severely active RA in adults who have failed one or more DMARDs. It can be used alone or in combination with any of the other DMARDs except for TNF-blocking agents. In 6-month clinical trials, response rates were 38% in patients given anakinra and 22% in patients receiving placebo.
- Injection-site reactions were the most common adverse effect (e.g., redness, swelling, pain). Infection risk and precautions are similar to those for the TNF inhibitors.

Corticosteroids

- **Corticosteroids** have anti-inflammatory and immunosuppressive properties. They interfere with antigen presentation to T lymphocytes, inhibit prostaglandin and leukotriene synthesis, and inhibit neutrophil and monocyte superoxide radical generation.
- Oral corticosteroids (e.g., prednisone, methylprednisolone) can be used to control pain and synovitis while DMARDs are taking effect ("bridging therapy").

This is often used in patients with debilitating symptoms when DMARD therapy is initiated.

- Low-dose, long-term corticosteroid therapy may be used to control symptoms in patients with difficult-to-control disease. Prednisone doses below 7.5 mg/day (or equivalent) are well tolerated but are not devoid of the long-term corticosteroid adverse effects. The lowest dose that controls symptoms should be used. Alternate-day dosing of low-dose oral corticosteroids is usually ineffective in rheumatoid arthritis.

- High-dose oral or intravenous bursts may be used for several days to suppress disease flares. After symptoms are controlled, the drug should be tapered to the lowest effective dose.

- The intramuscular route is preferable in nonadherent patients. Depot forms (**triamcinolone acetonide, triamcinolone hexacetonide, methylprednisolone acetate**) provide 2 to 8 weeks of symptomatic control. The onset of effect may be delayed for several days. The depot effect provides a physiologic taper, avoiding hypothalamic-pituitary axis suppression.

- Intra-articular injections of depot forms may be useful when only a few joints are involved. If effective, injections may be repeated every 3 months. No one joint should be injected more than 2 or 3 times per year.

- Adverse effects of systemic glucocorticoids limit their long-term use. Dosage tapering and eventual discontinuation should be considered at some point in patients receiving chronic therapy.

▶ EVALUATION OF THERAPEUTIC OUTCOMES

- Clinical signs of improvement include reduction in joint swelling, decreased warmth over actively involved joints, and decreased tenderness to joint palpation.

- Symptom improvement includes reduction in joint pain and morning stiffness, longer time to onset of afternoon fatigue, and improvement in ability to perform daily activities.

- Joint radiographs may be of some value in assessing disease progression.

- Laboratory monitoring is of little value in monitoring response to therapy but is essential for detecting and preventing adverse drug effects (Table 4–2).

- Patients should be questioned about the presence of symptoms that may be related to adverse drug effects (Table 4–3).

See Chapter 89, Rheumatoid Arthritis, authored by Arthur A. Schuna, for a detailed discussion of this topic.

Chapter 5

▶ ACUTE CORONARY SYNDROMES

▶ DEFINITION

- Acute coronary syndromes (ACSs) include all clinical syndromes compatible with acute myocardial ischemia resulting from an imbalance between myocardial oxygen demand and supply.
- In contrast to stable angina, an ACS results primarily from diminished myocardial blood flow secondary to an occlusive or partially occlusive coronary artery thrombus.
- ACSs are classified according to electrocardiographic (ECG) changes into (1) ST-segment-elevation ACS (ST-elevation myocardial infarction [STEMI]) and (2) non-ST-segment-elevation ACS (non–ST-elevation myocardial infarction [NSTEMI] and unstable angina [UA]).
- After an STEMI, pathologic Q waves are seen frequently on the ECG and usually indicate transmural MI. Q waves are less commonly seen after NSTEMI.
- NSTEMI differs from UA in that ischemia is severe enough to produce myocardial necrosis, resulting in release of detectable amounts of biochemical markers (primarily troponins T or I and creatine kinase myocardial band [CK-MB]) from the necrotic myocytes into the bloodstream.

▶ PATHOPHYSIOLOGY

- The formation of atherosclerotic plaques is the underlying cause of coronary artery disease (CAD) and ACS in most patients. Endothelial dysfunction leads to the formation of fatty streaks in the coronary arteries and eventually to atherosclerotic plaques. Factors responsible for development of atherosclerosis include hypertension, age, male gender, tobacco use, diabetes mellitus, obesity, elevated plasma homocysteine concentrations, and dyslipidemia.
- The cause of ACS in more than 90% of patients is rupture of an atheromatous plaque. Plaques most susceptible to rupture have an eccentric shape, thin fibrous cap, large fatty core, high content of inflammatory cells such as macrophages and lymphocytes, and limited amounts of smooth muscle.
- A partially or completely occlusive clot forms on top of the ruptured plaque. Exposure of collagen and tissue factor induce platelet adhesion and activation, which promote release of adenosine diphosphate (ADP) and thromboxane A_2 (TXA_2) from platelets. These produce vasoconstriction and potentiate platelet activation. A change in the conformation of the glycoprotein (GP) IIb/IIIa surface receptors of platelets occurs that cross-links platelets to each other through fibrinogen bridges (the final common pathway of platelet aggregation).
- Simultaneously, activation of the extrinsic coagulation cascade occurs as a result of exposure of blood to the thrombogenic lipid core and endothelium, which are rich in tissue factor. This pathway ultimately leads to the formation of a fibrin clot composed of fibrin strands, cross-linked platelets, and trapped red blood cells.
- Ventricular remodeling occurs after an MI and is characterized by changes in the size, shape, and function of the left ventricle that may lead to cardiac failure. Factors contributing to ventricular remodeling include neurohormonal factors (e.g., activation of the renin-angiotensin-aldosterone and sympathetic nervous systems), hemodynamic factors, mechanical factors, and changes in gene expression. This process may lead to cardiomyocyte hypertrophy, loss of

cardiomyocytes, and increased interstitial fibrosis, which promote both systolic and diastolic dysfunction.

- Complications of MI include cardiogenic shock, heart failure, valvular dysfunction, various arrhythmias, pericarditis, stroke secondary to left ventricular (LV) thrombus embolization, venous thromboembolism, and LV free wall rupture.

▶ CLINICAL PRESENTATION

- The predominant symptom of ACS is midline anterior chest discomfort (most often occurring at rest), severe new-onset, or increasing angina that is at least 20 minutes in duration. The discomfort may radiate to the shoulder, left arm, back, or jaw. Accompanying symptoms may include nausea, vomiting, diaphoresis, or shortness of breath. Elderly patients, patients with diabetes, and women are less likely to present with classic symptoms.
- There are no specific features indicative of ACS on physical examination.

▶ DIAGNOSIS

- A 12-lead ECG should be obtained within 10 minutes of patient presentation. Key findings indicating myocardial ischemia or MI are ST-segment elevation, ST-segment depression, and T-wave inversion (see Figure 5–1). These changes in certain groupings of leads help to identify the location of the involved coronary artery. The appearance of a new left bundle branch block accompanied by chest discomfort is highly specific for acute MI. Some patients with myocardial ischemia have no ECG changes, so biochemical markers and other risk factors for CAD should be assessed to determine the patient's risk for experiencing a new MI or other complications.
- Biochemical markers of myocardial cell death are important for confirming the diagnosis of MI. An evolving MI is defined as a typical rise and gradual fall in troponin I or T or a more rapid rise and fall of CK-MB (Figure 5–2). Typically, blood is obtained immediately and two additional times in the first 12 to 24 hours after presentation. An MI is identified if at least one troponin value or two CK-MB values are greater than the MI decision limit set by the hospital. Both troponins and CK-MB are detectable within 6 hours of MI. Troponins remain elevated for up to 10 days, whereas CK-MB returns to normal within 48 hours.
- Patient symptoms, past medical history, ECG, and troponin or CK-MB determinations are used to stratify patients into low, medium, or high risk of death or MI or likelihood of needing urgent coronary angiography and percutaneous coronary intervention (PCI).

▶ DESIRED OUTCOME

Short-term goals of therapy include (1) early restoration of blood flow to the occluded artery to prevent infarct expansion (in the case of MI) or prevent complete occlusion and MI (in UA), (2) prevention of complications and death, (3) prevention of coronary artery reocclusion, and (4) relief of ischemic chest discomfort.

▶ TREATMENT

GENERAL APPROACH

- General treatment measures include hospital admission, oxygen administration if saturation is less than 90%, continuous multilead ST-segment monitoring for arrhythmias and ischemia, frequent measurement of vital signs, bedrest for 12 hours in hemodynamically stable patients, use of stools softeners to avoid Valsalva maneuver, and pain relief.

- A fasting lipid panel should be obtained within the first 24 hours of hospitalization because values for cholesterol (an acute phase reactant) may be falsely low beyond that period. However, initiation of statin therapy is common for all ACS patients regardless of the lipid panel results.
- It is important to triage and treat patients according to their risk category (Figure 5–1).
  - Patients with ST-segment-elevation ACS are at high risk of death, and efforts to reestablish coronary perfusion should be initiated immediately (without evaluation of biochemical markers).
  - Patients with non–ST-segment-elevation ACS who are considered to be at low risk (based on TIMI risk score) should have serial biochemical markers obtained; if they are negative, the patient may be admitted to a general medical floor with ECG telemetry monitoring, undergo a noninvasive stress test, or may be discharged.
  - High-risk non–ST-segment-elevation ACS patients should undergo early coronary angiography with revascularization if a significant coronary artery stenosis is found. Moderate-risk patients with positive biochemical markers typically also undergo angiography and revascularization, if indicated.
  - Moderate-risk patients with negative biochemical markers may initially undergo a noninvasive stress test, with only those having a positive test proceeding to angiography.

NONPHARMACOLOGIC THERAPY

- For patients with ST-segment-elevation ACS, either fibrinolysis or primary PCI (with either balloon angioplasty or stent placement) is the treatment of choice for reestablishing coronary artery blood flow when the patient presents within 3 hours of symptom onset. Primary PCI may be associated with a lower mortality rate than fibrinolysis, possibly because PCI opens more than 90% of coronary arteries compared with less than 60% opened with fibrinolytics. The risks of intracranial hemorrhage and major bleeding are also lower with PCI than with fibrinolysis. Primary PCI is generally preferred if institutions have skilled interventional cardiologists and other necessary facilities, in patients with cardiogenic shock, in patients with contraindications to fibrinolytics, and in patients presenting with symptom onset more than 3 hours prior.
- In patients with non–ST-segment-elevation ACS, clinical practice guidelines recommend either PCI or coronary artery bypass grafting (CABG) revascularization as an early treatment for high- and moderate-risk patients. An early invasive approach results in fewer MIs, less need for revascularization procedures over the next year after hospitalization, and lower cost than a conservative medical stabilization approach.

EARLY PHARMACOTHERAPY FOR ST-SEGMENT-ELEVATION ACS

See Figure 5–3.

According to the American College of Cardiology/American Heart Association (ACC/AHA) practice guidelines, early pharmacologic therapy should include (1) intranasal oxygen (if oxygen saturation is less than 90%), (2) sublingual followed by intravenous (IV) nitroglycerin, (3) aspirin, (4) an IV β blocker, (5) unfractionated heparin, and (6) fibrinolysis in eligible candidates. Morphine is administered to patients with refractory angina as an analgesic and venodilator

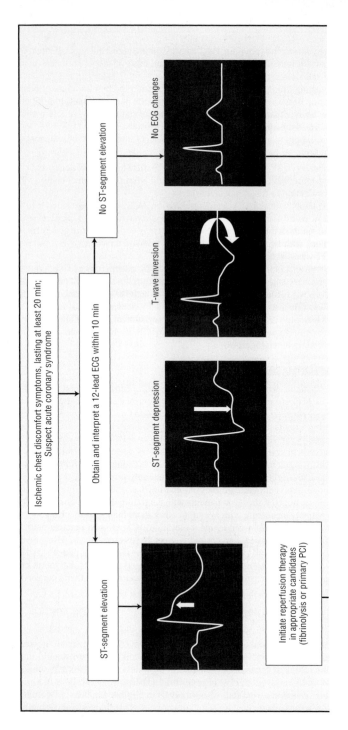

Ischemic chest discomfort symptoms, lasting at least 20 min; Suspect acute coronary syndrome

Obtain and interpret a 12-lead ECG within 10 min

ST-segment elevation

No ST-segment elevation

ST-segment depression

T-wave inversion

No ECG changes

Initiate reperfusion therapy in appropriate candidates (fibrinolysis or primary PCI)

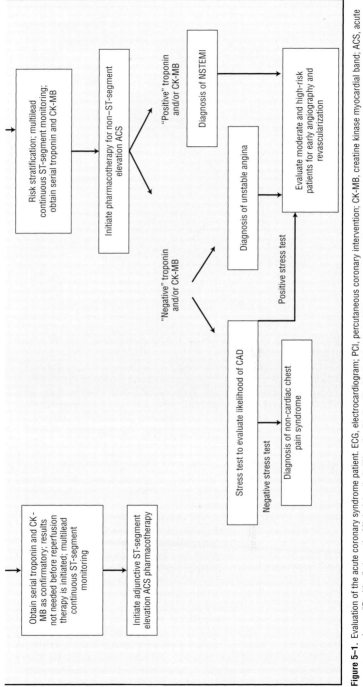

Figure 5–1. Evaluation of the acute coronary syndrome patient. ECG, electrocardiogram; PCI, percutaneous coronary intervention; CK-MB, creatine kinase myocardial band; ACS, acute coronary syndrome; "Positive," above the MI decision limit; "Negative," below the MI decision limit; CAD, coronary artery disease.

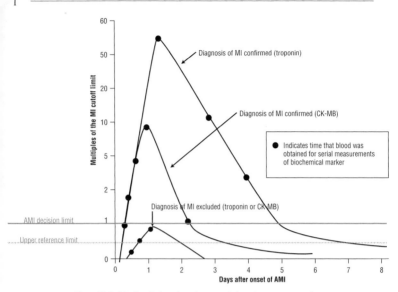

Figure 5–2. Biochemical markers in suspected acute coronary syndrome.

that lowers preload. These agents should be administered early, while the patient is still in the emergency department.

Fibrinolytic Therapy
- A fibrinolytic is indicated in patients presenting within 24 hours of the onset of chest discomfort who have at least 1 mm of ST-segment elevation in two or more contiguous ECG leads. Fibrinolysis is preferred over primary PCI in patients presenting within 3 hours of symptoms onset when there would be a delay in performing primary PCI.
- It is not necessary to obtain the results of biochemical markers before initiating fibrinolytic therapy.
- Absolute contraindications to fibrinolytic therapy include (1) active internal bleeding, (2) previous intracranial hemorrhage at any time, (3) ischemic stroke within 3 months, (4) known intracranial neoplasm, (5) known structural vascular lesion, (6) suspected aortic dissection, and (7) significant closed head or facial trauma within 3 months. Primary PCI is preferred in these situations.
- Patients with relative contraindications to fibrinolytics may receive therapy if the perceived risk of death from MI is higher than the risk of major hemorrhage. These situations include (1) severe, uncontrolled hypertension (BP greater than 180/110 mm Hg); (2) history of prior ischemic stroke longer than 3 months prior, dementia, or known intracranial pathology not considered an absolute contraindication; (3) current anticoagulant use; (4) known bleeding diathesis; (5) traumatic or prolonged cardiopulmonary resuscitation or major surgery within 3 weeks; (6) noncompressible vascular puncture; (7) recent (within 2 to 4 weeks) internal bleeding; (8) pregnancy; (9) active peptic ulcer; (10) history of severe, chronic poorly controlled hypertension; and (11) for streptokinase, prior administration (5 days to 2 years) or prior allergic reactions.

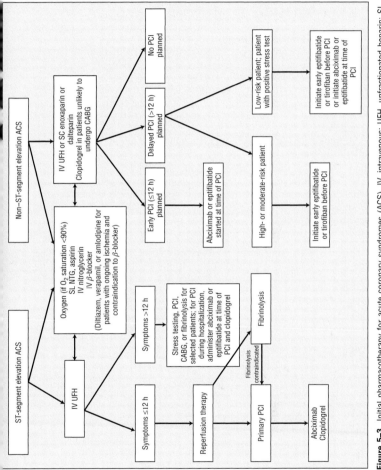

Figure 5–3. Initial pharmacotherapy for acute coronary syndromes (ACS). IV, intravenous; UFH, unfractionated heparin; SL, sublingual; NTG, nitroglycerin; SC, subcutaneous; CABG, coronary artery bypass graft; PCI, percutaneous coronary intervention.

- Practice guidelines indicate that a more fibrin-specific agent (alteplase, reteplase, tenecteplase) is preferred over the non–fibrin-specific agent streptokinase. Fibrin-specific agents open a greater percentage of infarct arteries, which results in smaller infarcts and lower mortality.
- Eligible patients should be treated as soon as possible, but preferably within 30 minutes from the time they present to the emergency department, with one of the following regimens:
  - **Alteplase** (recombinant tissue-type plasminogen activator, or tPA [Activase]): 15-mg IV bolus followed by 0.75-mg/kg infusion (maximum 50 mg) over 30 minutes, followed by 0.5-mg/kg infusion (maximum 35 mg) over 1 hour (maximum dose 100 mg)
  - **Reteplase** (recombinant plasminogen activator, or rPA [Retavase]): 10 units IV over 2 minutes, followed 30 minutes later with another 10 units IV over 2 minutes
  - **Tenecteplase** (TNK-tPA [TNKase])—a single IV bolus dose given over 5 seconds based on patient weight: 30 mg if less than 60 kg; 35 mg if 60 to 69.9 kg; 40 mg if 70 to 79.9 kg; 45 mg if 80 to 89.9 kg; and 50 mg if 90 kg or greater
  - **Streptokinase** (Streptase): 1.5 million units in 50 mL of normal saline or D_5W IV over 60 minutes
- Intracranial hemorrhage and major bleeding are the most serious side effects. The risk of intracranial hemorrhage is higher with fibrin-specific agents than with streptokinase. However, the risk of systemic bleeding other than intracranial hemorrhage is higher with streptokinase than with fibrin-specific agents.

Aspirin

- **Aspirin** should be administered to all patients without contraindications within the first 24 hours of hospital admission. It provides an additional mortality benefit in patients with ST-segment-elevation ACS when given with fibrinolytic therapy.
- In patients experiencing an ACS, non–enteric-coated aspirin, 160 to 325 mg, should be chewed and swallowed as soon as possible after the onset of symptoms or immediately after presentation to the emergency department regardless of the reperfusion strategy being considered.
- A daily maintenance dose of 75 to 160 mg is recommended thereafter and should be continued indefinitely.
- Low-dose aspirin is associated with a reduced risk of major bleeding, particularly gastrointestinal bleeding. In order to further minimize bleeding risk, concomitant use of other agents that can induce bleeding (including clopidogrel and warfarin) should be avoided, unless the combination is clinically indicated and the increased risk of bleeding has been considered. Other gastrointestinal disturbances (e.g., dyspepsia, nausea) are infrequent with low-dose aspirin. Ibuprofen should not be administered on a regular basis concurrently with aspirin because it may block aspirin's antiplatelet effects.

Thienopyridines

- **Clopidogrel** is recommended for patients with ST-segment-elevation ACS if they have an aspirin allergy. A 300- to 600-mg loading dose is given on the first hospital day, followed by a maintenance dose of 75 mg daily. It should be continued indefinitely.
- For patients undergoing PCI, clopidogrel is administered as a 300- to 600-mg loading dose followed by a 75 mg/day maintenance dose, in combination with

aspirin, to prevent subacute stent thrombosis and long-term events (e.g., MI, death, need to undergo repeat PCI).

- The most frequent side effects of clopidogrel are nausea, vomiting, and diarrhea (5% of patients). Thrombotic thrombocytopenia purpura has been reported rarely. The most serious side effect of clopidogrel is hemorrhage.
- **Ticlopidine** is associated with neutropenia that requires frequent monitoring of the complete blood count (CBC) during the first 3 months of use. For this reason, clopidogrel is the preferred thienopyridine for ACS and PCI patients.

Glycoprotein IIb/IIIa Inhibitors

- **Abciximab** is a first-line glycoprotein IIb/IIIa inhibitor for patients undergoing primary PCI who have not received fibrinolytics. It should not be administered to ST-segment-elevation ACS patients who will not be undergoing PCI.
- Abciximab is preferred over **eptifibatide** and **tirofiban** in this setting because it is the most widely studied agent in primary PCI trials.
- Abciximab, in combination with aspirin, a thienopyridine, and unfractionated heparin (administered as an infusion for the duration of the procedure), reduces the risk of reinfarction and need for repeat PCI in ST-segment-elevation ACS.
- The dose of abciximab is 0.25 mg/kg IV bolus given 10 to 60 minutes before the start of PCI, followed by 0.125 mcg/kg/min (maximum 10 mcg/min) for 12 hours.
- GP IIb/IIIa inhibitors increase the risk of bleeding, especially if given in the setting of recent (less than 4 hours) administration of fibrinolytic therapy. An immune-mediated thrombocytopenia occurs in about 5% of patients.

Heparin

- **Unfractionated heparin** (UFH), administered as a continuous infusion, is a first-line anticoagulant for ST-segment-elevation ACS, both for medical therapy and PCI.
- UFH should be initiated in the emergency department and continued for 24 hours or longer in patients who will receive chronic warfarin after acute MI. UFH typically is continued until the patient has undergone PCI during the hospitalization for ST-segment-elevation ACS. UFH is discontinued immediately after the PCI procedure.
- If a fibrinolytic agent is administered, UFH is given concomitantly with alteplase, reteplase, and tenecteplase, but UFH is not administered with streptokinase because no benefit of combined therapy has been demonstrated. Rates of reinfarction are higher if UFH is not given with the fibrin-selective agents.
- For ST-segment-elevation ACS, the dose of UFH is 60 units/kg IV bolus (maximum 4000 units) followed by a continuous IV infusion of 12 units/kg/h (maximum 1000 units/h).
- The dose is titrated to maintain the activated partial thromboplastin time (aPTT) between 50 and 70 seconds. The first aPTT should be measured at 3 hours in patients with ST-segment-elevation ACS who are treated with fibrinolytics and at 4 to 6 hours in patients not receiving thrombolytics.
- Besides bleeding, the most frequent adverse effect of UFH is immune-mediated thrombocytopenia, which occurs in up to 5% of patients.
- **Low-molecular-weight heparins** (LMWHs) may be an alternative to UFH in ST-segment-elevation ACS based on limited data. Pooled data from smaller trials with **enoxaparin** suggest that it is associated with similar safety and reduced reinfarction when coadministered with fibrinolytics (and aspirin). LMWHs have not been studied in the setting of primary PCI.

Nitrates

- Immediately upon presentation, one sublingual **nitroglycerin** (NTG) tablet should be administered every 5 minutes for up to three doses to relieve chest pain and myocardial ischemia.
- Intravenous NTG should be initiated in all patients with an ACS who do not have a contraindication and who have persistent ischemic symptoms, heart failure, or uncontrolled high blood pressure. The usual dose is 5 to 10 mcg/min by continuous infusion, titrated up to 75 to 100 mcg/min until relief of symptoms or limiting side effects (e.g., headache or hypotension). Treatment should be continued for approximately 24 hours after ischemia is relieved.
- NTG causes venodilation, which lowers preload and myocardial oxygen demand. In addition, arterial vasodilation may lower blood pressure, thereby reducing myocardial oxygen demand. Arterial dilation also relieves coronary artery vasospasm and improves myocardial blood flow and oxygenation.
- Oral nitrates play a limited role in ACS because clinical trials have failed to show a mortality benefit for IV followed by oral nitrate therapy in acute MI. Therefore, other life-saving therapy, such as ACE inhibitors and β blockers, should not be withheld.
- The most significant adverse effects of nitrates are tachycardia, flushing, headache, and hypotension. Nitrates are contraindicated in patients who have taken the oral phosphodiesterase-5 inhibitors sildenafil or vardenafil within the prior 24 hours and tadalafil within the prior 48 hours.

β-Adrenergic Blockers

- IV bolus or oral doses of a β blocker should be administered early in the care of patients with ST-segment-elevation ACS (within the first 24 hours), and then an oral β blocker should be continued indefinitely.
- The benefits result from blockade of β_1 receptors on the myocardium, which produces a reduction in heart rate, myocardial contractility, and blood pressure, thereby decreasing myocardial oxygen demand. The reduced heart rate increases diastolic time, thus improving ventricular filling and coronary artery perfusion.
- Because of these effects, β blockers reduce the risk for recurrent ischemia, infarct size, risk of reinfarction, and occurrence of ventricular arrhythmias.
- The usual doses of β blockers are as follows:
  - **Metoprolol:** 5 mg by slow (over 1 to 2 minutes) IV bolus, repeated every 5 minutes for a total initial dose of 15 mg. If a conservative regimen is desired, initial doses can be reduced to 1 to 2 mg. This is followed in 1 to 2 hours by 25 to 50 mg orally every 6 hours. If appropriate, initial IV therapy may be omitted.
  - **Propranolol:** 0.5 to 1 mg slow IV push, followed in 1 to 2 hours by 40 to 80 mg orally every 6 to 8 hours. If appropriate, the initial IV therapy may be omitted.
  - **Atenolol:** 5 mg IV dose, followed 5 minutes later by a second 5-mg IV dose; then 50 to 100 mg orally every day beginning 1 to 2 hours after the IV dose. The initial IV therapy may be omitted.
  - **Esmolol:** Starting maintenance dose of 0.1 mg/kg/min IV, with titration in increments of 0.05 mg/kg/min every 10 to 15 minutes as tolerated by blood pressure until the desired therapeutic response is obtained, limiting symptoms develop, or a dose of 0.2 mg/kg/min is reached. An optional loading dose of 0.5 mg/kg may be given by slow IV administration (2 to 5 minutes) for more rapid onset of action. Alternatively, the initial IV therapy may be omitted.

- The target resting heart rate is 50 to 60 beats/min. The most serious side effects early in ACS are hypotension, bradycardia, and heart block. Initial acute administration of β blockers is not appropriate for patients presenting with decompensated heart failure. However, therapy may be attempted in most patients before hospital discharge after treatment of acute heart failure. Diabetes mellitus is not a contraindication to β-blocker use. If possible intolerance to β blockers is a concern (e.g., due to chronic obstructive pulmonary disease), a short-acting drug such as metoprolol or esmolol should be administered IV initially.

Calcium Channel Blockers

- In the setting of ST-segment-elevation ACS, calcium channel blockers are reserved for patients who have contraindications to β blockers. They are used for relief of ischemic symptoms only.
- Patients who had been prescribed calcium channel blockers for hypertension, who are not receiving β blockers, and who do not have a contraindication should have the calcium channel blocker discontinued and a β blocker initiated.
- Dihydropyridine channel blockers (e.g., **nifedipine**) have little benefit on clinical outcomes beyond symptom relief. The role of **verapamil** and **diltiazem** appears to be limited to symptom relief or control of heart rate in patients with supraventricular arrhythmias in whom β blockers are contraindicated or ineffective.
- Patients with variant (Prinzmetal's) angina or cocaine-induced ACS may benefit from calcium channel blockers as initial therapy because they can reverse coronary vasospasm. β Blockers generally should be avoided in these situations because they may worsen vasospasm through an unopposed β_2-blocking effect on smooth muscle.

EARLY PHARMACOTHERAPY FOR NON–ST-SEGMENT-ELEVATION ACS

See Figure 5–3.

- Early pharmacotherapy for non–ST-segment-elevation ACS is similar to that for ST-segment-elevation ACS except that (1) fibrinolytic therapy is not administered; (2) clopidogrel should be given in addition to aspirin to most patients, and (3) GP IIb/IIIa receptor blockers are administered to high-risk patients for medical therapy as well as to PCI patients.
- According to ACC/AHA practice guidelines, early pharmacotherapy should include (1) intranasal oxygen (if oxygen saturation is less than 90%), (2) sublingual followed by IV nitroglycerin, (3) an IV β blocker, and (4) UFH or, preferably, LMWH. Morphine is also administered to patients with refractory angina, as described previously. These agents should be administered early, while the patient is still in the emergency department.

Fibrinolytic Therapy

Fibrinolytics are not indicated in any patient with non–ST-segment-elevation ACS, even those who have positive biochemical markers that indicate infarction. The risk of death from MI is lower in these patients, and the hemorrhagic risks of fibrinolytic therapy outweigh the benefit.

Aspirin

Aspirin reduces the risk of death or developing MI by about 50% compared with no antiplatelet therapy in patients with non–ST-segment-elevation ACS. Dosing of aspirin is the same as for ST-segment-elevation ACS, and aspirin is continued indefinitely.

Thienopyridines
- The addition of clopidogrel started on the first day of hospitalization as a 300- to 600-mg loading dose followed the next day by 75 mg/day orally is recommended for most patients. Although aspirin is the mainstay of antiplatelet therapy in ACS, addition of clopidogrel may further reduce morbidity and mortality.
- On the basis of clinical trial results, clopidogrel is indicated for at least 9 months in non–ST-segment-elevation ACS patients who do not undergo PCI or CABG (medical management only) and for at least 30 days in patients receiving bare metal intracoronary stents.
- Because of the potential increased risk for bleeding with combination antiplatelet therapy, a low dose of aspirin (75 to 100 mg/day) is recommended for maintenance therapy with clopidogrel.
- In patients undergoing CABG, clopidogrel (but not aspirin) should be withheld at least 5 days and preferably 7 days before the procedure.

Glycoprotein IIb/IIIa Inhibitors
- Administration of tirofiban or eptifibatide is recommended for high-risk non–ST-segment-elevation ACS patients as medical therapy without planned revascularization.
- Administration of either abciximab or eptifibatide is recommended for non–ST-segment-elevation ACS patients undergoing PCI.
- Tirofiban and eptifibatide are also indicated in patients with continued or recurrent ischemia despite treatment with aspirin and an anticoagulant.

Heparin
- Either UFH or LMWHs should be administered to patients with non–ST-segment-elevation ACS. Therapy should be continued for up to 48 hours or until the end of the angiography or PCI procedure.
- In patients initiating warfarin therapy, UFH or LMWHs should be continued until the INR with warfarin is in the therapeutic range.
- For non–ST-segment-elevation ACS, the dose of UFH is 60 to 70 units/kg IV bolus (maximum 5000 units) followed by a continuous IV infusion of 12 to 15 units/kg/h (maximum 1000 units/h). The dose is titrated to maintain the aPTT between 1.5 and 2.5 times control.
- LMWHs are administered by a fixed, weight-based dose:
  - **Enoxaparin:** 1 mg/kg subcutaneously every 12 hours (extend the interval to 24 hours if creatinine clearance is less than 30 mL/min)
  - **Dalteparin:** 120 IU/kg subcutaneously every 12 hours (maximum single bolus dose of 10,000 units)

Nitrates
In the absence of contraindications, sublingual followed by IV NTG should be administered to all patients with non–ST-segment-elevation ACS. IV NTG is continued for approximately 24 hours after ischemia relief.

β Blockers
In the absence of contraindications, IV followed by oral β blockers should be administered to all patients with non–ST-segment-elevation ACS. The drugs are continued indefinitely.

Calcium Channel Blockers
As described previously, calcium channel blockers should not be administered to most patients with ACS.

► SECONDARY PREVENTION FOLLOWING MI

DESIRED OUTCOME

- The long-term goals after MI are to (1) control modifiable CHD risk factors, (2) prevent the development of systolic heart failure, (3) prevent recurrent MI and stroke, and (4) prevent death, including sudden cardiac death.

PHARMACOTHERAPY

General Approach

- Drug therapy that has been proven to decrease mortality, heart failure, reinfarction, or stroke should be started before hospital discharge for secondary prevention.
- The ACC/AHA guidelines suggest that after MI from either ST-segment-elevation or non–ST-segment-elevation ACS, patients should receive indefinite treatment with aspirin, a β blocker, and an ACE inhibitor.
- Most patients with non–ST-segment-elevation ACS should receive clopidogrel in addition to aspirin for up to 9 months. Selected patients also will be treated with long-term warfarin anticoagulation.
- For all ACS patients, treatment and control of modifiable risk factors such as hypertension, dyslipidemia, and diabetes mellitus are essential.

Aspirin

- Aspirin decreases the risk of death, recurrent MI, and stroke after MI. All patients should receive aspirin indefinitely (or clopidogrel if there are aspirin contraindications).
- The risk of major bleeding from chronic aspirin therapy is approximately 2% and is dose related. Therefore, chronic low doses of 75 to 162 mg are recommended.

Anticoagulation

Warfarin should be considered in selected patients after an ACS, including those with a left ventricular thrombus, extensive ventricular wall motion abnormalities on cardiac echocardiogram, and a history of thromboembolic disease or chronic atrial fibrillation.

β Blockers, Nitrates, and Calcium Channel Blockers

- After an ACS, patients should received a β blocker indefinitely, regardless of whether they have residual symptoms of angina. Therapy should continue indefinitely in the absence of contraindications or intolerance.
- A calcium channel blocker can be used to prevent anginal symptoms in patients who cannot tolerate or have a contraindication to a β blocker but should not be used routinely in the absence of such symptoms.
- All patients should be prescribed a short-acting sublingual NTG or lingual NTG spray to relieve anginal symptoms when necessary. Chronic long-acting nitrates have not been shown to reduce CHD event after MI. Therefore, chronic nitrates are not used in ACS patients who have undergone revascularization unless the patient has chronic stable angina or significant coronary stenosis that was not revascularized.

ACE Inhibitors and Angiotensin Receptor Blockers

- ACE inhibitors should be initiated in all patients after MI to reduce mortality, decrease reinfarction, and prevent the development of heart failure. On the basis of extensive benefits of ACE inhibitors in patients with CAD, their routine use should be considered in all patients following an ACS (even those without infarction) in the absence of a contraindication. Their benefit is most likely related to prevention of cardiac remodeling.

- The dose should be low initially and titrated to the dose used in clinical trials if tolerated. Example doses include the following:
  - **Captopril:** 6.25 to 12.5 mg initially; target dose 50 mg two or three times daily
  - **Enalapril:** 2.5 to 5 mg initially; target dose 10 mg twice daily
  - **Lisinopril:** 2.5 to 5 mg initially; target dose 10 to 20 mg once daily
  - **Ramipril:** 1.25 to 2.5 mg initially; target dose 5 mg twice daily or 10 mg once daily
  - **Trandolapril:** 1 mg initially; target dose 4 mg once daily
- An angiotensin receptor blocker may be prescribed for patients with ACE inhibitor cough and either clinical signs of heart failure or LVEF less than 40%. Example doses include the following:
  - **Candesartan**: 4 to 8 mg initially; target dose 32 mg once daily
  - **Valsartan**: 40 mg initially; target dose 160 mg twice daily

Lipid-Lowering Agents
- All patients with CAD should receive dietary counseling and pharmacotherapy in order to reach an LDL cholesterol concentration of less than 100 mg/dL. Newer recommendations from the NCEP give an optional LDL goal of less than 70 mg/dL in selected patients.
- Statins are the preferred agents for lowering LDL cholesterol and should be prescribed at or near discharge in most patients.
- A fibrate derivative or niacin should be considered in selected patients with a low HDL cholesterol (less than 40 mg/dL) and/or a high triglyceride level (greater than 200 mg/dL).

▶ EVALUATION OF THERAPEUTIC OUTCOMES

- Monitoring parameters for efficacy of therapy for both ST-segment-elevation and non–ST-segment-elevation ACS include (1) relief of ischemic discomfort, (2) return of ECG changes to baseline, and (3) absence or resolution of heart failure signs.
- Monitoring parameters for adverse effects are dependent upon the individual drugs used. In general, the most common adverse reactions from ACS therapies are hypotension and bleeding.

See Chapter 16, Acute Coronary Syndromes, authored by Sarah A. Spinler and Simon de Denus, for a more detailed discussion of this topic.

Chapter 6

▶ ARRHYTHMIAS

▶ DEFINITION

Arrhythmia is defined as loss of cardiac rhythm, especially irregularity of heartbeat. This chapter covers the group of conditions caused by an abnormality in the rate, regularity, or sequence of cardiac activation.

▶ PATHOPHYSIOLOGY

SUPRAVENTRICULAR ARRHYTHMIAS

Common supraventricular tachycardias requiring drug treatment are atrial fibrillation or atrial flutter, paroxysmal supraventricular tachycardia, and automatic atrial tachycardias. Other common supraventricular arrhythmias that usually do not require drug therapy (e.g., premature atrial complexes, wandering atrial pacemaker, sinus arrhythmia, sinus tachycardia) are not included in this chapter.

Atrial Fibrillation and Atrial Flutter

- Atrial fibrillation is characterized as an extremely rapid (400 to 600 atrial beats/min) and disorganized atrial activation. There is a loss of atrial contraction (atrial kick), and supraventricular impulses penetrate the atrioventricular (AV) conduction system in variable degrees, resulting in irregular ventricular activation and irregularly irregular pulse (120 to 180 beats/min).
- Atrial flutter is characterized by rapid (270 to 330 atrial beats/min) but regular atrial activation. The ventricular response usually has a regular pattern and a pulse of 300 beats/min. This arrhythmia occurs less frequently than atrial fibrillation but has similar precipitating factors, consequences, and drug therapy.
- The predominant mechanism of atrial fibrillation and atrial flutter is reentry, which is usually associated with organic heart disease that causes atrial distention (e.g., ischemia or infarction, hypertensive heart disease, valvular disorders). Additional associated disorders include acute pulmonary embolus and chronic lung disease, resulting in pulmonary hypertension and cor pulmonale; and states of high adrenergic tone such as thyrotoxicosis, alcohol withdrawal, sepsis, or excessive physical exertion.

Paroxysmal Supraventricular Tachycardia Caused by Reentry

Paroxysmal supraventricular tachycardia (PSVT) arising by reentrant mechanisms includes arrhythmias caused by AV nodal reentry, AV reentry incorporating an anomalous AV pathway, sinoatrial (SA) nodal reentry, and intra-atrial reentry.

Automatic Atrial Tachycardias

Automatic atrial tachycardias such as multifocal atrial tachycardia appear to arise from supraventricular foci with enhanced automatic properties. Severe pulmonary disease is the underlying precipitating disorder in 60% to 80% of patients.

VENTRICULAR ARRHYTHMIAS

Premature Ventricular Complexes

Premature ventricular complexes (PVCs) are common ventricular rhythm disturbances that occur in patients with or without heart disease and may be elicited

II experimentally by abnormal automaticity, triggered activity, or reentrant mechanisms.

Ventricular Tachycardia

- Ventricular tachycardia (VT) is defined by three or more repetitive PVCs occurring at a rate greater than 100 beats/min. It occurs most commonly in acute myocardial infarction (MI); other causes are severe electrolyte abnormalities (e.g., hypokalemia), hypoxemia, and digitalis toxicity. The chronic recurrent form is almost always associated with underlying organic heart disease (e.g., idiopathic dilated cardiomyopathy or remote MI with left ventricular [LV] aneurysm).
- Sustained VT is that which requires therapeutic intervention to restore a stable rhythm or that lasts a relatively long time (usually greater than 30 seconds). Nonsustained VT (NSVT) self-terminates after a brief duration (usually less than 30 seconds). Incessant VT refers to VT occurring more frequently than sinus rhythm, so that VT becomes the dominant rhythm. Exercise-induced VT occurs during high sympathetic tone (e.g., physical exertion). Monomorphic VT has a consistent QRS configuration, whereas polymorphic VT has varying QRS complexes. Torsades de pointes (TdP) is a polymorphic VT in which the QRS complexes appear to undulate around a central axis.

Ventricular Proarrhythmia

Proarrhythmia refers to development of a significant new arrhythmia (such as VT, ventricular fibrillation [VF], or TdP) or worsening of an existing arrhythmia. Proarrhythmia results from the same mechanisms that cause other arrhythmias or from an alteration in the underlying substrate due to the antiarrhythmic agent.

Incessant Monomorphic Ventricular Tachycardia

Although the proarrhythmia associated with type Ic agents was initially thought to occur within several days of drug initiation, risk may persist throughout treatment. Factors that predispose patients to this type of proarrhythmia include underlying ventricular arrhythmias, ischemic heart disease, and poor left ventricular function.

Torsades de Pointes

TdP is a rapid form of polymorphic VT associated with evidence of delayed ventricular repolarization due to blockade of potassium conductance. TdP may be hereditary or acquired. Acquired forms are associated with many clinical conditions and drugs, especially type Ia and type III I_{Kr} blockers. Quinidine-induced TdP or quinidine syncope occurs in 4% to 8% of patients treated with this agent.

Ventricular Fibrillation

VF is electrical anarchy of the ventricle resulting in no cardiac output and cardiovascular collapse. Sudden cardiac death occurs most commonly in patients with ischemic heart disease and primary myocardial disease associated with LV dysfunction. VF associated with acute MI may be classified as either (1) primary (an uncomplicated MI not associated with heart failure) or (2) secondary or complicated (an MI complicated by heart failure).

BRADYARRHYTHMIAS

- Asymptomatic sinus bradyarrhythmias (heart rate less than 60 beats/min) are common especially in young, athletically active individuals. However, some patients have sinus node dysfunction (sick sinus syndrome) because of underlying organic heart disease and the normal aging process, which attenuates

SA nodal function. Sinus node dysfunction is usually representative of diffuse conduction disease, which may be accompanied by AV block and by paroxysmal tachycardias such as atrial fibrillation. Alternating bradyarrhythmias and tachyarrhythmias are referred to as the tachy–brady syndrome.

- AV block or conduction delay may occur in any area of the AV conduction system. AV block may be found in patients without underlying heart disease (e.g., trained athletes) or during sleep when vagal tone is high. It may be transient when the underlying etiology is reversible (e.g., myocarditis, myocardial ischemia, after cardiovascular surgery, during drug therapy). β Blockers, digitalis, or calcium antagonists may cause AV block, primarily in the AV nodal area. Type I antiarrhythmics may exacerbate conduction delays below the level of the AV node. AV block may be irreversible if the cause is acute MI, rare degenerative disease, primary myocardial disease, or a congenital condition.

▶ CLINICAL PRESENTATION

- Supraventricular tachycardias may cause a variety of clinical manifestations ranging from no symptoms to minor palpitations and/or irregular pulse to severe and even life-threatening symptoms. Patients may experience dizziness or acute syncopal episodes; symptoms of heart failure; anginal chest pain; or, more often, a choking or pressure sensation during the tachycardia episode.
- Atrial fibrillation or flutter may be manifested by the entire range of symptoms associated with other supraventricular tachycardias, but syncope is not a common presenting symptom. An additional complication of atrial fibrillation is arterial embolization resulting from atrial stasis and poorly adherent mural thrombi, which accounts for the most devastating complication: embolic stroke. Patients with atrial fibrillation and concurrent mitral stenosis or severe systolic heart failure are at particularly high risk for cerebral embolism.
- PVCs often cause no symptoms or only mild palpitations. The presentation of VT may vary from totally asymptomatic to pulseless hemodynamic collapse. Consequences of proarrhythmia range from no symptoms to worsening of symptoms to sudden death. VF results in hemodynamic collapse, syncope, and cardiac arrest.
- Patients with bradyarrhythmias experience symptoms associated with hypotension such as dizziness, syncope, fatigue, and confusion. If LV dysfunction exists, symptoms of congestive heart failure may be exacerbated.

▶ DIAGNOSIS

- The surface electrocardiogram (ECG) is the cornerstone of diagnosis for cardiac rhythm disturbances.
- Less sophisticated methods are often the initial tools for detecting qualitative and quantitative alterations of heartbeat. For example, direct auscultation can reveal the irregularly irregular pulse that is characteristic of atrial fibrillation.
- Proarrhythmia can be difficult to diagnose because of the variable nature of underlying arrhythmias.
- TdP is characterized by long QT intervals or prominent U waves on the surface ECG.
- Specific maneuvers may be required to delineate the etiology of syncope associated with bradyarrhythmias. Diagnosis of carotid sinus hypersensitivity can be confirmed by performing carotid sinus massage with ECG and blood pressure monitoring. Vasovagal syncope can be diagnosed using the upright body-tilt test.

- On the basis of ECG findings, AV block is usually categorized into three different types (first-, second-, or third-degree AV block).

▶ DESIRED OUTCOME

The desired outcome depends on the underlying arrhythmia. For example, the ultimate treatment goals of treating atrial fibrillation or flutter are restoring sinus rhythm, preventing thromboembolic complications, and preventing further recurrences.

▶ TREATMENT

GENERAL PRINCIPLES

- The use of antiarrhythmic drugs in the United States is declining because of major trials that showed increased mortality with their use in several clinical situations, the realization of proarrhythmia as a significant side effect, and the advancing technology of nondrug therapies such as ablation and the internal cardioverter-defibrillator.

CLASSIFICATION OF ANTIARRHYTHMIC DRUGS

- Drugs may have antiarrhythmic activity by directly altering conduction in several ways. Drugs may depress the automatic properties of abnormal pacemaker cells by decreasing the slope of phase 4 depolarization and/or by elevating threshold potential. Drugs may alter the conduction characteristics of the pathways of a reentrant loop.
- The most frequently used classification system is that proposed by Vaughan Williams (Table 6–1). Type Ia drugs slow conduction velocity, prolong refractoriness, and decrease the automatic properties of sodium-dependent (normal and diseased) conduction tissue. Type Ia drugs are broad-spectrum antiarrhythmics, being effective for both supraventricular and ventricular arrhythmias.
- Although categorized separately, type Ib drugs probably act similarly to type Ia drugs, except that type Ib agents are considerably more effective in ventricular than supraventricular arrhythmias.
- Type Ic drugs profoundly slow conduction velocity while leaving refractoriness relatively unaltered. Although effective for both ventricular and supraventricular arrhythmias, their use for ventricular arrhythmias has been limited by the risk of proarrhythmia.
- Collectively, type I drugs can be referred to as sodium channel blockers. Antiarrhythmic sodium channel receptor principles account for drug combinations that are additive (e.g., **quinidine** and **mexiletine**) and antagonistic (e.g., **flecainide** and **lidocaine**), as well as potential antidotes to excess sodium–channel blockade (e.g., sodium bicarbonate, propranolol).
- Type II drugs include β-**adrenergic antagonists;** clinically relevant mechanisms result from their antiadrenergic actions. β Blockers are most useful in tachycardias in which nodal tissues are abnormally automatic or are a portion of a reentrant loop. These agents are also helpful in slowing ventricular response in atrial tachycardias (e.g., atrial fibrillation) by their effects on the AV node.

TABLE 6–1. Classification of Antiarrhythmic Drugs

Type	Drug	Conduction Velocity[a]	Refractory Period	Automaticity	Ion Block
Ia	Quinidine Procainamide Disopyramide	↓	↑	↓	Sodium (intermediate) Potassium
Ib	Lidocaine Mexiletine Tocainide	0/↓	↓	↓	Sodium (fast on/off)
Ic	Flecainide Propafenone[c] Moricizine[d]	↓↓	0	↓	Sodium (slow on/off) Potassium[e]
II[b]	β-Blockers	↓	↑	↓	Calcium (indirect)
III	Amiodarone[f] Bretylium[c] Dofetilide Sotalol[c] Ibutilide	0	↑↑	0	Potassium
IV[b]	Verapamil Diltiazem	↓	↑	↓	Calcium

[a]Variables for normal tissue models in ventricular tissue.
[b]Variables for SA and AV nodal tissue only.
[c]Also has type II β-blocking actions.
[d]Classification controversial.
[e]Not clinically manifest.
[f]Also has sodium, calcium, and β-blocking actions.

- Type III drugs specifically prolong refractoriness in atrial and ventricular fibers and include very different drugs that share the common effect of delaying repolarization by blocking potassium channels.
  - **Bretylium** prolongs repolarization by blocking potassium conductance independent of the sympathetic nervous system, increases the VF threshold, and seems to have selective antifibrillatory but not antitachycardic effects. Bretylium can be effective in VF but is often ineffective in VT.
  - In contrast, **amiodarone** and **sotalol** are effective in most tachycardias. Amiodarone displays electrophysiologic characteristics consistent with each type of antiarrhythmic drug. It is a sodium channel blocker with relatively fast on-off kinetics, has nonselective β-blocking actions, blocks potassium channels, and has slight calcium antagonist activity. The impressive effectiveness and low proarrhythmic potential of amiodarone have challenged the notion that selective ion channel blockade is preferable. **Sotalol** is a potent inhibitor of outward potassium movement during repolarization and also possesses β-blocking actions. **Ibutilide** and **dofetilide** block the rapid component of the delayed potassium rectifier current.
- Type IV drugs inhibit calcium entry into the cell, which slows conduction, prolongs refractoriness, and decreases SA and AV nodal automaticity. **Calcium channel antagonists** are effective for automatic or reentrant tachycardias that arise from or use the SA or AV nodes.
- Usual intravenous (IV) antiarrhythmic doses and common side effects are listed in Tables 6–2 and 6–3, respectively.

TABLE 6–2. Intravenous Antiarrhythmic Dosing

Drug	Clinical Situation	Dose
Amiodarone	Recurrent VT/VF	150 mg/10 min IV Push
		1 mg/min for 6 h, then 0.5 mg/min infusion
	Cardiac arrest	300 mg IV push
Bretylium	Acute VF	5 mg/min IV push (may repeat to total dose 30 mg/kg)
		1–2 mg/min infusion if needed
Diltiazem	PSVT; rate control AF	0.25 mg/kg IV push (may repeat with 0.35 mg/kg)
	5–15 mg/h infusion	
Ibutilide	Termination AF	1 mg/10 min IV push (may repeat if needed)
Lidocaine	VT/VF	100 mg IV push (may repeat up to total dose 300 mg) (limit total to 200 mg if CHF present)
		2–4 mg/min infusion (1–2 mg/min if liver disease or CHF)
Procainamide	AF, VT	15–18 mg/kg at 20–50 mg/min load
		1–6 mg/min infusion
Verapamil	PSVT; rate control AF	5 mg IV push (may repeat up to 20 mg)
		5–15 mg/h infusion

VT, ventricular tachycardia; VF, ventricular fibrillation; PSVT, paroxysmal supraventricular tachycardia; AF, atrial fibrillation/flutter.

ATRIAL FIBRILLATION OR ATRIAL FLUTTER

- Many methods are available for restoring sinus rhythm, preventing thromboembolic complications, and preventing further recurrences (Figure 6–1); however, treatment selection depends in part on onset and severity of symptoms.
- If symptoms are severe and of recent onset, patients may require direct-current cardioversion (DCC) to restore sinus rhythm immediately.
- If symptoms are tolerable, drugs that slow conduction and increase refractoriness in the AV node should be used as initial therapy. Many clinicians prefer IV calcium antagonists (**verapamil** or **diltiazem**). If a high adrenergic state is the precipitating factor, IV β blockers (e.g., **propranolol, esmolol**) can be highly effective and should be considered first. Type Ia and III antiarrhythmic agents should not be administered initially because they may paradoxically increase ventricular response in the absence of drugs that slow AV nodal conduction. **Digoxin's** place in therapy has been questioned because it is sometimes ineffective and often slow in onset.
- After treatment with AV nodal blocking agents and a subsequent decrease in ventricular response, the patient should be evaluated for the possibility of restoring sinus rhythm if atrial fibrillation persists.
- If sinus rhythm is to be restored, anticoagulation should be initiated prior to cardioversion because return of atrial contraction increases risk of thromboembolism. Current recommendations are to initiate **warfarin** (international normalized ratio [INR] 2 to 3) for at least 3 weeks prior to cardioversion and continuing for at least 1 month after effective cardioversion. Anticoagulation

TABLE 6–3. Side Effects of Antiarrhythmic Drugs

Amiodarone	CNS, corneal microdeposites/blurred vision, optic neuropathy/neuritis, GI, aggravation of underlying ventricular arrhythmias, torsade de pointes, bradycardia or AV block, bruising without thrombocytopenia, pulmonary fibrosis, hepatitis, hypothyrodidism, hyperthyroidism, photosensitivity, blue-gray skin discoloration, myopathy, hypotension and phlebitis (IV use)
Bretylium	Hypotension, GI
Disopyramide	Anticholinergic symptoms, GI, torsade de pointes, heart failure, aggravation of underlying conductionn disturbances and/or ventricular arrhythmias, hypoglycemia, hepatic cholestasis
Dofetilide	Torsades de pointes
Flecainide	Blurred vision, dizziness, headache, GI, bronchospasm,[a] aggravation of underlying
Propafenone	heart failure, conduction disturbances or ventricular arrhythmias
Ibutilide	Torsades de pointes, hypotension
Lidocaine	CNS, siezures, psychosis, sinus arrest, aggravation of underlying conduction disturbances
Mexiletine	CNS, psychosis, GI, aggravation of underlying conduction disturbances or ventricular arrhythmias
Moricizine	Dizziness, headache, GI, aggravation of underlying conduction disturbances or ventricular arrhythmias
Procainamide	Systemic lupus erythematosus, GI, torsade de pointes, aggravaion of underlying heart failure, conduction disturbances or ventricular arrhythmias, agranulocytosis
Quinidine	Cinchonism, diarrhea, GI, hypotension, torsade de pointes, aggravation of underlying heart failure, conduction disturbances or ventricular arrhythimias, hepatitis, thrombocytopenia, hemolytic anemia
Sotalol	Fatigue, GI, depression, torsades de pointes, bronchospasm, aggravation of underlying heart failure, conduction disturbances or ventricular arrhythmias
Tocainide	CNS, psychosis, GI, aggravation of underlying conduction disturbances or ventricular arrhythmias, rash/arthralgias, pulmonary infiltrates, agranulocytosis, thrombocytopenia

[a]Propafenone only.
GI, nausea, anorexia; CNS, confusion, paresthesias, tremor, ataxia.

II

may not be necessary in patients with atrial fibrillation of less than 48 hours' duration and in the absence of atrial thrombus or severe stasis on transesophageal echocardiography (TEE).

- After prior anticoagulation or TEE, methods for restoring sinus rhythm in patients with atrial fibrillation or flutter are pharmacologic cardioversion and DCC. International consensus guidelines recommend that elective DCC be considered first. DCC is quick and more often successful, but it requires prior sedation or anesthesia and has a small risk of serious complications such as sinus arrest or ventricular arrhythmias. Although type Ia, Ic, and III agents have all been shown to be effective, there is strong evidence of efficacy only for type III pure I_k blockers (e.g., **ibutilide, dofetilide**) and type Ic drugs (e.g., **flecainide, propafenone**). Advantages of initial drug therapy are that an effective agent may be determined in case long-term therapy is required. Disadvantages are significant side effects such as drug-induced TdP, drug–drug interactions, and lower cardioversion rate for drugs compared with DCC.

- The American College of Chest Physicians Consensus Conference on antithrombotic therapy recommends chronic **warfarin** treatment (INR 2 to 3, target 2.5) for all patients with atrial fibrillation who are at high risk for stroke (i.e.,

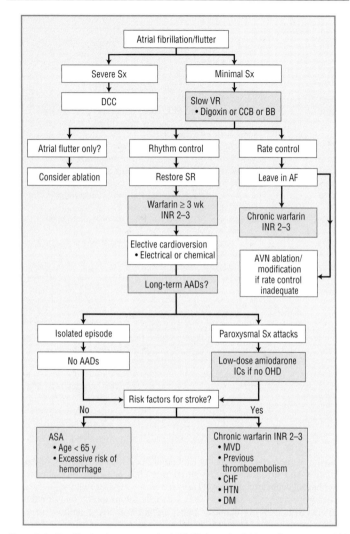

Figure 6–1. Algorithm for the treatment of atrial fibrillation and atrial flutter. Sx, symptoms; DCC, direct-current cardioversion; VR, ventricular rate; CCB, calcium channel antagonist (verapamil or diltiazem); BB, β blocker; SR, sinus rhythm; AF, atrial fibrillation or flutter; INR, international normalized ratio; AADs, antiarrhythmic drugs; AVN, atrioventricular node; ICs, type Ic antiarrhythmic drugs; OHD, organic heart disease; ASA, aspirin; MVD, mitral valve disease; CHF, congestive heart failure; HTN, hypertension; DM, diabetes mellitus.

those with prosthetic heart valves, rheumatic valvular disease, prior history of thromboembolism, age greater than 75 years, LV dysfunction, or hypertension). Those at low risk (i.e., age less than 65 years without discernible cardiovascular disease or lone atrial fibrillation) should receive **aspirin,** 325 mg/day. Warfarin or aspirin should be continued until sinus rhythm has been maintained for at least 4 weeks. Antithrombotic therapy should be continued indefinitely in patients with permanent atrial fibrillation or documented, recurrent paroxysms.

- Atrial fibrillation often recurs after initial cardioversion because most patients have irreversible underlying heart or lung disease. A meta-analysis confirmed that **quinidine** maintained sinus rhythm better than placebo; however, 50% of patients had recurrent atrial fibrillation within a year, and more importantly, quinidine increased mortality, presumably due in part to proarrhythmia. Type Ic (e.g., **flecainide, propafenone**) and type III (e.g., **amiodarone, sotalol, dofetilide**) antiarrhythmic agents may be alternatives to quinidine; however, these agents are also associated with proarrhythmia. Consequently, chronic antiarrhythmic drugs should be reserved for patients with documented paroxysmal atrial fibrillation associated with intolerable symptoms. Low-dose amiodarone is the preferred agent for most patients.

PAROXYSMAL SUPRAVENTRICULAR TACHYCARDIA

- The choice between pharmacologic and nonpharmacologic methods for treating PSVT depends on symptom severity (Figure 6–2). Synchronized DCC is the treatment of choice if symptoms are severe (e.g., syncope, near syncope, anginal chest pain, severe heart failure). Nondrug measures that increase vagal tone to the AV node (e.g., unilateral carotid sinus massage, Valsalva maneuver) can be used for mild to moderate symptoms. If these methods fail, drug therapy is the next option.
- The choice among drugs is based on the QRS complex (Figure 6–2). Drugs can be divided into three broad categories: (1) those that directly or indirectly increase vagal tone to the AV node (e.g., **digoxin**); (2) those that depress conduction through slow, calcium-dependent tissue (e.g., **adenosine, β blockers, calcium channel blockers**); and (3) those that depress conduction through fast, sodium-dependent tissue (e.g., **quinidine, procainamide, disopyramide, flecainide**).
- **Adenosine** has been recommended as the drug of first choice in patients with PSVT because its short duration of action will not cause prolonged hemodynamic compromise in patients with wide QRS complexes who actually have VT rather than PSVT.
- After acute PSVT is terminated, long-term preventive treatment is indicated if frequent episodes necessitate therapeutic intervention or if episodes are infrequent but severely symptomatic. Serial testing of antiarrhythmic agents can be evaluated in the ambulatory setting via ambulatory ECG recordings (Holter monitors) or telephonic transmissions of cardiac rhythm (event monitors) or by invasive electrophysiologic techniques in the laboratory.
- Chronic antiarrhythmic drug treatment in young, otherwise healthy patients is problematic because of possible need for lifelong daily medication, poor tolerability, occasional severe side effects, and frequent lack of efficacy.
- Transcutaneous catheter ablation using radiofrequency current on the PSVT substrate should be considered in any patient who would have previously been considered for chronic antiarrhythmic drug treatment. It is highly effective and curative, rarely results in complications, obviates the need for chronic antiarrhythmic drug therapy, and is cost-effective.

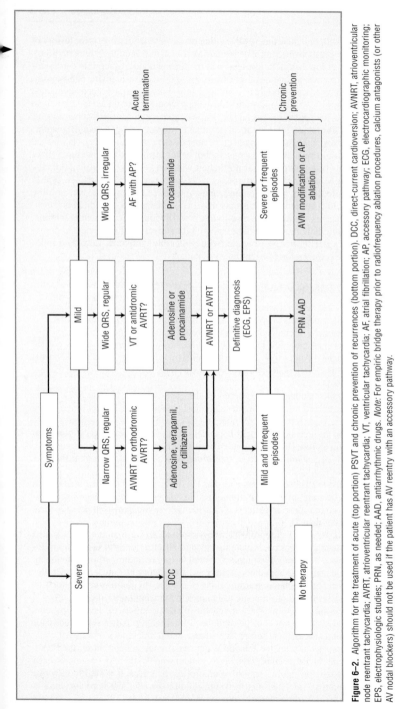

Figure 6–2. Algorithm for the treatment of acute (top portion) PSVT and chronic prevention of recurrences (bottom portion). DCC, direct-current cardioversion; AVNRT, atrioventricular node reentrant tachycardia; AVRT, atrioventricular reentrant tachycardia; VT, ventricular tachycardia; AF, atrial fibrillation; AP, accessory pathway; ECG, electrocardiographic monitoring; EPS, electrophysiologic studies; PRN, as needed; AAD, antiarrhythmic drugs. *Note:* For empiric bridge therapy prior to radiofrequency ablation procedures, calcium antagonists (or other AV nodal blockers) should not be used if the patient has AV reentry with an accessory pathway.

AUTOMATIC ATRIAL TACHYCARDIAS

- Underlying precipitating factors should be corrected by ensuring proper oxygenation and ventilation and by correcting acid-base or electrolyte disturbances.
- If tachycardia persists, the need for additional treatment is determined by symptoms. Patients with asymptomatic atrial tachycardia and relatively slow ventricular response usually require no drug therapy.
- In symptomatic patients, medical therapy can be tailored either to control ventricular response or to restore sinus rhythm. Calcium antagonists (e.g., **verapamil**) are considered first-line drug therapy for decreasing ventricular response. Type I agents (e.g., **procainamide, quinidine**) are only occasionally effective in restoring sinus rhythm. DCC is ineffective, and β blockers are usually contraindicated because of coexisting severe pulmonary disease or uncompensated heart failure.

PREMATURE VENTRICULAR COMPLEXES

- In apparently healthy individuals, drug therapy is unnecessary because PVCs without associated heart disease carry little or no risk. In patients with risk factors for arrhythmic death (recent MI, LV dysfunction, complex PVCs), chronic drug therapy should be restricted to β **blockers** because only they have been conclusively proven to prevent mortality in these patients.

VENTRICULAR TACHYCARDIA

Acute Ventricular Tachycardia

- If severe symptoms are present, DCC should be instituted to restore sinus rhythm immediately. Precipitating factors should be corrected if possible. If VT is an isolated electrical event associated with a transient initiating factor (e.g., acute myocardial ischemia, digitalis toxicity), there is no need for long-term antiarrhythmic therapy after precipitating factors are corrected.
- Patients with mild or no symptoms can be treated initially with antiarrhythmic drugs. IV **amiodarone** is usually the first step in this situation. **Procainamide** or **lidocaine** given IV are suitable alternatives. If lidocaine fails to terminate tachycardia, IV procainamide (loading dose and infusion) can be tried. DCC should be instituted or a transvenous pacing wire should be inserted if the patient's status deteriorates, VT degenerates to VF, or drug therapy fails.

Sustained Ventricular Tachycardia

- Patients with chronic recurrent sustained VT are at extremely high risk for death; trial-and-error attempts to find effective therapy are unwarranted. Neither electrophysiologic studies nor serial Holter monitoring with drug testing is ideal. These findings and the side-effect profiles of antiarrhythmic agents have led to nondrug approaches.
- The automatic implantable cardioverter defibrillator (ICD) may be the most effective method for preventing sudden death due to recurrent VT or VF. It resulted in better overall survival at 3 years than chronic antiarrhythmic with amiodarone, the most effective drug known.
- Patients with complex ventricular ectopy should not receive type I or III antiarrhythmic drugs.

Nonsustained Ventricular Tachycardia

The approach to NSVT is controversial. Patients with long symptomatic episodes require drug therapy, but most patients are asymptomatic. Patients with NSVT and coronary disease are at risk for sudden death, particularly if they have inducible

II sustained VT after programmed stimulation. Consequently, these patients should undergo electrophysiologic studies and be given chronic preventive therapy with an ICD or empiric **amiodarone** if sustained VT/VF is inducible.

Proarrhythmia

Proarrhythmia is resistant to resuscitation with cardioversion or overdrive pacing. Some clinicians have had success with IV **lidocaine** (competes for the sodium channel receptor) or **sodium bicarbonate** (reverses the excessive sodium channel blockade).

Torsades de Pointes

- For an acute episode, most patients require and respond to DCC. However, TdP tends to be paroxysmal and often recurs rapidly after countershock.
- IV **magnesium sulfate** is considered the drug of choice for preventing recurrences of TdP. If ineffective, strategies to increase heart rate and shorten ventricular repolarization should be instituted (i.e., temporary transvenous pacing at 105 to 120 beats/min or pharmacologic pacing with **isoproterenol** or **epinephrine** infusion). Agents that prolong the QT interval should be discontinued, and exacerbating factors (e.g., hypokalemia) corrected. Drugs that further prolong repolarization (e.g., IV procainamide) are contraindicated. Lidocaine is usually ineffective.

Ventricular Fibrillation

VF (with or without associated myocardial ischemia) should be managed according to the American Heart Association's recommendations for advanced cardiac life support (see Chapter 7). After successful resuscitation, antiarrhythmics should be continued until the patient's rhythm and overall status are stable. Long-term antiarrhythmics or ICD implantation may or may not be required.

BRADYARRHYTHMIAS

- Treatment of sinus node dysfunction involves elimination of symptomatic bradycardia and possibly managing alternating tachycardias such as atrial fibrillation. Asymptomatic sinus bradyarrhythmias usually do not require therapeutic intervention.
- In general, long-term therapy of choice for patients with significant symptoms is a permanent ventricular pacemaker.
- Drugs commonly employed to treat supraventricular tachycardias should be used with caution, if at all, in the absence of a functioning pacemaker.
- Symptomatic carotid sinus hypersensitivity also should be treated with permanent pacemaker therapy. Patients who remain symptomatic may benefit from adding an α-adrenergic stimulant such as **midodrine,** sometimes with a β **blocker** to maximize α-sympathetic stimulation.
- Vasovagal syncope can usually be treated successfully with oral β blockers to inhibit the sympathetic surge that causes forceful ventricular contraction and precedes the onset of hypotension and bradycardia. Other drugs that have been used successfully (with or without β blockers) include anticholinergics (**scopolamine patches, disopyramide**), α-adrenergic agonists (**midodrine**), adenosine analogs (**theophylline, dipyridamole**), and selective serotonin reuptake inhibitors (**sertraline, fluoxetine**).

Atrioventricular Block

- The cornerstone of acute treatment for acute, symptomatic bradycardia or AV block is temporary pacing through a transvenous wire or, in an emergency, by transcutaneous leads. **Atropine,** 0.5 to 1 mg IV, should be given as the pacing leads are being placed. **Epinephrine** or **dopamine** infusions can be used in the event of atropine failure. These agents will not help if AV block is below the AV node (Mobitz II or trifascicular AV block).

- Chronic symptomatic AV block warrants insertion of a permanent pacemaker. Patients without symptoms can sometimes be followed closely without the need for a pacemaker.

▶ EVALUATION OF THERAPEUTIC OUTCOMES

The most important monitoring parameters include (1) mortality (total and due to arrhythmic death), (2) arrhythmia recurrence (duration, frequency, symptoms), (3) hemodynamic consequences (rate, blood pressure, symptoms), and (4) treatment complications (need for alternative or additional drugs, devices, or surgery).

See Chapter 17, Arrhythmias, authored by Jerry L. Bauman and Marieke Dekker Schoen, for a more detailed discussion of this topic.

Chapter 7

► CARDIOPULMONARY RESUSCITATION

► DEFINITION

Cardiopulmonary arrest is the abrupt cessation of spontaneous and effective ventilation and circulation after a cardiac or respiratory event. Cardiopulmonary resuscitation (CPR) provides artificial ventilation and circulation until it is possible to provide advanced cardiac life support (ACLS) and reestablish spontaneous circulation.

► PATHOPHYSIOLOGY

- Cardiopulmonary arrest in adults usually results from arrhythmias. The most common arrhythmias are ventricular fibrillation (VF) and pulseless ventricular tachycardia (PVT). In children, cardiopulmonary arrest is often the terminal event of progressive shock or respiratory failure.
- Two theories exist regarding the mechanism of blood flow in CPR. The cardiac pump theory states that the active compression of the heart between the sternum and vertebrae creates an "artificial systole" in which intraventricular pressure increases, the atrioventricular valves close, the aortic valve opens, and blood is forced out of the ventricles. When ventricular compression ends, the decline in intraventricular pressure causes the mitral and tricuspid valves to open, and ventricular filling begins. The more recent thoracic pump theory is based on the belief that blood flow during CPR results from intrathoracic pressure alterations induced by chest compressions. During compression (systole), a pressure gradient develops between the intrathoracic arteries and extrathoracic veins, causing forward blood flow from the lungs into the systemic circulation. After compression ends (diastole), intrathoracic pressure declines and blood flow returns to the lungs. Components of both theories may apply during CPR.

► CLINICAL PRESENTATION

The onset of cardiopulmonary arrest may be characterized by symptoms of chest pain; diaphoresis, dyspnea, shortness of breath, or no respiration; cold, clammy extremities; anxiety, mental status changes, or unconsciousness; and nausea or vomiting. Physical signs may include hypotension; tachycardia, bradycardia, irregular or no pulse; cyanosis; hypothermia; and distant or absent heart and lung sounds.

► DIAGNOSIS

- Rapid diagnosis is vital to the success of CPR. Patients must receive early intervention to prevent cardiac rhythms from degenerating into less treatable arrhythmias.
- Cardiac arrest is diagnosed initially by observation of clinical manifestations consistent with cardiac arrest. The diagnosis is confirmed by evaluating vital signs, especially heart rate and respirations.
- Electrocardiography (ECG) is useful for determining the cardiac rhythm, which in turn determines drug therapy.
  - VF is electrical anarchy of the ventricle resulting in no cardiac output and cardiovascular collapse.

- Pulseless electrical activity (PEA) is the absence of a detectable pulse and the presence of some type of electrical activity other than VF or PVT.
- Asystole is the presence of a "flat line" on the ECG monitor.

II

▶ DESIRED OUTCOME

- The goal of CPR is to return effective ventilation and circulation as quickly as possible to minimize hypoxic damage to vital organs.
- After successful resuscitation, the primary goals include optimizing tissue oxygenation, identifying precipitating cause(s) of arrest, and preventing subsequent episodes.

▶ TREATMENT

GENERAL PRINCIPLES

- The philosophies for providing CPR and emergency cardiovascular care (ECC) have been organized and revised periodically by the American Heart Association (AHA). The latest recommendations for CPR and ECC resulted from the Guidelines 2000 Conference (Figure 7–1).
- The likelihood of a successful resuscitation outcome is enhanced if each of four critical elements in the "chain of survival" is implemented promptly: (1) early access, which encompasses the events initiated after patient collapse to arrival of paramedics; (2) early bystander basic life support and CPR; (3) early defibrillation, including use of automatic external defibrillators (AEDs) by paramedics or trained laypersons; and (4) early application of ACLS.
- Basic life support is based on the assessment and application of the ABCs: airway, breathing, and circulation. If spontaneous breathing is absent, the airway should be opened and rescue breathing attempted. If the victim is pulseless, closed-chest compressions should be combined with rescue breathing. Basic life support should be continued until spontaneous circulation returns, ACLS is obtained, or exhaustion prohibits continued efforts.
- ACLS incorporates CPR, electrical defibrillation, airway management, ECG monitoring, and drug administration.
- Use of a central venous catheter is the most efficacious method of drug administration and results in faster and higher peak drug concentrations than peripheral venous administration. Because it is not practical to interrupt CPR for central line placement, a peripheral venous line must be used if a central line is not already in place. The antecubital vein is the first target for peripheral IV access.
- If neither central nor peripheral access is available, atropine, lidocaine, and epinephrine may be administered endotracheally. The endotracheal dose should generally be 2 to 2.5 times larger than the IV dose. The endotracheal dose should be diluted with 10 mL of sterile water or normal saline to permit distribution over the largest possible surface area. CPR should be interrupted and the dose administered beyond the tip of the endotracheal tube. Immediately thereafter, three to five forceful insufflations should be given using a bag-valve device to aerosolize the drug and enhance bioavailability.
- In pediatric patients, the intraosseous route may be used temporarily if no other routes of drug administration are available.
- Intracardiac drug administration is no longer recommended because of potential complications such as myocardial laceration, coronary artery laceration, hemopericardium, and pneumopericardium.

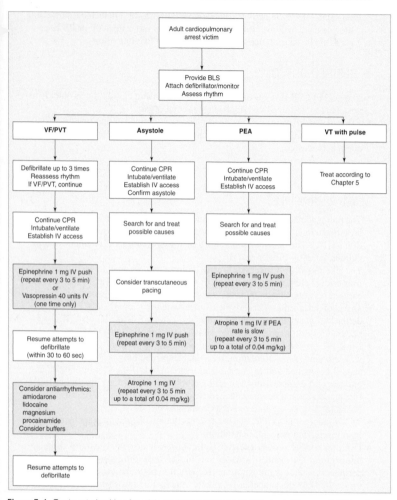

Figure 7–1. Treatment algorithm for adult cardiopulmonary arrest. BLS, basic life support; PEA, pulseless electrical activity; VT, ventricular tachycardia; VF, ventricular fibrillation; PVT, pulseless ventricular tachycardia; CPR, cardiopulmonary resuscitation; IV, intravenous.

TREATMENT OF VF AND PVT

Nonpharmacologic Therapy

- Persons in VF or PVT should receive electrical defibrillation with at least three shocks using 200 J with the first attempt and 200 to 360 J for the second and third attempts. After three unsuccessful attempts of defibrillation, the patient should receive about 1 minute of CPR. Endotracheal intubation and IV access should be obtained at this time. Once an airway is ensured, patients should be ventilated with 100% oxygen. Pharmacologic agents play a secondary role and are not recommended until an airway has been established and IV access attempted.

- Hypothermia can protect from cerebral injury by suppressing chemical reactions that occur after restoration of blood flow following cardiac arrest. On the basis of the results of two clinical trials, the Advanced Life Support Task Force of the International Liaison Committee on Resuscitation recommends that unconscious adult patients with spontaneous circulation after out-of-hospital cardiac arrest be cooled to 32 to 34°C for 12 to 24 hours if the initial rhythm was VF. Cooling may also benefit other rhythms or in-hospital cardiac arrest in adults; there is insufficient evidence to recommend therapeutic hypothermia in children.

Pharmacologic Therapy
Sympathomimetics

- The goal of sympathomimetic therapy is to augment both coronary and cerebral perfusion pressures during the low-flow state associated with CPR. These agents increase systemic arteriolar vasoconstriction, thereby improving coronary and cerebral perfusion pressure. They also maintain vascular tone, decrease arteriolar collapse, and shunt blood to the heart and brain.
- **Epinephrine** is a drug of first choice for treating VF, PVT, asystole, and PEA. It is an agonist of α_1, α_2, β_1, and β_2 receptors. Its effectiveness is thought to be primarily due to its α effects.
- The standard adult dose of epinephrine is 1 mg administered by intravenous push (IVP) every 3 to 5 minutes. If a 1-mg dose is unsuccessful, high-dose epinephrine (up to 0.2 mg/kg) may be considered. Although some studies have shown that higher doses (e.g., 5 mg) may increase the initial resuscitation rate, overall survival is not significantly improved.
- **Norepinephrine** (an α_1, α_2, and β_1 agonist) has demonstrated beneficial effects over epinephrine on myocardial oxygen balance and return of spontaneous circulation (ROSC), but there is no difference in survival to hospital discharge. Consequently, epinephrine remains the first-line sympathomimetic for CPR.

Vasopressin

- **Vasopressin** may be used as the drug of first choice instead of epinephrine for VF or PVT. Vasopressin is a potent vasoconstrictor that increases blood pressure and systemic vascular resistance. It may have several advantages over epinephrine. First, the metabolic acidosis that frequently accompanies cardiopulmonary arrest can blunt the vasoconstrictive effect of epinephrine; this does not occur with vasopressin. Second, stimulation of β receptors by epinephrine can increase myocardial oxygen demand and complicate the postresuscitative phase of CPR. Clinical studies suggest that vasopressin have a beneficial effect in out-of-hospital cardiac arrests or arrests secondary to asystole, situations in which the effect of catecholamines may be diminished because of profound acidosis. Its usefulness for in-hospital cardiac arrest secondary to VF or PVT remains questionable.
- A single 40-unit IV dose of vasopressin may be used in place of epinephrine after the initial three unsuccessful defibrillation attempts. If there is no response to vasopressin after 5 to 10 minutes, epinephrine therapy may resume.

Antiarrhythmics

- The primary reason for using antiarrhythmic agents after unsuccessful defibrillation and vasopressor administration is to prevent the development or recurrence of VF and PVT by raising the fibrillation threshold. Because there is conflicting evidence of their efficacy, these agents are categorized by the

Guidelines 2000 Conference as either possibly beneficial without causing harm (**amiodarone**, **magnesium**, **procainamide**) or indeterminate (**lidocaine**).

- **Amiodarone** is considered by many experts to be the antiarrhythmic of choice for secondary intervention. The initial adult dose is 300 mg diluted in 20 to 30 mL of normal saline or 5% dextrose in water (D_5W) and infused rapidly IV (e.g., over 10 minutes). Supplementary doses of 150 mg may be given by rapid infusion for recurrent or refractory VF/PVT, followed by an infusion of 1 mg/min for 6 hours and then 0.5 mg/min, to a maximum daily dose of 2 g.

- Hypotension occurs in approximately 20% of patients but can generally be reversed by decreasing the infusion rate. Other acute effects include fever, elevated liver function tests, confusion, nausea, and thrombocytopenia.

- **Lidocaine** has been shown to increase the VF threshold in some studies and to decrease the amount of energy required to convert VF to a more stable rhythm. However, its efficacy has been categorized as indeterminate (insufficient evidence to support a final class decision) because clinical studies have shown conflicting results on ROSC, survival to hospital admission, and other endpoints.

- The initial adult dose of lidocaine is 1.5 mg/kg by IVP. If treatment is associated with restoration of a stable rhythm, a continuous infusion of 2 to 4 mg/min is reasonable. Reappearance of an arrhythmia during a continuous infusion should be treated with a small bolus dose of lidocaine (0.5 mg/kg) and an increase in the infusion rate.

Alternatives for Refractory VF or PVT

- Persistent or recurrent VF or PVT after antiarrhythmic administration may be associated with underlying electrolyte abnormalities, primarily hyperkalemia, hypokalemia, and hypomagnesemia.

- **Magnesium** administration is recommended only when a low serum magnesium concentration is the suspected cause of an arrhythmia or when the patient experiences torsades de pointes (TdP). Magnesium treatment is categorized as possibly beneficial without causing harm in polymorphic VT (TdP) and suspected hypomagnesemia. Magnesium sulfate, 1 to 2 g, is diluted in 100 mL of D_5W and administered IV over 1 to 2 minutes. For treatment of TdP, a loading dose of 1 to 2 g mixed in 50 to 100 mL of D_5W should be given over 5 to 60 minutes, followed by an infusion of 0.5 to 1 g/h.

TREATMENT OF PEA AND ASYSTOLE

Nonpharmacologic Therapy

- Successful treatment of PEA and asystole depends almost entirely on diagnosis of the underlying cause. Potentially reversible causes include (1) hypovolemia, (2) hypoxia, (3) preexisting acidosis, (4) hyperkalemia, (5) hypothermia, (6) drug overdose, (7) cardiac tamponade, (8) tension pneumothorax, (9) coronary thrombosis, and (10) pulmonary thrombosis.

- Treatment of PEA is similar to treatment of asystole. Both conditions require CPR, intubation, and IV access. Defibrillation should be avoided in asystole because the resulting parasympathetic discharge may reduce the chance of ROSC and worsen the chance of survival. If available, transcutaneous pacing can be attempted.

Pharmacologic Therapy

- **Epinephrine** may be given in doses identical to those used for the treatment of VF or PVT.

- **Atropine** is an antimuscarinic agent that blocks the depressant effect of acetylcholine on the sinus and atrioventricular nodes, thereby decreasing parasympathetic tone. During asystole, parasympathetic tone may increase because of vagal stimulation from intubation, hypoxia and acidosis, or alterations in the balance of parasympathetic and sympathetic control. There are no large randomized trials showing benefit from atropine for treatment of asystole; evidence is limited to small case series or retrospective reviews. Overall, the results show that although atropine may achieve ROSC in some instances, asystolic arrest is almost always fatal. Therefore, the use of atropine for this indication is not harmful, but the beneficial effect is limited. For the treatment of PEA, atropine may be used if the rate is slow. The recommended dose is 1 mg IV, repeated as needed every 3 to 5 minutes up to a total dose of 0.04 mg/kg. Doses less than 0.5 mg should be avoided to prevent paradoxical bradycardia.

ACID–BASE MANAGEMENT DURING CPR

- Acidosis occurs during cardiac arrest because of decreased blood flow and inadequate ventilation. Chest compressions generate only about 20% to 30% of normal cardiac output, leading to inadequate organ perfusion, tissue hypoxia, and metabolic acidosis. Furthermore, the lack of ventilation causes retention of carbon dioxide, leading to respiratory acidosis. The combined acidosis reduces myocardial contractility and may cause arrhythmias because of a lower fibrillation threshold.
- In early cardiac arrest, adequate alveolar ventilation is the primary means of limiting carbon dioxide accumulation and controlling the acid-base imbalance. With arrests of long duration, buffer therapy is often necessary.
- **Sodium bicarbonate** administration for cardiac arrest is controversial because there are few clinical data supporting its use and it may have some detrimental effects. According to the 2000 Guidelines, sodium bicarbonate is appropriate and efficacious for patients with known, preexisting hyperkalemia. It is considered to be probably beneficial and efficacious for preexisting bicarbonate-responsive acidosis and overdoses of tricyclic antidepressants and to alkalinize the urine in aspirin and other drug overdoses. It may also be of possible benefit in intubated and ventilated patients with a long arrest interval. Sodium bicarbonate may be harmful in hypercarbic acidosis, and it should not be given in this situation.
- The initial recommended dose of sodium bicarbonate is 1 mEq/kg IV. Therapy should be guided by the bicarbonate concentration or calculated base deficit obtained from blood gas analysis or laboratory measurement. Complete correction of the base deficit should be avoided to minimize the risk of iatrogenically induced alkalosis.

▶ EVALUATION OF THERAPEUTIC OUTCOMES

- To gauge the success of CPR, therapeutic outcome monitoring should occur both during the resuscitation attempt and in the postresuscitation phase. The optimal outcome following CPR is an awake, responsive, spontaneously breathing patient. Ideally, patients must remain neurologically intact with minimal morbidity after the resuscitation.
- Heart rate, cardiac rhythm, and blood pressure should be assessed and documented throughout the resuscitation attempt and after each intervention. Determination of the presence or absence of a pulse is paramount to deciding

II

which interventions may be appropriate. Nonresponse to an array of suitable interventions may indicate that resuscitation is impossible.

- Clinicians should consider the precipitating cause of the cardiac arrest, such as an acute myocardial infarction, electrolyte imbalance, or primary arrhythmia. Prearrest status should be carefully reviewed, particularly if the patient was receiving drug therapy.
- Laboratory investigations are necessary, including a 12-lead ECG, portable chest x-ray, measurement of arterial blood gases, and blood chemistry determinations.
- Altered cardiac, hepatic, and renal function resulting from ischemic damage during the arrest may warrant special attention.
- Neurologic function should be assessed by means of the Glasgow Coma Scale and the Cerebral Performance Category.

See Chapter 12, Cardiopulmonary Resuscitation, authored by Jeffrey F. Barletta, for a more detailed discussion of this topic.

Chapter 8

▶ HEART FAILURE

▶ DEFINITION

Heart failure (HF) is a clinical syndrome caused by the inability of the heart to pump sufficient blood to meet the metabolic needs of the body. Heart failure can result from any disorder that reduces ventricular filling (diastolic dysfunction) and/or myocardial contractility (systolic dysfunction).

▶ PATHOPHYSIOLOGY

- Causes of systolic dysfunction (decreased contractility) are reduction in muscle mass (e.g., myocardial infarction [MI]), dilated cardiomyopathies, and ventricular hypertrophy. Ventricular hypertrophy can be caused by pressure overload (e.g., systemic or pulmonary hypertension, aortic or pulmonic valve stenosis) or volume overload (e.g., valvular regurgitation, shunts, high-output states).
- Causes of diastolic dysfunction (restriction in ventricular filling) are increased ventricular stiffness, ventricular hypertrophy, infiltrative myocardial diseases, myocardial ischemia and infarction, mitral or tricuspid valve stenosis, and pericardial disease (e.g., pericarditis, pericardial tamponade).
- The most common underlying etiologies are ischemic heart disease, hypertension, or both.
- As cardiac function decreases, the heart relies on the following compensatory mechanisms: (1) tachycardia and increased contractility through sympathetic nervous system activation; (2) the Frank-Starling mechanism, whereby increased preload increases stroke volume; (3) vasoconstriction; and (4) ventricular hypertrophy and remodeling. Although these compensatory mechanisms initially maintain cardiac function, they are responsible for the symptoms of heart failure and contribute to disease progression.
- The neurohormonal model of HF recognizes that an initiating event (e.g., acute MI) leads to decreased cardiac output but that the HF state then becomes a systemic disease whose progression is mediated largely by neurohormones and autocrine/paracrine factors. These substances include angiotensin II, norepinephrine, aldosterone, natriuretic peptides, arginine vasopressin, and proinflammatory cytokines (e.g., tumor necrosis factor α, interleuleins-6 and interleukins-1β), endothelin-1.
- Common precipitating factors that may cause a previously compensated patient to decompensate include noncompliance with diet or drug therapy, coronary ischemia, inappropriate medication use, cardiac events (e.g., MI, atrial fibrillation), and pulmonary infections.
- Drugs may precipitate or exacerbate HF because of their negative inotropic, cardiotoxic, or sodium-retaining properties.

▶ CLINICAL PRESENTATION

- The patient presentation may range from asymptomatic to cardiogenic shock.
- The primary symptoms are dyspnea (particularly on exertion) and fatigue, which lead to exercise intolerance. Other pulmonary symptoms include orthopnea, paroxysmal nocturnal dyspnea, tachypnea, and cough.
- Fluid overload results in pulmonary congestion and peripheral edema.
- Nonspecific symptoms may include nocturia, hemoptysis, abdominal pain, anorexia, nausea, bloating, ascites, and mental status changes.

II

- Physical examination findings may include pulmonary crackles, an S_3 gallop, pleural effusions, Cheyne-Stokes respiration, tachycardia, cardiomegaly, peripheral edema, jugular venous distention, hepatojugular reflux, and hepatomegaly.

▶ DIAGNOSIS

- A diagnosis of HF should be considered in patients exhibiting characteristic signs and symptoms. A complete history and physical examination with appropriate laboratory testing are essential in the initial evaluation of patients suspected of having HF.
- Ventricular hypertrophy can be demonstrated on chest x-ray or electrocardiogram (ECG).
- The New York Heart Association (NYHA) Functional Classification System is intended primarily to classify *symptomatic* HF patients according to the physician's subjective evaluation. Functional class (FC)-I patients have no limitation of physical activity, FC-II patients have slight limitation, FC-III patients have marked limitation, and FC-IV patients are unable to carry on physical activity without discomfort.
- The recent American College of Cardiology/American Heart Association (ACC/AHA) staging system provides a more comprehensive framework for evaluating, preventing, and treating HF (Figure 8–1).

▶ DESIRED OUTCOME

The therapeutic goals for chronic HF are to improve symptoms and quality of life, reduce symptoms, reduce hospitalizations, slow disease progression, and prolong survival.

▶ TREATMENT OF CHRONIC HEART FAILURE

GENERAL PRINCIPLES

- The first step in managing chronic HF is to determine the etiology or precipitating factors. Treatment of underlying disorders (e.g., anemia, hyperthyroidism) may obviate the need for treatment of HF.
- Nonpharmacologic interventions include cardiac rehabilitation and restriction of fluid intake (maximum 2 L/day from all sources) and dietary sodium (approximately 1.5 to 2 g of sodium per day).
- **Stage A:** The emphasis is on identifying and modifying risk factors to prevent development of structural heart disease and subsequent HF. Strategies include smoking cessation and control of hypertension, diabetes mellitus, and dyslipidemia according to current treatment guidelines. ACE inhibitors should be strongly considered for antihypertensive therapy in patients with multiple atherosclerotic vascular risk factors.
- **Stage B:** In these patients with structural heart disease but no symptoms, treatment is targeted at minimizing additional injury and preventing or slowing the remodeling process. In addition to treatment measures outlined for stage A, patients with a previous MI should receive both ACE inhibitors and β blockers regardless of the ejection fraction (EF). Patients with reduced EFs (less than 40%) should also receive both agents, regardless of whether they have had an MI.
- **Stage C:** Patients with structural heart disease and previous or current HF symptoms may also have their symptoms classified according to the NYHA

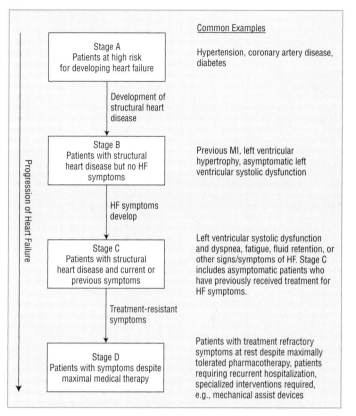

Figure 8–1. ACC/AHA heart failure staging system.

system. Most patients should be treated routinely with four medications: an ACE inhibitor, a diuretic, a β blocker, and digoxin (see Figure 8–2). Aldosterone receptor antagonists, angiotensin-receptor blockers (ARBs), and hydralazine/isosorbide dinitrate are useful in selected patients. Other general measures include moderate sodium restriction, daily weight measurement, immunization against influenza and pneumococcus, modest physical activity, and avoidance of medications that can exacerbate HF.

- **Stage D:** Patients with symptoms at rest despite maximal medical therapy should be considered for specialized therapies, including mechanical circulatory support, continuous positive inotropic therapy, cardiac transplantation, or hospice care.

PHARMACOLOGIC THERAPY

Standard First-Line Therapies
Angiotensin-Converting Enzyme Inhibitors
- ACE inhibitors (see Table 8–1) decrease angiotensin II and aldosterone, attenuating many of their deleterious effects, including reducing ventricular remodeling, myocardial fibrosis, myocyte apoptosis, cardiac hypertrophy,

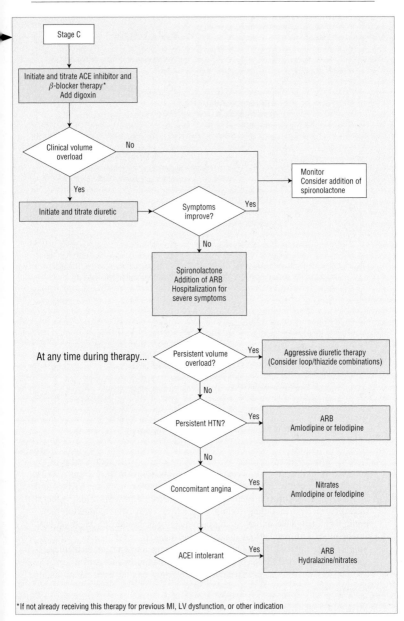

Figure 8–2. Treatment algorithm for patients with ACC/AHA stage C heart failure. ACE, angiotensin-converting enzyme; ARB, angiotensin II receptor blocker; HTN, hypertension; ACEI, ACE inhibitor.

TABLE 8–1. ACE Inhibitors Approved for Use in Heart Failure

Generic Name	Brand Name	Initial Dose	Survival Benefit[a]	Prodrug	Elimination[b]
Captopril	Capoten	6.25 mg t.i.d.	50 mg t.i.d.	No	Renal
Enalapril	Vasotec	2.5–5 mg b.i.d.	10 mg b.i.d.	Yes	Renal
Lisinopril	Zestril, Prinivil	2.5–5 mg q.d.	20–40 mg q.d.[c]	No	Renal
Quinapril	Accupril	10 mg b.i.d.	20–40 mg b.i.d.[d]	Yes	Renal
Ramipril	Altace	1.25–2.5 mg b.i.d.	5 mg b.i.d.	Yes	Renal
Fosinopril	Monopril	5–10 mg q.d.	40 mg q.d.[d]	Yes	Renal/hepatic
Trandolapril	Mavik	0.5–1 mg q.d.	4 mg q.d.	Yes	Renal/hepatic

Abbreviations: t.i.d., three times daily; b.i.d., twice daily; q.d., once daily.
[a]Target doses associated with survival benefits in clinical trials.
[b]Primary route of elimination.
[c]Note that in the ATLAS trial no significant difference in mortality was found between low dose (~5 mg/day) and high dose (~35 mg/day) lisinopril therapy.
[d]Effects on mortality have not been evaluated.

norepinephrine release, vasoconstriction, and sodium and water retention. Hemodynamic effects observed with long-term therapy include significant increases in cardiac index, stroke work index, and stroke volume index, as well as significant reductions in left ventricular filling pressure, systemic vascular resistance (SVR), mean arterial pressure (MAP), and heart rate. Significant improvements in clinical status, functional class, exercise tolerance, left ventricular size, and mortality are also well documented.

- Clinical trials have demonstrated a 20% to 30% reduction in mortality compared with placebo. ACE inhibitors also reduce the combined risk of death or hospitalization, slow progression of HF, and reduce rates of reinfarction. ACE inhibitors are superior to vasodilator therapy with hydralazine/isosorbide dinitrate. ACE inhibitors are also effective for prevention of HF.
- All patients with documented left ventricular dysfunction, irrespective of symptoms, should receive ACE inhibitors, unless a contraindication or intolerance is present.

β Blockers
- Beneficial effects β blockers may result from slowing or reversing the detrimental ventricular remodeling caused by sympathetic simulation, decreased myocyte death from catecholamine-induced necrosis or apoptosis, antiarrhythmic effects, and prevention of other effects of sympathetic nervous system activation. These drugs consistently increase left ventricular ejection fraction, decrease ventricular mass, and reduce systolic and diastolic volumes.
- There is overwhelming evidence that stable patients initiated on low doses of a β blocker with slow upward dose titration over several weeks derive significant benefits, including slowed disease progression and reduced hospitalizations and mortality. Many studies (but not all) have also shown improvement in NYHA functional class, patient symptom scores or quality-of-life assessments, and exercise performance.
- The ACC/AHA guidelines recommend use of β blockers in all patients with stable systolic HF unless they have a contraindication or have been shown clearly to be unable to tolerate β blockers. Patients should receive a β blocker even if symptoms are well controlled with an ACE inhibitor and diuretic because they remain at risk for disease progression.
- Because greater benefit is seen at higher doses, patients should be titrated to target doses when possible. However, even lower doses have benefits over

II

placebo, so inability to titrate to the target dose is not justification to discontinue therapy.

- On the basis of clinical trial data, therapy should be limited to **carvedilol, metoprolol CR/XL**, or **bisoprolol**. It cannot be assumed that immediate-release metoprolol will provide benefits equivalent to metoprolol CR/XL. Because bisoprolol is not available in the necessary starting dose of 1.25 mg, the choice is typically limited to either carvedilol or metoprolol CR/XL. On the basis of regimens proven in large clinical trials to reduce mortality, initial and target oral doses are as follows:
  - Bisoprolol, 1.25 mg daily initially; target dose, 10 mg daily.
  - Carvedilol, 3.125 mg twice daily initially; target dose, 25 mg twice daily (the target dose for patients weighing more than 85 kg is 50 mg twice daily).
  - Metoprolol succinate CR/XL, 12.5 to 25 mg daily initially; target dose, 200 mg daily.
- Doses should be doubled approximately every 2 weeks or as tolerated until the target dose or the highest tolerated dose is reached.

Diuretics

- Compensatory mechanisms in HF stimulate excessive sodium and water retention, often leading to systemic and pulmonary congestion. Consequently, diuretic therapy is indicated for all patients with evidence of fluid retention. However, because they do not alter disease progression or prolong survival, they are not considered mandatory therapy for patients without fluid retention.
- Thiazide diuretics (e.g., **hydrochlorothiazide**) are relatively weak diuretics and are used alone infrequently in HF. However, thiazides or the thiazide-like diuretic **metolazone** can be used in combination with a loop diuretic if needed to promote effective diuresis.
- Loop diuretics (**furosemide, bumetanide, torsemide**) are the most widely used diuretics for HF. In addition to acting in the thick ascending limb of the loop of Henle, they induce a prostaglandin-mediated increase in renal blood flow that contributes to their natriuretic effect. Unlike thiazides, loop diuretics maintain their effectiveness in the presence of impaired renal function, although higher doses are necessary.
- Doses of loop diuretics above the recommended ceiling doses produce no additional diuresis in HF. Thus, once those doses are reached, more frequent dosing should be used for additional effect, rather than giving progressively higher doses.
- Ranges of doses and ceiling doses for loop diuretics in patients with varying degrees of renal function are listed in Table 8–2.

TABLE 8–2. Loop Diuretic Use in Heart Failure

	Furosemide	Bumetanide	Torsemide
Usual daily dose (PO)	20–160 mg/day	0.5–4 mg/day	10–80 mg/day
Ceiling dose[a]			
Normal renal function	80–160 mg	1–2 mg	20–40 mg
CL_{CR}: 20–50 mL/min	160 mg	2 mg	40 mg
CL_{CR}: <20 mL/min	400 mg	8–10 mg	100 mg
Bioavailability	10–100%	80–90%	80–100%
	Average, 50%		
Affected by food	Yes	Yes	No
Half-life	0.3–3.4 h	0.3–1.5 h	3–4 h

[a]Ceiling dose: single dose above which additional response is unlikely to be observed.

Digoxin

- In patients with HF and supraventricular tachyarrhythmias such as atrial fibrillation, digoxin should be considered early in therapy to help control ventricular response rate.

- For patients in normal sinus rhythm, digoxin does not improve survival, but its positive inotropic effects, symptom reduction, and its effect on symptom reduction and quality-of-life improvement are evident in patients with mild to severe HF. Therefore, it should be used together with other standard HF therapies (ACE inhibitors, β blockers, and diuretics) in patients with symptomatic HF. Consideration should be given to adding it after instituting β-blocker therapy so that digoxin-associated bradycardia does not preclude β-blocker use.

- Most of the benefit from digoxin is achieved at low plasma concentrations. For most patients, the target plasma digoxin concentration should be 0.5 to 1 ng/mL. Most patients with normal renal function can achieve this level with a dose of 0.125 mg/day. Patients with decreased renal function, the elderly, or those receiving interacting drugs (e.g., amiodarone) should receive 0.125 mg every other day. In the absence of supraventricular tachyarrhythmias, a loading dose is not indicated because digoxin is a mild inotropic agent that produces gradual effects over several hours, even after loading.

Other Heart Failure Therapies
Aldosterone Antagonists

- **Spironolactone** is an inhibitor of aldosterone that produces a weak potassium-sparing diuretic effect. It has been studied in HF because aldosterone is a neurohormone that plays an important role in ventricular remodeling particularly by causing increased collagen deposition and cardiac fibrosis. In a placebo-controlled trial, addition of spironolactone 25 mg/day to standard therapy in patients with class III or IV HF was associated with significant reductions in mortality and hospitalizations and improvement in symptoms. The most common adverse effect was gynecomastia, which occurred in 10% of men. There was a statistically significant (but probably clinically unimportant) mean increase in serum potassium concentration (0.3 mEq/L).

- **Eplerenone** is an aldosterone-selective receptor antagonist that has been associated with a reduction in death from any cause and a reduction in the risk of hospitalization from HF. Because of its receptor-selective nature, it was not associated with gynecomastia. However, serious hyperkalemia occurred in 5.5% of patients compared with 3.9% of patients receiving placebo.

- Data from clinical practice suggest that the risk of serious hyperkalemia and worsening renal function are much higher than observed in clinical trials. This may be due in part to failure of clinicians to consider renal impairment, to reduce or stop potassium supplementation, or to monitor renal function and potassium closely once the aldosterone antagonist is initiated. Even in closely monitored patients, the risk of hyperkalemia may remain high, particularly in the elderly and those with very low EFs. Thus, aldosterone antagonists must be used cautiously and with careful monitoring of renal function and potassium concentration. They should be avoided in patients with significant renal impairment or high-normal potassium levels.

- Although the place of aldosterone antagonists in therapy remains to be fully defined, it is reasonable to consider their addition to standard therapy in patients similar to those who participated in the controlled clinical trials of the drugs. It is also reasonable to consider addition of spironolactone to class II or III HF patients who remain symptomatic despite optimal therapy.

Cardiovascular Disorders

Angiotensin II Receptor Blockers (ARBs)

II
- The angiotensin II receptor blockers (e.g., **losartan, candesartan, valsartan**) block the angiotensin II receptor subtype AT_1, preventing the deleterious effects of angiotensin II, regardless of its origin. They do not appear to affect bradykinin and are not associated with the side effect of cough that sometimes results from ACE inhibitor–induced accumulation of bradykinin. Also, direct blockade of AT_1 receptors allows unopposed stimulation of AT_2 receptors, causing vasodilation and inhibition of ventricular remodeling.
- Although some data suggest that ARBs produce equivalent mortality benefits with fewer adverse effects than ACE inhibitors, the ACC/AHA guidelines indicate that ARBs should not be considered equivalent or superior to ACE inhibitors and that they should be considered in patients who are intolerant of ACE inhibitors.
- For patients unable to tolerate ACE inhibitors, usually because of intractable cough or angioedema, an ARB is a safe and effective alternative. However, angioedema has been reported with ARBs, including recurrence after angioedema due to an ACE inhibitor. ARBs are not reasonable alternatives in patients with hypotension, hyperkalemia, or renal insufficiency due to ACE inhibitors because they are just as likely to cause these adverse effects.
- The addition of an ARB to optimal HF therapy (e.g. ACE inhibitors, β blockers, diuretics) offers marginal benefits at best with increased risk of adverse effects. Until additional data are available, ACE inhibitor and β-blocker therapy should be optimized before considering the addition of an ARB.

Nitrates and Hydralazine

- Nitrates (e.g., **isosorbide dinitrate** [ISDN]) and **hydralazine** were combined originally in the treatment of HF because of their complementary hemodynamic actions. Nitrates are primarily venodilators, producing reductions in preload. Hydralazine is a direct vasodilator that acts predominantly on arterial smooth muscle to reduce SVR and increase stroke volume and cardiac output. Furthermore, nitrates may inhibit the ventricular remodeling process, and hydralazine prevents nitrate tolerance and may interfere with HF progression.
- In one study, the ACE inhibitor enalapril produced superior mortality reduction over the combination of hydralazine 75 mg q.i.d. and ISDN 40 mg q.i.d. Furthermore, adverse effects of hydralazine and nitrates limit their use in many patients, and the need for frequent dosing may reduce patient adherence.
- Current guidelines recommend that hydralazine/ISDN should not be used instead of ACE inhibitors as standard therapy in HF. The combination may be an option in patients unable to take ACE inhibitors or ARBs because of renal insufficiency, hyperkalemia, or possibly hypotension. However, compliance with the regimen is likely to be poor and the risk of adverse effects high. For these reasons, many clinicians prefer ARBs in patients intolerant of ACE inhibitors.

▶ TREATMENT OF ADVANCED OR DECOMPENSATED HEART FAILURE

GENERAL PRINCIPLES

- Patients should be admitted to an intensive care unit (ICU) when they show signs of significant systemic hypoperfusion (e.g., severe fatigue, shortness of breath as rest), develop pulmonary vascular congestion requiring mechanical ventilation, manifest symptomatic sustained tachyarrhythmias, or require potent IV vasoactive or inotropic drugs or mechanical ventricular assistance.

- Cardiopulmonary support must be instituted and adjusted rapidly. ECG monitoring, continuous pulse oximetry, urine flow monitoring, and automated sphygmomanometric blood pressure recording are necessary. Flow-directed pulmonary artery or Swan-Ganz catheters may also be placed to estimate the pulmonary venous (left atrial) pressure.
- Reversible or treatable causes of decompensation should be addressed and corrected. Drugs that may aggravate HF should be evaluated carefully and discontinued when possible.
- The first step in the management of advanced HF is to ascertain that optimal treatment with oral medications has been achieved. If there is evidence of fluid retention, aggressive diuresis, often with IV diuretics, should be accomplished. Most patients should be receiving digoxin at a low dose prescribed to achieve a trough serum concentration of 0.5 to 1 ng/mL. Optimal treatment with an ACE inhibitor should be a priority. Although β blockers should not be started during this period of instability, they should be continued, if possible, in patients who are already receiving them on a chronic basis.
- Appropriate management of advanced HF is aided by determination of whether the patient has signs and symptoms of fluid overload ("wet" HF) or low cardiac output ("dry" HF) (Figure 8–3).
- In addition to the clinical presentation, invasive hemodynamic monitoring helps guide treatment and classify patients into four specific hemodynamic subsets based on cardiac index and pulmonary artery occlusion pressure (PAOP). Refer to textbook Chapter 14 for more information.

PHARMACOTHERAPY OF ADVANCED OR DECOMPENSATED HEART FAILURE

Diuretics

- IV loop diuretics, including **furosemide, bumetanide,** and **torsemide,** are used for advanced HF, with furosemide being the most widely studied agent.
- Bolus diuretic administration decreases preload by functional venodilation within 5 to 15 minutes and later (>20 min) via sodium and water excretion, thereby improving pulmonary congestion. However, acute reductions in venous return may severely compromise effective preload in patients with significant diastolic dysfunction or intravascular depletion.
- Because diuretics can cause excessive preload reduction, they must be used judiciously to obtain the desired improvement in congestive symptoms while avoiding a reduction in cardiac output.
- Diuresis may be improved by adding a second diuretic with a different mechanism of action (e.g., combining a loop diuretic with a distal tubule blocker such as **metolazone** or **hydrochlorothiazide**). Combination therapy should generally be reserved for inpatients who can be monitored closely for the development of severe sodium, potassium, and volume depletion. Very low doses of the thiazide-type diuretic should be used in the outpatient setting to avoid serious adverse events.

Positive Inotropic Agents
Dobutamine

- **Dobutamine** is a β_1 and β_2 receptor agonist with some α_1 agonist effects (Table 8–3). The net vascular effect is usually vasodilation. It has a potent inotropic effect without producing a significant change in heart rate. Initial doses of 2.5 to 5 mcg/kg/min can be increased progressively to 20 mcg/kg/min or higher on the basis of clinical and hemodynamic responses.

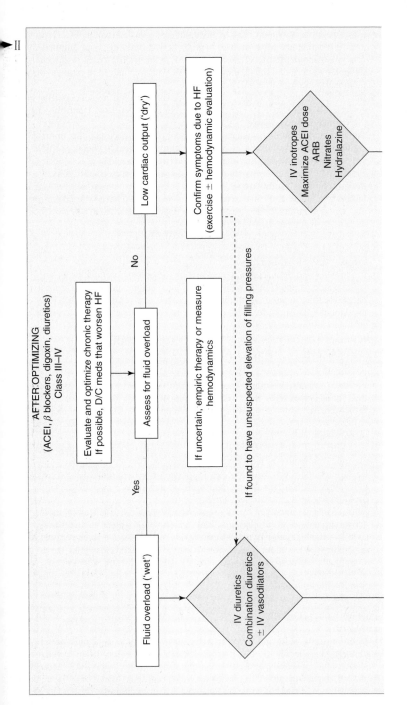

AFTER OPTIMIZING
(ACEI, β blockers, digoxin, diuretics)
Class III–IV

Evaluate and optimize chronic therapy
If possible, D/C meds that worsen HF

Assess for fluid overload

Yes

No

Fluid overload ('wet')

Low cardiac output ('dry')

IV diuretics
Combination diuretics
± IV vasodilators

Confirm symptoms due to HF
(exercise ± hemodynamic evaluation)

If uncertain, empiric therapy or measure hemodynamics

If found to have unsuspected elevation of filling pressures

IV inotropes
Maximize ACEI dose
ARB
Nitrates
Hydralazine

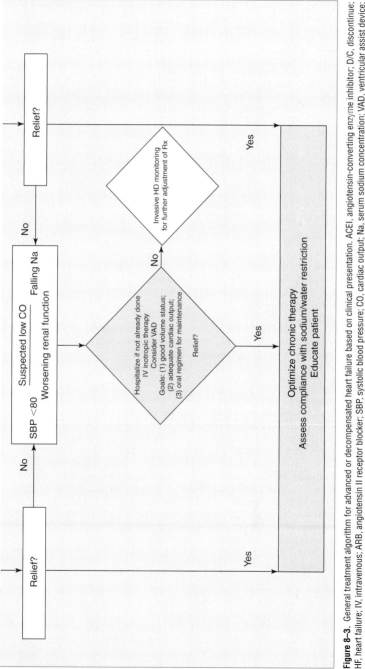

Figure 8–3. General treatment algorithm for advanced or decompensated heart failure based on clinical presentation. ACEI, angiotensin-converting enzyme inhibitor; D/C, discontinue; HF, heart failure; IV, intravenous; ARB, angiotensin II receptor blocker; CO, cardiac output; Na, serum sodium concentration; SBP, systolic blood pressure; VAD, ventricular assist device; HD, hemodynamic; Rx, therapy.

TABLE 8–3. Usual Hemodynamic Effects of Intravenous Agents Commonly Used for Treatment of Acute/Severe Heart Failure[a]

Drug	Dose	HR	MAP	PAOP	CO	SVR
Dopamine	0.5–3 mcg/kg/min	0	0	0	0/+	−
Dopamine	3–10 mcg/kg/min	+	+	0	+	0
Dopamine	>10 mcg/kg/min	+	+	+	+	+
Dobutamine	2.5–20 mcg/kg/min	0/+	0	−	+	−
Amrinone	5–10 mcg/kg/min	0/+	0/−	−	+	−
Milrinone	0.375–0.75 mcg/kg/min	0/+	0/−	−	+	−
Nitroprusside	0.25–3 mcg/kg/min	0/+	0/−	−	+	−
Nitroglycerin	5–200 mcg/min	0/+	0/−	−	0/+	0/−
Furosemide	20–80 mg; repeated as needed up to 4–6 times/day	0	0	−	0	0
Enalaprilat	0.25–2.5 mg every 6–8 h	0	0/−	−	+	+
Nesiritide	Bolus: 2 mcg/kg; infusion: 0.01 mcg/kg/min	0	0/−	−	+	−

Abbreviations: + = increase; − = decrease; 0 = no change; HR = heart rate; MAP = mean arterial pressure; PAOP = pulmonary artery occlusion pressure; CO = cardiac output; SVR = systemic vascular resistance.

- Dobutamine increases cardiac index because of inotropic stimulation, arterial vasodilation, and a variable increase in heart rate. It causes relatively little change in mean arterial pressure compared with the more consistent increases observed with dopamine.
- Attenuation of dobutamine's hemodynamic effects has been reported after 72 hours of continuous infusion. However, many patients (especially those awaiting transplantation) are "dobutamine dependent" and experience hemodynamic deterioration when discontinuation is attempted. Thus, therapy should be tapered rather than stopped abruptly when it is discontinued.

Amrinone and Milrinone
- **Amrinone** and **milrinone** are bipyridine derivatives that inhibit phosphodiesterase III and produce positive inotropic and vasodilating effects; hence, these drugs are referred to as *inodilators*.
- During IV administration, amrinone or milrinone increases stroke volume (and cardiac output) with little change in heart rate (Table 8–3). They also decrease PAOP by venodilation and thus are particularly useful in patients with a low cardiac index and an elevated left ventricular filling pressure. However, this decrease in preload can be hazardous for patients without excessive filling pressure, leading to a decrease in cardiac index.
- Amrinone and milrinone should be used cautiously as single agents in severely hypotensive HF patients because these drugs will not increase, and may even decrease, arterial blood pressure.
- The usual loading dose of amrinone is 0.75 mg/kg over 2 to 3 minutes, followed by a continuous infusion of 5 to 10 mcg/kg/min.
- The usual loading dose of milrinone is 50 mcg/kg over 10 minutes, followed by a continuous infusion of 0.5 mcg/kg/min (range, 0.375 to 0.75 mcg/kg/min).
- The usual loading dose of amrinone is 0.75 mg/kg over 2 to 3 minutes, followed by a continuous infusion of 5 to 10 mcg/kg/min.
- Other than undesirable hemodynamic effects, adverse events include arrhythmias and a dose-dependent, reversible thrombocytopenia. Milrinone is preferred over amrinone because of its better side-effect profile (thrombocytopenia less than 0.5% vs. 2.4% with amrinone). Patients receiving either drug

should be monitored for signs of bleeding and have platelet counts determined before and during therapy.

- Generally, milrinone should be considered for patients who are receiving chronic β-blocker therapy because its positive inotropic effect does not involve stimulation of β receptors.

Dopamine

- **Dopamine** should generally be avoided in advanced HF, but its pharmacologic actions may be preferable to dobutamine or milrinone in two circumstances: (1) in patients with marked systemic hypotension or cardiogenic shock in the face of elevated ventricular filling pressures, where dopamine in doses greater than 5 mcg/kg/min may be necessary to raise central aortic pressure; and (2) to directly attempt to improve renal function in patients with inadequate urine output despite volume overload and high ventricular filling pressures. Although controversial, low doses (1 to 3 mcg/kg/min) have been given for the latter indication.
- Dopamine produces dose-dependent hemodynamic effects because of its relative affinity for α_1, β_1, β_2, and D_1 (vascular dopaminergic) receptors. Positive inotropic effects mediated primarily by β_1 receptors become more prominent with doses of 3 to 10 mcg/kg/min. At doses above 10 mcg/kg/min, chronotropic and α_1-mediated vasoconstricting effects become more prominent. Especially at higher doses, dopamine alters several parameters that increase myocardial oxygen demand and potentially decrease myocardial blood flow, worsening ischemia in some patients with coronary artery disease.

Vasodilators

- Arterial vasodilators act as impedance-reducing agents and typically increase cardiac output. Venous vasodilators act as preload reducers by increasing venous capacitance, reducing symptoms of pulmonary congestion in patients with high cardiac filling pressures. Mixed vasodilators act on both arterial resistance and venous capacitance vessels, reducing congestive symptoms while increasing cardiac output.

Nitroprusside

- **Sodium nitroprusside** is a mixed arterial-venous vasodilator that acts directly on vascular smooth muscle to increase cardiac index and decrease venous pressure. Despite its lack of direct inotropic activity, nitroprusside exerts hemodynamic effects that are qualitatively similar to those of dobutamine, amrinone, and milrinone. However, nitroprusside generally decreases PAOP, SVR, and blood pressure more than those agents do.
- Hypotension is an important dose-limiting adverse effect of nitroprusside and other vasodilators. Therefore, nitroprusside is primarily used in patients who have a significantly elevated SVR.
- Nitroprusside is effective in the short-term management of severe HF in a variety of settings (e.g., acute MI, valvular regurgitation, after coronary bypass surgery, decompensated HF). Generally, it will not worsen, and may improve, the balance between myocardial oxygen demand and supply. However, an excessive decrease in systemic arterial pressure can decrease coronary perfusion and worsen ischemia.
- Nitroprusside has a rapid onset and a duration of action of less than 10 minutes, which necessitates use of continuous IV infusions. It should be initiated at a low dose (i.e., 0.1 to 0.2 mcg/kg/min) to avoid excessive hypotension, and then increased by small increments (0.1 to 0.2 mcg/kg/min) every 5 to 10 minutes as needed and tolerated. Usual effective doses range from 0.5 to

II

3 mcg/kg/min. Because of a rebound phenomenon after abrupt withdrawal of nitroprusside in patients with HF, doses should be tapered slowly when stopping therapy. Nitroprusside-induced cyanide and thiocyanate toxicity are unlikely when doses less than 3 mcg/kg/min are administered for less than 3 days, except in patients with serum creatinine levels above 3 mg/dL.

Nitroglycerin
- The major hemodynamic effects of IV **nitroglycerin** are decreased preload and PAOP because of functional venodilation and mild arterial vasodilation. It is used primarily as a preload reducer for patients with pulmonary congestion and low-normal cardiac output or in combination with inotropic agents for patients with severely depressed systolic function and pulmonary edema. Combination therapy with nitroglycerin and dobutamine or dopamine produces complementary effects to increase cardiac index and decrease PAOP.
- Nitroglycerin should be initiated at 5 to 10 mcg/min (0.1 mcg/kg/min) and increased every 5 to 10 minutes as necessary and tolerated. Maintenance doses usually vary from 35 to 200 mcg/min (0.5 to 3 mcg/kg/min). Hypotension and an excessive decrease in PAOP are important dose-limiting side effects. Some tolerance develops in most patients over 12 to 72 hours of continuous administration.

Nesiritide
- Nesiritide is manufactured using recombinant techniques and is identical to the endogenous B-type natriuretic peptide (BNP) secreted by the ventricular myocardium in response to volume overload. Consequently, nesiritide mimics the vasodilatory and natriuretic actions of the endogenous peptide, resulting in venous and arterial vasodilation, increased natriuresis and diuresis, and decreased cardiac filling pressures, blood pressure, and sympathetic nervous system and renin-angiotensin-aldosterone system activity.
- The precise role of nesiritide in the pharmacotherapy of decompensated HF remains to be defined. It has not been shown to improve mortality or other clinical outcomes when compared with nitroglycerin (or nitroprusside), and it is substantially more expensive than nitroglycerin. Its longer elimination half-life compared with that of nitroglycerin also poses a risk of sustained hypotension. Its advantages include beneficial neurohormonal effects, use without hemodynamic monitoring, administration in outpatient settings (e.g., emergency departments), and low proarrhythmic potential compared with inotropes.
- Nesiritide may be most useful in patients with volume overload and systolic blood pressure greater than 90 mm Hg who fail to respond adequately to IV diuretics and/or vasodilators such as nitroglycerin.

MECHANICAL CIRCULATORY SUPPORT

Intra-aortic Balloon Pump
- The intra-aortic balloon pump (IABP), typically, is employed in patients with advanced HF who do not respond adequately to drug therapy, those with intractable myocardial ischemia, or patients in cardiogenic shock.
- IABP support increases cardiac index, coronary artery perfusion, and myocardial oxygen supply, accompanied by decreased myocardial oxygen demand.
- IV vasodilators and inotropic agents are generally used in conjunction with the IABP to maximize hemodynamic and clinical benefits.

Ventricular Assist Devices
- Ventricular assist devices (VADs) are surgically implanted and assist, or in some cases replace, the pumping functions of the right and/or left ventricles.

- VADs are used to provide short-term hemodynamic support in patients experiencing an acute event (e.g., acute MI with cardiogenic shock or patients who cannot be weaned from cardiopulmonary bypass after cardiac surgery) in which ventricular recovery is anticipated.
- VADs are also being used as a bridge to cardiac transplantation in patients whose ventricular function is unlikely to recover and for palliative therapy in lieu of continuous inotropic therapy in patients who are not transplant candidates.

SURGICAL THERAPY

- Orthotopic cardiac transplantation is the best therapeutic option for patients with chronic irreversible NYHA Class IV HF, with a 5-year survival of approximately 60% to 70% in well-selected patients.
- The shortage of donor hearts has prompted development of new surgical techniques, including ventricular aneurysm resection, mitral valve repair, and myocardial cell transplantation, which have resulted in variable degrees of symptomatic improvement.

▶ EVALUATION OF THERAPEUTIC OUTCOMES

CHRONIC HEART FAILURE

- Patients should be asked about the presence and severity of symptoms and how the symptoms affect their daily activities.
- The efficacy of diuretic treatment is evaluated by disappearance of the signs and symptoms of excess fluid retention. Physical examination should focus on body weight, extent of jugular venous distention, presence of hepatojugular reflux, and presence and severity of pulmonary congestion (rales, dyspnea on exertion, orthopnea, paroxysmal nocturnal dyspnea).
- Other outcomes include improvement in exercise tolerance and fatigue, decreased nocturia, and a decrease in heart rate.
- Blood pressure should be monitored to ensure that symptomatic hypotension does not develop as a result of drug therapy.
- Body weight is a sensitive marker of fluid loss or retention, and patients should weigh themselves daily and report changes to their health care provider.
- Symptoms may worsen initially on β-blocker therapy, and it may take weeks to months before patients notice symptomatic improvement.
- Routine monitoring of serum electrolytes and renal function is mandatory in patients with HF.

ADVANCED OR DECOMPENSATED HEART FAILURE

- Initial stabilization requires achievement of adequate arterial oxygen saturation and content.
- Cardiac index and blood pressure must be sufficient to ensure adequate organ perfusion, as assessed by alert mental status, creatinine clearance sufficient to prevent metabolic azotemic complications, hepatic function adequate to maintain synthetic and excretory functions, a stable heart rate (generally between 50 and 110 beats/min) and rhythm, absence of ongoing myocardial ischemia or infarction, skeletal muscle and skin blood flow sufficient to prevent ischemic injury, and normal arterial pH (7.34 to 7.47) with a normal serum lactate concentration. These goals are most often achieved with a cardiac index greater than 2.2 (L/min)/m^2, a mean arterial blood pressure greater than 60 mm Hg, and PAOP of 25 mm Hg or greater.

II

- Discharge from the ICU requires maintenance of the preceding parameters in the absence of ongoing IV infusion therapy, mechanical circulatory support, or positive-pressure ventilation.

See Chapter 14, Heart Failure, authored by Robert B. Parker, J. Herbert Patter-son, and Julie A. Johnson, for a more detailed discussion of this topic.

Chapter 9

▶ HYPERLIPIDEMIA

▶ DEFINITION

Hyperlipidemia is defined as an elevation of one or more of the following: cholesterol, cholesterol esters, phospholipids, or triglycerides. Hyperlipoproteinemia describes an increased concentration of the lipoprotein macromolecules that transport lipids in the plasma. Abnormalities of plasma lipids can result in a predisposition to coronary, cerebrovascular, and peripheral vascular arterial disease.

▶ PATHOPHYSIOLOGY

- Cholesterol, triglycerides, and phospholipids are transported in the bloodstream as complexes of lipid and proteins known as lipoproteins. Elevated total and low-density lipoprotein (LDL) cholesterol and reduced high-density lipoprotein (HDL) cholesterol are associated with the development of coronary heart disease (CHD).
- The response-to-injury hypothesis states that risk factors such as oxidized LDL, mechanical injury to the endothelium, excessive homocysteine, immunologic attack, or infection-induced changes in endothelial and intimal function lead to endothelial dysfunction and a series of cellular interactions that culminate in atherosclerosis. The eventual clinical outcomes may include angina, myocardial infarction, arrhythmias, stroke, peripheral arterial disease, abdominal aortic aneurysm, and sudden death.
- Atherosclerotic lesions are thought to arise from transport and retention of plasma LDL through the endothelial cell layer into the extracellular matrix of the subendothelial space. Once in the artery wall, LDL is chemically modified through oxidation and nonenzymatic glycation. Mildly oxidized LDL then recruits monocytes into the artery wall. These monocytes then become transformed into macrophages that accelerate LDL oxidation.
- Oxidized LDL provokes an inflammatory response mediated by a number of chemoattractants and cytokines (e.g., monocyte colony-stimulating factor, intercellular adhesion molecule, platelet-derived growth factor, transforming growth factors, interleukin-1, interleukin-6).
- Repeated injury and repair within an atherosclerotic plaque eventually leads to a fibrous cap protecting the underlying core of lipids, collagen, calcium, and inflammatory cells such as T lymphocytes. Maintenance of the fibrous plaque is critical to prevent plaque rupture and subsequent coronary thrombosis.
- The extent of oxidation and the inflammatory response are under genetic control, and primary or genetic lipoprotein disorders are classified into six categories for the phenotypic description of hyperlipidemia. The types and corresponding lipoprotein elevations include the following: I (chylomicrons), IIa (LDL), IIb (LDL + very low density lipoprotein, or VLDL), III (intermediate-density lipoprotein, or IDL); IV (VLDL), and V (VLDL + chylomicrons). Secondary forms of hyperlipidemia also exist, and several drug classes may elevate lipid levels (e.g., progestins, thiazide diuretics, glucocorticoids, β blockers, isotretinoin, protease inhibitors, cyclosporine, mirtazapine, sirolimus).
- The primary defect in familial hypercholesterolemia is the inability to bind LDL to the LDL receptor (LDL-R) or, rarely, a defect of internalizing the LDL-R complex into the cell after normal binding. This leads to lack of LDL degradation by cells and unregulated biosynthesis of cholesterol, with total

cholesterol and LDL-C being inversely proportional to the deficit in LDL receptors.

▶ CLINICAL PRESENTATION

- Familial hypercholesterolemia is characterized by a selective elevation in plasma LDL and deposition of LDL-derived cholesterol in tendons (xanthomas) and arteries (atheromas).
- Familial lipoprotein lipase deficiency is characterized by a massive accumulation of chylomicrons and a corresponding increase in plasma triglycerides or a type I lipoprotein pattern. Presenting manifestations include repeated attacks of pancreatitis and abdominal pain, eruptive cutaneous xanthomatosis, and hepatosplenomegaly beginning in childhood. Symptom severity is proportional to dietary fat intake, and consequently to the elevation of chylomicrons. Accelerated atherosclerosis is not associated with this disease.
- Patients with familial type III hyperlipoproteinemia develop the following clinical features after age 20: xanthoma striata palmaris (yellow discolorations of the palmar and digital creases); tuberous or tuberoeruptive xanthomas (bulbous cutaneous xanthomas); and severe atherosclerosis involving the coronary arteries, internal carotids, and abdominal aorta.
- Type IV hyperlipoproteinemia is common and occurs in adulthood primarily in patients who are obese, diabetic, and hyperuricemic and do not have xanthomas. It may be secondary to alcohol ingestion and can be aggravated by stress, progestins, oral contraceptives, thiazides, or β blockers.
- Type V is characterized by abdominal pain, pancreatitis, eruptive xanthomas, and peripheral polyneuropathy. These patients are commonly obese, hyperuricemic, and diabetic; alcohol intake, exogenous estrogens, and renal insufficiency tend to be exacerbating factors. The risk of atherosclerosis is increased with this disorder.

▶ DIAGNOSIS

- A fasting lipoprotein profile (FLP) including total cholesterol, LDL, HDL, and triglycerides should be measured in all adults 20 years of age or older at least once every 5 years.
- Measurement of plasma cholesterol (which is about 3% lower than serum determinations), triglyceride, and HDL levels after a 12-hour or longer fast is important, because triglycerides may be elevated in nonfasted individuals; total cholesterol is only modestly affected by fasting.
- Two determinations, 1 to 8 weeks apart, with the patient on a stable diet and weight, and in the absence of acute illness, are recommended to minimize variability and to obtain a reliable baseline. If the total cholesterol is greater than 200 mg/dL, a second determination is recommended, and if the values are more than 30 mg/dL apart, the average of three values should be used.
- After a lipid abnormality is confirmed, major components of the evaluation are the history (including age, gender, and, if female, menstrual and estrogen replacement status), physical examination, and laboratory investigations.
- A complete history and physical examination should assess (1) presence or absence of cardiovascular risk factors or definite cardiovascular disease in the individual; (2) family history of premature cardiovascular disease or lipid disorders; (3) presence or absence of secondary causes of hyperlipidemia, including concurrent medications; and (4) presence or absence of xanthomas, abdominal pain, or history of pancreatitis, renal or liver disease, peripheral vascular

disease, abdominal aortic aneurysm, or cerebral vascular disease (carotid bruits, stroke, or transient ischemic attack).

- Diabetes mellitus is now regarded as a CHD risk equivalent. That is, the presence of diabetes in patients without known CHD is associated with the same level of risk as patients without diabetes but having confirmed CHD.
- If the physical examination and history are insufficient to diagnose a familial disorder, then agarose-gel lipoprotein electrophoresis is useful to determine which class of lipoproteins is affected. If the triglyceride levels are below 400 mg/dL and neither type III hyperlipidemia nor chylomicrons are detected by electrophoresis, then one can calculate VLDL and LDL concentrations: VLDL = triglyceride/5; LDL = total cholesterol − (VLDL + HDL). Initial testing uses total cholesterol for case finding, but subsequent management decisions should be based on LDL.
- Because total cholesterol is composed of cholesterol derived from LDL, VLDL, and HDL, determination of HDL is useful when total plasma cholesterol is elevated. HDL may be elevated by moderate alcohol ingestion (fewer than two drinks per day), physical exercise, smoking cessation, weight loss, oral contraceptives, phenytoin, and terbutaline. HDL may be lowered by smoking, obesity, a sedentary lifestyle, and drugs such as β blockers.
- Diagnosis of lipoprotein lipase deficiency is based on low or absent enzyme activity with normal human plasma or apolipoprotein C-II, a cofactor of the enzyme.

▶ DESIRED OUTCOME

The goals of treatment are to lower total and LDL cholesterol in order to reduce the risk of first or recurrent events such as myocardial infarction, angina, heart failure, ischemic stroke, or other forms of peripheral arterial disease such as carotid stenosis or abdominal aortic aneurysm.

▶ TREATMENT

GENERAL PRINCIPLES

- The National Cholesterol Education Program Adult Treatment Panel III (NCEP ATP III) recommends that a fasting lipoprotein profile and risk factor assessment be used in the initial classification of adults.
- If the total cholesterol is less than 200 mg/dL, then the patient has a desirable blood cholesterol level (Table 9–1). If the HDL is also above 40 mg/dL, no further follow-up is recommended for patients without known CHD and who have fewer than two risk factors (Table 9–2).
- In patients with borderline-high blood cholesterol (200 to 239 mg/dL), assessment of risk factors is needed to more clearly define disease risk.
- Decisions regarding classification and management are based on the LDL cholesterol levels as outlined in Table 9–3.
- There are three categories of risk that modify the goals and modalities of LDL-lowering therapy. The highest risk category is having known CHD or CHD risk equivalents; the risk for major coronary events is equal to or greater than that for established CHD (i.e., more than 20% per 10 years, or 2% per year). The intermediate category includes two or more risk factors, in which the 10-year risk for CHD is 20% or less. The lowest risk category is persons with zero to one risk factor, which is usually associated with a 10-year risk of CHD of less than 10%.

TABLE 9–1. Classification of Total, LDL, and HDL Cholesterol and Triglycerides

Total cholesterol	
< 200 mg/dL	Desirable
200–239 mg/dL	Borderline high
≥ 240 mg/dL	High
LDL cholesterol	
< 100 mg/dL	Optimal
100–129 mg/dL	Near or above optimal
130–159 mg/dL	Borderline high
160–189 mg/dL	High
≥ 190 mg/dL	Very high
HDL cholesterol	
< 40 mg/dL	Low
≥ 60 mg/dL	High
Triglycerides	
< 150 mg/dL	Normal
150–199 mg/dL	Borderline high
200–499 mg/dL	High
≥ 500 mg/dL	Very high

HDL, high-density lipoproteins; LDL, low-density lipoproteins.

TABLE 9–2. Major Risk Factors (Exclusive of LDL Cholesterol) that Modify LDL Goals[a]

Age
   Men: ≥ 45 years
   Women: ≥ 55 years or premature menopause without estrogen-replacement therapy
Family history of premature CHD (definite myocardial infarction or sudden death before 55 years of age in father or other male first-degree relative or before 65 years of age in mother or other female first-degree relative)
Cigarette smoking
Hypertension (≥140/90 mm Hg or on antihypertensive medication)
Low HDL cholesterol (< 40 mg/dL)[b]

[a] Diabetes is regarded as a coronary heart disease (CHD) risk equivalent; LDL, low-density lipoprotein; HDL, high-density lipoprotein.
[b] HDL cholesterol (≥ 60 mg/dL) counts as a "negative" risk factor; its presence removes one risk factor from the total count.

TABLE 9–3. LDL Cholesterol Goals and Cutpoints for Therapeutic Lifestyle Changes (TLCs) and Drug Therapy in Different Risk Categories

Risk Category	LDL Goal (mg/dL)	LDL Level at Which to Initiate TLCs (mg/dL)	LDL Level at Which to Consider Drug Therapy (mg/dL)
CHD or CHD risk equivalents (10-yr risk > 20%)	<100	≥100	≥130 (100–129: drug optional)[a]
2+ Risk factors (10-yr risk ≤ 20%)	<130	≥130	10-yr risk 10–20%: ≥130 10-yr risk < 10%: ≥160
0–1 Risk factor[b]	<160	≥160	≥190 (160–189: LDL-lowering drug optional)

LDL, low-density lipoprotein; CHD, coronary heart disease.
[a] Some authorities recommend use of LDL-lowering drugs in this category if an LDL cholesterol level of less than 100 mg/dL cannot be achieved by TLCs. Others prefer use of drugs that primarily modify triglycerides and HDL, e.g., nicotinic acid or fibrates. Clinical judgment also may call for deferring drug therapy in this subcategory.
[b] Almost all people with 0–1 risk factor have a 10-year risk of less than 10%; thus 10-year risk assessment in people with 0–1 risk factor is not necessary.

TABLE 9–4. Macronutrient Recommendations for the TLC Diet

II

Component[a]	Recommended Intake
Total fat	25–35% of total calories
Saturated fat	< 7% of total calories
Polyunsaturated fat	Up to 10% of total calories
Monounsaturated fat	Up to 20% of total calories
Carbohydrates[b]	50–60% of total calories
Cholesterol	< 200 mg/day
Dietary fiber	20–30 g/day
Plant sterols	2 g/day
Protein	Approximately 15% of total calories
Total calories	To achieve and maintain desirable body weight

[a]Calories from alcohol not included.
[b]Carbohydrates should derive from foods rich in complex carbohydrates, such as whole grains, fruits, and vegetables.

- ATP III recognizes the metabolic syndrome as a secondary target of risk reduction after LDL-C has been addressed. This syndrome is characterized by abdominal obesity, atherogenic dyslipidemia (elevated triglycerides, small LDL particles, low HDL cholesterol), increased blood pressure, insulin resistance (with or without glucose intolerance), and prothrombotic and proinflammatory states. If the metabolic syndrome is present, the patient is considered to have a CHD risk equivalent.

NONPHARMACOLOGIC THERAPY

- TLCs are begun on the first visit and include dietary therapy, weight reduction, and increased physical activity. Inducing a weight loss of 10% should be discussed with patients who are overweight. In general, physical activity of moderate intensity 30 minutes a day for most days of the week should be encouraged. All patients should be counseled to stop smoking and to meet the Seventh Joint National Committee on the Detection, Evaluation, and Treatment of High Blood Pressure (JNC 7) guidelines for control of hypertension.
- The objectives of dietary therapy are to progressively decrease the intake of total fat, saturated fat, and cholesterol and to achieve a desirable body weight (Table 9–4).
- Excessive dietary intake of cholesterol and saturated fatty acids leads to decreased hepatic clearance of LDL and deposition of LDL and oxidized LDL in peripheral tissues.
- Increased intake of soluble fiber in the form of oat bran, pectins, certain gums, and psyllium products can result in useful adjunctive reductions in total and LDL cholesterol (5% to 20%), but these dietary alterations or supplements should not be substituted for more active forms of treatment. They have little or no effect on HDL-C or triglyceride concentrations. These products may also be useful in managing constipation associated with the bile acid resins.
- Ingestion of 2 to 3 g/day of plant sterols and stanols will reduce LDL by 6% to 15%. They are usually available in commercial margarines.
- Fish oil supplementation has a fairly large effect in reducing triglycerides and VLDL cholesterol, but it either has no effect on total and LDL cholesterol or may cause elevations in these fractions.
- If all recommended dietary changes from NCEP were instituted, the estimated average reduction in LDL would range from 20% to 30%.

TABLE 9–5. Effects of Drug Therapy on Lipids and Lipoproteins

Drug	Mechanism of Action	Effects on Lipids	Effects on Lipoproteins
Cholestyramine, colestipol, and colesevelam	↑LDL catabolism ↓Cholesterol absorption	↓Cholesterol	↓LDL ↑VLDL
Niacin	↓LDL and VLDL Synthesis	↓Triglyceride and cholesterol	↓VLDL, ↓LDL, ↑HDL
Gemfibrozil, fenofibrate	↑VLDL clearance ↓VLDL synthesis	↓Triglyercide and cholesterol	↓VLDL, ↓LDL, ↑HDL
Lovastatin, pravastatin, simvastatin, fluvastatin, atorvastatin, rosuvastatin	↑LDL catabolism ↓LDL synthesis	↓Cholesterol	↓LDL
Ezetimibe	Inhibits cholesterol absorption across the intestinal border	↓Cholesterol	↓LDL

PHARMACOLOGIC THERAPY

- The effect of drug therapy on lipids and lipoproteins is shown in Table 9–5.
- Recommended drugs of choice for each lipoprotein phenotype are given in Table 9–6.
- Available products and their doses are provided in Table 9–7.

Bile Acid Resins (**Cholestyramine, Colestipol, Colesevelam**)

- The primary action of bile acid resins (BARs) is to bind bile acids in the intestinal lumen, with a concurrent interruption of enterohepatic circulation of bile acids, which decreases the bile acid pool size and stimulates hepatic synthesis of bile acids from cholesterol. Depletion of the hepatic pool of cholesterol results in an increase in cholesterol biosynthesis and an increase in the number

TABLE 9–6. Lipoprotein Phenotype and Recommended Drug Treatment

Lipoprotein Type	Drug of Choice	Combination Therapy
I	Not indicated	—
IIa	Statins	Niacin or BAR
	Cholestyramine or colestipol	Statins or niacin
	Niacin	Statins or BAR Ezetimibe
IIb	Statins	BAR or fibrates or niacin
	Fibrates	Statins or niacin or BAR[a]
	Niacin	Statins or fibrates Ezetimibe
III	Fibrates	Statins or niacin
	Niacin	Statins or fibrates Ezetimibe
IV	Fibrates	Niacin
	Niacin	Fibrates
V	Fibrates	Niacin
	Niacin	Fish oils

BAR, bile acid resins; fibrates include gemfibrozil or fenofibrate.
[a]BARs are not used as first-line therapy if triglycerides are elevated at baseline because hypertriglyceridemia may worsen with BARs alone.

TABLE 9-7. Comparison of Drugs Used in the Treatment of Hyperlipidemia

Drug	Dosage Forms	Usual Daily Dose	Maximum Daily Dose
Cholestyramine (Questran)	Bulk powder/4-g packets	8 g t.i.d.	32 g
Cholestyramine (Cholybar)	4 g resin per bar		
Colestipol hydrochloride (Colestid)	Bulk powder/5-g packets	10 g b.i.d.	30 g
Colesevelam (Welchol)	625-mg tablets	1875 mg b.i.d.	4375 mg
Niacin	50-, 100-, 250-, and 500-mg tablets; 125-, 250-, and 500-mg capsules	2 g t.i.d.	9 g
Extended-release niacin (Niaspan)	500-, 750-, and 1000-mg tablets	500 mg	2000 mg
Extended-release niacin + lovastatin (Advicor)	Niacin/lovastatin 500-mg/20-mg tablets Niacin/lovastatin 750-mg/20-mg tablets Niacin/lovastatin 1000-mg/20-mg tablets	500 mg/20 mg	1000 mg/20 mg
Fenofibrate (Tricor)	67-, 134-, and 200-mg capsules (micronized); 54- and 160-mg tablets	54 mg or 67 mg	201 mg
Gemfibrozil (Lopid)	300-mg capsules	600 mg b.i.d.	1.5 g
Lovastatin (Mevacor)	20- and 40-mg tablets	20–40 mg	80 mg
Pravastatin (Pravachol)	10- and 20-mg tablets	10–20 mg	40 mg
Simvastatin (Zocor)	5-, 10-, 20-, 40-, and 80-mg tablets	10–20 mg	80 mg
Atorvastatin (Lipitor)	10-mg tablets	10 mg	80 mg
Rosuvastatin (Crestor)	5- and 10-mg tablets	5 mg	40 mg
Ezetimibe (Zetia)	10-mg tablet	10 mg	10 mg
Simvastatin/ezetimibe (Vytorin)	Simvastatin/ezetimibe 10 mg/10 mg Simvastatin/ezetimibe 20 mg/10 mg Simvastatin/ezetimibe 40 mg/10 mg	Simvastatin/ezetimibe 20 mg/10 mg	Simvastatin/ezetimibe 40 mg/10 mg

Gemfibrozil, fenofibrate, and lovastatin are available as generic product.

II

II

of LDL receptors on the hepatocyte membrane, which stimulates an enhanced rate of catabolism from plasma and lowers LDL levels. The increase in hepatic cholesterol biosynthesis may be paralleled by increased hepatic VLDL production and, consequently, BARs may aggravate hypertriglyceridemia in patients with combined hyperlipidemia.

- BARs are useful in treating primary hypercholesterolemia (familial hypercholesterolemia, familial combined hyperlipidemia, type IIa hyperlipoproteinemia).

- Gastrointestinal complaints of constipation, bloating, epigastric fullness, nausea, and flatulence are most commonly reported. These adverse effects can be managed by increasing fluid intake, modifying the diet to increase bulk, and using stool softeners.

- The gritty texture and bulk may be minimized by mixing the powder with orange drink or juice. Colestipol may have better palatability than cholestyramine because it is odorless and tasteless. Tablet forms should help improve adherence with this form of therapy.

- Other potential adverse effects include impaired absorption of fat-soluble vitamins A, D, E, and K; hypernatremia and hyperchloremia; gastrointestinal obstruction; and reduced bioavailability of acidic drugs such as warfarin, nicotinic acid, thyroxine, acetaminophen, hydrocortisone, hydrochlorothiazide, loperamide, and possibly iron. Drug interactions may be avoided by alternating administration times with an interval of 6 hours or greater between the BAR and other drugs.

Niacin

- **Niacin** (nicotinic acid) reduces the hepatic synthesis of VLDL, which in turn leads to a reduction in the synthesis of LDL. Niacin also increases HDL by reducing its catabolism.

- The principal use of niacin is for mixed hyperlipidemia or as a second-line agent in combination therapy for hypercholesterolemia. It is a first-line agent or alternative for the treatment of hypertriglyceridemia and diabetic dyslipidemia.

- Niacin has many common adverse drug reactions; most of the symptoms and biochemical abnormalities seen do not require discontinuation of therapy.

- Cutaneous flushing and itching appear to be prostaglandin mediated and can be reduced by taking aspirin 325 mg shortly before niacin ingestion. Taking the niacin dose with meals and slowly titrating the dose upward may minimize these effects. Concomitant alcohol and hot drinks may magnify the flushing and pruritus from niacin, and they should be avoided at the time of ingestion. Gastrointestinal intolerance is also a common problem.

- Potentially important laboratory abnormalities occurring with niacin therapy include elevated liver function tests, hyperuricemia, and hyperglycemia. Niacin-associated hepatitis is more common with sustained-release preparations, and their use should be restricted to patients intolerant of regular-release products. Niacin is contraindicated in patients with active liver disease, and it may exacerbate preexisting gout and diabetes.

- Nicotinamide should not be used in the treatment of hyperlipidemia because it does not effectively lower cholesterol or triglyceride levels.

HMG-CoA Reductase Inhibitors (**Atorvastatin, Fluvastatin, Lovastatin, Pravastatin, Rosuvastatin, Simvastatin**)

- Statins inhibit 3-hydroxy-3-methylglutaryl coenzyme A (HMG-CoA) reductase, interrupting the conversion of HMG-CoA to mevalonate, the rate-limiting step in de novo cholesterol biosynthesis. Reduced synthesis of LDL and enhanced catabolism of LDL mediated through LDL receptors appear to be the principal mechanisms for lipid-lowering effects.

- When used as monotherapy, statins are the most potent total and LDL cholesterol-lowering agents and among the best tolerated. Total and LDL cholesterol are reduced in a dose-related fashion by 30% or more when added to dietary therapy.
- Combination therapy with a statin and BAR is rational as numbers of LDL receptors are increased, leading to greater degradation of LDL cholesterol; intracellular synthesis of cholesterol is inhibited; and enterohepatic recycling of bile acids is interrupted.
- Combination therapy with a statin and ezetimibe is also rational because ezetimibe inhibits cholesterol absorption across the gut border and adds 12% to 20% further reduction when combined with a statin or other drugs.
- Constipation occurs in fewer than 10% of patients taking statins. Other adverse effects include elevated serum aminotransferase levels (primarily alanine aminotransferase), elevated creatine kinase levels, myopathy, and rarely rhabdomyolysis.

Fibric Acids (**Gemfibrozil, Fenofibrate, Clofibrate**)

- Fibrate monotherapy is effective in reducing VLDL, but a reciprocal rise in LDL may occur and total cholesterol values may remain relatively unchanged. Plasma HDL concentrations may rise 10% to 15% or more with fibrates.
- Gemfibrozil reduces the synthesis of VLDL and, to a lesser extent, apolipoprotein B with a concurrent increase in the rate of removal of triglyceride-rich lipoproteins from plasma. Clofibrate is less effective than gemfibrozil or niacin in reducing VLDL production.
- Gastrointestinal complaints occur in 3% to 5% of patients, rash in 2%, dizziness in 2.4%, and transient elevations in transaminase levels and alkaline phosphatase in 4.5% and 1.3%, respectively. Clofibrate and, less commonly, gemfibrozil may enhance the formation of gallstones.
- A myositis syndrome of myalgia, weakness, stiffness, malaise, and elevations in creatine kinase and aspartate aminotransferase may occur and seems to be more common in patients with renal insufficiency.
- Fibrates may potentiate the effects of oral anticoagulants, and the international normalized ratio (INR) should be monitored very closely with this combination.

Ezetimibe

- **Ezetimibe** interferes with the absorption of cholesterol from the brush border of the intestine, a novel mechanism that makes it a good choice for adjunctive therapy. It is approved as both monotherapy and for use with a statin. The dose is 10 mg once daily, given with or without food. When used alone, it results in an approximate 18% reduction in LDL cholesterol. When added to a statin, ezetimibe lowers LDL by about an additional 12% to 20%. A combination product (Vytorin) containing ezetimibe 10 mg and simvastatin 10, 20, 40 or 80 mg is available. Ezetimibe is well tolerated; approximately 4% of patients experience gastrointestinal upset. Because cardiovascular outcomes with ezetimibe have not been evaluated, it should be reserved for patients unable to tolerate statin therapy or those who do not achieve satisfactory lipid lowering with a statin alone.

Fish Oil Supplementation

- Diets high in omega-3 polyunsaturated fatty acids (from **fish oil**), most commonly eicosapentaenoic acid (EPA), reduce cholesterol, triglycerides, LDL, and VLDL and may elevate HDL cholesterol.

- Fish oil supplementation may be most useful in patients with hypertrigly-ceridemia, but its role in treatment is not well defined.
- Complications of fish oil supplementation such as thrombocytopenia and bleeding disorders have been noted, especially with high doses (EPA, 15 to 30 g/day).

TREATMENT RECOMMENDATIONS

- Treatment of type I hyperlipoproteinemia is directed toward reduction of chylomicrons derived from dietary fat with the subsequent reduction in plasma triglycerides. Total daily fat intake should be no more than 10 to 25 g/day, or approximately 15% of total calories. Secondary causes of hypertriglyceridemia should be excluded, and, if present, the underlying disorder should be treated appropriately.
- Primary hypercholesterolemia (familial hypercholesterolemia, familial combined hyperlipidemia, type IIa hyperlipoproteinemia) is treated with **BARs, statins, niacin,** or **ezetimibe.**
- Combined hyperlipoproteinemia (type IIb) may be treated with **statins, niacin,** or **gemfibrozil** to lower LDL-C without elevating VLDL and triglycerides. Niacin is the most effective agent and may be combined with a BAR. A BAR alone in this disorder may elevate VLDL and triglycerides, and their use as single agents for treating combined hyperlipoproteinemia should be avoided.
- Type III hyperlipoproteinemia may be treated with fibrates or niacin. Although **clofibrate** has been suggested as the drug of choice, **niacin, gemfibrozil,** or **fenofibrate** should be considered first because of the lack of data supporting a cardiovascular mortality benefit from clofibrate and because of its potentially serious adverse effects. Fish oil supplementation may be an alternative therapy.
- Type V hyperlipoproteinemia requires stringent restriction of dietary fat intake. Drug therapy with **fibrates** or **niacin** is indicated if the response to diet alone is inadequate. **Medium-chain triglycerides,** which are absorbed without chylomicron formation, may be used as a dietary supplement for caloric intake if needed for both types I and V.

Combination Drug Therapy

- Combination therapy may be considered after adequate trials of monotherapy and for patients documented to be adherent to the prescribed regimen. Two or three lipoprotein profiles at 6-week intervals should confirm lack of response prior to initiation of combination therapy.
- Contraindications to and drug interactions with combined therapy should be screened carefully, and the extra cost of drug product and monitoring should be considered.
- In general, a **statin** plus a **BAR** or **niacin** plus a **BAR** provide the greatest reduction in total and LDL cholesterol.
- Regimens intended to increase HDL levels should include either **gemfibrozil** or **niacin,** and it should be remembered that **statins** combined with either of these drugs may result in a greater incidence of hepatotoxicity or myositis.
- Familial combined hyperlipidemia may respond better to a fibrate and a statin than to a fibrate and a BAR.

TREATMENT OF HYPERTRIGLYCERIDEMIA

- Lipoprotein pattern types I, III, IV, and V are associated with hypertriglyceridemia, and these primary lipoprotein disorders should be excluded prior to implementing therapy.
- A positive family history of CHD is important in identifying patients at risk for premature atherosclerosis. If a patient with CHD has elevated triglycerides, the

associated abnormality is probably a contributing factor to CHD and should be treated.

II

- High serum triglycerides (see Table 9–1) should be treated by achieving desirable body weight, consumption of a low saturated fat and cholesterol diet, regular exercise, smoking cessation, and restriction of alcohol (in selected patients).
- ATP III identifies the sum of LDL and VLDL (termed *non-HDL* [total cholesterol – HDL]) as a secondary therapeutic target in persons with high triglycerides (200 mg/dL or greater). The goal for non-HDL with high serum triglycerides is set at 30 mg/dL higher than that for LDL on the premise that a VLDL level of 30 mg/dL or less is normal.
- Drug therapy with **niacin** should be considered in patients with borderline-high triglycerides but with accompanying risk factors of established CHD, family history of premature CHD, concomitant LDL elevation or low HDL, and genetic forms of hypertriglyceridemia associated with CHD. Niacin may be used cautiously in persons with diabetes because a clinical trial found only a slight increase in glucose and no change in hemoglobin A_{1c}. Alternative therapies include **gemfibrozil, statins,** and **fish oil.** The goal of therapy is to lower triglycerides and VLDL particles that may be atherogenic, increase HDL, and reduce LDL.
- Very high triglycerides are associated with pancreatitis and other adverse consequences. Management includes dietary fat restriction (10% to 20% of calories as fat), weight loss, alcohol restriction, and treatment of coexisting disorders (e.g., diabetes). Drug therapy includes **gemfibrozil, niacin,** and higher-potency statins (**atorvastatin, rosuvastatin,** and **simvastatin**).

TREATMENT OF LOW HDL CHOLESTEROL

Low HDL cholesterol is a strong independent risk predictor of CHD. ATP III redefined low HDL cholesterol as less than 40 mg/dL but specified no goal for HDL cholesterol raising. In low HDL, the primary target remains LDL, but treatment emphasis shifts to weight reduction, increased physical activity, smoking cessation, and to **fibrates** and **niacin** if drug therapy is required.

TREATMENT OF DIABETIC DYSLIPIDEMIA

- Diabetic dyslipidemia is characterized by hypertriglyceridemia, low HDL, and minimally elevated LDL. Small, dense LDL (pattern B) in diabetes is more atherogenic than larger, more buoyant forms of LDL (pattern A).
- ATP III considers diabetes to be a CHD risk equivalent, and the primary target is to lower the LDL to less than 100 mg/dL. When LDL is greater than 130 mg/dL, most patients require simultaneous TLC and drug therapy. When LDL is between 100 and 129 mg/dL, intensifying glycemic control, adding drugs for atherogenic dyslipidemia (**fibrates, niacin**), and intensifying LDL-lowering therapy are options. **Statins** are considered by many to be the drugs of choice because the primary target is LDL.

▶ EVALUATION OF THERAPEUTIC OUTCOMES

- Short-term evaluation of therapy for hyperlipidemia is based on response to diet and drug treatment as measured in the clinical laboratory by total cholesterol, LDL cholesterol, HDL cholesterol, and triglycerides.
- Many patients treated for primary hyperlipidemia have no symptoms or clinical manifestations of a genetic lipid disorder (e.g., xanthomas), so monitoring is solely laboratory based.

- In patients treated for secondary intervention, symptoms of atherosclerotic cardiovascular disease, such as angina or intermittent claudication, may improve over months to years. Xanthomas or other external manifestations of hyperlipidemia should regress with therapy.
- Lipid measurements should be obtained in the fasted state to minimize interference from chylomicrons. Monitoring is needed every few months during dosage titration. Once the patient is stable, monitoring at intervals of 6 months to 1 year is sufficient.
- Patients on BAR therapy should have a fasting panel checked every 4 to 8 weeks until a stable dose is reached; triglycerides should be checked at a stable dose to ensure they have not increased.
- Niacin requires baseline tests of liver function (alanine aminotransferase [ALT]), uric acid, and glucose. Repeat tests are appropriate at doses of 1000 to 1500 mg/day. Symptoms of myopathy or diabetes should be investigated and may require creatine kinase or glucose determinations. Patients with diabetes may require more frequent monitoring.
- Patients receiving statins should have a fasting panel 4 to 8 weeks after the initial dose or dose changes. Liver function tests should be obtained at baseline and periodically thereafter based on package insert information. Some experts believe that monitoring for hepatotoxicity and myopathy should be triggered by symptoms.
- Patients with multiple risk factors and established CHD should also be monitored and evaluated for progress in managing their other risk factors such as blood pressure control, smoking cessation, exercise and weight control, and glycemic control (if diabetic).
- Evaluation of dietary therapy with diet diaries and recall survey instruments allows information about diet to be collected in a systematic fashion and may improve patient adherence to dietary recommendations.

See Chapter 21, Hyperlipidemia, authored by Robert L. Talbert, for a more detailed discussion of this topic.

Chapter 10

▶ HYPERTENSION

▶ DEFINITION

- Hypertension is defined by persistent elevation of arterial blood pressure. The Seventh Joint National Committee on the Detection, Evaluation, and Treatment of High Blood Pressure (JNC 7) classifies adult blood pressure as shown in Table 10–1.
- Patients with diastolic blood pressure (DBP) values less than 90 mm Hg and systolic blood pressure (SBP) values greater than or equal to 140 mm Hg have isolated systolic hypertension.
- A hypertensive crisis (blood pressure greater than 180/120 mm Hg) may be categorized as either a hypertensive emergency (extreme blood pressure elevation with acute or progressing target organ damage) or a hypertensive urgency (severe blood pressure elevation without acute or progressing target organ injury).

▶ PATHOPHYSIOLOGY

- Hypertension is a heterogeneous disorder that may result either from a specific cause (secondary hypertension) or from an underlying pathophysiologic mechanism of unknown etiology (primary or essential hypertension). Secondary hypertension accounts for fewer than 10% of cases, and most of these are caused by chronic kidney disease or renovascular disease. Other conditions causing secondary hypertension include pheochromocytoma, Cushing's syndrome, hyperthyroidism, hyperparathyroidism, primary aldosteronism, pregnancy, obstructive sleep apnea, and coarctation of the aorta. Some drugs that may increase blood pressure include corticosteroids, estrogens, nonsteroidal anti-inflammatory drugs (NSAIDs), amphetamines, sibutramine, cyclosporine, tacrolimus, erythropoietin, and venlafaxine.
- Multiple factors may contribute to the development of primary hypertension, including:
  - humoral abnormalities involving the renin-angiotensin-aldosterone system (RAS), natriuretic hormone, or hyperinsulinemia;
  - a pathologic disturbance in the central nervous system (CNS), autonomic nerve fibers, adrenergic receptors, or baroreceptors;
  - abnormalities in either the renal or tissue autoregulatory processes for sodium excretion, plasma volume, and arteriolar constriction;
  - a deficiency in the local synthesis of vasodilating substances in the vascular endothelium, such as prostacyclin, bradykinin, and nitric oxide, or an increase in production of vasoconstricting substances such as angiotensin II and endothelin I;

TABLE 10–1. Adult Blood Pressure Classification

Classification	Systolic (mm Hg)		Diastolic (mm Hg)
Normal	< 120	and	< 80
Prehypertension[b]	120–139	or	80–89
Stage 1 hypertension	140–159	or	90–99
Stage 2 hypertension	≥ 160	or	≥ 100

► II

- a high sodium intake and increased circulating natriuretic hormone inhibition of intracellular sodium transport, resulting in increased vascular reactivity and a rise in blood pressure; and
- increased intracellular concentration of calcium, leading to altered vascular smooth muscle function and increased peripheral vascular resistance.

- The main causes of death in hypertensive subjects are cerebrovascular accidents, cardiovascular events, and renal failure. The probability of premature death correlates with the severity of blood pressure elevation.

► CLINICAL PRESENTATION

- Patients with uncomplicated primary hypertension are usually asymptomatic initially.
- Patients with secondary hypertension may complain of symptoms suggestive of the underlying disorder. Patients with pheochromocytoma may have a history of paroxysmal headaches, sweating, tachycardia, palpitations, and orthostatic hypotension. In primary aldosteronism, hypokalemic symptoms of muscle cramps and weakness may be present. Patients with hypertension secondary to Cushing's syndrome may complain of weight gain, polyuria, edema, menstrual irregularities, recurrent acne, or muscular weakness.

► DIAGNOSIS

- Frequently, the only sign of primary hypertension on physical examination is elevated blood pressure. The diagnosis of hypertension should be based on the average of two or more readings taken at each of two or more clinical encounters.
- As hypertension progresses, signs of end-organ damage begin to appear, chiefly related to pathologic changes in the eye, brain, heart, kidneys, and peripheral blood vessels.
- The funduscopic examination may reveal arteriolar narrowing, focal arteriolar narrowing, arteriovenous nicking, and retinal hemorrhages, exudates, and infarcts. The presence of papilledema indicates hypertensive emergency requiring rapid treatment.
- Cardiopulmonary examination may reveal an abnormal heart rate or rhythm, left ventricular hypertrophy, precordial heave, third and fourth heart sounds, and rales.
- Peripheral vascular examination can detect evidence of atherosclerosis, which may present as aortic or abdominal bruits, distended veins, diminished or absent peripheral pulses, or lower extremity edema.
- Patients with renal artery stenosis may have an abdominal systolic-diastolic bruit.
- Patients with Cushing's syndrome may have the classic physical features of moon face, buffalo hump, hirsutism, and abdominal striae.
- Baseline hypokalemia may suggest mineralocorticoid-induced hypertension. The presence of protein, blood cells, and casts in the urine may indicate renovascular disease.
- Laboratory tests that should be obtained in all patients prior to initiating drug therapy include urinalysis, complete blood cell count, serum chemistries (sodium, potassium, creatinine, fasting glucose, fasting lipid panel), and a 12-lead electrocardiogram (ECG). These tests are used to assess other risk factors and to develop baseline data for monitoring drug-induced metabolic changes.

- More specific laboratory tests are used to diagnose secondary hypertension. These include plasma norepinephrine and urinary metanephrine levels for pheochromocytoma, plasma and urinary aldosterone levels for primary aldosteronism, and plasma renin activity, captopril stimulation test, renal vein renins, and renal artery angiography for renovascular disease.

▶ DESIRED OUTCOME

- The overall goal of treating hypertension is to reduce morbidity and mortality by the least intrusive means possible.
- Goal blood pressure values are less than 140/90 for uncomplicated hypertension and less than 130/80 for patients with diabetes mellitus and chronic kidney disease.
- SBP is a better predictor of cardiovascular risk than DBP and must be used as the primary clinical marker of disease control in hypertension.

▶ TREATMENT

NONPHARMACOLOGIC THERAPY

- All patients with prehypertension and hypertension should be prescribed lifestyle modifications, including (1) weight reduction if overweight, (2) adoption of the Dietary Approaches to Stop Hypertension (DASH) eating plan, (3) dietary sodium restriction to less than or equal to 2.4 g/day (6 g/day sodium chloride), (4) regular aerobic physical activity, (5) moderate alcohol consumption (less than or equal to 1 oz ethanol per day), and (6) smoking cessation.
- Patients diagnosed with stage 1 or 2 hypertension should be placed on lifestyle modifications and drug therapy concurrently.

PHARMACOLOGIC THERAPY

- Initial drug selection depends on the degree of blood pressure elevation and the presence of compelling indications for selected drugs.
- Most patients with stage 1 hypertension should be treated initially with a **thiazide diuretic** (Figure 10–1). Patients with stage 2 disease should generally be prescribed combination therapy, with one of the agents being a thiazide-type diuretic unless contraindications exist.
- There are six compelling indications where specific antihypertensive drug classes have shown evidence of unique benefits (Figure 10–2).
- **Diuretics, β blockers, angiotensin-converting enzyme (ACE) inhibitors, angiotensin II receptor blockers (ARBs), and calcium channel blockers (CCBs)** are the primary agents based on outcome data demonstrating reductions in target organ damage or cardiovascular morbidity and mortality (Table 10–2).
- α **Blockers, central α_2-agonists, adrenergic inhibitors**, and **vasodilators** are alternatives that may be used in select patients after primary agents (Table 10–3).

Diuretics

- **Thiazides** are the preferred type of diuretic for treating hypertension, and all are equally effective in lowering blood pressure. In patients with adequate renal function (i.e., glomerular filtration rate [GFR] greater than 30 mL/min), thiazides are the most effective diuretics for lowering blood pressure. However, as renal function declines, sodium and fluid accumulate, and the use of a more

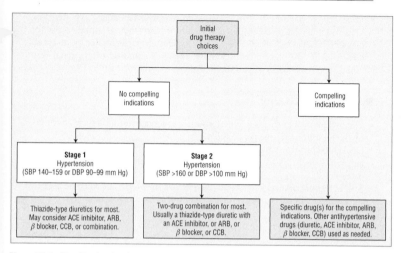

Figure 10–1. Algorithm for the pharmacologic treatment of hypertension. SBP, systolic blood pressure; DBP, diastolic blood pressure; ACE, angiotensin-converting enzyme; ARB, angiotensin-receptor blocker; CCB, calcium channel blocker.

potent loop diuretic is necessary to counter the effects that volume and sodium expansion have on arterial blood pressure.

- **Potassium-sparing diuretics** are weak antihypertensives when used alone but provide an additive hypotensive effect when combined with thiazide or loop diuretics. Moreover, they counteract the potassium- and magnesium-losing properties of other diuretics.

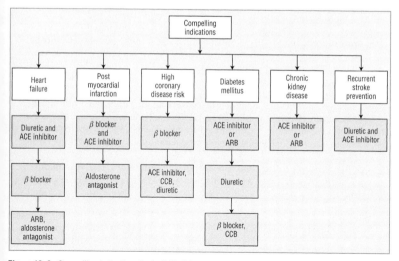

Figure 10–2. Compelling indications for individual drug classes. The order of therapies should be considered a guide that must be balanced with clinical judgment and patient response.

TABLE 10–2. Primary Antihypertensive Agents

Class/Subclass/Drug (Brand Name)	Usual Dose Range, mg/day	Daily Frequency
Diuretics		
Thiazides		
Chlorthalidone (Hygroton)	6.25–25	1
Hydrochlorothiazide (Esidrix, HydroDiuril, Microzide, Oretic)	12.5–50	1
Indapamide (Lozol)	1.25–2.5	1
Metolazone (Mykrox)	0.5	1
Metolazone (Zaroxolyn)	2.5	1
Loops		
Bumetanide (Bumex)	0.5–4	2
Furosemide (Lasix)	20–80	2
Torsemide (Demadex)	5	1
Potassium sparing		
Amiloride (Midamor)	5–10	1 or 2
Amiloride/hydrochlorothiazide (Moduretic)	5–10/50–100	1
Triamterene (Dyrenium)	50–100	1 or 2
Triamterene/hydrochlorothiazide (Dyazide)	37.5–75/25–50	1
Aldosterone antagonists		
Eplerenone (Inspra)	50–100	1 or 2
Spironolactone (Aldactone)	25–50	1 or 2
Spironolactone/hydrochlorothiazide (Aldactazide)	25–50/25–50	1
Agiotensin-converting enzyme inhibitors		
Benazepril (Lotensin)	10–40	1 or 2
Captopril (Capoten)	12.5–150	2 or 3
Enalapril (Vasotec)	5–40	1 or 2
Fosinopril (Monopril)	10–40	1
Lisinopril (Prinivil, Zestril)	10–40	1
Moexipril (Univasc)	7.5–30	1 or 2
Perindopril (Aceon)	4–16	1
Quinapril (Accupril)	10–80	1 or 2
Ramipril (Altace)	2.5–10	1 or 2
Trandolapril (Mavik)	1–4	1
Angiotensin II receptor blockers		
Candesartan (Atacand)	8–32	1 or 2
Eprosartan (Teveten)	600–800	1 or 2
Irbesartan (Avapro)	150–300	1
Losartan (Cozaar)	50–100	1 or 2
Olmesartan (Benicar)	20–40	1
Telmisartan (Micardis)	20–80	1
Valsartan (Diovan)	80–320	1
β-Blockers		
Cardioselective		
Atenolol (Tenormin)	25–100	1
Betaxolol (Kerlone)	5–20	1
Bisoprolol (Zebeta)	2.5–10	1
Metoprolol (Lopressor)	50–200	2
Metoprolol extended release (Toprol XL)	50–200	1
Nonselective		
Nadolol (Corgard)	40–120	1
Propranolol (Inderal)	160–480	2
Propranolol long-acting (Inderal LA, InnoPran XL)	80–320	1

continued

TABLE 10–2. (*Continued*)

Class/Subclass/Drug (Brand Name)	Usual Dose Range, mg/day	Daily Frequency
Timolol (Blocadren)	10–40	1
Intrinsic sympathomimetic activity		
Acebutolol (Sectral)	200–800	2
Carteolol (Cartrol)	2.5–10	1
Penbutolol (Levatol)	10–40	1
Pindolol (Visken)	10–60	2
Mixed α- and β-blockers		
Carvedilol (Coreg)	12.5–50	2
Labetolol (Normodyne, Trandate)	200–800	2
Calcium channel blockers		
Dihydropyridines		
Amlodipine (Norvasc)	2.5–10	1
Felodipine (Plendil)	5–20	1
Isradipine (DynaCirc)	5–10	2
Isradipine SR (DynaCirc SR)	5–20	1
Nicardipine sustained release (Cardene SR)	60–120	2
Nifedipine long-acting (Adalat CC, Procardia XL)	30–90	1
Nisoldipine (Sular)	10–40	1
Non-Dihydropyridines		
Diltiazem sustained-release (Cardizem SR)	180–360	2
Diltiazem sustained-release	120–480	1
(Cardizem CD, Cartia XT, Dilacor XR, Diltia XT, Tiazac, Taztia XT)		
Diltiazem extended-release	120–540	1 (morning or evening)
(Cardizem LA)		
Verapamil sustained-release	180–480	1 or 2
(Calan SR, Isoptin SR, Verelan)		
Verapamil controlled-onset extended-release	180–420	1 (in the evening)
(Covera HS)		
Verapamil chronotherapeutic oral drug absorption system (Verelan PM)	100–400	1 (in the evening)

TABLE 10–3. Alternative Antihypertensive Agents

Class Drug (Brand Name)	Usual Dose Range, mg/day	Daily Frequency
α_1-Blockers		
Doxazosin (Cardura)	1–8	1
Prazosin (Minipress)	2–20	2 or 3
Terazosin (Hytrin)	1–20	1 or 2
Central α_2-agonists		
Clonidine (Catapres)	0.1–0.8	2
Clonidine patch (Catapres-TTS)	0.1–0.3	1 weekly
Methyldopa (Aldomet)	250–1000	2
Peripheral adrenergic antagonist		
Reserpine (generic only)	0.05–0.25	1
Direct arterial vasodilators		
Minoxidil (Loniten)	10–40	1 or 2
Hydralazine (Apresoline)	20–100	2 to 4

- **Aldosterone antagonists** are also potassium-sparing diuretics but are more potent antihypertensives with a slow onset of action (up to 6 weeks with spironolactone).

II

- Acutely, diuretics lower blood pressure by causing diuresis. The reduction in plasma volume and stroke volume associated with diuresis decreases cardiac output and, consequently, blood pressure. The initial drop in cardiac output causes a compensatory increase in peripheral vascular resistance. With chronic diuretic therapy, the extracellular fluid volume and plasma volume return almost to pretreatment levels, and peripheral vascular resistance falls below its pretreatment baseline. The reduction in peripheral vascular resistance is responsible for the long-term hypotensive effects. Thiazides lower blood pressure by mobilizing sodium and water from arteriolar walls, which may contribute to decreased peripheral vascular resistance.
- When diuretics are combined with other antihypertensive agents, an additive hypotensive effect is usually observed because of independent mechanisms of action. Furthermore, many nondiuretic antihypertensive agents induce salt and water retention, which is counteracted by concurrent diuretic use.
- Side effects of thiazides include hypokalemia, hypomagnesemia, hypercalcemia, hyperuricemia, hyperglycemia, hyperlipidemia, and sexual dysfunction. Loop diuretics have less effect on serum lipids and glucose, but hypocalcemia may occur.
- Hypokalemia and hypomagnesemia may cause muscle fatigue or cramps. Serious cardiac arrhythmias may occur, especially in patients receiving digitalis therapy, patients with left ventricular hypertrophy, and those with ischemic heart disease. Low-dose therapy (e.g., 25 mg **hydrochlorothiazide** or 12.5 mg **chlorthalidone** daily) rarely causes significant electrolyte disturbances.
- Potassium-sparing diuretics may cause hyperkalemia, especially in patients with chronic kidney disease or diabetes, and in patients receiving concurrent treatment with an ACE inhibitor, ARB, NSAID, or potassium supplement. **Eplerenone** has an increased risk for hyperkalemia and is contraindicated in patients with impaired renal function or type 2 diabetes with proteinuria. **Spironolactone** may cause gynecomastia in up to 10% of patients, but this effect occurs rarely with eplerenone.

Angiotensin-Converting Enzyme Inhibitors

- ACE facilitates production of angiotensin II, which has a major role in regulating arterial blood pressure. ACE is distributed in many tissues and is present in several different cell types, but its principal location is in endothelial cells. Therefore, the major site for angiotensin II production is in the blood vessels, not the kidney. ACE inhibitors block the conversion of angiotensin I to angiotensin II, a potent vasoconstrictor and stimulator of aldosterone secretion. ACE inhibitors also block the degradation of bradykinin and stimulate the synthesis of other vasodilating substances including prostaglandin E_2 and prostacyclin. The fact that ACE inhibitors lower blood pressure in patients with normal plasma renin activity suggests that bradykinin and perhaps tissue production of ACE are important in hypertension.
- Starting doses of ACE inhibitors should be low with slow dose titration. Acute hypotension may occur at the onset of ACE inhibitor therapy, especially in patients who are sodium- or volume-depleted, in heart failure exacerbation, very elderly, or on concurrent vasodilators or diuretics. Patients with these risk factors should start with half the normal dose followed by slow dose titration (e.g., 6-week intervals).

- All 10 ACE inhibitors available in the United States can be dosed once daily for hypertension except captopril, which is usually dosed 2 or 3 times daily. The absorption of captopril (but not enalapril or lisinopril) is reduced by 30% to 40% when given with food.
- ACE inhibitors decrease aldosterone and can increase serum potassium concentrations. Hyperkalemia occurs primarily in patients with chronic kidney disease or diabetes and in those also taking ARBs, NSAIDs, potassium supplements, or potassium-sparing diuretics.
- The most serious adverse effects of the ACE inhibitors are neutropenia and agranulocytosis, proteinuria, glomerulonephritis, and acute renal failure; these effects occur in less than 1% of patients. Bilateral renal artery stenosis or unilateral stenosis of a solitary functioning kidney renders patients dependent on the vasoconstrictive effect of angiotensin II on efferent arterioles, making these patients particularly susceptible to acute renal failure.
- The GFR decreases in patients receiving ACE inhibitors because of inhibition of angiotensin II vasoconstriction on efferent arterioles. Serum creatinine concentrations often increase, but modest elevations (e.g., absolute increases of less than 1 mg/dL) do not warrant changes. Therapy should be stopped or the dose reduced if larger increases occur.
- Angioedema is a serious potential complication that occurs in less than 2% of patients. It may be manifested as lip and tongue swelling and possibly difficulty breathing. Drug withdrawal is appropriate for all patients with angioedema, and some patients may also require drug treatment and/or emergent intubation. Cross-reactivity between ACE inhibitors and ARBs has been reported.
- A persistent dry cough occurs in up to 20% of patients and is thought to be due to inhibition of bradykinin breakdown. If an ACE inhibitor is indicated because of compelling indications, patients should be switched to an ARB.
- ACE inhibitors are absolutely contraindicated in pregnancy because serious neonatal problems, including renal failure and death in the infant, have been reported when mothers took these agents during the second and third trimesters.

Angiotensin II Receptor Blockers

- Angiotensin II is generated by the renin-angiotensin pathway (which involves ACE) and an alternative pathway that uses other enzymes such as chymases. ACE inhibitors block only the renin-angiotensin pathway, whereas ARBs antagonize angiotensin II generated by either pathway. The ARBs directly block the angiotensin type 1 (AT_1) receptor that mediates the known effects of angiotensin II (vasoconstriction, aldosterone release, sympathetic activation, antidiuretic hormone release, and constriction of the efferent arterioles of the glomerulus).
- Unlike ACE inhibitors, ARBs do not block the breakdown of bradykinin. While this accounts for the lack of cough as a side effect, there may be negative consequences because some of the antihypertensive effect of ACE inhibitors may be due to increased levels of bradykinin. Bradykinin may also be important for regression of myocyte hypertrophy and fibrosis, and increased levels of tissue plasminogen activator.
- All drugs in this class have similar antihypertensive efficacy and fairly flat dose-response curves. The addition of low doses of a thiazide diuretic can increase efficacy significantly.
- In patients with type 2 diabetes and nephropathy, ARB therapy has been shown to significantly reduce progression of nephropathy. For patients with systolic heart failure, ARB therapy has also been shown to reduce the risk

of cardiovascular events when added to a stable regimen of a diuretic, ACE inhibitor, and β blocker or as alternative therapy in ACE inhibitor-intolerant patients.

- ARBs appear to have the lowest incidence of side effects compared with other antihypertensive agents. Cough is very uncommon. Like ACE inhibitors, they may cause renal insufficiency, hyperkalemia, and orthostatic hypotension. Angioedema is less likely to occur than with ACE inhibitors, but cross-reactivity has been reported. ARBs should not be used in pregnancy.

β Blockers

- The exact hypotensive mechanism of β blockers is not known but may involve decreased cardiac output through negative chronotropic and inotropic effects on the heart and inhibition of renin release from the kidney.
- Even though there are important pharmacodynamic and pharmacokinetic differences among the various β blockers, there is no difference in clinical antihypertensive efficacy.
- **Atenolol, betaxolol, bisoprolol,** and **metoprolol** are cardioselective at low doses and bind more avidly to β_1 receptors than to β_2 receptors. As a result, they are less likely to provoke bronchospasm and vasoconstriction and may be safer than nonselective β blockers in patients with asthma, chronic obstructive pulmonary disease (COPD), diabetes, and peripheral arterial disease. Cardioselectivity is a dose-dependent phenomenon, and the effect is lost at higher doses.
- **Acebutolol, carteolol, penbutolol,** and **pindolol** possess intrinsic sympathomimetic activity (ISA) or partial β-receptor agonist activity. When sympathetic tone is low, as in resting states, β receptors are partially stimulated, so resting heart rate, cardiac output, and peripheral blood flow are not reduced when receptors are blocked. Theoretically, these drugs may have advantages in patients with heart failure, sinus bradycardia, or perhaps peripheral arterial disease. Unfortunately, they do not reduce cardiovascular events as well as other β blockers and may increase risk after myocardial infarction or in those with high coronary disease risk. Thus, agents with ISA are rarely needed.
- There are pharmacokinetic differences among β blockers in first-pass metabolism, serum half-lives, degree of lipophilicity, and route of elimination. **Propranolol** and **metoprolol** undergo extensive first-pass metabolism. **Atenolol** and **nadolol** have relatively long half-lives and are excreted renally; the dosage may need to be reduced in patients with moderate to severe renal insufficiency. Even though the half-lives of the other β blockers are much shorter, once-daily administration still may be effective. β Blockers vary in their lipophilic properties and thus CNS penetration.
- Side effects from β blockade in the myocardium include bradycardia, atrioventricular (AV) conduction abnormalities, and acute heart failure. Pulmonary β_2 blockade may cause acute exacerbations of bronchospasm in patients with asthma or COPD. Blocking β_2 receptors in arteriolar smooth muscle may cause cold extremities and aggravate intermittent claudication or Raynaud's phenomenon because of decreased peripheral blood flow.
- Abrupt cessation of β-blocker therapy may produce unstable angina, myocardial infarction, or even death in patients predisposed to ischemic myocardial events. In patients without coronary artery disease, abrupt discontinuation of β-blocker therapy may be associated with sinus tachycardia, increased sweating, and generalized malaise. For these reasons, it is always prudent to taper the dose gradually over 1 to 2 weeks before discontinuation.
- Increases in serum lipids and glucose appear to be transient and of little clinical importance. β Blockers increase serum triglyceride levels and decrease HDL

II

cholesterol levels slightly. β Blockers with α-blocking properties (carvedilol and labetalol) do not affect serum lipid concentrations.

Calcium Channel Blockers

- The calcium channel blockers (CCBs) cause relaxation of cardiac and smooth muscle by blocking voltage-sensitive calcium channels, thereby reducing the entry of extracellular calcium into cells. Vascular smooth muscle relaxation leads to vasodilation and a corresponding reduction in blood pressure. Dihydropyridine calcium channel antagonists may cause reflex sympathetic activation, and all agents (except amlodipine) may demonstrate negative inotropic effects.
- **Verapamil** decreases heart rate, slows AV nodal conduction, and produces a negative inotropic effect that may precipitate heart failure in patients with borderline cardiac reserve. **Diltiazem** decreases AV conduction and heart rate to a lesser extent than verapamil.
- Diltiazem and verapamil can cause cardiac conduction abnormalities such as bradycardia, AV block, and heart failure. Both can cause anorexia, nausea, peripheral edema, and hypotension. Verapamil causes constipation in about 7% of patients.
- Dihydropyridines cause a baroreceptor-mediated reflex increase in heart rate because of their potent peripheral vasodilating effects. Dihydropyridines usually do not decrease AV node conduction.
- Nifedipine rarely may cause an increase in the frequency, intensity, and duration of angina in association with acute hypotension. This effect may be obviated by using sustained-released formulations of nifedipine or other dihydropyridines. Other side effects of dihydropyridines include dizziness, flushing, headache, gingival hyperplasia, peripheral edema, mood changes, and gastrointestinal complaints. Side effects due to vasodilation such as dizziness, flushing, headache, and peripheral edema occur more frequently with dihydropyridines than with verapamil or diltiazem.

α_1-Receptor Blockers

- **Prazosin, terazosin,** and **doxazosin** are selective α_1-receptor blockers that inhibit catecholamine uptake in smooth muscle cells of the peripheral vasculature, resulting in vasodilation. They do not alter α_2-receptor activity and therefore do not cause reflex tachycardia.
- A potentially severe side effect is a first-dose phenomenon characterized by orthostatic hypotension accompanied by transient dizziness or faintness, palpitations, and even syncope within 1 to 3 hours of the first dose or after later dosage increases. These episodes can be obviated by having the patient take the first dose, and subsequent first increased doses, at bedtime. Occasionally, orthostatic dizziness persists with chronic administration.
- Sodium and water retention can occur with higher doses and sometimes with chronic administration of low doses. These agents are most effective when given with a diuretic to maintain hypotensive efficacy and minimize potential edema.
- CNS side effects include lassitude, vivid dreams, and depression.
- Because data suggest that doxazosin (and probably other α_1-receptor blockers) are not as protective against cardiovascular events as other therapies, their use should be reserved for unique cases such as men with benign prostatic hyperplasia if they are already receiving other standard antihypertensive therapy (diuretic, β blocker, or ACE inhibitor).

Central α_2-Agonists

- **Clonidine, guanabenz, guanfacine,** and **methyldopa** lower blood pressure primarily by stimulating α_2-adrenergic receptors in the brain, which reduces sympathetic outflow from the vasomotor center and increases vagal tone. Stimulation of presynaptic α_2 receptors peripherally may contribute to the reduction in sympathetic tone. Consequently, there may be decreases in heart rate, cardiac output, total peripheral resistance, plasma renin activity, and baroreceptor reflexes.

- Chronic use results in sodium and fluid retention, which is most prominent with methyldopa. Low doses of clonidine, guanfacine, or guanabenz can be used to treat mild hypertension without the addition of a diuretic.

- Sedation and dry mouth are common side effects that may diminish or disappear with chronic low doses. As with other centrally acting antihypertensives, they may cause depression.

- Abrupt cessation may lead to rebound hypertension (sudden increase in blood pressure to the pretreatment level) or overshoot hypertension (increase in blood pressure higher than the pretreatment level). This is thought to occur secondary to a compensatory increase in norepinephrine release that follows discontinuation of presynaptic α-receptor stimulation.

- **Methyldopa** rarely may cause hepatitis or hemolytic anemia. A transient elevation in hepatic transaminases occasionally occurs with methyldopa and is clinically unimportant. A persistent increase in serum transaminases or alkaline phosphatase may herald the onset of fulminant hepatitis, which can be fatal. A Coombs-positive hemolytic anemia occurs in less than 1% of patients receiving methyldopa, although 20% exhibit a positive direct Coombs test without anemia. For these reasons, methyldopa has limited usefulness.

- **Transdermal clonidine** may be associated with fewer side effects and better adherence than oral clonidine. The patch is applied to the skin and replaced once a week. It reduces blood pressure while avoiding the high peak serum drug concentrations that are thought to contribute to adverse effects. Its disadvantages are high cost, a 20% incidence of local skin rash or irritation, and a 2- or 3-day delay in onset of effect.

Reserpine

- **Reserpine** depletes norepinephrine from sympathetic nerve endings and blocks the transport of norepinephrine into its storage granules. When the nerve is stimulated, less than the usual amount of norepinephrine is released into the synapse. This reduces sympathetic tone, decreasing peripheral vascular resistance and blood pressure.

- Reserpine has a long half-life that allows for once-daily dosing, but it may take 2 to 6 weeks before the maximal antihypertensive effect is seen.

- Reserpine can cause significant sodium and fluid retention, and it should be given with a diuretic (preferably a thiazide).

- Reserpine's strong inhibition of sympathetic activity allows increased parasympathetic activity to occur, which is responsible for side effects of nasal stuffiness, increased gastric acid secretion, diarrhea, and bradycardia.

- The most serious side effect is dose-related mental depression resulting from CNS depletion of catecholamines and serotonin. This can be minimized by not exceeding 0.25 mg daily.

- The combination of a diuretic and reserpine is an effective, inexpensive antihypertensive regimen.

Direct Arterial Vasodilators

II
- **Hydralazine** and **minoxidil** cause direct arteriolar smooth muscle relaxation. Compensatory activation of baroreceptor reflexes results in increased sympathetic outflow from the vasomotor center, producing an increase in heart rate, cardiac output, and renin release. Consequently, the hypotensive effectiveness of direct vasodilators diminishes over time unless the patient is also taking a sympathetic inhibitor and a diuretic.
- Patients who are candidates for these drugs generally should receive prior therapy with both a diuretic and a β-adrenergic blocker. Direct vasodilators can precipitate angina in patients with underlying coronary artery disease unless the baroreceptor reflex mechanism is completely blocked with a sympathetic inhibitor. Clonidine can be used in patients with contraindications to β blockers.
- Hydralazine may cause a dose-related, reversible lupus-like syndrome, which is more common in slow acetylators. Lupus-like reactions can usually be avoided by using total daily doses of less than 200 mg. Other hydralazine side effects include dermatitis, drug fever, peripheral neuropathy, hepatitis, and vascular headaches. For these reasons, hydralazine has limited usefulness in the treatment of hypertension.
- Minoxidil is a more potent vasodilator than hydralazine, and the compensatory increases in heart rate, cardiac output, renin release, and sodium retention are more dramatic. Severe sodium and water retention may precipitate congestive heart failure. Minoxidil also causes reversible hypertrichosis on the face, arms, back, and chest. Other side effects include pericardial effusion and a nonspecific T-wave change on the ECG. Minoxidil generally is reserved for very difficult to control hypertension.

Postganglionic Sympathetic Inhibitors

- **Guanethidine** and **guanadrel** deplete norepinephrine from postganglionic sympathetic nerve terminals and inhibit the release of norepinephrine in response to sympathetic nerve stimulation. This reduces cardiac output and peripheral vascular resistance.
- Orthostatic hypotension is common due to blockade of reflex-mediated vasoconstriction. Other side effects include erectile dysfunction, diarrhea, and weight gain. Because of these adverse effects, postganglionic sympathetic inhibitors have little role in the management of hypertension.

COMPELLING INDICATIONS

- The six compelling indications identified by JNC 7 represent specific comorbid conditions for which clinical trial data support using specific antihypertensive drug classes to treat both hypertension and the compelling indication (Figure 10–2).
- Drug therapy recommendations are either in combination with or in place of a thiazide diuretic.

Heart Failure

- Diuretics are part of first-line therapy because they provide symptomatic relief of edema by diuresis. Loop diuretics may be needed, especially in patients with advanced systolic failure.
- ACE inhibitors are the first drugs of choice based on numerous outcome studies showing reduced morbidity and mortality. Because of the high renin and angiotensin II status of patients with heart failure, therapy should be initiated at low doses to avoid orthostatic hypotension.

- β-Blocker therapy is appropriate to further modify disease in systolic heart failure. Because of the risk of exacerbating heart failure, they must be started in very low doses and titrated slowly to high doses based on tolerability.
- ARBs are acceptable as alternative therapy for patients who cannot tolerate ACE inhibitors and possibly as add-on therapy for those already receiving a standard three-drug regimen.
- Aldosterone antagonists may be considered in symptomatic systolic heart failure but only in addition to diuretics, ACE inhibitors or ARBS, and β blockers.

Postmyocardial Infarction

- β Blockers decrease cardiac adrenergic stimulation and reduce the risk of a subsequent myocardial infarction or sudden cardiac death.
- ACE inhibitors improve cardiac function and reduce cardiovascular events after myocardial infarction.
- The aldosterone antagonist eplerenone was shown to be beneficial soon after myocardial infarction in patients with systolic heart failure. It should only be used in selected patients.

High Coronary Disease Risk

- β blockers are the first-line therapy in chronic stable angina and are beneficial in unstable angina and myocardial infraction.
- CCBs (especially the nondihydropyridines verapamil and diltiazem) lower blood pressure and reduce myocardial oxygen demand. Dihydropyridine CCBs may cause cardiac stimulation and should be reserved as second- or third-line therapy.

Diabetes Mellitus

- The blood pressure goal in diabetes is less than 130/80 mm Hg.
- All patients with diabetes and hypertension should be treated with a regimen that includes either an ACE inhibitor or an ARB. Both classes provide nephro-protection and reduced cardiovascular risk.
- A thiazide diuretic is recommended if a second drug is needed.
- β Blockers reduce cardiovascular risk in patients with diabetes, and they are especially indicated in patients with diabetes who have experienced a myocardial infarction or who have high coronary disease risk. However, they may mask most of the symptoms of hypoglycemia (tremor, tachycardia, and palpitations but not sweating) in tightly controlled patients, delay recovery from hypo-glycemia, and produce elevations in blood pressure due to vasoconstriction caused by unopposed α-receptor stimulation during the hypoglycemic recovery phase. Despite these potential problems, β blockers are highly beneficial in diabetes after ACE inhibitors, ARBs, and diuretics.
- CCBs are useful add-on agents for blood pressure control in hypertensive patients with diabetes.

Chronic Kidney Disease

- ACE inhibitors and ARBs lower blood pressure and also reduce intragomerular pressure, which further reduces the decline in renal function. Some data indicate that the combination of an ACE inhibitor and ARB may be more effective than either agent alone.
- Because these patients usually require multiple-drug therapy, diuretics and a third class (β blocker or CCB) are often needed.

Recurrent Stroke Prevention

II One clinical trial showed that the combination of an ACE inhibitor and thiazide diuretic reduces the incidence of recurrent stroke in patients with a history of stroke or transient ischemic attacks.

SPECIAL POPULATIONS

Selection of drug therapy should follow the JNC 7 guidelines, but the treatment approach in some patient populations may be slightly different. In these situations, alternative agents may have unique properties that benefit a coexisting condition, but the data may not be based on evidence from outcome studies in hypertension.

Hypertension in Older People

- Elderly patients may present with either isolated systolic hypertension or an elevation in both SBP and DBP. Epidemiologic data indicate that cardiovascular morbidity and mortality are more closely related to SBP than to DBP in patients 50 years of age and older.
- Elderly patients are usually more sensitive to volume depletion and sympathetic inhibition, and treatment generally should be initiated with a small dose of a diuretic (e.g., hydrochlorothiazide, 12.5 mg) and increased gradually.
- If a diuretic alone does not achieve the desired reduction in SBP, an ACE inhibitor can be added at low doses with gradual increases. β Blockers are the first drugs of choice in elderly patients with both hypertension and angina, and ACE inhibitors are strongly preferred for hypertensive patients with diabetes or heart failure.

Hypertension in Children and Adolescents

- In most cases, the factors associated with hypertension in children are identical to those in adults. However, secondary hypertension is much more common in children than in adults.
- Renal diseases (e.g., pyelonephritis, glomerulonephritis, renal artery stenosis, renal cysts) are the most common causes of secondary hypertension in children. Medical or surgical management of the underlying disorder usually restores normal blood pressure.
- Nonpharmacologic treatment is the cornerstone of therapy of primary hypertension. Diuretics, β blockers, and ACE inhibitors are very effective.
- ACE inhibitors and ARBs are contraindicated in sexually active girls because of potential teratogenic effect and in those who might have bilateral renal artery stenosis or unilateral stenosis in a solitary kidney.
- Long-acting dihydropyridine CCBs have been used successfully in children, but long-term safety is unknown.

Hypertension in Pregnancy

- Preeclampsia can lead rapidly to life-threatening complications for both the mother and fetus; it usually presents after 20 weeks' gestation in primigravid women. The diagnosis is based on the appearance of hypertension (greater than 140/90 mm Hg) after 20 weeks' gestation with proteinuria.
- Definitive treatment of preeclampsia is delivery, and this is indicated if pending or frank eclampsia (preeclampsia and convulsions) is present. Otherwise, measures such as restriction of activity, bedrest, and close monitoring are in order. Salt restriction or other measures that contract blood volume should be avoided. Antihypertensives are used prior to induction of labor if the DBP is greater than 105 or 110 mm Hg, with a target DBP of 95 to 105 mm Hg. The

II

most commonly used drug is intravenous hydralazine; intravenous labetalol is also effective.

- Chronic hypertension occurs before 20 weeks' gestation. Methyldopa is considered the drug of choice because of experience with its use. β Blockers, labetalol, and CCBs are also reasonable alternatives. ACE inhibitors and ARBs are absolutely contraindicated.

Hypertension in African Americans

- Hypertension is more common and more severe in black persons than in those of other races. Differences in electrolyte homeostasis, glomerular filtration rate, sodium excretion and transport mechanisms, plasma renin activity, and blood pressure response to plasma volume expansion have been noted.
- Thiazide diuretics are first-line therapy for most patients, and CCBs are also particularly effective.
- Addition of a β blocker, ACE inhibitor, or ARB to a thiazide diuretic or CCB significantly increases the antihypertensive response.

Hypertension with Pulmonary Disease and Peripheral Arterial Disease

- Nonselective β blockers should be avoided in hypertensive patients with asthma, COPD, and peripheral vascular disease.
- The α/β blockers carvedilol and labetalol may be used in peripheral arterial disease because they do not result in unopposed α constriction like pure β blockers. However, they should be avoided in patients with asthma or COPD.
- A β_1-selective agent should be selected if a hypertensive patient with mild to moderate asthma or COPD requires a β blocker to treat a compelling indication.

Hypertension with Dyslipidemia

- Dyslipidemia is a major cardiovascular risk factor, and it should be controlled in hypertensive patients.
- Thiazide diuretics and β blockers without ISA may affect serum lipids adversely, but these effects generally are transient and of no clinical consequence.
- The α blockers have been shown to have favorable effects (decreased low-density lipoprotein cholesterol and increased high-density lipoprotein cholesterol levels). Because they do not reduce cardiovascular risk as effectively as thiazide diuretics, this benefit is not clinically applicable.
- ACE inhibitors and CCBs have no effect on serum cholesterol.

HYPERTENSIVE URGENCIES AND EMERGENCIES

- Hypertensive urgencies are ideally managed by adjusting maintenance therapy by adding a new antihypertensive and/or increasing the dose of a present medication.
- Acute administration of a short-acting oral drug (captopril, clonidine, or labetalol) followed by careful observation for several hours to ensure a gradual blood pressure reduction is an option.
  - Oral captopril doses of 25 to 50 mg may be given at 1- to 2-hour intervals. The onset of action is 15 to 30 minutes.
  - For treatment of hypertensive rebound after withdrawal of clonidine, 0.2 mg is given initially, followed by 0.2 mg hourly until the DBP falls below 110 mm Hg or a total of 0.7 mg has been administered; a single dose may be sufficient.
  - Labetalol can be given in a dose of 200 to 400 mg, followed by additional doses every 2 to 3 hours.
- Hypertensive emergencies require immediate blood pressure reduction to limit new or progressing target-organ damage. The goal is not to lower blood pressure

to normal; instead, a reduction in mean arterial pressure (MAP) of up to 25% within minutes to hours is the initial target. If blood pressure is then stable, it can be reduced toward 160/100 mm Hg within the next 2 to 6 hours. Precipitous drops in blood pressure may cause end-organ ischemia or infarction. If blood pressure reduction is well tolerated, additional gradual decrease toward the goal blood pressure can be attempted after 24 to 48 hours.

- **Nitroprusside** is the agent of choice for minute-to-minute control in most cases. It is usually given as a continuous intravenous (IV) infusion at a rate of 0.25 to 10 mcg/kg/min. Its onset of hypotensive action is immediate and disappears within 2 to 5 minutes of discontinuation. When the infusion must be continued longer than 72 hours, serum thiocyanate levels should be measured, and the infusion should be discontinued if the level exceeds 12 mg/dL. The risk of thiocyanate toxicity is increased in patients with impaired renal function. Other side effects of nitroprusside include nausea, vomiting, muscle twitching, and sweating. Nitroprusside administration requires constant intra-arterial pressure monitoring.
- **Nitroglycerin** may be given at a rate of 5 to 100 mcg/min intravenously. As with other nitrates, nitroglycerin is associated with tolerance over 24 to 48 hours.
- **Nicardipine** is administered at 5 to 15 mg/h intravenously, adjusted by 1 to 2.5 mg/h after 15 minutes. Common side effects include headache, tachycardia, flushing, nausea, and vomiting.
- **Felodopam**, 0.1 to 0.3 mcg/kg/min, is given by intravenous infusion. It may cause tachycardia, flushing, and headache.
- **Labetalol** may be given at an initial dose of 20 mg by slow IV injection over a 2-minute period, followed by repeated injections of 40 to 80 mg at 10-minute intervals, up to a total dose of 300 mg. It can also be administered by continuous infusion at an initial rate of 0.5 to 2 mg/min and adjusted according to blood pressure response. Labetalol can cause orthostatic hypotension because of its α-blocking effects. Other side effects include nausea, vomiting, scalp tingling, sweating, dizziness, flushing, and headaches.
- **Hydralazine** may be given intravenously by diluting 10 to 20 mg in 20 mL of 5% dextrose in water (D_5W) and administering it at a rate of 0.5 to 1.0 mL/min. Its onset of action ranges from 10 to 30 minutes, and its effects last 2 to 4 hours. Because the hypotensive response is less predictable than with other parenteral agents, its major role is in the treatment of eclampsia or hypertensive encephalopathy associated with renal insufficiency.

▶ EVALUATION OF THERAPEUTIC OUTCOMES

- The goal of antihypertensive treatment is to maintain arterial blood pressure below 140/90 mm Hg to prevent cardiovascular morbidity and mortality. Lowering blood pressure to less than 130/80 mm Hg should be targeted in patients with diabetes or chronic kidney disease.
- Self-reported measurements or automatic ambulatory blood pressure monitoring can be used to establish effective 24-hour control. Readings should be taken 2 to 4 weeks after initiating or making changes in therapy. Once the goal level is achieved, readings need to be evaluated only every 3 to 6 months in asymptomatic patients.
- A careful history should be taken for chest pain, palpitations, dizziness, dyspnea, orthopnea, slurred speech, and loss of balance to assess the likelihood of cardiovascular and cerebrovascular hypertensive complications.

- Other parameters used to assess therapeutic efficacy include changes in funduscopic findings, left ventricular hypertrophy regression on ECG or echocardiogram, reduction in proteinuria, and improvement in renal function.
- Patient adherence with the therapeutic regimen should be assessed regularly. They should be questioned periodically about changes in their general health perception, energy level, physical functioning, and overall satisfaction with treatment. Patients should be monitored routinely for adverse drug effects, as discussed previously in this chapter.

See Chapter 13, Hypertension, authored by Joseph J Saseen and Barry L. Carter, for a more detailed discussion of this topic.

Chapter 11 _____

▶ ISCHEMIC HEART DISEASE

▶ DEFINITION

Ischemic heart disease (IHD), also known as coronary artery disease (CAD), is defined as a lack of oxygen and decreased or no blood flow to the myocardium resulting from coronary artery narrowing or obstruction. IHD may present as an acute coronary syndrome (ACS), which includes unstable angina pectoris and acute myocardial infarction (AMI) associated with ECG changes of either ST-segment elevation (STEMI) or non-ST-segment elevation (NSTEMI). IHD may also present as myocardial infarction (MI) diagnosed by biochemical markers only, chronic stable exertional angina, ischemia without symptoms, or ischemia due to coronary artery vasospasm (variant or Prinzmetal's angina).

▶ PATHOPHYSIOLOGY

- The major determinants of myocardial oxygen demand (MVo_2) are heart rate, contractility, and intramyocardial wall tension during systole. Wall tension is thought to be the most important factor. Because the consequences of IHD usually result from increased demand in the face of a fixed oxygen supply, alterations in MVo_2 are important in producing ischemia and for interventions intended to alleviate it.
- A clinically useful indirect estimate of MVo_2 is the double product (DP), which is heart rate (HR) multiplied by systolic blood pressure (SBP) (DP = HR × SBP). The DP does not consider changes in contractility (an independent variable), and because only changes in pressure are considered, volume loading of the left ventricle and increased MVo_2 related to ventricular dilation are underestimated.
- The caliber of the resistance vessels delivering blood to the myocardium and MVo_2 are the prime determinants in the occurrence of ischemia.
- The normal coronary system consists of large epicardial or surface vessels (R_1) that offer little resistance to myocardial flow and intramyocardial arteries and arterioles (R_2) that branch into a dense capillary network to supply basal blood flow (Figure 11–1). Under normal circumstances, the resistance in R_2 is much greater than that in R_1. Myocardial blood flow is inversely related to arteriolar resistance and directly related to the coronary driving pressure.
- Atherosclerotic lesions occluding R_1 increase arteriolar resistance, and R_2 can vasodilate to maintain coronary blood flow. With greater degrees of obstruction, this response is inadequate, and the coronary flow reserve afforded by R_2 vasodilation is insufficient to meet oxygen demand. Relatively severe stenosis (greater than 70%) may provoke ischemia and symptoms at rest, whereas less severe stenosis may allow a reserve of coronary blood flow for exertion.
- The diameter and length of obstructing lesions and the influence of pressure drop across an area of stenosis also affect coronary blood flow and function of the collateral circulation. Dynamic coronary obstruction can occur in normal vessels and vessels with stenosis in which vasomotion or spasm may be superimposed on a fixed stenosis. Persisting ischemia may promote growth of developed collateral blood flow.
- Critical stenosis occurs when the obstructing lesion encroaches on the luminal diameter and exceeds 70%. Lesions creating obstruction of 50% to 70% may reduce blood flow, but these obstructions are not consistent, and vasospasm and thrombosis superimposed on a "noncritical" lesion may lead to clinical

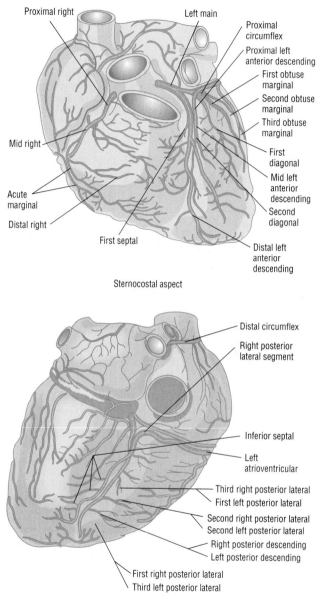

Sternocostal aspect

Diaphragmatic aspect

Figure 11–1. Coronary artery anatomy with sternocostal and diaphragmatic views.

► II

events such as AMI. If the lesion enlarges from 80% to 90%, resistance in that vessel is tripled. Coronary reserve is diminished at about 85% obstruction due to vasoconstriction.

- Abnormalities of ventricular contraction can occur, and regional loss of contractility may impose a burden on the remaining myocardial tissue, resulting in heart failure, increased MV_{O_2}, and rapid depletion of blood flow reserve. Zones of tissue with marginal blood flow may develop that are at risk for more severe damage if the ischemic episode persists or becomes more severe. Nonischemic areas of myocardium may compensate for the severely ischemic and border zones of ischemia by developing more tension than usual in an attempt to maintain cardiac output. The left or right ventricular dysfunction that ensues may be associated with clinical findings of an S_3 gallop, dyspnea, orthopnea, tachycardia, fluctuating blood pressure, transient murmurs, and mitral or tricuspid regurgitation. Impaired diastolic and systolic function leads to elevation of the filling pressure of the left ventricle.

CLINICAL PRESENTATION

- Many episodes of ischemia do not cause anginal symptoms (silent ischemia). Patients often have a reproducible pattern of pain or other symptoms that appear after a specific amount of exertion. Increased frequency, severity, duration, and symptoms at rest suggest an unstable pattern that requires immediate medical evaluation.
- Symptoms may include a sensation of pressure or burning over the sternum or near it, which often radiates to the left jaw, shoulder, and arm. Chest tightness and shortness of breath may also occur. The sensation usually lasts from 30 seconds to 30 minutes.
- Precipitating factors include exercise, cold environment, walking after a meal, emotion upset, fright, anger, and coitus. Relief occurs with rest and within 45 seconds to 5 minutes of taking nitroglycerin.
- Patients with variant or Prinzmetal's angina secondary to coronary spasm are more likely to experience pain at rest and in the early morning hours. Pain is not usually brought on by exertion or emotional stress nor relieved by rest; the ECG pattern is that of current injury with ST-segment elevation rather than depression.
- Unstable angina is stratified into categories of low, intermediate, or high risk for short-term death or nonfatal MI. Features of high-risk unstable angina include (but are not limited to): (1) accelerating tempo of ischemic symptoms in the preceding 48 hours; (2) pain at rest lasting more than 20 minutes; (3) age greater than 75 years; (4) ST-segment changes; and (5) clinical findings of pulmonary edema, mitral regurgitation, S_3, rales, hypotension, bradycardia, or tachycardia.
- Episodes of ischemia may also be painless, or "silent," in at least 60% of patients, perhaps due to a higher threshold and tolerance for pain than in patients who have pain more frequently.

DIAGNOSIS

- Important aspects of the clinical history include the nature or quality of the chest pain, precipitating factors, duration, pain radiation, and the response to nitroglycerin or rest. There appears to be little relationship between the historical features of angina and the severity or extent of coronary artery vessel involvement. Ischemic chest pain may resemble pain arising from a variety of noncardiac sources, and the differential diagnosis of anginal pain from other etiologies may be difficult based on history alone.

- The patient should be asked about existing personal risk factors for coronary heart disease (CHD) including smoking, hypertension, and diabetes mellitus.
- A detailed family history should be obtained that includes information about premature CHD, hypertension, familial lipid disorders, and diabetes mellitus.
- There are few signs on physical examination to indicate the presence of CAD. Findings on the cardiac examination may include abnormal precordial systolic bulge, decreased intensity of S_1, paradoxical splitting of S_2, S_3, S_4, apical systolic murmur, and diastolic murmur. Elevated heart rate or blood pressure can yield an increased DP and may be associated with angina. Noncardiac physical findings suggesting significant cardiovascular disease include abdominal aortic aneurysms or peripheral vascular disease.
- Recommended laboratory tests include hemoglobin (to ensure adequate oxygen-carrying capacity), fasting glucose (to exclude diabetes), and fasting lipoprotein panel. Important risk factors in some patients may include C-reactive protein, homocysteine level, evidence of *Chlamydia* infection, and elevations in lipoprotein (a), fibrinogen, and plasminogen activator inhibitor. Cardiac enzymes should all be normal in stable angina. Troponin T or I, myoglobin, and CK-MB may be elevated in unstable angina.
- The resting ECG is normal in about one-half of patients with angina who are not experiencing an acute attack. Typical ST-T-wave changes include depression, T-wave inversion, and ST-segment elevation. Variant angina is associated with ST-segment elevation, whereas silent ischemia may produce elevation or depression. Significant ischemia is associated with ST-segment depression of greater than 2 mm, exertional hypotension, and reduced exercise tolerance.
- Exercise tolerance (stress) testing (ETT) is recommended for patients with an intermediate probability of CAD. Results correlate well with the likelihood of progressing to angina, occurrence of AMI, and cardiovascular death. Ischemic ST-segment depression during ETT is an independent risk factor for cardiovascular events and mortality. Thallium (^{201}Tl) myocardial perfusion scintigraphy may be used in conjunction with ETT to detect reversible and irreversible defects in blood flow to the myocardium.
- Radionuclide angiocardiography is used to measure ejection fraction (EF), regional ventricular performance, cardiac output, ventricular volumes, valvular regurgitation, asynchrony or wall motion abnormalities, and intracardiac shunts.
- Ultrarapid computed tomography may minimize artifact from heart motion during contraction and relaxation and provides a semiquantitative assessment of calcium content in coronary arteries.
- Echocardiography is useful if the history or physical findings suggest valvular pericardial disease or ventricular dysfunction. In patients unable to exercise, pharmacologic stress echocardiography (e.g., dobutamine, dipyridamole, or adenosine) may identify abnormalities that would occur during stress.
- Cardiac catheterization and coronary angiography are used in patients with suspected CAD to document the presence and severity of disease as well as for prognostic purposes. Interventional catheterization is used for thrombolytic therapy in patients with AMI and for managing patients with significant CAD to relieve obstruction through percutaneous transluminal coronary angioplasty (PTCA), atherectomy, laser treatment, or stent placement.

▶ DESIRED OUTCOME

The short-term goals of therapy for IHD are to reduce or prevent anginal symptoms that limit exercise capability and impair quality of life. Long-term goals are

II

to prevent CHD events such as MI, arrhythmias, and heart failure and to extend the patient's life.

▶ TREATMENT

RISK-FACTOR MODIFICATION

- Primary prevention through the modification of risk factors should significantly reduce the prevalence of IHD. Secondary intervention is effective in reducing subsequent morbidity and mortality.
- Risk factors for IHD are additive and can be classified as alterable or unalterable. Unalterable risk factors include gender, age, family history or genetic composition, environmental influences, and, to some extent, diabetes mellitus. Alterable risk factors include smoking, hypertension, hyperlipidemia, obesity, sedentary lifestyle, hyperuricemia, psychosocial factors such as stress and type A behavior patterns, and the use of drugs that may be detrimental (e.g., progestins, corticosteroids, and cyclosporine). Although thiazide diuretics and β blockers (nonselective without intrinsic sympathomimetic activity) may elevate both cholesterol and triglycerides by 10% to 20%, and these effects may be detrimental, no objective evidence exists from prospective well-controlled studies to support avoiding these drugs.

PHARMACOLOGIC THERAPY

β-Adrenergic Blocking Agents

- Decreased heart rate, contractility, and blood pressure reduce MVo_2 and oxygen demand in patients with effort-induced angina. β Blockers do not improve oxygen supply and, in certain instances, unopposed α-adrenergic stimulation may lead to coronary vasoconstriction.
- β Blockers improve symptoms in about 80% of patients with chronic exertional stable angina, and objective measures of efficacy demonstrate improved exercise duration and delay in the time at which ST-segment changes and initial or limiting symptoms occur. β Blockade may allow angina patients previously limited by symptoms to perform more exercise and ultimately improve overall cardiovascular performance through a training effect.
- Ideal candidates for β blockers include patients in whom physical activity is a prominent cause of attacks; those with coexisting hypertension, supraventricular arrhythmias, or post-MI angina; and those with anxiety associated with anginal episodes. β Blockers may be used safely in angina and heart failure.
- β Blockade is effective in chronic exertional angina as monotherapy and in combination with nitrates and/or calcium channel antagonists. β Blockers are the first-line drugs in chronic angina requiring daily maintenance therapy because they are more effective in reducing episodes of silent ischemia and early morning peak of ischemic activity and improving mortality after Q-wave MI than nitrates or calcium channel blockers.
- If β blockers are ineffective or not tolerated, then monotherapy with a calcium channel blocker or combination therapy may be instituted. Reflex tachycardia from nitrates can be blunted with β-blocker therapy, making this a useful combination. Patients with severe angina, rest angina, or variant angina may be better treated with calcium channel blockers or long-acting nitrates.
- Initial doses of β blockers should be at the lower end of the usual dosing range and titrated to response. Treatment objectives include lowering the resting heart rate to 50 to 60 beats/min and limiting maximal exercise heart rate to about 100 beats/ min or less. Heart rate with modest exercise should be no more than

about 20 beats/min above resting heart rate (or a 10% increment over resting heart rate).

- There is little evidence to suggest superiority of any particular β blocker. Those with longer half-lives may be administered less frequently, but even **propranolol** may be given twice a day in most patients. Membrane stabilizing activity is irrelevant in the treatment of angina. Intrinsic sympathomimetic activity appears to be detrimental in patients with rest or severe angina because the reduction in heart rate would be minimized, therefore limiting a reduction in MVo_2. Cardioselective β blockers may be used in some patients to minimize adverse effects such as bronchospasm, intermittent claudication, and sexual dysfunction. Combined nonselective β and α blockade with **labetolol** may be useful in some patients with marginal left ventricular (LV) reserve.

- Adverse effects of β blockade include hypotension, heart failure, bradycardia, heart block, bronchospasm, peripheral vasoconstriction and intermittent claudication, altered glucose metabolism, fatigue, malaise, and depression. Abrupt withdrawal in patients with angina has been associated with increased severity and number of pain episodes and MI. Tapering of therapy over about 2 days should minimize the risk of withdrawal reactions if therapy is to be discontinued.

Nitrates

- The action of nitrates appears to be mediated indirectly through reduction of myocardial oxygen demand secondary to venodilation and arterial-arteriolar dilation, leading to a reduction in wall stress from reduced ventricular volume and pressure. Direct actions on the coronary circulation include dilation of large and small intramural coronary arteries, collateral dilation, coronary artery stenosis dilation, abolition of normal tone in narrowed vessels, and relief of spasm.

- Pharmacokinetic characteristics common to nitrates include a large first-pass effect of hepatic metabolism, short to very short half-lives (except for **isosorbide mononitrate** [ISMN]), large volumes of distribution, high clearance rates, and large interindividual variations in plasma or blood concentrations. The half-life of **nitroglycerin** is 1 to 5 minutes regardless of the route, hence the potential advantage of sustained-release and transdermal products. **Isosorbide dinitrate** (ISDN) is metabolized to isosorbide 2- and 5-mononitrate (ISMN). ISMN has a half-life of about 5 hours and may be given once or twice daily, depending on the product chosen.

- Nitrate therapy may be used to terminate an acute anginal attack, to prevent effort- or stress-induced attacks, or for long-term prophylaxis, usually in combination with β blockers of calcium channel blockers. Sublingual, buccal, or spray nitroglycerin products are preferred for alleviation of anginal attacks because of rapid absorption (Table 11–1). Symptoms may be prevented by prophylactic oral or transdermal products (usually in combination with β blockers or calcium channel blockers), but development of tolerance may be problematic.

- **Sublingual nitroglycerin,** 0.3 to 0.4 mg, relieves pain in about 75% of patients within 3 minutes, with another 15% becoming pain free in 5 to 15 minutes. Pain persisting beyond 20 to 30 minutes after use of two or three nitroglycerin tablets suggests acute coronary syndrome, and the patient should be instructed to seek emergency aid.

- Chewable, oral, and transdermal products are acceptable for long-term prophylaxis of angina. Dosing of long-acting preparations should be adjusted to provide a hemodynamic response. This may require doses of oral ISDN ranging

121

Cardiovascular Disorders

TABLE 11–1. Nitrate Products

Product	Onset (min)	Duration	Initial Dose
Nitroglycerin			
IV	1–2	3–5 min	5 mcg/min
Sublingual/lingual	1–3	30–60 min	0.3 mg
PO	40	3–6 h	2.5–9 mg t.i.d.
Ointment	20–60	2–8 h	1/2–1 in
Patch	40–60	>8 h	1 patch
Erythritol tetranitrate	5–30	4–6 h	5–10 mg t.i.d.
Pentaerythritol tetranitrate	30	4–8 h	10–20 mg t.i.d.
Isosorbide dinitrate			
Sublingual/chewable	2–5	1–2 h	2.5–5 mg t.i.d.
PO	20–40	4–6 h	5–20 mg t.i.d.
Isosorbide mononitrate	30–60	6–8 h	20 mg qd, b.i.d.[a]

[a]Product-dependent.

from 10 to 60 mg as often as every 3 to 4 hours due to tolerance or first–pass metabolism. Intermittent (10 to 12 hours on, 12 to 14 hours off) transdermal nitroglycerin therapy may produce modest but significant improvement in exercise time in chronic stable angina.

- Adverse effects include postural hypotension with associated central nervous system symptoms, reflex tachycardia, headaches and flushing, and occasional nausea. Excessive hypotension may result in MI or stroke. Noncardiovascular adverse effects include rash (especially with transdermal nitroglycerin) and methemoglobinemia with high doses given for extended periods.
- Because both the onset and offset of tolerance to nitrates occurs quickly, one strategy to circumvent it is to provide a daily nitrate-free interval of 8 to 12 hours. For example, ISDN should not be used more often than 3 times a day to avoid tolerance.
- Nitrates may be combined with other drugs with complementary mechanisms of action for chronic prophylactic therapy. Combination therapy is generally used in patients with more frequent symptoms or symptoms that do not respond to β blockers alone (nitrates plus β blockers or calcium channel blockers), in patients intolerant of β blockers or calcium channel blockers, and in patients having an element of vasospasm leading to decreased supply (nitrates plus calcium channel blockers).

Calcium Channel Antagonists
- Direct actions include vasodilation of systemic arterioles and coronary arteries, leading to a reduction of arterial pressure and coronary vascular resistance as well as depression of myocardial contractility and the conduction velocity of the SA and AV nodes. Reflex β-adrenergic stimulation overcomes much of the negative inotropic effect, and depression of contractility becomes clinically apparent only in the presence of LV dysfunction and when other negative inotropic drugs are used concurrently.
- **Verapamil** and **diltiazem** cause less peripheral vasodilation than dihydropyridines such as **nifedipine,** but greater decreases in AV node conduction. They must be used with caution in patients with preexisting conduction abnormalities or in patients taking other drugs with negative chronotropic properties.
- MVo_2 is reduced with all calcium channel antagonists primarily because of reduced wall tension secondary to reduced arterial pressure. Overall, the benefit

provided by calcium channel antagonists is related to reduced MVo$_2$ rather than improved oxygen supply.

II

- In contrast to the β blockers, calcium channel antagonists have the potential to improve coronary blood flow through areas of fixed coronary obstruction by inhibiting coronary artery vasomotion and vasospasm.
- Good candidates for calcium channel antagonists include patients with contraindications or intolerance to β blockers, coexisting conduction system disease (excluding the use of verapamil and possibly diltiazem), Prinzmetal's angina, peripheral vascular disease, severe ventricular dysfunction, and concurrent hypertension. **Amlodipine** is probably the agent of choice in severe ventricular dysfunction, and the other dihydropyridines should be used with caution if the EF is less than 40%.

TREATMENT OF STABLE EXERTIONAL ANGINA PECTORIS

See Figure 11–2.

- After assessing and manipulating alterable risk factors, a regular exercise program should be undertaken with caution in a graduated fashion and with adequate supervision to improve cardiovascular and muscular fitness.
- Nitrate therapy should be the first step in managing acute attacks of chronic stable angina if the episodes are infrequent. If angina occurs no more often than once every few days, then sublingual **nitroglycerin** tablets or spray or buccal products may be sufficient.
- For prophylaxis when undertaking activities that predictably precipitate attacks, nitroglycerin 0.3 to 0.4 mg sublingually may be used about 5 minutes prior to the time of the activity. Nitroglycerin spray may be useful when inadequate saliva is produced to rapidly dissolve sublingual nitroglycerin or if a patient has difficulty opening the tablet container. The response usually lasts about 30 minutes.
- When angina occurs more frequently than once a day, chronic prophylactic therapy should be instituted. **β-Adrenergic blocking agents** may be preferable because of less frequent dosing and other desirable properties (e.g., potential cardioprotective effects, antiarrhythmic effects, lack of tolerance, antihypertensive efficacy). The appropriate dose should be determined by the goals outlined for heart rate and DP. An agent should be selected that is well tolerated by individual patients at a reasonable cost. Patients most likely to respond well to β blockade are those with a high resting heart rate and those with a relatively fixed anginal threshold (i.e., their symptoms appear at the same level of exercise or workload on a consistent basis).
- **Calcium channel antagonists** have the potential advantage of improving coronary blood flow through coronary artery vasodilation as well as decreasing MVo$_2$ and may be used instead of β blockers for chronic prophylactic therapy. They are as effective as β blockers and are most useful in patients who have a variable threshold for exertional angina. Calcium antagonists may provide better skeletal muscle oxygenation, resulting in decreased fatigue and better exercise tolerance. They can be used safely in many patients with contraindications to β-blocker therapy. The available drugs have similar efficacy in the management of chronic stable angina. Patients with conduction abnormalities and moderate to severe LV dysfunction (EF less than 35%) should not be treated with **verapamil,** whereas **amlodipine** may be used safely in many of these patients. **Diltiazem** has significant effects on the AV node and can produce heart block in patients with preexisting conduction disease or when other drugs with effects on conduction (e.g., digoxin, β blockers) are used

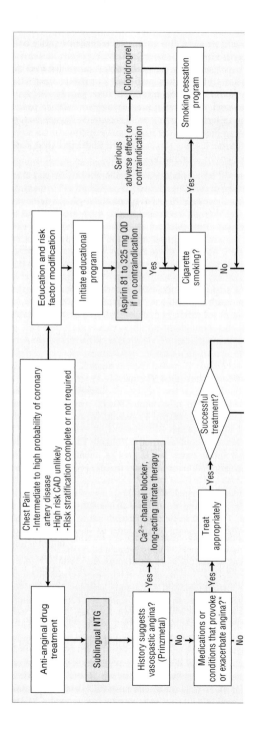

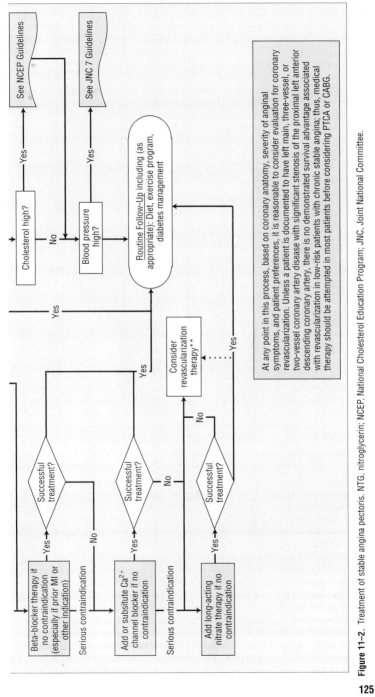

At any point in this process, based on coronary anatomy, severity of anginal symptoms, and patient preferences, it is reasonable to consider evaluation for coronary revascularization. Unless a patient is documented to have left main, three-vessel, or two-vessel coronary artery disease with significant stenosis of the proximal left anterior descending coronary artery, there is no demonstrated survival advantage associated with revascularization in low-risk patients with chronic stable angina; thus, medical therapy should be attempted in most patients before considering PTCA or CABG.

Figure 11–2. Treatment of stable angina pectoris. NTG, nitroglycerin; NCEP, National Cholesterol Education Program; JNC, Joint National Committee.

125

II

concurrently. **Nifedipine** may cause excessive heart rate elevation, especially if the patient is not receiving a β blocker, and this may offset its beneficial effect on MV_{O_2}. The combination of calcium channel blockers and β blockers is rational because the hemodynamic effect of calcium antagonists is complementary to β blockade. However, combination therapy may not always be more effective than single-agent therapy.

- Chronic prophylactic therapy with long-acting forms of **nitroglycerin** (oral or transdermal), **ISDN, ISMN,** and **pentaerythritol trinitrate** may also be effective when angina occurs more than once a day. Monotherapy with nitrates should not be first-line therapy unless β blockers and calcium channel blockers are contraindicated or not tolerated. A nitrate-free interval of 8 h/day or longer should be provided to maintain efficacy. Dose titration should be based on changes in the DP. The choice among nitrate products should be based on experience, cost, and patient acceptance.

TREATMENT OF CORONARY ARTERY SPASM AND VARIANT ANGINA PECTORIS

- All patients should be treated for acute attacks and maintained on prophylactic treatment for 6 to 12 months after the initial episode. Aggravating factors such as alcohol or cocaine use and cigarette smoking should be stopped.
- **Nitrates** are the mainstay of therapy, and most patients respond rapidly to sublingual **nitroglycerin** or **ISDN.** Intravenous (IV) and intracoronary nitroglycerin may be useful for patients not responding to sublingual preparations.
- Because calcium channel antagonists may be more effective, have few serious adverse effects, and can be given less frequently than nitrates, some authorities consider them the agents of choice for variant angina. **Nifedipine, verapamil,** and **diltiazem** are all equally effective as single agents for initial management. Patients unresponsive to calcium channel antagonists alone may have nitrates added. Combination therapy with nifedipine plus diltiazem or nifedipine plus verapamil has been reported to be useful in patients unresponsive to single-drug regimens.
- β Blockers have little or no role in the management of variant angina as they may induce coronary vasoconstriction and prolong ischemia.

▶ EVALUATION OF THERAPEUTIC OUTCOMES

- Subjective measures of drug response include the number of painful episodes, amount of rapid-acting nitroglycerin consumed, and patient-reported alterations in activities of daily living (e.g., time to walk two blocks, number of stairs climbed without pain).
- Objective clinical measures of response include heart rate, blood pressure, and the DP as a measure of MV_{O_2}. Nitrates may increase heart rate but lower SBP, whereas calcium channel blockers and β blockers reduce the DP.
- Objective assessment also includes the resolution of ECG changes at rest, during exercise, or with ambulatory ECG monitoring.
- Monitoring for major adverse effects should be undertaken; they include headache and dizziness with nitrates; fatigue and lassitude with β blockers; and peripheral edema, constipation, and dizziness with calcium channel blockers.
- The ECG is very useful, particularly if the patient is experiencing chest pain or other symptoms thought to be of ischemic origin. ST-segment deviations are very important, and the extent of their deviation is related to the severity of ischemia.

- ETT may also be used to evaluate the response to therapy, but the expense and time needed to perform this test preclude its routine use.
- Cardiac catheterization, radionuclide scans, and echocardiography are used primarily for risk stratification and selecting patients for more invasive procedures rather than for monitoring therapy.
- A comprehensive plan includes ancillary monitoring of lipid profiles, fasting plasma glucose, thyroid function tests, hemoglobin/hematocrit, and electrolytes.
- For variant angina, reduction in symptoms and nitroglycerin consumption as documented by a patient diary can assist the interpretation of objective data obtained from ambulatory ECG recordings. Evidence of efficacy includes the reduction of ischemic events, both ST-segment depression and elevation. Additional evidence is a reduced number of attacks of angina requiring hospitalization, and the absence of MI and sudden death.

See Chapter 15, Ischemic Heart Disease, authored by Robert L. Talbert, for a more detailed discussion of this topic.

Chapter 12

▶ SHOCK

▶ DEFINITION

Shock refers to conditions manifested by hemodynamic alterations (e.g., hypotension, tachycardia, low cardiac output [CO], and oliguria) caused by intravascular volume deficit (hypovolemic shock), myocardial pump failure (cardiogenic shock), or peripheral vasodilation (septic, anaphylactic, or neurogenic shock). The underlying problem in these situations is inadequate tissue perfusion resulting from circulatory failure.

▶ PATHOPHYSIOLOGY

- Shock results in failure of the circulatory system to deliver sufficient oxygen (O_2) to body tissues despite normal or reduced O_2 consumption. General pathophysiologic mechanisms of different forms of shock are similar except for initiating events.
- Hypovolemic shock is characterized by acute intravascular volume deficiency due to external losses or internal redistribution of extracellular water. This type of shock can be precipitated by hemorrhage, burns, trauma, surgery, intestinal obstruction, and dehydration from considerable insensible fluid loss, overaggressive loop-diuretic administration, and severe vomiting or diarrhea. Relative hypovolemia leading to hypovolemic shock occurs during significant vasodilation, which accompanies anaphylaxis, sepsis, and neurogenic shock.
- Regardless of the etiology, fall in blood pressure (BP) is compensated by an increase in sympathetic outflow, activation of the renin-angiotensin system, and other humoral factors that stimulate peripheral vasoconstriction. Compensatory vasoconstriction redistributes blood away from the skin, skeletal muscles, kidneys, and gastrointestinal (GI) tract toward vital organs (e.g., heart, brain) in an attempt to maintain oxygenation, nutrition, and organ function.
- Severe metabolic lactic acidosis often develops secondary to tissue ischemia and causes localized vasodilation, which further exacerbates the impaired cardiovascular state.

▶ CLINICAL PRESENTATION

- Shock presents with a diversity of signs and symptoms. Patients with hypovolemic shock may present with thirst, anxiousness, weakness, lightheadedness, and dizziness. Patients may also report scanty urine output and dark-yellow-colored urine.
- Hypotension, tachycardia, tachypnea, confusion, and oliguria are common symptoms. Myocardial and cerebral ischemia, pulmonary edema (cardiogenic shock), and multisystem organ failure often follow.
- Significant hypotension (systolic blood pressure (SBP) less than 90 mm Hg) with reflex sinus tachycardia (greater than 120 beats/min) and increased respiratory rate (more than 30 breaths/min) are often observed in hypovolemic patients. Clinically, the patient presents with extremities cool to the touch and a "thready" pulse. If coronary hypoxia persists, cardiac arrhythmias may occur, which eventually lead to irreversible myocardial pump failure, pulmonary edema, and cardiovascular collapse.
- In a patient with extensive myocardial damage, chest auscultation may reveal heart sounds consistent with valvular heart disease (regurgitation, outflow

obstruction) or significant ventricular dysfunction (S_3). Chest roentgenogram may detect dissecting ascending aortic aneurysm (widened mediastinum) or cardiomegaly.

- Mental status changes associated with volume depletion may range from subtle fluctuations in mood to agitation to unconsciousness.
- Respiratory alkalosis secondary to hyperventilation is usually observed secondary to central nervous system (CNS) stimulation of ventilatory centers as a result of trauma, sepsis, or shock. Lung auscultation may reveal crackles (pulmonary edema) or absence of breath sounds (pneumothorax, hemothorax). Chest roentgenogram can confirm early suspicions or disclose an undetected abnormality such as pneumonia (pulmonary infiltrates). Continued insult to the lungs may result in adult respiratory distress syndrome (ARDS).
- Kidneys are exquisitely sensitive to changes in perfusion pressures. Moderate alterations can lead to significant changes in glomerular filtration rate (GFR). Oliguria, progressing to anuria, occurs because of vasoconstriction of afferent arterioles.
- Skin is often cool, pale, or cyanotic (bluish) due to hypoxemia. Sweating results in a moist, clammy feel. Digits will have severely slowed capillary refill.
- Redistribution of blood flow away from the GI tract may cause stress gastritis, gut ischemia, and, in some cases, infarction, resulting in GI bleeding.
- Reduced hepatic blood flow, especially in vasodilatory forms of shock, can alter metabolism of endogenous compounds and drugs. Progressive liver damage (shock liver) manifests as elevated serum hepatic transaminases and unconjugated bilirubin. Impaired synthesis of clotting factors may increase prothrombin time (PT), international normalized ratio (INR), and activated partial thromboplastin time (aPTT).

DIAGNOSIS AND MONITORING

- Information from noninvasive and invasive monitoring (Table 12–1) and evaluation of past medical history, clinical presentation-, and laboratory findings are key components in establishing the diagnosis as well as in assessing general mechanisms responsible for shock. Regardless of the etiology, consistent findings include hypotension (SBP less than 90 mm Hg), depressed cardiac index (CI less than 2.2 L/min/m^2), tachycardia (heart rate [HR] greater than 100 beats/min), and low urine output (less than 20 mL/h).
- Noninvasive assessment of BP using the sphygmomanometer and stethoscope may be inaccurate in the shock state.
- Pulmonary artery catheterization using the Swan-Ganz catheter is frequently performed for invasive monitoring of multiple cardiovascular parameters. A Swan-Ganz catheter can be used to determine central venous pressure (CVP); pulmonary artery pressure; cardiac output; and pulmonary artery occlusive pressure (PAOP), an approximate measure of the left ventricular end-diastolic volume and a major determinant of left ventricular preload.
- Cardiac output (2.5 to 3 L/min) and Svo$_2$ (70% to 75%) may be very low in a patient with extensive myocardial damage.
- Respiratory alkalosis is associated with low partial pressure of O$_2$ (Pao$_2$) (25 to 35 mm Hg) and alkaline pH, but normal bicarbonate. The first two values are measured by arterial blood gas, which also yields partial pressure of carbon dioxide (Paco$_2$) and Sao$_2$. Circulating Sao$_2$ can also be measured by an oximeter, which is a noninvasive method that is fairly accurate and useful at the patient's bedside.
- Renal function can be grossly assessed by hourly measurements of urine output, but estimation of creatinine clearance based on isolated serum creatinine values

TABLE 12–1. Hemodynamic and Oxygen Transport Monitoring Parameters

Parameter	Normal Value
Blood pressure (systolic/diastolic)	100–130/70–85 mm Hg
Mean arterial pressure (MAP)	80–100 mm Hg
Pulmonary artery pressure (PAP)	25/10 mm Hg
Mean pulmonary artery pressure (MPAP)	12–15 mm Hg
Central venous pressure (CVP)	2–6 mm Hg
Pulmonary artery occlusion pressure (PAOP)	8–12 mm Hg (normal), 15–18 (ICU) mm Hg
Heart rate (HR)	60–80 beats/min
Cardiac output (CO)	4–7 L/min
Cardiac index (CI)	2.8–3.6 L/min/m^2
Stroke volume index (SVI)	30–50 mL/m^2
Systemic vascular resistance index (SVRI)	1300–2100 dyne · sec/m^{2}cm^5
Pulmonary vascular resistance index (PVRI)	45–225 dyne · sec/m^{2}cm^5
Arterial oxygen saturation (Sao$_2$)	97% (range, 95%–100%)
Mixed venous oxygen saturation (Svo$_2$)	75% (range, 60%–80%)
Arterial oxygen content (Cao$_2$)	20.1 vol% (range, 19–21)
Venous oxygen content (Cvo$_2$)	15.5 vol% (range, 11.5–16.5)
Oxygen content difference (C(a-v)o$_2$)	5 vol% (range, 4–6)
Oxygen consumption index (Vo$_2$)	131 mL/min/m^2 (range, 100–180)
Oxygen delivery index (Do$_2$)	578 mL/min/m^2 (range, 370–730)
Oxygen extraction ratio (O$_2$ER)	25% (range, 22%–30%)
Intramucosal pH (pHi)	7.40 (range, 7.35–7.45)
Index	Parameter indexed to body surface area

in critically ill patients may yield erroneous results. Decreased renal perfusion and aldosterone release result in sodium retention, and thus, low urinary sodium (U_{Na} less than 30 mEq/L).

- In normal individuals, oxygen consumption (Vo_2) is dependent on oxygen delivery (Do_2) up to a certain critical level (Vo_2 flow dependency). At this point, tissue oxygen requirements have apparently been satisfied and further increases in Do_2 will not alter Vo_2 (flow independency). However, studies in critically ill patients show a continuous, pathologic dependence relationship of Vo_2 on Do_2. These indexed parameters are calculated as: $Do_2 = CI \times Cao_2$ and $Vo_2 = CI \times (Cao_2 - Cvo_2)$, where CI = cardiac index, Cao_2 = arterial oxygen content, and Cvo_2 = mixed venous oxygen content. Currently available data do not support the concept that patient outcome or survival is altered by treatment measures directed to achieve supranormal levels of Do_2 and Vo_2.
- The Vo_2 to Do_2 ratio (oxygen extraction ratio, or O_2ER) can be used to assess adequacy of perfusion and metabolic response. Patients who are able to increase Vo_2 when Do_2 is increased are more likely to survive. However, low Vo_2 and o_2ER values are indicative of poor oxygen utilization and lead to greater mortality.
- Serum lactate concentrations may be used as another measure of tissue oxygenation and may show better correlation with outcome than oxygen transport parameters in some patients.
- Gastric tonometry measures gut luminal Pco_2 at equilibrium by placing a saline-filled gas-permeable balloon in the gastric lumen. Increases in mucosal Pco_2 and calculated decreases in intramucosal pH (pHi) are associated with mucosal hypoperfusion and perhaps increased mortality. However, the presence of respiratory acid-base disorders, systemic bicarbonate administration,

arterial blood gas measurement errors, enteral feeding solutions, and blood or stool in the gut may confound pHi determinations. Many clinicians believe that gastric mucosal P_{CO_2} may be more accurate than pHi.

II

▶ DESIRED OUTCOME

The initial goal is to support oxygen delivery through the circulatory system by assuring effective intravascular plasma volume, optimal oxygen-carrying capacity, and adequate BP while definitive diagnostic and therapeutic strategies are being determined. The ultimate goals are to prevent further progression of the disease with subsequent organ damage and, if possible, to reverse organ dysfunction that has already occurred.

▶ TREATMENT

GENERAL PRINCIPLES

- Figure 12–1 contains an algorithm summarizing one approach to an adult patient presenting with hypovolemia.
- Supplemental oxygen should be initiated at the earliest signs of shock, beginning with 4 to 6 L/min via nasal cannula or 6 to 10 L/min by face mask.
- Adequate fluid resuscitation to maintain circulating blood volume is essential in managing all forms of shock. Different therapeutic options are discussed below.
- If fluid challenge does not achieve desired end points, pharmacologic support is necessary with inotropic and vasoactive drugs.

FLUID RESUSCITATION FOR HYPOVOLEMIC SHOCK

- Initial fluid resuscitation consists of isotonic crystalloid (**0.9% sodium chloride** or **lactated Ringer's solution**), colloid (**5% plasmanate** or **albumin, 6% hetastarch**), or **whole blood.** Choice of solution is based on oxygen-carrying capacity (e.g., hemoglobin, hematocrit), cause of hypovolemic shock, accompanying disease states, degree of fluid loss, and required speed of fluid delivery.
- Most clinicians agree that crystalloids should be the initial therapy of circulatory insufficiency. Crystalloids are preferred over colloids as initial therapy for burn patients because they are less likely to cause interstitial fluid accumulation. If volume resuscitation is suboptimal following several liters of crystalloid, colloids should be considered. Some patients may require blood products to assure maintenance of oxygen-carrying capacity, as well as clotting factors and platelets for blood hemostasis.

Crystalloids

- Crystalloids consist of electrolytes (e.g., Na^+, Cl^-, K^+) in water solutions, with or without dextrose. **Lactated Ringer's solution** may be preferred because it is unlikely to cause the hyperchloremic metabolic acidosis seen with infusion of large amounts of normal saline.
- Crystalloids are administered at a rate of 500 to 2000 mL/h, depending on the severity of the deficit, degree of ongoing fluid loss, and tolerance to infusion volume. Usually 2 to 4 L of crystalloid normalizes intravascular volume.
- Advantages of crystalloids include rapidity and ease of administration, compatibility with most drugs, absence of serum sickness, and low cost.
- The primary disadvantage is the large volume necessary to replace or augment intravascular volume. Approximately 4 L of normal saline must be infused to replace 1 L of blood loss. In addition, dilution of colloid oncotic pressure

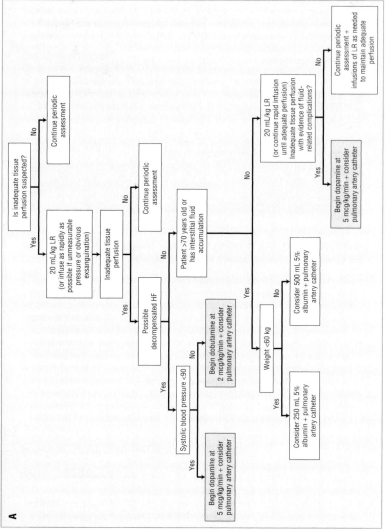

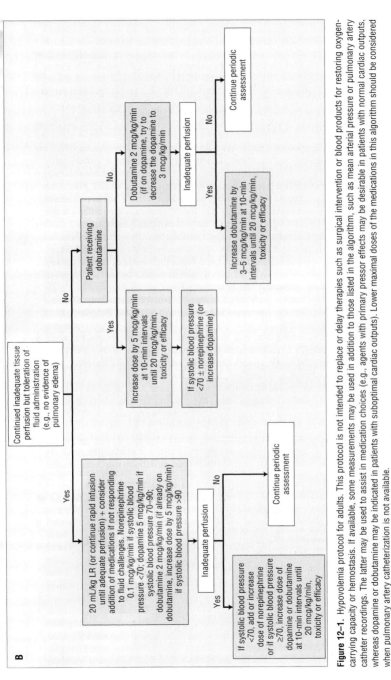

Figure 12–1. Hypovolemia protocol for adults. This protocol is not intended to replace or delay therapies such as surgical intervention or blood products for restoring oxygen-carrying capacity or hemostasis. If available, some measurements may be used in addition to those listed in the algorithm, such as mean arterial pressure or pulmonary artery catheter recordings. The latter may be used to assist in medication choices (e.g., agents with primary pressor effects may be desirable in patients with normal cardiac outputs, whereas dopamine or dobutamine may be indicated in patients with suboptimal cardiac outputs). Lower maximal doses of the medications in this algorithm should be considered when pulmonary artery catheterization is not available.

HF, heart failure; LR, lactated Ringer's solution. Colloids that may be substituted for albumin are hetastarch 6% and dextran 40.

II

leading to pulmonary edema is more likely to follow crystalloid than colloid resuscitation.

Colloids

- Colloids are larger molecular weight solutions (more than 30,000 daltons) that have been recommended for use in conjunction with or as replacements for crystalloid solutions. **Albumin** is a monodisperse colloid because all of its molecules are of the same molecular weight, whereas **hetastarch** and **dextran** solutions are polydisperse compounds with molecules of varying molecular weights. Colloids are useful because their increased molecular weight corresponds to an increased intravascular retention time (in the absence of increased capillary permeability). However, even with intact capillary permeability, the colloid molecules will eventually leak through capillary membranes.

- **Albumin 5%** and **25%** concentrations are available. It takes approximately 3 to 4 times as much lactated Ringer's or normal saline solution to yield the same volume expansion as 5% albumin solution. However, albumin is much more costly than crystalloid solutions. The 5% albumin solution is relatively iso-oncotic, whereas 25% albumin is hyperoncotic and tends to pull fluid into the compartment containing the albumin molecules. In general, 5% albumin is used for hypovolemic states. The 25% solution should not be used for acute circulatory insufficiency unless diluted with other fluids or unless it is being used in patients with excess total body water but intravascular depletion, as a means of pulling fluid into the intravascular space.

- **Hetastarch 6%** has comparable plasma expansion to 5% albumin solution but is usually less expensive, which accounts for much of its use. Hetastarch should be avoided in situations in which short-term impairments in hemostasis could have adverse consequences (e.g., cardiopulmonary bypass surgery, intracranial hemorrhage), since it may aggravate bleeding due to mechanisms such as decreased factor VIII activity. Hetastarch may cause elevations in serum amylase concentrations but does not cause pancreatitis.

- **Dextran-40, dextran-70,** and **dextran-75** are available for use as plasma expanders (the number indicates the average molecular weight × 1000). These solutions are not used as often as albumin or hetastarch for plasma expansion, possibly due to concerns related to aggravation of bleeding (i.e., anticoagulant actions related to inhibiting stasis of microcirculation) and anaphylaxis, which is more likely to occur with the higher molecular weight solutions.

- The theoretical advantage of colloids is their prolonged intravascular retention time compared to crystalloid solutions. In contrast to isotonic crystalloid solutions, which have substantial interstitial distribution within minutes of intravenous (IV) administration, colloids remain in the intravascular space for hours or days depending on factors such as capillary permeability.

- However, colloids (especially albumin) are expensive solutions, and a large study involving almost 7000 critically ill patients found no significant difference in 28-day mortality between patients resuscitated with either normal saline or 4% albumin. For these reasons, crystalloids should be considered first-line therapy in patients with hypovolemic shock.

- Adverse effects of colloids are generally extensions of their pharmacologic activity (e.g., fluid overload, dilutional coagulopathy). **Albumin** and **dextran** may be associated with anaphylactoid reactions or anaphylaxis. Bleeding may occur in certain patients receiving **hetastarch** and **dextran.**

Blood Products

- **Whole blood** could be used for large volume blood loss, but most institutions use component therapy, with crystalloids or colloids used for plasma expansion.

- **Packed red blood cells** contain hemoglobin that increases the oxygen-carrying capacity of blood, thereby increasing oxygen delivery to tissues. This is a function not performed by crystalloids or colloids. Packed red cells are usually indicated in patients with continued deterioration after volume replacement or obvious exsanguination. The product needs to be warmed before administration, especially when used in children.

- **Fresh frozen plasma** replaces clotting factors. Although it is often overused, the product is indicated if there is ongoing hemorrhage in patients with a PT or aPTT greater than 1.5 times normal, severe hepatic disease, or other bleeding disorders.

- **Platelets** are used for bleeding due to severe thrombocytopenia (platelet counts less than $10,000/mm^3$) or in patients with rapidly dropping platelet counts, as seen in massive bleeding.

- **Cryoprecipitate** and **Factor VIII** are generally not indicated in acute hemorrhage but may be used once specific deficiencies have been identified.

- Risks associated with infusion of blood products include transfusion-related reactions, virus transmission (rare), hypocalcemia resulting from added citrate, elevations in serum potassium and phosphorus concentrations from use of stored blood that has hemolyzed, increased blood viscosity from supranormal hematocrit elevations, and hypothermia from failure to appropriately warm solutions before administration.

PHARMACOLOGIC THERAPY FOR SHOCK

Inotropic agents and vasopressors are generally not indicated in the initial treatment of hypovolemic shock (assuming that fluid therapy is adequate), as the body's normal response is to increase cardiac output and constrict blood vessels to maintain BP. However, once the cause of circulatory insufficiency has been stopped or treated and fluids have been optimized, medications may be needed in patients who continue to have signs and symptoms of inadequate tissue perfusion. Pressor agents such as **norepinephrine** and **high-dose dopamine** should be avoided if possible because they may increase BP at the expense of peripheral tissue ischemia. In patients with unstable BP despite massive fluid replacement and increasing interstitial fluid accumulation, inotropic agents such as **dobutamine** are preferred if BP is adequate (SBP 90 mm Hg or greater) because they should not aggravate the existing vasoconstriction. When pressure cannot be maintained with inotropes, or when inotropes with vasodilatory properties cannot be used due to concerns about inadequate BP, pressors may be required as a last resort.

- The choice of vasopressor or inotropic agent in septic shock should be made according to the needs of the patient. An algorithm for the use of these agents in septic shock is shown in Figure 12–2. The traditional approach is to start with **dopamine,** then **norepinephrine; dobutamine** is added for low cardiac output states, and occasionally **epinephrine** and **phenylephrine** are used when necessary. However, recent observations of improved outcomes with norepinephrine and decreased regional perfusion with dopamine are calling into question the use of dopamine as a first-line agent.

- The receptor selectivities of vasopressors and inotropes are listed in Table 12–2. In general, these drugs act rapidly with short durations of action and are given as continuous infusions. Potent vasoconstrictors such as norepinephrine and phenylephrine should be given through central veins due to the possibility of extravasation and tissue damage with peripheral administration. Careful monitoring and calculation of infusion rates is advised because dosing adjustments

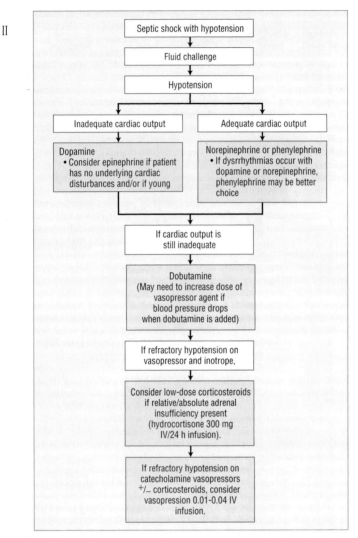

Figure 12–2. Algorithmic approach to the use of vasopressors and inotropes in septic shock. Approach is intended to be used in conjunction with clinical judgment, hemodynamic monitoring parameters, and therapy end points.

are made frequently and varying admixture concentrations are used in volume-restricted patients.

- **Dopamine** is often the initial vasopressor used in septic shock because it increases BP by increasing myocardial contractility and vasoconstriction. Although dopamine has been reported to have dose-related receptor activity at dopamine (DA_1), β_1, and α_1 receptors, this dose-response relationship has not

TABLE 12–2. Receptor Pharmacology of Selected Inotropic and Vasopressor Agents Used in Septic Shock[a]

Agent	α_1	α_2	β_1	β_2	DA[b]
Dobutamine (500 mg/250 mL D$_5$W or NS)					
2–10 mcg/kg/min	+	0	+ + ++	++	0
>10–20 mcg/kg/min	++	0	+ + ++	+ + +	0
Dopamine (800 mg/250 mL D$_5$W or NS)					
1–3 mcg/kg/min	0	0	+	0	+ + ++
3–10 mcg/kg/min	0/+	0	+ + ++	++	+ + ++
>10–20 mcg/kg/min	+ + +	0	+ + ++	+	0
Epinephrine (2 mg/250 mL D$_5$W or NS)					
0.01–0.05 mcg/kg/min	++	++	+ + ++	+ + +	0
>0.05 mcg/kg/min	+ + ++	+ + ++	+ + +	+	
Norepinephrine (4 mg/250 mL D$_5$W or NS)					
0.02–3 mcg/kg/min (2–20 mcg/min)	+ + +	+ + +	+ + +	+/ + +	0
Phenylephrine (50 mg/250 mL D$_5$W or NS)					
0.5–9 mcg/kg/min	+ + +	+	?	0	0

[a]Activity ranges from no activity (0) to maximal (+ + ++) activity or ? when activity is not known.
[b]dopaminergic.

been confirmed in critically ill patients. In patients with septic shock, there is overlap of hemodynamic effects with doses as low as 3 mcg/kg/min. Doses of 5 to 10 mcg/kg/min are initiated to improve mean arterial pressure (MAP). In septic shock, these doses increase CI by improving ventricular contractility, heart rate, arterial pressure, and systemic vascular resistance. The clinical utility of dopamine in septic shock is limited because large doses are frequently necessary to maintain CO and BP. At doses above 20 mcg/kg/min, there is limited further improvement in cardiac performance and regional hemodynamics. The use of dopamine is also hampered frequently by tachycardia and tachydysrhythmias. Other adverse effects limiting its use in septic shock include increases in PAOP, pulmonary shunting, and decreases in Pao$_2$. Dopamine should be used with caution in patients with elevated preload, as it may worsen pulmonary edema. Low doses of dopamine (1 to 3 mcg/kg/min) sometimes are used in patients with septic shock receiving vasopressor with or without oliguria. The goal of therapy is to prevent or reverse renal vasoconstriction caused by other pressors, to prevent oliguric renal failure, or to convert it to nonoliguric renal failure. Dopamine is often added in low doses to other vasopressors or inotropes (e.g., norepinephrine). More commonly, pressor doses of dopamine are found to be ineffective or not tolerated and an additional agent is given. At this point, dopamine is titrated to a low dose. There is little evidence to support use of low-dose dopamine in preserving kidney function in oliguria, with or without septic shock, or in reversing vasopressor-induced vasoconstriction in septic shock.

• **Dobutamine** is primarily a selective β_1 agonist with mild β_2 and vascular α_1 activity, resulting in strong positive inotropic activity without concomitant vasoconstriction. Dobutamine produces a larger increase in CO and is less dysrhythmogenic than dopamine. Clinically, the increased myocardial contractility and subsequent reflex reduction in sympathetic tone lead to a decrease in systemic vascular resistance (SVR). Even though dobutamine is optimally used for low CO states with high filling pressures or in cardiogenic shock, vasopressors may be needed to counteract arterial vasodilation. The addition

II

of dobutamine (held constant at 5 mcg/kg/min) to epinephrine regimens can improve mucosal perfusion as measured by improvements in pHi and arterial lactate concentrations. Dobutamine should be started with doses ranging from 2.5 to 5 mcg/kg/min. Doses above 5 mcg/kg/min provide limited beneficial effects on oxygen transport values and hemodynamics and may increase adverse cardiac effects. Infusion rates should be guided by clinical end points. Decreases in Pao$_2$ and increases in Pvo$_2$, as well as myocardial adverse effects such as tachycardia, ischemic changes on ECG, tachydysrhythmias, and hypotension, are seen.

- **Norepinephrine** is a combined α and β agonist, but it primarily produces vasoconstriction, thereby increasing SVR. It generally produces either no change or a slight decrease in CO. Norepinephrine is initiated after vasopressor doses of dopamine (4 to 20 mcg/kg/min), alone or in combination with dobutamine (2 to 40 mcg/kg/min), fail to achieve the desired goals. Doses of dopamine and dobutamine are kept constant or stopped altogether or, in some instances, dopamine is kept at low doses for purported renal protection. Norepinephrine, 0.01 to 2 mcg/kg/min, reliably and predictably improves hemodynamic parameters to normal or supranormal values in most patients with septic shock. Recent data suggest that norepinephrine should potentially be repositioned as the vasopressor of choice in septic shock.

- **Phenylephrine** is a pure α_1 agonist and is thought to increase BP through vasoconstriction. It may also increase contractility and CO. Phenylephrine may be beneficial in septic shock because of its selective α agonism, vascular effects, rapid onset, and short duration. Phenylephrine should be used when a pure vasoconstrictor is desired in patients who may not require or do not tolerate the β effects of dopamine or norepinephrine with or without dobutamine. It is generally initiated at dosages of 0.5 mcg/kg/min and may be titrated quickly to the desired effect. Adverse effects such as tachydysrhythmias are infrequent when it is used as a single agent or with higher doses.

- **Epinephrine** has combined α and β agonist effects and has traditionally been reserved as the vasopressor of last resort because of reports of peripheral vasoconstriction, particularly in the splanchnic and renal beds. At the high infusion rates used in septic shock, α-adrenergic effects are predominantly seen, and SVR and MAP are increased. It is an acceptable single agent in septic shock due to its combined vasoconstrictor and inotropic effects. Epinephrine may be particularly useful when used earlier in the course of septic shock in young patients and those without known cardiac abnormalities. Infusion rates of 0.04 to 1 mcg/kg/min alone increase hemodynamic and oxygen transport variables to supranormal levels without adverse effects in patients without coronary heart disease. Large doses (0.05 to 1 mcg/kg/min) may be required when epinephrine is added to other agents. Smaller doses (0.1 to 0.5 mcg/kg/min) are effective if dobutamine and dopamine infusions are kept constant. Although Do$_2$ increases mainly as a function of consistent increases in CI (and a more variable increase in SVR), Vo$_2$ may not increase and o$_2$ER may fall. Lactate concentrations may rise during the first few hours of epinephrine therapy but normalize over the ensuing 24 hours in survivors. Caution must be used before considering epinephrine for managing hypoperfusion in hypodynamic patients with coronary artery disease to avoid ischemia, chest pain, and myocardial infarction.

EVALUATION OF THERAPEUTIC OUTCOMES

- The initial monitoring of a patient with suspected volume depletion should include vital signs, urine output, mental status, and physical examination.

- Placement of a CVP line provides a useful (although indirect and insensitive) estimate of the relationship between increased right atrial pressure and cardiac output.
- The indications for pulmonary artery catheterization are controversial. Because there is a lack of well-defined outcome of data associated with this procedure, its use is presently best reserved for complicated cases of shock not responding to conventional fluid and medication therapies. Complications related to catheter insertion, maintenance, and removal include damage to vessels and organs during insertion, arrhythmias, infections, and thromboembolic damage.
- Laboratory tests indicated for the ongoing monitoring of shock include electrolytes and renal function tests (BUN, serum creatinine); complete blood count to assess possible infection, oxygen-carrying capacity of the blood, and ongoing bleeding; PT and aPTT to assess clotting ability; and lactate concentration and base deficit to detect inadequate tissue perfusion.
- Cardiovascular and respiratory parameters should be monitored continuously (see Table 12–1). Trends, rather than specific CVP or PAOP numbers, should be monitored because of interpatient variability in response.
- Successful fluid resuscitation should increase SBP (greater than 90 mm Hg), CI (greater than 2.2 L/min/m^2), and urine output (0.5 to 1 mL/kg/h) while decreasing SVR to the normal range (900 to 1200 dyne/s/cm^5). MAP greater than 60 mm Hg should be achieved to ensure adequate cerebral and coronary perfusion pressure.
- Intravascular volume overload is characterized by high filling pressures (CVP greater than 12 to 15 mm Hg, PAOP greater than 20 to 24 mm Hg) and decreased CO (less than 3.5 L/min). If volume overload occurs, furosemide, 20 to 40 mg, should be administered by slow IV push to produce rapid diuresis of intravascular volume and "unload" the heart through venous dilation.
- Coagulation problems are primarily associated with low levels of clotting factors in stored blood as well as dilution of endogenous clotting factors and platelets following administration of the blood. As a result, a coagulation panel (PT, INR, aPTT) should be checked in patients undergoing replacement of 50% to 100% of blood volume in 12 to 24 hours.

See Chapter 23, Use of Vasopressors and Inotropes in the Pharmacotherapy of Shock, authored by Maria I. Rudis and Joseph F. Dasta, and Chapter 24, Hypovolemic Shock, authored by Brian L. Erstad, for a more detailed discussion of this topic.

Chapter 13

▶ STROKE

▶ DEFINITION

Stroke is a term used to describe an abrupt onset of focal neurologic deficit that lasts at least 24 hours and is presumed to be of vascular origin. Transient ischemic attacks (TIAs) are focal ischemic neurologic deficits lasting less than 24 hours and usually less than 30 minutes.

▶ PATHOPHYSIOLOGY

RISK FACTORS FOR STROKE

- Nonmodifiable risk factors for stroke include increased age, male gender, race (African American, Asian, Hispanic), and heredity.
- The major modifiable risk factors include hypertension and cardiac disease (e.g., coronary artery disease, heart failure, left ventricular hypertrophy, atrial fibrillation).
- Other major risk factors include transient ischemic attacks, diabetes mellitus, dyslipidemia, and cigarette smoking.

ISCHEMIC STROKE

- Ischemic strokes account for 88% of all strokes and are due either to local thrombus formation or to emboli that occlude a cerebral artery. Cerebral atherosclerosis is a causative factor in most cases of ischemic stroke, although 30% are of unknown etiology. Emboli can arise either from intra- or extra-cranial arteries. Twenty percent of embolic strokes arise from the heart.
- In carotid atherosclerosis, plaques may rupture resulting in collagen exposure, platelet aggregation, and thrombus formation. The clot may cause local occlusion or may dislodge and travel distally, eventually occluding a cerebral vessel.
- In the case of cardiogenic embolism, stasis of blood flow in the atria or ventricles leads to formation of local clots that can dislodge and travel through the aorta to the cerebral circulation.
- The final result of both thrombus formation and embolism is arterial occlusion, decreasing cerebral blood flow and causing ischemia and ultimately infarction distal to the occlusion.

HEMORRHAGIC STROKE

- Hemorrhagic strokes account for 12% of strokes, and include subarachnoid hemorrhage, intracerebral hemorrhage, and subdural hematomas. Subarachnoid hemorrhage may result from trauma or rupture of an intracranial aneurysm or arteriovenous malformation. Intracerebral hemorrhage occurs when a ruptured blood vessel within the brain parenchyma causes formation of a hematoma. Subdural hematomas are most often caused by trauma.
- The presence of blood in the brain parenchyma causes damage to surrounding tissue through a mass effect and the neurotoxicity of blood components and their degradation products. Compression of tissue surrounding hematomas may lead to secondary ischemia. Much of the early mortality of hemorrhagic stroke

is due to the abrupt increase in intracranial pressure that can lead to herniation and death.

► CLINICAL PRESENTATION

- The patient may not be able to give a reliable history because of cognitive or language deficits. This information may need to be obtained from family members or other witnesses.
- The patient may experience weakness on one side of the body, inability to speak, loss of vision, vertigo, or falling. Ischemic stroke is not usually painful, but headache may occur and may be severe in hemorrhagic stroke.
- Patients usually have multiple signs of neurologic dysfunction on physical examination. The specific deficits observed depend upon the area of the brain involved. Hemi- or monoparesis and hemisensory deficits are common. Patients with posterior circulation involvement may present with vertigo and diplopia. Anterior circulation strokes commonly result in aphasia. Patients may also experience dysarthria, visual field defects, and altered levels of consciousness.

► DIAGNOSIS

- Computerized tomography (CT) head scan will reveal an area of hyperintensity (white) in an area of hemorrhage and will be normal or hypointense (dark) in an area of infarction. The area of infarction may not be visible on CT scan for 24 hours (and rarely longer).
- Magnetic resonance imaging (MRI) of the head will reveal areas of ischemia with higher resolution and earlier than the CT scan. Diffusion-weighted imaging (DWI) will reveal an evolving infarct within minutes.
- Carotid Doppler studies will determine whether there is a high degree of stenosis in the carotid arteries.
- The electrocardiogram (ECG) will determine whether atrial fibrillation is present.
- A transthoracic echocardiogram (TTE) can detect valve or wall motion abnormalities that are sources of emboli to the brain.
- A transesophageal echocardiogram (TEE) is a more sensitive tests for left atrial thrombus. It is also effective in examining the aortic arch for atheroma, another potential source of emboli.
- Transcranial Doppler (TCD) can determine the presence of intracranial arterial sclerosis (e.g., middle cerebral artery stenosis).
- Laboratory tests for hypercoagulable states should only be done when the cause of the stroke cannot be determined based on the presence of well-known risk factors. Protein C, protein S, and antithrombin III are best measured in steady state rather than in the acute stage. Antiphospholipid antibodies are of higher yield but should be reserved for patients aged less than 50 years and those who have had multiple venous or arterial thrombotic events or livedo reticularis.

► DESIRED OUTCOME

The goals of treatment for acute stroke are to: (1) reduce the ongoing neurologic injury and decrease mortality and long-term disability; (2) prevent complications secondary to immobility and neurologic dysfunction; and (3) prevent stroke recurrence.

► TREATMENT

GENERAL PRINCIPLES

- The initial approach is to ensure adequate respiratory and cardiac support and to determine quickly whether the lesion is ischemic or hemorrhagic based on a CT scan.
- Ischemic stroke patients presenting within hours of symptom onset should be evaluated for reperfusion therapy.
- Elevated blood pressure should remain untreated in the acute period (first 7 days) after ischemic stroke because of the risk of decreasing cerebral blood flow and worsening symptoms. The pressure should be lowered if it exceeds 220/120 mm Hg or there is evidence of aortic dissection, acute myocardial infarction, pulmonary edema, or hypertensive encephalopathy. If blood pressure is treated in the acute phase, short-acting parenteral agents (e.g., labetalol, nicardipine, nitroprusside) are preferred.
- Patients with hemorrhagic stroke should be assessed to determine whether they are candidates for surgical intervention via an endovascular or craniotomy approach.
- After the hyperacute phase has passed, attention is focused on preventing progressive deficits, minimizing complications, and instituting appropriate secondary prevention strategies.

NONPHARMACOLOGIC THERAPY

- In acute ischemic stroke, surgical interventions are limited. However, surgical decompression can be lifesaving in cases of significant swelling associated with cerebral infarction. An interdisciplinary approach to stroke care that includes early rehabilitation is very effective in reducing long-term disability. Carotid endarterectomy is effective in reducing stroke incidence and recurrence in appropriate patients. Carotid stenting may be effective in reducing recurrent stroke risk in patients at high risk of complications during endarterectomy.
- In subarachnoid hemorrhage due to a ruptured intracranial aneurysm or arteriovenous malformation, surgical intervention to clip or ablate the vascular abnormality substantially reduces mortality from bleeding. The benefits of surgery are less well documented in cases of primary intracerebral hemorrhage. In patients with intracerebral hematomas, insertion of an intraventricular drain with monitoring or intracranial pressure is commonly performed. Surgical decompression of a hematoma is a controversial exception as a last resort in life-threatening situations.

PHARMACOLOGIC THERAPY OF ISCHEMIC STROKE

The American Stroke Association's Stroke Council guidelines for the management of acute ischemic stroke give grade A recommendations (i.e., evidence supported by data from randomized trials with low false-positive and false-negative errors) only to use of intravenous tissue plasminogen activator (tPA, alteplase) within 3 hours of onset and aspirin within 48 hours of onset. Recommendations for pharmacotherapy of ischemic stroke are given in Table 13-1.

- **Alteplase** initiated within 3 hours of symptom onset has been shown to reduce the ultimate disability due to ischemic stroke. A head CT scan must be obtained to rule out hemorrhage before beginning therapy. The patient must also meet specific inclusion criteria and no exclusionary criteria (Table 13-2). The dose is 0.9 mg/kg (maximum 90 mg) infused intravenously (IV) over 1 hour after

TABLE 13–1. Recommendations for Pharmacotherapy of Ischemic Stroke

	Primary Agents	Alternatives
Acute Treatment	Alteplase 0.9 mg/kg IV (maximum 90 kg) over 1 h in selected patients within 3 h of onset. Aspirin 160–325 mg daily started within 48 h of onset	Alteplase (various doses) intraarterially up to 6 h after onset in selected patients
Secondary Prevention		
Noncardioembolic	Aspirin 50–325 mg daily Clopidogrel 75 mg daily Asprin 25 mg + extended-release dipyridamole 200 mg twice daily	Ticlopidine 250 mg twice daily
Cardioembolic (esp. atrial fibrillation)	Warfarin (INR = 2.5)	
All	ACE inhibitor + diuretic or ARB blood pressure lowering Statin	

INR, international normalized ratio; ACE, angiotensin-converting enzyme; ARB, angiotensin receptor blocker

a bolus of 10% of the total dose given over 1 minute. Anticoagulant and antiplatelet therapy should be avoided for 24 hours, and the patient should be monitored closely for hemorrhage.

- **Aspirin** 50 to 325 mg/day started between 24 and 48 hours after completion of alteplase has also been shown to reduce long-term death and disability.
- The American College of Chest Physicians (ACCP) guidelines for use of antithrombotic therapy in the secondary prevention of ischemic stroke recommend antiplatelet therapy as the cornerstone for secondary prevention

TABLE 13–2. Inclusion and Exclusion Criteria for Alteplase Use in Acute Ischemic Stroke

Inclusion Criteria (all YES boxes must be checked before treatment)
YES
- ☐ Age 18 yr or older
- ☐ Clinical diagnosis of ischemic stroke causing a measurable neurologic deficit
- ☐ Time of symptom onset well established to be less than 180 min before treatment would begin

Exclusion Criteria (all NO boxes must be checked before treatment)
NO
- ☐ Evidence of intracranial hemorrhage on noncontrast head CT
- ☐ Only minor or rapidly improving stroke symptoms
- ☐ High clinical suspicion of subarachnoid hemorrhage even with normal CT
- ☐ Active internal bleeding (e.g., GI/GU bleeding within 21 days)
- ☐ Known bleeding diathesis, including but not limited to platelet count <100,000/mm³
- ☐ Patient has received heparin within 48 h and had an elevated APTT
- ☐ Recent use of anticoagulant (e.g., warfarin) and elevated PT (>15 s)/INR
- ☐ Intracranial surgery, serious head trauma, or previous stroke within 3 months
- ☐ Major surgery or serious trauma within 14 days
- ☐ Recent arterial puncture at noncompressible site
- ☐ Lumbar puncture within 7 days
- ☐ History of intracranial hemorrhage, arteriovenous malformation, or aneurysm
- ☐ Witnessed seizure at stroke onset
- ☐ Recent acute myocardial infarction
- ☐ SBP > 185 mm Hg or DBP > 110 mm Hg at time of treatment

II

in noncardioembolic strokes. **Aspirin**, **clopidogrel**, and **extended-release dipyridamole plus aspirin** are all considered first-line antiplatelet agents (see Table 13-1). **Ticlopidine** should be reserved for patients who fail or are intolerant of other therapies because of its side effect profile (neutropenia, aplastic anemia, thrombotic thrombocytopenic purpura, rash, diarrhea, hypercholesterolemia). The combination of aspirin and clopidogrel can only be recommended in patients with ischemic stroke and a recent history of myocardial infarction or other coronary events and then only with ultra-low-dose aspirin to minimize bleeding risk.

- **Warfarin** is the antithrombotic agent of first choice for secondary prevention in patients with atrial fibrillation and a presumed cardiac source of embolism.
- Elevated blood pressure is common after ischemic stroke, and its treatment is associated with a decreased risk of stroke recurrence. The Joint National Committee (JNC 7) recommends an ACE inhibitor and a diuretic for reduction of blood pressure in patients with stroke or TIA after the acute period (first 7 days). Angiotensin II receptor blockers (ARBs) have been shown to reduce the risk of stroke and should be considered in patients unable to tolerate ACE inhibitors after acute ischemic stroke.
- The National Cholesterol Education Program (NCEP) considers ischemic stroke or TIA to be a coronary risk equivalent and recommends the use of statins to achieve a low-density lipoprotein (LDL) cholesterol concentration of less than 100 mg/dL.
- **Low-molecular-weight heparin** or **low-dose subcutaneous unfractionated heparin** (5000 units twice daily) is recommended for prevention of deep venous thrombosis in hospitalized patients with decreased mobility due to stroke and should be used in all but the most minor strokes.
- The use of **full-dose unfractionated heparin** in the acute stroke period has not been proven to positively affect stroke outcome, and it significantly increases the risk of intracerebral hemorrhage. Trials of low-molecular-weight heparins and heparinoids have been largely negative and do not support their routine use in stroke patients.

PHARMACOLOGIC THERAPY OF HEMORRHAGIC STROKE

- There are currently no proven pharmacologic strategies for treating intracerebral hemorrhage. Medical guidelines for managing blood pressure, increased intracranial pressure, and other medical complications in acutely ill patients in neurointensive care units should be followed.
- Subarachnoid hemorrhage due to aneurysm rupture is associated with a high incidence of delayed cerebral ischemia in the two weeks after the bleeding episode. Vasospasm of the cerebral vasculature is thought to be responsible for the delayed ischemia and occurs between 4 and 21 days after the bleed. The calcium channel blocker **nimodipine** is recommended to reduce the incidence and severity of neurologic deficits resulting from delayed ischemia. Nimodipine 60 mg every 4 hours should be initiated on diagnosis and continued for 21 days in all subarachnoid hemorrhage patients. If hypotension occurs, the dose may be reduced to 30 mg every 4 hours while maintaining intravascular volume.

▶ EVALUATION OF THERAPEUTIC OUTCOMES

Patients with acute stroke should be monitored intensely for the development of neurologic worsening, complications of thromboembolism or infections, and

TABLE 13–3. Monitoring the Stroke Patient

	Treatment	Parameter(s)	Frequency	Comments
Ischemic stroke	Alteplase	BP, neurologic function, bleeding	Every 15 min × 1 h; every 0.5 h × 6 h; every 1 h × l 7 h; every shift after	
	Aspirin	Bleeding	Daily	
	Clopidogrel	Bleeding	Daily	
	ERDP/ASA	Headache, bleeding	Daily	
	Ticlopidine	CBC, bleeding, diarrhea	CBC every 2 weeks × 3 months; other, daily	
	Warfarin	Bleeding, INR, Hb/Hct	INR daily × 3 days; weekly until stable; monthly	
Hemorrhagic stroke		BP, neurologic function, ICP	Every 2 h in ICU	Many patients require intervention with short-acting agents to reduce BP to <180 mm Hg systolic
	Nimodipine (for SAH)	BP, neurologic function, fluid status	Every 2 h in ICU	
All		Temperature, CBC	Temp. every 8 h; CBC daily	For infectious complications such as UTI or pneumonia
		Pain (calf or chest)	Every 8 h	For DVT, MI, acute headache
		Electrolytes and ECG	Up to daily	For fluid and electrolyte imbalances, cardiac rhythm abnormalities
	Heparins for DVT prophylaxis	Bleeding, platelets	Bleeding daily, platelets if suspected thrombocytopenia	

BP, blood pressure; ERDP/ASA, extended-release dipyridamole plus aspirin; CBC, complete blood count; INR, internation normalized ratio; Hb, hemoglobin; Hct, hematocrit; ICP, intracranial pressure; ICU, intensive care unit; SAH, subarachnoid hemorrhage; UTI, urinary troct infection; DVT, deep venous thrombosis; MI, myocardial infraction; ECG, electrocardiogram

adverse effects from pharmacologic or nonpharmacologic interventions. The approach to monitoring stroke patients is summarized in Table 13-3. The plan should be individualized for each patient based on comorbidities and ongoing disease processes.

See Chapter 20, Stroke, authored by Susan C. Fagan and David C. Hess, for a more detailed discussion of this topic.

Chapter 14

► VENOUS THROMBOEMBOLISM

► DEFINITION

Venous thromboembolism (VTE) results from clot formation in the venous circulation and is manifested as deep vein thrombosis (DVT) and pulmonary embolism (PE). A DVT is a thrombus composed of cellular material (red and white blood cells, platelets) bound together with fibrin strands. A PE is a thrombus that arises from the systemic circulation and lodges in the pulmonary artery or one of its branches, causing complete or partial obstruction of pulmonary blood flow.

► PATHOPHYSIOLOGY

- The coagulation cascade is a stepwise series of enzymatic reactions that results in the formation of a fibrin mesh (Figure 14–1). It can be triggered through either the intrinsic or extrinsic pathways. The intrinsic pathway is activated when negatively charged surfaces in contact with the blood activate factor XII, and activated platelets convert factor XI. The extrinsic pathway is activated when damaged vascular tissue releases tissue thromboplastin. Vascular injury also exposes the subendothelium, causing adherence, activation, and aggregation of platelets. The intrinsic and extrinsic pathways meet at a common point with the activation of factor X. With its partner, factor Va, factor Xa converts prothrombin (II) to thrombin (IIa), which then cleaves fibrinogen-forming fibrin monomers. Factor XIII covalently bonds fibrin strands together. The fibrinolytic protein plasmin ultimately degrades the fibrin mesh into soluble end products known as fibrin split products.
- Three primary components—venous stasis, vascular injury, and hypercoagulability (Virchow's triad)—play a role in the development of a pathogenic thrombus.
- Venous stasis is slowed blood flow in the deep veins of the legs resulting from damage to venous valves, vessel obstruction, prolonged periods of immobility, or increased blood viscosity. Conditions associated with venous stasis include major medical illness (e.g., heart failure, myocardial infarction), major surgery, paralysis (e.g., stroke, spinal cord injury), polycythemia vera, obesity, or varicose veins.
- Vascular injury may result from major orthopedic surgery (e.g., knee and hip replacement), trauma (especially fractures of the pelvis, hip, or leg), or indwelling venous catheters.
- Hypercoagulable states include malignancy; activated protein C resistance; deficiency of protein C, protein S, or antithrombin; factor VIII or XI excess; antiphospholipid antibodies; and other situations. Estrogens and selective estrogen receptor modulators (SERMs) have been linked to venous thrombosis, perhaps due in part to increased serum clotting factor concentrations.
- Although a thrombus can form in any part of the venous circulation, the majority of thrombi begin in the lower extremities. Once formed, a venous thrombus may: (1) remain asymptomatic; (2) lyse spontaneously; (3) obstruct the venous circulation; (4) propagate into more proximal veins; (5) embolize; or (6) act in any combination of these ways. Even asymptomatic patients may experience long-term consequences, such as the postthrombotic syndrome and recurrent VTE.

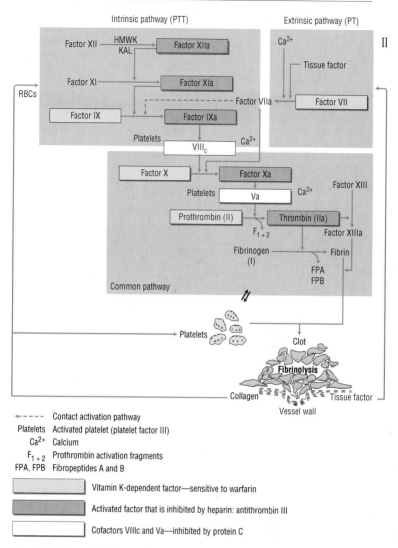

Figure 14–1. Scheme of the hemostatic system, showing interaction of vessel wall, platelets, coagulation pathways, and fibrinolytic system. Important features of the coagulation pathways include the contact activation phase, vitamin K-dependent factors (affected by warfarin), the activated serine proteases that are inhibited by heparin: antithrombin III, and the role of platelets and calcium. Factors VIIIc and Va are nonenzymatic cofactors that are inactivated by protein C. The prothrombin time (PT) measures the function of the extrinsic and common pathways; the partial thromboplastin time (PTT or aPTT) measures the function of the intrinsic and common pathways. HMWK, high-molecular-weight kininogen; KAL, kallikrein.

II

▶ CLINICAL PRESENTATION

- Most patients with VTE never develop symptoms from the acute event.
- Symptoms of DVT include unilateral leg swelling, pain, tenderness, erythema, and warmth. Physical signs may include a palpable cord and a positive Homan's sign.
- Postthrombotic syndrome (a long-term complication of DVT caused by damage to venous valves) may produce chronic lower extremity swelling, pain, tenderness, skin discoloration, and ulceration.
- Symptoms of PE include dyspnea, tachypnea, pleuritic chest pain, tachycardia, palpitations, cough, diaphoresis, and hemoptysis. Cardiovascular collapse, characterized by cyanosis, shock, and oliguria, is an ominous sign.

▶ DIAGNOSIS

- Assessment of the patient's status should focus on the search for risk factors (e.g., increased age, major surgery, previous VTE, trauma, malignancy, hypercoagulable states, and drug therapy). Signs and symptoms of DVT are nonspecific, and objective tests are required to confirm or exclude the diagnosis.
- Radiographic contrast studies are the most accurate and reliable method for diagnosis of VTE. Contrast venography allows visualization of the entire venous system in the lower extremity and abdomen. Pulmonary angiography allows visualization of the pulmonary arteries. The diagnosis of VTE can be made if there is a persistent intraluminal filling defect on multiple x-ray films.
- Because contrast studies are expensive, invasive, and technically difficult to perform and evaluate, noninvasive tests (e.g., ultrasonography and the ventilation-perfusion [V/Q] scan) are used frequently for the initial evaluation of patients with suspected VTE.
- Doppler ultrasonography can sensitively detect large thrombi occluding proximal veins but is relatively insensitive to smaller nonocclusive thrombi and calf vein thrombi. Doppler ultrasonography is also useful to assess venous valve competence.
- The V/Q scan is a principal screening test for PE. Small defects in perfusion to lung tissue can be detected, but pulmonary perfusion defects are nonspecific. Ventilation to lung tissue is determined by inhalation of aerosolized radiolabeled particles; an x-ray image of air flow distribution in the alveoli is taken. If a large section of lung tissue is ventilated but not perfused (a V/Q mismatch), there is a high probability of a PE. The results are interpreted as normal or high probability, intermediate probability, or low probability for PE. A normal scan reasonably excludes the diagnosis of PE, but patients with an intermediate probability should have ultrasonography of the lower extremities because most patients with a PE have an antecedent DVT.
- Clinical assessment improves the diagnostic accuracy of objective noninvasive tests. Major features suggestive for DVT include: (1) active cancer; (2) prolonged immobility or paralysis; (3) recent surgery or major medical illness; and (4) clinical features of DVT.
- If the results of the clinical assessment and ultrasonogram are discordant, venography or angiography should be performed to make the definitive diagnosis.

▶ DESIRED OUTCOME

The objectives of treating VTE are to prevent the development of PE and the postthrombotic syndrome, to reduce morbidity and mortality from the acute event, and to minimize adverse effects and cost of treatment.

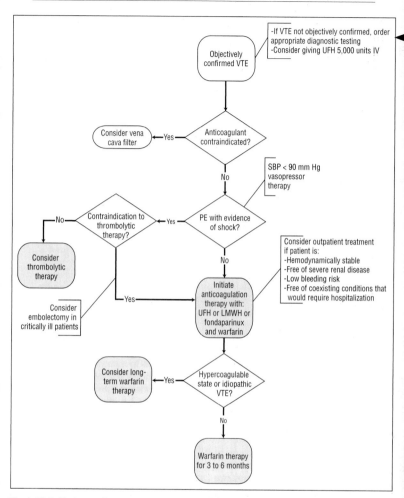

Figure 14–2. Treatment of venous thromboembolism (VTE). SBP, systolic blood pressure; PE, pulmonary embolism; UFH, unfractionated heparin; LMWH, low-molecular-weight heparin.

▶ TREATMENT

See Figure 14–2.

UNFRACTIONATED HEPARIN

- **Unfractionated heparin** (UFH) is a heterogeneous mixture of sulfated glycosaminoglycans of variable lengths and pharmacologic properties. The molecular weight of these molecules ranges from 5000 to 30,000 daltons (mean 15,000 daltons).
- The anticoagulant effect of UFH is mediated through a specific pentasaccharide sequence on the heparin molecule that binds to antithrombin, provoking a

▶ II

conformational change. The UFH-antithrombin complex is 100 to 1000 times more potent as an anticoagulant than antithrombin alone. Antithrombin inhibits the activity of factors IXa, Xa, XIIa, and thrombin (IIa). It also inhibits thrombin-induced activation of factors V and VIII.

- UFH prevents the growth and propagation of a formed thrombus and allows the patient's own thrombolytic system to degrade the clot.
- Contraindications to heparin therapy include hypersensitivity to the drug, active bleeding, hemophilia, severe liver disease with elevated prothrombin time (PT), severe thrombocytopenia, malignant hypertension, and inability to meticulously supervise and monitor treatment.
- UFH must be given parenterally, preferably by the intravenous (IV) or subcutaneous (SC) route. Intramuscular administration is discouraged because absorption is erratic and it may cause large hematomas.
- IV administration is needed when rapid anticoagulation is required. Continuous IV infusion is preferable because intermittent boluses produce high peaks in anticoagulation activity and have been associated with a greater risk of major bleeding.
- Doses should be based on actual body weight; adjusted body weight may be used for obese patients (greater than 130% of ideal body weight). A loading dose of 80 to 100 units/kg (maximum 10,000 units) is followed by a continuous IV infusion at an initial rate of 17 to 20 units/kg/h (maximum 2300 units/h).
- The aPTT should be checked no sooner than 6 h after beginning the infusion or after any dosage change. The therapeutic range is 1.5 to 2.5 times the mean normal control value. Recommended adjustments in UFH dose based upon aPTT measurements are given in Table 14–1. Once the target aPTT is achieved, daily monitoring is indicated for minor dosing adjustments.
- Bleeding is the primary adverse effect associated with UFH. The most common bleeding sites are the gastrointestinal tract, urinary tract, and soft tissues. Critical areas include intracranial, pericardial, and intraocular sites as well as the adrenal gland. Symptoms of bleeding may include severe headache, joint pain, chest pain, abdominal pain, swelling, tarry stools, hematuria, or the passing of bright red blood through the rectum.
- If major bleeding occurs, UFH should be discontinued immediately and IV **protamine sulfate** should be given by slow IV infusion over 10 minutes (1 mg/100 units of UFH infused during the previous 4 hours; maximum 50 mg).
- Thrombocytopenia (platelet count less than 150,000/mm^3) is common and two distinct types can occur:

TABLE 14–1. Adjusted Heparin Dose Based on Activated Partial Thromboplastin Time (aPTT) Measurements

aPTT (s)	Dose Adjustment
<37 (or > 12 s below institution-specific therapeutic range)	80 units/kg bolus then increase infusion by 4 units/kg/h
37–47 (or 1–12 s below institution-specific therapeutic range)	40 units/kg bolus then increase infusion by 2 units/kg/h
48–71 (or within institution-specific therapeutic range)	No change
72–93 (or 1–22 s above institution-specific therapeutic range)	Decrease infusion by 2 units/kg/h
>93 (or >22 s above institution-specific therapeutic range)	Hold infusion for 1 h then decrease by 3 units/kg/h

- Heparin-associated thrombocytopenia (HAT) is a benign, transient, and mild phenomenon that usually occurs within the first few days of treatment. Platelet counts rarely drop below 100,000/mm^3 and recover with continued therapy.
- Heparin-induced thrombocytopenia (HIT) is a serious problem that requires immediate intervention. Platelet counts must be monitored every 1 to 2 days, and the patient's condition should be carefully evaluated for HIT if the platelet count drops by more than 50% or to less than 100,000/mm^3. With HIT, platelet counts typically begin to fall after 5 or more days of continuous heparin use. Platelet counts can nadir as low as 20,000/mm^3. The immune-mediated platelet activation and thrombin generation seen during HIT can lead to severe thrombotic complications in arteries or veins (i.e., limb artery occlusion, stroke, myocardial infarction, DVT, PE). Skin lesions occur in 10% to 20% of patients and range from painful, localized erythematous plaques to widespread dermal necrosis that may require amputation. Laboratory testing to detect heparin antibodies must be performed to confirm the diagnosis of HIT. Prompt discontinuation of heparin and initiation of an alternative anticoagulant are imperative to prevent thrombotic complications. Anticoagulants that rapidly inhibit thrombin activity are required. The direct thrombin inhibitors **lepirudin** and **argatroban** are FDA-approved for this use (see below).
- Bruising, local irritation, mild pain, erythema, histamine-like reactions, and hematoma can occur at the site of injection. Hypersensitivity reactions involving chills, fever, urticaria, and rarely bronchospasm, nausea, vomiting, and shock have been reported in patients with HIT. Long-term UFH has been reported to cause alopecia, priapism, hyperkalemia, and osteoporosis.

LOW-MOLECULAR-WEIGHT HEPARINS

- Low-molecular-weight heparins (LMWHs) are fragments of UFH that are heterogeneous mixtures of sulfated glycosaminoglycans with approximately one-third the molecular weight of UFH.
- Advantages of LMWHs over UFH include: (1) more predictable anticoagulation dose response; (2) improved subcutaneous bioavailability; (3) dose-independent clearance; (4) longer biologic half-life; (5) lower incidence of thrombocytopenia; and (6) less need for routine laboratory monitoring.
- Like UFH, the LMWHs enhance and accelerate the activity of antithrombin and prevent the growth and propagation of formed thrombi. The peak anticoagulant effect is seen in 3 to 5 hours after subcutaneous dosing.
- The usefulness of LMWHs has been evaluated extensively for many indications, including acute coronary syndromes, DVT, PE, and prevention of VTE in several high-risk populations.
- Subcutaneous dosage regimens are based on body weight and vary depending upon the product and indication. The recommended doses for treatment of DVT with or without PE are:
  - **Enoxaparin** (Lovenox) 1 mg/kg every 12 hours or 1.5 mg/kg every 24 hours
  - **Dalteparin** (Fragmin) 100 units/kg every 12 hours or 200 units/kg every 24 hours
  - **Tinzaparin** (Innohep) 175 units/kg every 24 hours
- Because the LMWHs achieve predictable anticoagulant response when given subcutaneously, routine laboratory monitoring is unnecessary to guide dosing. The PT and aPTT are minimally affected by LMWH. Prior to the initiation of therapy, a baseline PT/INR, aPTT, complete blood count (CBC) with platelet count, and serum creatinine should be obtained. Periodic monitoring

II

of the CBC and platelet counts and occult fecal blood is recommended during therapy.

- Measuring antifactor Xa activity may be helpful in patients who have significant renal impairment, weigh less than 50 kg, are morbidly obese, require prolonged therapy (e.g., more than 14 days), are pregnant, or are at a very high risk for bleeding or thrombotic recurrence. Samples for antifactor Xa activity should be drawn approximately 4 hours after the subcutaneous injection. For the treatment of VTE, an acceptable target range is 0.5 to 1 unit/mL.

- As with UFH, bleeding is the most common adverse effect of the LMWHs. Although not demonstrated consistently in clinical trials, major bleeding may be less common than with UFH. Minor bleeding occurs frequently, particularly at the site of injection. If major bleeding occurs, **protamine sulfate** should be administered IV, although it cannot neutralize the anticoagulant effect completely. The recommended dose of protamine sulfate is 1 mg per 1 mg of enoxaparin or 1 mg per 100 antifactor Xa units of dalteparin or tinzaparin administered in the previous 8 hours. If the LMWH dose was given in the previous 8 to 12 hours, the protamine sulfate dose is 0.5 mg per 100 antifactor Xa units. Protamine sulfate is not recommended if the LMWH was given more than 12 hours earlier.

DANAPAROID

Danaparoid sodium (Orgaran) is structurally distinct from but mechanistically related to heparin. It is a mixture of three sulfated glycosaminoglycans: heparan, dermatan, and chondroitin. Like heparin, its anticoagulant activity is mediated in part through its interaction with antithrombin. It is FDA-approved for VTE prophylaxis in patients undergoing elective hip replacement surgery, but in 2002 the manufacturer discontinued its distribution in the United States.

FONDAPARINUX

Fondaparinux sodium (Arixtra) is a selective inhibitor of factor Xa. Similar to UFH and the LMWHs, it binds to antithrombin, greatly accelerating its activity. However, it has no direct effect on thrombin activity at therapeutic plasma concentrations. It is approved for prevention of VTE in patients undergoing surgery for hip fracture and hip or knee replacements; the dose is 2.5 mg subcutaneously once daily starting 6 to 8 hours after surgery. Fondaparinux is also approved for treatment of DVT and PE; the usual dose for these indications is 7.5 mg subcutaneously once daily.

DIRECT THROMBIN INHIBITORS

- These agents interact directly with thrombin and do not require antithrombin to have antithrombotic activity. They are capable of inhibiting both circulating and clot-bound thrombin, which is a potential advantage over UFH and the LMWHs. They also do not induce immune-mediated thrombocytopenia and have been used for the treatment of HIT.

- **Lepirudin** (Refludan) is indicated for anticoagulation in patients with HIT and associated thromboembolic disease in order to prevent further thromboembolic complications. The recommended dose is 0.4 mg/kg slow IV bolus, followed by a 0.15-mg/kg/h continuous IV infusion. After obtaining a baseline aPTT, an aPTT should be obtained at least 4 hours after starting the infusion and then at least daily thereafter. The dose should be titrated to achieve an aPTT 1.5 to 2.5 times control.

- **Argatroban** is indicated as an anticoagulant for patients with HIT and for patients at risk for HIT undergoing percutaneous coronary intervention (PCI).

The recommended dose for the treatment of HIT is 2 mcg/kg/min by continuous IV infusion. The first aPTT should be obtained 2 hours after initiation. The dose can be adjusted as clinically indicated (maximum 10 mcg/kg/min) until the aPTT is 1.5 to 3 times control.

- **Bivalirudin** (Angiomax, formerly known as hirulog) is indicated for use as an anticoagulant in patients with unstable angina undergoing PTCA. The recommended dose is an IV bolus of 1 mg/kg followed by a 4-hour infusion at a rate of 2.5 mg/kg/h. An additional IV infusion may be initiated at a rate of 0.2 mg/kg/h for up to 20 hours if needed. Bivalirudin is intended for use with aspirin 300 to 325 mg/day.

- **Desirudin** (Iprivask) is indicated for prophylaxis of DVT in patients undergoing hip replacement surgery. The recommended dose is 15 mg subcutaneously every 12 hours beginning 5 to 15 minutes prior to surgery and for up to 12 days thereafter. Daily aPTT monitoring is recommended for patients on desirudin.

- **Ximelagatran** (investigational at the time of this writing) is a prodrug converted in the liver to the active moiety melagatran. Oral bioavailability is good and does not appear to be affected by food. Its elimination half-life is 3 to 5 hours, making twice-daily administration necessary. Routine anticoagulation monitoring is not required. Ximelagatran was associated with a 6% to 9% incidence of elevated liver function tests in phase III clinical trails, and less than 1% of patients may have had severe irreversible liver injury. In 2004, the FDA denied approval of ximelagatran until more safety data are available and an effective risk management strategy is developed.

- Contraindications are similar to those of other antithrombotic drugs, and hemorrhage is the most common and serious adverse effect. For all agents in this class, a CBC should be obtained at baseline and periodically thereafter to detect potential bleeding. There are no known agents that reverse the activity of direct thrombin inhibitors.

WARFARIN

- **Warfarin** inhibits the enzymes responsible for the cyclic interconversion of vitamin K in the liver. Reduced vitamin K is a cofactor required for the carboxylation of the vitamin K-dependent coagulation proteins prothrombin (II); factors VII, IX, and X; and the endogenous anticoagulant proteins C and S. By reducing the supply of vitamin K available to serve as a cofactor in the production of these proteins, warfarin indirectly slows their rate of synthesis. By suppressing the production of clotting factors, warfarin prevents the initial formation and propagation of thrombi. Warfarin has no direct effect on previously circulating clotting factors or previously formed thrombi. The time required to achieve its anticoagulant effect depends on the elimination half-lives of the coagulation proteins. Because prothrombin has a 2- to 3-day half-life, warfarin's full antithrombotic effect is not achieved for 8 to 15 days after initiation of therapy.

- Warfarin should begin concurrently with UFH or LMWH therapy. For patients with acute VTE, heparin and warfarin therapy should be overlapped for at least 4 to 5 days, regardless of whether the target international normalized ratio (INR) has been achieved earlier. The UFH or LMWH can then be discontinued once the INR is within the desired range for two consecutive days.

- Guidelines for initiating warfarin therapy are given in Figure 14–3. The usual initial dose is 5 to 10 mg. In older patients (age greater than 65 years) and those taking potentially interacting medications, a starting dose of 2.5 mg should be considered.

- Warfarin therapy is monitored by the INR (target: 2 to 3 for DVT or PE). After an acute thromboembolic event, the INR should be measured minimally

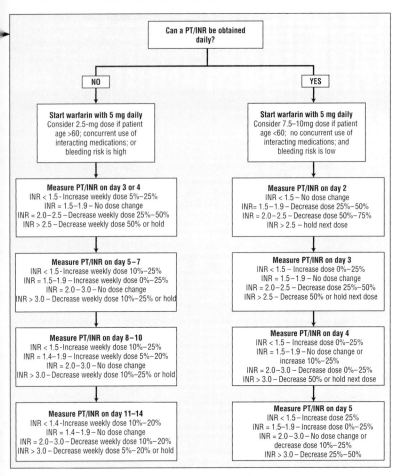

Figure 14–3. Initiation of warfarin therapy. PT, prothrombin time; INR, international normalized ratio.

every 3 days during the first week of therapy. In general, dose changes should not be made more frequently than every 3 days. Doses should be adjusted by calculating the weekly dose and reducing or increasing it by 5% to 25%. The effect of a small dose change may not become evident for 5 to 7 days. Once the patient's dose response is established, an INR should be determined every 7 to 14 days until it stabilizes and then every 4 weeks thereafter.

- Six to 12 weeks of warfarin therapy is sufficient for symptomatic isolated calf vein DVT. Treatment should be continued for at least 3 months for patients with a proximal vein DVT. Most experts recommend at least 6 months of therapy for large iliofemoral DVT or PE. A longer duration (e.g., more than 1 year) is recommended for patients who have persistent risk factors or who suffer a recurrent VTE event.
- Hemorrhagic complications ranging from mild to severe and life-threatening can occur at any body site. The gastrointestinal tract is the most frequent

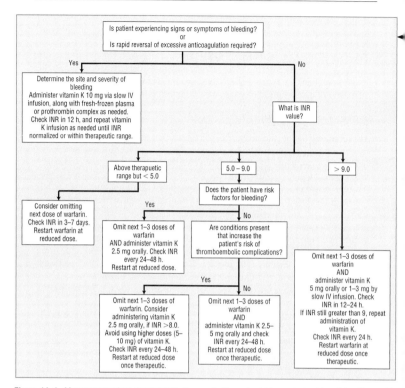

Figure 14–4. Management of an elevated INR. Dose reductions should be made by determining the weekly warfarin dose and reducing the weekly dose by 10% to 25% based on the degree of INR elevation.

site of bleeding. Bruising on the arms and legs is common, but a painful hematoma may necessitate temporary discontinuation of therapy. Intracranial hemorrhage is the most serious complication and often results in permanent disability and death. Figure 14–4 outlines guidelines for managing an elevated INR. Patients with a mildly elevated INR (3.5 to 5) and no signs or symptoms of bleeding can usually be managed by either reducing the dose or holding 1 or 2 warfarin doses. If rapid reduction of an elevated INR is required, oral or IV administration of vitamin K_1 (**phytonadione**) can be given. Oral administration is preferable in the absence of major bleeding. The IV route produces the most rapid reversal of anticoagulation, but it has been associated with anaphylactoid reactions. If the INR is 5 to 9, warfarin doses may be withheld or may be combined with phytonadione 1 to 5 mg. If the INR is greater than 9, a 5-mg oral dose is recommended. Low vitamin K doses reduce the INR consistently within 24 hours without making the patient refractory to warfarin. In the event of serious or life-threatening bleeding, IV vitamin K should be administered together with fresh frozen plasma or clotting factor concentrates.

- Nonhemorrhagic adverse effects include the rare "purple toe syndrome" and skin necrosis.
- Absolute contraindications to warfarin include active bleeding, hemorrhagic tendencies, pregnancy, and a history of warfarin-induced skin necrosis. It

II

should be used with great caution in patients with a history of gastrointestinal bleeding, recent neurosurgery, alcoholic liver disease, severe renal impairment, or inability to keep follow-up appointments for monitoring.

- Because of the large number of food-drug and drug-drug interactions with warfarin, close monitoring and additional INR determinations may be indicated whenever other medications are initiated, or discontinued, or an alteration in consumption of vitamin K–containing foods is noted.

THROMBOLYSIS AND THROMBECTOMY

- Thrombolytic agents are proteolytic enzymes that enhance the conversion of plasminogen to plasmin, which subsequently degrades the fibrin matrix.
- In the management of PE, thrombolytics have been shown to restore pulmonary artery patency more rapidly when compared to UFH alone, but this early benefit does not improve long-term patient outcomes. Thrombolytic therapy has not been shown to improve morbidity or mortality and is associated with a substantial risk of hemorrhage. For these reasons, thrombolytics should be reserved for patients with PE who are most likely to benefit. Patients who had thrombus in the right atrium or ventricle or who have hemodynamic compromise as evidenced by significant hypotension or severe right ventricular strain may benefit from thrombolytic therapy. Patients with massive DVT and limb gangrene despite anticoagulation are also candidates for thrombolysis.
- Three thrombolytic agents and regimens are available for treatment of DVT and PE:
  - **Alteplase** (Activase): For PE, 100 mg by IV infusion over 2 h. For DVT, 0.05-mg/kg/h continuous infusion over 24 hours (maximum, 150 mg) or 80- to 100-mg infusion over 2 hours.
  - **Reteplase** (Retavase): For PE, 10 units IV bolus followed 30 minutes later by a second 10 units IV bolus.
  - **Streptokinase** (Streptase): 250,000 units bolus infusion over 30 minutes followed by a continuous IV infusion of 100,000 units/h for 24 hours (PE) or 24 to 72 hours (DVT).
- The thrombin time or aPTT should be performed prior to and 3 to 4 hours after the initiation of treatment. As long as test values during the infusion are prolonged beyond the control value, it can be assumed that systemic fibrinolysis has been achieved.
- During the thrombolytic infusion, UFH or LMWH therapy should be temporarily withheld. Continuous infusion with UFH should be restarted without a bolus dose after administration of the thrombolytic when the aPTT returns to less than twice normal. UFH may be administered immediately after completion of an alteplase infusion.
- Venous thrombectomy may be performed to remove a massive obstructive thrombus in a patient with significant iliofemoral venous thrombosis, particularly if the patient is either not a candidate for or has not responded to thrombolysis. Full-dose anticoagulation therapy is essential during the entire operative and postoperative period. These patients still need chronic anticoagulation given orally for the usual recommended duration of treatment.

PREVENTION OF VENOUS THROMBOEMBOLISM

- Nonpharmacologic methods improve venous blood flow by mechanical means and include early ambulation, electrical stimulation of calf muscles during prolonged surgery, graduated compression stockings, intermittent pneumatic compression (IPC) devices, and inferior vena cava (IVC) filters.

TABLE 14–2. Risk Classification and Consensus Guidelines for VTE Prevention

Level of Risk	Prevention Strategies
Low	
Minor surgery, age <40 yr, and no clinical risk factors	Ambulation
Moderate	
Major or minor surgery, age 40–60 yr, and no clinical risk factors	UFH 5000 units SC q 1 2 h
Major surgery, age <40 yr and no clinic risk factors	Dalteparin 2500 units SC q 2 4 h
Minor surgery, with clinical risk factor(s)	Enoxaparin 40 mg SC q 2 4 h
Acutely ill (e.g., MI, ischemic stroke, CHF exacerbation), and no clinical risk factors	Tinzaparin 3500 units SC q 2 4 h
	IPC
	Graduated compression stockings
High	
Major surgery, age >60 yr, and no clinical risk factors	UFH 5000 units SC q8h
Major surgery, age 40–60 yr, with clinical risk factor(s)	Dalteparin 5000 units SC q 2 4 h
Acutely ill (e.g., MI, ischemic stroke, CHF exacerbation), with risk factor(s)	Enoxaparin 40 mg SC q 2 4 h
	Tinzaparin 75 units/kg SC q 2 4 h
	IPC
Highest	
Major lower extremity orthopedic surgery	Adjusted dose UFH SC q 8 h (aPTT >36 s)
Hip fracture	Dalteparin 5000 units SC q 2 4 h
Multiple trauma	Desirudin 15 mg SC q 1 2 h
Major surgery, age >40 yr, and prior history of VTE	Enoxaparin 30 mg SC q 1 2 h
Major surgery, age >40 yr and malignancy	Fondaparinux 2.5 mg SC q 2 4 h
Major surgery, age >40 yr, and hypercoagulable state	Tinzaparin 75 units/kg SC q 2 4 h
Spinal cord injury or stroke with limb paralysis	Warfarin (INR = 2.0–3.0)
	IPC with UFH 5000 units SC q 8 h

UFH, unfractionated heparin; SC, subcutaneously; IPC, intermittent pneumatic compression

- Pharmacologic techniques counteract the propensity for thrombosis formation by dampening the coagulation cascade. Appropriately selected therapy can dramatically reduce the incidence of VTE after hip or knee replacement, general surgery, myocardial infarction, and ischemic stroke. The **LMWHs** and **fondaparinux** provide superior protection against VTE compared with **low-dose UFH**. Even so, UFH is a highly effective, cost-conscious choice for many patients, provided that it is given in the appropriate dose (Table 14–2). Adjusted-dose subcutaneous UFH with doses adjusted to maintain the aPTT at high-normal is more effective in the highest risk patients (hip and knee replacement surgery). There is no evidence that one LMWH is superior to another for the prevention of VTE. **Warfarin** is commonly used for VTE prevention after orthopedic surgeries of the lower extremities, but evidence is equivocal regarding its relative effectiveness compared to LMWH for preventing clinically important VTE events in the highest risk populations.
- Prophylaxis should be continued throughout the period of risk. For general surgical procedures and medical conditions, prophylaxis can be discontinued

157

II

once the patient is able to ambulate regularly and other risk factors are no longer present. Most clinical trial support the use of antithrombotic therapy for 21 to 35 days after total hip replacement, hip fracture repair, and knee replacement surgery.

▶ EVALUATION OF THERAPEUTIC OUTCOMES

- Patients should be monitored for resolution of symptoms, the development of recurrent thrombosis, and symptoms of the postthrombotic syndrome, as well as for adverse effects from the treatments described in this chapter.
- Hemoglobin, hematocrit, and blood pressure should be monitored carefully to detect bleeding from anticoagulant therapy.
- Coagulation tests (aPTT, PT, INR) should be performed prior to initiating therapy to establish the patient's baseline values and guide later anticoagulation.
- Outpatients taking warfarin should be questioned about medication adherence and symptoms related to bleeding and thromboembolic complications. Any changes in concurrent medications should be carefully explored.

See Chapter 19, Venous Thromboembolism, authored by Stuart T. Haines, Mario Zeolla, and Daniel M. Witt, for a more detailed discussion of this topic.

Dermatologic Disorders
Edited by Terry L. Schwinghammer

Chapter 15

▶ ACNE

▶ DEFINITION

Acne vulgaris is a common, usually self-limiting, multifactorial disease involving inflammation of the sebaceous follicles of the face and upper trunk.

▶ PATHOPHYSIOLOGY

- The primary factors involved in the formation of acne lesions are increased sebum production, sloughing of keratinocytes, bacterial growth, and inflammation.
- The primary lesion, the comedo, forms as a result of plugging of the pilosebaceous follicle. The follicular canal widens, and cell production increases. Sebum mixes with excess loose cells in the follicular canal to form a keratinous plug. This appears as an open comedo, or "blackhead" (because of melanin accumulation). Inflammation or trauma to the follicle may lead to formation of a closed comedo, or "whitehead." Closed comedones may presage larger, inflammatory lesions.
- If the follicular wall is damaged or ruptured, follicle contents may extrude into the dermis and present as a pustule.
- Increased androgen activity at puberty triggers growth of sebaceous glands and enhanced sebum production. Sebum consists of glycerides, wax esters, squalene, and cholesterol. Glyceride is converted to free fatty acids and glycerol by lipases, which are products of *Propionibacterium acnes*. Free fatty acids may irritate the follicular wall and cause increased cell turnover and inflammation. *P. acnes* is a resident anaerobic organism that proliferates in the environment created by the mixture of excessive sebum and keratinocytes. It is antigenic and can increase antibody formation leading to an inflammatory response.
- A primary factor in the development of acne is an alteration in the pattern of keratinization within the follicle. Increased production and sloughing of keratinocytes correlates with comedo formation.

▶ CLINICAL PRESENTATION

- Acne lesions typically occur on the face, back, upper chest, and shoulders. Lesions are classified primarily as either inflammatory or noninflammatory.
- The presentation can range from a mild comedonal form to severe inflammatory necrotic acne.
- Lesions may take months to heal completely, and fibrosis associated with healing may lead to permanent scarring.

▶ DIAGNOSIS

Diagnosis is established by observation of acne lesions (e.g., comedones, pustules, papules, nodules, cysts) on the face, back, or chest. The presence of 5 to 10 comedones is usually considered to be diagnostic.

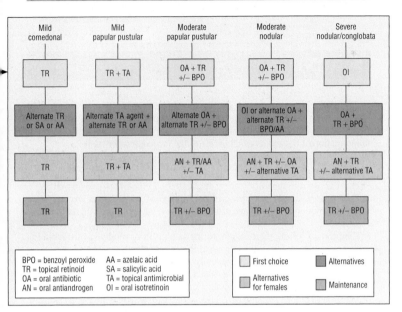

Figure 15–1. Algorithms for acne treatment.

▶ DESIRED OUTCOME

The goals of treatment are to prevent the formation of new acne lesions, heal existing lesions, and prevent or minimize scarring.

▶ TREATMENT

Figure 15–1 provides treatment algorithms based on acne severity.

NONPHARMACOLOGIC THERAPY

- Surface skin cleansing with soap and water has a relatively small effect on acne because it has minimal impact within follicles.
- Skin scrubbing or excessive face washing does not necessarily open or cleanse pores and may lead to skin irritation.
- Use of gentle, nondrying cleansing agents is important to avoid skin irritation and dryness during some acne therapies.

TOPICAL PHARMACOLOGIC THERAPY

Benzoyl Peroxide

- **Benzoyl peroxide** may be used to treat superficial inflammatory acne. It is a nonantibiotic antibacterial that is bacteriostatic against *P. acnes*. It is decomposed on the skin by cysteine, liberating free oxygen radicals that oxidize bacterial proteins. It increases the sloughing rate of epithelial cells and loosens the follicular plug structure, resulting in some degree of comedolytic activity.

- Soaps, lotions, creams, washes, and gels are available in concentrations of 2.5% to 10%. The 10% concentration is not significantly more effective but may be more irritating. Gel formulations are usually most potent, whereas lotions, creams, and soaps have weaker potency. Alcohol-based gel preparations generally cause more dryness and irritation. III◄
- To limit irritation and increase tolerability, begin with a low-potency formulation (2.5%) and increase either the strength (5% to 10%) or application frequency (every other day, each day, then twice daily).
- Apply the formulation chosen to cool, clean, dry skin no more often than twice daily to minimize irritation. Fair or moist skin is more sensitive; advise patients to apply the medication to dry skin at least 30 minutes after washing.
- Side effects include dryness, irritation, and allergic contact dermatitis. It may bleach or discolor some fabrics (e.g., clothing, bed linen, towels).

Tretinoin

- **Tretinoin** (a retinoid; topical vitamin A acid) is a comedolytic agent that increases cell turnover in the follicular wall and decreases cohesiveness of cells, leading to extrusion of comedones and inhibition of new comedo formation. It also decreases the number of cell layers in the stratum corneum from about 14 to about 5.
- Tretinoin is available as 0.05% solution (most irritating), 0.01% and 0.025% gels, and 0.025%, 0.05%, and 0.1% creams (least irritating).
- Treatment initiation with 0.025% cream is recommended for mild acne in people with sensitive and nonoily skin, 0.01% gel for moderate acne on easily irritated skin in people with oily complexions, and 0.025% gel for moderate acne in those with nonsensitive and oily skin.
- Patients should be advised to apply the medication to dry skin approximately 30 minutes after washing to minimize erythema and irritation. Slowly increasing the application frequency from every other day to daily and then twice daily may also increase tolerability.
- A flare of acne may appear suddenly after initiation of treatment, followed by clinical clearing in 8 to 12 weeks. Once control is established, continue therapy at the lowest effective concentration and the longest effective interval that minimizes acne exacerbations.
- Side effects include skin irritation, erythema, peeling, allergic contact dermatitis (rare), and increased sensitivity to sun exposure, wind, cold, and other irritants.
- **Retin-A Micro** (microsphere vehicle of porous beads) and **Avita** (liquid polymer vehicle) are less irritating formulations than products with standard vehicles.
- Concomitant use of an antibacterial agent with tretinoin can decrease keratinization, inhibit *P. acnes,* and decrease inflammation. A combination of benzoyl peroxide each morning and tretinoin at bedtime may enhance efficacy and be less irritating than either agent used alone.

Adapalene

- **Adapalene** (Differin) is a third-generation retinoid with comedolytic, keratolytic, and anti-inflammatory activity. It is available as 0.1% gel, cream, alcoholic solution, and pledgets.
- Adapalene is indicated for mild to moderate acne vulgaris. The 0.1% gel can be used as an alternative to tretinoin 0.025% gel to achieve better tolerability in some patients.
- Coadministration with a topical or oral antibiotic is reasonable for moderate forms of acne.

Tazarotene

- **Tazarotene** (Tazorac) is a synthetic acetylenic retinoid that is converted to its active form, tazarotenic acid, after topical application.
- It is used in the treatment of mild to moderate acne vulgaris and has comedolytic, keratolytic, and anti-inflammatory action.
- The product is available as a 0.05% and 0.1% gel or cream.
- Dose-related adverse effects include erythema, pruritus, stinging, and burning.

Erythromycin

- **Erythromycin** with or without zinc is effective against inflammatory acne. Zinc combination products may enhance penetration of erythromycin into the pilosebaceous unit.
- Commonly used erythromycin formulations include 2% gel, lotion, solution, and disposable pads that are usually applied twice daily.
- Development of *P. acnes* resistance to erythromycin may be reduced by combination therapy with benzoyl peroxide.

Clindamycin

- **Clindamycin** inhibits *P. acnes* and provides comedolytic and anti-inflammatory activity.
- It is available as 1% or 2% concentrations in gel, lotion, solution, and disposable pad formulations and is usually applied twice daily. Combination with benzoyl peroxide increases efficacy.

Azelaic Acid

- **Azelaic acid** (Azelex) has antibacterial, anti-inflammatory, and comedolytic activity.
- It is available as a 20% cream, which is usually applied twice daily on clean, dry skin.
- Azelaic acid is useful for mild to moderate acne in patients who do not tolerate benzoyl peroxide. It is also useful for postinflammatory hyperpigmentation because it has skin-lightening properties.
- Although uncommon, mild transient burning, pruritus, stinging, and tingling may occur.

Salicylic Acid, Sulfur, and Resorcinol

- **Salicylic acid, sulfur,** and **resorcinol** are keratolytic and mildly antibacterial agents. Salicylic acid has comedolytic and anti-inflammatory action.
- Each agent has been classified as safe and effective by an FDA advisory panel. Some combinations may be synergistic (e.g., sulfur and resorcinol).
- Keratolytics may be less irritating than benzoyl peroxide and tretinoin, but they are not as effective comedolytic agents.
- Disadvantages include the odor created by hydrogen sulfide on reaction of sulfur with skin, the brown scale from resorcinol, and (rarely) salicylism from long-term use of high concentrations of salicylic acid on highly permeable (inflamed or abraded) skin.

SYSTEMIC THERAPY

Isotretinoin

- **Isotretinoin** (Accutane) decreases sebum production, changes sebum composition, inhibits *P. acnes* growth within follicles, inhibits inflammation, and alters patterns of keratinization within follicles.
- It is indicated for severe nodular or inflammatory acne in patients unresponsive to conventional therapies, for scarring acne, for those with chronic relapsing acne, and for acne associated with severe psychological distress.

- Dosing guidelines range from 0.5 to 1 mg/kg/day, but the cumulative dose taken during a treatment course may be the major factor influencing long-term outcome. Optimal results are usually attained with cumulative doses of 120 to 150 mg/kg.
- A 6-month course is sufficient for most patients. Alternatively, an initial dose of 1 mg/kg/day for 3 months followed by 0.5 mg/kg/day (or 0.2 mg/kg/day if possible) for 3 to 9 more months may optimize the therapeutic outcome.
- Adverse effects are frequent and often dose-related. About 90% of patients experience mucocutaneous effects; drying of the mouth, nose, and eyes is most common. Cheilitis and skin desquamation occur in more than 80% of patients. The conjunctiva and nasal mucosa are affected less frequently. Systemic effects include transient increases in serum cholesterol and triglycerides, increased creatine kinase, hyperglycemia, photosensitivity, pseudotumor cerebri, excess granulation tissue, hepatomegaly with abnormal liver injury tests, bone abnormalities, arthralgias, muscle stiffness, headache, and a high incidence of teratogenicity. Patients should be counseled about and screened for depression during therapy, although a causal relationship to isotretinoin therapy is controversial.
- Because of teratogenicity, contraception is required in female patients beginning 1 month before therapy, continuing throughout treatment, and for up to 3 months after discontinuation of therapy.

Oral Antibacterial Agents

- **Erythromycin** has efficacy similar to tetracycline, but it induces higher rates of bacterial resistance. Resistance may be reduced by combination therapy with benzoyl peroxide. Erythromycin can be used for patients who require systemic antibiotics but cannot tolerate tetracyclines, or those who acquire bacterial resistance to tetracyclines. The usual dose is 1 g/day with meals to minimize gastrointestinal intolerance.
- **Azithromycin** is a safe and effective alternative for moderate to severe inflammatory acne. Its long half-life permits intermittent dosing 3 times a week.
- Tetracyclines inhibit *P. acnes*, reduce the amount of keratin in sebaceous follicles, and inhibit chemotaxis, phagocytosis, complement activation, and cell-mediated immunity. Drawbacks to tetracyclines include gastrointestinal disturbances, hepatotoxicity, photosensitivity, predisposition to superinfections (e.g., vaginal candidiasis), tooth discoloration in children, and inhibition of skeletal growth in the developing fetus. Tetracyclines must not be combined with systemic retinoids because of the increase risk of intracranial hypertension. Women taking oral contraceptives and given tetracycline should be informed of the potential for contraceptive failure.
  - **Tetracycline** is the least expensive agent in this class and is often prescribed for initial therapy in moderate to severe acne vulgaris. A common initial dose is 500 mg twice daily given 1 hour before meals; after 1 or 2 months when marked improvement is observed, the dose may be reduced to 500 mg daily for another 1 or 2 months. Tetracycline administration must be separated from food and dairy products.
  - **Doxycycline** is commonly used for moderate to severe acne vulgaris. It is more effective and produces less resistance than tetracycline. The initial dose is 100 or 200 mg daily, followed by 50 mg daily as a maintenance dose after improvement is seen. Doxycycline may be given with food, but it is more effective when taken 30 minutes before meals.
  - **Minocycline** is also commonly used for moderate to severe acne vulgaris. It is more effective than tetracycline. It is dosed similar to doxycycline

(100 mg/day or 50 mg twice daily) and on an indefinite basis in selected patients. Minocycline has the most reported adverse effects of the tetracyclines, some of which may be serious.

- **Trimethoprim-sulfamethoxazole** may be used for patients who do not tolerate tetracyclines and erythromycin or in cases of resistance to these antibiotics. The adult dose is usually 800 mg sulfamethoxazole and 160 mg trimethoprim twice daily.
- **Clindamycin** use is limited by diarrhea and the risk of pseudomembranous colitis.

Oral Contraceptives

Ortho Tri-Cyclen is FDA-approved for moderate acne in women unresponsive to topical medications. This triphasic product contains a fixed dose of **ethinyl estradiol,** 0.035 mg, and increasing doses of **norgestimate,** 0.180, 0.215, and 0.250 mg. The combination increases sex hormone–binding globulin (SHBG), causing a decrease in unbound, biologically active testosterone.

▶ EVALUATION OF THERAPEUTIC OUTCOMES

- Information regarding pathogenic factors and the importance of medication compliance should be conveyed to patients.
- Patients should understand that effectiveness of any therapeutic regimen may require 6 to 8 weeks and that they may also notice an exacerbation of acne after initiation of topical comedolytic therapy.

See Chapter 95, Acne Vulgaris, authored by Dennis P. West, Lee E. West, Maria Letizia Musumeci, and Giuseppe Micali, for a more detailed discussion of this topic.

Chapter 16

▶ PSORIASIS

▶ DEFINITION

Psoriasis is a common chronic inflammatory disease characterized by recurrent exacerbations and remissions of thickened, erythematous, and scaling plaques.

▶ PATHOPHYSIOLOGY

- Cell-mediated immune mechanisms play a central role in psoriasis. Cutaneous inflammatory T-cell-mediated immune activation requires two T-cell signals mediated via cell-cell interactions by surface proteins and antigen-presenting cells (APC) such as dendritic cells or macrophages. The first signal is the interaction of the T-cell receptor with antigen presented by APC. The second signal (called *costimulation*) is mediated through various surface interactions.
- Once T cells are activated, they migrate from lymph nodes and the bloodstream into skin and secrete various cytokines (primarily interferon-Υ and interleukin-2) that induce the pathologic changes of psoriasis. Local keratinocytes and neutrophils are induced to produce other cytokines, including tumor necrosis factor-α (TNF-α) and interleukin-8 (IL-8).
- As a result of pathogenic T-cell production and activation, psoriatic epidermal cells proliferate at a rate sevenfold faster than normal epidermal cells. Epidermal proliferation is also elevated in apparently normal skin of psoriatic patients.
- There is a significant genetic component in psoriasis. Studies of histocompatibility antigens in psoriatic patients indicate a number of significant associations, especially with HLA-Cw6, where the relative likelihood for developing psoriasis is 9 to 15 times normal.
- Climate, stress, alcohol, smoking, infection, trauma, and drugs may aggravate psoriasis. Warm seasons and sunlight improve psoriasis in 80% of patients, whereas 90% of patients worsen in cold weather. Psoriatic lesions may develop at the site of injury (e.g., rubbing, venipuncture, bites, surgery) on normal-appearing skin (Koebner response). Lithium carbonate, β-adrenergic blockers, some antimalarials, nonsteroidal anti-inflammatory drugs, ACE inhibitors, tetracyclines, and interferons have been reported to exacerbate psoriasis.

▶ CLINICAL PRESENTATION

- Psoriatic lesions are relatively asymptomatic, but about 25% of patients complain of pruritus.
- Lesions are characterized by sharply demarcated, erythematous papules and plaques often covered with silver-white fine scales. Initial lesions are usually small papules that enlarge over time and coalesce into plaques. If the fine scale is removed, a salmon-pink lesion is exposed, perhaps with punctate bleeding from prominent dermal capillaries (Auspitz sign).
- Scalp psoriasis ranges from diffuse scaling on an erythematous scalp to thickened plaques with exudation, microabscesses, and fissures. Trunk, back, arm, and leg lesions may be generalized, scattered, discrete, droplike lesions or large plaques. Palms, soles, face, and genitalia may also be involved. Affected nails are often pitted and associated with subungual keratotic material. Yellowing under the nail plate may be seen.

III

- Psoriatic arthritis is a distinct clinical entity in which both psoriatic lesions and inflammatory arthritis-like symptoms occur. Distal interphalangeal joints and adjacent nails are most commonly involved, but knees, elbows, wrists, and ankles may also be affected.

▶ DIAGNOSIS

- The diagnosis is based on physical examination findings of the characteristic lesions of psoriasis.
- The medical history of a patient with psoriasis should include information about the onset and duration of lesions, family history of psoriasis, presence of exacerbating factors, previous history of antipsoriatic treatment (if any) along with efficacy and adverse effect data, exposure to chemicals and toxins, and allergies (food, drugs, and environmental).
- Skin biopsy of lesional skin is useful in confirming the diagnosis.

▶ DESIRED OUTCOME

The goal of therapy is to achieve resolution of lesions, but partial clearing using regimens with decreased toxicity and increased patient acceptability is acceptable in some cases.

▶ TREATMENT

NONPHARMACOLOGIC THERAPY

- **Emollients (moisturizers)** hydrate the stratum corneum and minimize water evaporation. They may enhance desquamation, eliminate scaling, and decrease pruritus. The lotions, creams, or ointments often need to be applied up to 4 times a day to achieve a beneficial response. Adverse effects include folliculitis and allergic or irritant contact dermatitis.
- **Balneotherapy** (and **climatotherapy**) involves bathing in waters containing certain salts, often combined with natural sun exposure. The salts in certain waters (e.g., the Dead Sea) reduce activated T cells in skin and may be remittive for psoriasis.
- **Ultraviolet B (UV-B) light exposure** (290 to 320 nm) is a beneficial intervention. Use of a "narrow-band" (NB) light sources, in which 83% of the UV-B emission is at 310 to 313 nm, focuses treatment within the most effective wavelength. NB-UVB has been demonstrated to be effective in plaque-type psoriasis. Many topical and systemic therapies (discussed below) are used adjunctively to hasten and improve the response to UV-B phototherapy (e.g., short-contact anthralin with UV-B, addition of topical calcipotriene, or adding systemic methotrexate or retinoids). Emollients enhance efficacy of UV-B and may be applied just prior to UV-B treatments.

FIRST-LINE TOPICAL PHARMACOTHERAPY

Keratolytics

- **Salicylic acid** is one of the most commonly used keratolytics. It causes a disruption in corneocyte-to-corneocyte cohesion in the abnormal horny layer of psoriatic skin. This serves to remove scales, smooth the skin, and decrease hyperkeratosis. The keratolytic effect enhances penetration and efficacy of some other topical agents such as corticosteroids.
- It is applied as a 2% to 10% gel or lotion 2 or 3 times a day.

- Salicylic acid produces local irritation. Application to large, inflamed areas may induce salicylism with symptoms of nausea, vomiting, tinnitus, or hyperventilation.

Corticosteroids
See Table 16–1.

III◄

- **Topical corticosteroids** may halt synthesis and mitosis of DNA in epidermal cells and appear to inhibit phospholipase A, lowering the amounts of arachidonic acid, prostaglandins, and leukotrienes in the skin. These effects, coupled with local vasoconstriction, reduce erythema, pruritus, and scaling. As antipsoriatic agents, they are best used adjunctively with a product that specifically functions to normalize epidermal hyperproliferation.
- Low-potency products (e.g., hydrocortisone 1%) have a weak anti-inflammatory effect and are safest for long-term application, for use on the face and intertriginous areas, for use with occlusion, and for use in infants and young children.
- Medium-potency products are used in moderate inflammatory dermatoses. They may be used on the face and intertriginous areas for a limited time.
- High-potency preparations are used primarily as alternatives to systemic corticosteroids when local therapy is feasible.
- Very high potency products may be used for thick, chronic psoriatic lesions but for only short periods of time and on relatively small surface areas.
- Ointments are the most effective formulations for psoriasis because they have an occlusive oily phase that conveys a hydrating effect and enhances penetration of the corticosteroid into the dermis. They are not suited for use in the axilla, groin, or other intertriginous areas where maceration and folliculitis may develop secondary to the occlusive effect.
- Creams are more cosmetically desirable for some patients. They may be used in intertriginous areas even though their lower oil content makes them more drying than ointments.
- Topical corticosteroids are applied 2 to 4 times daily during long-term therapy.
- Adverse effects include local tissue atrophy, skin degeneration, and striae. If detected early, these effects may be reversible with discontinuation. Thinning of the epidermis may result in visibly distended capillaries (telangiectasias) and purpura. Acneiform eruptions and masking of symptoms of bacterial or fungal skin infections have been reported. Systemic consequences include risk of suppression of the hypothalamic-pituitary-adrenal axis, hyperglycemia, and development of cushingoid features. Tachyphylaxis and rebound flare of psoriasis after abrupt cessation of therapy can also occur.

Vitamin D Analogs
- Vitamin D and its analogs inhibit keratinocyte differentiation and proliferation and have anti-inflammatory effects by reducing IL-8 and IL-2. Use of vitamin D itself is limited by its propensity to cause hypercalcemia.
- **Calcipotriene** (Dovonex) is a synthetic vitamin D analog used for mild to moderate plaque psoriasis. Improvement is usually seen within 2 weeks of treatment, and approximately 70% of patients demonstrate marked improvement after 8 weeks. Adverse effects occur in about 10% of patients and include lesional and perilesional burning and stinging. Calcipotriene 0.005% cream, ointment, or solution is applied 1 or 2 times a day (no more than 100 g/wk).

TABLE 16–1. Topical Corticosteroid Products for Treating Psoriasis

Corticosteroids	Dosage Forms/Strength (%)	USP Potency Ratings[a]	Vasoconstrictive Potency Rating[b]
Alclometasone dipropionate	Cream 0.05	Low	VI
	Ointment 0.05	Low	V
Amcinonide	Lotion, ointment 0.1	High	II
	Cream 0.1	High	III
Beclomethasone dipropionate	Cream, lotion, ointment 0.025	Medium	—
Betamethasone benzoate	Cream, gel 0.025	Medium	III
	Ointment 0.025	Medium	IV
Betamethasone dipropionate	Cream AF (optimized vehicle) 0.05	Very high	I
	Cream 0.05	High	III
	Gel, lotion, ointment (optimized vehicle) 0.05	Very high	I
	Lotion 0.05	High	V
	Ointment 0.05	High	II
	Topical aerosol 0.1	High	—
Betamethasone valerate	Cream 0.01, 0.05, 0.1	Medium	V
	Lotion, ointment 0.05, 0.1	Medium	III
	Foam 0.12	Medium	IV
Clobetasol propionate	Cream, ointment, solution, foam 0.05	Very high	I
Clobetasol butyrate	Cream, ointment 0.05	Medium	—
Clocortolone pivalate	Cream 0.1	Low	—
Desonide	Cream, lotion, ointment 0.05	Low	VI
Desoximetasone	Cream 0.05	Medium	II
	Cream, ointment 0.25	High	II
	Gel 0.05	High	II
Dexamethasone	Gel 0.1	Low	VII
	Topical aerosol 0.01, 0.04	Low	VII
Dexamethasone sodium phosphate	Cream 0.1	Low	VII
Diflorasone diacetate	Cream 0.05	High	III
	Ointment 0.05	High	II
	Ointment (optimized vehicle) 0.05	Very high	II
Diflucortolone valerate	Cream, ointment 0.1	Medium	—
Flumethasone pivalate	Cream, ointment 0.03	Low	—
Fluocinolone acetonide	Cream 0.01	Medium	VI
	Cream 0.025	Medium	V
	Cream 0.2	High	—
	Ointment 0.025	Medium	IV
	Solution 0.01	Medium	VI
Fluocinonide	Gel, cream, ointment 0.05	High	II
	Solution 0.05	High	II
Flurandrenolide	Cream, ointment 0.0125	Low	—
	Ointment 0.05	Medium	IV
	Cream, lotion 0.05	Medium	V
	Tape 4 mcg/cm²	Medium	I
Fluticasone propionate	Cream 0.05	Medium	IV
	Ointment 0.05	Medium	III
Halcinonide	Cream 0.025, 0.1	High	II
	Ointment 0.1	High	III
	Solution 0.1	High	—

Continued

TABLE 16–1. (Continued)

Corticosteroids	Dosage Forms/Strength (%)	USP Potency Ratings[a]	Vasoconstrictive Potency Rating[b]
Halobetasol propionate	Cream, ointment 0.05	Very high	I
Hydrocortisone	Cream, lotion, ointment All strengths	Low	VII
Hydrocortisone acetate	Cream, lotion, ointment All strengths	Low	VII
Hydrocortisone butyrate	Cream 0.1	Medium	V
	Ointment 0.1	Medium	—
Hydrocortisone valerate	Cream 0.2	Medium	V
	Ointment 0.2	Medium	IV
Methylprednisolone acetate	Cream, ointment 0.25	Low	VII
	Ointment 1	Low	VII
Mometasone furoate	Cream 0.1	Medium	IV
	Lotion, ointment 0.1	Medium	II
Triamcinolone acetonide	Cream, ointment 0.1	Medium	IV
	Cream, lotion, ointment 0.025	Medium	—
	Cream (Aristocort) 0.1	Medium	VI
	Cream (Kenalog) 0.1	High	IV
	Lotion 0.1	Medium	V
	Ointment (Aristocort, Kenalog) 0.1	High	III
	Cream, ointment 0.5	High	III
	Topical aerosol 0.015	Medium	—

[a]USP ratings are low, medium, high, and very high.
[b]Vasoconstriction potency scale is I (highest) to VII (lowest);—denotes unknown vasoconstrictive properties.

- Calcitriol and tacalcitol are other vitamin D derivatives that have been studied for treatment of psoriasis.

Tazarotene

- **Tazarotene** (Tazorac) is a synthetic retinoid that is hydrolyzed to its active metabolite, tazarotenic acid, which modulates keratinocyte proliferation and differentiation.
- It is available as a 0.05% or 0.1% gel and cream and is applied once daily (usually in the evening) for mild to moderate plaque psoriasis. The 0.1% gel is somewhat more effective, but the 0.05% gel causes less irritation.
- Adverse effects are dose- and frequency-related and include mild to moderate pruritus, burning, stinging, and erythema.
- Application of the gel to eczematous skin or to more than 20% of body surface area is not recommended because this may lead to extensive systemic absorption.
- Tazarotene is often used with topical corticosteroids to decrease local adverse effects and increase efficacy.

SECOND-LINE TOPICAL PHARMACOTHERAPY

Coal Tar

- **Coal tar** contains numerous hydrocarbon compounds formed from distillation of bituminous coal. Ultraviolet B (UV-B) light–activated coal tar photoadducts with epidermal DNA and inhibits DNA synthesis. This normalized epidermal replication rate reduces plaque elevation.

169

III

- Coal tar preparations of 2% to 5% tar are available in lotions, creams, shampoos, ointments, gels, and solutions. It is usually applied directly to lesions in the evening and allowed to remain in skin contact through the night. It may also be used in bath water.
- Coal tar is an effective treatment, but it is time-consuming, causes local irritation, has an unpleasant odor, stains skin and clothing, and increases sensitivity to UV light (including the sun).
- The risk of carcinogenicity is low but there are cases indicating a higher rate of nonmyeloma skin cancers in patients chronically exposed to coal tar and UV light.

Anthralin

- **Anthralin** possesses antiproliferative activity on keratinocytes, inhibiting DNA synthesis by intercalation between DNA strands.
- Because anthralin exerts its clinical effects at low cellular concentrations, therapy usually starts with low concentrations (0.1% to 0.25%) with gradual increases to higher concentrations (0.5% to 1%). Cream and ointment formulations are usually applied in the evening and allowed to remain overnight.
- Alternatively, short-contact anthralin therapy (SCAT) with application for 10 to 20 minutes of higher concentrations (1% to 5%) in water-soluble vehicles is effective with decreased local adverse effects.
- Anthralin products must be applied only to affected areas because contact with uninvolved skin may result in excessive irritation and staining, which usually disappears within 1 to 2 weeks of discontinuation. Staining of affected plaques indicates a positive response because cell turnover has been slowed enough to take up the stain.
- Inflammation, irritation, and staining of skin and clothing are often therapy-limiting effects.

FIRST-LINE SYSTEMIC PHARMACOTHERAPY

See Table 16–2.

Acitretin

- **Acitretin** (Soriatane) is a retinoic acid derivative and the active metabolite of etretinate. It is indicated for severe psoriasis, including erythrodermic and generalized pustular types. However, it is more useful as an adjunct in the treatment of plaque psoriasis.
- It has shown good results when combined with other therapies, including PUVA and UV-B, cyclosporine, and methotrexate.
- The initial recommended dose is 25 or 50 mg; therapy is continued until lesions have resolved.
- Selected adverse effects are included in Table 16–2.
- Acitretin is a teratogen and is contraindicated in females who are pregnant or who plan pregnancy within 3 years after drug discontinuation.

SECOND-LINE SYSTEMIC PHARMACOTHERAPY

See Table 16–2.

- **Cyclosporine** demonstrates immunosuppressive activity by inhibiting the first phase of T-cell activation. It also inhibits release of inflammatory mediators from mast cells, basophils, and polymorphonuclear cells. It is used in the treatment of both cutaneous and arthritis manifestations of severe psoriasis.

TABLE 16–2. Systemic Psoriasis Treatment Guidelines

Active Ingredient	Regimen	Selected Adverse Effects
Acitretin	25–50 mg/day until lesions have resolved. Food enhances absorption and tolerability	Hypervitaminosis A (dry lips/cheilitis, dry mouth, dry nose, dry eyes/conjunctivitis, dry skin, pruritus, scaling, and hair loss), hepatotoxicity, skeletal changes, hypercholesterolemia, hypertriglyceridemia
Cyclosporine	2.5–4 mg/kg/day in 2 divided doses; may increase to 5 mg/kg/day in 1 month if no response	Nephrotoxicity, malignancies, hypertension, hypomagnesemia, hyperkalemia, alterations in liver function tests, elevations of serum lipids, gastrointestinal intolerance, paresthesias, hypertrichosis, gingival hyperplasia
Methotrexate	7.5–15 mg/wk, increased incrementally by 2.5 mg every 2 to 4 wk until response; maximal doses are approximately 25 mg/wk	Anemia, leukopenia, thrombocytopenia, hepatotoxicity, gastrointestinal upset, nausea, vomiting, mucosal ulceration, stomatitis, malaise, headaches, pulmonary toxicity
Tacrolimus	0.05 mg/kg daily, with increases to 0.10 mg/kg daily at 3 wk and to 0.15 mg/kg daily at 6 wk, depending on results	Nephrotoxicity, immunosuppression, gastrointestinal upset, diarrhea, nausea, paresthesias, hypertension, tremor, insomnia
Mycophenolate mofetil	500 mg 4 times a day, up to maximum of 4 g/day	Gastrointestinal toxicity (diarrhea, nausea, vomiting), hematologic effects (anemia, neutropenia, thrombocytopenia), viral and bacterial infections; lymphoproliferative disease or lymphoma can occur
Sulfasalazine	3–4 g/day for 8 wk	Gastrointestinal upset
6-Thioguanine	80 mg twice weekly, increased by 20 mg every 2–4 wk; maximum dose 160 mg 3 times a week	Bone marrow suppression; gastrointestinal complications including nausea and diarrhea; elevation of liver function tests
Hydroxyurea	1 g/day; may increase to 2 g/day	Bone marrow toxicity with leukopenia or thrombocytopenia, cutaneous reactions, leg ulcers, megaloblastic anemia
Infliximab	5 or 10 mg/kg for three intravenous infusions at weeks 0, 2, and 6	Headaches, fever, chills, fatigue, diarrhea, pharyngitis, upper respiratory and urinary tract infections; hypersensitivity reactions (urticaria, dyspnea, hypotension); lymphoproliferative disorders
Etanercept	50 mg subcutaneously twice a week	Local reaction at the injection site (20% of patients); respiratory tract and gastrointestinal infections, abdominal pain, nausea and vomiting, headaches, rash; serious infections (including tuberculosis) and malignancies are rare
Alefacept	15 mg intramuscularly once weekly	Pharyngitis, influenza-like symptoms, chills, dizziness, nausea, headache, injection site pain and inflammation, and nonspecific infection; opportunistic infections and malignancy are rare
Efalizumab	1 mg/kg subcutaneously once weekly	Headache, nausea, chills, nonspecific infection, pain, fever, and asthenia; no evidence drug causes organ toxicity, serious infection, or malignancy

The dosage regimen and adverse effects are included in Table 16–2. Cumulative treatment for more than 2 years may increase the risk of malignancy, including skin cancers and lymphoproliferative disorders.

- **Methotrexate**, an antimetabolite, is indicated for moderate to severe psoriasis. It is particularly beneficial for psoriatic arthritis. It is also indicated for patients refractory to topical or ultraviolet therapy. Methotrexate can be administered orally, subcutaneously, or intramuscularly. The dosage regimen and adverse effects are included in Table 16–2. Nausea and macrocytic anemia can be ameliorated by giving oral folic acid 1 to 5 mg/day. Methotrexate should be avoided in patients with active infections and in those with liver disease. It is contraindicated in pregnancy because it is teratogenic.

- **Tacrolimus**, an immunosuppressant that inhibits T-cell activation, is a useful alternative in severe recalcitrant psoriasis. The dosage regimen and adverse effects are included in Table 16–2.

- **Mycophenolate mofetil** (CellCept) inhibits DNA and RNA synthesis and has been shown to have a specific lymphocyte antiproliferative effect. It is used as part of combination therapy in moderate to severe psoriasis and other autoimmune dermatoses. The dosage regimen and adverse effects are included in Table 16–2.

- **Sulfasalazine** is an anti-inflammatory agent that inhibits 5-lipoxygenase. It is used selectively as an alternative treatment, particularly in patients with concurrent psoriatic arthritis. When used alone, it is not as effective as methotrexate, PUVA, or acitretin. However, it has a relatively high margin of safety. The dosage regimen and adverse effects are included in Table 16–2.

- **6-Thioguanine** is a purine analog that has been used as an alternative treatment for psoriasis when conventional therapies have failed. See Table 16–2 for usual dosing and adverse effects. It may be less hepatotoxic and therefore more useful than methotrexate in hepatically compromised patients with severe psoriasis.

- **Hydroxyurea** inhibits cell synthesis in the S phase of the DNA cycle. It is used selectively in the treatment of psoriasis, especially in those with liver disease who would be at risk of adverse effects with other agents. However, it is less effective than methotrexate. Table 16–2 provides the usual dosing regimen and adverse effects.

BIOLOGIC THERAPY

- **Infliximab** (Remicade) is a chimeric monoclonal antibody directed against TNF-α. It was not FDA-approved for the treatment of psoriasis at the time of this writing. One study in moderate to severe psoriasis reported a good response in 82% and 91% of patients treated with 5 mg/kg or 10 mg/kg. Table 16–2 contains dosing recommendations and adverse effects of infliximab. An advantage over other systemic psoriasis treatment is that infliximab does not adversely affect blood counts, hepatic enzyme levels, or kidney function.

- **Etanercept** (Enbrel) is a fusion protein that binds TNF-α, competitively interfering with its interaction with cell-bound receptors. Unlike the chimeric infliximab, etanercept is fully humanized, thereby minimizing the risk of immunogenicity. Etanercept is FDA-approved for reducing signs and symptoms and inhibiting the progression of joint damage in patients with psoriatic arthritis. It can be used in combination with methotrexate in patients who do not respond adequately to methotrexate alone. It is also indicated for adult patients with chronic moderate to severe plaque psoriasis who are candidates for systemic therapy or phototherapy. The recommended dose for adults with psoriatic arthritis is 50 mg subcutaneously once a week. The recommended starting dose for adults with plaque psoriasis is 50 mg subcutaneously twice weekly (administered 3 or 4 days apart) for 3 months followed by a maintenance dose of 50 mg/wk. Selected adverse effects are listed in Table 16–2.

- **Alefacept** (Amevive) is a dimeric fusion protein that binds to CD2 on T cells to inhibit cutaneous T-cell activation and proliferation. It also produces a dose-dependent decrease in circulating total lymphocytes. Alefacept is approved for treatment of moderate to severe plaque psoriasis and is also effective for treatment of psoriatic arthritis. Significant response is usually achieved after about 3 months of therapy. The recommended dose is 15 mg intramuscularly once weekly for 12 weeks. See Table 16–2 for selected adverse effects.

- **Efalizumab** (Raptiva) is a humanized monoclonal antibody that inhibits CD11-α integrin, which is involved in T-cell activation, migration into skin, and cytotoxic function. It is approved for adults with chronic moderate to severe plaque psoriasis who are candidates for systemic therapy or phototherapy. The recommended dose is a single 0.7 mg/kg subcutaneous conditioning dose followed by weekly subcutaneous doses of 1 mg/kg (200 mg maximum single dose). Selective adverse effects are given in Table 16–2.

PHOTOCHEMOTHERAPY

- **UV-A combined with oral methoxsalen (PUVA)** is a photochemotherapeutic approach for selected patients. Candidates for PUVA therapy usually have moderate to severe, incapacitating psoriasis unresponsive to conventional topical and systemic therapies.

- Systemic PUVA consists of oral ingestion of a potent photosensitizer such as methoxsalen (8-methoxypsoralen) at a constant dose (0.6 to 0.8 mg/kg) and variable doses of ultraviolet A (UV-A) depending on patient skin type and history of previous response to UV radiation. Two hours after ingesting psoralen, the patient is exposed to UV-A light. Photochemotherapy is performed 2 or 3 times a week. Partial clearing occurs in most patients by the twenty-fifth treatment.

- Another method that may have less carcinogenic potential is to topically deliver the photosensitizer (methoxsalen) to the skin by adding it to bath water (bath PUVA) instead of through systemic administration. Advantages of this approach include minimal risk of systemic effects, overall reduction of PUVA dose to one-fourth of that required with conventional PUVA, and reduction in the risk of nonmelanoma skin cancer.

COMBINATIONAL, ROTATIONAL, AND SEQUENTIAL THERAPY

- If monotherapy with a systemic agent does not provide optimal outcomes, combining systemic therapies with other modalities may enhance benefit. The dose of each agent may often be reduced, resulting in lower toxicity. Combinations include:
  - Acitretin + UV-B
  - Acitretin + photochemotherapy using UV-A light (PUVA)
  - Methotrexate + UV-B
  - PUVA + UV-B
  - Methotrexate + cyclosporine

- Rotational therapy involves using a biologic regimen for a limited period and then switching to a nonbiologic regimen, continuing on a rotational basis. One objective of this approach is to minimize cumulative drug toxicity.

- Sequential therapy involves rapid clearing of psoriasis with aggressive therapy (e.g., cyclosporine), followed by a transitional period in which a safer drug such as acitretin is started at maximal dosing. Subsequently, a maintenance period using acitretin in lower doses or in combination with UV-B or PUVA is continued.

III ▶ EVALUATION OF THERAPEUTIC OUTCOMES

- Patients should understand the general concepts of therapy and the importance of adherence.
- Monitoring for disease resolution and side effects is critical to a successful therapy. A positive response is noted with the normalization of involved areas of skin, as measured by reduced erythema and scaling, as well as reduction of plaque elevation.
- Achievement of efficacy by any therapeutic regimen requires days to weeks. Initial dramatic response may be achieved with some agents such as corticosteroids; however, sustained benefit with pharmacologically specific antipsoriatic therapy may require 2 to 8 weeks or longer for clinically meaningful response.

See Chapter 96, Psoriasis, authored by Dennis P. West, Lee E. West, Laura Scuderi, and Giuseppe Micaldi, for a more detailed discussion of this topic.

Chapter 17

▶ SKIN DISORDERS AND CUTANEOUS DRUG REACTIONS

▶ DEFINITION

The word *dermatitis* is a general term denoting an inflammatory erythematous rash. The disorders discussed in this chapter include contact dermatitis, seborrheic dermatitis, diaper dermatitis, and atopic dermatitis. Drug-induced skin disorders have been associated with most commonly used medications and may present as maculopapular eruptions, fixed-drug eruptions, and photosensitivity reactions.

▶ PATHOPHYSIOLOGY

- *Contact dermatitis* is an acute or chronic inflammatory skin condition resulting from contact of an inciting factor with the skin. In *allergic contact dermatitis*, an antigenic substance triggers Langerhans cells, and their immunologic responses produce the allergic skin reaction, sometimes several days later. *Irritant contact dermatitis* is caused by an organic substance that usually results in a reaction within a few hours of exposure.
- *Diaper dermatitis* (diaper rash) is an acute, inflammatory dermatitis of the buttocks, genitalia, and perineal region. The reaction is a type of contact dermatitis, as it results from direct fecal and moisture contact with the skin in an occlusive environment.
- *Atopic dermatitis* is an inflammatory condition with genetic, environmental, and immunologic mechanisms. Many immune cells have demonstrated abnormalities, including Langerhans cells, monocytes, macrophages, lymphocytes, mast cells, and keratinocytes.
- *Drug-induced cutaneous reactions* tend to be immunologic in origin and relate to hypersensitivity, but some reactions are nonallergic. The pathogenesis of fixed-drug reactions is not well understood.
- Drug-induced photosensitivity reactions are divided into *phototoxicity* (a nonimmunologic reaction) and *photoallergic reactions* (an immunologic reaction). The latter form is far less common. Medications associated with photosensitivity reactions include fluoroquinolones, nonsteroidal anti-inflammatory drugs, phenothiazines, antihistamines, estrogens, progestins, sulfonamides, sulfonylureas, thiazide diuretics, and tricyclic antidepressants.

▶ CLINICAL PRESENTATION

- The skin lesions of dermatitis may or may not be painful or pruritic. Typically, lesions are described as being less than or greater than 0.5 cm in diameter.
- *Macules* are circumscribed, flat lesions of any shape or size that differ from surrounding skin because of their color. They may result from hyperpigmentation, hypopigmentation, vascular abnormalities, capillary dilatation (erythema), or purpura.
- *Papules* are small, solid, elevated lesions less than 1 cm in diameter. They may result from metabolic deposits in the dermis, from localized dermal cellular infiltrates, or from localized hyperplasia of cellular elements in the dermis and epidermis.

III ◄

- *Plaques* are mesa-like elevations that occupy a relatively large surface area in comparison with their height above the skin surface.
- *Seborrheic dermatitis* typically occurs around the areas of skin rich in sebaceous follicles (e.g., the face, ears, scalp, and upper trunk). In infants with involvement of the scalp, the condition is commonly referred to as cradle cap.
- *Diaper dermatitis* results in erythematous patches, skin erosions, vesicles, and ulcerations. Although commonly seen in infants, it can occur in adults who wear diapers for incontinence.
- *Atopic dermatitis* in its acute phase is associated with intensely pruritic, erythematous papules and vesicles over erythematous skin. Scratching may result in excoriations and exudates. Subacute lesions are thicker, paler, scaly, erythematous and excoriated plaques. Chronic lesions are characterized by thickened plaques, accentuated skin markings (lichenification), and fibrotic papules. In all phases, the atopic skin has a dry luster.
- *Drug-induced cutaneous reactions* are unpredictable, ranging from mild, self-limiting episodes to more severe, life-threatening conditions. Selected drugs implicated in various types of skin eruptions are included in Table 17–1. *Maculopapular eruptions* are most common and often involve the trunk or pressure areas in a symmetrical fashion. Early eruptions appear within a few hours to 3 days after drug ingestion, whereas late eruptions occur up to 9 days after exposure.
- A *fixed-drug reaction* usually presents as an erythematous or hyperpigmented round or oval lesion usually between a few millimeters to 20 cm in diameter. The oral mucosa and genitalia are the most common sites involved, but lesions can appear anywhere on the body. If the patient takes the drug again, the reaction tends to recur within 30 minutes to 8 hours, often in the same location. Although this is highly indicative of a fixed-drug reaction, rechallenge should be avoided when possible.
- *Sun-induced drug eruptions* appear similar to a sunburn and present with erythema, papules, edema, and sometimes vesicles. They appear in areas exposed to sunlight (e.g., the ears, nose, cheeks, forearms, and hands).

► DIAGNOSIS

- Patient age and hormonal status in women should be considered in the initial evaluation of patients with skin disorders. Older patients are predisposed to developing psoriasis, seborrhea, and other skin conditions. Atopic dermatitis is most likely to occur in children. Menopausal women tend to develop brown hyperpigmentation, or melasma. Pregnant women may develop hyperpigmentation of the areola and genitalia as well as melasma.
- Patients presenting with a rash or skin lesion should be evaluated for potential anaphylaxis or angioedema (e.g., symptoms of difficulty in breathing, fever, nausea, vomiting).
- The area involved and the number of lesions present are important considerations. A rash involving only the arms and legs suggests a nonsystemic cause, whereas involvement of the arms, legs, and trunk indicates a systemic cause.
- Lesions should be inspected for color, texture, size, and temperature. Areas that are oozing, erythematous, and warm to the touch may be infected.
- The duration of the skin condition should be determined, and the temporal relationship with any new medications should be established.
- Assessment for potential drug-induced skin disorders begins with a comprehensive medication history, including episodes of previous drug allergies.

TABLE 17–1. Types of Drug-Induced Skin Eruptions

Clinical Presentation	Pattern and Distribution of Skin Lesions	Mucous Membrane Involvement	Implicated Drugs	Treatment
Erythema multiforme	Target lesions, limbs	Absent	Anticonvulsants (including lamotrigine), sulfonamide antibiotics, allopurinol, NSAIDs, dapsone	Supportive[a]
Stevens–Johnson syndrome	Atypical targets, widespread	Present	As above	Intravenous immunoglobulins, cyclosporine
Toxic epidermal necrolysis	Epidermal necrosis with skin detachment	Present	As above	Supportive[a]
Pseudoporphyria	Skin fragility, blister formation in photodistribution	Absent	Tetracycline, furosemide, naproxen	Supportive[a]
Linear IgA disease	Bullous dermatosis	Present or absent	Vancomycin, lithium, diclofenac, piroxicam, amiodarone	Supportive[a]
Pemphigus	Flaccid bullae, chest	Present or absent	Penicillamine, captopril, piroxicam, penicillin, rifampin	Supportive[a]
Bullous pemphigoid	Tense bullae, widespread	Present or absent	Furosemide, penicillamine, penicillins, sulfasalazine, captopril	Supportive[a]

[a]Supportive care includes administration of systemic glucocorticoids until all symptoms of active disease disappear. NSAIDs, nonsteroidal anti-inflammatory drugs.

III

- Diagnostic criteria for atopic dermatitis include the presence of pruritus with three or more of the following: (1) history of flexural dermatitis, or facial dermatitis in children younger than 10 years of age; (2) history of asthma or allergic rhinitis in the child or a first-degree relative; (3) history of generalized xerosis (dry skin) within the past year; (4) visible flexural eczema; (5) onset of rash before 2 years of age.

▶ DESIRED OUTCOME

- The goals of treatment for contact dermatitis are to relieve the patient's symptoms, identify the underlying cause, identify and remove offending agents, and avoid future exposure to likely offending agents.
- Therapeutic goals for seborrheic dermatitis are to loosen and remove scales, prevent yeast colonization, control secondary infections, and reduce itching and erythema.
- General treatment goals for patients with skin disorders are to relieve bothersome symptoms, remove precipitating factors, prevent recurrences, avoid adverse treatment effects, and improve quality of life.

▶ TREATMENT

CONTACT DERMATITIS

- Initial treatment should focus on identification and removal of the offending agent.
- Products that relieve itching, rehydrate the skin, and decrease the weeping of lesions provide some immediate relief.
- In the acute inflammatory stage, wet dressings are preferred because ointments and creams further irritate the tissue.
- Astringents such as **aluminum acetate** or **witch hazel** decrease weeping from lesions, dry out the skin, and relieve itching. They are applied as wet dressing for no longer than 7 days.
- For chronic dermatitis, lubricants, emollients, or moisturizers should be applied after bathing. Soap-free cleansers and colloidal oatmeal products also alleviate itching and soothe the skin.
- If the reaction does not subside within a few days, **topical corticosteroids** may be needed.

SEBORRHEIC DERMATITIS

- Depending on the area of the body that is affected, topical solutions or scalp shampoos may be used.
- **Selenium sulfide**, **salicylic acid**, and **coal tar** can help soften and remove scales.
- The condition responds quickly to low-potency topical corticosteroids, but judicious use is necessary to avoid long-term side effects.
- **Topical ketoconazole 2%** can help control yeast colonization.

DIAPER DERMATITIS

- Effective treatment involves frequent diaper changes and keeping the area dry.
- Lukewarm water and mild soap can be used to clean the area thoroughly, which should then be allowed to dry.
- Occlusive agents (e.g., **zinc oxide**, **titanium dioxide**, **petrolatum**) should be generously applied to the area before the clean diaper is applied.

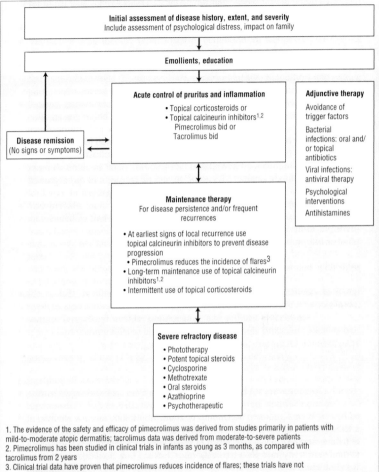

Figure 17–1. Treatment of atopic dermatitis.

ATOPIC DERMATITIS

- An algorithm for the treatment of atopic dermatitis is provided in Figure 17–1.
- Possible aggravating factors that may trigger a flare-up should be identified and avoided.
- Moisturizers, including emollients, occlusives, and humectants should be recommended based on the needs of individual patients.
- Topical corticosteroids may be used for short-term treatment of acute flare-ups (see Table 16–1 in the chapter on *Psoriasis*). Most corticosteroids are applied once or twice daily. High-potency agents are used for less than 3 weeks for flare-ups or for lichenified (thickened) lesions. Moderate-potency steroids may

be used for more chronic conditions, and low-potency steroids are usually used in children. When used in combination with other topical agents such as moisturizers, the corticosteroid should be applied first, rubbed in well, and followed by the other product.

III
- Antihistamines are frequently used, but few clinical studies support their efficacy. A sedating antihistamine (e.g., **hydroxyzine**, **diphenhydramine**) can offer an advantage by facilitating sleep because pruritus is often worse at night.
- **Doxepin** is a tricyclic antidepressant that inhibits histamine receptors. It may be helpful in atopic patients who have a component of depression. Doses of 10 to 75 mg at night and up to 75 mg twice daily have been used.
- The topical immunomodulators **tacrolimus** (Protopic) and **pimecrolimus** (Elidel) inhibit calcineurin, which normally initiatives T-cell activation. These agents can be used on all parts of the body for prolonged periods without producing corticosteroid-induced adverse effects. Tacrolimus ointment 0.03% and 0.1% is applied twice daily; the lower strength is preferred in children with moderate to severe atopic dermatitis. The most common adverse effect is transient itching and burning at the site of application. Pimecrolimus cream 1% is applied twice daily for mild to moderate atopic dermatitis in adults and children older than age 2.
- Coal tar preparations reduce itching and skin inflammation and are available as **crude coal tar** (1% to 3%) or **liquor carbonis detergens** (5% to 20%). They have been used in combination with topical corticosteroids, as adjuncts to permit effective use of lower corticosteroid strengths, and in conjunction with ultraviolet light therapies. Patients can apply the product at bedtime and wash it off in the morning. Factors limiting coal tar use include its strong odor and staining of clothing. Coal tar preparations should not be used on acute oozing lesions, which would result in stinging and irritation.

CUTANEOUS DRUG REACTIONS

- Most maculopapular reactions disappear within a few days after discontinuing the agent, so symptomatic control of the affected area is the primary intervention. Topical corticosteroids and oral antihistamines can relieve pruritus. In severe cases, a short course of systemic corticosteroids may be warranted.
- Treatment of fixed drug reactions involves removal of the offending agent. Other therapeutic measures include corticosteroids, antihistamines to relieve itching, and perhaps cool water compresses on the affected area.
- Photosensitivity reactions typically resolve with drug discontinuation. Some patients benefit from topical corticosteroids and oral antihistamines, but these are often ineffective. In some cases, systemic corticosteroids (e.g., oral **prednisone** 1 mg/kg/day tapered over 3 weeks) is more effective.

▶ EVALUATION OF THERAPEUTIC OUTCOMES

- Information regarding causative factors, avoidance of substances that trigger skin reactions, and the potential benefits and limitations of nondrug and drug therapy should be conveyed to patients.
- Patients with chronic skin conditions should be evaluated periodically to assess disease control, the efficacy of current therapy, and the presence of possible adverse effects.

See Chapter 94, Dermatologic Drug Reactions, Self-Treatable Skin Disorders, and Skin Cancer; and Chapter 97, Atopic Dermatitis, both authored by Nina H. Cheigh, for a more detailed discussion of this topic.

Endocrinologic Disorders
Edited by Terry L. Schwinghammer

Chapter 18

▶ DIABETES MELLITUS

▶ DEFINITION

Diabetes mellitus (DM) is a group of metabolic disorders characterized by hyperglycemia and abnormalities in carbohydrate, fat, and protein metabolism. It results from defects in insulin secretion, insulin sensitivity, or both. Chronic microvascular, macrovascular, and neuropathic complications may ensue.

▶ PATHOPHYSIOLOGY

- Type 1 DM accounts for up to 10% of all diabetes cases. It generally develops in childhood or early adulthood and results from immune-mediated destruction of pancreatic β cells, resulting in an absolute deficiency of insulin. There is a long preclinical period (up to 9 to 13 years) marked by the presence of immune markers when β-cell destruction is thought to occur. Hyperglycemia occurs when 80% to 90% of β cells are destroyed. There is a transient remission ("honeymoon" phase) followed by established disease with associated risks for complications and death. The factors that initiate the autoimmune process are unknown, but the process is mediated by macrophages and T lymphocytes with circulating autoantibodies to various β-cell antigens (e.g., islet cell antibody, insulin antibodies).

- Type 2 DM accounts for as many as 90% of DM cases and is usually characterized by the presence of both insulin resistance and relative insulin deficiency. Insulin resistance is manifested by increased lipolysis and free fatty acid production, increased hepatic glucose production, and decreased skeletal muscle uptake of glucose. β-Cell dysfunction is progressive and contributes to worsening blood glucose control over time. Type 2 DM occurs when a diabetogenic lifestyle (excessive calories, inadequate exercise, and obesity) is superimposed upon a susceptible genotype.

- Uncommon causes of diabetes (1% to 2% of cases) include endocrine disorders (e.g., acromegaly, Cushing's syndrome), gestational diabetes mellitus (GDM), diseases of the exocrine pancreas (e.g., pancreatitis), and medications (e.g., glucocorticoids, pentamidine, niacin, and α-interferon).

- Impaired fasting glucose and impaired glucose tolerance are terms used to describe patients whose plasma glucose levels are higher than normal but not diagnostic of DM (see DIAGNOSIS). These disorders are risk factors for developing DM and cardiovascular disease and are associated with the insulin-resistance syndrome.

- Microvascular complications include retinopathy, neuropathy, and nephropathy. Macrovascular complications include coronary heart disease, stroke, and peripheral vascular disease.

▶ CLINICAL PRESENTATION

TYPE 1 DM

- Individuals with type 1 DM are often thin and are prone to develop diabetic ketoacidosis (DKA) if insulin is withheld or under conditions of severe stress with an excess of insulin counterregulatory hormones.

- Between 20% and 40% of patients present with DKA after several days of polyuria, polydipsia, polyphagia, and weight loss.

TYPE 2 DM

- Patients with type 2 DM are often asymptomatic and may be diagnosed secondary to unrelated blood testing. However, the presence of complications may indicate that they have had DM for several years.
- Lethargy, polyuria, nocturia, and polydipsia can be seen on diagnosis; significant weight loss is less common.

IV

▶ DIAGNOSIS

- Screening for type 2 DM should be performed every 3 years in all adults beginning at the age of 45. Testing should be considered at an earlier age and more frequently in individuals with risk factors (e.g., family history of DM, obesity, habitual physical inactivity).
- The recommended screening test is a fasting plasma glucose (FPG). Normal FPG is less than 100 mg/dL.
- Impaired fasting glucose (IFG) is defined as FPG of at least 110 mg/dL but less than 126 mg/dL.
- Impaired glucose tolerance (IGT) is diagnosed when the 2-hour postload sample of the oral glucose tolerance test (OGTT) is 140 mg/dL or greater but less than 200 mg/dL.
- The diagnostic criteria for DM are contained in Table 18–1.
- Pregnant women should undergo risk assessment for GDM at their first prenatal visit and proceed with glucose testing if at high risk (e.g., marked obesity, personal history of GDM, glycosuria, or a strong family history of DM).

▶ DESIRED OUTCOME

- The goals of therapy in DM are to ameliorate symptoms of hyperglycemia, reduce the onset and progression of microvascular and macrovascular complications, reduce mortality, and improve quality of life. Desirable plasma glucose and glycosylated hemoglobin (HbA$_{1c}$) levels are listed in Table 18–2.

TABLE 18–1. Criteria for the Diagnosis of Diabetes Mellitus[a]

Symptoms of diabetes plus casual[b] plasma glucose concentration ≥200 mg/dL
or
Fasting[c] plasma glucose ≥126 mg/dL
or
2-h postload glucose ≥200 mg/dL during an OGTT[d]

[a]In the absence of unequivocal hyperglycemia, these criteria should be confirmed by repeat testing on a different day. The third measure (oral glucose tolerance test; OGTT) is not recommended for routine clinical use.
[b]Casual is defined as any time of day without regard to time since last meal. The classic symptoms of diabetes include polyuria, polydipsia, and unexplained weight loss.
[c]Fasting is defined as no caloric intake for at least 8 h.
[d]The test should be performed as described by the World Health Organization, using a glucose load containing the equivalent of 75 g anhydrous glucose dissolved in water.

TABLE 18–2. Glycemic Goals of Therapy

Biochemical Index	ADA	ACE and AACE
Hemoglobin A_{1c}	<7%[a]	≤6.5%
Preprandial plasma glucose	90–130 mg/dL	<110 mg/dL
Postprandial plasma glucose	<180 mg/dL[b]	<140 mg/dL

[a]Referenced to a nondiabetic range of 4.0%–6.0% using a DCCT-based assay. More stringent glycemic goals (i.e., a normal HbA_{1c}, <6%) may further reduce complications at the cost of increased risk of hypoglycemia (particularly in those with type 1 diabetes).

[b]Postprandial glucose measurements should be made 1–2 h after the beginning of the meal, generally the time of peak levels in patients with diabetes.

ADA, American Diabetes Association; ACE, American College of Endocrinology; AACE, American Association of Clinical Endocrinologists; DCCT, Diabetes Control and Complications Trial.

IV

▶ TREATMENT

GENERAL PRINCIPLES

- Near-normal glycemia reduces the risk of microvascular disease complications, but aggressive management of traditional cardiovascular risk factors (i.e., smoking cessation, treatment of dyslipidemia, intensive blood pressure control, antiplatelet therapy) is needed to reduce macrovascular disease risk.
- Appropriate care requires goal setting for glycemia, blood pressure, and lipid levels; regular monitoring for complications; dietary and exercise modifications; appropriate self-monitoring of blood glucose (SMBG); and appropriate assessment of laboratory parameters.

NONPHARMACOLOGIC THERAPY

- Medical nutrition therapy is recommended for all patients. For individuals with type 1 DM, the focus is on regulating insulin administration with a balanced diet to achieve and maintain a healthy body weight. Most patients require a meal plan that is moderate in carbohydrates and low in saturated fat, with a focus on balanced meals. In addition, patients with type 2 DM often require caloric restriction to promote weight loss. Bedtime and between-meal snacks are not usually needed if pharmacologic management is appropriate.
- Most patients benefit from increased physical activity. Aerobic exercise can improve insulin resistance and glycemic control and may reduce cardiovascular risk factors, contribute to weight loss or maintenance, and improve well-being. Exercise should be started slowly in previously sedentary patients. Older patients and those with atherosclerotic disease should have a cardiovascular evaluation prior to beginning a substantial exercise program.

PHARMACOLOGIC THERAPY

Insulin

- Characteristics commonly used to categorize insulins include source, strength, onset time, and duration of action (Tables 18–3 and 18–4). Manufacturers in the United States exclusively use recombinant DNA techniques to manufacture insulin. Insulin analogs are preparations that have amino acids within the insulin molecule modified to impart particular physiochemical and pharmacokinetic advantages.
- **Regular insulin** has a relatively slow onset of action when given subcutaneously, requiring injection 30 minutes prior to meals to achieve optimal postprandial glucose control and to prevent delayed postmeal hypoglycemia.

TABLE 18–3. Available Insulin Preparations

Generic Name	Analog[a]	Administration Options
Rapid-acting insulins		
Humalog (insulin lispro)	Yes	Insulin pen, vial, or 1.5-mL and 3-mL pen cartridge
NovoLog (insulin aspart)	Yes	Insulin pen, vial, or 3-mL pen cartridge
Apidra (insulin glulisine[c])	Yes	Vial
Short-acting insulins		
Humulin R (regular)	No	U-100, 10-mL vial
Available in: U-100 and U-500		U-500, 20-mL vial
Novolin R (regular)	No	Insulin pen, vial, or 3-mL pen cartridge, and InnoLet[c]
Intermediate-acting insulins		
NPH		
Humulin N	No	Vial, prefilled pen
Novolin N	No	Vial, prefilled pen, and InnoLet[c]
Lente		
Humulin L	No	Vial
Long-acting insulins		
Humulin U (ultralente)	No	Vial
Lantus (insulin glargine)	Yes	Vial
Pre-mixed insulins		
Pre-mixed insulin analogs		
Humalog Mix 75/25 (75% neutral protamine lispro, 25% lispro)	Yes	Vial, prefilled pen
Novolog Mix 70/30 (70% aspart protamine suspension, 30% aspart)	Yes	Vial, prefilled pen, 3-mL pen cartridge
NPH-regular combinations		
Humulin 70/30	No	Vial, prefilled pen
Novolin 70/30	No	Vial, pen cartridge, innoLet[c]
Humulin 50/50	No	Vial

[a]All insulins available in the US are now made by human recombinant DNA technology. An insulin analog is a modified human insulin molecule that imparts particular pharmacokinetic advantages.

[b]Room temperature defined as 59–86°F.

[c]InnoLet: A prefilled insulin pen with a "kitchen timer" type of dial for determining the number of insulin units. May be useful in patients with impaired eyesight or dexterity.

TABLE 18–4. Pharmacokinetics of Various Insulins Administered Subcutaneously

Type of Insulin	Onset (h)	Peak (h)	Duration (h)	Maximum Duration (h)	Appearance
Rapid-acting					
Aspart	15–30 min	1–2	3–5	5–6	Clear
Lispro	15–30 min	1–2	3–4	4–6	Clear
Glulisine	15–30 min	1–2	3–4	5–6	Clear
Short-acting					
Regular	0.5–1.0	2–3	3–6	6–8	Clear
Intermediate-acting					
NPH	2–4	4–6	8–12	14–18	Cloudy
Lente	3–4	6–12	12–18	20	Cloudy
Long-acting					
Ultralente	6–10	10–16	18–20	24	Cloudy
Glargine	4–5	—	22–24	24	Clear

- **Lispro, aspart,** and **glulisine insulins** are analogs that are more rapidly absorbed, peak faster, and have shorter durations of action than regular insulin. This permits more convenient dosing within 10 minutes of meals (rather than 30 minutes prior), produces better efficacy in lowering postprandial blood glucose than regular insulin in type 1 DM, and minimizes delayed postmeal hypoglycemia.
- **NPH** and **Lente insulins** are intermediate-acting and **Ultralente insulin** is long-acting. Variability in absorption, inconsistent preparation by the patient, IV◄ and inherent pharmacokinetic differences may contribute to a labile glucose response, nocturnal hypoglycemia, and fasting hyperglycemia.
- **Insulin glargine** is a long-acting "peakless" human insulin analog that was developed to obviate the disadvantages of other intermediate- and long-acting insulins. It results in less nocturnal hypoglycemia than NPH insulin when given at bedtime.
- In type 1 DM, the average daily insulin requirement is 0.5 to 0.6 units/kg. Requirements may fall to 0.1 to 0.4 units/kg in the honeymoon phase. Higher doses (0.5 to 1 unit/kg) are warranted during acute illness or ketosis. In type 2 DM, a dosage range of 0.7 to 2.5 units/kg is often required for patients with significant insulin resistance.
- Hypoglycemia and weight gain are the most common adverse effect of insulin. Treatment of hypoglycemia is as follows:
  - **Glucose** (10 to 15 g) given orally is the recommended treatment in conscious patients.
  - **Dextrose** IV may be required in individuals who have lost consciousness.
  - **Glucagon,** 1 g IM, is the treatment of choice in unconscious patients when IV access cannot be established.

Sulfonylureas
See Table 18–5.

- Sulfonylureas exert a hypoglycemic action by stimulating pancreatic secretion of insulin. All sulfonylureas are equally effective in lowering blood glucose when administered in equipotent doses. On average, the HbA_{1c} will fall by 1.5% to 2% with FPG reductions of 60 to 70 mg/dL.
- The most common side effect is hypoglycemia, which is more problematic with long half-life drugs. Individuals at high risk include the elderly, those with renal insufficiency or advanced liver disease, and those who skip meals, exercise vigorously, or lose a substantial amount of weight. Weight gain is common; less common adverse effects include skin rash, hemolytic anemia, gastrointestinal upset, and cholestasis. Hyponatremia is most common with chlorpropamide but has also been reported with tolbutamide.
- The recommended starting doses (Table 18–5) should be reduced in elderly patients who may have compromised renal or hepatic function. Dosage can be titrated every 1 to 2 weeks (longer interval with chlorpropamide) to achieve glycemic goals.

Short-Acting Insulin Secretagogues (Meglitinides)
- Similar to sulfonylureas, meglitinides lower glucose by stimulating pancreatic insulin secretion, but insulin release is glucose dependent and diminishes at low blood glucose concentrations. Hypoglycemic risk appears to be less with meglitinides than with sulfonylureas. The average reduction in HbA_{1c} is 0.6% to 1%. These agents can be used to provide increased insulin secretion during meals (when it is needed) in patients who are close to glycemic goals. They

TABLE 18–5. Oral Agents for the Treatment of Type 2 Diabetes Mellitus

Generic Name (generic version available? Y = yes, N = no)	Brand	Dose (mg)	Recommended Starting Dosage (mg/day) Nonelderly	Recommended Starting Dosage (mg/day) Elderly	Equivalent Therapeutic Dose (mg)	Maximum Dose (mg/day)	Duration of Action	Metabolism or Therapeutic Notes
Sulfonylureas								
Acetohexamide (Y)	Dymelor	250, 500	250	125–250	500	1500	Up to 16 h	Metabolized in liver; metabolite potency equal to parent compound; renally eliminated
Chlorpropamide (Y)	Diabinese	100, 250	250	100	250	500	Up to 72 h	Metabolized in liver; also excreted unchanged renally
Tolazamide (Y)	Tolinase	100, 250, 500	100–250	100	250	1000	Up to 24 h	Metabolized in liver; metabolite less active than parent compound; renally eliminated
Tolbutamide (Y)	Orinase	250, 500	1000–2000	500–1000	1000	3000	Up to 12 h	Metabolized in liver to inactive metabolites that are renally excreted
Glipizide (Y)	Glucotrol	5, 10	5	2.5–5	5	40	Up to 20 h	Metabolized in liver to inactive metabolites
Glipizide (N)	Glucotrol XL	2.5, 5, 10, 20	5	2.5–5	5	20	24 h	Slow-release form; do not cut tablet
Glyburide (Y)	DiaβBeta Micronase	1.25, 2.5, 5	5	1.25–2.5	5	20	Up to 24 h	Metabolized in liver; elimination 1/2 renal. 1/2 feces
Glyburide, micronized (Y)	Glynase	1.5, 3, 6	3	1.5–3	3	12	Up to 24 h	Equal control, but better absorption from micronized preparation
Glimepiride (N)	Amaryl	1, 2, 4	1–2	0.5–1	2	8	24 h	Metabolized in liver to inactive metabolites
Short-acting insulin secretagogues								
Nateglinide (N)	Starlix	60, 120	120 with meals	120 with meals	NA	120 mg 3 times a day	Up to 4 h	Metabolized by cytochrome P450 (CYP450) 2C9 and 3A4 to weakly active metabolites; renally eliminated
Repaglinide (N)	Prandin	0.5, 1, 2	0.5–1 with meals	0.5–1 with meals	NA	16	Up to 4 h	Metabolized by CYP 3A4 to inactive metabolites; excreted in bile

Biguanides								
Metformin (Y)	Glucophage	500, 850, 1000	500 mg twice a day	Assess renal function	NA	2550	Up to 24 h	No metabolism; renally secreted and excreted
Metformin extended-release (N)	Glucophage XR	500, 750 (generic available for 500 mg)	500–1000 mg with evening meal	Assess renal function	NA	2550	Up to 24 h	Take with evening meal or may split dose; may consider trial if intolerant to immediate-release
Thiazolidinediones								
Pioglitazone (N)	Actos	15, 30, 45	15	15	NA	45	24 h	Metabolized by CYP 2C8 and 3A4; two metabolites have longer half-lives than parent compound
Rosiglitazone (N)	Avandia	2, 4, 8	2–4	2	NA	8 mg/day or 4 mg twice a day	24 h	Metabolized by CYP2C8 and 2C9 to inactive metabolites that are renally excreted
α-Glucosidase inhibitors								
Acarbose (N)	Precose	25, 50, 100	25 mg 1 to 3 times a day	25 mg 1 to 3 times a day	NA	25–100 mg 3 times a day	1–3 h	Eliminated in bile
Miglitol (N)	Glyset	25, 50, 100	25 mg 1 to 3 times a day	25 mg 1 to 3 times a day	NA	25–100 mg 3 times a day	1–3 h	Eliminated renally
Combination products								
Glyburide/metformin (Y)	Glucovance	1.25/250, 2.5/500, 5/500	2.5–5/500 twice a day	1.25/250 twice a day; assess renal function	NA	20 of glyburide, 2000 of metformin	Combination medication	Use as initial therapy 1.25/250 mg twice a day
Glipizide/metformin (N)	Metaglip	2.5/250, 2.5/500, 5/500	2.5–5/500 twice a day	2.5/250; assess renal function	NA	20 of glipizide, 2000 of metformin	Combination medication	Use as initial therapy 2.5/250 mg twice a day
Rosiglitazone/metformin (N)	Avandamet	1/500, 2/500, 4/500, 2/1000, 4/1000	1–2/500 twice a day	1/500 twice a day	NA	8 of rosiglitazone; 2000 of metformin	Combination medication	FDA-approved for secondline therapy, but could be used as initial therapy

should be administered before each meal (up to 30 minutes prior). If a meal is skipped, the medication should also be skipped.

- **Repaglinide** (Prandin) is initiated at 0.5 to 2 mg with a maximum dose of 4 mg per meal (up to four meals per day or 16 mg/day).
- **Nateglinide** (Starlix) dosing is 120 mg three times daily before each meal. The dose may be lowered to 60 mg per meal in patients who are near goal HbA_{1c} when therapy is initiated.

IV Biguanides

- **Metformin** is the only biguanide available in the United States. It enhances insulin sensitivity of both hepatic and peripheral (muscle) tissues. This allows for increased uptake of glucose into these insulin-sensitive tissues. Metformin consistently reduces HbA_{1c} levels by 1.5% to 2%, FPG levels by 60 to 80 mg/dL, and retains the ability to reduce FPG levels when they are very high (greater than 300 mg/dL). It reduces plasma triglycerides and low-density lipoprotein (LDL) cholesterol by 8% to 15% and modestly increases high-density lipoprotein (HDL) cholesterol (2%). It does not induce hypoglycemia when used alone.
- Metformin should be included in the therapy for all type 2 DM patients (if tolerated and not contraindicated) because it is the only oral antihyperglycemic medication proven to reduce the risk of total mortality and cardiovascular death.
- The most common adverse effects are abdominal discomfort, stomach upset, diarrhea, anorexia, and a metallic taste. These effects can be minimized by titrating the dose slowly and taking it with food. Extended-release metformin (glucophage XR) may reduce some of the gastrointestinal side effects. Lactic acidosis occurs rarely and can be minimized by avoiding its use in patients with renal insufficiency (serum creatinine 1.4 mg/dL or greater in women and 1.5 mg/dL or greater in men), congestive heart failure, or conditions predisposing to hypoxemia or inherent lactic acidosis. Metformin should be discontinued 2 to 3 days prior to IV radiographic dye studies and withheld until normal renal function has been documented post study.
- **Metformin immediate-release** is initiated at 500 mg twice daily with meals (or 850 mg once daily) and increased by 500 mg weekly (or 850 mg every 2 weeks) to a total of 2000 mg/day. The maximum recommended dose is 2550 mg/day.
- **Metformin extended-release** (Glucophage XR) can be initiated with 500 mg with the evening meal and increased by 500 mg weekly to a maximum dose of 2000 mg/day. Administration 2 to 3 times a day may help minimize gastrointestinal side effects and improve glycemic control.

Thiazolidinediones (Glitazones)

- These agents activate PPARγ, a nuclear transcription factor important in fat cell differentiation and fatty acid metabolism. PPARγ agonists enhance insulin sensitivity in muscle, liver, and fat tissues indirectly. Insulin must be present in significant quantities for these actions to occur.
- When given for about 6 months, pioglitazone and rosiglitazone reduce HbA_{1c} values approximately by 1.5% and FPG levels by about 60 to 70 mg/dL at maximal doses. Maximal glycemic-lowering effects may not be seen until 3 to 4 months of therapy. Monotherapy is often ineffective unless the drugs are given early in the disease course when sufficient β-cell function and hyperinsulinemia are present.
- Pioglitazone decreases plasma triglycerides by 10% to 20%, whereas rosiglitazone tends to have no effect. Pioglitazone does not cause significant increases in LDL cholesterol, whereas LDL cholesterol may increase by 5% to 15% with rosiglitazone.

- Fluid retention may occur, perhaps as a result of peripheral vasodilation and/or improved insulin sensitization with a resultant increase in renal sodium and water retention. A dilutional anemia may result, which does not require treatment. Edema is reported in 4% to 5% of patients when glitazones are used alone or with other oral agents. When used in combination with insulin, the incidence of edema is about 15%. Glitazones are contraindicated in patients with NYHA Class III and IV heart failure and should be used with great caution in patients with Class I or II heart failure or other underlying cardiac disease. IV◄

- Weight gain is dose-related, and an increase of 1.5 to 4 kg is not uncommon. Rarely, rapid gain of a large amount of weight may necessitate discontinuation of therapy. Weight gain positively predicts a larger HbA$_{1c}$ reduction but must be balanced with the potential adverse effects of long-term weight gain.

- Several case reports of hepatotoxicity with pioglitazone or rosiglitazone have been reported, but improvement in ALT was consistently observed upon drug discontinuation. Baseline ALT should be obtained prior to therapy and then periodically thereafter at the practitioner's discretion. Neither drug should be started if the baseline ALT exceeds 2.5 times the upper limit of normal. The drugs should be discontinued if the ALT is more than 3 times the upper limit of normal.

- **Pioglitazone** (Actos) is started at 15 mg once daily. The maximum dose is 45 mg/day.

- **Rosiglitazone** (Avandia) is initiated with 2 to 4 mg once daily. The maximum dose is 8 mg/day. A dose of 4 mg twice daily may reduce HbA$_{1c}$ by 0.2% to 0.3%, more than a dose of 8 mg taken once daily.

α-Glucosidase Inhibitors

- These agents prevent the breakdown of sucrose and complex carbohydrates in the small intestine, thereby prolonging the absorption of carbohydrates. The net effect is a reduction in the postprandial glucose concentrations (40 to 50 mg/dL) while fasting glucose levels are relatively unchanged (about 10% reduction). Efficacy on glycemic control is modest, with average reductions in HbA$_{1c}$ of 0.3% to 1%. Good candidates for these drugs are patients who are near target HbA$_{1c}$ levels with near-normal FPG levels but high postprandial levels.

- The most common side effects are flatulence, bloating, abdominal discomfort, and diarrhea, which can be minimized by slow dosage titration. If hypoglycemia occurs when used in combination with a hypoglycemic agent (sulfonylurea or insulin), oral or parenteral glucose (dextrose) products or glucagon must be given because the drug will inhibit the breakdown and absorption of more complex sugar molecules (e.g., sucrose).

- **Acarbose** (Precose) and **miglitol** (Glyset) are dosed similarly. Therapy is initiated with a very low dose (25 mg with one meal a day) and increased very gradually (over several months) to a maximum of 50 mg three times daily for patients weighing 60 kg or more, or 100 mg three times daily for patients above 60 kg. The drugs should be taken with the first bite of the meal so that the drug is present to inhibit enzyme activity.

PHARMACOTHERAPY OF TYPE 1 DM

- All patients with type I DM require insulin, but the type and manner of delivery differ considerably among individual patients and clinicians.

- Therapeutic strategies should attempt to match carbohydrate intake with glucose-lowering processes (usually insulin) and exercise. Dietary intervention should allow the patient to live as normal a life as possible.

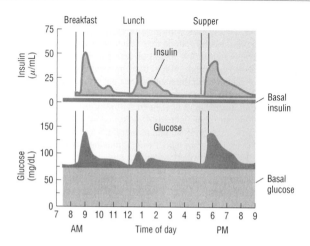

Intensive insulin therapy regimens

	7AM	11AM	5PM	HS
1. 2 doses, R + N or L	R + N or L		R + N or L	
2. 3 doses, R or rapid + N or L	R, Lis or A + N or L	R, Lis or A	R, Lis or A + N or L	
3. 4 doses, R or rapid acting + intermediate or ultralente	R, Lis or A + N, L or UL	R, Lis or A	R, Lis or A	N, L or UL
4. 4 doses, R or rapid acting + long acting	R, Lis or A	R, Lis or A	R, Lis or A	G
	←————— Adjusted Basal —————→			
5. CS-II pump	Bolus	Bolus	Bolus	

Figure 18–1. Relationship between insulin and glucose over the course of a day and how various insulin regimens could be given. A, aspart; CS-II, continuous subcutaneous insulin infusion; G, glargine; L, lente; Lis, lispro; N, NPH; R, regular; UL, ultralente.

- Figure 18–1 depicts the relationship between glucose concentrations and insulin secretion over the course of a day and how various insulin regimens may be given.
- The timing of insulin onset, peak, and duration of effect must match meal patterns and exercise schedules to achieve near-normal blood glucose values throughout the day.
- A regimen of two daily injections that may roughly approximate physiologic insulin secretion is split-mixed injections of a morning dose of **NPH insulin** and **regular insulin** before breakfast and again before the evening meal (see Figure 18–1, no. 1). This assumes that the morning NPH insulin provides basal insulin for the day and covers the midday meal, the morning regular insulin covers breakfast, the evening NPH insulin gives basal insulin for the rest of the day, and the evening regular insulin covers the evening meal. Patients may

be started on 0.6 units/kg/day, with two thirds given in the morning and one third in the evening. Intermediate-acting insulin (e.g., NPH) should comprise two thirds of the morning dose and one half of the evening dose. However, most patients are not sufficiently predictable in their schedule and food intake to allow tight glucose control with this approach. If the fasting glucose in the morning is too high, the evening NPH dose may be moved to bedtime (now three total injections per day). This may provide sufficient intensification of therapy for some patients.

IV◄

- The basal-bolus injection concept attempts to replicate normal insulin physiology by giving intermediate- or long-acting insulin as the basal component and short-acting insulin as the bolus portion (see Figure 18–1, nos. 2, 3, and 4). Intensive therapy using this approach is recommended for all adult patients at the time of diagnosis to reinforce the importance of glycemic control from the outset of treatment. Because children and prepubescent adolescents are relatively protected from microvascular complications and must be managed with a regimen that is practical for them, less intensive therapy (two injections per day of premixed insulins) is reasonable until they are postpubertal.
- The basal insulin component may be provided by once- or (more commonly) twice-daily **NPH, Lente,** or **Ultralente insulin** or once-daily **insulin glargine.** Insulin glargine is a feasible basal insulin supplement for most patients because it does not have a peak effect that must be considered in planning meals and activity with other long-acting insulins.
- The bolus insulin component is given before meals with **regular insulin, insulin lispro,** or **insulin aspart.** The rapid onset and short duration of insulin lispro and insulin aspart more closely replicate normal physiology than regular insulin, allowing the patient to vary the amount of insulin injected based on the preprandial SMBG level, upcoming activity level, and anticipated carbohydrate intake. Most patients have a prescribed dose of insulin preprandially that they vary based on an insulin algorithm. Carbohydrate counting is an effective tool for determining the amount of insulin to be injected preprandially.
- As an example, patients may begin on about 0.6 units/kg/day of insulin, with basal insulin 50% of the total dose and prandial insulin 20% of the total dose before breakfast, 15% before lunch, and 15% before dinner. Most patients require total daily doses between 0.5 and 1 unit/kg/day.
- Continuous subcutaneous insulin infusion (CSII) pump therapy (generally using **insulin lispro** to diminish aggregation) is the most sophisticated form of basal-bolus insulin delivery (see Figure 18–1, no. 5). The basal insulin dose may be varied, consistent with changes in insulin requirements throughout the day. In selected patients, this feature of CSII allows greater glycemic control. However, it requires greater attention to detail and frequency of SMBG than four injections daily.
- All patients receiving insulin should have extensive education in the recognition and treatment of hypoglycemia.

PHARMACOTHERAPY OF TYPE 2 DM

See Figure 18–2.

- Symptomatic patients may initially require insulin or combination oral therapy to reduce glucose toxicity (which may reduce β-cell insulin secretion and worsen insulin resistance).
- Patients with HbA_{1c} of about 7% or less are usually treated with therapeutic lifestyle measures with or without an insulin sensitizer. Those with HbA_{1c} above 7% but less than 8% are initially treated with a single oral agent. Patients

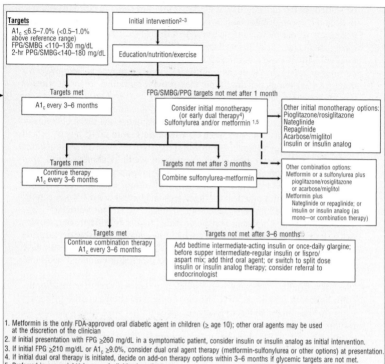

Targets
A1$_c$ ≤6.5–7.0% (<0.5–1.0% above reference range)
FPG/SMBG<110–130 mg/dL
2-hr PPG/SMBG<140–180 mg/dL

Initial intervention[2–3]

Education/nutrition/exercise

Targets met
A1$_c$ every 3–6 months

FPG/SMBG/PPG targets not met after 1 month

Consider initial monotherapy
(or early dual therapy)[4]
Sulfonylurea and/or metformin [1,5]

Other initial monotherapy options:
Pioglitazone/rosiglitazone
Nateglinide
Repaglinide
Acarbose/miglitol
Insulin or insulin analog

Targets met
Continue therapy
A1$_c$ every 3–6 months

Targets not met after 3 months
Combine sulfonylurea-metformin

Other combination options:
Metformin or a sulfonylurea plus
    pioglitazone/rosiglitazone
    or acarbose/miglitol
Metformin plus
    Nateglinide or repaglinide; or
    insulin or insulin analog (as
    mono—or combination therapy)

Targets met
Continue combination therapy
A1$_c$ every 3–6 months

Targets not met after 3–6 months

Add bedtime intermediate-acting insulin or once-daily glargine;
before supper intermediate-regular insulin or lispro/
aspart mix; add third oral agent; or switch to split dose
insulin or insulin analog therapy; consider referral to
endocrinologist

1. Metformin is the only FDA-approved oral diabetic agent in children (≥ age 10); other oral agents may be used
   at the discretion of the clinician
2. If initial presentation with FPG ≥260 mg/dL in a symptomatic patient, consider insulin or insulin analog as initial intervention.
3. If initial FPG ≥210 mg/dL or A1$_c$ ≥9.0%, consider dual oral agent therapy (metformin-sulfonylurea or other options) at presentation.
4. If initial dual oral therapy is initiated, decide on add-on therapy options within 3–6 months if glycemic targets are not met.
5. Preferred in overweight/obese or dyslipidemic patients.

Figure 18–2. Glycemic control algorithm for type 2 DM in children and adults. See *www.texasdiabetescouncil. org* for current algorithms.

with higher initial HbA$_{1c}$ values may benefit from initial therapy with two oral agents. Most patients with HbA$_{1c}$ values greater than 9% to 10% require two or more agents to reach glycemic goals.

- Obese patients (more than 120% ideal body weight) without contraindications should be started on **metformin** initially, titrated to at least 2000 mg/day. A thiazolidinedione **(rosiglitazone, pioglitazone)** may be used in patients intolerant of or having a contraindication to metformin.
- Near-normal-weight patients may be treated with **insulin secretagogues.**
- α-**Glucosidase inhibitors** may be used in patients at risk for hypoglycemia, in patients manifesting primarily postprandial hyperglycemia, and in combination with virtually any other drug.
- Failure of initial therapy should result in addition of another class of drug. Substitution of a drug from another class should be reserved for drug intolerance. Metformin and an insulin secretagogue are often first- and second-line therapy.
- Initial combination therapy should be considered for patients with HbA$_{1c}$ greater than 9% to 10%. Several oral combination products (Glucovance and Metaglip) are approved as first-line treatments.
- After a patient fails two drugs, adding a third class (usually **rosiglitazone** or **pioglitazone**) can be considered, although this triple therapy is not currently

FDA-approved. An alternative is to add **bedtime insulin,** using an intermediate- or long-acting insulin.

- Virtually all patients ultimately become insulinopenic and require insulin therapy. Patients are often transitioned to insulin by using a bedtime injection of an intermediate- or long-acting insulin with oral agents used primarily for glycemic control during the day. This results in less hyperinsulinemia during the day and less weight gain than more traditional insulin strategies. Insulin sensitizers are commonly used with insulin because most patients are insulin resistant.
- When the combination of bedtime insulin plus daytime oral medications fails, a conventional multiple daily dose insulin regimen with an insulin sensitizer can be used.
- Because of the variability of insulin resistance, insulin doses may range from 0.7 to 2.5 units/kg/day or more.
- Elderly patients with newly diagnosed type 2 DM may have less stringent glycemic goals because of the increased risk of hypoglycemia. Thinner, older patients may be treated with shorter-acting insulin secretagogues, low-dose shorter-acting sulfonylureas or α-glucosidase inhibitors. Metformin may be problematic because the risk for lactic acidosis increases with age and there is an age-related decline in renal function. Simple insulin regimens may be a desirable approach in elderly patients with newly diagnosed DM.

TREATMENT OF COMPLICATIONS

Retinopathy

- Patients with established retinopathy should be examined by an ophthalmologist at least every 6 to 12 months.
- Early background retinopathy may reverse with improved glycemic control. More advanced disease will not regress with improved control and may actually worsen with short-term improvements in glycemia.
- Laser photocoagulation has markedly improved sight preservation in diabetic patients.

Neuropathy

- Peripheral neuropathy is the most common complication in type 2 DM outpatients. Paresthesias, numbness, or pain may be predominant symptoms. The feet are involved far more often than the hands. Improved glycemic control may alleviate some of the symptoms. Pharmacologic therapy is symptomatic and empiric, including low-dose **tricyclic antidepressants,** anticonvulsants **(phenytoin, gabapentin, carbamazepine), duloxetine, venlafaxine, topical capsaicin,** and various analgesics, including **tramadol** and **nonsteroidal anti-inflammatory drugs** (NSAIDs).
- Gastroparesis can be severe and debilitating. Improved glycemic control, discontinuation of medications that slow gastric motility, and use of **metoclopramide** (preferably for only a few days at a time) or **erythromycin** may be helpful.
- Patients with orthostatic hypotension may require mineralocorticoids or adrenergic agonists.
- Diabetic diarrhea is commonly nocturnal and frequently responds to a 10- to 14-day course of an antibiotic such as **doxycycline** or **metronidazole. Octreotide** may be useful in unresponsive cases.
- Erectile dysfunction is common, and initial treatment should include one of the oral medications currently available (e.g., **sildenafil, vardenafil, tadalafil**).

Nephropathy

- Glucose and blood pressure control are most important for prevention of nephropathy, and blood pressure control is most important for retarding the progression of established nephropathy.
- **Angiotensin-converting enzyme (ACE) inhibitors** and **angiotensin receptor blockers** have shown efficacy in preventing the clinical progression of renal disease in patients with type 2 DM. **Diuretics** are frequently necessary due to volume-expanded states and are recommended second-line therapy.

IV

Peripheral Vascular Disease and Foot Ulcers

- Claudication and nonhealing foot ulcers are common in type 2 DM.
- Smoking cessation, correction of dyslipidemia, and antiplatelet therapy are important treatment strategies.
- **Pentoxifylline** (Trental) or **cilostazol** (Pletal) may be useful in selected patients.
- Revascularization is successful in selected patients.
- Local debridement and appropriate footwear and foot care are important in the early treatment of foot lesions. Topical treatments may be beneficial in more advanced lesions.

Coronary Heart Disease

- Multiple-risk-factor intervention (treatment of dyslipidemia and hypertension, smoking cessation, antiplatelet therapy) reduces macrovascular events.
- The NCEP ATP III guidelines (see Chapter 8) classify the presence of DM as a coronary heart disease (CHD) risk equivalent, and the goal LDL cholesterol is less than 100 mg/dL. After this goal is reached (usually with a **statin**), treatment of high triglycerides (200 mg/dL or higher) is considered. The non-HDL goal for patients with DM is less than 130 mg/dL. **Niacin** or a **fibrate** can be added to reach that goal if triglycerides are 201 to 499 mg/dL or if the patient has low HDL cholesterol (less than 40 mg/dL).
- The American Diabetes Association and the National Kidney Foundation recommend a goal blood pressure of less than 130/80 mm Hg in patients with DM. In patients with more than 1 g/day proteinuria and renal insufficiency, a goal of less than 125/75 mm Hg is advocated. **ACE inhibitors** and **angiotensin receptor blockers** are generally recommended for initial therapy. Many patients require multiple agents, so **diuretics**, **calcium channel blockers**, and β **blockers** are useful as second and third agents.

▶ EVALUATION OF THERAPEUTIC OUTCOMES

- The HbA_{1c} is the current standard for following long-term glycemic control for the previous 3 months. It should be measured at least twice a year in patients meeting treatment goals on a stable therapeutic regimen.
- Regardless of the insulin regimen chosen, gross adjustments in the total daily insulin dose can be made based on HbA_{1c} measurements and symptoms such as polyuria, polydipsia, and weight gain or loss. Finer insulin adjustments can be determined on the basis of the results of frequent SMBG.
- Patients receiving insulin should be questioned about the recognition of hypoglycemia at least annually. Documentation of frequency of hypoglycemia and the treatment required should be recorded.
- Patients receiving bedtime insulin should be monitored for hypoglycemia by asking about nocturnal sweating, palpitations, and nightmares, as well as the results of SMBG.

- Patients with type 2 DM should have a routine urinalysis at diagnosis as the initial screening test for albuminuria. If positive, a 24-hour urine for quantitative assessment will assist in developing a treatment plan. If the urinalysis is negative for protein, a test to evaluate the presence of microalbuminuria is recommended.
- Fasting lipid profiles should be obtained at each follow-up visit if not at goal, annually if stable and at goal, or every 2 years if the profile suggests low risk.
- Regular frequency of foot exams (each visit), urine albumin assessment (annually), dilated ophthalmologic exams (yearly or more frequently with abnormalities) should also be documented.
- Assessment for influenza and pneumococcal vaccine administration and assessment and management of other cardiovascular risk factors (e.g., smoking and antiplatelet therapy) are components of sound preventive medicine strategies.

See Chapter 72, Diabetes Mellitus, authored by Curtis L. Triplitt, Charles A. Reasner, and William L. Isley, for a more detailed discussion of this topic.

IV

Chapter 19

► THYROID DISORDERS

► DEFINITION

Thyroid disorders encompass a variety of disease states affecting thyroid hormone production or secretion that result in alterations in metabolic stability. Hyperthyroidism and hypothyroidism are the clinical and biochemical syndromes resulting from increased and decreased thyroid hormone production, respectively.

► THYROID HORMONE PHYSIOLOGY

- The thyroid hormones thyroxine (T_4) and triiodothyronine (T_3) are formed on thyroglobulin, a large glycoprotein synthesized within the thyroid cell. Inorganic iodide enters the thyroid follicular cell and is oxidized by thyroid peroxidase and covalently bound (organified) to tyrosine residues of thyroglobulin.
- The iodinated tyrosine residues monoiodotyrosine (MIT) and diiodotyrosine (DIT) combine (couple) to form iodothyronines in reactions catalyzed by thyroid peroxidase. Thus, two molecules of DIT combine to form T_4, and MIT and DIT form T_3.
- Thyroid hormone is liberated into the bloodstream by the process of proteolysis within thyroid cells. T_4 and T_3 are transported in the bloodstream by three proteins: thyroid-binding globulin (TBG), thyroid-binding prealbumin (TBPA), and albumin. Only the unbound (free) thyroid hormone is able to diffuse into the cell, elicit a biologic effect, and regulate thyroid-stimulating hormone (TSH) secretion from the pituitary.
- T_4 is secreted solely from the thyroid gland, but less than 20% of T_3 is produced there; the majority of T_3 is formed from the breakdown of T_4 catalyzed by the enzyme 5'-monodeiodinase found in peripheral tissues. T_3 is about 5 times more active than T_4.
- T_4 may also be acted on by the enzyme 5'-monodeiodinase to form reverse T_3, which has no significant biologic activity.
- Thyroid hormone production is regulated by TSH secreted by the anterior pituitary, which in turn is under negative feedback control by the circulating level of free thyroid hormone and the positive influence of hypothalamic thyrotropin-releasing hormone (TRH). Thyroid hormone production is also regulated by extrathyroidal deiodination of T_4 to T_3, which can be affected by nutrition, nonthyroidal hormones, drugs, and illness.

► THYROTOXICOSIS (HYPERTHYROIDISM)

PATHOPHYSIOLOGY

- Thyrotoxicosis results when tissues are exposed to excessive levels of T_4, T_3, or both.
- TSH-secreting pituitary tumors release biologically active hormone that is unresponsive to normal feedback control. The tumors may co-secrete prolactin or growth hormone; therefore, patients may present with amenorrhea, galactorrhea, or signs of acromegaly.
- In Graves' disease, hyperthyroidism results from the action of thyroid-stimulating antibodies (TSAb) directed against the thyrotropin receptor on the surface of the thyroid cell. These immunoglobulin G (IgG) antibodies bind

to the receptor and activate the enzyme adenylate cyclase in the same manner as TSH.

- An autonomous thyroid nodule (toxic adenoma) is a discrete thyroid mass whose function is independent of pituitary control. Hyperthyroidism usually occurs with larger nodules (i.e., those greater than 4 cm in diameter).
- In multinodular goiters (Plummer's disease), follicles with a high degree of autonomous function coexist with normal or even nonfunctioning follicles. Thyrotoxicosis occurs when the autonomous follicles generate more thyroid hormone than is required.
- Painful subacute (DeQuervain's) thyroiditis is believed to be caused by viral invasion of thyroid parenchyma.
- Painless (silent, lymphocytic, postpartum) thyroiditis is a common cause of thyrotoxicosis; its etiology is not fully understood and may be heterogeneous.
- Thyrotoxicosis factitia is hyperthyroidism produced by the ingestion of exogenous thyroid hormone. This may occur when **thyroid hormone** is used for inappropriate indications, when excessive doses are used for accepted medical indications, or when it is used surreptitiously by patients.
- **Amiodarone** may induce thyrotoxicosis (2% to 3% of patients) or hypothyroidism. It interferes with type I $5'$-deiodinase, leading to reduced conversion of T_4 to T_3, and iodide release from the drug may contribute to iodine excess. Amiodarone also causes a destructive thyroiditis with loss of thyroglobulin and thyroid hormones.

CLINICAL PRESENTATION

- Symptoms of thyrotoxicosis include nervousness, anxiety, palpitations, emotional lability, easy fatigability, heat intolerance, loss of weight concurrent with an increased appetite, increased frequency of bowel movements, proximal muscle weakness (noted on climbing stairs or arising from a sitting position), and scanty or irregular menses in women.
- Physical signs of thyrotoxicosis may include warm, smooth, moist skin and unusually fine hair; separation of the ends of the fingernails from the nail beds (onycholysis); retraction of the eyelids and lagging of the upper lid behind the globe upon downward gaze (lid lag); tachycardia at rest, a widened pulse pressure, and a systolic ejection murmur; occasional gynecomastia in men; a fine tremor of the protruded tongue and outstretched hands; and hyperactive deep tendon reflexes.
- Graves' disease is manifested by hyperthyroidism, diffuse thyroid enlargement, and the extrathyroidal findings of exophthalmos, pretibial myxedema, and thyroid acropachy. The thyroid gland is usually diffusely enlarged, with a smooth surface and consistency varying from soft to firm. In severe disease, a thrill may be felt and a systolic bruit may be heard over the gland.
- In subacute thyroiditis, patients complain of severe pain in the thyroid region, which often extends to the ear on the affected side. Low-grade fever is common, and systemic signs and symptoms of thyrotoxicosis are present. The thyroid gland is firm and exquisitely tender on physical examination.
- Painless thyroiditis has a triphasic course that mimics that of painful subacute thyroiditis. Most patients present with mild thyrotoxic symptoms; lid retraction and lid lag are present but exophthalmos is absent. The thyroid gland may be diffusely enlarged, but thyroid tenderness is absent.
- Thyroid storm is a life-threatening medical emergency characterized by severe thyrotoxicosis, high fever (often greater than 103°F), tachycardia, tachypnea, dehydration, delirium, coma, nausea, vomiting, and diarrhea. Precipitating

TABLE 19–1. Thyroid Function Test Results in Different Thyroid Conditions

	Total T_4	Free T_4	Total T_3	T_3 Resin Uptake	Free Thyroxine Index	TSH
Normal	4.5–12.5 mcg/dL	0.8–1.5 ng/dL	80–220 ng/dL	22%% to 34%	1.0–4.3 units	0.25–6.7 mIu/L
Hyperthyroid	↑↑	↑↑	↑↑↑	↑	↑↑↑	↓↓
Hypothyroid	↓↓	↓↓	↓	↓↓	↓↓↓	↑↑
Increased TBG	↑	Normal	↑	↓	Normal	Normal

TBG, thyroid-binding globulin; TSH, thyroid-stimulating hormone.

factors include infection, trauma, surgery, radioactive iodine treatment, and withdrawal from antithyroid drugs.

DIAGNOSIS

- An elevated 24-hour radioactive iodine uptake (RAIU) indicates true hyperthyroidism: the patient's thyroid gland is overproducing T_4, T_3, or both (normal RAIU 10% to 30%). Conversely, a low RAIU indicates that the excess thyroid hormone is not a consequence of thyroid gland hyperfunction.
- TSH-induced hyperthyroidism is diagnosed by evidence of peripheral hypermetabolism, diffuse thyroid gland enlargement, elevated free thyroid hormone levels, and elevated serum immunoreactive TSH concentrations. Because the pituitary gland is extremely sensitive to even minimal elevations of free T_4, a detectable TSH level in any thyrotoxic patient indicates inappropriate production of TSH.
- TSH-secreting pituitary adenomas are diagnosed by demonstrating lack of response to TRH stimulation, elevated TSH α-subunit levels, and radiologic imaging.
- In thyrotoxic Graves' disease, there is an increase in the overall hormone production rate with a disproportionate increase in T_3 relative to T_4 (Table 19–1). Saturation of TBG is increased due to the elevated levels of serum T_4 and T_3 which is reflected in an elevated T_3 resin uptake. As a result, the concentrations of free T_4, free T_3, and the free T_4 and T_3 indices are increased to an even greater extent than are the measured serum total T_4 and T_3 concentrations. The TSH level is undetectable due to negative feedback by elevated levels of thyroid hormone at the pituitary. The diagnosis of thyrotoxicosis is confirmed by measurement of the serum T_4 concentration, T_3 resin uptake (or free T_4), and TSH. An increased 24-hour RAIU (obtained in nonpregnant individuals) documents that the thyroid gland is inappropriately using the iodine to produce more thyroid hormone when the patient is thyrotoxic.
- Toxic adenomas may result in hyperthyroidism with larger nodules. Because there may be isolated elevation of serum T_3 with autonomously functioning nodules, a T_3 level must be measured to rule out T_3 toxicosis if the T_4 level is normal. After a radioiodine scan demonstrates that the toxic thyroid adenoma collects more radioiodine than the surrounding tissue, independent function is documented by failure of the autonomous nodule to decrease its iodine uptake during exogenous T_3 administration.
- In multinodular goiters, a thyroid scan shows patchy areas of autonomously functioning thyroid tissue.
- A low RAIU indicates the excess thyroid hormone is not a consequence of thyroid gland hyperfunction. This may be seen in painful subacute thyroiditis,

painless thyroiditis, struma ovarii, follicular cancer, and factitious ingestion of exogenous thyroid hormone.

- In subacute thyroiditis, thyroid function tests typically run a triphasic course in this self-limited disease. Initially, serum thyroxine levels are elevated due to release of preformed thyroid hormone from disrupted follicles. The 24-hour RAIU during this time is less than 2% owing to thyroid inflammation and TSH suppression by the elevated thyroxine level. As the disease progresses, intrathyroidal hormone stores are depleted, and the patient may become mildly hypothyroid with an appropriately elevated TSH level. During the recovery phase, thyroid hormone stores are replenished and serum TSH elevation gradually returns to normal.

- During the thyrotoxic phase of painless thyroiditis, the 24-hour RAIU is suppressed to less than 2%. Antithyroglobulin and antimicrosomal antibody levels are elevated in more than 50% of patients.

- Thyrotoxicosis factitia should be suspected in a thyrotoxic patient without infiltrative ophthalmopathy or thyroid enlargement. The RAIU is low because thyroid gland function is suppressed by the exogenous thyroid hormone. Measurement of plasma thyroglobulin reveals the presence of very low levels.

DESIRED OUTCOME

The therapeutic objectives for hyperthyroidism are to normalize the production of thyroid hormone; minimize symptoms and long-term consequences; and provide individualized therapy based on the type and severity of disease, patient age and gender, existence of nonthyroidal conditions, and response to previous therapy.

TREATMENT

Nonpharmacologic Therapy

- Surgical removal of the thyroid gland is the treatment of choice for coexisting cold nodules, extremely large goiters, lack of remission on antithyroid drug treatment, and patients with contraindications to thionamides (i.e., allergy or adverse effects) and RAI (i.e., pregnancy).

- If thyroidectomy is planned, **PTU** or **methimazole** is usually given until the patient is biochemically euthyroid (usually 6 to 8 weeks), followed by the addition of iodides (500 mg/day) for 10 to 14 days before surgery to decrease the vascularity of the gland. **Levothyroxine** may be added to maintain the euthyroid state while the thionamides are continued.

- **Propranolol** has been used for several weeks preoperatively and 7 to 10 days after surgery to maintain a pulse rate less than 90 beats/min. Combined pretreatment with propranolol and 10 to 14 days of **potassium iodide** also has been advocated.

- Complications of surgery include persistent or recurrent hyperthyroidism (0.6% to 18%), hypothyroidism (up to about 49%), hypoparathyroidism (up to 4%), and vocal cord abnormalities (up to 5%). The frequent occurrence of hypothyroidism requires periodic follow-up for identification and treatment.

Antithyroid Pharmacotherapy
Thioureas (Thionamides)

- **Propylthiouracil** (PTU) and **methimazole** (MMI) block thyroid hormone synthesis by inhibiting the peroxidase enzyme system of the thyroid gland, thus preventing oxidation of trapped iodide and subsequent incorporation into iodotyrosines and ultimately iodothyronine ("organification"), and by inhibiting coupling of monoiodotyrosine and diiodotyrosine to form T_4 and T_3. PTU (but not MMI) also inhibits the peripheral conversion of T_4 to T_3.

- Usual initial doses include PTU 300 to 600 mg daily (usually in three or four divided doses) or MMI 30 to 60 mg daily given in three divided doses. Evidence exists that both drugs can be given as a single daily dose.
- Improvement in symptoms and laboratory abnormalities should occur within 4 to 8 weeks, at which time a tapering regimen to maintenance doses can be started. Dosage changes should be made on a monthly basis because the endogenously produced T_4 will reach a new steady-state concentration in this interval. Typical daily maintenance doses are PTU 50 to 300 mg and MMI 5 to 30 mg.
- Antithyroid drug therapy should continue for 12 to 24 months to induce a long-term remission.
- Patients should be monitored every 6 to 12 months after remission. If a relapse occurs, alternate therapy with radioactive iodine (RAI) is preferred to a second course of antithyroid drugs, as subsequent courses of therapy are less likely to induce remission.
- Minor adverse reactions include pruritic maculopapular rashes, arthralgias, fever, and a benign transient leukopenia (WBC less than 4000/mm^3). The alternate thiourea may be tried in these situations, but cross-sensitivity occurs in about 50% of patients.
- Major adverse effects include agranulocytosis (with fever, malaise, gingivitis, oropharyngeal infection, and a granulocyte count less than 250/mm^3), aplastic anemia, a lupus-like syndrome, polymyositis, gastrointestinal intolerance, hepatotoxicity, and hypoprothrombinemia. Agranulocytosis, if it occurs, almost always develops in the first 3 months of therapy; routine monitoring is not recommended because of its sudden onset. Patients who have experienced a major adverse reaction to one thiourea should not be converted to the alternate drug because of cross-sensitivity.

Iodides

- **Iodide** acutely blocks thyroid hormone release, inhibits thyroid hormone biosynthesis by interfering with intrathyroidal iodide utilization, and decreases the size and vascularity of the gland.
- Symptom improvement occurs within 2 to 7 days of initiating therapy, and serum T_4 and T_3 concentrations may be reduced for a few weeks.
- Iodides are often used as adjunctive therapy to prepare a patient with Graves' disease for surgery, to acutely inhibit thyroid hormone release and quickly attain the euthyroid state in severely thyrotoxic patients with cardiac decompensation, or to inhibit thyroid hormone release after RAI therapy.
- **Potassium iodide** is available as a saturated solution (**SSKI,** 38-mg iodide per drop) or as **Lugol's solution,** containing 6.3 mg of iodide per drop.
- The typical starting dose of SSKI is 3 to 10 drops daily (120 to 400 mg) in water or juice. When used to prepare a patient for surgery, it should be administered 7 to 14 days preoperatively.
- As an adjunct to RAI, SSKI should not be used before but rather 3 to 7 days after RAI treatment so that the radioactive iodine can concentrate in the thyroid.
- Adverse effects include hypersensitivity reactions (skin rashes, drug fever, rhinitis, conjunctivitis); salivary gland swelling; "iodism" (metallic taste, burning mouth and throat, sore teeth and gums, symptoms of a head cold, and sometimes stomach upset and diarrhea); and gynecomastia.

Adrenergic Blockers

- β Blockers have been used widely to ameliorate thyrotoxic symptoms such as palpitations, anxiety, tremor, and heat intolerance. They have no effect on peripheral thyrotoxicosis and protein metabolism and do not reduce TSAb or prevent thyroid storm. **Propranolol** and **nadolol** partially block the conversion of T_4 to T_3, but this contribution to the overall therapeutic effect is small.

- β Blockers are usually used as adjunctive therapy with antithyroid drugs, RAI, or iodides when treating Graves' disease or toxic nodules; in preparation for surgery; or in thyroid storm. β Blockers are primary therapy only for thyroiditis and iodine-induced hyperthyroidism.
- **Propranolol** doses required to relieve adrenergic symptoms vary, but an initial dose of 20 to 40 mg four times daily is effective for most patients (heart rate less than 90 beats/min). Younger or more severely toxic patients may require as much as 240 to 480 mg/day.
- β Blockers are contraindicated in patients with decompensated heart failure unless it is caused solely by tachycardia (high output). Other contraindications include sinus bradycardia, concomitant therapy with monoamine oxidase inhibitors or tricyclic antidepressants, and patients with spontaneous hypoglycemia. Side effects include nausea, vomiting, anxiety, insomnia, lightheadedness, bradycardia, and hematologic disturbances.
- Centrally acting sympatholytics (e.g., **clonidine**) and calcium channel antagonists (e.g., **diltiazem**) may be useful for symptom control when contraindications to β blockade exist.

Radioactive Iodine
- **Sodium iodide 131** (^{131}I) is an oral liquid that concentrates in the thyroid and initially disrupts hormone synthesis by incorporating into thyroid hormones and thyroglobulin. Over a period of weeks, follicles that have taken up RAI and surrounding follicles develop evidence of cellular necrosis and fibrosis of the interstitial tissue.
- RAI is the agent of choice for Graves' disease, toxic autonomous nodules, and toxic multinodular goiters. Pregnancy is an absolute contraindication to the use of RAI.
- β **Blockers** are the primary adjunctive therapy to RAI, since they may be given anytime without compromising RAI therapy.
- Patients with cardiac disease and elderly patients are often treated with thionamides prior to RAI ablation because thyroid hormone levels will transiently increase after RAI treatment due to release of preformed thyroid hormone.
- Antithyroid drugs are not routinely used after RAI because their use is associated with a higher incidence of posttreatment recurrence or persistence of hyperthyroidism.
- If iodides are administered, they should be given 3 to 7 days after RAI to prevent interference with the uptake of RAI in the thyroid gland.
- The goal of therapy is to destroy overactive thyroid cells, and a single dose of 4000 to 8000 rad results in a euthyroid state in 60% of patients at 6 months or less. A second dose of RAI should be given 6 months after the first RAI treatment if the patient remains hyperthyroid.
- Hypothyroidism commonly occurs months to years after RAI. The acute, short-term side effects include mild thyroidal tenderness and dysphagia. Long-term follow-up has not revealed an increased risk for development of thyroid carcinoma, leukemia, or congenital defects.

Treatment of Thyroid Storm
- The following therapeutic measures should be instituted promptly: suppression of thyroid hormone formation and secretion, antiadrenergic therapy,

TABLE 19–2. Drug Dosages Used in the Management of Thyroid Storm

Drug	Regimen
Propylthiouracil	900–1200 mg/day orally in 4 or 6 divided doses
Methimazole	90–120 mg/day orally in 4 or 6 divided doses
Sodium iodide	Up to 2 g/day IV in single or divided doses
Lugol's solution	5–10 drops 3 times a day in water or juice
Saturated solution of potassium iodide	1–2 drops 3 times a day in water or juice
Propranolol	40–80 mg every 6 h
Dexamethasone	5–20 mg/day orally or IV in divided doses
Prednisone	25–100 mg/day orally in divided doses
Methylprednisolone	20–80 mg/day IV in divided doses
Hydrocortisone	100–400 mg/day IV in divided doses

IV

administration of corticosteroids, and treatment of associated complications or coexisting factors that may have precipitated the storm (Table 19–2).

- **PTU** in large doses is the preferred thionamide because it interferes with the production of thyroid hormones and blocks the peripheral conversion of T_4 to T_3.
- **Iodides,** which rapidly block the release of preformed thyroid hormone, should be administered after PTU is initiated to inhibit iodide use by the overactive gland.
- General supportive measures, including **acetaminophen** as an antipyretic (aspirin or other NSAIDs may displace bound thyroid hormone), **fluid** and **electrolyte replacement, sedatives, digitalis, antiarrhythmics, insulin,** and **antibiotics** should be given as indicated. Plasmapheresis and peritoneal dialysis have been used to remove excess hormone in patients not responding to more conservative measures.

EVALUATION OF THERAPEUTIC OUTCOMES

- After therapy (thionamides, RAI, or surgery) for hyperthyroidism has been initiated, patients should be evaluated on a monthly basis until they reach a euthyroid condition.
- Clinical signs of continuing thyrotoxicosis or the development of hypothyroidism should be noted.
- After thyroxine replacement is initiated, the goal is to maintain both the free thyroxine level and the TSH concentration in the normal range. Once a stable dose of thyroxine is identified, the patient may be followed every 6 to 12 months.

▶ HYPOTHYROIDISM

PATHOPHYSIOLOGY

- The vast majority of hypothyroid patients have thyroid gland failure (primary hypothyroidism). The causes include chronic autoimmune thyroiditis (Hashimoto's disease), iatrogenic hypothyroidism, iodine deficiency, enzyme defects, thyroid hypoplasia, and goitrogens.
- Pituitary failure (secondary hypothyroidism) is an uncommon cause resulting from pituitary tumors, surgical therapy, external pituitary radiation, postpartum pituitary necrosis, metastatic tumors, tuberculosis, histiocytosis, and autoimmune mechanisms.

CLINICAL PRESENTATION

- Adult manifestations of hypothyroidism include dry skin, cold intolerance, weight gain, constipation, weakness, lethargy, fatigue, muscle cramps, myalgia, stiffness, and loss of ambition or energy. In children, thyroid hormone deficiency may manifest as growth retardation.
- Physical signs include coarse skin and hair, cold or dry skin, periorbital puffiness, bradycardia, and slowed or hoarse speech. Objective weakness (with proximal muscles being affected more than distal muscles) and slow relaxation of deep tendon reflexes are common. Reversible neurologic syndromes such as carpal tunnel syndrome, polyneuropathy, and cerebellar dysfunction may also occur.
- Most patients with pituitary failure (secondary hypothyroidism) have clinical signs of generalized pituitary insufficiency such as abnormal menses and decreased libido, or evidence of a pituitary adenoma such as visual field defects, galactorrhea, or acromegaloid features.
- Myxedema coma is the end stage of long-standing uncorrected hypothyroidism and is manifested by hypothermia, advanced stages of hypothyroid symptoms, and altered sensorium ranging from delirium to coma. Untreated disease is associated with a high mortality rate.

DIAGNOSIS

- A rise in the TSH level is the first evidence of primary hypothyroidism. Many patients have a T_4 level within the normal range (compensated hypothyroidism) and few, if any, symptoms of hypothyroidism. As the disease progresses, the T_4 concentration drops below the normal level. The T_3 concentration is often maintained in the normal range despite a low T_4. Antithyroid peroxidase antibodies and antithyroglobulin antibodies are likely to be elevated. The RAIU is not a useful test in the evaluation of hypothyroidism.
- Pituitary failure (secondary hypothyroidism) should be suspected in a patient with decreased levels of thyroxine and inappropriately normal or low TSH levels.

DESIRED OUTCOME

The treatment goals for hypothyroidism are to normalize thyroid hormone concentrations in tissue, provide symptomatic relief, prevent neurologic deficits in newborns and children, and reverse the biochemical abnormalities of hypothyroidism.

TREATMENT OF HYPOTHYROIDISM

See Table 19–3.

- **Levothyroxine** (L-thyroxine) is the drug of choice for thyroid hormone replacement and suppressive therapy because it is chemically stable, relatively inexpensive, free of antigenicity, and has uniform potency; however, any of the commercially available thyroid preparations can be used. Once a particular product is selected, therapeutic interchange is discouraged.
- Because T_3 (and not T_4) is the biologically active form, levothyroxine administration results in a pool of thyroid hormone that is readily and consistently converted to T_3.
- Young patients with long-standing disease and patients older than 45 years without known cardiac disease should be started on 50 mcg daily of levothyroxine and increased to 100 mcg daily after 1 month.

TABLE 19–3. Thyroid Preparations Used in the Treatment of Hypothyroidism

Drug/Dosage Form	Content	Relative Dose
Thyroid USP Armour Thyroid (T_4:T_3 ratio) 9.5 mcg:2.25 mcg, 19 mcg:4.5 mcg, 38 mcg:9 mcg, 57 mcg:13.5 mcg, 76 mcg:18 mcg, 114 mcg:27 mcg, 152 mcg:36 mcg, 190 mcg:45 mcg tablets	Desiccated beef or pork thyroid gland	1 grain (equivalent to 60 mcg of T_4)
Thyroglobulin Proloid 32-mg, 65-mg, 100-mg, 130-mg, 200-mg tablets	Partially purified pork thyroglobulin	1 grain
Levothyroxine Synthroid, Levothroid, Levoxyl, Unithroid and other generics 25-, 50-, 75-, 88-, 100-, 112-, 125-, 137-, 150-, 175-, 200-, 300-mcg tablets; 200- and 500-mcg/vial injection	Synthetic T_4	50–60 mcg
Liothyronine Cytomel 5-, 25-, and 50-mcg tablets	Synthetic T_3	15–37.5 mcg
Liotrix Thyrolar 1/4-, 1/2, 1-, 2-, and 3-strength tablets	Synthetic T_4:T_3 in 4:1 ratio	50–60 mcg T_4 and 12.5–15 mcg T_3

IV

- The recommended initial daily dose for older patients or those with known cardiac disease is 25 mcg/day titrated upward in increments of 25 mcg at monthly intervals to prevent stress on the cardiovascular system.
- The average maintenance dose for most adults is about 125 mcg/day, but there is a wide range of replacement doses, necessitating individualized therapy and appropriate monitoring to determine an appropriate dose.
- Patients with subclinical hypothyroidism and marked elevations in TSH (greater than 10 mIU/L) and high titers of TSAb or prior treatment with ^{131}I may benefit from treatment with levothyroxine.
- Levothyroxine is the drug of choice for pregnant women, and the objective of the treatment is to decrease TSH to 1 mIU/L and to maintain free T_4 concentrations in the normal range.
- Cholestyramine, calcium carbonate, sucralfate, aluminum hydroxide, ferrous sulfate, soybean formula, and dietary fiber supplements may impair the absorption of levothyroxine from the gastrointestinal tract. Drugs that increase nondeiodinative T_4 clearance include rifampin, carbamazepine, and possibly phenytoin. Amiodarone may block the conversion of T_4 to T_3.
- **Thyroid USP** (or desiccated thyroid) is derived from hog, beef, or sheep thyroid gland. It may be antigenic in allergic or sensitive patients. Inexpensive generic brands may not be bioequivalent.
- **Thyroglobulin** is a purified hog-gland extract that is standardized biologically to give a T_4:T_3 ratio of 2.5:1. It has no clinical advantages and is not widely used.

- **Liothyronine** (synthetic T_3) has uniform potency but has a higher incidence of cardiac adverse effects, higher cost, and difficulty in monitoring with conventional laboratory tests.
- **Liotrix** (synthetic T_4:T_3 in a 4:1 ratio) is chemically stable, pure, and has a predictable potency but is expensive. It lacks therapeutic rationale because about 35% of T_4 is converted to T_3 peripherally.
- Excessive doses of thyroid hormone may lead to heart failure, angina pectoris, and myocardial infarction. Allergic or idiosyncratic reactions can occur with the natural animal-derived products such as desiccated thyroid and thyroglobulin, but they are extremely rare with the synthetic products used today. Excess exogenous thyroid hormone may reduce bone density and increase the risk of fracture.

TREATMENT OF MYXEDEMA COMA

- Immediate and aggressive therapy with intravenous (IV) bolus **thyroxine,** 300 to 500 mcg, is needed to prevent mortality.
- Glucocorticoid therapy with IV **hydrocortisone** 100 mg every 8 hours should be given until coexisting adrenal suppression is ruled out.
- Consciousness, lowered TSH concentrations, and normal vital signs are expected within 24 hours.
- Maintenance thyroxine doses are typically 75 to 100 mcg IV until the patient stabilizes and oral therapy is begun.
- Supportive therapy must be instituted to maintain adequate ventilation, euglycemia, blood pressure, and body temperature. Underlying disorders such as sepsis and myocardial infarction must be diagnosed and treated.

EVALUATION OF THERAPEUTIC OUTCOMES

- Serum TSH concentration is the most sensitive and specific monitoring parameter for adjustment of levothyroxine dose. Concentrations begin to fall within hours and are usually normalized within 2 to 6 weeks.
- TSH and T_4 concentrations should both be checked every 6 weeks until a euthyroid state is achieved. An elevated TSH level indicates insufficient replacement. Serum T_4 concentrations can be useful in detecting noncompliance, malabsorption, or changes in levothyroxine product bioequivalence. TSH may also be used to help identify noncompliance.
- In patients with hypothyroidism caused by hypothalamic or pituitary failure, alleviation of the clinical syndrome and restoration of serum T_4 to the normal range are the only criteria available for estimating the appropriate replacement dose of levothyroxine.

See Chapter 73, Thyroid Disorders, authored by Robert L. Talbert, for a more detailed discussion of this topic.

Gastrointestinal Disorders

Edited by Joseph T. DiPiro

Chapter 20

▶ CIRRHOSIS AND PORTAL HYPERTENSION

▶ DEFINITIONS

- Cirrhosis is defined as a diffuse process characterized by fibrosis and a conversion of the normal hepatic architecture into structurally abnormal nodules. The end result is destruction of hepatocytes and their replacement by fibrous tissue.
- The resulting resistance to blood flow results in portal hypertension and the development of varices and ascites. Hepatocyte loss and intrahepatic shunting of blood results in diminished metabolic and synthetic function, which leads to hepatic encephalopathy and coagulopathy.
- Cirrhosis has many causes (Table 20–1). In the United States, excessive alcohol intake and chronic viral hepatitis (types B and C) are the most common causes.

▶ PATHOPHYSIOLOGY

Cirrhosis and the pathophysiologic abnormalities that cause it result in the commonly encountered problems of ascites, portal hypertension and esophageal varices, hepatic encephalopathy, and coagulation disorders.

ASCITES

- Ascites is the pathologic accumulation of lymph fluid within the peritoneal cavity. It is one of the earliest and most common presentations of cirrhosis.
- The development of ascites is related to systemic arterial vasodilation that leads to the activation of the baroreceptors in the kidney and an activation of the rennin-angiotensis system, with sodium and water retention.

PORTAL HYPERTENSION AND VARICES

- Portal hypertension exists when the portal venous pressure is 5 to 10 mm Hg.
- The most important sequelae of portal hypertension are the development of varices and alternative routes of blood flow. Patients with cirrhosis are at risk for varices when portal pressures exceed the vena cava pressure by greater than or equal to 2 mm Hg.

TABLE 20–1. Etiology of Cirrhosis

Category	Example
Drugs and toxins	Alcohol, methotrexate, isoniazid, methyldopa, organic hydrocarbons
Infections	Viral hepatitis (types B and C), schistosomiasis
Immune-mediated	Primary biliary cirrhosis, autoimmune hepatitis, primary sclerosing cholangitis
Metabolic	Hemochromatosis, porphyria, α_1-antitrypsin deficiency, Wilson's disease
Biliary obstruction	Cystic fibrosis, atresia, strictures, gallstones
Cardiovascular	Chronic right heart failure, Budd-Chiari syndrome, veno-occlusive disease
Cryptogenic	Unknown
Other	Nonalcoholic steatohepatitis, sarcoidosis, gastric bypass

From Williams and Iredale.

- Hemorrhage from varices occurs in 25% to 40% of patients with cirrhosis, and each episode of bleeding carries a 5% to 50% risk of death.

HEPATIC ENCEPHALOPATHY/PORTAL SYSTEMIC ENCEPHALOPATHY

- Hepatic Encephalopathy (HE) is a complex neuropsychiatric syndrome with a broad spectrum of clinical signs and symptoms of neurologic impairment that occurs in cirrhotic patients.
- The symptoms are thought to result from an accumulation of gut-derived nitrogenous substances in the systemic circulation as a consequence of shunting through portosystemic collaterals. These substances then enter the central nervous system and result in alterations of neurotransmitters that affect conciousness and behavior.
- Serum ammonia levels are poorly correlated with the grade of HE.
- HE presents in one of three forms: acute, chronic, and subclinical.
- Acute HE is defined as a distinct event of altered sensorium lasting less than 4 weeks, followed by complete recovery to baseline mental status.
- Chronic encephalopathy is defined as a cognitive or neuropsychiatric abnormality that persists for at least 4 weeks.
- Subclinical encephalopathy refers to subtle alterations in neuropsychiatric function that are not clinically apparent.

COAGULATION DEFECTS

- Complex coagulation derangements can occur in cirrhosis. These derangements include the reduction in the synthesis of coagulation factors and the clearance of activated clotting factors.
- Portal hypertension is accompanied by a qualitative and quantitative reduction in platelets.
- The net effect of these events is the development of bleeding diathesis.

▶ CLINICAL PRESENTATION

- The range of presentation of patients with cirrhosis may be from asymptomatic with abnormal laboratory tests to acute life-threatening hemorrhage.
- Table 20–2 describes the presenting signs and symptoms of cirrhosis.

TABLE 20–2. Clinical Presentation of Cirrhosis

Signs and symptoms (percent of patients)[a]
    Fatigue (65%), pruritus (55%)
    Hyperpigmentation (25%), jaundice (10%)
    Hepatomegaly (25%), splenomegaly (15%)
    Palmar erythema, spider angiomata, gynecomastia
    Ascites, edema, pleural effusion, and respiratory difficulties
    Malaise, anorexia, and weight loss
    Encephalopathy
Laboratory tests
    Hypoalbuminemia
    Elevated prothrombin time
    Thrombocytopenia
    Elevated alkaline phosphatase
    Elevated aspartate transaminase (AST), alanine transaminase (ALT), and γ-glutamyl transpeptidase (GGT)

[a]From Talwalkar and Lindor.

- Jaundice is often a late manifestation of cirrhosis, and its absence does not exclude the diagnosis.
- On questioning, a patient who abuses alcohol will often underestimate the amount of alcohol consumed.
- An elevation of prothrombin time is the single most reliable manifestation of cirrhosis. The combination of thrombocytopenia, encephalopathy, and ascites had the highest predictive value for sepsis.
- The clinical manifestations of HE can range from subtle mental status abnormalities to deep coma.
- HE associated with acute fulminant liver failure has a rapid onset and a short prodrome. Patients can progress from drowsiness to delirium, convulsions, and coma in 24 hours.

LABORATORY ABNORMALITIES

- Routine liver assessment tests include alkaline phosphatase, bilirubin, aspartate transaminase (AST), alanine transaminase (ALT), and γ-glutamyl transpeptidase (GGT). Additional markers of hepatic synthetic activity include albumin and prothrombin time.
- The aminotransferases, AST and ALT, are enzymes that have increased concentrations in plasma following hepatocellular injury.
- Alkaline phosphatase levels and GGT are elevated in plasma with obstructive disorders that disrupt the flow of bile from hepatocytes to the bile ducts or from the biliary tree to the intestines.
- The levels of GGT in plasma correlate well with elevations of alkaline phosphatase and thus are a sensitive marker for biliary tract disease.
- Elevations of serum bilirubin are common in end-stage liver disease, but other causes of hyperbilirubinemia are numerous.
- Figure 20–1 describes a general algorithm for the interpretation of liver function tests.

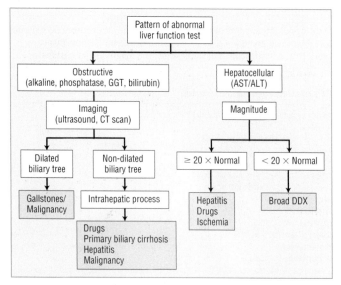

Figure 20–1. Interpretation of liver function tests.

TABLE 20–3. Criteria and Scoring for the Child-Pugh Grading of Chronic Liver Disease

Score	1	2	3
Bilirubin (mg/dL)	1–2	2–3	>3
Albumin (mg/dL)	>3.5	2.8–3.5	<2.8
Ascites	None	Mild	Moderate
Encephalopathy (grade)	None	1 and 2	3 and 4
Prothrombin time (seconds prolonged)	1–4	4–6	>6

Grade A, points; grade B, 7–9 points; grade C, 10–15 points.

V

- Albumin and coagulation factors are markers of hepatic synthetic activity and are used to estimate hepatocyte functioning in cirrhosis.
- Thrombocytopenia is a relatively common feature in both acute and chronic liver disease and is proportional to the extent of liver disease.
- Liver biopsy plays a central role in the diagnosis and staging of liver disease.
- The Child–Pugh classification system uses a combination of physical and laboratory findings to assess and define the severity of cirrhosis and is a predictor of patient survival, surgical outcome, and risk of variceal bleeding (Table 20–3).

▶ TREATMENT

DESIRED OUTCOME

- Clinical improvement or resolution of acute complications, such as variceal bleeding, and resolution of hemodynamic instability for an episode of acute variceal hemorrhage.
- Prevention of complications, achieving adequate lowering of portal pressure with medical therapy using β-adrenergic blocker therapy, or supporting abstinence from alcohol.

GENERAL APPROACHES

- Identify and eliminate the causes of cirrhosis (e.g., alcohol abuse).
- Assess the risk for variceal bleeding and begin pharmacologic prophylaxis where indicated, reserving endoscopic therapy for high-risk patients or acute bleeding episodes.
- The patient should be evaluated for clinical signs of ascites and managed with pharmacologic treatment (e.g., diuretics) and paracentesis. Careful monitoring for spontaneous bacterial peritonitis should be employed in patients with ascites who undergo acute deterioration.
- Hepatic encephalopathy is a common complication of cirrhosis and requires clinical vigilance and treatment with dietary restriction, elimination of central nervous system depressants, and therapy to lower ammonia levels.
- Frequent monitoring for signs of hepatorenal syndrome, pulmonary insufficiency, and endocrine dysfunction is necessary.

MANAGEMENT OF PORTAL HYPERTENSION AND VARICEAL BLEEDING

The management of varices involves three strategies: (1) primary prophylaxis to prevent rebleeding, (2) treatment of variceal hemorrhage, and (3) secondary prophylaxis to prevent rebleeding in patients who have already bled.

Primary Prophylaxis

- The mainstay of primary prophylaxis is the use of nonselective β-adrenergic blocking agents such as **propranolol** or **nadolol**. These agents decrease blood flow to the mesenteric vascular system and deceased portal vein pressure. They prevent bleeding, and there is a trend toward reduced mortality.

- β-Adrenergic blocker therapy should be continued for life, unless it is not tolerated, because bleeding can occur when therapy is abruptly discontinued.
- All patients with cirrhosis and portal hypertension should be considered for endoscopic screening, and patients with large varices should receive primary prophylaxis with β-adrenergic blockers.
- Therapy should be initiated with **propranolol**, 10 mg thrice daily, or **nadolol**, 20 mg once daily, and titrated to a reduction in resting heart rate of 20% to 25%, an absolute heart rate of 55 to 60 beats/min, or the development of adverse effects.
- Nitrates may be considered for patients with contraindications or intolerance to β-adrenergic blockers.
- Combination therapy with β blockers is recommended for patients with inadequate lowering of portal pressure from β-blockers alone.

Acute Variceal Hemorrhage
Figure 20–2 presents an algorithm for the management of variceal hemorrhage.

- Initial treatment goals include: (1) adequate fluid resuscitation, (2) correction of coagulopathy and thrombocytopenia, (3) control of bleeding, (4) prevention of rebleeding, and (5) preservation of liver function.
- Prompt stabilization and aggressive fluid resuscitation of patients with active bleeding is followed by endoscopic examination.
- The American College of Gastroenterology recommends esophagogastroduodenoscopy employing endoscopic injection sclerotherapy (EIS) or endoscopic band ligation (EBL) of varices as the primary diagnostic and treatment strategy

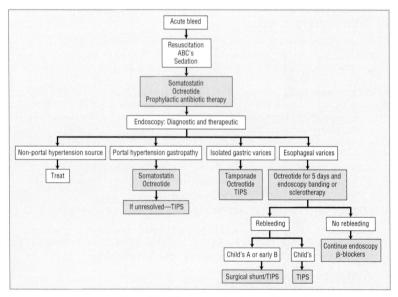

Figure 20–2. Management of acute variceal hemorrhage.

for upper gastrointestinal (GI) tract hemorrhage secondary to portal hypertension and varices.

- Fluid resuscitation involves colloids initially and subsequent blood products.
- Vasoactive drug therapy (somatostatin, octreotide, or terlipessin) to stop or slow bleeding is routinely employed early in patient management to allow stabilization of the patient and to permit endoscopy to proceed under more favorable conditions. These agents decrease splanchnic blood flow and reduce portal and variceal pressures, without significant adverse effects.
- Patients experiencing variceal hemorrhage require prompt resuscitation with colloids and blood products to correct intravascular losses and to reverse coagulopathies.
- Treatment with octreotide of somatostatin should be initiated early to control bleeding and facilitate endoscopy. Octreotide is preferred and is administered as an IV bolus of 50 to 100 mcg and is followed by a continuous infusion of 25 mcg/h, up to a maximum rate of 50 mcg/h. Patients should be monitored for hypo- or hyperglycemia.
- **Vasopressin,** alone or in combination with nitroglycerin, can no longer be recommended as first-line therapy for the management of variceal hemorrhage. Vasopressin causes nonselective vasoconstriction and can result in hypertension, severe headaches, coronary ischemia, myocardial infarction, and arrhythmias.
- Antibiotic therapy should be used early to prevent sepsis in patients with signs of infection or ascites.
- EIS or EBL is often used for upper GI tract hemorrhage secondary to portal hypertension and varices. Sclerosing agents used in EIS include **ethanolamine, sodium tetradecyl sulfate, polidocanol**, and **sodium morrhuate**.
- If standard therapy fails to control bleeding, a salvage procedure such as balloon tamponade (with a Sengstaken-Blakemore tube), transjugular intrahepatic portosystemic shunt (TIPS), or surgical shunting is necessary.

Prevention of Rebleeding

- β-Adrenergic blockers have traditionally been used for prevention of rebleeding; however, EIS or EBL is emerging as the preferred treatment option.
- In patients without contraindications, β-adrenergic blocking agents should be the initial step in prevention of rebleeding, along with EIS or EBL. Use of a long-acting β-adrenergic blocker (such as nadolol) is usually recommended to improve compliance, and gradual, individualized dose escalation may help to minimize side effects. **Propranolol** may be given at 20 mg three times daily (or **nadolol**, 20 to 40 mg once daily) and titrated weekly to achieve a goal of heart rate 55 to 60 beats/min or a heart rate that is 25% lower than the baseline heart rate. Patients should be monitored for evidence of heart failure, bronchospasm, or glucose intolerance.
- For patients who fail to achieve sufficient reductions in portal pressure with β-blocker therapy alone, combination therapy with **nitrates** or **spironolactone** may more effectively lower portal pressures.

ASCITES

- For patients with ascites, a serum-ascites albumin gradient (SAG) should be determined. If SAG is greater than 1.1, portal hypertension is present with 97% accuracy.
- The treatment of ascites secondary to portal hypertension includes abstinence from alcohol, sodium restriction, and diuretics. Sodium chloride should be restricted to 2 g/day.

TABLE 20–4. Treatment Goals; Acute and Chronic HE

Acute HE	Chronic HE
Control precipitating factor	Reverse encephalopathy
Reverse encephalopathy	Avoid recurrence
Hospital/inpatient therapy	Home/outpatient therapy
Maintain fluid and hemodynamic support	Manage persistent neuropsychiatric abnormalities
	Manage chronic liver disease
Expect normal mentation after recovery	High prevalence of abnormal mentation after recovery

V

- Diuretic therapy should be initiated with single morning doses of **spirono-lactone**, 100 mg, and **furosemide**, 40 mg, with a goal of 0.5-kg maximum daily weight loss. The dose of each can be increased together, maintaining the 100:40 mg ratio, to a maximum daily dose of 400 mg spironolactone and 160 mg furosemide.
- If tense ascites is present, a 4- to 6-L paracentesis should be performed prior to institution of diuretic therapy and salt restriction.
- Patients who experience encephalopathy, severe hyponatremia despite fluid restriction, or renal insufficiency should have diuretic therapy discontinued.
- Liver transplantation should be considered in patients with refractory ascites.

SPONTANEOUS BACTERIAL PERITONITIS (SBP)

- Patients with documented or suspected SBP should receive broad-spectrum antibiotic therapy to cover *Escherichia coli, Klebsiella pneumoniae,* and *Streptococcus pneumoniae*.
- **Cefotaxime**, 2 g every 8 hours, or a similar third-generation cephalosporin is considered the drug of choice.
- **Oral ofloxacin**, 400 mg every 12 hours, is equivalent to intravenous cefotaxime in terms of resolution of infection as well as survival.

TABLE 20–5. Portosystemic Encephalopathy: Precipitating Factors and Therapy

Factor	Therapy Alternatives
Gastrointestinal bleeding	
Variceal	Band ligation/sclerotherapy
	Octreotide
Nonvariceal	Endoscopic therapy
	Proton pump inhibitors
Infection/sepsis	Antibiotics
	Paracentesis
Electrolyte abnormalities	Discontinue diuretics
	Fluid and electrolyte replacement
Sedative ingestion	Discontinue sedatives/tranquilizers
	Consider reversal (flumazenil/naloxone)
Dietary excesses	Limit daily protein
	Lactulose
Constipation	Cathartics
	Bowel cleansing/enema
Renal insufficiency	Discontinue diuretics
	Discontinue NSAIDs, nephrotoxic antibiotics
	Fluid resuscitation

TABLE 20–6. Management Approach and Outcome Assessments

Complication	Treatment Approach	Monitoring Parameter	Outcome Assessment
Ascites	Diet, diuretics, paracentesis, TIPS	Daily assessment of weight	Prevent or eliminate ascites and its secondary complications
Spontaneous bacterial peritonitis	Antibiotic therapy, prophylaxis if undergoing paracentesis	Evidence of clinical deterioration (e.g., abdominal pain, fever, anorexia, malaise, fatigue)	Prevent/treat infection to decrease mortality
Varical bleeding	Pharmacologic prophylaxis	Child-Pugh score, endoscopy, CBC	Appropriate reduction in heart rate and portal pressure
	Endoscopy, vasoactive drug therapy (octreotide), sclerotherapy, volume resuscitation, pharmacologic prophylaxis	CBC, evidence of overt bleeding	Acute: control acute bleed Chronic: variceal obliteration, reduce portal pressures
Coagulation disorders	Blood products (PPF, platelets), vitamin K	CBC, prothrombin time, platelet count	Normalize PT time, maintain/improve hemostasis
Hepatic encephalopathy	Ammonia reduction (lactulose, cathartics), elimination of drugs causing CNS depression, limit excess protein in diet	Grade of encephalopathy, EEG, psychological testing, mental status changes, concurrent drug therapy	Maintain functional capacity, prevent hospitalization for encephalopathy, decrease ammonia levels, provide adequate nutrition
Hepatorenal syndrome	Eliminate concurrent nephrotoxins (NSAIDs), decrease or discontinue diuretics, volume resuscitation, liver transplantation	Serum and urine electrolytes, concurrent drug therapy	Prevent progressive renal injury by preventing dehydration and avoiding other nephrotoxins Liver transplantation for refractory hepatorenal syndrome
Hepatopulmonary syndrome	Paracentesis, O$_2$ therapy	Dyspnea, presence of ascites	Acute: relief of dyspnea and hypoxia Chronic: manage ascites as above

CBC, complete blood cell count; CNS, central nervous system; EEG, electroencephalogram; PT, prothrombin time; NSAID, nonsteroidal anti-inflammatory drug; PPF, plasma protein fraction; TIPS, transjugular intrahepatic portosystemic shunt.

V

213

- Short term fluoroquinolone therapy for the prevention of sbp should be considered in all patients at high risk of this complication, including those who have experienced a prior episode of sbp or variceal hemorrhage, and those with low-protein ascites (less than 1 g/dl).

Hepatic Encephalopathy

Table 20–4 describes the treatment goals for HE.

- The first approach to treatment of HE is to identify any precipitating causes. Precipitating factors and therapy alternatives are presented in Table 20–5.
- Treatment approaches include: (1) reduction of blood ammonia concentrations by dietary restrictions and drug therapy aimed at inhibiting ammonia production or enhancing its removal (lactulose), (2) inhibition of γ-aminobutyric acid–benzodiazepine receptors by flumazenil, and (3) inhibition of false neurotransmitters by optimizing amino acid balance.
- Approaches to reducing blood ammonia concentrations include: In patients with acute HE, limit protein intake to 10 to 20 g/day while maintaining the total caloric intake. Protein intake can be titrated by increasing 10 to 20 g/day every 3 to 5 days to a total of 0.8 to 1 g/kg/day. With chronic HE, restrict protein intake to 40 g/day.
  - In acute HE, lactulose is initiated at 45 mL every hour (or 300 mL lactulose syrup with 700 mL water given as a retention enema) until catharsis begins. The dose is then decreased to 15 to 30 mL orally 4 times daily and titrated to produce two to four soft, acidic stools per day.
  - With chronic HE, initiate lactulose at 30 to 60 mL/day with titration to the same end point.
  - Antibiotic therapy with **metronidazole** or **neomycin** is reserved for patients who have not responded to diet and lactulose.

▶ EVALUATION OF THERAPEUTIC OUTCOMES

Table 20–6 summarizes the management approach for patients with cirrhosis, including monitoring parameters and therapeutic outcomes.

See Chapter 37, Portal Hypertension and Cirrhosis, authored by Edward G. Timm and James J. Stragand, for a more detailed discussion of this topic.

Chapter 21

▶ CONSTIPATION

▶ DEFINITION

Constipation does not have a single, generally agreed upon definition Normal people pass at least three stools per week. Some of the definitions of constipation include: fewer than three stools per week for women and five for men despite a high-residue diet or a period of greater than 3 days without a bowel movement; straining at stool greater than 25% of the time and/or two or fewer stools per week; or straining at defecation and less than one stool daily with minimal effort.

▶ PATHOPHYSIOLOGY

- Constipation is not a disease but a symptom of an underlying disease or problem.
- Disorders of the gastrointestinal (GI) tract (e.g., irritable bowel syndrome or diverticulitis), metabolic disorders (e.g., diabetes), or endocrine disorders (e.g., hypothyroidism) may cause constipation.
- Constipation commonly results from a diet low in fiber or from use of constipating drugs such as opiates.
- Constipation may sometimes be psychogenic in origin.

Diseases or conditions that may cause constipation are:

- Gastrointestinal disorders
  - Gastroduodenal obstruction from ulceration or cancer
  - Irritable bowel syndrome
  - Diverticulitis
  - Hemorrhoids, anal fissures
  - Ulcerative proctitis
  - Tumors
- Metabolic and endocrine disorders
  - Diabetes mellitus
  - Hypothyroidism
  - Panhypopituitarism
  - Pheochromocytoma
  - Hypercalcemia
- Pregnancy
- Neurogenic constipation
  - Head trauma
  - Central nervous system tumors
  - Stroke
  - Parkinson's disease
- Psychogenic constipation
  - Psychiatric disorders
  - Inappropriate bowel habits
- Causes of drug-induced constipation are listed in Table 21–1.
- All opiate derivatives are associated with constipation, but the degree of intestinal inhibitory effects seems to differ between agents. Orally administered opiates appear to have greater inhibitory effect than parenterally administered agents; oral codeine is well known as a potent antimotility agent.

TABLE 21–1. Drugs Causing Constipation

Analgesics
    Inhibitors of prostaglandin synthesis
    Opiates
Anticholinergics
    Antihistamines
    Antiparkinsonian agents (e.g., benztropine or trihexaphenidyl)
    Phenothiazines
    Tricyclic antidepressants
Antacids containing calcium carbonate or aluminum hydroxide
Barium sulfate
Calcium channel blockers
Clonidine
Diuretics (non–potassium-sparing)
Ganglionic blockers
Iron preparations
Muscle blockers (D-tubocurarine, succinylcholine)
Nonsteroidal anti-inflammatory agents
Polystyrene sodium sulfonate

- Agents with anticholinergic properties inhibit bowel function by parasympatholytic actions on innervation to many regions of the GI tract, particularly the colon and rectum. Many types of drugs possess anticholinergic action, and these agents are used commonly in hospitalized and nonhospitalized patients.

▶ CLINICAL PRESENTATION

See Table 21–2.

- The patient should be asked about the frequency of bowel movements and the chronicity of constipation. The patient should also be carefully questioned about usual diet and laxative regimens. Does the patient have a diet consistently deficient in high-fiber items and containing mainly highly refined foods? What laxatives or cathartics has the patient used to attempt relief of constipation?
- The patient should be questioned about other concurrent medications, with interest toward agents that might cause constipation.

TABLE 21–2. Clinical Presentation of Constipation

Signs and symptoms
- It is important to ascertain whether the patient perceives the problem as infrequent bowel movements, stools of insufficient size, a feeling of fullness, or difficulty and pain on passing stool.
- Signs and symptoms include hard, small or dry stools, bloated stomach, cramping abdominal pain and discomfort, straining or grunting, sensation of blockade, fatigue, headache, and nausea and vomiting.

Laboratory tests
- A series of examinations, including proctoscopy, sigmoidoscopy, colonoscopy, or barium enema, may be necessary to determine the presence of colorectal pathology.
- Thyroid function studies may be performed to determine the presence of metabolic or endocrine disorders.
- With laxative abuse, fluid and electrolyte imbalances (most commonly hypokalemia), protein-losing gastroenteropathy with hypoalbuminemia may be present.

- The laxative abuser may present with contradictory findings, sometimes diarrhea or weight loss. Laxative abusers may also have vomiting, abdominal pain, lassitude, thirst, edema, and bone pain (due to osteomalacia). With prolonged abuse, patients may have fluid and electrolyte imbalances (most commonly hypokalemia), protein-losing gastroenteropathy with hypoalbuminemia, and syndromes resembling colitis. Laxative abusers frequently deny laxative use.

▶ DESIRED OUTCOME

A major goal for treatment of constipation is prevention of constipation by alteration of lifestyle (particularly diet) to prevent further episodes of constipation. For acute constipation, the goal is to relieve symptoms and restore normal bowel function.

▶ TREATMENT

GENERAL APPROACH TO TREATMENT

- General measures believed to be beneficial in managing constipation include dietary modification to increase the amount of fiber consumed daily, exercise, adjustment of bowel habits so that a regular and adequate time is made to respond to the urge to defecate, and increasing fluid intake.
- If an underlying disease is recognized as the cause of constipation, attempts should be made to correct it. GI malignancies may be removed through a surgical resection. Endocrine and metabolic derangements are corrected by the appropriate methods.
- Potential drug causes of constipation should be identified. For some medications (e.g., antacids), nonconstipating alternatives exist. If no reasonable alternatives exist to the medication thought to be responsible for constipation, consideration should be given to lowering the dose. If a patient must remain on constipating medications, then more attention must be paid to general measures for prevention of constipation, as discussed next.

DIETARY MODIFICATION AND BULK-FORMING AGENTS

- The most important aspect of the therapy for constipation for the majority of patients is dietary modification to increase the amount of fiber consumed. Patients should be advised to include at least 10 g of crude fiber in their daily diets. Fruits, vegetables, and cereals have the highest fiber content.
- A trial of dietary modification with high-fiber content should be continued for at least 1 month before effects on bowel function are determined.
- The patient should be cautioned that abdominal distention and flatus may be particularly troublesome in the first few weeks, particularly with high bran consumption.

SURGERY

- In a small percentage of patients presenting with complaints of constipation, surgical procedures (such as intestinal resection) are necessary. Surgery is usually necessary with most colonic malignancies and with GI obstruction from a number of causes.

BIOFEEDBACK

- The majority of patients with constipation related to pelvic floor dysfunction can benefit from electromyogram-guided biofeedback therapy.

TABLE 21–3. Dosage Recommendations for Laxatives and Cathartics

Agent	Recommended Dose
Agents that cause softening of feces in 1–3 days	
Bulk-forming agents	
Methylcellulose	4–6 g/day
Polycarbophil	4–6 g/day
Psyllium	Varies with product
Emollients	
Docusate sodium	50–360 mg/day
Docusate calcium	50–360 mg/day
Docusate potassium	100–300 mg/day
Lactulose	15–30 mL orally
Sorbitol	30–50 g/day orally
Mineral oil	15–30 mL orally
Agents that result in soft or semifluid stool in 6–12 h	
Bisacodyl (oral)	5–15 mg orally
Phenolphthalein	30–270 mg orally
Cascara sagrada	Dose varies with formulation
Senna	Dose varies with formulation
Magnesium sulfate (low dose)	<10 g orally
Agents that cause watery evacuation in 1–6 h	
Magnesium citrate	18 g 300 mL water
Magnesium hydroxide	2.4–4.8 g orally
Magnesium sulfate (high dose)	10–30 g orally
Sodium phosphates	Varies with salt used
Bisacodyl	10 mg rectally
Polyethylene glycol-electrolyte preparations	4 L

PHARMACOLOGIC THERAPY

- The various types of laxatives are discussed in this section. The agents are divided into three general classifications: (1) those causing softening of feces in 1 to 3 days (bulk-forming laxatives, **docusates**, and **lactulose**); (2) those that result in soft or semifluid stool in 6 to 12 hours (diphenylmethane derivatives and anthraquinone derivatives); and (3) those causing water evacuation in 1 to 6 hours (**saline** cathartics, **castor oil**, and **polyethylene glycol-electrolyte lavage solution**).
- Dosage recommendations for laxatives and cathartics are provided in Table 21–3.

Recommendations

- The basis for treatment and prevention of constipation should consist of bulk-forming agents in addition to dietary modifications that increase dietary fiber.
- For most nonhospitalized persons with acute constipation, the infrequent use (less than every few weeks) of most laxative products is acceptable; however, before more potent laxative or cathartics are used, relatively simple measures may be tried. For example, acute constipation may be relieved by the use of a **tap- water enema** or a **glycerin** suppository; if neither is effective, the use of oral **sorbitol**, low doses of diphenylmethane or anthraquinone derivatives, or saline laxatives (e.g., **milk of magnesia**) may provide relief.
- If laxative treatment is required for longer than 1 week, the person should be advised to consult a physician to determine if there is an underlying cause of constipation that requires treatment with agents other than laxatives.

- For some bedridden or geriatric patients, or others with chronic constipation, bulk-forming laxatives remain the first line of treatment, but the use of more potent laxatives may be required relatively frequently. Agents that may be used in these situations include diphenylmethane and anthraquinone derivatives, **milk of magnesia**, and **lactulose**.
- In the hospitalized patient without GI disease, constipation may be related to the use of general anesthesia and/or opiate substances. Most orally or rectally administered laxatives may be used. For prompt initiation of a bowel movement, a **tap–water enema** or **glycerin** suppository is recommended, or **milk of magnesia**.
- The approach to the treatment of constipation in infants and children should consider neurologic, metabolic, or anatomic abnormalities when constipation is a persistent problem. When not related to an underlying disease, the approach to constipation is similar to that in an adult. High-fiber diet should be emphasized.

Emollient Laxatives (Docusates)

- These surfactant agents, **docusate** in its various salts, work by facilitating the mixing of aqueous and fatty materials within the intestinal tract. They may increase water and electrolyte secretion in the small and large bowel.
- These products result in a softening of stools within 1 to 3 days.
- Emollient laxatives are not effective in treating constipation but are used mainly to prevent constipation. They may be helpful in situations where straining at stool should be avoided, such as after recovery from myocardial infarction, with acute perianal disease, or after rectal surgery.
- It is unlikely that these agents are very effective in preventing constipation if major causative factors (e.g., heavy opiate use, uncorrected pathology, inadequate dietary fiber) are not concurrently addressed.

Lubricants

- **Mineral oil** is the only lubricant laxative in routine use and acts by coating stool and allowing easier passage. It inhibits colonic absorption of water, thereby increasing stool weight and decreasing stool transit time. Generally, the effect on bowel function is noted after 2 or 3 days of use.
- Mineral oil is helpful in situations similar to those suggested for docusates: to maintain a soft stool and avoid straining for relatively short periods of time (a few days to 2 weeks).
- Mineral oil may be absorbed systemically and cause a foreign-body reaction in lymphoid tissue. Also, in debilitated or recumbent patients, mineral oil may be aspirated, causing lipoid pneumonia.

Lactulose and Sorbitol

- **Lactulose** is a disaccharide that causes an osmotic effect retained in the colon.
- Lactulose is generally not recommended as a first-line agent for the treatment of constipation because it is costly and not necessarily more effective than agents such as milk of magnesia. It may be justified as an alternative for acute constipation and has been found to be particularly useful in elderly patients.
- Occasionally, the use of lactulose may result in flatulence, cramps, diarrhea, and electrolyte imbalances.
- **Sorbitol**, a monosaccharide, has been recommended as a primary agent in the treatment of functional constipation in cognitively intact patients. It is as effective as lactulose and much less expensive.

Diphenylmethane Derivatives

- The two commonly used agents in this class are **bisacodyl** and **phenolph-thalein**.
- Bisacodyl stimulates the mucosal nerve plexus of the colon; the mechanism of action of phenolphthalein is poorly understood.
- The dose of these agents for effective use in various individuals appears to vary greatly. A dose that causes no effects in one patient may result in excessive cramping and fluid evacuation in another.
- These agents are not recommended for regular daily use. Their use is acceptable intermittently (every few weeks) to treat constipation or as a bowel preparation before diagnostic procedures in which cleansing of the colon is necessary.
- A patient taking phenolphthalein-containing laxatives should be cautioned that it may turn urine pink.

Anthraquinone Derivatives

- The agents in this class are **cascara sagrada, sennosides**, and **casanthrol**. Effects are limited to the colon, and stimulation of Auerbach's plexus may be involved.
- Recommendations for the use of these agents are similar to those for the diphenylmethane derivatives. In most cases, intermittent use is acceptable; daily use should be strongly discouraged.

Saline Cathartics

- Saline cathartics are composed of relatively poorly absorbed ions such as magnesium, sulfate, phosphate, and citrate, which produce their effects primarily by osmotic action to retain fluid in the GI tract. These agents may be given orally or rectally.
- A bowel movement may result within a few hours of oral doses and in 1 hour or less after rectal administration.
- These agents should be used primarily for acute evacuation of the bowel, which may be necessary before diagnostic examinations, after poisonings, and in conjunction with some anthelmintics to eliminate parasites.
- Agents such as **milk of magnesia** (an 8% suspension of magnesium hydroxide) may be used occasionally (every few weeks) to treat constipation in otherwise healthy adults.
- Saline cathartics should not be used on a routine basis to treat constipation. With fecal impactions, the enema formulations of these agents may be helpful.

Castor Oil

- **Castor oil** is metabolized in the GI tract to an active compound, ricinoleic acid, which stimulates secretory processes, decreases glucose absorption, and promotes intestinal motility, primarily in the small intestine. Castor oil usually results in a bowel movement within 1 to 3 hours of administration. Because the agent has such a strong purgative action, it should not be used for the routine treatment of constipation.

Glycerin

- This agent is usually administered as a 3-g suppository and exerts its effect by osmotic action in the rectum. As with most agents given as suppositories, the onset of action is usually less than 30 minutes.
- **Glycerin** is considered a safe laxative, although it may occasionally cause rectal irritation. Its use is acceptable on an intermittent basis for constipation, particularly in children.

Polyethylene Glycol-Electrolyte Lavage Solution

- Whole-bowel irrigation with **polyethylene glycol-electrolyte lavage solution** (PEG-ELS) has become popular for colon cleansing before diagnostic procedures or colorectal operations.
- Four liters of this solution is administered over 3 hours to obtain complete evacuation of the GI tract. The solution is not recommended for the routine treatment of constipation, and its use should be avoided in patients with intestinal obstruction.

Other Agents

- Tap-water enemas may be used to treat simple constipation. The administration of 200 mL of water by enema to an adult often results in a bowel movement within 1.5 hours. Soapsuds are no longer recommended for use in enemas because their use may result in proctitis or colitis.

See Chapter 36, Diarrhea and Constipation, authored by William J. Spruill and William E. Wade, for a more detailed discussion of this topic.

Chapter 22

▶ DIARRHEA

▶ DEFINITION

Diarrhea is an increased frequency and decreased consistency of fecal discharge as compared with an individual's normal bowel pattern. Frequency and consistency are variable within and between individuals. For example, some individuals defecate as many as 3 times a day, while others defecate only 2 or 3 times per week.

▶ PATHOPHYSIOLOGY

- Diarrhea is an imbalance in absorption and secretion of water and electrolytes. Diarrhea may be associated with a specific disease of the gastrointestinal tract or with a disease outside the gastrointestinal tract.
- Four general pathophysiologic mechanisms disrupt water and electrolyte balance, leading to diarrhea. These four mechanisms are the basis of diagnosis and therapy. They are (1) a change in active ion transport by either decreased sodium absorption or increased chloride secretion; (2) a change in intestinal motility; (3) an increase in luminal osmolarity; and (4) an increase in tissue hydrostatic pressure.

    These mechanisms have been related to four broad clinical diarrheal groups: secretory, osmotic, exudative, and altered intestinal transit.

- Secretory diarrhea occurs when a stimulating substance (e.g., vasoactive intestinal peptide [VIP], laxatives, or bacterial toxin) increases secretion or decreases absorption of large amounts of water and electrolytes.
- Poorly absorbed substances retain intestinal fluids, resulting in osmotic diarrhea.
- Inflammatory diseases of the gastrointestinal tract can cause exudative diarrhea by discharge of mucus, proteins, or blood into the gut.
- Intestinal motility can be altered by reduced contact time in the small intestine, premature emptying of the colon, and by bacterial overgrowth.

▶ CLINICAL PRESENTATION

The clinical presentation of diarrhea is shown in Table 22–1.

- Many agents, including antibiotics and other drugs, cause diarrhea (Table 21–2). Laxative abuse for weight loss may also result in diarrhea.

▶ DESIRED OUTCOME

The therapeutic goals of diarrhea treatment are to manage the diet; prevent excessive water, electrolyte, and acid-base disturbances; provide symptomatic relief; treat curable causes of diarrhea; and manage secondary disorders causing diarrhea. Clinicians must clearly understand that diarrhea, like a cough, may be a body defense mechanism for ridding itself of harmful substances or pathogens. The correct therapeutic response is not necessarily to stop diarrhea at all costs!

TABLE 22–1. Clinical Presentation of Diarrhea

General
- Usually, acute diarrheal episodes subside within 72 h of onset, whereas chronic diarrhea involves frequent attacks over extended time periods.

Signs and symptoms
- Abrupt onset of nausea, vomiting, abdominal pain, headache, fever, chills, and malaise.
- Bowel movements are frequent and never bloody, and diarrhea lasts 12 to 60 h.
- Intermittent periumbilical or lower right quadrant pain with cramps and audible bowel sounds is characteristic of small intestinal disease.
- When pain is present in large intestinal diarrhea, it is a gripping, aching sensation with tenesmus (straining, ineffective and painful stooling). Pain localizes to the hypogastric region, right or left lower quadrant, or sacral region.
- In chronic diarrhea, a history of previous bouts, weight loss, anorexia, and chronic weakness are important findings.

Physical examination
- Typically demonstrates hyperperistalsis with borborygmi and generalized or local tenderness.

Laboratory tests
- Stool analysis studies include examination for microorganisms, blood, mucus, fat, osmolality, pH, electrolyte and mineral concentration, and cultures.
- Stool test kits are useful for detecting gastrointestinal viruses, particularly rotavirus.
- Antibody serologic testing shows rising titers over a 3- to 6-day period, but this test is not practical and is nonspecific.
- Occasionally, total daily stool volume is also determined.
- Direct endoscopic visualization and biopsy of the colon may be undertaken to assess for the presence of conditions such as colitis or cancer.
- Radiographic studies are helpful in neoplastic and inflammatory conditions.

TABLE 22–2. Drugs Causing Diarrhea

Laxatives
Antacids containing magnesium
Antineoplastics
Auranofin (gold salt)
Antibiotics
    Clindamycin
    Tetracyclines
    Sulfonamides
    Any broad-spectrum antibiotic
Antihypertensives
    Reserpine
    Guanethidine
    Methyldopa
    Guanabenz
    Guanadrel
Cholinergics
    Bethanechol
    Neostigmine
Cardiac agents
    Quinidine
    Digitalis
    Digoxin
Nonsteroidal anti-inflammatory drugs
Prostaglandins
Colchicine

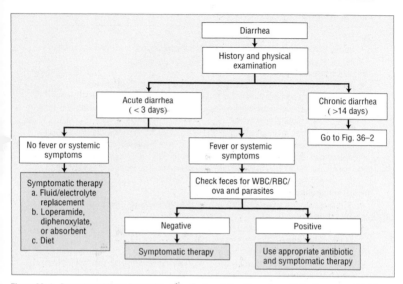

Figure 22–1. Recommendations for treating acute diarrhea. Follow these steps: (1) Perform a complete history and physical examination. (2) Is the diarrhea acute or chronic? If chronic diarrhea, go to Fig 36–2. (3) If acute diarrhea, check for fever and/or systemic signs and symptoms (i.e., toxic patient). If systemic illness (fever, anorexia, or volume depletion), check for an infectious source. If positive for infectious diarrhea, use appropriate antibiotic/anthelmintic drug and symptomatic therapy. If negative for infectious cause, use only symtomatic treatment. (4) If no systemic findings, then use symptomatic therapy based on severity of volume depletion, oral or parenteral fluid/electrolytes, antidiarrheal agents (see Table 36–4), and diet.

▶ TREATMENT

GENERAL PRINCIPLES

- Management of the diet is a first priority for treatment of diarrhea (Figures 22–1 and 22–2). Most clinicians recommend stopping solid foods for 24 hours and avoiding dairy products.
- When nausea or vomiting is mild, a digestible low-residue diet is administered for 24 hours.
- If vomiting is present and is uncontrollable with antiemetics, nothing is taken by mouth. As bowel movements decrease, a bland diet is begun. Feeding should continue in children with acute bacterial diarrhea.
- Overzealous laxative use in the elderly, whether self- or physician-prescribed, is a common cause of diarrhea and must be identified and stopped. Other drugs that may cause or worsen diarrhea should be stopped or the dosage reduced.
- Rehydration and maintenance of water and electrolytes are the primary treatment measures until the diarrheal episode ends. If vomiting and dehydration are not severe, enteral feeding is the less costly and preferred method. In the United States, many commercial oral rehydration preparations are available (Table 22–3).

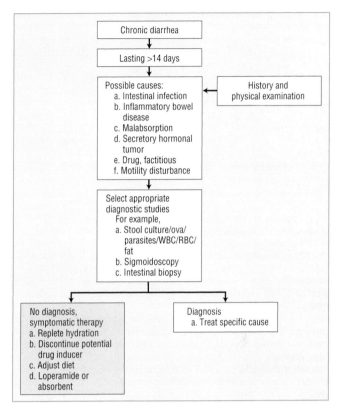

Figure 22–2. Recommendations for treating chronic diarrhea. Follow these steps: (1) Perform a careful history and physical examination. (2) The possible causes of chronic diarrhea are many. These can be classified into intestinal infections (bacterial or protozoal), inflammatory disease (Crohn's disease or ulcerative colitis), malabsorption (lactose intolerance), secretory hormonal tumor (intestinal carcinoid tumor or VIPoma), drug (antacid), factitious (laxative abuse), or motility disturbance (diabetes mellitus, irritable bowel syndrome, or hyperthyroidism). (3) If the diagnosis is uncertain, selected appropriate diagnostic studies should be ordered. (4) Once diagnosed, treatment is planned for the underlying cause with symptomatic antidiarrheal therapy. (5) If no specific cause can be identified, symptomatic therapy is prescribed.

PHARMACOLOGIC THERAPY

- Various drugs have been used to treat diarrhea (Table 22–4). These drugs are grouped into several categories: antimotility, adsorbents, antisecretory compounds, antibiotics, enzymes, and intestinal microflora. Usually, these drugs are not curative but palliative.
- Opiates and opioid derivatives delay the transit of intraluminal content or increase gut capacity, prolonging contact and absorption. The limitations of the opiates are addiction potential (a real concern with long-term use) and worsening of diarrhea in selected infectious diarrheas.

TABLE 22–3. Oral Rehydration Solutions

	WHO-ORS[a]	Pedialyte[b] (Ross)	Rehydralyte[b] (Ross)	Infalyte (Mead Johnson)	Resol[b] (Wyeth)
Osmolality (mOsm/L)	333	249	304	200	269
Carbohydrates[b] (g/L)	20	25	25	30[c]	20
Calories (cal/L)	85	100	100	126	80
Electrolytes (mEq/L)					
Sodium	90	45	75	50	50
Potassium	20	20	20	25	20
Chloride	80	35	65	45	50
Citrate	—	30	30	34	34
Bicarbonate	30	—	—	—	—
Calcium	—	—	—	—	4
Magnesium	—	—	—	—	4
Sulfate	—	—	—	—	—
Phosphate	—	—	—	—	5

[a]World Health Organization Oral Rehydration Solution
[b]Carbohydrate is glucose.
[c]Rice syrup solids are carbohydrate source.

- **Loperamide** is often recommended for managing acute and chronic diarrhea. Diarrhea lasting 48 hours beyond initiating loperamide warrants medical attention.
- Adsorbents (such as **kaolin-pectin**) are used for symptomatic relief (see Table 22–4). Adsorbents are nonspecific in their action; they adsorb nutrients, toxins, drugs, and digestive juices. Coadministration with other drugs reduces their bioavailability.
- **Bismuth subsalicylate** is often used for treatment or prevention of diarrhea (traveler's diarrhea) and has antisecretory, anti-inflammatory, and antibacterial effects.
- *Lactobacillus* preparation is intended to replace colonic microflora. This supposedly restores intestinal functions and suppresses the growth of pathogenic microorganisms. However, a dairy product diet containing 200 to 400 g of lactose or dextrin is equally effective in recolonization.
- Anticholinergic drugs, such as **atropine**, block vagal tone and prolong gut transit time. Their value in controlling diarrhea is questionable and limited by side effects.
- **Octreotide**, a synthetic octapeptide analog of endogenous somatostatin, is prescribed for the symptomatic treatment of carcinoid tumors and VIP-secreting tumors (VIPomas). Octreotide is used in selected patients with carcinoid syndrome. Octreotide blocks the release of serotonin and other active peptides and is effective in controlling diarrhea and flushing. Dosage range for managing diarrhea associated with carcinoid tumors is 100 to 600 mcg/day in two to four divided doses subcutaneously. Octreotide is associated with an adverse effects such as cholelithiasis, nausea, diarrhea, and abdominal pain.

▶ EVALUATION OF THERAPEUTIC OUTCOMES

- Therapeutic outcomes are directed to key symptoms, signs, and laboratory studies. The constitutional symptoms usually improve within 24 to 72 hours.
- One should check the frequency and character of bowel movements each day along with the vital signs and improving appetite.

TABLE 22–4. Selected Antidiarrheal Preparations

	Dose Form	Adult Dose
Antimotility		
Diphenoxylate	2.5 mg/tablet 2.5 mg/5 mL	5 mg four times daily; do not exceed 20 mg/day
Loperamide	2 mg/capsule	Initially 4 mg, then 2 mg after each loose stool; do not exceed 16 mg/day
	1 mg/5 mL	
Paregoric	2 mg/5 mL (morphine)	5–10 mL 1–4 times daily
Opium tincture	5 mg/mL (morphine)	0.6 mL four times daily
Difenoxin	1 mg/tablet	Two tablets, then one tablet after each loose stool; up to 8 tablets/day
Adsorbents		
Kaolin–pectin mixture	5.7 g kaolin + 130.2 mg pectin/30 mL	30–120 mL after each loose stool
Polycarbophil	500 mg/tablet	Chew 2 tablets four times daily or after each loose stool; do not exceed 12 tablets/day
Attapulgite	750 mg/15 mL 300 mg/7.5 mL 750 mg/tablet 600 mg/tablet 300 mg/tablet	1200–1500 mg after each loose bowel movement or every 2 hours; up to 9000 mg/day
Antisecretory		
Bismuth subsalicylate	1050 mg/30 mL 262 mg/15 mL 524 mg/15 mL 262 mg/tablet	Two tablets or 30 mL every 30 min to 1 h as needed up to 8 doses/day
Enzymes (lactase)	1250 neutral lactase units/4 drops	3–4 drops taken with milk or dairy product
	3300 FCC lactase units per tablet	1 or 2 tablets as above
Bacterial replacement (*Lactobacillus acidophilus, Lactobacillus bulgaricus*)		2 tablets or 1 granule packet 3 to 4 times daily; give with milk, juice, or water
Octreotide	0.05 mg/mL 0.1 mg/mL 0.5 mg/mL	Initial: 50 mcg subcutaneously 1–2 times per day and titrate dose based on indication up to 600 mcg/day in 2–4 divided doses

- The clinician also needs to monitor body weight, serum osmolality, serum electrolytes, complete blood cell count, urinalysis, and cultures (if appropriate). With an urgent or emergency situation, evaluation of the volume status of the patient is the most important outcome.
- Toxic patients (those with fever, dehydration, and hematochezia and those who are hypotensive) require hospitalization; they need intravenous electrolyte solutions and empiric antibiotics while awaiting cultures. With quick management, they usually recover within a few days.

See Chapter 36, Diarrhea and Constipation, authored by William J. Spruill and William E. Wade, for a more detailed discussion of this topic.

Chapter 23

▶ GASTROESOPHAGEAL REFLUX DISEASE

▶ DEFINITION

Gastroesophageal reflux refers to the retrograde movement of gastric contents from the stomach into the esophagus. Gastroesophageal reflux disease (GERD) refers to any symptomatic clinical condition or histologic alteration that results from episodes of gastroesophageal reflux. When the esophagus is repeatedly exposed to refluxed material for prolonged periods, inflammation of the esophagus (reflux esophagitis) can occur and in some cases it progresses to erosion of the esophagus (erosive esophagitis).

▶ PATHOPHYSIOLOGY

- In many patients with GERD, the problem is not excessive acid production but that the acid produced spends too much time in contact with the esophageal mucosa.
- Gastroesophageal reflux is often caused by defective lower esophageal sphincter (LES) pressure or function. Patients may have decreased LES pressures related to spontaneous transient LES relaxations, transient increases in intra-abdominal pressure, or an atonic LES. A variety of foods and medications may decrease LES pressure (Table 23–1).

TABLE 23–1. Foods and Medications that May Worsen GERD Symptoms

Decreased lower esophageal sphincter pressure	
Foods	
Fatty meal	Garlic
Carminatives (peppermint, spearmint)	Onions
Chocolate	Chili peppers
Coffee, cola, tea	
Medications	
Anticholinergics	Isoproterenol
Barbiturates	Narcotics (meperidine, morphine)
Benzodiazepines (diazepam)	
Caffeine	Nicotine (smoking)
Dihydropyridine calcium channel blockers	Nitrates
Dopamine	Phentolamine
Estrogen	Progesterone
Ethanol	Theophylline
Direct irritants to the esophageal mucosa	
Foods	
Spicy foods	Tomato juice
Orange juice	Coffee
Medications	
Alendronate	Quinidine
Aspirin	Potassium chloride
Iron	
Nonsteroidal anti-inflammatory drugs	

- Problems with other normal mucosal defense mechanisms may also contribute to the development of GERD, including prolonged acid clearance time from the esophagus, delayed gastric emptying, and reduced mucosal resistance.
- Aggressive factors that may promote esophageal damage upon reflux into the esophagus include gastric acid, pepsin, bile acids, and pancreatic enzymes. The composition and volume of the refluxate and the duration of exposure are the most important aggressive factors in determining the consequences of gastroesophageal reflux.

▶ CLINICAL PRESENTATION

- The hallmark symptom of gastroesophageal reflux and esophagitis is heartburn, or pyrosis. It is classically described as a substernal sensation of warmth or burning that may radiate to the neck. It is waxing and waning in character and is often aggravated by activities that worsen gastroesophageal reflux (e.g., recumbent position, bending over, eating a high-fat meal). Other symptoms include water brash (hypersalivation), belching, and regurgitation.
- Atypical symptoms include nonallergic asthma, chronic cough, hoarseness, pharyngitis, dental erosions, and chest pain that mimics angina.
- Inadequately treated GERD may lead to complications from long-term acid exposure such as continual pain, dysphagia, and odynophagia. Other severe complications include esophageal strictures, hemorrhage, Barrett's esophagus, and esophageal adenocarcinoma.

▶ DIAGNOSIS

- The most useful tool in the diagnosis of gastroesophageal reflux is the clinical history, including both presenting symptoms and associated risk factors.
- Endoscopy is the preferred technique for assessing the mucosa for esophagitis and complications such as Barrett's esophagus. It allows visualization and biopsy of the esophageal mucosa, but the mucosa may appear relatively normal in mild cases of GERD.
- Barium radiography is less expensive than endoscopy but lacks the sensitivity and specificity needed to accurately determine the presence of mucosal injury or to distinguish Barrett's esophagus from esophagitis.
- Twenty-four-hour ambulatory pH monitoring is useful in patients who continue to have symptoms without evidence of esophageal damage, patients who are refractory to standard treatment, and patients who present with atypical symptoms (e.g., chest pain or pulmonary symptoms). The test helps to correlate symptoms with abnormal esophageal acid exposure, documents the percentage of time the intraesophageal pH is low, and determines the frequency and severity of reflux.
- **Omeprazole** given empirically as a "therapeutic trial" for diagnosing GERD may be as beneficial as ambulatory pH monitoring while also being less expensive, more convenient, and more readily available. However, there is no standard dosing regimen; standard doses or double-dose omeprazole have been used.
- Esophageal manometry to evaluate motility should be performed in any patient who is a candidate for antireflux surgery. It is useful in determining which surgical procedure is best for the patient.

▶ DESIRED OUTCOME

The goals of treatment are to alleviate or eliminate symptoms, decrease the frequency and duration of gastroesophageal reflux, promote healing of the injured mucosa, and prevent the development of complications.

▶ TREATMENT

GENERAL PRINCIPLES

V

- Therapeutic modalities are targeted at reversing the pathophysiologic abnormalities. These include decreasing the acidity of the refluxate, decreasing the gastric volume available to be refluxed, improving gastric emptying, increasing LES pressure, enhancing esophageal acid clearance, and protecting the esophageal mucosa (Figure 23–1).
- Treatment is categorized into the following modalities:
  - Phase I: lifestyle changes and patient-directed therapy with **antacids** and/or over-the-counter (OTC) **H$_2$-receptor antagonists (H$_2$RA)** or **proton pump inhibitors (PPIs)**.
  - Phase II: pharmacologic interventions primarily with standard or high-dose acid-suppressing agents.
  - Phase III: interventional therapies (antireflux surgery or endoluminal therapies).
- The initial therapeutic modality depends in part on the patient's condition (symptom frequency, degree of esophagitis, presence of complications). Historically, a step-up approach has been used, starting with phase I and then progressing through phases II and III if necessary (Table 23–2). A step-down

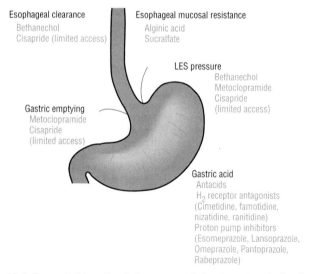

Figure 23–1. Therapeutic interventions in the management of gastroesophageal reflux disease. Pharmacologic interventions are targeted at improving defense mechanisms or decreasing aggressive factors. LES = lower esophageal sphincter.

approach is also effective, starting with a PPI once or twice daily instead of an H_2RA and then stepping down to the lowest acid suppression needed to control symptoms.

- Lifestyle modifications should be started initially and continued throughout the treatment course (Table 23–3).

ANTACIDS AND ANTACID-ALGINIC ACID PRODUCTS

- **Antacids** provide immediate, symptomatic relief for mild GERD and are often used concurrently with other acid-suppressing therapies. Patients who require frequent use for chronic symptoms should receive prescription-strength acid-suppressing therapy instead.
- An **antacid with alginic acid** (Gaviscon) is not a potent acid neutralizing agent but it does form a viscous solution that floats on the surface of the gastric contents. This serves as a protective barrier for the esophagus against reflux of gastric contents and reduces the frequency of reflux episodes. Efficacy data indicating endoscopic healing are lacking.
- Antacids have a short duration, which necessitates frequent administration throughout the day to provide continuous acid neutralization. Typical doses are 2 tablets or 1 tablespoonful 4 times daily (after meals and at bedtime). Nighttime acid suppression cannot be maintained with bedtime doses of antacids.

H_2-RECEPTOR ANTAGONISTS: CIMETIDINE, RANITIDINE, FAMOTIDINE, AND NIZATIDINE

- The H_2RAs in divided doses are effective for treating mild to moderate GERD. Low-dose OTC products may be beneficial for symptomatic relief of intermittent heartburn and for preventing meal-provoked heartburn in patients with mild disease. For nonerosive disease, H_2RAs are given in standard doses twice daily. For nonresponding patients and those with erosive disease, higher doses and/or 4 times daily dosing provide better acid control (see Table 23–2).
- The efficacy of H_2RAs in GERD is highly variable; although standard doses produce symptomatic improvement in about 60% of patients, endoscopic healing rates average only about 50%. The more severe the esophageal damage, the poorer the response. Higher doses and prolonged courses (8 weeks or more) are frequently required.
- The H_2RAs are generally well tolerated. The most common adverse effects are headache, somnolence, fatigue, dizziness, and either constipation or diarrhea. Cimetidine may inhibit the metabolism of theophylline, warfarin, phenytoin, nifedipine, and propranolol, among other drugs.
- Because all of the H_2RAs are equally efficacious, selection of the specific agent should be based on differences in pharmacokinetics, safety profile, and cost.

PROTON PUMP INHIBITORS: ESOMEPRAZOLE, LANSOPRAZOLE, OMEPRAZOLE, PANTOPRAZOLE, AND RABEPRAZOLE

- PPIs block gastric acid secretion by inhibiting H^+/K^+-ATPase in gastric parietal cells, which results in profound and long-lasting antisecretory effects.
- PPIs are superior to H_2RAs in patients with moderate to severe GERD, including those with erosive esophagitis, complicated symptoms (Barrett's esophagus, strictures), and nonerosive GERD with moderate to severe symptoms. Relapse is common in these patients, and long-term maintenance therapy is generally indicated. Symptomatic relief is seen in approximately 83% of patients, and endoscopic healing rates are about 78% at 8 weeks.

TABLE 23–2. Therapeutic Approach to GERD

Patient Presentation	Recommended Treatment Regimen	Comments
Phase I Intermittent, mild heartburn	A. Lifestyle Changes **PLUS** B. Antacids - Maalox or Mylanta 30 mL as needed or after meals and at bedtime - Maalox TC 5–10 mL as needed or after meals and at bedtime - Gaviscon 2 tabs after meals and at bedtime - Calcium carbonate (500 mg) 2–4 tablets as needed **AND/OR** C. Low-dose OTC H$_2$–receptor antagonists (each taken up to twice daily) - Cimetidine 200 mg - Famotidine 10 or 20 mg - Nizatidine 75 mg - Ranitidine 75 mg **OR** OTC proton pump inhibitor (taken once daily) - Omeprazole 20 mg	Lifestyle changes should be started initially and continued throughout the course of treatment. If symptoms are unrelieved with lifestyle changes and OTC medications after 2 wk, begin pharmacologic therapy (phase II therapy).
Phase II Symptomatic relief of GERD	A. Lifestyle modifications **PLUS** B. Standard doses of H$_2$–receptor antagonists for 6–12 wk - Cimetidine 400 mg twice daily - Famotidine 20 mg twice daily - Nizatidine 150 mg twice daily - Ranitidine 150 mg twice daily	For typical symptoms, treat empirically with phase II therapy. Mild GERD can usually be treated effectively with H$_2$–receptor antagonists. Patients with moderate to severe symptoms should receive a proton pump inhibitor as initial therapy. If symptoms are relieved, treat recurrences on an as-needed basis.

OR

B. Proton pump inhibitors for 4–8 wk. All are given once daily.
- Esomeprazole 20 mg
- Lansoprazole 15 mg
- Omeprazole 20 mg
- Pantoprazole 40 mg
- Rabeprazole 20 mg

If symptoms recur frequently, consider maintenance therapy (MT) with the lowest effective dose. Note: Most patients will require standard doses for MT.

Healing of erosive esophagitis or treatment of patients presenting with moderate to severe symptoms or complications

A. Lifestyle modifications

PLUS

B. Proton pump inhibitors for 4–16 wk (up to twice daily)
- Esomeprazole 20–40 mg daily
- Lansoprazole 30 mg daily
- Omeprazole 20 mg daily
- Rabeprazole 20 mg daily
- Pantoprazole 40 mg daily

OR

B. High–dose H$_2$-receptor antagonist for 8–12 weeks
- Cimetidine 400 mg four times daily or 800 mg twice daily
- Famotidine 40 mg twice daily
- Nizatidine 150 mg 4 times daily
- Ranitidine 150 mg 4 times daily

Interventional therapies (antireflux surgery or endoluminal therapies)

For atypical symtoms, obtain endoscopy (if possible) to evaluate mucosa. Give a trial of a proton pump inhibitor or an H$_2$-receptor antagonist. If symptoms are relieved, consider MT. Proton pump inhibitors are the most effective maintenance therapy in patients with atypical symptoms, complicated symptoms, and erosive disease.

Phase III

Patients not responding to phase II therapy, including those with persistent atypical symptoms, should be evaluated via ambulatory 24-h pH monitoring to confirm the diagnosis of GERD (if possible). If GERD is present, consider phase III therapy.

Manometry should be performed in anyone who is a candidate for surgery.

TABLE 23–3. Nonpharmacologic Treatment of GERD with Lifestyle Modifications

- Elevate the head of the bed (increases esophageal clearance). Use 6- to 8-inch blocks under the head of the bed. Sleep on a foam wedge
- Dietary changes

  Avoid foods that may decrease lower esophageal sphincter pressure (fats, chocolate, alcohol, peppermint, and spearmint)

  Avoid foods that have a direct irritant effect on the esophageal mucosa (spicy foods, orange juice, tomato juice, and coffee)

  Include protein-rich meals in diet (augments lower esophageal sphincter pressure)

  Eat small meals and avoid eating immediately prior to sleeping (within 3 h if possible) (decreases gastric volume)

  Weight reduction (reduces symtoms)
- Stop smoking (decreases spontaneous esophageal sphincter relaxation)
- Avoid alcohol (increases amplitude of the lower esophageal sphincter, peristaltic waves, and frequency of contraction)
- Avoid tight-fitting clothes
- Discontinue, if possible, drugs that may promote reflux (calcium channel blockers, β blockers, nitrates, theophylline)
- Take drugs that have a direct irritant effect on the esophageal mucosa with plenty of liquid if they cannot be avoided (tetracyclines, quinidine, and KCI, iron salts, aspirin, nonsteroidal anti-inflammatory drugs)

- PPIs are also efficacious in patients refractory to H_2RAs and are more cost effective than H_2RAs in patients with severe disease.
- PPIs are usually well tolerated. Potential adverse effects include headache, dizziness, somnolence, diarrhea, constipation, and nausea. All PPIs can decrease the absorption of drugs such as **ketoconazole** or **itraconazole** that require an acidic environment for absorption. Other drug interactions vary with each agent.
- The PPIs degrade in acidic environments and are therefore formulated in delayed-release capsules or tablets. **Lansoprazole, esomeprazole**, and **omeprazole** contain enteric-coated (pH-sensitive) granules in a capsule form. In patients unable to swallow the capsules, the contents can be mixed in applesauce or placed in orange juice. In patients with nasogastric tubes, the contents should be mixed in 8.4% sodium bicarbonate solution. **Esomeprazole** can be mixed with water. **Lansoprazole** is also available in packets for oral suspension and delayed-release orally disintegrating tablets; neither product should be placed through nasogastric tubes. Patients taking **pantoprazole** or **rabeprazole** should be instructed not to crush, chew, or split the delayed-release tablets.
- **Pantoprazole** and **lansoprazole intravenous (IV) injection** are indicated for the short-term treatment of GERD (e.g., up to 7 to 10 days) in patients unable to take oral therapy. However, IV formulations are not more effective than oral PPIs and are more expensive.
- Patients should be instructed to take oral PPIs in the morning 15 to 30 minutes before breakfast to maximize efficacy, because these agents inhibit only actively secreting proton pumps. If dosed twice daily, the second dose should be taken approximately 10 to 12 hours after the morning dose and prior to a meal or snack.
- All of the PPIs are safe and effective, and the choice of a particular agent is likely to be based on cost.

PROKINETIC AGENTS

- **Cisapride** has efficacy that is similar to that of the H$_2$RAs in mild esophagitis. However, it costs more than H$_2$RAs and offers no real advantage, especially in patients with normal GI motility. It is no longer available for routine use because of life-threatening arrhythmias when combined with certain medications and other disease states. Physicians must register as investigators with the manufacturer (Janssen), and patients must be enrolled just as with any other study protocol.
- **Metoclopramide**, a dopamine antagonist, increases LES pressure in a dose-related manner and accelerates gastric emptying. Unlike cisapride, it does not improve esophageal clearance.
- Metoclopramide may provide symptomatic improvement for some patients with GERD, but substantial evidence of endoscopic healing is lacking.
- Tachyphylaxis and side effects limit the usefulness of metoclopramide. Commonly reported adverse reactions include somnolence, nervousness, fatigue, dizziness, weakness, depression, diarrhea, and rash.
- Prokinetic agents have been used as adjunctive therapy with an H$_2$RA. This combination is only appropriate in patients with known or suspected motility disorders or in those who have failed high-dose PPI therapy.

MUCOSAL PROTECTANTS

- **Sucralfate** is a nonabsorbable aluminum salt of sucrose octasulfate that has limited value in the treatment of GERD.
- It has similar healing rates as H$_2$RAs in mild esophagitis, but it is less effective than higher doses of H$_2$RAs in patients with refractory esophagitis. Based on available data, sucralfate cannot be recommended for treating anything but the mildest cases of GERD.

COMBINATION THERAPY

- Combination therapy with an acid-suppressing agent and a prokinetic agent or mucosal protectant seems logical, but data supporting such therapy are limited. This approach should be reserved for patients who have esophagitis plus concurrent motor dysfunction or for those who have failed high-dose PPI therapy.
- Because combination therapy offers only modest improvement over standard doses of H$_2$RAs alone, patients not responding to standard H$_2$RA doses should have the dose increased or be switched to a PPI instead of adding a prokinetic agent.

MAINTENANCE THERAPY

- Although healing and/or symptomatic improvement may be achieved via many different therapeutic modalities, 70% to 90% of patients relapse within 1 year of discontinuation of therapy.
- Long-term maintenance therapy should be considered to prevent complications and worsening of esophageal function in patients who have symptomatic relapse after discontinuation of therapy or dosage reduction, including patients with complications such as Barrett's esophagus, strictures, or hemorrhage.
- Most patients require standard doses to prevent relapses. **H$_2$RAs** may be an effective maintenance therapy in patients with mild disease. The **PPIs** are the drugs of choice for maintenance treatment of moderate to severe esophagitis. Usual once-daily doses are **omeprazole** 20 mg, **lansoprazole** 30 mg,

rabeprazole 20 mg, or **esomeprazole** 20 mg. Lower doses of a PPI or alternate-day regimens may be effective in some patients with less severe disease.

INTERVENTIONAL APPROACHES

- Antireflux surgery (Nissen, Belsey, Toupet, or Hill fundoplication operations) should be considered in patients who fail to respond to pharmacologic treatment, opt for surgery because of lifestyle considerations, have complications (Barrett's esophagus, strictures, or grade 3 or 4 esophagitis), or have atypical symptoms and reflux documented on ambulatory pH monitoring.
- Endoluminal therapies (endoscopic gastroplastic plication, endoluminal application of radiofrequency heat energy, and endoscopic injection of a biopolymer) are FDA-approved therapies, but their precise role in the management of GERD remains to be determined.

▶ EVALUATION OF THERAPEUTIC OUTCOMES

- The short-term goals are to relieve symptoms such as heartburn and regurgitation so that they do not impair the patient's quality of life.
- The frequency and severity of symptoms should be monitored, and patients should be counseled on symptoms that suggest the presence of complications requiring immediate medical attention, such as dysphagia or odynophagia.
- Patients should also be monitored for the presence of atypical symptoms such as cough, nonallergic asthma, or chest pain. These symptoms require further diagnostic evaluation.

See Chapter 32, Gastroesophageal Reflux Disease, authored by Dianne B. Williams and Robert R. Schade, for a more detailed discussion of this topic.

Chapter 24

▶ HEPATITIS, VIRAL

▶ DEFINITION

Viral hepatitis refers to the clinically important hepatotrophic viruses responsible for hepatitis A (HAV), hepatitis B (HBV), delta hepatitis (HDV), hepatitis C (HCV), and hepatitis E (HEV). Viral hepatitis has acute, fulminant, and chronic clinical forms defined by duration or severity of infection.

Acute viral hepatitis is a systemic viral infection of up to but not exceeding 6 months in duration that produces inflammatory necrosis of the liver. Chronic viral hepatitis describes prolongation or continuation of the hepatic necroinflammatory process 6 months or more beyond the onset of the acute illness.

▶ HEPATITIS A

- HAV infection is one of the most frequently reported vaccine-preventable diseases in the United States.
- The incidence of HAV correlates directly with poor sanitary conditions and hygienic practices. HAV infection occurs primarily from person-to-person transmission.
- HAV infection usually produces a self-limited disease with a low case-fatality rate. The disease may last up to 6 months in three phases: incubation, acute hepatitis, and convalescence. Most patients have full clinical and biochemical recovery within 12 weeks.
- The minimal degree of liver cell damage with HAV is reflected by mild elevations of serum transaminases values to about twice normal.
- The clinical presentation of HAV infection is given in Table 24–1. The average incubation period is 28 days, with a range of 15 to 50 days.
- No cases of a chronic carrier state or chronic hepatitis have been reported with HAV.

TABLE 24–1. Clinical Presentation of Acute Hepatitis A

Signs and symptoms
- The preicteric phase brings nonspecific influenza-like symptoms consisting of anorexia, nausea, fatigue, and malaise
- Abrupt onset of anorexia, nausea, vomiting, malaise, fever, headache, and right upper quadrant abdominal pain with acute illness
- Icteric hepatitis is generally accompanied by dark urine, acholic (light-colored) stools, and worsening of systemic symptoms
- Pruritus is often a major complaint of icteric patients

Physical examination
- Icteric sclera, skin, and secretions
- Mild weight loss of 2 to 5 kg
- Hepatomegaly

Laboratory tests
- Positive serum IgM anti-HAV
- Mild elevations of serum bilirubin, γ-globulin, and hepatic transaminase (alanine transaminase [ALT], and aspartate transaminase [AST] values to about twice normal in acute anicteric disease
- Elevations of alkaline phosphatase, γ-glutamyl transferase, and total bilirubin in patients with cholestatic illness

- The diagnosis of acute HAV infection depends on clinical suspicion, characteristic symptoms, elevated aminotransferases and bilirubin, and a positive anti-HAV IgM. The antibody peaks during the early phase of convalescence and remains positive for 4 to 6 months after the onset of the disease.

TREATMENT

- Management of HAV infection is primarily supportive, including a healthy diet, rest, maintenance of fluid balance, avoidance of hepatotoxic drugs and alcohol.
- Pharmacologic agents offer no clear benefit in the treatment of HAV.

PREVENTION

- The spread of HAV can be best controlled by avoiding exposure. The most important measures to avoid exposure include good hand-washing techniques and good personal hygiene practices.
- The current vaccination strategy in the United States includes vaccinating: (1) children in states, counties, and communities with consistently elevated rates of hepatitis A, (2) persons in groups at increased risk for HAV infections, such as international travelers, and (3) persons at risk of adverse outcomes, such as those with chronic liver disease.
- HAV vaccines given preexposure demonstrate protective efficacy in 94% to 100% of vaccines within 1 month after primary vaccination. When a booster dose is given 6 months later, essentially 100% of recipients develop high antibody levels.
- Immunization is indicated for individuals aged 2 years or older who are at increased risk of hepatitis A infection. Groups who should receive HAV vaccine are shown in Table 24–2. Approved dosing recommendations are shown in Table 24–3.
- Prevention of HAV has traditionally focused on avoiding exposure as well as preexposure and postexposure prophylaxis with IG.
- A single dose of IG of 0.02 mL/kg intramuscularly (IM) is recommended for travelers to high-risk areas if travel is for less than 3 months. For lengthy stays,

TABLE 24–2. Groups at Increased Risk of Hepatitis A and Recommended for Preexposure Hepatitis A Vaccination

---

Children living in states, counties, or communities where rates of hepatitis A are at least twice the national average ≥20 cases per 100,000 population). For 1987–1997, these states included Arizona, Alaska, Oregon, New Mexico, Utah, Washington, Oklahoma, South Dakota, Idaho, Nevada, and California.

Children living in states, counties, or communities where rates of hepatitis A are greater than the national average but lower than twice the national average should be considered for routine vaccination (≥10 cases but <20 cases per 100,000 population). For 1987–1997, these states included Missouri, Texas, Colorado, Arkansas, Montana, and Wyoming.

Persons traveling to or working in countries that have high or intermediate endemicity of infection.[a]

Men who have sex with men.

Illegal-drug users.

Persons who have occupational risk for infection (e.g., persons who work with HAV-infected primates or HAV in a research laboratory setting).

Persons who have clotting-factor disorders.

Persons who have chronic liver disease (e.g., persons with chronic liver disease caused by hepatitis B or C and persons awaiting liver transplants).

---

[a]Travelers to Canada, Western Europe, Japan, Australia, or New Zealand are at no greater risk for HAV infection than they are while in the United States. All other travelers should be assessed for hepatitis A risk.
From Centers for Disease Control.[2]

TABLE 24–3. Recommended Dosing of Havrix and Vaqta

Vaccine	Vaccinee's Age (years)	Dose	Volume (mL)	Number Doses	Schedule (months)[b]
Havrix	2 to 18	720 ELISA units[a]	0.5	2	0, 6–12
	>18	1440 ELISA units	1	2	0, 6–12
Vaqta	2 to 17	25 units	0.5	2	0, 6–18
	>17	50 units	1	2	0, 6

[a]Havrix previously was also available as 360 ELISA units per dose. This formulation was administered as a three-dose schedule for persons 2 to 18 years of age. It is no longer available.
[b]0 months represents the timing of the initial dose; subsequent numbers represent months after the initial dose.
From Centers for Disease Control.[2]

0.06 mL/kg IM should be given every 3 to 5 months. Dosing is the same for adults and children.

- The postexposure prophylactic benefit from IG is greatest early in the incubation period and is of no benefit more than 2 weeks after exposure. A single IG dose of 0.02 mL/kg IM is used for postexposure prophylaxis of hepatitis A.
- The vaccines are known to produce protective levels of antibody for at least 5 to 8 years.
- Vaccine side effects include injection site reactions and headache.

▶ HEPATITIS B

- Hepatitis B is a leading cause of chronic hepatitis, cirrhosis, and hepatocellular carcinoma.
- Transmission of HBV in the United States occurs predominantly through contact with infected blood products or body secretions (saliva, vaginal fluids, and semen) or sharing of needles by intravenous drug abusers.
- The incubation period for HBV is 1 to 6 months. This is followed by a symptomatic prodromal phase consisting of malaise, fatigue, weakness, anorexia, myalgias, and arthralgias. Jaundice occurs in about one-third of patients and may persist for several weeks.
- The sequence of serologic markers for HBV are given in Table 24–4.
- Clinical manifestations of acute HBV infection are age dependent. Infants infected with HBV are generally asymptomatic, while about 85% to 95% of children aged 1 –to 5 years are asymptomatic.

TABLE 24–4. Interpretation of the Laboratory Profile in Hepatitis B Virus (HBV) Infection

Pattern	Is Patient Infectious?	HBsAg	HBeAg	Anti-HBc Total	Anti-HBs	Anti-HBe
Not infected/early incubation	No	—	—	—	—	—
Early acute HBV infection	Yes	+	—	—	—	—
Acute HBV infection	Yes	+	+	+	—	—
Chronic HBV infection[a]	Yes	+	+/–	+	—	—
Resolved infection	No	—	—	+	—	+
"Window" period following acute HBV infection	No	—	—	+	—	+

[a]Patient should be evaluated for complications of chronic infection such as cirrhosis and hepatocellular carcinoma. anti-HBc, antibody to HbcAg; anti-Hbe, antibody to HbeAg; anti-HBs, antibody to HbsAg; HBcAg, hepatitis B core antigen; HbeAg, hepatitis B e antigen; HBsAg: hepatitis B surface antigen.
From Lee.[10]

TABLE 24–5. Clinical Presentation of Chronic Hepatitis B[a]

Signs and symptoms
- Easy fatigability, anxiety, anorexia, and malaise
- Ascites, jaundice, variceal bleeding, and hepatic encephalopathy can manifest with liver decompensation
- Hepatic encephalopathy is associated with hyperexcitability, impaired mentation, confusion, obtundation, and eventually coma
- Vomiting and seizures

Physical examination
- Icteric sclera, skin, and secretions
- Decreased bowel sounds, increased abdominal girth, and detectable fluid wave
- Asterixis
- Spider angiomata

Laboratory tests
- Presence of hepatitis B surface antigen for at least 6 months
- Intermittent elevations of hepatic transaminase (alanine transaminase [ALT] and aspartate transaminase [AST]) and hepatitis B virus DNA greater than 10^5 copies/mL
- Liver biopsies for pathologic classification as chronic persistent hepatitis, chronic active hepatitis, or cirrhosis

[a]Chronic hepatitis B can be present even without all the signs, symptoms, and physical examination findings listed being apparent.

- Acute symptomatic infections vary in severity and include fever, anorexia, nausea, vomiting, jaundice, dark urine, clay-colored or pale stools, and abdominal pain.
- Approximately 90% of infants but 10% of adolescents or adults develop chronic HBV. Chronic HBV predisposes patients to chronic liver disease, cirrhosis, and hepatocellular carcinoma.
- The clinical presentation of chronic HBV is given in Table 24–5.

TREATMENT

- The key goal of therapy is to eradicate or permanently suppress HBV. The short-term goal is to limit hepatic inflammation and to reduce the risk of fibrosis and/or decompensation. The long-term goal is to prevent transaminase flares and the development of complications, and to prolong survival.
- No specific therapy is available for the management of acute HBV infection.
- **Interferon alpha2b** (IFN-alpha2B), **lamivudine**, and **adefovir dipivoxil** are approved in the US for treatment of HBV.
- Drug therapy is not recommended for patients with normal ALT values.
- Patients with persistent ALT levels greater than twice the upper limit of normal should be considered for treatment.
- Patients with ALT levels greater than 5 times the upper limit of normal are experiencing an exacerbation and should receive lamivudine.
- Patients considered for treatment are those who are HBsAg-positive for greater than 6 months with persistent elevations in serum aminotransferases, detectable markers of viral replication (HBeAg and HBV DNA) in serum and signs of chronic hepatitis on liver biopsy. Patients should not have decompensated liver disease.
- In patients with chronic HBV who are HBeAg-positive and have intermittent or persistent elevation of ALT, either interferon or lamivudine may be used as first-line therapy.
- Specific recommendations for treatment of chronic HBV are as follows (Figure 24–1):

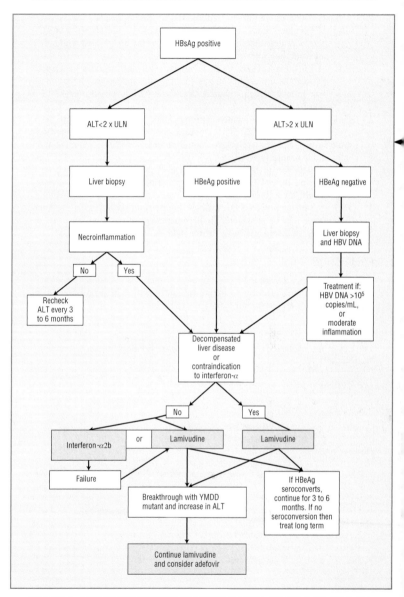

Figure 24–1. Treatment algorithm for the management of patients with chronic hepatitis B virus infection. ALT, alanine transaminase; HBeAg, hepatitis B e antigen; ULN, upper limit of normal.

1. Patients with HBeAg-positive chronic HBV
   (a) ALT greater than 2 times the upper limit of normal (ULN) or moderate/severe hepatitis on biopsy: Treatment may be initiated with either lamivudine or interferon-α
   (b) ALT less than 2 times ULN: Treatment with lamivudine or interferon-α should be limited to patients with significant necroinflammation on liver biopsy. Patients should have their ALT assessed every 3 to 6 months.
2. Patients with HBeAg-negative chronic HBV: Only patients with ALT greater than 2 times ULN, HBV DNA greater than 10^5 copies/mL, or moderate/severe hepatitis on biopsy should be considered for treatment with lamivudine or interferon-α.
3. Patients who fail to respond to a course of interferon-α and have ALT greater than 2 times ULN, HBV DNA greater than 10^5 copies/mL, or moderate/severe hepatitis on biopsy may be treated with a course of lamivudine.
4. Patients with decompensated cirrhosis: Interferon-α should not be used and lamivudine may be considered in these patients.
5. Patients in an inactive HBsAg carrier state: No treatment is indicated.

PREVENTION

- Two products are available for prevention of hepatitis B infection: **hepatitis B vaccine**, which provides active immunity, and **hepatitis B immune globulin (HBIG)**, which provides temporary passive immunity.

TABLE 24–6. Recommended Schedule of Immunoprophylaxis to Prevent Perinatal or Sexual Transmission of HBV Infection

Vaccine Recipient	Immunoprophylaxis	Timing
Infant born to HBsAg-positive mother	Vaccine dose 1	Within 12 h of birth
	HBIg (0.5 mL intramuscularly at a site different from that used for the vaccine)	Within 12 h of birth
	Vaccine doses 2 and 3	Usual schedule
Infant born to mother not screened for HBsAg	Vaccine dose 1[a]	Within 12 h of birth
	HBIg (0.5 mL intramuscularly at a site different from that used for the vaccine)	If mother is found to be HBsAg-positive, administer dose to infant as soon as possible, but no later than 1 wk after birth
	Vaccine doses 2 and 3[a]	Usual schedule
Sexual exposure	HBIg (0.06 mL/kg intramuscularly at a site different from that used for the vaccine)	Single dose within 14 days of sexual contact
	Vaccine dose 1	At time of HBIg treatment
	Vaccine doses 2 and 3	Usual schedule

[a]The first dose of vaccine is the same as that for the infant of an HBsAg-positive mother. If the mother is found to be HBsAg-positive, that dose is continued. If the mother is found to be HBsAg-negative, the remaining vaccine doses are those appropriate for other infants and children.

HBIg, hepatitis B immunoglobulin; HBsAg: hepatitis B surface antigen. From Centers for Disease Control and Prevention. Protection against viral hepatitis: Recommendations of the Immunization Practices Advisory Committee (ACIP). Morb Mortal Wkly Rep 1990;39:1–26; Centers for Disease Control and Prevention.

Recommendations of the Advisory Committee on Immunization Practices: Use of vaccines and immune globulins in persons with altered immunocompetence. Morb Mortal Wkly Rep 1993;42(RR-1):1–18; and Centers for Disease Control and Prevention. Hepatitis B virus: A comprehensive strategy for eliminating transmission in the United States through universal childhood vaccination. Morb Mortal Wkly Rep 1991;40(RR-13):1–25.

TABLE 24–7. Recommendations for Hepatitis B Prophylaxis Following Percutaneous or Permucosal Exposure

Vaccination Status of Exposed Person	Treatment According to HBsAg Status of Source		
	HBsAg-Positive	HBsAg-Negative	Source Not Tested or Unknown
Unvaccinated	HBIg (one dose of 0.06 mL/kg IM), plus initiate vaccine[a]	Initiative vaccine[a]	Initiate vaccine[a]
Previously vaccinated, known responder	Test exposed person for anti-HBs level. If adequate,[b] no treatment. If inadequate or titer unknown, I vaccine booster dose	No treatment	No treatment
Previously vaccinated, known nonresponder	HBIg (two doses 1 month apart) or HBIg one dose, plus dose of vaccine	No treatment	If known high-risk source, may treat as if source were HBsAg-positive
Previously vaccinated, response unknown	Test exposed person for anti-HBs level. If inadequate,[b] HBIg one dose, plus one vaccine booster dose. If adequate, no treatment. If titer unknown, one vaccine booster dose	No treatment	Test exposed for anti-HBs level. If inadequate,[b] vaccine booster dose. If adequate, no treatment

[a]Vaccine dosage is given in Table 40–8.
[b]Adequate anti-HBs is ≥10 milli-international units per milliliter by radioimmunoassay or enzyme immunoassay.
anti-HBs, antibody to HBsAg; HBIg, hepatitis B immunoglobulin; HBsAg, hepatitis B surface antigen.
From Centers for Disease Control and Prevention. Protection against viral hepatitis:
Recommendations of the Immunization Practices Advisory Committee (ACIP). Morb Mortal Wkly Rep 1990;391–26, Centers for Disease Control and Prevention. Recommendations of the Advisory Committee on Immunization Practices: Use of vaccines and immune globulins in persons with altered immunocompetence. Morb Mortal Wkly Rep 1993;42(RR-4);1–18, and Centers for Diseases Control and Prevention. Hepatitis B virus: A comprehensive strategy for eliminating transmission in the United States through universal childhood vaccination. Morb Mortal Wkly Rep 1991;40(RR–13):1–25.

- The goals of immunization against viral hepatitis include prevention of the short-term viremia that can lead to transmission of infection, clinical disease, and chronic HBV infection.

Hepatitis B Immune Globulin

- HBIg is used only for postexposure prophylaxis for HBV for perinatal exposure of infants of HBV-carrier mothers, sexual exposure to HBsAg-positive persons, percutaneous or permucosal exposure to HBsAg-positive blood, and exposure of an infant to a caregiver who has acute hepatitis B.
- The recommended dose is 0.06 mL/kg administered intramuscularly. Guidelines for use are listed in Tables 24–6 and 24–7.

Hepatitis B Vaccine

- The most effective measure for prevention of hepatitis B is universal precaution.
- Persons who should receive HBV vaccine are listed in Table 24–8. Recommended doses and schedules for hepatitis B vaccines are given in Table 24–9.
- Side effects of the vaccines are soreness at the injection site, headache, fatigue, irritability, and fever.

TABLE 24–8. Groups Recommended for Preexposure Hepatitis B Vaccination

All infants via routine infant vaccination

Unvaccinated 11- to 12-year-old children

Unvaccinated children ages <11 years of age who are Pacific Islanders of who reside in households of first-generation immigrants from countries where HBV is of high or intermediate endemicity

Health care and public safety workers who have occupational exposure to blood

HIV-infected individuals

Injection drug users

Heterosexual individuals who have had more than one sexual partner in the previous 6 months and/or those with a recent episode of a sexually transmitted disease

Sexually active homosexual or bisexual males

Hemodialysis patients

Recipients of certain blood products (i.e., patients with hemophilia and other clotting disorders)

Clients and staff of institutions for the developmentally disabled

Household, sexual, and blood exposure contacts of either HBsAg-positive persons or those with acute HBV infection

Household contacts of adoptees from countries where HBV is highly endemic

Populations where HBV is highly endemic (e.g., Alaskan Eskimos)

Inmates of long-term correctional facilities

International travelers to highly endemic HBV regions for >6 months and who have close contact with the local population; also short-term travelers who have contact with blood, or sexual contact with residents in high- or intermediate-risk areas

Unvaccinated infants under 12 months of age exposed to acute HBV infection through primary caregiver

HBsAg, hepatitis B surface antigen; HBV, hepatitis B virus; HIV, human immunodeficiency virus.
From Centers for Disease Control and Prevention. Protection against viral hepatitis: Recommendations of the Immunization Practices Advisory Committee (ACIP). Morb Mortal Wkly Rep 1990;39:1–26 and Centers for Disease Control and Prevention. 1999 USPHS/IDSA guidelines for the prevention of opportunistic infections in persons infected with human immunodeficiency virus. Morb Mortal Wkly Rep 1999;48(RR-10):1–66.

TABLE 24–9. Recommended Doses and Schedules of Currently Licensed Hepatitis B Vaccines

	Vaccine		
Group	Recombivax HB[a] dose, mcg (mL)	Engerix-B[a,b] dose, mcg (mL)	Comvax[c] dose, mcg (mL)
Infants of HBsAg-positive mothers	5 (0.5)	10 (0.5)	Not indicated
All other infants, children and adolescents ≤19 years of age	5 (0.5)[d]	10 (0.5)	5 (0.5)[e]
Adults age 20 years and older	10 (1)	20 (1)	Not indicated
Dialysis patients and other immunocompromised persons	40 (1)[f]	40 (2)[g, h]	Not indicated

[a]Usual schedules: Infants: Three doses given at birth, at 1 to 2 months, and at 6 to 18 months of age; or, for infants, with other routine immunizations at 1 to 2 months, 4 months, and 6 to 18 months of age. Older children and adults: Three doses given at 0-, 2-, and 6-month or, at 0-, 2-, and 4-month intervals. Higher titers of HBsAg are achieved with the last two doses of vaccine being spaced at least 4 months apart.
[b]Alternative approved schedule: Four doses, one given at 0, then one each given at 1-, 2-, and 12-month intervals. HBsAg, hepatitis B surface antigen.
[c]Contains 5 mcg 0.5 mL HBsAg and 7.5 mcg Haemophilus influenzae type B purified capsular polysaccharide fragments conjugated to 125 mcg Neisseria meningitidis outer membrane protein complex. [d]An alternate two-dose schedule can be used for adolescents aged 11 to 15 years. If the two-dose schedule is used, the adult dose (1 mL containing 10 mcg of HBsAg) is administered with the second dose given 4 to 6 months after the first dose. [e]Usually given at 2, 4 and 12 to 15 months of age. Comvax is not used when immunizing older children or adolescents. [f]Special formulation for dialysis patients. [g]Two 1-mL doses given at different sites. [h]Four-dose schedule recommended at 0 then at 1-, 2-, 6-month intervals.

TABLE 24–10. Side Effects of Interferon-α

Early (in First 2 Weeks of Therapy)	Hematologic	Neuropsychiatric	Autoimmune	Miscellaneous
Fever	Neutropenia	Irritability	Development of autoantibodies	Chronic fatigue
Chills	Thrombocytopenia	Mood lability		Infections
Myalgias	Anemia	Depression	Hepatitis	Increased sleep requirement
Fatigue		Tearfulness	Thyroid dysfunction	
Malaise		Delirium	Thyroiditis	Anorexia
Nausea		Paresthesias	Arthropathy	Weight loss
Sleep disturbance		Seizures	Type I diabetes mellitus	Myalgias
Abdominal pain		Psychosis	Exacerbation of psoriasis or lichen planus	Low-grade fevers
Diarrhea			Exacerbation of other autoimmune phenomena	Decreased libido
Headache				Alopecia
Appetite changes				Hypertriglyceridemia
				Irritability
				Anxiety
				Depression
				Attention span deficits

Absolute contraindications to use of interferon include current or past psychosis or severe depression, neutropenia or thrombocytopenia, organ transplant (except liver), symptomatic heart disease, decompensated cirrhosis, and uncontrolled seizures. Relative contraindications to interferon include uncontrolled diabetes and autoimmune disorders.

▶ HEPATITIS C

- Chronic hepatitis as a consequence of HCV has reached epidemic proportions worldwide.
- Hepatitis C is most often acquired through intravenous drug use; sexual contact; hemodialysis; or household, occupational, or perinatal exposure.
- Patients with acute hepatitis C are often asymptomatic. The clinical course is generally mild with less than 25% of patients developing malaise, anorexia, and jaundice.
- Serum transaminase values are elevated within 4 to 12 weeks after exposure.
- Seventy percent of cases eventually develop chronic hepatitis.
- Ten percent to 30% of patients with HCV infection develop cirrhosis, 1% to 5% develop hepatocellular carcinoma.

TREATMENT

- The goal of treating HCV is to return the individual to the previous state of health and prevent development of chronic infection, which can lead to morbidity and mortality from end-stage liver disease.
- Management of acute HCV is primarily supportive. General measures include a healthy diet, rest, maintenance of fluid balance, and avoidance of hepatotoxic drugs and alcohol.
- Patients seropositive for HCV with elevated ALT and inflammation on liver biopsy are candidates for antiviral therapy.
- First-line treatment for acute HCV includes pegylated interferon plus ribavirin. The dosing regimen varies with the specific product and the duration of therapy varies with the product and HCV genotype.
- Adverse effects of interferon are given in Table 24–10.

PREVENTION

- No HCV vaccine is currently available.
- Current recommendations for prevention of HCV include universal precautions for the prevention of blood-borne infections and anti-HCV screening of blood, organ, and tissue donors.

See Chapter 40, Viral Hepatitis, authored by Manjunath P. Pai, Renee-Claude Mercier, and Marsha A. Raebel for a more detailed discussion of this topic.

Chapter 25

▶ INFLAMMATORY BOWEL DISEASE

▶ DEFINITION

There are two forms of idiopathic inflammatory bowel disease (IBD): ulcerative colitis, a mucosal inflammatory condition confined to the rectum and colon, and Crohn's disease, a transmural inflammation of gastrointestinal (GI) mucosa that may occur in any part of the GI tract. The etiologies of both conditions are unknown, but they may have a common pathogenetic mechanism.

▶ PATHOPHYSIOLOGY

- The major theories of the cause of IBD involve infectious or immunologic causes. Microorganisms are a likely factor in the initiation of inflammation in IBD. The immunologic theory assumes that IBD is caused by an inappropriate reaction of the immune system (both autoimmune and nonautoimmune phenomenon) Proposed etiologies for IBD are found in Table 25–1.
- Smoking appears to be protective for ulcerative colitis but associated with increased frequency of Crohn's disease.
- Ulcerative colitis and Crohn's disease differ in two general respects: anatomic sites and depth of involvement within the bowel wall. There is, however, overlap between the two conditions, with a small fraction of patients showing features of both diseases (Table 25–2).

ULCERATIVE COLITIS

- Ulcerative colitis is confined to the colon and rectum and affects primarily the mucosa and the submucosa. The primary lesion occurs in the crypts of the mucosa (crypts of Lieberkuhn) in the form of a crypt abscess.
- Local complications (involving the colon) occur in the majority of ulcerative colitis patients. Relatively minor complications include hemorrhoids, anal fissures, or perirectal abscesses.

TABLE 25–1. Proposed Etilogies for Inflammatory Bowel Disease

Infectious agents
    Viruses (e.g., measles)
    L-Forms of bacteria
    Mycobacteria
    Chlamydia
Genetics
    Metabolic defects
    Connective tissue disorders
Environmental Factors
    Diet
    Smoking (Crohn's disease)
Immune defects
    Altered host suceptibility
    Immune-mediated mucosal damage
Psychologic factors
    Stress
    Emotional or physical trauma
    Occupation

TABLE 25–2. Comparison of the Clinical and Pathologic Features of Crohn's Disease and Ulcerative Colitis

Feature	Crohn's Disease	Ulcerative Colitis
Clinical		
Malaise, fever	Common	Uncommon
Rectal bleeding	Common	Common
Abdominal tenderness	Common	May be present
Abdominal mass	Common	Absent
Abdominal pain	Common	Unusual
Abdominal wall and internal fistulas	Common	Absent
Distribution	Discontinuous	Continuous
Aphthous or linear ulcers	Common	Rare
Pathologic		
Rectal involvement	Rare	Common
Ileal involvement	Very common	Rare
Strictures	Common	Rare
Fistulas	Common	Rare
Transmural involvement	Common	Rare
Crypt abscesses	Rare	Very common
Granulomas	Common	Rare
Linear clefts	Common	Rare
Cobblestone appearance	Common	Absent

V

- A major complication is toxic megacolon, a severe condition that occurs in up to 7.9% of ulcerative colitis patients admitted to hospitals. The patient with toxic megacolon usually has a high fever, tachycardia, distended abdomen, elevated white blood cell count, and a dilated colon.
- The risk of colonic carcinoma is much greater in patients with ulcerative colitis as compared with the general population.
- Approximately 11% of patients with ulcerative colitis have hepatobiliary complications including fatty liver, pericholangitis, chronic active hepatitis, cirrhosis, sclerosing cholangitis, cholangiocarcinoma, and gallstones.
- Arthritis commonly occurs in IBD patients and is typically asymptomatic and migratory. Arthritis typically involves one or a few large joints such as the knees, hips, ankles, wrists, and elbows.
- Ocular complications (iritis, episcleritis, and conjunctivitis) occur in up to 10% of patients. Five percent to 10% of patients experience dermatologic or mucosal complications (erythema nodosum, pyoderma ganrenosum, aphthous stomatitis).

CROHN'S DISEASE

- Crohn's disease is a transmural inflammatory process. The terminal ileum is the most common site of the disorder but it may occur in any part of the GI tract.
- About two thirds of patients have some colonic involvement, and 15% to 25% of patients have only colonic disease.
- Patients often have normal bowel separating segments of diseased bowel; that is, the disease is often discontinuous.
- Complications of Crohn's disease may involve the intestinal tract or organs unrelated to it. Small-bowel stricture and subsequent obstruction is a complication

TABLE 25–3. Clinical Presentation of Ulcerative Colitis

Signs and symptoms
- Abdominal cramping
- Frequent bowel movements, often with blood in the stool
- Weight loss
- Fever and tachycardia in severe disease
- Blurred vision, eye pain, and photophobia with ocular involvement
- Arthritis
- Raised, red, tender nodules that vary in size from 1 cm to several centimeters

Physical examination
- Hemorrhoids, and fissures, or perirectal abscesses may be present
- Iritis, uveitis, episcleritis, and conjunctivitis with ocular involvement
- Dermatologic findings with erythema nodosum, pyoderma gangrenosum, or aphthous ulceration

Laboratory tests
- Decreased hematocrit/hemoglobin
- Increased erythrocyte sedimentation rate
- Leukocytosis and hypoalbuminemia with severe disease

that may require surgery. Fistula formation is common and occurs much more frequently than with ulcerative colitis.
- Systemic complications of Crohn's disease are common and similar to those found with ulcerative colitis. Arthritis, iritis, skin lesions, and liver disease often accompany Crohn's disease.
- Nutritional deficiencies are common with Crohn's disease.

▶ CLINICAL PRESENTATION

ULCERATIVE COLITIS

- There is a wide range of ulcerative colitis presentation. Symptoms may range from mild abdominal cramping with frequent small-volume bowel movements to profuse diarrhea (Table 25–3).
- Most patients with ulcerative colitis experience intermittent bouts of illness after varying intervals of no symptoms.
- Mild disease has been defined as fewer than four stools daily, with or without blood, with no systemic disturbance and a normal erythrocyte sedimentation rate (ESR).
- Patients with moderate disease have more than four stools per day but with minimal systemic disturbance.
- With severe disease, the patient has more than six stools per day with blood, with evidence of systemic disturbance as shown by fever, tachycardia, anemia, or ESR greater than 30.

CROHN'S DISEASE

- As with ulcerative colitis, the presentation of Crohn's disease is highly variable (Table 25–4). A single episode may not be followed by further episodes, or the patient may experience continuous, unremitting disease. A patient may present with diarrhea and abdominal pain or a perirectal or perianal lesion.
- The course of Crohn's disease is characterized by periods of remission and exacerbation. Some patients may be free of symptoms for years, while others experience chronic problems in spite of medical therapy.

TABLE 25–4. Clinical Presentation of Crohn's Disease

Signs and symptoms
- Malaise and fever
- Abdominal pain
- Frequent bowel movements
- Hemotachezia
- Fistula
- Weight loss
- Arthritis

Physical examination
- Abdominal mass and tenderness
- Perianal fissure or fistula

Laboratory tests
- Increased white blood cell count and erythrocyte sedimentation rate

▶ DESIRED OUTCOME

Goals of treatment include resolution of acute inflammatory processes, resolution of attendant complications (e.g., fistulas, abscesses), alleviation of systemic manifestations (e.g., arthritis), maintenance of remission from acute inflammation, or surgical palliation or cure.

▶ TREATMENT

GENERAL APPROACH

- Treatment of IBD centers on agents used to relieve the inflammatory process. Salicylates, glucocorticoids, antimicrobials, and immunosuppressive agents such as azathioprine and mercaptopurine are commonly used to treat active disease and, for some agents, to lengthen the time of disease remission.
- In addition to the use of drugs, surgical procedures are sometimes performed when active disease is not adequately controlled or when the required drug dosages pose an unacceptable risk of adverse effects.

NONPHARMACOLOGIC TREATMENT

Nutritional Support
- Patients with moderate to severe disease IBD are often malnourished.
- The nutritional needs of the majority of patients can be adequately addressed with enteral supplementation. Patients who have severe disease may require a course of parenteral nutrition.
- Probiotic formulas have been effective in maintaining remission in ulcerative colitis.

Surgery
- For ulcerative colitis, colectomy may be performed when the patient has disease uncontrolled by maximum medical therapy or when there are complications of the disease such as colonic perforation, toxic dilatation (megacolon), uncontrolled colonic hemorrhage, or colonic strictures.
- The indications for surgery with Crohn's disease are not as well established as they are for ulcerative colitis, and surgery is usually reserved for the

complications of the disease. There is a high recurrence rate of Crohn's disease after surgery.

PHARMACOLOGIC THERAPY

- The major types of drug therapy used in IBD include **aminosalicylates, glucocorticoids,** immunosuppressive agents (**azathioprine, mercaptopurine, cyclosporine,** and **methotrexate**), antimicrobials (**metronidazole and ciprofloxacin**), and agents to inhibit tumor necrosis factor α (TNF α) (anti-TNFα antibodies).
- **Sulfasalazine**, an agent that combines a sulfonamide (sulfapyridine) antibiotic and mesalamine (5-aminosalicylic acid) in the same molecule, has been used for many years to treat IBD. Mesalamine-based products are listed in Table 25–5.
- Glucocorticoids and adrenocorticotropic hormone (ACTH) have been widely used for the treatment of ulcerative colitis and Crohn's disease and are used in moderate to severe disease. Prednisone is most commonly used. Budesonide is an oral controlled-release formulation that minimizes systemic effects.
- Immunosuppressive agents such as **azathioprine** and **mercaptopurine** (a metabolite of azathioprine) are sometimes used for the treatment of IBD. These agents are generally reserved for cases that are refractory to steroids and may be associated with serious adverse effects such as lymphomas, pancreatitis, or nephrotoxicity. Cyclosporine has been of short-term benefit in acute, severe ulcerative colitis when used in a continuous infusion.
- Methotrexate given 15 to 25 mg intramuscularly once weekly is useful for treatment and maintenance of Crohn's disease.
- Antimicrobial agents, particularly **metronidazole**, are frequently used in attempts to control Crohn's disease particularly when it involves the perineal area or fistulas.
- Infliximab is useful in steroid-dependent or fistulizing disease but the cost far exceeds that of other regimens.

Ulcerative Colitis
Mild to Moderate Disease
- The first line of drug therapy for the patient with mild to moderate colitis is oral **sulfasalazine** or an oral **mesalamine** derivative, or topical mesalamine or steroids for distal disease (Figure 25–1).
- When given orally, usually 4 g/day, up to 8 g/day of sulfasalazine is required to attain control of active inflammation. **Sulfasalazine** therapy should be instituted at 500 mg/day and increased every few days up to 4 g/day or the maximum tolerated.
- Oral **mesalamine** derivatives (such as those listed in Table 25–5) are reasonable alternatives to sulfasalazine for treatment of ulcerative colitis but they are not more effective than sulfasalazine (Figure 25–2).
- Steroids have a place in the treatment of moderate to severe ulcerative colitis that is unresponsive to maximal doses of oral and topical mesalamine. **Prednisone** up to 1 mg/kg/day may be used for patients who do not have an adequate response to sulfasalazine or mesalamine.
- Steroids and sulfasalazine appear to be equally efficacious; however, the response to steroids may be evident sooner.
- Rectally administered steroids or mesalamine can be used as initial therapy for patients with ulcerative proctitis or distal colitis.
- Transdermal **nicotine** in the highest tolerated dose improved symptoms of patients with active ulcerative.

TABLE 25–5. Mesalamine Derivatives for Treatment of Inflammatory Bowel Disease

Product	Trade Name(s)	Formulation	Dose/Day	Site of Action
Sulfasalazine	Azulfidine	Tablet	4–6 g	Colon
Mesalamine	Rowasa, Salofalk, Claversal, Pentasa	Enema	1–4 g	Rectum, terminal colon
	Asacol	Mesalamine tablet coated with Eudragit-S (delayed-release acrylic resin)	2.4–4.8 g	Distal ileum and colon
	Pentasa	Mesalamine capsules encapsulated in ethylcellulose microgranules	2–4 g	Small bowel and colon
Olsalazine	Dipentum	Dimer of 5-aminosalicylic acid oral	1.5–3 g	Colon
Balsalazide	Colazal	capsule	6.75 g	Colon

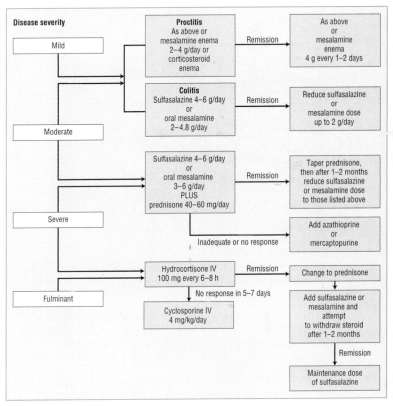

Figure 25–1. Treatment approaches for ulcerative colitis.

Severe or Intractable Disease

- Patients with uncontrolled severe colitis or incapacitating symptoms require hospitalization for effective management. Most medication is given by the parenteral route.
- With severe colitis, there is a much greater reliance on parenteral steroids and surgical procedures. Sulfasalazine or mesalamine derivatives have not been proven beneficial for treatment of severe colitis.
- Steroids have been valuable in the treatment of severe disease because the use of these agents may allow some patients to avoid colectomy. A trial of steroidsis is warranted in most patients before proceeding to colectomy, unless the condition is grave or rapidly deteriorating.
- Continuous intravenous infusion of **cyclosporine** (4 mg/kg/day) is recommended for patients with acute severe ulcerative colitis refractory to steroids.

Maintenance of Remission

- Once remission from active disease has been achieved, the goal of therapy is to maintain the remission.

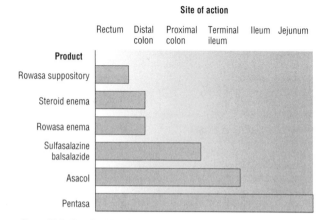

Figure 25–2. Site of activity of various agents to treat inflammatory bowel disease.

- The major agents used for maintenance of remission are **sulfasalazine** (2 g/day) and the **mesalamine** derivatives, although mesalamine is not as effective as sulfasalazine.
- Steroids do not have a role in the maintenance of remission with ulcerative colitis because they are ineffective. Steroids should be gradually withdrawn after remission is induced (over 3 to 4 weeks). If they are continued, the patient will be exposed to steroid side effects without likelihood of benefits.
- Maintenance of remission is well documented up to 1 year and may last as long as 3 years.
- **Azathioprine** is effective in preventing relapse of ulcerative colitis for periods of up to 2 years. However, 3 to 6 months may be required for beneficial effect.

Crohn's Disease (Figure 25–3)
Active Crohn's Disease

- The goal of treatment for active Crohn's disease is to achieve remission; however, in many patients, reduction of symptoms so that the patient may carry out normal activities or reduction of the steroid dose required for control is a significant accomplishment.
- In the majority of patients, active Crohn's disease is treated with **sulfasalazine, mesalamine** derivatives, or **steroids**, although **azathioprine, mercaptopurine**, or **metronidazole** is frequently used.
- **Sulfasalazine** is more effective when Crohn's disease involves the colon.
- Mesalamine derivatives (such as **Pentasa** or **Asacol**) that release mesalamine in the small bowel may be more effective than sulfasalazine for ileal involvement.
- **Steroids** are frequently used for the treatment of active Crohn's disease, particularly with more severe presentations. Steroids are preferred for treatment of severe Crohn's disease, mainly because these agents can be given parenterally and response to therapy may occur sooner than with other agents. Once remission is achieved, however, it may prove difficult to reduce steroid dosage without reintroduction of active disease.
- **Metronidazole** (given orally up to 20 mg/kg/day) may be useful in some patients with Crohn's disease, particularly in patients with colonic involvement or those with perineal disease.

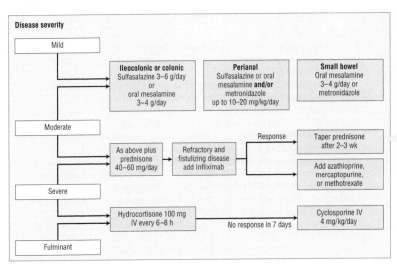

Figure 25–3. Treatment approaches for Crohn's disease.

- The immunosuppressive agents (**azathioprine** and **mercaptopurine**) are generally limited to use in patients not achieving adequate response to standard medical therapy, or to reduce steroid doses when toxic doses are required. The usual dose of azathioprine is 2 to 2.5 mg/kg/day and 1 to 1.5 mg/kg/day for mercaptopurine. Up to 6 months may be required to observe a response.
- A genetic polymorphism causes deficiency of the enzyme thiopurine S-methyltransferase in some people, reduces mercaptopurine metabolism and increases the risk of bone marrow suppression.
- **Cyclosporine** is not recommended for Cronn's disease except for patients with symptomatic and severe perianal or cutaneous fistulas. The dose of cyclosporine is important in determining efficacy. An oral dose of 5 mg/kg/day was not effective, whereas 7.9 mg/kg/day was effective. However, toxic effects limit application of the higher dosage.
- **Methotrexate**, given as a weekly injection of 5 to 25 mg has demonstrated efficacy for induction of remission in Crohn's disease as well as for maintenance therapy.
- **Infliximab**, 5 mg/kg single infusion, is effective for refractory or fistulizing Crohn's disease when given everyday for 8 weeks.

Maintenance of Remission
- Prevention of recurrence of disease is clearly more difficult with Crohn's disease than with ulcerative colitis. **Sulfasalazine** and oral **mesalamine** derivatives are effective in preventing acute recurrences in quiescent Crohn's disease.
- **Steroids** also have no place in the prevention of recurrence of Crohn's disease; these agents do not appear to alter the long-term course of the disease.
- Although the published data are not consistent, there is evidence to suggest that **azathioprine** and **mercaptopurine** are effective in maintaining remission in Crohn's disease.

SELECTED COMPLICATIONS

Toxic Megacolon

- The treatment required for toxic megacolon includes general supportive measures to maintain vital functions, consideration for early surgical intervention, and antimicrobials.
- Aggressive fluid and electrolyte management are required for dehydration.
- When the patient has lost significant amounts of blood (through the rectum), blood replacement is also necessary.
- Steroids in high dosages should be administered intravenously to reduce acute inflammation. Doses as high as 2 mg/kg/day of prednisone equivalent have been recommended (generally administered as hydrocortisone).
- Antimicrobial regimens that are effective against enteric aerobes and anaerobes (e.g., **aminoglycoside** with **clindamycin** or **metronidazole, imipenem, meropenem**, or **extended-spectrum penicillin with a** β**-lactamase inhibitor**) should be administered from the time of diagnosis and continued until patient improvement is assured.

Systemic Manifestations

- The common systemic manifestations of IBD include arthritis, anemia, skin manifestations such as erythema nodosum and pyoderma gangrenosum, uveitis, and liver disease.
- Anemia may be a common problem where there is significant blood loss from the GI tract. When the patient can consume oral medication, **ferrous sulfate** should be administered. Vitamin B_{12} or folic acid may also be required.

▶ SPECIAL CONSIDERATIONS

PREGNANCY

- Drug therapy for IBD is not a contraindication for pregnancy, and most pregnancies are well managed in patients with these diseases. The indications for medical and surgical treatment are similar to those in the nonpregnant patient. If a patient has an initial bout of IBD during pregnancy, a standard approach to treatment should be initiated.
- **Metronidazole** or **methotrexate** should not be used during pregnancy.

ADVERSE DRUG REACTIONS TO AGENTS USED FOR TREATMENT OF IBD

- Sulfasalazine is often associated with either dose-related or idiosyncratic adverse drug effects. Dose-related side effects usually include GI disturbances such as nausea, vomiting, diarrhea, or anorexia, but may also include headache and arthralgia.
- Patients receiving sulfasalazine should receive oral **folic acid** supplementation since sulfasalazine inhibits folic acid absorption.
- Non–dose-related adverse effects of sulfasalazine include rash, fever, or hepatotoxicity most commonly, as well as relatively uncommon but serious reactions such as pancreatitis and hepatitis.
- Oral mesalamine derivatives may impose a lower frequency of adverse effects compared with sulfasalazine. Eighty percent to 90% of patients who are intolerant to sulfasalazine will tolerate oral mesalamine derivatives.
- The well-appreciated adverse effects of glucocorticoids include hyperglycemia, hypertension, osteoporosis, fluid retention and electrolyte disturbances, myopathies, psychosis, and reduced resistance to infection. In addition,

glucocorticoid use may cause adrenocortical suppression. Specific regimens for withdrawal of glucocorticoid therapy have been suggested.

- Immunosuppressants such as azathioprine and mercaptopurine have a significant potential for adverse reactions, including bone marrow suppression, and have been associated with lymphomas (in renal transplant patients) and pancreatitis. Myelosuppression resulting in leucopenia is related to a deficiency in thiopurine S-methyltransferase in some patients.
- Infliximab has been associated with infusion reactions, serum sickness, sepsis, and tuberculosis.

▶ EVALUATION OF THERAPEUTIC OUTCOMES

- The success of therapeutic regimens to treat IBDs can be measured by patient-reported complaints, signs and symptoms, direct physician examination (including endoscopy), history and physical examination, selected laboratory tests, and quality of life measures.
- To create more objective measures, disease-rating scales or indices have been created. The Crohn's Disease Activity Index (CDAI) is a commonly used scale, particularly for evaluation of patients during clinical trials. The scale incorporates eight elements: (1) number of stools in the past 7 days; (2) sum of abdominal pain ratings from the past 7 days; (3) rating of general well-being in the past 7 days; (4) use of antidiarrheals; (5) body weight; (6) hematocrit; (7) finding of abdominal mass; and (8) a sum of symptoms present in the past week. Elements of this index provide a guide for those measures that may be useful in assessing the effectiveness of treatment regimens.
- Standardized assessment tools have also been constructed for ulcerative colitis. Elements in these scales include (1) stool frequency; (2) presence of blood in the stool; (3) mucosal appearance (from endoscopy); and (4) physician's global assessment based on physical examination, endoscopy, and laboratory data.

See Chapter 34, Inflammatory Bowel Disease, authored by Joseph T. DiPiro, PharmD, FCCP, and Robert R. Schade, MD, for a more detailed discussion of this topic.

Chapter 26

▶ NAUSEA AND VOMITING

▶ DEFINITION

Nausea is usually defined as the inclination to vomit or as a feeling in the throat or epigastric region alerting an individual that vomiting is imminent. Vomiting is defined as the ejection or expulsion of gastric contents through the mouth, often requiring a forceful event.

▶ PATHOPHYSIOLOGY

- Specific etiologies associated with nausea and vomiting are presented in Table 26–1.
- Table 26–2 presents specific cytotoxic agents categorized by their emetogenic potential. Although some agents may have greater emetogenic potential than others, combinations of agents, high doses, clinical settings, psychological conditions, prior treatment experiences, and unusual stimuli to sight, smell, or taste may alter a patient's response to a drug treatment.

TABLE 26–1. Specific Etiologies of Nausea and Vomiting

Gastrointestinal Mechanisms	**Neurologic Processes**
Mechanical gastric outlet obstruction	Midline cerebellar hemorrhage
Peptic ulcer disease	Increased intracranial pressure
Gastric carcinoma	Migraine headache
Pancreatic disease	Vestibular disorders
Motility disorders	Head trauma
Gastroparesis	**Metabolic Disorders**
Drug-induced gastric stasis	Diabetes mellitus (diabetic ketoacidosis)
Chronic intestinal pseudo-obstruction	Addison's disease
Postviral gastroenteritis	Renal disease (uremia)
Irritable bowel syndrome	**Psychogenic Causes**
Postgastric surgery	Self-induced
Idiopathic gastric stasis	Anticipatory
Anorexia nervosa	**Therapy-induced Causes**
Intra-abdominal emergencies	Cytotoxic chemotherapy
Intestinal obstruction	Radiation therapy
Acute pancreatitis	Theophylline preparations (intolerance, toxic)
Acute pyelonephritis	Anticonvulsant preparations (toxic)
Acute cholecystitis	Digitalis preparations (toxic)
Acute cholangitis	Opiates
Acute viral hepatitis	Amphotericin B
Acute gastroenteritis	Antibiotics
Viral gastroenteritis	**Drug Withdrawal**
Salmonellosis	Opiates
Shigellosis	Benzodiazepines
Staphylococcal gastroenteritis (enterotoxins)	**Miscellaneous Causes**
Cardiovascular Diseases	Pregnancy
Acute myocardial infarction	Any swallowed irritant (foods, drugs)
Congestive heart failure	Noxious odors
Shock and circulatory collapse	Operative procedures

TABLE 26–2. Emetogenicity of Chemotherapeutic Agents

Level 1 (less than 10% frequency)	Level 3 (30%–60% frequency)
Androgens	Aldesleukin
Bleomycin	Cyclophosphamide (IV, $\leq$ 750 mg/m^2)
Busulfan (oral < 4 mg/kg per day)	Dactinomycin ($\leq$ 1.5 mg/m^2)
Capecitabine (oral)	Doxorubicin HCl (20–60 mg/m^2)
Chlorambucil (oral)	Epirubicin HCl ($\leq$ 90 mg/m^2)
Cladribine	Idarubicin
Corticosteroids	Ifosfamide
Doxorubicin (liposomal)	Methotrexate (250–1000 mg/m^2)
Fludarabine	Mitoxantrone ($\leq$ 15 mg/m^2)
Hydroxyurea	**Level 4 (60%–90% frequency)**
Interferon	Carboplatin
Melphalan (oral)	Carmustine (< 250 mg/m^2)
Mercaptopurine	Cisplatin (<50 mg/m^2)
Methotrexate ($50mg/m2$)	Cisplatin (< 50 mg/m^2)
Thioguanine (oral)	Cyclophosphamide (> 750 mg/m^2 to $\leq$ 1500 mg/m^2)
Tretinoin	Cytarabine ($\geq$1 g/m^2)
Vinblastine	Dactinomycin (> 1.5 mg/m^2)
Vincristine	Doxorubicin HCl (> 60 mg/m^2)
Vinorelbine	Irinotecan
Level 2 (10%–30% frequency)	Melphalan (IV)
Asparaginase	Methotrexate (>1 g/m^2)
Cytarabine (< 1 g/m^2)	Mitoxantrone (> 15 mg/m^2)
Docetaxel	Oxaliplatin
Doxorubicin HCl (< 20 mg/m^2)	Procarbazine (oral)
Etoposide	**Level 5 (> 90% frequency)**
Fluorouracil (< 1 g/m^2)	Carmustine (>250 mg/m^2)
Gemcitabine	Cisplatin (> 50 mg/m^2)
Methotrexate (>50 mg/m^2; < 250 mg/m^2)	Cyclophosphamide (> 1500 mg/m^2)
Mitomycin	Dacarbazine ($\geq$ 500 mg/m^2)
Paclitaxel	Lomustine (> 604 mg/m^2)
Teniposide	Mechlorethamine
Thiotepa	Pentostatin
Topotecan	Streptozocin

- A variety of other common etiologies have been proposed for the development of nausea and vomiting in cancer patients. These are presented in Table 26–3.
- The three consecutive phases of emesis include nausea, retching, and vomiting. Nausea, the imminent need to vomit, is associated with gastric stasis. Retching is the labored movement of abdominal and thoracic muscles before vomiting. The final phase of emesis is vomiting, the forceful expulsion of gastric contents due to gastrointestinal (GI) retroperistalsis.
- Vomiting is triggered by afferent impulses to the vomiting center, a nucleus of cells in the medulla. Impulses are received from sensory centers, such as the chemoreceptor trigger zone (CTZ), cerebral cortex, and visceral afferents from the pharynx and GI tract. When excited, afferent impulses are integrated by the vomiting center, resulting in efferent impulses to the salivation center, respiratory center, and the pharyngeal, GI, and abdominal muscles, leading to vomiting.
- The CTZ, located in the area postrema of the fourth ventricle of the brain, is a major chemosensory organ for emesis and is usually associated with chemically induced vomiting.

TABLE 26–3. Nonchemotherapy Etiologies of Nausea and Vomiting in Cancer Patients

Fluid and electrolyte abnormalities
   Hypercalcemia
   Volume depletion
   Water intoxication
   Adrenocortical insufficiency
Drug-induced   Opiates
   Antibiotics
Gastrointestinal obstruction
Increased intracranial pressure
Peritonitis
Metastases
   Brain
   Meninges
   Hepatic
Uremia
Infections (septicemia, local)
Radiation therapy

- Numerous neurotransmitter receptors are located in the vomiting center, CTZ, and GI tract. Examples of such receptors include cholinergic and histaminic, dopaminergic, opiate, serotonin, neurokinin, and benzodiazepine receptors. It is theorized that chemotherapeutic agents, their metabolites, or other emetic compounds trigger the process of emesis through stimulation of one or more of these receptors.

▶ CLINICAL PRESENTATION

- Nausea and vomiting may be classified as either simple or complex. The term simple applies to those episodes of nausea and/or vomiting described by one of the following criteria: (1) occur occasionally and are self-limiting or relieved by the minimal use of antiemetic methods or medications; (2) account for slight patient deterioration such as fluid–electrolyte imbalances, pain, or noncompliance with prescribed therapies; or (3) are not related to the administration of or exposure to noxious agents.
- The term complex is used when describing a patient's clinical course as including symptoms that are not adequately or readily relieved by the administration of a single antiemetic method or medication; that lead to progressive patient deterioration secondary to fluid–electrolyte imbalances, pain, or noncompliance with prescribed therapies; or that are caused by noxious agents or psychogenic events.
- Nausea and vomiting occur frequently after operative procedures; those of the abdomen, eye, ear, nose, and throat are generally associated with higher incidences of nausea and vomiting than other procedures. Women experience a threefold higher incidence of nausea and vomiting compared to men, independent of the type of operation or anesthetic. Children are about twice as susceptible as adults.
- Other risk factors that may be associated with an increase in postoperative symptoms include patient variables such as obesity, increased age, a history of motion sickness or prior postoperative emesis, as well as drug therapy variables such as the choice of premedication or general anesthetic agent.

- Many women experience nausea and vomiting during pregnancy; however, the etiology of hyperemesis gravidarum is not well understood.

▶ DESIRED OUTCOME

The overall goal of antiemetic therapy is to prevent or eliminate nausea and vomiting; this should be accomplished without adverse effects or with clinically acceptable adverse effects.

▶ TREATMENT

GENERAL PRINCIPLES

- Most cases of nausea and vomiting are self-limiting, resolve spontaneously, and require only symptomatic therapy.
- Antiemetic therapy is indicated in patients with electrolyte disturbances secondary to vomiting, severe anorexia or weight loss, or progression of disease either owing to refusal of continued therapy or poor nutritional status.

NONPHARMACOLOGIC MANAGEMENT

- For patients with simple complaints, perhaps related to food or beverage consumption, avoidance or moderation of dietary intake may be preferable.
- Nonpharmacologic interventions are classified as behavioral interventions and include relaxation, biofeedback, self-hypnosis, cognitive distraction, guided imagery, and systematic desensitization.
- Psychogenic vomiting may benefit from psychological interventions.

PHARMACOLOGIC MANAGEMENT

- Antiemetic drugs (over-the-counter [OTC] and prescription) are most often recommended to treat nausea and vomiting. Provided that a patient can and will adhere to oral dosing, a suitable and effective agent can often be selected; however, for certain other patients, oral medications may be inappropriate because of their inability to retain any appreciable oral ingestion. In these patients, the rectal or injectable route of administration might be preferred.
- Information concerning commonly available antiemetic preparations is compiled in Table 26–4.
- For most conditions, a single-agent antiemetic is preferred; however, for those patients not responding to such therapy and those receiving highly emetogenic chemotherapy, multiple-agent regimens are usually required.
- The treatment of simple nausea and vomiting usually requires minimal therapy. Both OTC and prescription drugs useful in the treatment of simple nausea and vomiting are usually effective in small, infrequently administered doses.
- The management of complex nausea and vomiting may require aggressive drug therapy, possibly with more than one antiemetic agent.

DRUG CLASS INFORMATION

Antacids

- Single or combination OTC antacid products, especially those containing magnesium hydroxide, aluminum hydroxide, and/or calcium carbonate, may provide sufficient relief from simple nausea or vomiting, primarily through gastric acid neutralization.

TABLE 26–4. Presentation of Nausea and Vomiting

General
Depending on severity of symptoms, patients may present in mild to severe distress
Symptoms
Simple: Self-limiting, resolves spontaneously and requires only symptomatic therapy
Complex: Not relieved after administration of antiemetics; progressive deterioration of patient secondary to
　fluid-electrolyte imbalances; usually associated with noxious agents or psychogenic events
Signs
Simple: Patient complaint of queasiness or discomfort
Complex: Weight loss; fever; abdominal pain
Laboratory tests
Simple: None
Complex: Serum electrolyte concentrations; upper/lower GI evaluation
Other information
Fluid input and output
Medication history
Recent history of behavioral or visual changes, headache, pain, or stress
Family history positive for psychogenic vomiting

- Common antacid dosage regimens for the relief of nausea and vomiting include one or more small doses of single- or multiple-agent products.

Antihistamines, Anticholinergics

- Histamine$_2$ antagonists (cimetidine, famotidine, nizatidine, ranitidine) may be used in low doses to manage simple nausea and vomiting associated with heartburn.
- Antiemetic drugs from the antihistaminic–anticholinergic category may be appropriate in the treatment of simple symptomology.
- Adverse reactions that may be apparent with the use of the antihistaminic–anticholinergic agents primarily include drowsiness or confusion, blurred vision, dry mouth, urinary retention, and possibly tachycardia, particularly in elderly patients.

Phenothiazines

- **Phenothiazines** are most useful in patients with simple nausea and vomiting or in those receiving mildly emetogenic doses of chemotherapy.
- Rectal administration is most preferred when parenteral administration is impractical or oral medications cannot be retained and are therefore ineffective.
- In many patients, low doses of phenothiazine drugs may not be effective, while larger doses may produce unacceptable risks.
- Problems associated with these drugs include troublesome and potentially dangerous side effects, including extrapyramidal reactions, hypersensitivity reactions with possible liver dysfunction, marrow aplasia, and excessive sedation.

Corticosteroids

- **Corticosteroids** have been used successfully in the management of chemotherapy-induced nausea and vomiting (CINV) and postoperative nausea and vomiting (PONV) with few problems.
- Reported adverse effects included mood changes ranging from anxiety to euphoria as well as headache, a metallic taste in the mouth, abdominal discomfort, and hyperglycemia

Metoclopramide

- **Metoclopramide** increases lower esophageal sphincter tone, aids gastric emptying, and accelerates transit through the small bowel, possibly through the release of acetylcholine.
- Because the adverse reactions to metoclopramide include extrapyramidal effects, IV diphenhydramine, 25 to 50 mg, should be administered prophylactically or provided on-call for its anticipated need.

Cannabinoids

- When compared with conventional antiemetics, oral **nabilone** and oral **dronabinol** were slightly more effective than active comparators in patients receiving moderately emetogenic chemotherapy regimens.
- The efficacy of cannabinoids as compared to SSRIs for CINV has not been studied. They should be considered for the treatment of refractory nausea and vomiting in patients receiving chemotherapy.
- Adverse reactions include euphoria, drowsiness, sedation, somnolence, dysphoria, depression, hallucinations, and paranoia.

Substance P/Neurokinin 1 Receptor Antagonists

- Substance P is a peptide neurotransmitter in the neurokinin (NK) family whose preferred receptor is the NK_1 receptor. Substance P is believed to be the primary mediator of the delayed phase of CINV and one of two mediators of the acute phase of CINV.
- Aprepitant is the first approved member of this class of drugs and is indicated as part of a multiple drug regimen for prophylaxis of nausea and vomiting associated with high-dose cisplatin-based chemotherapy.
- Numerous potential drug interactions are possible; clinically significant drug interactions with oral contraceptives, warfarin and oral dexamethasone have been described.

Selective Serotonin Receptor Inhibitors (Ondansetron, Granisetron, Dolasetron, and Palonosetron)

SSRIs act by blocking presynaptic serotonin receptors on sensory vagal fibers in the gut wall.

CHEMOTHERAPY-INDUCED NAUSEA AND VOMITING (CINV)

- The emetogenic potential of the chemotherapeutic agent or regimen (see Table 35–2) is the primary factor to consider when selecting an antiemetic for **prophylaxis** of CINV.
- Patients receiving level 2 regimens can receive dexamethasone 8 to 20 mg IV or PO as a prophylactic agent. Prochlorperazine 10 mg IV or PO is also an option for adult patients.
- Adult and pediatric patients receiving level 3 through 5 regimens should receive a corticosteroid in combination with a SSRI.
- Ondansetron can be administered intravenously 30 minutes prior to chemotherapy. The least effective IV dose should be used, with a range of 8 to 32 mg. Oral therapy is preferred; 8 to 24 mg should be given 30 minutes prior to chemotherapy.
- In adults and children, at least 2 years of age, granisetron should be infused IV in a dose of 10 mcg/kg for 5 minutes, beginning within 30 minutes before the initiation of chemotherapy, only on the day(s) chemotherapy is given. Oral doses of 1 to 2 mg may be used in adults.

- Dolasetron may be administered to adults as a single dose of 1.8 mg/kg, or as a fixed dose of 100 mg intravenously for 30 seconds, or infused (diluted) for 15 minutes. For children 2 to 16 years of age, dolasetron may be given 1.8 mg/kg up to 100 mg.
- Aprepitant, a substance P/NK$_1$ receptor antagonist given in combination with an SSRI and a corticosteroid (125 mg PO day 1, 80 mg PO days 2 and 3) has been shown to effectively control acute and delayed nausea and vomiting associated with high dose cisplatin-based chemotherapy.
- Palonestron 0.25 mg IV for 30 seconds, 30 minutes prior to chemotherapy is another SSRI option for prophylaxis of CINV.
- Adult patients who experience nausea and vomiting despite prophylaxis should receive prochlorperazine, lorazepam or a corticosteroid as treatment for breakthrough symptoms. Chlorpromazine, lorazepam or corticosteroids are recommended for pediatric patients. SSRIs are not superior to conventional antiemetics in the treatment of breakthrough nausea or vomiting.
- Dexamethasone with metoclopramide or a SSRI is recommended for the prevention of delayed emesis in adults.

Benzodiazepines
- Benzodiazepines (particularly **lorazepam**) represent the best of the therapeutic alternatives in the treatment of anticipatory nausea and vomiting. Dosage regimens include one dose the night before chemotherapy and multiple doses after each treatment with cytotoxic chemotherapy.

POSTOPERATIVE NAUSEA AND VOMITING (PONV)
- A variety of pharmacologic approaches are available and may be prescribed as single or combination therapy for prophylaxis of PONV. See Table 26–5 for doses of specific agents.
- With or without antiemetic therapy, nonpharmacologic methods (including assisting patients with movement and providing particularly close attention to adequate hydration and pain management) may be effective in reducing the potential for emesis and should be universally applied.
- Selective serotonin antagonists are very effective in the prevention of postoperative nausea and vomiting but are much more expensive than alternative agents.

RADIATION-INDUCED NAUSEA AND VOMITING (RINV)
Patients receiving total or hemibody irradiation or single-exposure, high-dose radiation therapy to the upper abdomen should receive prophylactic doses of granisetron 2 mg or ondansetron 8 mg.

TABLE 26–5. Recommended Prophylactic Doses of Antiemetics for PONV

Drug	Adult Dose (IV)	Pediatric Dose (IV)	Timing of Dose[a]
Dolasetron	12.5 mg	350 mcg/kg up to 12.5 mg	At end of surgery
Cranisetron	0.35–1 mg		At end of surgery
Ondansetron	4–8 mg	50–100 mcg/kg up to 4 mg	At end of surgery
Dexamethasone	5–10 mg	150 mcg/kg up to 8 mg	Before induction
Droperidol	0.625–1.25 mg	50–70 mcg/kg up to 1.25 mg	At end of surgery
Dimenhydrinate	1–2 mg/kg	0.5 mg/kg	

[a]Based on recommendations from consensus guidelines; may differ from manufacturer's recommendations. PONV, postoperative nausea and vomiting.

DISORDERS OF BALANCE

- Beneficial therapy for patients with nausea and vomiting associated with disorders of balance can reliably be found among the antihistaminic–anticholinergic agents, particularly transdermal **scopolamine.**
- Neither the antihistaminic nor the anticholinergic potency appears to correlate well with the ability of these agents to prevent or treat the nausea and vomiting associated with motion sickness.

ANTIEMETIC USE DURING PREGNANCY

- Agents that have commonly been prescribed during pregnancy include phenothiazines (**prochlorperazine** and **promethazine**), the antihistaminic–anticholinergic agents (**dimenhydrinate, diphenhydramine, meclizine,** and **scopolamine**), **metoclopramide,** and **pyridoxine.**
- The efficacy of antiemetics has been questioned, while the importance of other management plans (including emphasis on fluid and electrolyte management, vitamin supplements, and efforts aimed at reducing psychosomatic complaints) has been addressed.
- Teratogenicity is a major consideration for the use of antiemetic drugs during pregnancy and is the primary factor that dictates the drug of choice. Of the agents commonly used, dimenhydrinate, diphenhydramine, doxylamine, hydroxyzine and meclizine have no human teratogenic potential.
- Studies using SSRIs in nausea and vomiting of pregnancy are limited.

ANTIEMETIC USE IN CHILDREN

- The safety and efficacy of SSRIs for the prophylaxis of CINV in children has been established but the best doses or dosing strategy have not been determined.
- For nausea and vomiting associated with pediatric gastroenteritis, there is greater emphasis on rehydration measures than on pharmacologic intervention.

▶ EVALUATION OF THERAPEUTIC OUTCOMES

- Monitoring criteria for drug therapy includes the subjective assessment of the severity of nausea as well as objective parameters such as the number of vomiting episodes each day, the volume of vomitus lost, and evaluation of fluid, acid-base balance, and electrolyte status, with particular attention to serum sodium, potassium, and chloride concentrations. In addition, evaluation of renal function may become important, particularly in patients with volume contraction and progressive electrolyte disturbances. Specific parameters include daily urine volume, urine specific gravity, and urine electrolyte concentrations.
- Physical assessment of patients should include evaluation of mucous membranes and skin turgor, since dryness of these tissues may be indicative of significant volume loss.

See Chapter 35, Nausea and Vomiting, authored by Cecily V. DiPiro and A. Thomas Taylor, PharmD, for a more detailed discussion of this topic.

Chapter 27

▶ PANCREATITIS

▶ DEFINITION

- Acute pancreatitis (AP) is an inflammatory disorder of the pancreas characterized by severe pain in the upper abdomen and increased serum concentrations of pancreatic lipase and amylase. Most patients with mild AP recover completely, but severe AP is associated with local complications such as acute fluid collection, pancreatic necrosis, abscess, and pseudocyst. Exocrine and endocrine pancreatic functions may remain impaired for variable periods after an acute attack, but AP rarely progresses to chronic pancreatitis (CP).
- Chronic pancreatitis is a syndrome of destructive and inflammatory conditions resulting from long-standing pancreatic injury. It is characterized by irreversible fibrosis and destruction of exocrine and endocrine tissue but is not invariably progressive. Most patients have periods of intractable abdominal pain. Progressive pancreatic insufficiency leads to maldigestion and diabetes mellitus.

▶ PATHOPHYSIOLOGY

ACUTE PANCREATITIS

- Gallstone-associated biliary tract disease and ethanol use account for most cases in the United States. A cause cannot be identified in some patients (idiopathic pancreatitis).
- Many medications have been implicated, but a causal association is difficult to confirm because ethical and practical considerations prevent rechallenge.
- Table 27–1 lists medications according to their certainty of causing AP. A definite association implies a temporal relationship of drug administration to abdominal pain and hyperamylasemia or to a positive response to rechallenge. Suggestive evidence exists for drugs with a probable association, whereas evidence is inadequate or contradictory for drugs having a possible association.
- AP is initiated by premature activation of pancreatic zymogens (inactive enzymes) within the acinar cells, pancreatic ischemia, or pancreatic duct obstruction.
- Release of active pancreatic enzymes directly causes local or distant tissue damage. Trypsin digests cell membranes and leads to the activation of other pancreatic enzymes. Lipase damages fat cells, producing noxious substances that cause further pancreatic and peripancreatic injury.
- Release of cytokines injures the acinar cell and enhances the inflammatory response. Injured acinar cells liberate chemoattractants that attract neutrophils, macrophages, and other cells to the area of inflammation, and increased vascular permeability promotes tissue edema.
- Pancreatic infection may result from increased intestinal permeability and translocation of colonic bacteria.
- Local complications include acute fluid collection, pancreatic necrosis, abscess, pseudocyst formation, and pancreatic ascites.
- Systemic complications include cardiovascular, renal, pulmonary, metabolic, hemorrhagic, and central nervous system abnormalities.

TABLE 27–1. Medications Associated with Acute Pancreatitis

Definite Association	Probable Association	Possible Association	
5-Aminosalicylic acid	Ampicillin	Acetaminophen	Ibuprofen
Asparaginase	Angiotensin-converting	Amiodarone	Indomethacin
Azathioprine	enzyme inhibitors	Amoxapine	Interleukin-2
Didanosine	Bumetamide	Angiotensin II	Isoniazid
Estrogens	Calcium	receptor antagonists	Isotretinoin
Furosemide	Cimetidine	Carbamazepine	Ketoprofen
Pentamidine	Chlorthalidone	Cholestyramine	Ketorolac
Mercaptopurine	Cisplatin	Clarithromycin	Lipid emulsion
Methyldopa	Clozapine	Clonidine	Mefenamic acid
Metronidazole	Corticosteroids	Cyclosporine	Metolazone
Sulfonamides	Cytarabine	Cyproheptadine	Nitrofurantoin
Sulindac	Ethacrynic acid	Danazol	Octreotide
Tetracycline	Interferon alfa-2b	Diazoxide	Ondansetron
Thiazides	Ifosfamide	Diphenoxylate	Opiates
Valproic acid/salts	Losartan	Ergotamine	Oxyphenbutazone
	Meglumine	Erythromycin	Paclitaxel
	antimoniate	Glyburide	Penicillin
	Piroxicam	Famciclovir	Propoxyphene
	Procainamide	Granisetron	Ranitidine
	Salicylates	Gold therapy	Tryptophan
	Sodium	Hepatitis A vaccination	Warfarin
	stibogluconate		
	Zalcitabine		

CHRONIC PANCREATITIS

- In most individuals, CP is progressive and loss of pancreatic function is irreversible. Permanent destruction of pancreatic tissue usually leads to exocrine and endocrine insufficiency.
- Prolonged ethanol consumption accounts for 70% of all cases in the United States; 10% result from other causes, and 20% are idiopathic.
- Ethanol-induced pancreatitis appears to progress from inflammation to cellular necrosis, and fibrosis occurs over time. Chronic alcohol ingestion causes changes in pancreatic fluid that create intraductal protein plugs that block small ductules. This results in progressive structural damage in the ducts and acinar tissue. Calcium complexes with the protein plugs, eventually resulting in destruction of pancreatic tissue.
- Abdominal pain may be related in part to increased intraductal pressure secondary to continued pancreatic secretion, pancreatic inflammation, and abnormalities of pancreatic nerves.
- Malabsorption of protein and fat occurs when the capacity for enzyme secretion is reduced by 90%. Lipase secretion decreases more rapidly than the proteolytic enzymes. Reduced bicarbonate secretion may lead to a duodenal pH of less than 4.
- A minority of patients develop complications including pancreatic pseudocyst, abscess, and ascites or common bile duct obstruction leading to cholangitis or secondary biliary cirrhosis.

▶ CLINICAL PRESENTATION

ACUTE PANCREATITIS

- The clinical presentation depends on the severity of the inflammatory process and whether damage is confined to the pancreas or involves contiguous organs.
- The initial presentation ranges from moderate abdominal discomfort to excruciating pain, shock, and respiratory distress. Abdominal pain occurs in 95% of patients and is usually epigastric, often radiating to the upper quadrants or back. The onset is usually sudden and the intensity is often described as "knifelike" or "boring." The pain tends to be steady and usually persists for several days. Nausea and vomiting occur in 85% of patients and usually follow the onset of pain.
- Clinical signs associated with widespread pancreatic inflammation and necrosis include marked epigastric tenderness, abdominal distention, hypotension, and low-grade fever. In severe disease, bowel sounds are diminished or absent. Dyspnea and tachypnea are signs of acute respiratory complications.

CHRONIC PANCREATITIS

- The main features are abdominal pain, malabsorption, weight loss, and diabetes. Jaundice occurs in about 10% of patients.
- Patients typically report dull epigastric or abdominal pain that radiates to the back. It may be either consistent or episodic. The pain is deep-seated, positional, frequently nocturnal, and unresponsive to medication. Nausea and vomiting often accompany the pain. Severe attacks last from several days to weeks and may be aggravated by eating and relieved by abstinence from alcohol.
- Steatorrhea (excessive loss of fat in the feces) and azotorrhea (excessive loss of protein in the feces) are seen in most patients. Steatorrhea is often associated with diarrhea and bloating. Weight loss may occur.
- Pancreatic diabetes is usually a late manifestation that is commonly associated with pancreatic calcification. Neuropathy is sometimes seen.

▶ DIAGNOSIS

ACUTE PANCREATITIS

- A definitive diagnosis of AP is made by surgical examination of the pancreas or pancreatic histology. In the absence of these procedures, the diagnosis depends on recognition of an etiologic factor, clinical signs and symptoms, abnormal laboratory tests, and imaging techniques that predict disease severity.
- Acute pancreatitis and its complications may be associated with leukocytosis, hyperglycemia, hypoalbuminemia, mild hyperbilirubinemia, and elevations in serum alkaline phosphatase and hepatic transaminases.
- Dehydration may lead to hemoconcentration with elevated hemoglobin, hematocrit, BUN, and serum creatinine.
- Marked hypocalcemia indicates severe necrosis and is a poor prognostic sign.
- Some patients with severe pancreatitis develop thrombocytopenia and a prolonged prothrombin time.
- C-reactive protein increases by 48 hours after the onset of symptoms and may be useful in distinguishing mild from severe pancreatitis.
- The serum amylase concentration usually rises 4 to 8 hours of symptom onset, peaks at 24 hours, and returns to normal over the next 8 to 14 days. Serum amylase elevations do not correlate with disease etiology or severity.

- Serum lipase is specific to the pancreas, and concentrations are usually elevated. Serum lipase elevations persist longer than serum amylase elevations and can be detected after the amylase has returned to normal.
- Contrast-enhanced computed tomography (CT) distinguishes interstitial from necrotizing pancreatitis. Endoscopic retrograde cholangiopancreatography (ERCP) is used to visualize and remove bile duct stones in patients with gallstone pancreatitis.

CHRONIC PANCREATITIS

- Most patients have a history of heavy ethanol use and attacks of recurrent upper abdominal pain. The classic triad of calcification, steatorrhea, and diabetes usually confirms the diagnosis.
- Serum amylase and lipase concentrations usually remain normal unless the pancreatic duct is blocked or a pseudocyst is present.
- The white blood cell count, fluid balance, and electrolyte concentrations usually remain normal unless fluids and electrolytes are lost due to vomiting and diarrhea.
- Malabsorption of fat can be detected by Sudan staining of the feces or a 72-hour quantitative measurement of fecal fat.
- Surgical biopsy of pancreatic tissue through laparoscopy or laparotomy is the gold standard for confirming the diagnosis of CP.
- In the absence of histologic samples, imaging techniques are helpful in detecting calcification of the pancreas and other causes of pain (ductal obstruction secondary to stones, strictures, or pseudocysts) and in differentiating CP from pancreatic cancer. Ultrasound is the simplest and least expensive technique, and abdominal CT is often used if the ultrasound examination is negative or unsatisfactory.
- ERCP is the most sensitive and specific diagnostic test, but it is reserved for patients in whom the diagnosis cannot be established by imaging techniques because of its expense and the potential for complications.

▶ DESIRED OUTCOME

- Treatment of AP is aimed at relieving abdominal pain, replacing fluids, minimizing systemic complications, and preventing pancreatic necrosis and infection.
- The goal of treatment of uncomplicated CP is directed at control of chronic pain and correction of malabsorption and glucose intolerance.

▶ TREATMENT

ACUTE PANCREATITIS
Figure 27–1.

- Medications listed in Table 27–1 should be discontinued whenever possible.
- Initial treatment usually involves withholding food or liquids to minimize exocrine stimulation of the pancreas.
- Nasogastric (NG) aspiration is beneficial in patients with profound pain, severe disease, paralytic ileus, and intractable vomiting.
- Patients predicted to follow a severe course require treatment of any cardiovascular, respiratory, renal, and metabolic complications. Aggressive fluid resuscitation is essential to correct intravascular volume depletion and maintain

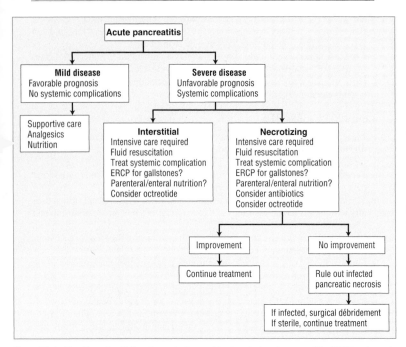

Figure 27–1. Algorithm of guidelines for evaluation and treatment of acute pancreatitis. ERCP, endoscopic retrograde cholangiopancreatography.

blood pressure. **Intravenous colloids** may be required because fluid losses are rich in protein. **Drotrecogin alfa** may benefit patients with pancreatitis and systemic inflammatory response syndrome. Intravenous **potassium, calcium, and magnesium** are used to correct deficiency states. **Insulin** is used to treat hyperglycemia. Patients with necrotizing pancreatitis may require antibiotics and surgical intervention.

- Nutritional support with enteral or parenteral nutrition should be initiated if it is anticipated that oral nutrition will be withheld for more than 1 week.
- Analgesics are given to reduce abdominal pain. In the past, treatment was usually initiated with parenteral **meperidine** (50 to 100 mg) every 3 to 4 hours because it causes less spasm of the sphincter of Oddi than other narcotics. Meperidine is used less frequently today because it is not as effective as other opioids and is contraindicated in renal failure. Parenteral **morphine** is sometimes used, but it can cause spasm of the sphincter of Oddi, increase serum amylase and rarely pancreatitis. Although it is less well studied, **hydromorphone** has a longer half-life than meperidine and can be given parenterally by a patient-controlled analgesia (PCA) pump.
- There is no evidence that inhibition of gastric acid secretion by antisecretory drugs prevents exacerbations of abdominal pain, but they may be used to prevent stress-related mucosal bleeding.
- Although there are conflicting data, **octreotide,** 0.1 mg subcutaneously every 8 hours, may decrease sepsis, length of hospital stay, and perhaps mortality in patients with severe AP.

- Only patients with severe AP complicated by necrosis should receive infection prophylaxis with broad-spectrum antibiotics. Agents that cover the range of enteric aerobic gram-negative bacilli and anaerobic organisms should be started within the first 48 hours and continued for 2 to 3 weeks. Imipenem-cilastatin (500 mg every 8 hours) may be most effective; a fluoroquinolone (e.g., ciprofloxacin, levofloxacin) with metronidazole should be considered for penicillin-allergic patients.

CHRONIC PANCREATITIS

- In patients with ethanol-induced CP, abstinence is the most important factor in preventing abdominal pain in the early stages of the disease.
- Small and frequent meals (6 meals/day) and a diet restricted in fat (50 to 75 g/day) are recommended to minimize postprandial pancreatic secretion and pain.
- Pain management should begin with nonnarcotic analgesics such as **acetaminophen** or **nonsteroidal anti-inflammatory drugs** given on a scheduled basis before meals to prevent postprandial exacerbation of pain. If these agents are ineffective, consideration should be given to using **tramadol** or adding a low-dose opioid (e.g., **acetaminophen and codeine**). If pain persists, the response to exogenous pancreatic enzymes should be evaluated in patients with mild to moderate CP. If these measures fail, an oral opioid should be added to the regimen. Parenteral opioids are reserved for patients with severe pain unresponsive to oral analgesics. In patients with pain that is difficult to manage, nonnarcotic modulators of chronic pain (e.g., selective serotonin reuptake inhibitors, tricyclic antidepressants) may be considered.
- Most patients with malabsorption require pancreatic enzyme supplementation (Figure 27–2). The combination of pancreatic enzymes (lipase, amylase, and protease) and a reduction in dietary fat (to less than 25 g/meal) enhances nutritional status and reduces steatorrhea. An initial dose containing about 30,000 IU of lipase and 10,000 IU of trypsin should be given with each meal.
- Oral pancreatic enzyme supplements are available as powders, uncoated or coated tablets, capsules, enteric-coated spheres (ECS) and microspheres (ECMS), or enteric-coated microtablets (ECMT) encased in a cellulose or gelatin capsule (Table 27–2). Microencapsulated enteric-coated products are not superior to recommended doses of conventional nonenteric-coated enzyme preparations. The quantity of active lipase delivered to the duodenum appears to be a more important determinant in pancreatic enzyme replacement therapy than the dosage form. Gastrointestinal side effects appear to be dose-related but occur less frequently with enteric-coated products.
- The concurrent use of antisecretory drugs (H_2-receptor antagonists or proton pump inhibitors) may improve the efficacy of pancreatic enzyme supplementation by both increasing pH and decreasing intragastric volume. Antacids appear to have little or no added effect in reducing steatorrhea. Addition of an H_2-receptor antagonist may be beneficial for symptomatic patients whose steatorrhea is not corrected by enzyme replacement therapy and reducing dietary fat. A proton pump inhibitor should be considered in patients who fail to benefit from an H_2-receptor antagonist.

SURGERY

- Removal of an underlying biliary tract gallstone with ERCP or surgery usually resolves AP and reduces the risk of recurrence. Surgery may be indicated in

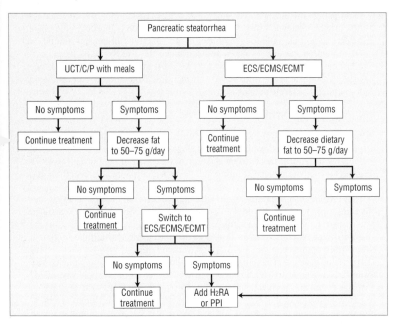

Figure 27–2. Algorithm of guidelines for the treatment of pancreatic steatorrhea in chronic pancreatitis. UCT, uncoated tablet; C, capsule; P, powder; ECS, enteric-coated sphere; ECMS, enteric-coated microsphere; ECMT, enteric-coated microtablet; H_2RA, H_2-receptor antagonist; PPI, proton pump inhibitor.

AP to treat pseudocyst, pancreatic abscess, and to drain the pancreatic bed if hemorrhagic or necrotic material is present.

- The most common indication for surgery in CP is abdominal pain refractory to medical therapy. Surgical procedures that alleviate pain include a subtotal pancreatectomy, decompression of the main pancreatic duct, or interruption of the splanchnic nerves.

▶ EVALUATION OF THERAPEUTIC OUTCOMES

ACUTE PANCREATITIS

- In patients with mild AP, pain control, fluid and electrolyte status, and nutrition should be assessed periodically depending on the degree of abdominal pain and fluid loss.
- Patients with severe AP should be transferred to an intensive care unit for close monitoring of vital signs, prothrombin time, fluid and electrolyte status, white blood cell count, blood glucose, lactate dehydrogenase, aspartate aminotransferase, serum albumin, hematocrit, BUN, and serum creatinine. Continuous hemodynamic and arterial blood gas monitoring is essential. Serum lipase, amylase, and bilirubin require less frequent monitoring. The patient should be monitored for signs of infection, relief of abdominal pain, and adequate nutritional status.

TABLE 27–2. Enzyme content of selected pancreatic enzyme preparations

Product	Dosage Form	Enzyme Content (Units)[a]		
		Lipase	Amylase	Protease
Creon-10	ECMS	10,000	33,200	37,500
Creon-20	ECMS	20,000	66,400	75,000
Ku-Zyme HP	C	8000	30,000	30,000
Lipram-CR10	ECMS	10,000	33,200	37,500
Lipram-PN16	ECMS	16,000	48,000	48,000
Lipram-CR20	ECMS	20,000	66,400	75,000
Lipram-PN20	ECMS	20,000	56,000	44,000
Lipram-UL12	ECMS	12,000	39,000	39,000
Lipram-PN10	ECMS	10,000	30,000	30,000
Lipram-UL18	ECMS	18,000	58,500	58,500
Lipram-UL20	ECMS	20,000	65,000	65,000
Pancrease	ECMS	4500	20,000	25,000
Pancrease MT-4	ECMT	4000	12,000	12,000
Pancrease MT-10	ECMT	10,000	30,000	30,000
Pancrease MT-16	ECMT	16,000	48,000	48,000
Pancrease MT-20	ECMT	20,000	56,000	44,000
Ultrase MT 12	ECMT	12,000	39,000	39,000
Ultrase MT 18	ECMT	18,000	58,500	58,500
Ultrase MT 20	ECMT	20,000	65,000	65,000
Viokase[b]	P	16,800	70,000	70,000
Viokase 8	UCT	8000	30,000	30,000
Viokase 16	UCT	16,000	60,000	60,000

[a]All listed products contain pancrelipase. Pancrelipase contains not less than 24 USP units of lipase activity, not less than 100 USP units of amylase activity, and not less than 100 USP units of protease activity per mg.
[b]Units of 0.7 g of powder.
C, powder encased in a cellulose capsule; ECS, enteric-coated sphere encased in a cellulose capsule; ECMS, enteric-coated microspheres encased in a cellulose or gelatin capsule; ECMT, enteric-coated microtablets encased in a cellulose capsule; UCT, uncoated tablet; P, powder.

CHRONIC PANCREATITIS

- The severity and frequency of abdominal pain should be assessed periodically to determine the efficacy of the analgesic regimen.
- The effectiveness of pancreatic enzyme supplementation is measured by improvement in body weight and stool consistency or frequency. The 72-hour stool test for fecal fat may be used when the adequacy of treatment is in question.
- Serum uric acid and folic acid concentrations should be monitored yearly in patients prone to hyperuricemia or folic acid deficiency. Blood glucose must be monitored carefully in diabetic patients.

See Chapter 39, Pancreatitis, authored by Rosemary R. Berardi and Patricia A. Montgomery, for a more detailed discussion of this topic.

Chapter 28

▶ PEPTIC ULCER DISEASE

▶ DEFINITION

Peptic ulcer disease (PUD) refers to a group of ulcerative disorders of the upper gastrointestinal (GI) tract that require acid and pepsin for their formation. Ulcers differ from gastritis and erosions in that they extend deeper into the muscularis mucosa. The three common forms of peptic ulcers include *Helicobacter pylori* (HP)–associated ulcers, nonsteroidal anti-inflammatory drug (NSAID)–induced ulcers, and stress-related mucosal damage (also called stress ulcers).

▶ PATHOPHYSIOLOGY

- The pathogenesis of duodenal ulcers (DU) and gastric ulcers (GU) is multifactorial and most likely reflects a combination of pathophysiologic abnormalities and environmental and genetic factors.
- Most peptic ulcers occur in the presence of acid and pepsin when *H. pylori,* NSAIDs, or other factors disrupt normal mucosal defense and healing mechanisms. Acid is an independent factor that contributes to disruption of mucosal integrity. Increased acid secretion has been observed in patients with DU and may result from HP infection. Patients with GU usually have normal or reduced rates of acid secretion.
- Alterations in mucosal defense induced by HP or NSAIDs are the most important cofactors in peptic ulcer formation. Mucosal defense mechanisms include mucus and bicarbonate secretion, intrinsic epithelial cell defense, and mucosal blood flow. Maintenance of mucosal integrity and repair is mediated by endogenous prostaglandin production.
- *H. pylori* infection causes gastritis in all infected individuals and is causally linked to PUD. However, only about 20% of infected persons develop symptomatic PUD. Most non-NSAID ulcers are infected with HP, and HP eradication markedly decreases ulcer recurrence. *H. pylori* may cause ulcers by direct mucosal damage, impairing mucosal defense via elaboration of toxins and enzymes, altering the immune/inflammatory response, and by increasing antral gastrin release, which leads to increased acid secretion.
- Nonselective NSAIDs (including aspirin) cause gastric mucosal damage by two mechanisms: (1) a direct or topical irritation of the gastric epithelium, and (2) systemic inhibition of the cyclooxygenase-1 (COX-1) enzyme, which results in decreased synthesis of protective prostaglandins.
- Use of corticosteroids alone does not increase the risk of ulcer or complications, but ulcer risk is doubled in corticosteroid users taking NSAIDs concurrently.
- Epidemiologic evidence links cigarette smoking to PUD, impaired ulcer healing, and ulcer-related GI complications. The risk is proportional to the amount smoked per day. Smoking does not increase ulcer recurrence after HP eradication.
- Although clinical observation suggests that ulcer patients are adversely affected by stressful life events, controlled studies have failed to document a cause-and-effect relationship.
- Coffee, tea, cola beverages, beer, milk, and spices may cause dyspepsia but do not increase PUD risk. Ethanol ingestion in high concentrations is associated with acute gastric mucosal damage and upper GI bleeding but is not clearly the cause of ulcers.

▶ CLINICAL PRESENTATION

- Abdominal pain is the most frequent symptom of PUD. The pain is often epigastric and described as burning but can present as vague discomfort, abdominal fullness, or cramping. A typical nocturnal pain may awaken patients from sleep, especially between 12 AM and 3 AM.
- Pain from DU often occurs 1 to 3 hours after meals and is usually relieved by food, whereas food may precipitate or accentuate ulcer pain in GU. Antacids provide rapid pain relief in most ulcer patients.
- Heartburn, belching, and bloating often accompany the pain. Nausea, vomiting, and anorexia are more common in GU.
- The severity of symptoms varies from patient to patient and may be seasonal, occurring more frequently in the spring or fall.
- Pain does not always correlate with the presence of an ulcer. Asymptomatic patients may have an ulcer at endoscopy, and patients may have persistent symptoms even with endoscopically proven healed ulcers. Many patients (especially older adults) with NSAID-induced ulcer-related complications have no prior abdominal symptoms.
- Complications of ulcers caused by HP and NSAIDs include upper GI bleeding, perforation into the peritoneal cavity, penetration into an adjacent structure (e.g., pancreas, biliary tract, or liver), and gastric outlet obstruction. Bleeding may be occult or present as melena or hematemesis. Perforation is associated with sudden, sharp, severe pain, beginning first in the epigastrium but quickly spreading over the entire abdomen. Symptoms of gastric outlet obstruction typically occur over several months and include early satiety, bloating, anorexia, nausea, vomiting, and weight loss.

▶ DIAGNOSIS

- The physical examination may reveal epigastric tenderness between the umbilicus and the xiphoid process that less commonly radiates to the back.
- Routine laboratory tests are not helpful in establishing a diagnosis of uncomplicated PUD. The hematocrit, hemoglobin, and stool hemoccult tests are used to detect bleeding.
- The diagnosis of HP infection can be made using endoscopic or nonendoscopic tests. The tests that require upper endoscopy are more expensive, uncomfortable, and require a mucosal biopsy for histology, culture, or detection of urease activity. The nonendoscopic tests include serologic antibody detection tests, the urea breath test (UBT), and the stool antigen test. Serologic tests detect circulating IgG directed against HP but are of limited value in evaluating post-treatment eradication. The UBT is based on urease production by HP.
- Testing for HP is only recommended if eradication therapy is considered. If endoscopy is not planned, serologic antibody testing is reasonable to determine HP status. The UBT is the preferred nonendoscopic method to verify HP eradication after treatment.
- The diagnosis of PUD depends on visualizing the ulcer crater either by upper GI radiography or endoscopy. Radiography may be the preferred initial diagnostic procedure in patients with suspected uncomplicated PUD. If complications are thought to exist or if an accurate diagnosis is warranted upper endoscopy should be performed. If a gastric ulcer is found on radiography, malignancy should be excluded by direct endoscopic visualization and histology.

Gastrointestinal Disorders

▶ DESIRED OUTCOME

The goals of treatment are relieving ulcer pain, healing the ulcer, preventing ulcer recurrence, and reducing ulcer-related complications. In HP–positive patients, the goals are to eradicate the organism, heal the ulcer, and cure the disease with a cost-effective drug regimen.

▶ TREATMENT

NONPHARMACOLOGIC TREATMENT

- Patients with PUD should eliminate or reduce psychological stress, cigarette smoking, and the use of NSAIDs (including aspirin). If possible, alternative agents such as **acetaminophen,** a nonacetylated salicylate (e.g., **salsalate**), or COX-2 selective inhibitor should be used for pain relief.
- Although there is no need for a special diet, patients should avoid foods and beverages that cause dyspepsia or exacerbate ulcer symptoms (e.g., spicy foods, caffeine, alcohol).

PHARMACOLOGIC TREATMENT

- An algorithm for the evaluation and management of a patient with dyspeptic or ulcer-like symptoms is presented in Figure 28–1.
- Eradication of HP is recommended for HP–infected patients with GU, DU, ulcer-related complications, and in some other situations. Treatment should be effective, well tolerated, easy to comply with, and cost-effective (Table 28–1).
- First-line eradication therapy is a proton pump inhibitor (PPI)-based three-drug regimen containing two antibiotics. Most clinicians prefer **clarithromycin** and **amoxicillin,** reserving **metronidazole** for back-up therapy. The PPI should be taken 15 to 30 minutes before meals along with the two antibiotics. Although an initial 7-day course provides minimally acceptable eradication rates, longer treatment periods (10 to 14 days) are associated with higher eradication rates and less antimicrobial resistance.
- First-line treatment with quadruple therapy using a PPI (with **bismuth,** **metronidazole,** and **tetracycline**) achieves similar eradication rates as PPI-based triple therapy and permits a shorter treatment duration (7 days). However, this regimen is often recommended as second-line treatment when a clarithromycin-amoxicillin regimen is used initially. All medications except the PPI should be taken with meals and at bedtime.
- If the initial treatment fails to eradicate HP, second-line empiric treatment should: (1) use antibiotics that were not included in the initial regimen; (2) include antibiotics that do not have resistance problems; (3) use a drug that has a topical effect (e.g., bismuth); (4) be extended to 10 to 14 days. Thus, if a PPI-clarithromycin-amoxicillin regimen fails, therapy should be instituted with a PPI, bismuth subsalicylate, metronidazole, and tetracycline for 10 to 14 days.
- Conventional treatment with standard dosages of H_2-receptor antagonists (H_2RA) or sucralfate alone (without antibiotics) relieves ulcer symptoms and heals most gastric and duodenal ulcers in 6 to 8 weeks (Table 28–2). PPIs provide comparable healing rates over 4 weeks. However, when conventional antiulcer therapy is discontinued after ulcer healing, most HP-positive patients develop a recurrent ulcer within 1 year.

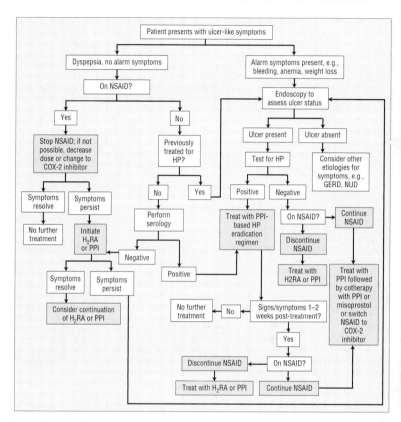

Figure 28–1. Algorithm for the evaluation and management of a patient who presents with dyspeptic or ulcer-like symptoms. COX-2, cyclooxygenase-2; GERD, gastroesophageal reflux disease; HP, *Helicobacter pylori*; H$_2$RA, H$_2$-receptor antagonist; PPI, proton pump inhibitor; NSAID, nonsteroidal anti-inflammatory drug; NUD, nonulcer dyspepsia.

• Maintenance therapy with a PPI, low-dose H$_2$RA, or sucralfate (see Table 28–2) may be indicated for patients who have a history of ulcer-related complications, a healed refractory ulcer, failed HP eradication therapy, or who are heavy smokers or NSAID users.

• Most uncomplicated NSAID-induced ulcers heal with standard regimens of an H$_2$RA, PPI, or sucralfate (Table 28–2) if the NSAID is discontinued. If the NSAID must be continued, consideration should be given to reducing the NSAID dose or switching to acetaminophen, a nonacetylated salicylate, a partially selective COX-2 inhibitor, or a selective COX-2 inhibitor. PPIs are the drugs of choice when NSAIDs must be continued because potent acid suppression is required to accelerate ulcer healing. If HP is present, treatment should be initiated with an eradication regimen that contains a PPI. Patients at risk of developing serious ulcer-related complications while on NSAIDs should receive prophylactic cotherapy with misoprostol or a PPI.

TABLE 28–1. Drug Regimens to Eradicate *Helicobacter pylori*[a]

Drug #1	Drug #2	Drug #3	Drug #4
Proton pump inhibitor-based three-drug regimens			
Omeprazole 20 mg twice daily **or** lansoprazole 30 mg twice daily **or** pantoprazole 40 mg twice daily **or** esomeprazole 40 mg daily **or** rabeprazole 20 mg daily	Clarithromycin 500 mg twice daily	Amoxicillin 1 g twice daily **or** metronidazole 500 mg twice daily	
Bismuth-based four-drug regimens[b]			
Omeprazole 40 mg twice daily **or** lansoprazole 30 mg twice daily **or** pantoprazole 40 mg twice daily **or** esomeprazole 40 mg daily **or** rabeprazole 20 mg daily **or** Standard ulcer-healing dosages of an H_2-receptor antagonist taken for 4–6 wk (see Table 28–2)	Bismuth subsalicylate 525 mg 4 times daily	Metronidazole 250–500 mg 4 times daily	Tetracycline 500 mg four times daily **or** amoxicillin 500 mg four times daily, **or** clarithromycin 250–500 mg 4 times daily

[a]Although treatment is minimally effective if used for 7 days, 10–14 days of treatment is recommended. The antisecretory drug may be continued beyond antimicrobial treatment in the presence of an active ulcer.
[b]In the setting of an active ulcer, acid suppression is added to hasten pain relief.

- Patients with ulcers refractory to treatment should undergo upper endoscopy to confirm a nonhealing ulcer, exclude malignancy, and assess HP status. HP-positive patients should receive eradication therapy. In HP-negative patients, higher PPI doses (e.g., omeprazole 40 mg/day) heal the majority of ulcers. Continuous PPI treatment is often necessary to maintain healing.

TABLE 28–2. Oral Drug Regimens Used to Heal Peptic Ulcers or Maintain Ulcer Healing

Drug	Duodenal or Gastric Ulcer Healing (mg/dose)	Maintenance of Duodenal or Gastric Ulcer Healing (mg/dose)
Proton pump inhibitors		
Omeprazole	20–40 daily	20–40 daily
Lansoprazole	15–30 daily	15–30 daily
Rabeprazole	20 daily	20 daily
Pantoprazole	40 daily	40 daily
Esomeprazole	20–40 daily	20–40 daily
H_2-receptor antagonists		
Cimetidine	300 four times daily 400 twice daily 800 at bedtime	400–800 at bedtime
Famotidine	20 twice daily 40 at bedtime	20–40 at bedtime
Nizatidine	150 twice daily 300 at bedtime	150–300 at bedtime
Ranitidine	150 twice daily 300 at bedtime	150–300 at bedtime
Promote mucosal defense		
Sucralfate (g/dose)	1 four times daily 2 twice daily	1–2 twice daily 1 four times daily

▶ EVALUATION OF THERAPEUTIC OUTCOMES

- Patients should be monitored for symptomatic relief of ulcer pain as well as potential adverse effects and drug interactions related to drug therapy.
- Ulcer pain typically resolves in a few days when NSAIDs are discontinued and within 7 days upon initiation of antiulcer therapy. Most patients with uncomplicated PUD will be symptom-free after treatment with any one of the recommended antiulcer regimens.
- The persistence or recurrence of symptoms after several weeks of treatment suggests failure of ulcer healing or HP eradication, or an alternative diagnosis such as gastroesophageal reflux disease.
- Most patients with uncomplicated HP–positive ulcers do not require confirmation of ulcer healing or HP eradication.
- High-risk patients on NSAIDs should be closely monitored for signs and symptoms of bleeding, obstruction, penetration, and perforation.
- Follow-up endoscopy is justified in patients with frequent symptomatic recurrence, refractory disease, complications, or suspected hypersecretory states.

See Chapter 33, Peptic Ulcer Disease, authored by Rosemary R. Berardi and Lynda S. Welage, for a more detailed discussion of this topic.

Gynecologic and Obstetric Disorders
Edited by Barbara G. Wells

Chapter 29

▶ CONTRACEPTION

▶ DEFINITION

- Contraception is the prevention of pregnancy following sexual intercourse by inhibiting sperm from reaching a mature ovum (i.e., methods that act as barriers or prevent ovulation) or by preventing a fertilized ovum from implanting in the endometrium (i.e., mechanisms that create an unfavorable uterine environment).
- Method failure (perfect-use failure) is a failure inherent to the proper use of the contraceptive alone.
- User failure (typical use failure) takes into account the user's ability to follow directions correctly and consistently.

▶ THE MENSTRUAL CYCLE

- The median length of the menstrual cycle is 28 days (range 21 to 40).
- The first day of menses is day 1 of the follicular phase.
- Ovulation usually occurs on day 14 of the menstrual cycle.
- After ovulation, the luteal phase lasts until the beginning of the next cycle.
- Epinephrine and norepinephrine stimulate the hypothalamus to secrete gonadotropin-releasing hormone (GnRH), which stimulates the anterior pituitary to secrete bursts of gonadotropins, follicle-stimulating hormone (FHS) and luteinizing hormone (LH).
- In the follicular phase, FSH causes recruitment of a small group of follicles for continued growth. Between 5 and 7 days, one of these becomes the dominant follicle, which later ruptures to release the oocyte. The dominant follicle develops increasing amounts of estradiol and inhibin, which cause a negative feedback on the secretion of GnRH and FSH, causing atresia of the remaining follicles recruited earlier.
- The dominant follicle continues to grow and synthesizes estradiol, progesterone, and androgen. Estradiol stops the menstrual flow from the previous cycle, thickens the endometrial lining, and produces thin, watery cervical mucus. FSH regulates aromatase enzymes that induce conversion of androgens to estrogens in the follicle.
- The pituitary releases a mid-cycle LH surge which stimulates the final stages of follicular maturation and ovulation, which occurs 24 to 36 hours after the estradiol peak and 10 to 16 hours after the LH peak.
- The LH surge occurring 28 to 32 hours before a follicle ruptures is the most clinically useful predictor of approaching ovulation. Conception is most successful when intercourse takes place from 2 days before ovulation to the day of ovulation.
- After ovulation, the remaining luteinized follicles become the corpus luteum, which synthesizes androgen, estrogen, and progesterone (Figure 29–1).
- If pregnancy occurs, human chorionic gonadotropin (hCG) prevents regression of the corpus luteum and stimulates continued production of estrogen and progesterone. If pregnancy does not occur, the corpus luteum degenerates, and progesterone declines. As progesterone levels decline, menstruation occurs.

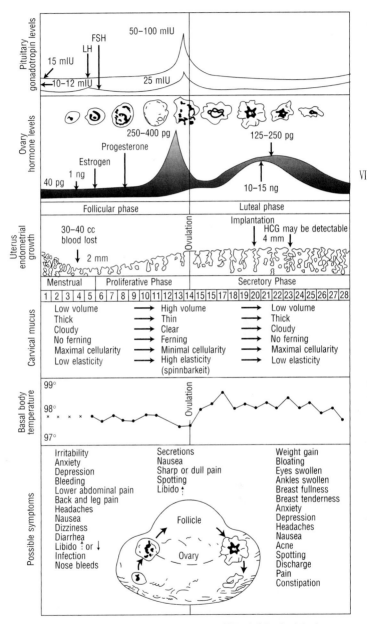

Figure 29–1. Menstrual cycle events—idealized 28-day cycle. FSH = follicle-stimulating hormone, HCG = human chorionic gonadotropin, LH = luteining hormone. *(Reproduced courtesy of Hatcher RA, Nelson AL, Zieman M, et al. A pocket Guide to Managing Contraception. Tiger, GA, Bridging the Gap Foundation, 2003:1–146. This figure may be reproduced at no cost to the reader.)*

► TREATMENT: Contraception

Table 29–1 provides a comparison of reversible methods of contraception with regard to absolute contraindications, advantages, disadvantages and percent of women with pregnancy.

NONPHARMACOLOGIC THERAPY

Periodic Abstinence

• The abstinence (rhythm) method is not well accepted as it is associated with relatively high pregnancy rates and necessitates avoidance of intercourse for several days in each cycle.

Barrier Techniques

• Barrier methods, including the diaphragm, cervical cap, sponge, condom, and spermicides, can reduce the rate of sexually transmitted disease (STD) transmission.

• The effectiveness of the diaphragm depends on its function as a barrier and on the spermicidal cream or jelly placed in the diaphragm before insertion.

• The Prentif cervical cap, smaller and less messy than the diaphragm, fits over the cervix like a thimble. It is filled one-third full with spermicide prior to insertion. Women should not wear the cap for longer than 48 hours to reduce the risk of toxic shock syndrome.

• Most condoms made in the United States are latex rubber, which is impermeable to viruses, but about 5% are made from lamb intestine, which is not. When used with another barrier method, the effectiveness of condoms approaches 95%. Mineral oil-based lotions, lubricants, or vaginal drug formulations (e.g., Cleocin vaginal cream, Premarin vaginal cream, Vagistat 1, Femstat, and Monistat Vaginal suppositories) can decrease barrier strength of latex by 90% in 60 seconds.

• The female condom (Reality) covers the labia as well as the cervix, thus it may be more effective than the male condom in preventing transmission of diseases such as herpes. However, the pregnancy rate is reported to be 26% per year, based on a 6-month follow-up study of 200 women.

PHARMACOLOGIC THERAPY

Spermicides

Spermicides, most of which contain nonoxynol-9, are surfactants that destroy sperm cell walls. They offer some protection against STDs and cervical cancer. Tablets and suppositories require 10 to 30 minutes to dissolve. Additional spermicide must be used each time intercourse is repeated.

Spermicide-implanted Barrier Techniques

The vaginal contraceptive sponge (Today) contains 1 g of nonoxynol-9 and provides protection for 24 hours. After intercourse, the sponge must be left in place for at least 6 hours before removal. It is now being reviewed by the Food and Drug Administration (FDA) for re-release in the United States.

Oral Contraceptives (OCs)
Composition and Formulations

• OCs contain either a combination of synthetic estrogen and synthetic progestin or a progestin alone.

  • Estrogens suppress FSH and thus prevents development of a dominant follicle. They also stabilize the endometrial lining and potentiate the action of the progestin.

TABLE 29–1. Comparison of Reversible Methods of Contraception

Method	Absolute Contraindications	Advantages	Disadvantages	Lowest Expected	Typical Use
Episodic Contraceptive Methods					
Spermicides alone	Allergy to spermicide	Inexpensive No office visit required Some protection against STDs	High user failure rate Must be reapplied before each act of intercourse May cause local irritation in either partner May enhance HIV transmission	3	21
Condoms, male	Allergy to latex or rubber	Inexpensive Readily available No office visit required STD protection, including HIV (latex only)	High user failure rate Poor acceptance Possibility of breakage Efficacy decreased by oil-based lubricants Possible-allergic reactions to latex in either partner	2	12
Condoms, female (Reality)	Allergy to polyurethane History of toxic shock syndrome	Can be inserted just before intercourse or ahead of time; provides protection for 8 h STD protection, including HIV	High user failure rate Dislike ring hanging outside vagina Cumbersome	5	21
Diaphragm with spermicide	Allergy to latex, rubber, or spermicide Recurrent UTIs History of toxic shock syndrome Abnormal gynecologic anatomy	Low cost Decreased incidence of cervical neoplasia Some protection against STDs Can be inserted for up to 6 h before intercourse	High user failure rate Office visit required Decreased efficacy with increased frequency of intercourse Must be refitted after significant change in weight (+/–10 pounds)	6	18

(Continued)

TABLE 29–1. Continued

Method	Absolute Contraindications	Advantages	Disadvantages	Lowest Expected	Typical Use
			Increased incidence of vaginal yeast and UTIs		
			Increased incidence of toxic shock syndrome		
			Efficacy affected by oil-based lubricants		
			Cervical irritation		
Cervical cap (Prentif)	Allergy to rubber or spermicide	Low cost	High user failure rate	6	18
	Recurrent UTIs	Some protection against STDs	Office visit required		
	History of toxic shock syndrome	Can be inserted just before or ahead of time; provides protection for 48 h	May be difficult for patient to use correctly		
	Abnormal gynecologic anatomy		Decreased efficacy with parity		
	Abnormal Papanicolaou smear		Cannot be used during menses		
Sponge (Today)	Allergy to spermicide	Inexpensive	High user failure rate	Parous 9	Parous 28
	Recurrent UTIs	No office visit required	Problems removing the sponge due to vaginal dryness	Nulliparous 6	Nulliparous 18
	History of toxic shock syndrome	Some protection against STDs	Cannot be used during menses		
	Abnormal gynecologic anatomy	Can be inserted just before or ahead of time; provides protection for 24 h	Not yet available in United States		
Hormonal Methods					
Oral contraceptives	Hepatic adenomas	Decreased risk of PID, ovarian and endometrial cancer	Office visit required	0.1	3
	Thromboembolic disorders or history thereof	Improvement in endometriosis (probably)	Increased risk of benign hepatocellular adenomas		
	Cerebrovascular or coronary artery disease	Fewer functional ovarian cysts (possibly)	Mild increased risk of thromboembolism and stroke		
			May elevate blood pressure		

(Continued)

	Contraindications	Advantages	Disadvantages		
	Known or suspected breast cancer Undiagnosed abnormal gynecologic bleeding Jaundice with pregnancy or previous pill use	Less salpingitis and ectopic pregnancy Prevention of benign breast disease (fibroadenoma and fibrocystic changes) Less rheumatoid arthritis (possibly) Increased bone density (possibly) Improvement in acne/hirsutism Significant improvement in menstruation-related problems: fewer cramps, less flow for fewer days, less iron deficiency anemia, more predictable menses, elimination of mittelschmerz, less dysmenorrhea and premenstrual syndrome	No protection against most STDs Estrogenic side effects (nausea, breast tenderness, fluid retention) Progestin side effects (acne, increased appetite, depression) Increased risk of myocardial infarction in older women, smokers		
Progestin-only oral contraceptives	Undiagnosed abnormal gynecologic bleeding	May be used by lactating women and women with cardiovascular risk Allows avoidance of estrogen-related side effects Protection against PID, iron deficiency anemia, and dysmenorrhea	Frequent spotting and amenorrhea Increased risk of ectopic pregnancy Must take every day at the same time	0.5	3

(Continued)

TABLE 29–1. (Continued)

Method	Absolute Contraindications	Advantages	Disadvantages	Lowest Expected	Typical Use
				Percent of Women With Pregnancy[a]	
Transdermal contraceptives (Ortho-Evra)	Same as above for oral contraceptives	Same as above for oral contraceptives Convenience of weekly application	Same as above for oral contraceptives	1	Up to 9 in women >90 kg
Contraceptive rings (NuvaRing)	Same as above for oral contraceptives	Same as above for oral contraceptives Convenience of monthly insertion	Same as above for oral contraceptives	1	?
Progestin implants: levonorgestrel (Norplant and Norplant II,[b] Jadelle,[b] Capronor[b]), 3 ketodesogestrel (Implanon[b]), nomegestrol acetate (uniplant[b])	Pregnancy Undiagnosed abnormal gynecologic bleeding Acute liver disease Benign or malignant liver tumors Known or suspected breast cancers Active thrombophlebitis or thromboembolic disease	Passive contraception Duration of efficacy varies; effective up to 5 yr with Norplant in women <154 pounds Effects are quickly reversible Less menstrual cramping and mittelschmerz pain No suppression of lactation No metabolic disturbances Can be considered for use in women who have diabetes, hypertension, gall bladder disease, history of cardiovascular or thromboembolic disease and in women who are smokers or lactating	Requires outpatient surgical procedure Irregular menstrual bleeding, headaches, weight gain, acne Progestin side effects Local infection or bruising on insertion; removal may be difficult Expensive initially High discontinuation rate Unacceptable in patients using some anticonvulsants	0.3	0.3

(Continued)

Depo-Provera	Pregnancy Undiagnosed abnormal gynecologic bleeding Known or suspected breast cancers Liver disease (relative contraindication) Severe depression (relative contraindication) Severe cardiovascular disease (relative contraindication)	Passive contraception No suppression of lactation No increased risk of thromboembolism May decrease seizure frequency Effective for 3 months Can be considered for use in women who have seizure disorders, diabetes, hypertension, gall bladder disease, history of cardiovascular or thromboembolic disease and in women who are smokers or lactating	Office visit required every 3 months Irregular menstrual bleeding, headache, weight gain, acne Delayed return of fertility Possible increased risk of breast cancer in younger users Decreased HDL Progestin side effects Decreased bone density in long-term users	0.3	0.3
Lunelle	Pregnancy Undiagnosed abnormal gynecologic bleeding Known or suspected breast cancers Thromboembolic disorders or history thereof Cerebrovascular or coronary artery disease Jaundice of pregnancy or with prior pill use	Effects quickly reversible Less menstrual cramping and mittelschmerz pain Less menstrual irregularity than other injectable or implantable methods	Office visit required monthly Progestin side effects Estrogen side effects	0.1	0.1

(Continued)

TABLE 29–1. Continued

Method	Absolute Contraindications	Advantages	Disadvantages	Lowest Expected	Typical Use[a]
Intrauterine Devices (Hormonal and Nonhormonal)					
Copper-T 380A (ParaGard)	Multiple sexual partners or partner with multiple partners (high risk for STDs) History of PID or ectopic pregnancy, acute pelvic infection Abnormal uterine cavity/pelvic surgery/undiagnosed gynecologic bleeding Uterine or cervical cancer Wilson's disease Allergy to copper	Passive contraception Long-term contraception (can remain in place for up to 10 yr) Less expensive per year and easier for some patients No delay in return of fertility after removal	Increased heavy bleeding Spotting between periods Increased cramping and dysmenorrhea Increased risk of ectopic pregnancy Office visit required Rarely, uterine perforation	0.8	3
Progesterone T (Progestasert)	Postpartum endometritis or infected abortion in previous 3 months Acute cervicitis or vaginitis (including BV) until infection controlled	Remains in place for 1 yr Decreased cramping and dysmenorrhea Decrease in menstrual blood loss No delay in return of fertility after removal	Office visit required Must be changed each year Increased risk of ectopic pregnancy Rarely, uterine perforation	1.5	2

(Continued)

Method	Contraindications	Noncontraceptive benefits/comments	Typical use failure rate[a]	Perfect use failure rate[a]
Levonorgestrel IUD (Mirena)	Conditions associated with increased susceptibility to infections, including leukemia, AIDS, IV drug abuse, and corticosteroid use Valvular heart disease (relative contraindication) Nulliparity (relative contraindication) Genital actinomyces Wilson's disease Allergy to copper	Constant rate of hormone release for 5 yr Possibly the single most effective reversible contraceptive method over 5-yr period Decreased cramping, dysmenorrhea, menorrhagia Combines benefits of Norplant and Copper-T Office visit required Irregular menstrual bleeding Rarely, uterine perforation	0.1	0.1

STD, sexually transmitted disease; HIV, human immunodeficiency virus; UTI, urinary tract infection; PID, pelvic inflammatory disease; HDL, high-density lipoprotein cholesterol; BV, bacterial vaginosis; AIDS, acquired immunodeficiency syndrome; IV, intravenous.

[a] Failure rates during first year of use, United States.

[b] Products in development.

- Progestins suppress the LH surge and thus block ovulation. They also thicken cervical mucus and causes the endometrium to atrophy.
- The low dose combination OCs contain approximately one third to one fourth the estrogen and one tenth the progestin dose that was in the earlier pills.
- Combination multiphasic (biphasic and triphasic) formulations have further lowered the total monthly hormonal dose without clearly demonstrating clinical advantage.
- The progestin-only "minipills" (28 days of active hormone per cycle) are also available, and they contain even lower doses of progestin than in the combination OCs. They are less effective than the combination OCs with typical use and are usually reserved for women who must avoid estrogen.

Components

VI
- Mestranol must be converted to ethinyl estradiol to be active. It is approximately 50% less potent than ethinyl estradiol.
- Progestins vary in their progestational activity and differ with respect to inherent estrogenic, antiestrogenic, and androgenic effects. Their estrogenic and antiestrogenic properties occur because progestins are metabolized to estrogenic substances. Androgenic properties occur because of the structural similarity of progestin to testosterone.
- Third generation OCs contain newer progestins (e.g., desogestrel, drospirenone, gestodene, and norgestimate), which appear to have no estrogenic effects and are less androgenic compared to levonorgestrel on a weight basis. Therefore, these agents are thought to be more effective in improving mild to moderate acne. Drospirenone may cause less weight gain compared with OCs containing levonorgestrel.
- Table 29–2 lists available OCs by brand name and hormonal composition.

Considerations with Oral Contraceptive Use

- The recommendation of the American College of Obstetrics is to allow provision of hormonal contraception after a simple medical history and blood pressure measurement.

WOMEN OVER 35 YEARS OF AGE

- OCs are an acceptable form of birth control for nonsmoking women up to the time of menopause, and women over 35 years should use the lowest dose estrogen products. Women who have not smoked for 1 year can be regarded as nonsmokers. (see Table 29–3 for precautions in the provision of combined OCs.)
- In healthy nonsmoking women over 35 years, OCs increased the risk of myocardial infarction (MI) and stroke.

SMOKING WOMEN

Women who smoke more than 1 pack a day over the ages of 35 should not use OCs containing estrogen. If they smoke fewer than 20 cigarettes a day and are over 35 years, they should use estrogen containing OCs only with caution. If smoking women use OCs, they should use the 20-mcg estrogen formulation.

HYPERTENSION

- Combination OCs, even those with less than 35 mcg estrogen, can cause small increases in blood pressure, but clinically significant increases are rare with low-dose agents. The use of low-dose OCs is acceptable in women with well-controlled and well-monitored hypertension. But if they have end organ disease or smoke, they should not use combination OCs.

DIABETES
- The new progestins are believed to have little, if any, effect on carbohydrate metabolism. Nonsmoking women with diabetes, but no vascular disease, can use OCs safely, but diabetic women with vascular disease should not use OCs.

DYSLIPIDEMIA
- Generally synthetic progestins decrease high-density lipoprotein (HDL) and increase low-density lipoprotein (LDL). Estrogens decrease LDL, increase HDL and triglycerides. Most low-dose combination OCs, with the possible exception of levonorgestrel pills, have no significant impact on HDL, LDL, triglycerides, or total cholesterol.
- However, the mechanism for the increased incidence of cardiovascular disease in OC users is believed to be secondary to thromboembolic and thrombotic changes, not atherosclerosis.
- Women with controlled dyslipidemias can use low-dose OCs, but they need frequent monitoring. Women with uncontrolled dyslipidemia (LDL greater than 160 mg/dL, HDL less than 35 mg/dL, triglycerides greater than 250 mg/dL) and additional risk factors (e.g., coronary artery disease, diabetes, hypertension, smoking, or a positive family history) should use an alternative method of contraception.

THROMBOEMBOLISM
- Estrogens have a dose-related effect in the development of venous thromboembolism (VTE) and pulmonary embolism, especially in women who smoke or have other inherited conditions that are risk factors for thrombosis, inherited or acquired. The risk of VTE is less with non–third-generation OCs than originally thought (less than a threefold increase in relative risk). The 20-mcg ethinyl estradiol formulations do not appear to have an effect on clotting parameters, even in smokers, but whether they lower the risk of thrombotic events is not known.
- Recent data have shown that third-generation OCs are associated with a small increase in the risk of VTE, but do not establish a cause-effect relationship. There have also been reports of VTE in patients taking OCs containing drospirenone.
- Currently, OCs are contraindicated in any woman with a history of VTE or pulmonary embolism. Some clinicians support the use of OCs in women with coagulation disorders who have been properly anticoagulated.

CEREBROVASCULAR DISEASE
Both thrombotic and hemorrhagic stroke have been associate with use of OCs. With low-dose OCs, the risk for stroke is extremely low in healthy young women. Data suggest that the effect of smoking in women younger than 35 years is minimal in the absence of hypertension, and that hypertension may be the major risk factor for stroke. Patients should be counseled to recognize warning signs of cerebrovascular accidents.

MIGRAINE HEADACHE
- OCs usually decrease the frequency of migraine headaches, but they can exacerbate them in some women. Migraines may be a risk factor for stroke.
- Combination OCs may be used in young (less than 35 years), healthy, nonsmoking women with migraines if they do not have focal neurologic signs.

VI

TABLE 29–2. Composition of Commonly Prescribed Oral Contraceptives

Product	Estrogen	mcg	Progestin	mg	Spotting and BTB
50 mcg Estrogen					
Necon 1/50M, Nelova 1/50M, Norinyl 1/50, Norethin 1/50M, Ortho–Novum 1/50	Mestranol	50	Norethindrone	1	10.6
Norlestrin 1/50	E. estradiol	50	Nor. acetate	1	103.6
Ovcon 50	E. estradiol	50	Norethindrone	1	11.9
Ovral, Ogestrel	E. estradiol	50	Norgestrel	0.5	4.5
Demulen 1/50, Zovia 1/50	E. estradiol	50	Ethy. diacetate	1	13.9
Sub-50 mcg Estrogen Monophasic					
Alesse, Levlite	E. estradiol	20	Levonorgestrel	0.1	26.5
Brevicon, Modicon, Necon 0.5/30	E. estradiol	35	Norethindrone	0.5	25.2
Demulen 1/35, Zovia 1/35	E. estradiol	35	Ethy. diacetate	1	37.4
Desogen, Ortho-Cept	E. estradiol	30	Desogestrel	0.15	13.1
Levlen, Levora 0.15/30, Nordette	E. estradiol	30	Levonorgestrel	0.15	14.0
Loestrin 1/20,[a] Microgestin 1/20	E. estradiol	20	Nor. acetate	1	29.7
Loestrin 1.5/30,[a] Microgestin 1.5/30	E. estradiol	30	Nor. acetate	1.5	25.2
Lo-Ovral, Low-Ogestrel	E. estradiol	30	Norgestrel	0.3	9.6
Necon 1/35, Norinyl 1/35, Norethin 1/35, Ortho–Novum 1/35	E. estradiol	35	Norethindrone	1	14.7
Ortho-Cyclen	E. estradiol	35	Norgestimate	0.25	14.3
Ovcon-35	E. estradiol	35	Norethindrone	0.4	11
Seasonale[b]	E. estradiol	30	Levonorgestrel	0.15	?
Yasmin	E. estradiol	30	Drospirenone	3	14.5
Sub-50 mcg Estrogen Multiphasic					
Cyclessa	E. estradiol	25 (7) 25 (7) 25 (7)	Desogestrel	0.1 (7) 0.125 (7) 0.150 (7)	11.1
Estrostep[a]	E. estradiol E. estradiol E. estradiol	20 (5) 30 (7) 35 (9)	Norethindrone Norethindrone Norethindrone	1 (5) 1 (7) 1 (9)	26.2

(Continued)

Mircette	E. estradiol	20 (21)	Desogestrel	0.15 (21)	19.7
	E. estradiol	10 (5)	Desogestrel		
Necon 10/11	E. estradiol	35 (10)	Norethindrone	0.5 (10)	17.6
Nelova 10/11	E. estradiol	35 (11)	Norethindrone	1 (11)	
Ortho-Novum 10/11					
Ortho-Novum 7/7/7	E. estradiol	35 (7)	Norethindrone	0.5 (7)	14.5
	E. estradiol	35 (7)	Norethindrone	0.75 (7)	
	E. estradiol	35 (7)	Norethindrone	1 (7)	
Ortho Tri-Cyclen	E. estradiol	35 (7)	Norgestimate	0.18 (7)	17.7
	E. estradiol	35 (7)	Norgestimate	0.215 (7)	
	E. estradiol	35 (7)	Norgestimate	0.25 (7)	
Tri-Levlen, Triphasil	E. estradiol	30 (6)	Levonorgestrel	0.05 (6)	15.1
Trivora	E. estradiol	40 (5)	Levonorgestrel	0.075 (5)	
	E. estradiol	30 (10)	Levonorgestrel	0.125 (10)	
Tri-Norinyl	E. estradiol	35 (7)	Norethindrone	0.5 (7)	25.5
Progestin Only					
Micronor/Nor-Q.D.	E. estradiol	—	Norethindrone	0.35	42.3
Ovrette	E. estradiol	—	Norgestrel	0.075	34.9

[a] OK; products approved but not yet available.
[b] 91-day regimen.

TABLE 29-3. Precautions in the Provision of Combined Oral Contraceptives (OCs)

Precautions	Rationale/Discussion
World Health Organization Category #4: Refrain from providing combined oral contraceptives for women with the following diagnoses.	
• Deep vein thrombosis or pulmonary embolism, or a history thereof	• Estrogens promote blood clotting. Thromboembolic events related to known trauma or an intravenous needle are not necessarily a reason to avoid use of pills
• Cerebrovascular accident (stroke), coronary artery or ischemic heart disease, or a history thereof	• Estrogens promote blood clotting
• Structural heart disease, complicated by pulmonary hypertension, atrial fibrillation, or history of subacute bacterial endocarditis	• Estrogens promote blood clotting
• Diabetes with nephropathy, retinopathy, neuropathy, or other vascular disease; diabetes of more than 20 yr duration	• Estrogens promote blood clotting
• Breast cancer	• Breast cancer is a hormonally sensitive tumor. In theory, the hormones in OCs might cause some masses to grow.
• Pregnancy	• Current data do not show that hormonal contraceptives taken during pregnancy cause any significant risk of birth defects. However, hormonal contraceptives should not be given to pregnant women
• Lactation (<6 wk postpartum)	• There is some theoretical concern that the neonate may be at risk owing to exposure to steroid hormones during the first 6 weeks postpartum. OCs can diminish the volume of breast milk
• Liver problems: benign hepatic adenoma or liver cancer, or a history thereof; active viral hepatitis; severe cirrhosis	• OCs are metabolized by the liver, and their use may adversely affect prognosis of existing disease
• Headaches, including migraine (with aural) with focal neurologic symptoms	• Focal neurologic symptoms such as blurred vision, seeing flashing lights or zigzag lines, or trouble speaking or moving may be an indication of an increased risk of stroke
• Major surgery with prolonged immobilization or any surgery on the legs	• Risk for deep vein thrombosis and pulmonary embolism is increased
• Older than 35 yr and currently a heavy smoker (20 or more cigarettes a day)	• Smoking increases the risk for cardiovascular disease
• Hypertension, 160 + mm Hg/100 + mm Hg or with vascular disease	• Hypertension is an important risk factor for cardiovascular disease
World Health Organization Category #3: Exercise caution if combined oral contraceptives are used or considered in the following situations and carefully monitor for adverse effects.	
• Postpartum <21 days	• There is some theoretical concern regarding the association between OC ≤3 wk postpartum and risk of thrombosis
• Lactation (6 wk to 6 months)	• In the first 6 months postpartum, use of OCs during breastfeeding diminishes the quantity of breast milk and may adversely affect the health of the infant
• Undiagnosed abnormal vaginal/uterine bleeding	• Although OCs are often used to manage heavy bleeding, clinicians should be sure that the cause of the bleeding is known before prescribing OCs
• Older than 35 yr and light smoker (fewer than 20 cigarettes/day)	• Smoking increases the risk for cardiovascular disease. All smokers should be warned of this risk and should be encouraged and advised to stop smoking
• Past history of breast cancer, but no evidence of recurrence for 5 yr	• Breast cancer is a hormonally sensitive tumor
• Use of drugs that affect liver enzymes (rifampicin, rifabutin, griseofulvin); anticonvulsants (phenytoin, carbamazepine, barbiturates, topiramate, and primidone)	• OCs are metabolized by the liver. Drugs that affect liver enzymes could reduce the contraceptive effectiveness of OCs

(Continued)

- Gallbladder disease: medically treated and current biliary tract disease and history of OC-related cholestasis

World Health Organization Category #2: Advantages generally outweigh theoretical or proven disadvantages and generally can be provided without restrictions in these conditions.

- Severe headaches that definitely start after initiation of OCs; migraine headaches without focal neurologic symptoms (without aura)
- Diabetes mellitus: gestational diabetes or diabetes without vascular disease

- Major surgery without prolonged immobilization

- Sickle cell disease or sickle C disease

- Moderate blood pressure (140–159 mm Hg/100–109 mm Hg)
- Undiagnosed breast mass

- Cervical cancer awaiting treatment and cervical intraepithelial neoplasia

- Over 50 yr of age
- Conditions likely to make it very difficult for a woman to take OCs consistently and correctly
- Family history of hyperlipidemia

- Family history of death of a parent or sibling due to myocardial infarction before age 50

World Health Organization Category #1: Do not restrict use of combined oral contraceptives for the following conditions.

- Postpartum ≥21 days
- Postabortion after first or second trimester or immediately after postseptic abortion
- History of gestational diabetes
- Varicose veins
- Mild headaches

- Recent reports show that OCs may be weakly associated with the development of gallbladder disease. There is also concern that OCs may worsen existing gallbladder disease

- Migraine headaches with focal neurologic symptoms clearly starting after initiation of pills may be related to pill use
- Women with diabetes are at increased risk of heart disease and stroke, particularly if the woman smokes. Estrogens and progestins may slightly decrease glucose tolerance, but this is unlikely to happen with low-dose OCs
- With the current low-dose pills, the problems associated with pill use and elective surgery have decreased
- Women with sickle cell disease are predisposed to occlusion of the microvasculature (because of abnormal, inflexible red blood cells). Studies of women with sickle cell disease have shown no significant differences between OC users and non-users with regard to coagulation studies, blood viscosity measurements, or incidence or severity of painful sickle cell crisis
- Monitor blood pressure periodically. Hypertension is an important risk factor for cardiovascular disease
- Some clinicians and clinical protocols suggest that women found to have a breast mass should not be provided combined OCs until cancer of the breast has been ruled out. Other clinicians are comfortable prescribing pills while the cause of the breast mass is being evaluated
- The risk of cervical cancer appears to be increased slightly in OC users. OC users may get Papanicolaou smears more regularly so that early dysplasia is more likely to be recognized. They also tend to have more sexual partners. Pill use may also alter susceptibility to infection with human papilloma virus a known risk factor for cancer of the cervix
- Women over 50 are at increased risk for heart and cerebrovascular disease
- Mental retardation, major psychiatric illness, alcoholism, or other chemical abuse, and/or a history of repeatedly taking OCs or other medications incorrectly, make compliance with OC regimens difficult
- Some types of hyperlipidemia increase a woman's risk for heart disease. Routine screening is not recommended by WHO because of the rarity of the conditions and the high cost of screening
- Myocardial infarction in a mother or sister is especially significant and suggests a need for lipid evaluation

(Continued)

TABLE 29-3. Precautions in the Provision of Combined Oral Contraceptives (OCs)

Precautions	Rationale/Discussion
• Irregular vaginal bleeding patterns, without or with heavy or prolonged bleeding and not anemia	
• Past history of pelvic inflammatory disease (PID)	
• Current or recent history of (within last 3 months) PID	
• Current or recent history of (within last 3 months) sexually transmitted infection (STI)	
• Vaginitis without purulent cervicitis	
• Increased risk of STI (i.e., multiple partners or partner who has multiple partners)	
• Infection with human immunodeficiency virus (HIV), high risk or HIV or acquired immunodeficiency syndrome (AIDS)	
• Benign breast disease.	
• Family history of breast cancer	
• Cervical ectropion	
• Endometrial or ovarian cancer	
• Viral hepatitis carrier	
• Uterine fibroids	
• Past ectopic pregnancy	
• Obesity	
• Thyroid conditions: simple goiter, hyperthyroidism, hypothyroidism	
• Benign or malignant gestational trophoblastic disease	
• Iron deficiency anemia	
• Epilepsy	
• Schistosomiasis (uncomplicated or with fibrosis of the liver)	
• Malaria	
• Current use of antibiotics	
• Nulliparity or parity	
• Severe dysmenorrhea	
• Tuberculosis, including pelvic	
• Endometriosis	
• Benign ovarian tumors	
• Prior pelvic surgery	

Compiled from refs. 4 and 18.

MYOCARDIAL INFARCTION
- MI in OC users usually occurs in those older than 35 years who have additional risk factors for cardiovascular disease (e.g., smoking, diabetes, hypertension, and obesity).
- Healthy, nonsmoking women can use OCs safely without an increased risk of MI. However, those with a history of coronary artery disease and smokers who have other risk factors for MI should not use combined OCs, but should use progestin-only or nonhormonal methods of contraception.

CANCER
- The risk for ovarian and endometrial cancer decreases by 40% to 50% with OC use, and the beneficial effect is believed to persist for at least 15 years after use ceases.
- Evidence supports that former or current use of OCs is not associated with an increased risk of breast cancer in women aged 35 to 64 years.
- The current recommendation is that a positive family history of breast cancer in a mother or sister, or both, or a history of benign breast disease should not be regarded as a contraindication to OC use.

SYSTEMIC LUPUS ERYTHEMATOSUS (SLE)
There appears to be an association between VTE and OC use in women with SLE and antiphospholipid antibodies. Progestin-only contraceptives should be used in women with SLE and in those with a history of vascular disease or antiphospholipid antibodies, and combination OCs should be avoided.

Choice of an Oral Contraceptive
- Progestin-only pills (minipills) tend to be less effective than combination OCs and are associated with unpredictable menstrual bleeding and increased frequency of functional ovarian cysts. Minipills are always begun on the first day of menses, and must be taken at approximately the same time each day to maintain contraceptive efficacy. With minipills, nearly 40% of women continue to ovulate normally.
- Multiphasic pills have a lower total hormone dose per cycle, but they may provide no real advantage.
- A reasonable first choice of an OC is a monophasic pill containing 30 to 35 mcg ethinyl estradiol.
- Products containing 20 mcg ethinyl estradiol may cause less bloating and breast tenderness, and women older than 40 years may prefer them. However, these low-estrogen OCs are associated with more breakthrough bleeding and an increased risk of contraceptive failure if doses are missed.
- All combination OCs may improve acne symptoms. Norgestimate-containing OCs also have been shown to improve acne symptoms, and Ortho Tri-Cyclen and Estrostep are approved by the FDA for this indication.
- Many symptoms occurring in the first cycle of OC use (e.g., breakthrough bleeding and symptoms of estrogen excess), improve by the second or third cycle of use. So, use should be reevaluated during the first 3 to 6 months of therapy to assess for side effects.
- Table 29–4 shows symptoms of a serious or potentially serious nature associated with OCs.
- Clinically significant differences between the low-dose OCs are difficult to distinguish.
- Women who continue to experience nausea after 3 months of OC use may benefit from a change to a pill with lower estrogenic activity. Taking the OC with food or at bedtime may also help.

Gynecologic and Obstetric Disorders

TABLE 29–4. Symptoms of a Serious or Potentially Serious Nature Associated With Oral Contraceptives (OCs)

Symptom	Possible Cause
Serious: OCs Should Be Stopped Immediately	
Loss of vision, proptosis, diplopia, papilledema	Retinal artery thrombosis
Unilateral numbness, weakness, or tingling	Hemorrhagic or thrombotic stroke
Severe pains in chest, left arm, or neck	Myocardial infarction
Hemoptysis	Pulmonary embolism
Severe pains, tenderness or swelling, warmth, or palpable cord in legs	Thrombophlebitis
Slurring of speech	Hemorrhagic or thrombotic stroke
Hepatic mass or tenderness	Liver neoplasm
Potentially Serious: OCs May Be Continued With Caution While Patient Is Being Evaluated	
Absence of menses	Pregnancy
Spotting or breakthrough bleeding	Cervical, endometrial, or vaginal cancer
Breast mass, pain, or swelling	Breast cancer
Right upper-quadrant pain	Cholecystitis, cholelithiasis, or liver neoplasm
Midepigastric pain	Thrombosis of abdominal artery or vein, myocardial infarction, or pulmonary embolism
Migraine (vascular or throbbing) headache	Vascular spasm which may precede thrombosis
Severe nonvascular headache	Hypertension, vascular spasm
Galactorrhea	Pituitary adenoma
Jaundice, pruritus	Cholestatic jaundice
Depression	Vitamin B_6 deficiency
Uterine size increase	Leiomyomata, adenomyosis, pregnancy

Drug Interactions

- Table 29–5 shows drug-drug interaction of OCs. Women should be told to use an alternative method of contraception if there is a possibility of a drug interaction compromising OC efficacy.
- Rifampin reduces the efficacy of OCs.
- Case reports have shown a reduction in ethinyl estradiol levels when taken with tetracyclines and penicillin derivatives.
- Phenobarbital, carbamazepine, and phenytoin reduce efficacy of OCs, and many anticonvulsants are known teratogens. The use of condoms in conjunction with high-estrogen OCs, injectable progestin-only contraceptives, or intrauterine devices may be considered for women taking these drugs.

Discontinuation of the Oral Contraceptive, Return of Fertility, and Breast-Feeding

- In several large cohort and case-controlled studies, infants conceived in the first month after an OC was discontinued had no greater chance of miscarriage or a birth defect than those born in the general population.
- Progestin-only formulations can be started immediately after delivery.
- Breast-feeding has generally been regarded as a relative contraindication to OC use, but this restriction may no longer be necessary with the newer formulations.
- Some clinicians recommend progestin-only contraceptives for breast-feeding women because progestins do not diminish the amount of breast milk. A recent Cochrane review concluded that existing randomized, controlled trials are insufficient to establish an effect of hormonal contraception, if any, on milk quality and quantity. That review further stated that current recommendations for breast-feeding women are to avoid combined OCs in the first 6 weeks postpartum and to use them with caution in the first 6 months postpartum.

TABLE 29–5. Interactions of Oral Contraceptives (OCs) With Other Drugs

Interacting Drugs	Adverse Effects (Probable Mechanism)	Comments and Recommendation
Acetaminophen (Tylenol and others)	Possible decreased pain-relieving effect (increased metabolism)	Monitor pain-relieving response
Alcohol	Possible increased effect of alcohol	Use with caution
Ampicillin	Decreased contraceptive effect	Low but unpredictable incidence; use backup method of contraception
Anticoagulants (oral)	Decreased anticoagulant effect	Use with caution, monitor INR
Anticonvulsants (barbiturates, including phenobarbital and primidone; carbamazepine; felbamate; phenytoin; topiramate; vigabatrin)	Possible decreased contraceptive effect	Avoid simultaneous use; use alternative contraceptive (DMPA) for patients with seizure disorder
Antidepressants (Elavil, Norpramin, Tofranil, and others)	Possible increased antidepressant pharmacologic effect	Monitor for adverse effects
Benzodiazepine tranquilizers (Ativan, Librium, Serax, Tranxene, Valium, Xanax, and others)	Possible increased or decreased tranquilizer effects including psychomotor impairment	Use with caution; greatest impairment during drug-free week in oral contraceptive dosage
β-Blockers (Corgard, Inderal, Lopressor, Tenormin)	Possible increased β-blocker pharmacologic effect	Monitor cardiovascular status
Corticosteroids (cortisone)	Possible increased corticosteroid toxicity	Clinical significance not established
Griseofulvin (Fulvicin, Grifulvin V, and others)	Decreased contraceptive effect	Use backup method of contraception
Hypoglycemics (Tolbutamide, Diabinese, Orinase, Tolinase)	Possible decreased hypoglycemic effect	Monitor blood glucose
Methyldopa (Aldoclor, Aldomet, and others)	Possible decreased antihypertensive effect, especially with high-dose OCs	Monitor blood pressure
Non-nucleoside reverse transcriptase inhibitors (Sustiva, Viramune)	Decreased contraceptive effect (Viramune), possible decreased contraceptive effect (Sustiva)	Use alternative method of contraception
Phenytoin (Dilantin)	Decreased contraceptive effect, possible increased phenytoin effect	Use alternative contraceptive (DMPA); monitor phenytoin concentration
Pioglitazone (Actos)	Decreased contraceptive effect documented with previous thiazolidinedione, troglitazone (Rezulin); no documented interaction with rosiglitazone (Avandia); interaction with pioglitazone (Actos) not studied	Use alternative method of contraception

VI

(Continued)

TABLE 29–5. (Continued)

Interacting Drugs	Adverse Effects (Probable Mechanism)	Comments and Recommendation
Protease inhibitors (Agenerase, Crixivan, Norvir, Viracept)	Decreased contraceptive effect (Agenerase, Norvir, Viracept), possible decreased contraceptive effect (Crixivan)	Use alternative method of contraception
Rifampin	Decreased contraceptive effect	Use backup method of contraception; use alternate method if planned concomitant use is long term
Sulfonamides	Decreased contraceptive effect	Use backup method of contraception
Tetracycline	Decreased contraceptive effect	Use backup method of contraception
Theophylline (Bronkotabs, Marax, Primatene, Quibron, Tedral, TheoDur, and others)	Decreased contraceptive effect, increased theophylline effect	Monitor theophylline concentration
Troleandomycin (TAO)	Jaundice (additive)	Avoid simultaneous use
Vitamin C	Increased serum concentration and possible increased adverse effects of estrogens with 1 g or more per day of vitamin C	Avoid high dose of vitamin C

INR, International Normalized Ratio; DMPA, depomedroxyprogesterone acetate.

Emergency Contraception (EC)
- The FDA has approved two hormonal contraceptives (Preven and Plan B) for EC. Some states allow pharmacists to dispense EC without a physician's prescription.
- Preven Emergency Contraceptive Kit contains 4 tablets (2 tablets/dose), each tablet with 50 mcg ethinyl estradiol and 0.25 mg levonorgestrel (similar to 4 tablets of Ovral), also known as the Yuzpe regimen. It also contains a urine pregnancy test to determine if the woman is already pregnant.
- Plan B contains two tablets, each containing 0.75 mg levonorgestrel (similar to two 10-tablet doses of Ovrette).
- The first dose of each regimen is to be taken within 72 hours of unprotected intercourse (the sooner, the more effective); the second dose is taken 12 hours later.
- The FDA has also approved the following regimens for EC (first dose within 72 hours of unprotected intercourse and a follow-up dose 12 hours later):
  - Ovral (2 tablets/dose)
  - Nordette, Levlen, Levora, Lo/Ovral, Triphasil, Tri-Levlen, or Trivora (4 tablets/dose)
  - Alesse or Levlite (5 tablets/dose)
- In addition, progestin-only pills can be used as EC (Ovrette (20 tablets/dose). Again, the first dose should be taken within 72 hours of unprotected intercourse and a follow-up dose 12 hours later.

VI

Transdermal Contraceptives
- A combination contraceptive is available as a transdermal patch (Ortho Evra), which may have improved adherence compared to an OC. Efficacy may be compromised as body weight increases. The patch should be applied to the abdomen, buttocks, upper torso, or upper outer arm at the beginning of the menstrual cycle and replaced every week for 3 weeks.

Contraceptive Rings
- The first vaginal ring (NuvaRing) is available. It releases approximately 15 mcg/day of ethinyl estradiol and 120 mcg/day of etonogestrel over a 3-week period. On first use, the ring should be inserted on or prior to the fifth day of the cycle, remain in place for 3 weeks, then be removed. One week should lapse before the new ring is inserted on the same day of the week as insertipon during the last cycle. A second form of contraception should be used for the first 7 days of ring use or if the ring has been expelled for more than 3 hours.

Long-Acting Injectable and Implantable Contraceptives
- Sustained progestins block the LH surge to prevent ovulation. They also reduce ovum motility in the fallopian tubes and thin the endometrium, reducing the chance of implantation.
- Women who particularly benefit from progestin-only methods, including minipills, are those who are breast-feeding, those who are intolerant to estrogens, those taking medications for medical conditions in which estrogen is not preferred, and those who smoke and are older than 35 years of age.
- Pregnancy failure rates with long-acting progestin contraception are comparable to that of female sterilization.

INJECTABLE PROGESTINS
- Depomedroxyprogesterone acetate 150 mg administered by deep intramuscular injection in the gluteal or deltoid muscle within 5 days of the onset of menstrual bleeding inhibits ovulation for more than 3 months, and the dose should be repeated every 12 weeks to ensure continuous contraception. The manufacturer recommends excluding pregnancy in women more than 1 week late for repeat injection.
- Depomedroxyprogesterone acetate can be used in women who are lactating, and it may increase the length of time that a woman can breast-feed.
- Women using medroxyprogesterone acetate have a lower incidence of *Candida* vulvovaginitis, ectopic pregnancy, pelvic inflammatory disease, and endometrial and ovarian cancer. The median time to conception from the first omitted dose is 10 months.
- The most frequent adverse effect of depomedroxyprogesterone is menstrual irregularities, which decrease after the first year. After two years, 68% of women report amenorrhea. Women can also lose bone density, the clinical significance of which is unknown. Breast tenderness, weight gain, and depression occur less frequently. A decrease in glucose tolerance has been observed in some patients. Overall, the risk of breast cancer in women who have used depomedroxyprogesterone acetate is not increased. However, one study found a slightly increased risk in the first 4 years of use, but not with a longer duration of use. Another study reported a possible increased risk in women initiating use at an early age.

INJECTABLE ESTROGEN/PROGESTINS
- Lunelle is a once-a-month injectable contraceptive agent containing 5 mg estradiol cypionate and 25 mg medroxyprogesterone acetate. The addition of

estrogen promotes regular bleeding patterns. It is given every 23 to 32 days, and efficacy is similar to that of other injectable or implantable contraceptives. Body weight does not appear to affect its efficacy. Fertility returns as early as 1 month after discontinuation.

SUBDERMAL PROGESTIN IMPLANTS

- Norplant is a set of six implantable , nonbiodegradable, soft silicone rubber capsules, each filled with 36 mg of crystalline levonorgestrel. They are inserted under the skin to provide continuous contraception for up to 5 years. Replacement after 3 years in heavier women helps to ensure effectiveness. Removal can be difficult because of poor insertion technique, broken capsules, or presence of fibrous tissue. Regular cyclic bleeding in a woman with Norplant implants signals the return of ovulation. Most women return to baseline ovulation patterns within one month after removal of the system.
- Norplant II or Jadelle, is a two-rod 150-mg levonorgestrel implantable system (unavailable in the United States) that provides 3 years of contraception and may be easier to insert and remove.
- Implanon (also unavailable in the United States) is a single rod implantable system containing 68 mg 3-keto-desogestrel that lasts for 3 years.

INTRAUTERINE DEVICES

- Intrauterine devices (IUDs) cause low-grade intrauterine inflammation and increased prostaglandin formation, thus having a spermicidal effect. They also interfere with implantation of the fertilized ovum.
- The risk of pelvic inflammatory disease among users ranges from 1% to 2.5%; the risk is highest during the first 2 days after the insertion procedure.
- The three IUDs available in the United States are shaped like a T and are medicated:
  - ParaGard (copper)—can be left in place for 10 years.
  - Progestasert (progesterone)—must be replaced annually.
  - Mirena (levonorgestrel)—releases drug over 5 years.

▶ EVALUATION OF THERAPEUTIC OUTCOMES

- All OC users should have at least annual blood pressure monitoring.
- Glucose levels should be monitored closely when OCs are started or stopped in patients with a history of glucose intolerance or diabetes mellitus.
- OC users should have annual cytologic screening, and they should also be regularly evaluated for problems that may relate to the OC.
- Women using Norplant should be regularly monitored for menstrual cycle disturbances, weight gain, local inflammation or infection at the implant site, acne, breast tenderness, headaches, and hair loss.
- Women using medroxyprogesterone acetate should be evaluated every 3-months for weight gain, menstrual cycle disturbances, and STD risks.
- Patients on depomedroxyprogesterone acetate also should be weighed, have their blood pressure monitored, and have a physical exam, and Papanicolaou smear annually, as well as mammogram as indicated based on the patient's age.

See Chapter 77, Contraception, authored by Lori M. Dickerson and Kathryn K. Bucci, for a more detailed discussion of this topic.

Chapter 30

▶ HORMONE THERAPY IN WOMEN

▶ DEFINITIONS AND INTRODUCTION

- Menopause is the permanent cessation of menses following the loss of ovarian follicular activity.
- Perimenopause is the transitional period prior to and the first year after menopause, which lasts a total of approximately 5 years.
- Approved indications of postmenopausal hormone therapy include the usually short-term treatment of menopausal symptoms (i.e., hot flushes, night sweats, and urogenital atrophy) and long-term treatment for osteoporosis prevention.

▶ PHYSIOLOGY

- The hypothalamic-pituitary-ovarian axis controls reproductive physiology through the reproductive years. Follicle-stimulating hormone (FSH) and luteinizing hormone (LH), produced by the pituitary in response to gonadotropin-releasing hormone (GnRH) from the hypothalamus, regulate ovarian function. Gonadotropins are also influenced by negative feedback from the sex steroids estradiol (produced by the dominant follicle) and progesterone (produced by the corpus luteum). Other sex steroids are androgens, primarily testosterone and androstenedione, secreted by the ovarian stroma and the adrenal gland.
- Pathophysiologic changes associated with menopause are caused by loss of ovarian follicular activity. The postmenopausal ovary is no longer the primary site of estradiol or progesterone synthesis.
- As women age, circulating FSH progressively rises and ovarian inhibin declines. Menopause is characterized by a 10- to 15-fold increase in circulating FSH compared with follicular phase concentrations, a four- to fivefold increase in LH, and 90% decrease in estradiol.

▶ CLINICAL PRESENTATION

- Vasomotor symptoms (e.g., hot flashes and night sweats) are common short-term symptoms of estrogen withdrawal, which usually disappear within 1 to 2 years but sometimes persist for 20 years.
- Vaginal dryness is also directly related to estrogen insufficiency.
- Other symptoms, including mood swings, depression, insomnia, migraine, formication, arthralgia, myalgia, and urinary frequency, are attributed to menopause, but the relationship between these symptoms and estrogen deficiency is controversial.
- Long-term morbidity associated with menopause includes accelerated bone loss, osteoporosis, and cardiovascular disease. Osteoporosis is covered in Chapter 3.

▶ DIAGNOSIS

- Menopause is determined retrospectively after 12 consecutive months of amenorrhea.
- The diagnosis of menopause should include a comprehensive medical history and physical examination, complete blood count, and measurement of serum

FSH. When ovarian function has ceased, serum FSH concentrations exceed 40 mIU/mL. Altered thyroid function and pregnancy must be excluded.

▶ TREATMENT

NONPHARMACOLOGIC TREATMENT

- Mild menopausal symptoms can often be alleviated by lifestyle modification, weight control, smoking cessation, exercise, and a healthy diet.
- Mild vaginal dryness can sometimes be relieved by nonestrogenic vaginal creams, but significant vaginal dryness often requires local or systemic estrogen therapy.
- Current data suggest that **phytoestrogens** are no more effective than placebo for hot flushes or other symptoms of menopause.
- Phytoestrogens decrease low-density lipoprotein (LDL) and triglyceride concentrations, do not change high-density lipoprotein (HDL) concentrations, and may improve bone density. Adverse effects include constipation, bloating, and nausea.
- The three main classes of phytoestrogens (and common food sources) are **isoflavones** (soybeans), **lignans** (cereals and oilseeds such as flaxseed), and **coumestans** (alfalfa sprouts). The biologic potency of phytoestrogens varies and is less than that of synthetic estrogen.
- **Black cohosh** has been shown to be effective for vasomotor symptoms in some randomized controlled trials, but it does not appear to have strong intrinsic estrogenic properties and may act through the serotonergic system.

HORMONAL REGIMENS

- In women with intact uterus, hormone therapy consists of an estrogen plus a progestogen. In women who have undergone hysterectomy, estrogen therapy is given unopposed by a progestogen.
- The **continuous combined oral estrogen-progestogen** arm of the Women's Health Initiative (WHI) study was terminated prematurely after a mean of 5.2-year follow-up because of the occurrence of a prespecified level of invasive breast cancer. The study also found increased coronary disease events, stroke, and pulmonary embolism. Beneficial effects included decreases in hip fracture and colorectal cancer.
- The **oral estrogen-alone** arm was stopped early after a mean of 7 years of follow-up. Estrogen-only therapy had no effect on coronary heart disease risk and caused no increase in breast cancer risk.
- A subsequent large epidemiologic study found a greater risk for breast cancer with **combined estrogen-progestogen** use, as well as increased risk for **estrogen-only** therapy and tibolone.

ESTROGENS

- Preparations suitable for replacement therapy are shown in Table 30–1. The oral and transdermal routes are used most frequently. There is no evidence that one **strogen** compound is more effective than another in relieving menopausal symptoms or preventing osteoporosis.
- **Conjugated equine estrogens** is composed of **estrone sulfate** (50% to 60%) and other estrogens such as **equilin** and **17α-dihydroequilin**.

VI

TABLE 30–1. Systemic Estrogen Products[a,b]

Estrogen	Dosage Strength	Comments
Oral estrogens		
Conjugated equine estrogens	0.3, 0.45, 0.625, 0.9, 1.25 mg	Orally administered estrogens stimulate the synthesis of hepatic proteins and increase the circulating concentrations of sex hormone-binding globulin, which, in turn, may compromise the bioavailability of androgens and estrogens.
Synthetic conjugated estrogens	0.3, 0.45, 0.625, 0.9, 1.25 mg	
Esterified estrogens	0.3, 0.625, 1.25, 2.5 mg	
Estropipate (piperazine estrone sulfate)	0.625, 1.5, 2.5 mg	
Micronized estradiol	0.5, 1, 1.5, 2 mg	
Parenteral estrogens		
Transdermal 17β-estradiol (patch)	14, 25, 37.5, 50, 75, 100 mcg per 24 h	Women with elevated triglyceride concentrations or significant liver function abnormalities may benefit from parenteral therapy
Estradiol vaginal ring	0.05, 0.1 mg/24 h (replaced every 3 months)	
Estradiol topical emulsion	4.35 mg of estradiol hemihydrate	
Estradiol topical gel	0.75 mg of estradiol	
Intranasal estradiol[c]	One spray per nostril delivers 150 mcg	

[a]Systemic oral and transdermal estrogen and progestogen combination products are available in the United States.
[b]Systemic oral estrogen and androgen combination products are available in the United States.
[c]Not available in the United States.

- **Estradiol** is the predominant and most active form of endogenous estrogens. Given orally, it is metabolized, and only 10% reaches the circulation as free estradiol, and estrone concentrations are 3 to 6 times those of estradiol.
- **Ethinyl estradiol** is a semisynthetic estrogen that has similar activity following administration by the oral and parenteral routes.
- **Parenteral estrogens**, including transdermal, intranasal, and vaginal, avoid first-pass metabolism and result in a more physiologic estradiol-to-estrone ratio, i.e., estradiol concentrations greater than estrone concentrations. These routes also are less likely to affect sex hormone-binding globulin, circulating lipids, coagulation parameters, or C-reactive protein levels.
- Variability in absorption is common with the **percutaneous preparations** (gels, creams, and emulsions).
- **Estradiol pellets** (implants) contain pure **crystalline 17 β-estradiol** and are placed subcutaneously into the anterior abdominal wall or buttock. They are difficult to remove.
- **Intranasal 17 β-estradiol** spray is given once or twice daily, and is clinically equivalent to oral or transdermal estradiol, but causes less mastalgia.
- **Vaginal creams, tablets, and rings** are used for treatment of urogenital atrophy. Systemic estrogen absorption is lower with the vaginal tablets and rings, compared to the vaginal creams.

TABLE 30–2. Estrogen for the Treatment of Menopausal Symptoms and Osteoporosis Prevention

Regimen	Standard Dose	Low Dose	Route	Frequency
Conjugated equine estrogens	0.625 mg	0.3 or 0.45 mg	Oral	Once daily
Synthetic conjugated estrogens	0.625 mg	0.3 mg	Oral	Once daily
Esterified estrogens	0.625 mg	0.3 mg	Oral	Once daily
Estropipate (piperazine estrone sulfate)	1.5 mg	0.625 mg	Oral	Once daily
Ethinyl estradiol	5 mcg	2.5 mcg	Oral	Once daily
Micronized 17β-estradiol	1–2 mg	0.25–0.5 mg	Oral	Once daily
Transdermal 17β-estradiol	50 mcg	25 mcg	Transdermal (patch)	Once or twice weekly
Intranasal 17β-estradiol[a]	150 mcg, per nostril	—	Intranasally	Once daily
Implanted 17β-estradiol	50-100 mg pellets	25-mg pellets	Pellets implanted subcutaneously	Every 6 months
Percutaneous 17β-estradiol	0.04 mg (gel) 0.05 mg (emulsion)		Transdermal (emulsion, gel)	Once daily

[a]Not available in the United States.

- New evidence indicates that lower doses of estrogens are effective in controlling postmenopausal symptoms and reducing bone loss (see Table 30–2). Even ultralow doses of 17β-estradiol delivered by vaginal ring improved serum lipid profiles and prevented bone loss in elderly women.
- Adverse effects of **estrogen** include nausea, headache, breast tenderness, and heavy bleeding. More serious adverse effects include increased risk for coronary heart disease, stroke, venous thromboembolism, breast cancer, and gallbladder disease. Transdermal estrogen is less likely than oral estrogen to cause nausea, headache, breast tenderness, and deep vein thrombosis.

PROGESTOGENS

- In women who have not undergone hysterectomy, **progestin** should be added because estrogen monotherapy is associated with endometrial hyperplasia and cancer.
- The most commonly used oral progestogens are **medroxyprogesterone acetate, micronized progesterone, and norethisterone acetate.**
- Several progestogen regimens to prevent endometrial hyperplasia are shown in Table 30–3.
- Four **combination estrogen and progestogen** regimens are currently in use. (Table 30–4).
  - Continuous-cyclic (sequential)—results in scheduled vaginal bleeding in 90% of women.
  - Continuous-combined—prevents monthly bleeding. It may initially cause unpredictable spotting or bleeding; thus, it is best reserved for women who are at least 2 years postmenopause.
  - Continuous long-cycle (cyclic withdrawal)—reduces monthly bleeding. Estrogen is given daily, and progestogen is given 6 times yearly (every other month) for 12 to 14 days, resulting in 6 periods/year.

TABLE 30–3. Progestogen Doses for Endometrial Protection (Oral Cyclic Administration)

Progestogen	Dose
Dydrogesterone[a]	10–20 mg for 12 to 14 days per calender month
Medroxyprogesterone acetate	5–10 mg for 12 to 14 days per calender month
Micronized progesterone	200 mg for 12 to 14 days per calender month
Norethisterone[a]	0.7–1 mg for 12 to 14 days per calender month
Norethindrone acetate	5 mg for 12 to 14 days per calender month
Norgestrel	0.15 mg for 12 to 14 days per calender month
Levonorgestrel[a]	150 mcg for 12 to 14 days per calender month

[a]Not available in the United States in a progestogen-only oral dosage form.

- Intermittent-combined (continuous-pulsed)—prevents monthly bleeding. It consists of 3 days of estrogen therapy alone, followed by 3 days of combined estrogen and progestogen, which is then repeated without interruption. It may cause fewer side effects than regimens with higher progestogen doses.

- Adverse effects of progestogens are irritability, depression, headache, mood swings, fluid retention, and sleep disturbance.

- Low-dose hormone therapy (**conjugated equine estrogen 0.45 mg and medroxyprogesterone acetate 1.5 mg/day**) has demonstrated equivalent symptom relief and bone density preservation without an increase in endometrial hyperplasia. Whether such lower doses will be safer (cause less venous thromboembolism and breast cancer) remains to be seen.

TABLE 30–4. Common Combination Postmenopausal Hormone Therapy Regimens

Regimen	Doses
Oral Continuous-Cyclic Regimens	
CEE + MPA[a]	0.625 mg + 5 mg; 0.625 mg + 10 mg
Oral Continuous-Combined Regimens	
CEE + MPA	0.625 mg + 2.5 mg; 0.625 mg + 5 mg; 0.45 mg + 2.5 mg; 0.3 mg + 1.5 mg/day
17β-Estradiol + NETA	1 mg + 0.1 mg; 1 mg + 0.25 mg; 1 mg + 0.5 mg/day
Ethinyl estradiol + NETA	1 mcg + 0.2 mg; 2.5 mcg + 0.5 mg; 5 mcg + 1 mg; 10 mcg + 1.0 mg/day
Transdermal Continuous-Cyclic Regimens	
17β-Estradiol + NETA[a]	50 mcg + 0.14 mg; 50 mcg + 0.25 mg
Transdermal Continuous-Combined Regimens	
17β-Estradiol + NETA	50 mcg + 0.14 mg; 50 mcg + 0.25 mg; 25 mcg + 0.125 mg

[a]Estrogen alone for days 1–14, followed by estrogen-progestogen on days 15–28. CEE, conjugated equine estrogens; MPA, medroxyprogesterone acetate; NETA, norethindrone acetate.

TABLE 30–5. Androgen Regimens Used for Women

Regimen	Dose	Frequency	Route
Methyltestosterone in combination with esterfied estrogen	1.25–2.5 mg	Daily	Oral
Mixed testosterone esters	50–100 mg	Every 4 to 6 wk	Intramuscular
Testosterone pellets	50 mg	Every 6 months	Subcutaneous (implanted)
Transdermal testosterone system[a]	150–300 mcg/day	Every 3 to 4 days	Transdermal patch
Nandrolone decanoate	50 mg	Every 8 to 12 wk	Intramuscular

[a]Undergoing clinical trials in the United States.

VI ANDROGENS

- The therapeutic use of **testosterone** in women, although controversial, is becoming more widespread. There is evidence that androgen therapy, usually testosterone, is effective in alleviating some symptoms of androgen insufficiency including loss of sexual desire, diminished well-being, loss of energy, decreased bone mass, and reduced muscle strength.
- Androgen regimens now available are shown in Table 30–5.
- Testosterone treatment should not be given to postmenopausal women who are not receiving concurrent **estrogen**.
- Testosterone is generally accepted for women who have had surgical menopause, but may also be considered for naturally menopausal women and those with premature ovarian failure.
- Estrogen combined with androgen improves sexual activity and satisfaction and increases bone density sooner and to a greater degree than does estrogen monotherapy.
- **Testosterone** appears safe when given in doses that achieve circulating serum free testosterone concentrations within the physiologic range for young reproductive women. There are no data on the effects of exogenous androgen therapy on the incidence of breast cancer.
- Relative contraindications to testosterone therapy are moderate to severe acne, clinical hirsutism, and androgenic alopecia. Absolute contraindications to androgen replacement include pregnancy or lactation and known or suspected androgen-dependent neoplasia.
- Adverse effects from excessive dosage include virilization, fluid retention, and adverse lipoprotein lipid effects, which are more likely with oral administration.

SELECTIVE ESTROGEN-RECEPTOR MODULATORS (SERMS)

- SERMS prevent bone loss and spinal fractures. Serms bind to estrogen receptors and function as tissue-specific estrogen antagonists or agonists.
- **Tamoxifen** is discussed in Chapter 59, "Breast Cancer"; **raloxifene** is discussed in Chapter 3, "Osteoporosis."

TIBOLONE

- **Tibolone** has combined estrogenic, progestogenic, and androgenic activity. Its effects depend on metabolism and activation in peripheral tissues. Tibolone has beneficial effects on mood and libido and improves menopausal symptoms and vaginal atrophy. It protects against bone loss, and causes endometrial atrophy, thus it usually does not cause withdrawal bleeding in women who have had amenorrhea for at least 1 year. It is associated with a low rate of bleeding, about 4% after 6 months of treatment. It reduces total cholesterol, triglyceride, lipoprotein (a), and, unfortunately, HDL concentrations. It may increase cardiovascular and breast cancer risk.

- Major adverse effects include weight gain and bloating.

TREATMENT CONSIDERATIONS

- **Hormone therapy** is contraindicated in women with endometrial or breast cancer, undiagnosed vaginal bleeding, thromboembolism (including presence of thrombophilia), or active liver disease. Relative contraindications include uterine leiomyoma, migraine headaches, and seizure disorder. Oral **estrogen** should also be avoided in women with hypertriglyceridemia, liver disease, and gallbladder disease. For these women, transdermal administration is safer.
- Before initiating hormone therapy, Papanicolaou cervical cytologic examination and screening mammography negative for malignancy are required. VI

BENEFITS OF HRT

Relief of Menopausal Symptoms

- Most women with vasomotor symptoms need hormone treatment for less than 5 years. Without treatment, hot flushes usually disappear within 1 to 2 years. Hormone therapy can usually be tapered and stopped after about 2 or 3 years.
- **Estrogen** is more effective than any other therapy in relieving vasomotor symptoms, and all types and routes of systemic administration are equally effective in a dose-dependent fashion.
- Alternatives to estrogen for hot flushes are shown in Table 30–6. Selective serotonin reuptake inhibitors and venlafaxine are considered by some to be a first-line therapy for hot flushes when hormone therapy is contraindicated. Progesterone alone may be an option in women with a history of breast cancer or venous thrombosis, but side effects limit their use. Data supporting use of these agents are limited and equivocal.
- Significant vaginal dryness because of vaginal atrophy requires use of local or systemic estrogen therapy. It can be treated with topical estrogen cream, tablet, or vaginal ring. Creams may be more effective.

TABLE 30–6. Alternatives to Estrogen for Treatment of Hot Flushes

Drug	Dose (Oral)	Interval	Comments
Tibolone	2.5–5 mg	Once daily	Tibolone is not recommended during the perimenopause because it may cause irregular bleeding
Venlafaxine	37.5–150 mg	Once daily	Side effects include dry mouth, decreased appetite, nausea, and constipation
Paroxetine	12.5–25 mg	Once daily	12.5 mg is an adequate and well-tolerated starting dose for most women; adverse effects include headache, nausea, and insomnia
Fluoxetine	20 mg	Once daily	Modest improvement seen in hot flushes
Megestrol acetate	20–40 mg	Once daily	Progesterone may be linked to breast cancer etiology; also, there is concern regarding the safety of progestational agents in women with preexisting breast cancer
Clonidine	0.1 mg	Once daily	Can be administered orally or transdermally; drowsiness and dry mouth can occur, especially with higher doses
Gabapentin	900 mg	Divided in three daily doses	Adverse effects include somnolence and dizziness; these symptoms often can be obviated with a gradual increase in dosing

- Concomitant progestogen therapy generally is unnecessary with **low-dose micronized 17 β-estradiol**, but regular use of **conjugated equine estrogen creams** and other products that may promote endometrial proliferation in women with an intact uterus requires intermittent progestogen challenges (i.e., for 10 days every 12 weeks).
- The benefits of hormonal therapies for osteoporosis prevention are discussed in Chapter 3. Although prevention of postmenopsusal osteoporosis is an indication for hormone therapy, consideration should be given to approved nonestrogen products, such as **raloxifene** and **bisphosphonates**.
- The Womens Health Initiative (WHI) was the first randomized, controlled trial to confirm that hormone therapy reduces colon cancer risk.

VI ▶ RISKS OF HORMONE THERAPY

- The American Heart Association recommends against postmenopausal hormone therapy for reducing the risk of coronary heart disease.
- The WHI trial showed an overall increase in the risk of coronary heart disease (most apparent at 1 year) in healthy postmenopausal women aged 50 to 79 years taking **estrogen-progestogen therapy** compared with those taking placebo. The estrogen-alone arm of the WHI showed no effect (either increase or decrease) in the risk of coronary heart disease. The increased risk for ischemic stroke and venous thromboembollism continued throughout the 5 years of therapy. In the estrogen-alone arm, there was a similar increase in risk for stroke.
- In women at high risk for coronary heart disease, those receiving **raloxifene** has a statistically significant reduction in risk of cardiovascular events, but these findings must be confirmed in a randomized controlled trial.
- In the WHI study, **estrogen plus progestogen therapy** had an increased risk for invasive breast cancer. The estrogen-only arm of the WHI showed no increased risk for breast cancer during the 7-year follow-up.
- The Million Women Study reported that current use of hormone therapy increased breast cancer risk and breast cancer mortality. Increased incidence was observed for **estrogen only**, **estrogen plus progestin**, and for **tibolone**.
- In a reanalysis of 51 studies, less than 5 years of therapy with **combined estrogen and progestogen** was associated with a 15% increase in risk for breast cancer, and the risk increased with greater duration of treatment. Five years after discontinuation of hormone replacement therapy, the risk of breast cancer was no longer increased.
- Addition of progestogen to estrogen may increase breast cancer risk beyond that observed with estrogen alone.
- **Raloxifene** treatment of osteoporosis was associated with a 76% risk reduction for estrogen-receptor positive breast cancer.
- **Estrogen alone** given to women with an intact uterus increases uterine cancer risk. This increased risk begins within 2 years of treatment and persists for many years after estrogen is discontinued. The sequential addition of **progestin** to estrogen for at least 10 days of the cycle or continuous combined estrogen-progestogen does not increase the risk of endometrial cancer. A 4-year trial of **raloxifene** in women with osteoporosis showed no increased risk of endometrial cancer.
- **Combined hormone therapy** may increase the risk of ovarian cancer, but more study is needed to confirm these findings.
- Women taking hormone therapy have a twofold increase in risk for thromboembolic events, with the highest risk occurring in the first year of use. The increased risk is dose dependent.

- The age-adjusted relative risk for cholecystectomy is 2.2 for women taking **0.625 mg of conjugated equine estrogen**. Risk is increased with duration of therapy. Transdermal estrogen is an alternative to oral therapy for women at high risk for cholelithiasis.

OTHER EFFECTS OF HORMONE THERAPY

- Women with vasomotor symptoms taking hormone therapy have better mental health and less depressive symptoms compared to those taking placebo, but hormone therapy may worsen quality of life in women without vasomotor symptoms.
- The WHI study found that postmenopausal women 65 years or older taking **estrogen plus progestogen** therapy had twice the rate of dementia, including Alzheimer's disease. Combined therapy also did not prevent mild cognitive impairment.

VI

▶ EVALUATION OF THERAPEUTIC OUTCOMES

- After initiating hormone therapy, follow-up at 6 months is advisable to assess for efficacy, side effects, and patterns of withdrawal bleeding.
- With estrogen-based therapy, there should be yearly breast exams and periodic mammograms.
- Women on hormonal therapy should undergo annual monitoring, including pelvic examination, blood pressure checks, and routine endometrial cancer surveillance.
- Women 65 years or younger with risk factors for osteoporosis should have their bone mineral density measured, with repeat testing as indicated.

▶ PREMATURE OVARIAN FAILURE AND PREMENOPAUSAL HORMONE REPLACEMENT

DEFINITION

- Premature ovarian failure (POF) is a condition characterized by sex-steroid deficiency, amenorrhea, and infertility in women younger than 40 years of age.
- POF is associated with a significantly higher risk for osteoporosis and cardiovascular disease and increased mortality.
- The goal of therapy in young women with POF is to provide a hormone-replacement regimen that maintains sex steroid status as effectively as the normal, functioning ovary.
- Young women with primary amenorrhea (i.e., absence of menses in a girl who is 16 years or older) in whom secondary sex characteristics have failed to develop should receive initially very **low doses of estrogen, e.g., 0.3 mg of conjugated equine estrogen** (with no pregestogen) daily for 6 months, with dose increases at 6-month intervals until the required dose is achieved. Toward the end of the second year of treatment, **cyclic progestogen therapy** can be given 12 to 14 days/month.
- Women with secondary amenorrhea (i.e., cessation of menses in a woman who was previously menstruating for 6 months or more) who have been estrogen deficient for 12 months or longer should also receive **low-dose estrogen** initially, but the dose can be increased up to maintenance levels over a 6-month period, and **progestin therapy** can be instituted with the initiation of estrogen therapy.

- An **estrogen** dose equivalent to at least 1.25 mg conjugated equine estrogen (or 100 mcg transdermal estradiol) is needed to achieve adequate replacement in young women, and **progestin** should be given for 12 to 14 days per calendar month to prevent endometrial hyperplasia.
- If these patients miss an expected menses, they should be tested for pregnancy and discontinue hormone therapy.
- Androgen replacement (**testosterone**) should also be considered for women with fatigue, poor well-being, and low libido despite adequate **estrogen** replacement.
- Hormone therapy must be continued at least until the average age of natural menopause, and long-term follow-up is necessary.

See Chapter 80, Hormone Therapy in Women, authored by Sophia N. Kalantari-dou, Susan R. Davis, and Karim Anton Calis, for a more detailed discussion of this topic.

VI

Chapter 31

▶ PREGNANCY AND LACTATION

Therapeutic considerations associated with pregnancy and lactation encompass many complex issues that affect both the mother and her child, beginning with planning for pregnancy and lasting through lactation. A comprehensive review is beyond the scope of the chapter. Additional resources on pregnancy and lactation include computerized databases (e.g., the Canadian database, www.motherisk.org) and textbooks with information from large cohorts of treated women, as well as the primary literature.

▶ NATURAL COURSE OF PREGNANCY

- The duration of pregnancy is approximately 280 days; this time period extends from the first day of the last menstrual period to birth. Pregnancy is divided into three periods of three calendar months; each 3-month period is called a trimester.
- Drug absorption during pregnancy can be affected by a decrease in gastrointestinal motility, an increase in gastric pH, and an increase in pulmonary alveolar drug uptake.
- Drug distribution during pregnancy may change because maternal plasma volume increases by 50%. However, the net impact on drug distribution for many (not all) drugs is an unaltered free-drug serum concentration. Notable exceptions of drugs for which the unbound fraction increases significantly include **salicylic acid**, **sulfisoxazole**, **diazepam**, **valproic acid**, and **phenytoin**.
- Drug elimination during pregnancy is affected in various ways. Maternal hormones enhance the hepatic metabolism for some drugs (e.g., **phenytoin**) and inhibit it for others (e.g., **theophylline**). In addition, the clearance of drugs excreted into the biliary system may be slow. Renal drug clearance may be affected by an increase in renal flood flow and glomerular filtration rate. Fortunately, these changes usually do not result in a clinically significant alteration requiring a change in drug dosing.
- The placenta is the organ of exchange between the mother and fetus for a number of substances, including drugs. It is generally thought that drug exposure during the embryonic period (the fifth through tenth week of gestation) has the greatest potential influence on organ development. Drug exposure at other times during pregnancy may be associated with subtle changes in function or behavior.

▶ DRUG SELECTION DURING PREGNANCY

- The incidence of congenital malformation is approximately 3% to 5%, and it is estimated that 1% of all birth defects are caused by medication exposure.
- Adverse fetal drug effects depend on dosage, route of administration, concomitant exposure to other agents, and stage of pregnancy.
- Medications associated with teratogenic effects in the period of organogenesis (18 to 60 days postconception) include **methotrexate**, **cyclophosphamide**, **diethylstilbesterol**, **lithium**, **retinoids**, **thalidomide**, certain antiepileptic drugs, and **coumarin** derivatives.
- Medications which may cause adverse fetal effects in the second or third trimesters include angiotensin-converting enzyme inhibitors, nonsteroidal antiinflammatory agents, and **tetracycline** derivatives.

- Principles that may be helpful in selecting medications for use during pregnancy include selecting drugs that have been used safely for long periods of time and prescribing drug doses at the lower end of the dosing range. Also, pregnant women should be discouraged from self-medication.

▶ PRECONCEPTION PLANNING

Preconception interventions have been shown to improve pregnancy outcomes.

- Ingestion of **folic acid** (400 mcg/day) by all women of childbearing potential reduces the risk for neural tube defects in offspring.
- Women who have had a child with a neural tube defect or who use certain seizure medications should receive 4000 mcg of folic acid daily beginning 1 to 3 months prior to conception and continuing throughout the first trimester.
- Screening and immunization for rubella and varicella; screening for and treatment of sexually transmitted diseases (STDs); and assessment and reduction in the use of alcohol, tobacco, and other substances prior to pregnancy all improve outcomes.
- Behavioral therapy with or without nicotine replacement therapy may help women quit smoking before and during pregnancy.

▶ PREGNANCY-INFLUENCED ISSUES

GASTROINTESTINAL TRACT
Constipation
- Constipation commonly occurs during pregnancy. Nondrug modalities such as education, physical exercise, biofeedback, and increased intake of dietary fiber and fluid should be instituted first.
- If additional therapy is warranted, the use of supplemental fiber with or without a stool softener is appropriate.
- **Castor oil** and **mineral oil** should be avoided.

Gastroesophageal Reflux Disease
- Therapy includes lifestyle and dietary modifications such as small, frequent meals; caffeine avoidance; food avoidance 3 hours before bedtime; and elevation of the head of the bed.
- Drug therapy, if necessary, may be initiated with **aluminum**, **calcium**, or **magnesium antacids**; **sucralfate**; or **cimetidine** or **ranitidine. Lansoprazole** and **metoclopramide** are also options if the patient does not respond to histamine-2 receptor blockers.
- **Sodium bicarbonate** and **magnesium trisilicate** should be avoided.

Hemorrhoids
- Hemorrhoids during pregnancy are common.
- Therapy includes high intake of dietary fiber, adequate oral fluid intake, use of sitz baths; topical anesthetics, skin protectants and astringents may also be used. Treatment for refractory hemorrhoids includes rubber band ligation, sclerotherapy, and surgery.

Nausea and Vomiting
- Up to 80% of all pregnant women experience some degree of nausea and vomiting. Hyperemesis gravidarum (i.e., severe nausea and vomiting requiring

hospitalization for hydration and nutrition) occurs in only about 0.5% of pregnant women.
- Nonpharmacologic treatments include eating small, frequent meals; avoiding fatty and fibrous foods; acupressure and acustimulation. Pharmacotherapy may include the following: antihistamines (e.g., **doxylamine**), vitamins (e.g., **pyridoxine, cyanocobalamin**), anticholinergics (e.g., **dicyclomine, scopolamine**), dopamine antagonists (e.g., **phenothiazines, metoclopramide**), ondansetron, and **ginger**.

GESTATIONAL DIABETES MELLITUS

- Screening for gestational diabetes mellitus utilizes the oral glucose challenge test.
- First-line therapy includes nutritional and exercise interventions for all women, and caloric restrictions for obese women. If first-line therapy fails to achieve fasting whole blood glucose levels less than or equal to 95 mg/dL and 2-hour postprandial levels less than or equal to 120 mg/dL, then therapy with **recombinant human insulin** should be instituted; **glyburide** may be considered after 11 weeks of gestation.
- Goals for self-monitored blood glucose levels while on insulin therapy are a preprandial plasma glucose level between 80 and 110 mg/dL, and a 2-hour postprandial plasma glucose level less than 155 mg/dL.

HYPERTENSION

- Hypertension during pregnancy includes chronic hypertension, gestational hypertension, preeclampsia-eclampsia, and preeclampsia superimposed on chronic hypertension. Preeclampsia-eclampsia is a syndrome consisting of gestational blood pressure elevation with proteinuria (i.e., greater than or equal to 300 mg in a 24-hour urine collection). Preeclampsia-eclampsia is suspected in the absence of proteinuria if the woman has gestational blood pressure elevation with blurred vision, abdominal pain, headache, thrombocytopenia, or elevated liver enzymes. Eclampsia is preeclampsia with seizures.
- For women at high risk for preeclampsia, **aspirin**, 50 to 150 mg/day, reduced rates of perinatal death and preeclampsia, reduced rates of spontaneous preterm birth and increased mean birth weight. **Calcium** may also benefit these high-risk women.
- Antihypertensive drug therapy for gestational hypertension or preeclampsia has not been shown to improve fetal outcomes. First-line therapy for mild to moderate hypertension in pregnancy is **methyldopa.** Alternatives include **labetolol** and other β blockers (except **atenolol**), **prazosin, nifedipine, isradipine, hydralazine,** and **clonidine.**
- The cure for preeclampsia is delivery of the fetus if the pregnancy is at term. Parenteral **hydralazine** and **labetolol** in addition to **oral nifedipine** for hypertension and **magnesium sulfate** for seizure prevention are standard therapy for acute severe hypertension in preeclampsia.

VENOUS THROMBOEMBOLISM

- Risk factors for venous thromboembolism in pregnancy include increasing age, history of thromboembolism, hypercoaguable conditions, operative vaginal delivery or cesarean section, obesity, and a family history of thrombosis.
- **Low-molecular-weight heparins** are the preferred treatment for prophylaxis or treatment of venous thromboembolism during pregnancy. Unfractionated

heparin may also be used, but is associated with more side effects. **Warfarin** should be avoided after the first 6 weeks of gestation because it may cause fetal bleeding, malformations of the nose, stippled epiphyses, or central nervous system anomalies.

▶ ACUTE CARE ISSUES IN PREGNANCY

HEADACHE

- For tension headaches during pregnancy, nonpharmacologic approaches are first-line therapies, including rest, reassurance, and ice applications.
- For migraine and tension headaches, **acetaminophen** is the drug of first choice for pain.
- Nonsteroidal anti-inflammatory drugs are contraindicated after 37 weeks' gestation. For refractory migraines, narcotics may be used. The use of **Sumatriptan** is controversial. Nausea of migraines may be treated with **metoclopramide**.

URINARY TRACT INFECTION

- The principle infecting organism is *Escherichia coli,* but *Proteus mirabilis* and *Klebsiella pneumoniae* account for some infections. Untreated bacteriuria may result in pyelonephritis, preterm labor, and low birth weight.
- Group B *Streptococcus* bacteriuria should be treated when discovered to reduce the rate of preterm delivery. These women should also receive antibiotics at delivery to prevent infection in the newborn.
- **Ampicillin** or **amoxicillin** are considered safe medications during pregnancy, but resistance to these drugs may occur in up to 20% to 30% of isolates. Alternatives include **nitrofurantoin** and **cephalexin.**
- Sulfa-containing drugs should be avoided during the third trimester; folate antagonists, such as **trimethoprim,** are relatively contraindicated during the first trimester; and fluoroquinolones and **tetracyclines** are contraindicated throughout pregnancy. Courses of treatment of 7 to 10 days are common, and a repeat culture to confirm cure is recommended.

SEXUALLY TRANSMITTED DISEASE

- It is important to distinguish STDs that are bacterial in origin from those that are viral in origin because microbiologic cure is the usual end point of therapy for bacterial infections, whereas control of outbreaks at the time of delivery is the end point for viral infections.

Chlamydia

- The current recommendation for the treatment of *Chlamydia* cervicitis is **erythromycin** base, 500 mg four times daily for 7 days, or **amoxicillin,** 500 mg three times daily for 7 days.
- Other options include **azithromycin** 1 g as a single dose.

Syphilis

- Penicillin is the drug of choice, and it is effective for preventing transmission to the fetus and treating the already infected fetus. No alternatives to penicillin are available for the pregnant woman who is allergic to penicillin.

VI

N. Gonorrhoeae
- N. Gonorrhoeae is a risk factor for preterm delivery.
- The treatment of choice is **ceftriaxone** 125 mg intramuscularly as a single dose. **Spectinomycin** 2 g intramuscularly as a single dose is appropriate as a second choice.

Genital Herpes
- The overriding concern with genital herpes is transmission of the virus to the neonate during birth.
- **Acyclovir** has been used safely, and most women will receive oral acyclovir therapy for first episodes or for recurrence. **Valacyclovir** and **famciclovir** are newer, and safety data are more limited.

Bacterial Vaginosis
- Bacterial vaginosis is a risk factor for premature rupture of membranes, preterm labor, preterm birth, and spontaneous abortion.
- The recommended regimen for treatment is **metronidazole,** 250 mg three times daily for 7 days or **clindamycin,** 300 mg twice daily for 7 days.

VI

▶ CHRONIC ILLNESSES IN PREGNANCY

ALLERGIC RHINITIS, ASTHMA
- Pregnant women with asthma who need anti-inflammatory therapy should be given inhaled **cromolyn**. If the asthma is unresponsive to cromolyn, inhaled **budesonide** or **beclomethasone** is recommended. for women using other inhaled corticosteroids effectively when they become pregnant, continuation of that therapy is reasonable.
- Inhaled β agonists (e.g., **terbutaline**, **metaproterenol**, and **albuterol**) are considered safe in pregnancy. Oral **theophylline** may be added to inhaled corticosteroids for moderate or severe persistent asthma, or **salmeterol** may be used.
- Leukotriene antagonists may be continued if required before pregnancy, but they are not considered drugs of choice in other pregnant patients.
- Oral corticosteroids are essential therapy for severe, acute asthma.
- **Cromolyn** nasal spray is first-line therapy for chronic allergic rhinitis.
- **Chlorpheniramine** and **tripelenamine** are safe in pregnancy, but nonsedating antihistamines, **loratidine** or **cetirizine** can be used if the older drugs are not tolerated.
- **Pseudoephedrine** may be used, but a rare gastrointestinal birth defect has been linked to its use.
- Nasal corticosteroids (e.g., **budesonide** and **beclomethasone**) may be considered for pregnant women unresponsive to other modalities.

DERMATOLOGIC CONDITIONS
- Of all the dermatologic agents commonly used during pregnancy, only topical **nystatin** has been shown to have no fetal risk in controlled studies.
- **Bacitracin, benzoyl peroxide, ciclopirox, clindamycin, erythromycin, metronidazole, mupirocin, permethrin, terbinafine**, and topical corticosteroids are considered to have minimal pregnancy risk.
- Systemic agents that are considered safe in pregnancy include **acyclovir, amoxicillin, azithromhycin, cephalosporins, clorpheniramine, cyproheptadine, dicloxacillin, diphenhydramine, erythromycin** (except estolates), **nystatin**, and **penicillin**.

- **Lidocaine** and **lidocaine with epinephrine** are also considered safe during pregnancy.

DIABETES

- **Insulin** is the drug treatment of choice for patients with either type 1 or type 2 diabetes during pregnancy; **glyburide** can be used for type 2 diabetes after the eleventh week of gestation.
- Goals for self-monitoring of blood glucose are the same as for gestational diabetes.

EPILEPSY

VI

- Major malformations occur in 4% to 6% of the offspring of women taking **benzodiazepines**, **carbamazepine**, **phenobarbital**, **phenytoin**, and **valproic acid**.
- Minor malformations occur in 6% to 20% of pregnancies affected by epilepsy; this is twice the rate in the general population. The increase is considered to be a result of fetal exposure to antiepileptic drugs. Regimens consisting of combinations of antiepileptic drugs are associated with higher malformation rates.
- Medication change exclusively to minimize teratogenic risk is no longer recommended. Drug therapy should be optimized prior to conception, and antiepileptic drug monotherapy is recommended when possible.
- If drug withdrawal is planned, it should be done at least 6 months prior to conception.
- All women with epilepsy should take a **folic acid** supplement, 0.4 to 5 mg daily.
- To correct vitamin K deficiency in newborns, women should take 10 mg oral **vitamin K**$_1$ daily during the last month of gestation.

HUMAN IMMUNODEFICIENCY VIRUS (HIV) INFECTIONS

- **Zidovudine** (100 mg five times daily, 200 mg three times daily, or 300 mg twice daily) should be initiated at 14 to 34 weeks' gestation and continued throughout pregnancy. It is also recommended during labor, delivery, and the postpartum period.
- Continuation of other therapies during pregnancy (except **efavirenz** and **hydroxyurea**) should be strongly considered. Inclusion of **zidovudine** is recommended after 14 weeks' gestation whether it is added to the other agents or replaces another nucleoside analog.
- The infant should receive **zidovudine** beginning 8 to 12 hours after birth and continued for the first 6 weeks of life.
- A single dose of **nevirapine** administered to women at the beginning of labor and to newborns at 72 hours after birth may be an alternative to zidovudine, especially in developing countries.

HYPERTENSION

- For women with 140 to 179 mm Hg systolic or 90 to 109 mm Hg diastolic, the decision to continue or stop antihypertensive therapy during pregnancy is controversial. Antihypertensive drugs may be continued during pregnancy except for angiotensin converting enzyme inhibitors (ACEIs) and angiotensin II receptor blockers.

- If discontinued, therapy should be restarted if blood pressure exceeds 150 to 160 mm Hg systolic or 100 to 110 mm Hg diastolic or if target-organ damage is present.
- The Working Group on High Blood Pressure in Pregnancy determined that diuretic use is acceptable.
- No evidence exists for the superior efficacy of one antihypertensive agent versus another.
- Patients receiving an ACEI should be switched to a different agent before beginning the second trimester of pregnancy.

DEPRESSION

- If antidepressants are used, the lowest possible dose should be used for the shortest possible time to minimize adverse fetal and maternal pregnancy outcomes. Doses may need to be increased during pregnancy due to changes in plasma volume, liver metabolism, and renal clearance.
- Tricyclic antidepressants are considered safe during pregnancy, and **desipramine** and **nortriptyline** are commonly used.
- Although less information is available for the use of selective serotonin reuptake inhibitors, they are emerging as first-line agents for use during pregnancy, and an increased risk for birth defects has not been identified. Evaluations to date suggest a possible association of **fluoxetine** with premature birth and decreased fetal growth rate.
- When TCAs are withdrawn during pregnancy, they should be tapered gradually to avoid withdrawal symptoms. If possible, drug tapering is usually begun 5 to 10 days before the estimated day of confinement.
- Many of the selective serotonin reuptake inhibitors are well tolerated by breast-fed infants, but **fluoxetine** has resulted in some reports of gastrointestinal problems, irritability, and insomnia.

THYROID DISORDERS

- Thyroid replacement therapy should be instituted if hypothyroidism is diagnosed during pregnancy.
- Women who receive thyroid replacement therapy prior to pregnancy can expect an increased dosage requirement of 25% to 50% during pregnancy.
- Therapy for hyperthyroidism includes **propylthiouracil, methimazole,** or surgery. Propylthiouracil historically was the preferred agent because it was thought to cross the placenta less readily and is less likely than methimazole to cause fetal malformations, however, recent evidence does not support this tenet.

▶ LABOR AND DELIVERY

PRETERM LABOR

Preterm labor is labor that occurs before 37 weeks' gestation.

Tocolytic Therapy

- The goal of tocolytic therapy is to postpone delivery long enough to reduce the incidence of problems associated with prematurity. Tocolytic drugs may prolong pregnancy from 48 hours to 1 week.
- Drugs most commonly used for acute tocolysis include **magnesium sulfate,** β-adrenergic agonists, nonsteroidal anti-inflammatory agents, and non-dihydropyridine calcium channel blockers.

- Recommended doses of **terbutaline** are 250 to 500 mcg subcutaneously every 3 to 4 hours. Its use is associated with a higher incidence of maternal side effects (e.g., hyperkalemia, arrhythmias, hyperglycemia, hypotension, and pulmonary edema) than the other drugs.
- **Nifedipine** is associated with fewer side effects than magnesium or β–agonist therapy. Five to 10 mg nifedipine may be administered sublingually every 15 to 20 minutes for 3 doses. Once stabilized, 10 to 20 mg may be administered by mouth every 4 to 6 hours for preterm contractions.

Antenatal Glucocorticoids

- The benefit of administering antenatal glucocorticoids includes prevention of respiratory distress syndrome, intraventricular hemorrhage, and death in infants delivered prematurely.
- Current recommendations are to administer **betamethasone,** 12 mg intramuscularly (IM) every 24 hours for 2 doses, or **dexamethasone,** 6 mg IM every 12 hours for 4 doses, to pregnant women between 24 and 34 weeks' gestation who are at risk for preterm delivery within the next 7 days. Benefits from antenatal glucocorticoid administration are believed to begin within 24 hours and continue for up to 1 week.
- Repeat administration of antenatal glucocorticoids does not improve fetal outcomes and may cause harm.

GROUP B *STREPTOCOCCUS* INFECTION

- The Centers for Disease Control and Prevention recommends prenatal screening (vaginal and rectal cultures) for group B *Streptococcus* colonization of all pregnant women at 35 to 37 weeks' gestation. If cultures are positive, and if the woman had a previous infant with invasive group B *Spreptococcus* disease, or if the woman had group B *Streptococcus* bacteriuria, antibiotics are given.
- The currently recommended regimen for group B *Streptococcus* disease is **penicillin G,** 5 million units intravenously (IV), followed by 2.5 million units IV every 4 hours until delivery. Alternatives include **ampicillin,** 2 g IV, followed by 1 g IV every 4 hours; cefazolin 2 g IV, followed by 1 g every 8 hours; **clindamycin,** 900 mg IV every 8 hours; or **erythromycin,** 500 mg IV every 6 hours. In women who are penicillin-allergic, and in whom sensitivity testing shows the organism to be resistant to clindamycin and erythromycin, vancomycin 1 g IV every 12 hours until delivery can be used.

CERVICAL RIPENING AND LABOR INDUCTION

- Prostaglandin E$_2$ analogs (e.g., **dinoprostone, Prepidil, Cervidil**) are the most commonly used pharmacologic agents for cervical ripening. Fetal heart rate monitoring is required when Cervidil is used. **Misoprostol,** a prostaglandin E$_1$ analog, is effective and inexpensive, but it is not approved for cervical ripening and has been associated with uterine rupture.
- **Oxytocin** is the most commonly used agent for labor induction after cervical ripening.

LABOR ANALGESIA

- The IV or IM administration of narcotics **(meperidine, morphine, fentanyl)** is commonly used to treat the pain associated with labor; **promethazine** or **hydroxyzine** may be added to augment the effects.

- Epidural administration of analgesics can also be used to provide pain relief during labor, especially during the first and second stages. Epidural analgesia is associated with more oxytocin augmentation, longer stages of labor, and more instrumental deliveries than parenteral narcotic analgesia.
- Other options for labor analgesia include spinal analgesia and nerve blocks.

▶ POSTPARTUM ISSUES

DRUG USE DURING LACTATION

- Medications enter breast milk via passive diffusion of nonionized and non–protein-bound medication. Drugs with high molecular weights, lower lipid solubility, or higher protein binding are less likely to cross into breast milk.
- Most of the medications listed by the American Academy of Pediatrics are compatible with breast-feeding (Spencer JP, Gonzalez LS, Barnhart DJ. Am Fam Phys 2001; 64:119–126).

MASTITIS

- Mastitis is usually caused by *Staphylococcus aureus.*
- Treatment includes 10 to 14 days of antibiotic therapy for the mother (**cloxacillin, dicloxacillin, oxacillin,** or **cephalexin**), bedrest, adequate oral fluid intake, analgesia, and frequent evacuation of breast milk.

POSTPARTUM DEPRESSION

- Nondrug therapies include emotional support from family and friends, education about the condition, and psychotherapy. Bright-light therapy may also provide benefit.
- Drug therapies include tricyclic antidepressants and serotonin reuptake inhibitors.
- Antidepressants can be detected in the infants of breast-feeding mothers; most infants do not experience adverse effects.

RELACTATION

- Recommended pharmacologic therapy for relactation is **metoclopramide,** 10 mg three times daily for 7 to 14 days. It should be used only if nondrug therapy is ineffective.

See Chapter 76, Pregnancy and Lactation: Therapeutic Considerations, authored by Denise L. Walbrandt Pigarelli, Connie K. Kraus, and Beth E. Potter for a more detailed discussion of this topic.

Hematologic Disorders

Edited by Cindy W. Hamilton

Chapter 32

▶ ANEMIAS

▶ DEFINITION

Anemias are a group of diseases characterized by a decrease in hemoglobin or red blood cells (RBCs), resulting in decreased oxygen-carrying capacity of blood.

▶ PATHOPHYSIOLOGY

- Anemias can be classified on the basis of RBC morphology, etiology, or pathophysiology (Table 32–1). The most common anemias are included in this chapter.
- Morphologic classifications are based on cell size. Macrocytic cells are larger than normal and are associated with deficiencies of vitamin B_{12} or folate. Microcytic cells are smaller than normal and are associated with iron deficiency or a genetic anomaly (see Chapter 33); corresponding iron concentrations are decreased (hypochromic).
- Iron-deficiency anemia can be caused by inadequate dietary intake, inadequate gastrointestinal absorption, increased iron demand (e.g., pregnancy), blood loss, and chronic diseases.
- Vitamin B_{12}- and folate-deficiency anemias can be caused by inadequate dietary intake, decreased absorption, and inadequate utilization. Deficiency of intrinsic factor can cause decreased absorption of vitamin B_{12} (i.e., pernicious anemia). Folate-deficiency anemia can be caused by hyperutilization due to pregnancy, hemolytic anemia, myelofibrosis, malignancy, chronic inflammatory disorders, long-term dialysis, or growth spurt. Drugs can cause anemia by reducing absorption of folate (e.g., **phenytoin**), or by interfering with corresponding metabolic pathways (e.g., **methotrexate**).
- Anemia of chronic disease is a hypoproliferative anemia associated with chronic infectious or inflammatory processes, tissue injury, or conditions that release proinflammatory cytokines. The pathogenesis is based on shortened RBC survival, impaired marrow response, and disturbance of iron metabolism. For information on anemia of chronic kidney disease see Chapter 74.
- In anemia of critical illness, the mechanism for RBC replenishment and homeostasis is altered by, for example, blood loss or cytokines, which can blunt the erythropoietic response and inhibit RBC production.
- Age-related reductions in bone marrow reserve can render the elderly patient more susceptible to anemia that is caused by multiple minor and often unrecognized diseases (e.g., nutritional deficiencies) that negatively affect erythropoiesis.
- Anemias in children are often due to a primary hematologic abnormality. The risk of iron-deficiency anemia is increased by rapid growth spurts and dietary deficiency.
- Hemolytic anemia results from decreased RBC survival time due to destruction in the spleen or circulation. The most common etiologies are RBC membrane defects (e.g., hereditary spherocytosis), altered hemoglobin solubility or stability (e.g., sickle cell anemia [see Chapter 32] and thalassemias), and changes in intracellular metabolism (e.g., glucose-6-phosphate dehydrogenase

TABLE 32–1. Classification Systems for Anemias

1. Morphology
   Macrocytic anemias
      Megaloblastic anemias
         Vitamin B_{12} deficiency
         Folic acid deficiency anemia
   Microcytic, hypochromic anemias
      Iron deficiency anemia
      Genetic anomaly
         Sickle cell anemia
         Thalassemia
         Other hemoglobinopathies (abnormal
            hemoglobins)
   Normocytic anemias
      Recent blood loss
      Hemolysis
      Bone marrow failure
      Anemias of chronic disease
      Renal failure
      Endocrine disorders
      Myeloplastic anemias
II. Etiology
   Deficiency
      Iron
      Vitamin B_{12}
      Folic acid
      Pyridoxine
   Central—caused by impaired bone marrow
      function
         Anemia of chronic disease
         Anemia of the elderly
         Malignant bone marrow disorders
   Peripheral
      Bleeding (hemorrhage)
      Hemolysis (hemolytic anemias)
III. Pathophysiology
   Excessive blood loss
      Recent hemorrhage
      Trauma
      Peptic ulcer

Gastritis
Hemorrhoids
Chronic hemorrhage
   Vaginal bleeding
   Peptic ulcer
   Intestinal parasites
   Aspirin and other nonsteroidal
      anti-inflammatory agents
Excessive RBC destruction
   Extracorpuscular (outside the cell) factors
      RBC antibodies
      Drugs
      Physical trauma to RBC (artifical valves)
      Excessive sequestration in the spleen
   Intracorpuscular factors
      Heredity
      Disorders of hemoglobin synthesis
Inadequate production of mature RBCs
   Deficiency of nutrients (B_{12}, folic acid, iron,
      protein)
   Deficiency of erythroblasts
      Aplastic anemia
      Isolated (often transient) erythroblastopenia
      Folic acid antagonists
      Antibodies
   Conditions with infiltration of bone marrow
      Lymphoma
      Leukemia
      Myelofibrosis
      Carcinoma
   Endocrine abnormalities
      Hypothyroidism
      Adrenal insufficiency
      Pituitary insufficiency
   Chronic renal disease
   Chronic inflammatory disease
      Granulomatous diseases
      Collagen vascular diseases
   Hepatic disease

RBC, red blood cell.

[G6PD] deficiency). Some drugs cause direct oxidative damage to RBCs (see Appendix 2).

▶ CLINICAL PRESENTATION

- Signs and symptoms depend on the onset and cause of the anemia, and on the individual. Acute-onset anemia is characterized by cardiorespiratory symptoms such as tachycardia, light-headedness, and breathlessness. Chronic anemia is characterized by weakness, fatigue, headache, vertigo, faintness, cold sensitivity, pallor, and loss of skin tone. Otherwise healthy adults may tolerate anemia better than elderly patients.

Hematologic Disorders

- Iron-deficiency anemia is characterized by glossal pain, smooth tongue, reduced salivary flow, pica (compulsive eating of nonfood items), and pagophagia (compulsive eating of ice).
- Vitamin B_{12}- and folate-deficiency anemias are characterized by pallor, icterus, and gastric mucosal atrophy. Vitamin B_{12} anemia is distinguished by neuropsychiatric abnormalities (e.g., numbness and paresthesias), which are absent in patients with folate-deficiency anemia.

▶ DIAGNOSIS

- Rapid diagnosis is essential because anemia is often a sign of underlying pathology.
- Laboratory evaluation of anemia involves a complete blood count including RBC indices (Table 32–2), reticulocyte index, and examinations of the peripheral blood smear and of the stool for occult blood.
- The earliest and most sensitive laboratory change for iron-deficiency anemia is decreased serum ferritin (storage iron), which should be interpreted in conjunction with decreased transferrin saturation and increased total iron-binding concentration (TIBC). Hemoglobin, hematocrit, and RBC indices usually remain normal until later stages of iron-deficiency anemia. Symptoms do not appear until hemoglobin concentrations fall below 8 or 9 g/dL.
- Macrocytic anemias are characterized by increased mean corpuscular volume (MCV) (110 to 140 fL). One of the earliest and most specific indications of

TABLE 32–2. Normal Hematologic Values

Test	Reference Range (y)			
	2–6	6–12	12–18	18–49
Hemoglobin (R/dL)	11.5–15.5	11.5–15.5	M 13.0–16.0	M 13.5–17.5
			F 12.0–16.0	F 12.0–16.0
Hematocrit (%)	34–40	35–45	M 37–49	M 41–53
			F 36–46	F 36–46
MCV (fL)	75–87	77–95	M 78–98	80–100
			F 78–102	
MCHC (%)	—	31–37	31–37	31–37
MCH (pg)	24–30	25–33	25–35	26–34
RBC (million/mm³)	3.9–5.3	4.0–5.2	M 4.5–5.3	M 4.5–5.9
Reticulocyte count, absolute (%)				0.5–1.5
Serum iron (mcg/dL)		50–120	50–120	M 50–160
				F 40–150
TIBC (mcg/dL)	250–400	250–400	250–400	250–400
RDW (%)				11–16
Ferritin (ng/mL)	7–140	7–140	7–140	M 15–200
				F 12–150
Folate (ng/mL)				1.8–16.0
Vitamin B_{12} (pg/mL)				100–900[a]
Erythropoietin (mU/mL)				0–19
Serum MMA				75–270 mM
Total homocysteine				5–14 MCM

[a]Varies by assay method.

F_1 female; M, male; MCHC, mean corpuscular hemoglobin concentration; MCH, mean corpuscular hemoglobin; MCV, mean corpuscular volume; MMA, methylmalonic acid; RDW, red blood cell distribution; TIBC, total Iron-binding capacity.

macrocytic anemia is hypersegmented polymorphonuclear leukocytes on the peripheral blood smear.

- Vitamin B_{12} and folate concentrations can be measured to differentiate between the two deficiency anemias. A vitamin B_{12} value of less than 150 pg/mL, together with appropriate peripheral smear and clinical symptoms, is diagnostic of vitamin B_{12}-deficiency anemia. A decreased RBC folate concentration (less than 150 ng/mL) appears to be a better indicator of folate-deficiency anemia than a decreased serum folate concentration (less than 3 ng/mL).
- Diagnosis of anemia of chronic disease is usually one of exclusion, with consideration of coexisting iron and folate deficiencies. Serum iron is usually decreased but, unlike iron-deficiency anemia, serum ferritin is normal or increased and TIBC is decreased. The bone marrow reveals an abundance of iron; the peripheral smear reveals normocytic anemia.
- Laboratory findings of anemia of critical illness disease are similar to those of anemia of chronic disease.
- Elderly patients with symptoms of anemia should undergo complete blood cell count, including peripheral smear and reticulocyte count, and other laboratory studies as needed to determine the etiology of anemia.
- Diagnosis of anemia in pediatric populations requires the use of age- and sex-adjusted norms for laboratory values.
- Hemolytic anemias tend to be normocytic and normochromic and to have increased levels of reticulocytes, lactic dehydrogenase, and indirect bilirubin.

VII

▶ DESIRED OUTCOME

The ultimate goals of treatment in the anemic patient are to alleviate signs and symptoms, correct the underlying etiology (e.g., restore substrates needed for RBC production), and prevent recurrence of anemia.

▶ TREATMENT

IRON-DEFICIENCY ANEMIA

- **Oral iron** therapy with soluble ferrous iron salts, which are not enteric coated and not slow- or sustained-release, is recommended at a daily dosage of 200 mg elemental iron in two or three divided doses (Table 32–3).
- Diet plays a significant role because iron is poorly absorbed from vegetables, grain products, dairy products, and eggs; iron is best absorbed from meat, fish, and poultry. Administration of iron therapy with a meal decreases absorption by more than 50% but can be needed to improve tolerability.
- **Parenteral iron** may be required for patients with iron malabsorption, intolerance of oral iron therapy, or noncompliance. Parenteral administration, however, does not hasten the onset of hematologic response. The replacement dose depends on etiology of anemia and hemoglobin concentration (Table 32–4).
- Available parenteral iron preparations have similar efficacy but different pharmacologic, pharmacokinetic, and safety profiles (Table 32–5). The newer products, **sodium ferric gluconate** and **iron sucrose**, appear to be better tolerated than **iron dextran**.
- Iron dextran can be given intramuscularly (IM) by Z-tract administration, or intravenously (IV) by multiple slow injections of the undiluted solution or by infusion of the diluted solution. After an initial test dose of 25 mg IM or IV (or a 5 to 10 minute infusion of the diluted IV solution), patients should be

Hematologic Disorders

TABLE 32–3. Oral Iron Products

Salt	Elemental Iron (%)	Elemental Iron Provided
Ferrous sulfate	20	60–65 mg/324–325 mg tablet
		18 mg iron/5 mL syrup
		44 mg iron/5 mL elixir
		15 mg iron/0.6 mL drop
Ferrous sulfate (exsiccated)	30	65 mg/200 mg tablet
		60 mg/187 mg tablet
		50 mg/160 mg tablet
Ferrous gluconate	12	36 mg/325 mg tablet
		27 mg/240 mg tablet
Ferrous fumarate	33	33 mg/100 mg tablet
		63–66 mg/200 mg tablet
		106 mg/324–325 mg tablet
		15 mg/0.6 mL drop
		33 mg/5 mL suspension
Polysaccharide iron complex	100	150 mg capsule
		50 mg tablet
		100 mg/5 mL elixir
Carbonyl iron	100	50 mg caplet

monitored for 1 hour for adverse reactions such as allergic reactions, including anaphylaxis.

VITAMIN B$_{12}$-DEFICIENCY ANEMIA

- Oral vitamin B$_{12}$ supplementation appears to be as effective as parenteral, even in patients with pernicious anemia, because the alternate vitamin B$_{12}$ absorption pathway is independent of intrinsic factor. Oral **cobalamin** is initiated at 1 to 2 mg daily for 1 to 2 weeks, followed by 1 mg daily.
- Parenteral therapy is more rapid acting than oral therapy and should be used if neurologic symptoms are present. A popular regimen is **cyanocobalamin**

TABLE 32–4. Equations for Calculating Doses of Parenteral Iron

In patients with iron deficiency anemia:

Adults + children over 15 kg

Dose (mL) = 0.0442 (desired Hgb − observed Hgb)
$\times$ LBW + (0.26 $\times$ LBW)

LBW males = 50 kg + (2.3 $\times$ inches over 5 ft)

LBW females = 45.5 kg + (2.3 $\times$ inches over 5 ft)

Children 5–15 kg

Dose (mL) = 0.0442 (desired Hgb − observed Hgb)
$\times$ W + (0.26 $\times$ W)

Hgb = hemoglobin
mL = milliliter
W = weight
LBW = lean body weight

In patients with anemia secondary to blood loss (hemorrhagic diathesis or long-term dialysis):

mg of iron = blood loss $\times$ hematocrit

where blood loss is in milliliters and hematocrit is expressed as a decimal fraction.

TABLE 32–5. Parenteral Iron Preparations

	Sodium Ferric Gluconate	Iron Dextran	Iron Sucrose
Elemental iron Molecular weight	62.5 mg iron/5 mL Ferrlecit: 289,000–444,000 daltons	50 mg iron/mL InFeD: 165,000 daltons DexFerrum: 267,000 daltons	20 mg iron/mL Venofer: 34,000–60,000 daltons
Composition	Ferric oxide hydrate bonded to sucrose chelates with gluconate in a molar rate of 2 iron molecules to 1 gluconate molecule	Complex of ferric hydroxide and dextran	Complex of polynuclear iron hydroxide in sucrose
Preservative	Benzyl alcohol 9 mg/5 mL 20% (975 mg in 62.5 mg iron)	None	None
Indication	Iron deficiency anemia in patients undergoing chronic hemodialysis and receiving supplemental erythropoietin therapy	Patients with documented iron deficiency in whom oral therapy is unsatisfactory or impossible	Iron deficiency anemia in patients undergoing chronic hemodialysis and receiving supplemental epoetin alfa therapy
Warning	No black box warning; hypersensitivity reactions	Black box warning: anaphylactic-type reactions	Black box warning: anaphylactic-type reactions
IM injection	No	Yes	No
Usual dose	125 mg (10 mL) diluted in 100 mL normal saline, infused over 60 minutes; or as a slow IV injection (rate of 12.5 mg/min)	100 mg undiluted at a rate not to exceed 50 mg (1 mL) per min	100 mg into the dialysis line at a rate of 1 mL (20 mg of iron) undiluted solution per min
Treatment	8 doses × 125 mg = 1,000 mg	10 doses × 100 mg = 1,000 mg	Up to 10 doses × 100 mg = 1,000 mg
Common adverse effects	Cramps, nausea and vomiting, flushing, hypotension, rash, pruritus	Pain and brown staining at injection site, flushing, hypotension, fever, chills, myalgia, anaphylaxis	Leg cramps, hypotension

VII

1000 μg daily for a week, then weekly for a month, and then monthly. When symptoms resolve, daily oral administration can be initiated.

- An intranasal gel formulation can be advantageous for patients who are home-bound, have cognitive impairment, or experience dysphagia.
- Adverse events are rare with vitamin B_{12} therapy.

FOLATE-DEFICIENCY ANEMIA

- For treatment of folate-deficiency anemia, oral **folate** 1 mg daily for 4 months is usually sufficient, unless the etiology cannot be corrected. If malabsorption is present, the daily dose should be increased to 5 mg.

ANEMIA OF CHRONIC DISEASE

- Treatment of anemia of chronic disease is less specific than that of other anemias and should focus on correcting reversible causes. Iron therapy is not effective when inflammation is present. RBC transfusions are effective but should be limited to episodes of inadequate oxygen transport and hemoglobin of 8 to 10 g/dL.
- **Epoetin alfa** can be considered, especially if cardiovascular status is compromised; but the response can be impaired in patients with anemia of chronic disease. The initial dosage is 50 to 100 units/kg three times weekly. If hemoglobin does not increase after 6 to 8 weeks the dosage can be increased to 150 units/kg three times weekly or, in patients with AIDS, to 300 units/kg three times weekly.
- Epoetin alfa is usually well tolerated. The hypertension seen in patients with end-stage kidney disease is less common in patients with AIDS.

OTHER TYPES OF ANEMIA

- Patients with other types of anemia require appropriate supplementation depending on the etiology of anemia.
- In patients with anemia of critical illness, parenteral iron is often utilized but is associated with a theoretical risk of infection. Routine use of epoetin alfa or RBC transfusions is not supported by clinical studies.
- Anemia of prematurity is usually treated with RBC transfusions. The use of epoetin alfa is controversial.
- In the pediatric population, the daily dose of elemental iron, administered as iron sulfate, is 3 mg/kg for infants and 6 mg/kg for older children. The dose and schedule of vitamin B_{12} should be titrated according to clinical and laboratory response. The daily dose of folate is 1 to 3 mg.
- Treatment of hemolytic anemia should focus on correcting the underlying cause. There is no specific therapy for G6PD deficiency, so treatment consists of avoiding oxidant medications and chemicals. Steroids, other immunosuppressants, and even splenectomy can be indicated to reduce RBC destruction.

▶ EVALUATION OF THERAPEUTIC OUTCOMES

- In patients with iron-deficiency anemia, **iron** therapy should cause reticulocytosis in 5 to 7 days and raise hemoglobin by 2 to 4 g/dL every 3 weeks. The patient should be reevaluated if reticulocytosis does not occur or if hemoglobin does not increase by 2 g/dL within 3 weeks. Iron therapy is continued until iron stores are replenished, which usually requires at least 3 to 6 months.
- In patients with megaloblastic anemia, signs and symptoms usually improve within a few days after starting **vitamin B_{12}** or **folate** therapy. Neurologic symptoms can take longer to improve or can be irreversible, but they should not progress during therapy. Reticulocytosis should occur within 2 to 5 days. A

week after starting vitamin B_{12} therapy, hemoglobin should rise and leukocyte and platelet counts should normalize. Hematocrit should rise 2 weeks after starting folate therapy.

- In patients with anemia of chronic disease, reticulocytosis should occur a few days after starting **epoetin alfa** therapy. Iron, TIBC, transferring saturation, or ferritin levels should be monitored at baseline and periodically because iron depletion is a major reason for treatment failure. The optimal form and schedule of iron supplementation is unknown. If clinical response does not occur by 12 weeks, epoetin alfa should be discontinued.

See Chapter 99, Anemias, authored by Beata Ineck, Barbara J. Mason, and E. Gregory Thompson, for a more detailed discussion of this topic.

VII

Chapter 33

▶ SICKLE CELL DISEASE

▶ DEFINITION

Sickle cell syndromes are hereditary disorders characterized by the presence of sickle hemoglobin (HbS) in red blood cells (RBCs).

▶ PATHOPHYSIOLOGY

- The most common abnormal hemoglobin in the United States is hemoglobin S. Two genes for hemoglobin S (HbSS) result in sickle cell disease or sickle cell anemia, which occurs in 0.3% of African Americans. One gene for hemoglobin S (HbS) results in sickle cell trait, which occurs in 8% of African Americans. Hemoglobin C, another abnormality, occurs in 2% to 3% of African Americans.
- Pathology is more likely to occur with HbSS but can occur with HbS, especially if it coexists with hemoglobin C or thalassemia.
- The clinical manifestations of sickle cell disease are attributable to impaired circulation, RBC destruction, and stasis of blood flow. These problems are attributable to disturbances in RBC polymerization and to membrane damage.
- Polymerization allows deoxygenated hemoglobin to exist as a semisolid gel that protrudes into the cell membrane, distorting RBCs into sickle shapes. Sickle-shaped RBCs increase blood viscosity and encourage sludging in the capillaries and small vessels. Such obstructive events lead to local tissue hypoxia and accentuate the pathologic process.
- Repeated cycles of sickling, upon deoxygenation, and unsickling, upon oxygenation, damage the RBC membrane and cause irreversible sickling. Rigid, sickled RBCs are easily trapped, shortening their circulatory survival and resulting in chronic hemolysis.
- Additional contributing factors include functional asplenia (and increased risk of bacterial infection), deficient opsonization, and coagulation abnormalities.

▶ CLINICAL PRESENTATION

- Sickle cell disease involves many organ systems. Clinical manifestations depend on the genotype (Table 33–1).
- The feature presentations of sickle cell disease are hemolytic anemia and vasoocclusion. Symptoms are delayed until 4 to 6 months of age when HbS replaces fetal hemoglobin (HbF). Common findings include pain with fever, pneumonia, splenomegaly and, in infants, pain and swelling of the hands and feet (e.g., hand-and-foot syndrome or dactylitis).
- The usual clinical signs and symptoms of sickle cell disease are chronic anemia; fever; pallor; arthralgia; scleral icterus; abdominal pain; weakness; anorexia; fatigue; enlarged liver, spleen, and heart; and hematuria.
- Children experience delayed growth and sexual maturation, and characteristic physical findings such as protuberant abdomen and exaggerated lumbar lordosis.
- Acute complications of sickle cell disease include fever and infection (e.g., sepsis caused by encapsulated pathogens such as *Streptococcus pneumoniae*), stroke, acute chest syndrome, and priapism. Acute chest syndrome is characterized by pulmonary infiltration, respiratory symptoms, and equivocal response to antibiotic therapy.

TABLE 33–1. Clinical Features of Sickle Cell Trait and Common Sickle Cell Disease

Type	Clinical Features
Sickle cell trait (SCT)	Rare painless hematuria; normal Hgb level; heavy exercise under extreme conditions may provoke gross hematuria and complications
Sickle cell anemia (SCA)	Pain crises, microvascular disruption of organs (spleen, liver, bone marrow, kidney, brain, and lung), gallstone, priapism, leg ulcers, anemia (Hgb 7–10 g/dL)
Sickle hemoglobin C	Painless hematuria and rare aseptic necrosis of bone; vaso-occlusive crises are less common and occur later in life; other complications are ocular disease and pregnancy-related problems; mild anemia (Hgb 10–12 g/dL)
Sickle β^+-thalassemia	Rare crises; milder severity than sickle cell disease because of production of HbA; Hgb 10–14 g/dL with microcytosis
Sickle β°-thalassemia	No HbA production; severity similar to SCA; Hgb 7–10 g/dL with microcytosis

Hgb, hemoglobin

- Sickle cell crisis can be precipitated by fever, infection, dehydration, hypoxia, acidosis, sudden temperature change, or a combination of factors. The most common type is vasoocclusive or infarctive crisis, which is manifested by pain over the involved areas without change in hemoglobin. Aplastic crisis is characterized by decreased reticulocyte count and rapidly developing severe anemia, with or without pain. Splenic sequestration crisis is a massive enlargement of the spleen and a major cause of mortality in young patients.
- Chronic complications involve many organs and include pulmonary hypertension, bone and joint destruction, ocular problems, cholelithiasis, cardiovascular abnormalities, and hematuria and other renal complications.
- Patients with sickle cell trait are usually asymptomatic, except for impaired renal function and dilute urine, increased risk of dehydration, and hematuria.

▶ DIAGNOSIS

- Sickle cell disease is usually identified by routine neonatal screening programs using isoelectric focusing.
- Laboratory findings include low hemoglobin; increased reticulocyte, platelet, and leukocyte counts; and sickle forms on the peripheral smear.

▶ DESIRED OUTCOME

The goal of treatment is to reduce hospitalizations, complications, and mortality.

▶ TREATMENT

GENERAL PRINCIPLES

- Patients with sickle cell disease require lifelong multidisciplinary care. Interventions include general measures, preventive strategies, and treatment of complications and acute crises.
- Patients with sickle cell disease should receive routine immunizations plus influenza, meningococcal, and pneumococcal vaccinations.
- Prophylactic **penicillin** is recommended for children with sickle cell disease until they are 5 years old. The dosage is penicillin V potassium, 125 mg orally

twice daily until 3 years of age and then 250 mg twice daily, or benzathine penicillin, 600,000 units intramuscularly every 4 weeks.

- **Folic acid,** 1 mg daily, is recommended in adult patients, pregnant women, and patients of all ages with chronic hemolysis.

FETAL HEMOGLOBIN STIMULATORS AND OTHER STRATEGIES

- **Hydroxyurea**, a chemotherapeutic agent, is indicated for patients with frequent painful episodes, severe symptomatic anemia, acute chest syndrome, or other severe vasoocclusive complications. The dosage should be individualized based on response and toxicity (Figure 33–1).
- Strategies being considered to induce fetal hemoglobin include **butyrate** and **5-aza-2-deoxycytidine.**
- Chronic transfusion is indicated to prevent stroke and stroke recurrence in children. Transfusion frequency is usually every 3 to 4 weeks and should be adjusted to maintain HbS of less than 30% of total hemoglobin. The optimal duration is unknown. Risks include alloimmunization, hyperviscosity, viral transmission (requiring hepatitis A and B vaccination), volume and iron overload, and transfusion reactions.
- Allogeneic hematopoietic stem cell transplantation is the only therapy that is curative. The best candidates are younger than 16 years of age, have severe complications, and have HLA-matched donors. Risks must be carefully considered and include mortality, graft rejection, and secondary malignancies.

TREATMENT OF COMPLICATIONS

- Patients should be educated to recognize conditions that require urgent evaluation. To avoid exacerbation during acute illness, patients should maintain balanced fluid status and oxygen saturation of at least 92%.
- RBC transfusions are indicated for acute exacerbation of baseline anemia (e.g., aplastic crisis, hepatic or splenic sequestration, severe hemolysis), severe vasoocclusive episodes, and procedures requiring general anesthesia or ionic contrast. Transfusions might be beneficial in patients with complicated obstetric problems, refractory leg ulcers, refractory and protracted painful episodes, and severe priapism.
- Fever of 38.5°C or higher should be evaluated promptly. A low threshold for empiric antibiotic therapy with coverage against encapsulated organisms is recommended (e.g., **ceftriaxone** for outpatients and **cefotaxime** for inpatients).
- Patients with acute chest syndrome should receive incentive spirometry; appropriate fluid therapy; broad-spectrum antibiotics including a **macrolide** or **quinolone**; and, for hypoxia or acute distress, oxygen therapy. Steroids and nitric oxide are being evaluated.
- Priapism has been treated with analgesics, antianxiety agents, vasoconstrictors to force blood out of the corpus cavernosum (e.g., **phenylephrine, epinephrine**), and vasodilators to relax smooth muscle (e.g., **terbutaline, hydralazine**).

TREATMENT OF SICKLE CELL CRISIS

- Treatment of *aplastic crisis* is primarily supportive. Blood transfusions may be indicated for severe or symptomatic anemia. Antibiotic therapy is not warranted because the most common etiology is viral, not bacterial, infection.
- Treatment options for *splenic sequestration* include observation alone, especially for adults because they tend to have milder episodes; chronic transfusion

VII

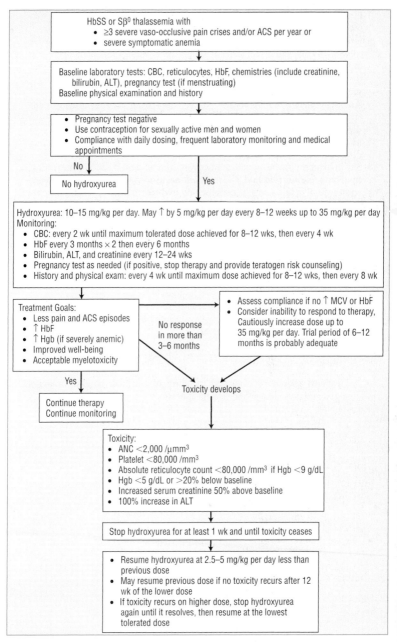

Figure 33–1. Hydroxyurea use in sickle cell disease. ACS, acute chest syndrome; ALT, alanine aminotransferase; ANC, absolute neutrophil count; CBC, complete blood cell count; HbF, fetal hemoglobin; Hgb, hemoglobin; HbSS, homozygous sickle hemoglobin; MCV, mean corpuscular volume.

to delay splenectomy; and splenectomy after a life-threatening crisis, after repetitive episodes, or for chronic hypersplenism.

- Hydration and analgesics are the mainstays of treatment for *vasoocclusive (painful) crisis*. Fluid replacement should be 1.5 times the maintenance requirement, can be administered intravenously or orally, and should be monitored to avoid volume overload. An infectious etiology should be considered; if appropriate, empiric therapy should be initiated.
- Analgesic therapy should be tailored to the individual because of the variable frequency and severity of pain. Pain scales should be used to quantify the degree of pain.
- Mild to moderate pain should be treated with nonsteroidal anti-inflammatory drugs or acetaminophen.
- Severe pain should be treated aggressively with an opioid, such as **morphine, hydromorphone, fentanyl**, and **methadone.** Moderate pain should be treated with a weak opioid, such as **codeine** and **hydrocodone. Meperidine** should be used sparingly because accumulation of the normeperidine metabolite can cause neurotoxicity, especially in patients with impaired renal function.
- Severe pain should be treated with an intravenous opioid titrated to pain relief and then administered on a scheduled basis with as-needed dosing for breakthrough pain. Patient-controlled analgesia is commonly utilized.
- Suspicion of addiction commonly leads to suboptimal pain control. Factors that minimize dependence include aggressive pain control, frequent monitoring, and tapering medication according to response.
- **Poloxamer** 188 (Flocor) is being evaluated for vasoocclusive crisis. This surfactant returns RBCs to a nonadhesive state and blocks RBC aggregation to enhance blood flow in ischemic areas.

▶ EVALUATION OF THERAPEUTIC OUTCOMES

- All patients should be evaluated regularly to establish baseline, monitor changes, and provide age-appropriate education.
- Laboratory evaluations include complete blood cell and reticulocyte counts, and hemoglobin F level. Renal, hepatobiliary, and pulmonary function should be evaluated. Patients should be screened for retinopathy.
- The efficacy of hydroxyurea can be assessed by monitoring the number, severity, and duration of sickle cell crises.

See Chapter 101, Sickle Cell Disease, authored by C. Y. Jennifer Chan and Reginald Moore, for a more detailed discussion of this topic.

Infectious Diseases
Edited by Joseph T. DiPiro

Chapter 34 _____

► INTRODUCTION

A generally accepted systematic approach to the selection and evaluation of an antimicrobial regimen is shown in Table 34–1. An "empiric" antimicrobial regimen is begun before the offending organism is identified, while a "definitive" regimen is instituted when the causative organism is known.

► CONFIRMING THE PRESENCE OF INFECTION

FEVER

• Fever is defined as a controlled elevation of body temperature above the normal range of 36.7 to 37.0°C. Fever is a manifestation of many disease states other than infection.

• Many drugs have been identified as causes of fever. Drug-induced fever is defined as persistent fever in the absence of infection or other underlying condition. The fever must coincide temporally with the administration of the offending agent and disappear promptly upon its withdrawal, after which it remains normal.

SIGNS AND SYMPTOMS

White Blood Cell Count

• Most infections result in elevated white blood cell (WBC) counts (leukocytosis) because of the mobilization of granulocytes and/or lymphocytes to destroy invading microbes. The generally accepted range of normal values for WBC counts is between 4000 and 10,000/mm^3.

TABLE 34–1. Systematic Approach for Selection of Antimicrobials

Confirm the presence of infection
   Careful history and physical
   Signs and symptoms
   Predisposing factors
Identification of the pathogen
   Collection of infected material
   Stains
   Serologies
   Culture and sensitivity
Selection of presumptive therapy considering every infected site
   Host factors
   Drug factors
Monitor therapeutic response
   Clinical assessment
   Laboratory tests
   Assessment of therapeutic failure

- Bacterial infections are associated with elevated granulocyte counts (neutrophils, basophils), often with increased numbers of immature forms (band neutrophils) seen in peripheral blood smears (left-shift). With infection, peripheral leukocyte counts may be very high, but are rarely higher than 30,000 to 40,000/mm^3. Low neutrophil counts (neutropenia) after the onset of infection indicate an abnormal response and are generally associated with a poor prognosis for bacterial infection.
- Relative lymphocytosis, even with normal or slightly elevated total WBC counts, is generally associated with viral or fungal infections. Lymphocytopenia occurs with AIDS.
- Many types of infections, however, may be accompanied by a completely normal WBC count and differential.

Pain and Inflammation

- Pain and inflammation may accompany infection and are sometimes manifested by swelling, erythema, tenderness, and purulent drainage. Unfortunately, these signs may be apparent only if the infection is superficial or in a bone or joint.
- The manifestations of inflammation with deep-seated infections such as meningitis, pneumonia, endocarditis, and urinary tract infection must be ascertained by examining tissues or fluids. For example, the presence of polymorphonuclear leukocytes (neutrophils) in spinal fluid, lung secretions (sputum), and urine is highly suggestive of bacterial infection.

VIII

▶ IDENTIFICATION OF THE PATHOGEN

- Infected body materials must be sampled, if at all possible or practical, before the institution of antimicrobial therapy, for two reasons. First, Gram stain of the material may rapidly reveal bacteria or acid-fast stain may detect mycobacteria or actinomycetes. Second, a delay in obtaining infected fluids or tissues until after therapy is started may result in false-negative culture results or alterations in the cellular and chemical composition of infected fluids.
- Blood cultures should be performed in the acutely ill, febrile patient. Less accessible fluids or tissues must be obtained based on localized signs or symptoms (e.g., spinal fluid in meningitis, joint fluid in arthritis). Abscesses and cellulitic areas should also be aspirated.
- Caution must be used in the evaluation of positive culture results from normally sterile sites (e.g., blood, cerebrospinal fluid, joint fluid). The recovery of bacteria normally found on the skin in large quantities (e.g., coagulase-negative staphylococci, diphtheroids) from one of these sites may be a result of contamination of the specimen rather than a true infection.

▶ SELECTION OF PRESUMPTIVE THERAPY

- To select rational antimicrobial therapy for a given infection, a variety of factors must be considered. These include the severity and acuity of the disease, host factors, factors related to the drugs used, and the necessity for use of multiple agents.
- There are generally accepted drugs of choice for the treatment of most pathogens (Table 34–2). The drugs of choice are compiled from a variety of sources and are intended as guidelines rather than specific rules for antimicrobial use.

TABLE 34–2. Drugs of Choice, First Choice, *Alternative(s)*

GRAM-POSITIVE COCCI

Enterococcus faecalis (generally not as resistant to antibiotics as *E. faecium*)
    Serious infection (endocarditis, meningitis, pyelonephritis with bacteremia)
    Ampicillin (or penicillin G) + (gentamicin or streptomycin)
    Vancomycin + (gentamicin or streptomycin), linezolid
    Urinary tract infection (UTI)
    Ampicillin, amoxicillin
    Doxycycline[a] fosfomycin, or nitrofurantoin
E. faecium (generally more resistant to antibiotics than *E. faecalis*)
    Recommend consultation with infectious disease specialist.
    Linezolid, quinupristin/dalfopristin
Staphylococcus aureus/Staphylococcus epidermidis
    Methicillin (oxacillin)-sensitive
    PRP[c]
    FGC,[d,e] trimethoprim-sulfamethoxazole, clindamycin,[f] ampicillin-sulbactam, amoxicillin-clavulante, or
        fluoroquinolone
    Methicillin (oxacillin)–resistant
    Vancomycin + (gentamicin or rifampin)
    Linezolid, quinupristin-dalfopristin, daptomycin
    Per sensitivities: Trimethoprim-sulfamethoxazole, doxycycline,[a] or clindamycin
Streptococcus (groups A, B, C, G, and *S. bovis*)
    Penicillin G[h] or V[i] or ampicillin
    FGC,[d,e] erythromycin, azithromycin, clarithromycin,[i] S. pneumoniae
    Penicillin-sensitive (MIC < 0.1 mcg/mL)
    Penicillin G or V or ampicillin
    Erythromycin, FGC,[d,e] azithromycin, or clarithromycin[i]
    Penicillin intermediate (MIC 0.1 – 1.0 mcg/mL)
    High-dose penicillin (12 million units/day for adults) or ceftriaxone[e] or cefotaxime[e]
    Gatifloxacin[b], levofloxacin[b], moxifloxacin[b], or vancomycin
    Penicillin-resistant (MIC ≥ 1.0 mcg/mL)
    Recommend consultation with infectious disease specialist.
    Vancomycin ± rifampin
    Per sensitivities: TGC,[e,k] levofloxacin,[b] gatifloxacin,[b] or moxifloxacin[b]
Streptococcus, viridans group
    Penicillin G ± gentamicin[f]
    TGC,[d,e] erythromycin, azithromycin, clarithromycin,[i] or vancomycin ± gentamicin

VIII

GRAM-NEGATIVE COCCI

Moraxella (Branhamella) catarrhalis
    Amoxicillin-clavulanate, ampicillin-sulbactam
    Trimethoprim-sulfamethoxazole, erythromycin, azithromycin, clarithromycin,[i] doxycycline,[a] SGC,[e,m] TGC,[e,k] or
        TGCpo[e,n]
Neisseria gonorrhoeae (also give concomitant treatment for *Chlamydia trachomatis*)
    Disseminated gonococcal infection
    Ceftriaxone[e] or cefotaxime[e]
    Oral follow-up: Cefixime,[e] cefpodoxime,[e] ciprofloxacin,[b] or ofloxacin[b]
    Uncomplicated infection
    Ceftriaxone[e] or cefotaxime,[e] cefixime,[e] or cefpodoxime[e]
    Ciprofloxacin[b] or ofloxacin[b]
N. meningitides
    Penicillin G
    TGC[e,k]

GRAM-POSITIVE BACILLI

Clostridium perfringens
    Penicillin G ± clindamycin
    Metronidazole, clindamycin, doxycycline,[a] cefazolin,[e] imipenem,[o] meropenem,[o] or ertapenem[o]

(Continued)

TABLE 34–2. (Continued)

C. difficile
Oral metronidazole
Oral vancomycin

GRAM-NEGATIVE BACILLI

Acinetobacter spp.
Imipenem or meropenem either ± aminoglycoside[p] (amikacin usually most effective)
Ciprofloxacin,[b] trimethoprim-sulfamethoxazole, or ampicillin-sulbactam
Bacteroides fragilis (and others)
Metronidazole
BLIC,[g] clindamycin, cephamycin,[e,q] or carbapenem[o]
Enterobacter spp.
Imipenem, meropenem, ertapenem, or cefepime ± aminoglycoside[p]
Ciprofloxacin,[b] levofloxacin,[b] piperacillin-tazobactam, ticarcillin-clavulanate, or trimethoprim-sulfamethoxazole
Escherichia coli
Meningitis
TGC[e,k] or meropenem
Systemic infection
TGC[e,k]

VIII   *Ampicillin-sulbactam, FGC,[d,e] BL/BLI,[g] trimethoprim-sulfamethoxazole, SGC,[e,m] fluoroquinolone,[b,o,r] imipenem,[o] meropenem[o]*
Urinary tract infection
Most oral agents: Check sensitivities.
Ampicillin, amoxicillin-clavulanate, trimethoprim-sulfamethoxazole, or cephalexin[e]
Aminoglycoside, FGC[d,e] nitrofurantoin, fluoroquinolone[b,o,r]
Gardnerella vaginalis
Metronidazole
Clindamycin
Hemophilus influenzae
Meningitis
Cefotaxime[e] or ceftriaxone[e]
Meropenem[o] or chloramphenicol[f]
Other infections
BLIC,[g] or if β-lactamase-negative, ampicillin or amoxicillin
Trimethoprim-sulfamethoxazole, cefuroxime,[e] erythromycin, azithromycin, clarithromycin,[j] or fluoroquinolone[b,o,r]
Klebsiella pneumoniae
TGC[e,k] (if UTI only: Aminoglycoside[p])
Trimethoprim-sulfamethoxazole, cefuroxime,[e] fluoroquinolone,[b,r] BLIC,[g] imipenem,[o] or meropenem[o]
Legionella spp.
Erythromycin ± rifampin or fluoroquinolone[b,r]
Trimethoprim-sulfamethoxazole, clarithromycin,[j] azithromycin, or doxycycline[a]
Pasteurella multocida
Penicillin G, ampicillin, amoxicillin
Doxycycline,[a] BLIC,[g] trimethoprim-sulfamethoxazole or ceftriaxone[e,k]
Proteus mirabilis
Ampicillin
Trimethoprim-sulfamethoxazole, most antibiotics except PRP[c]
Proteus (indole-positive) (including *Providencia rettgeri, Morganella morganii*, and *Proteus vulgaris*)
TGC[e,k] or fluoroquinolone[b,r]
Trimethoprim-sulfamethoxazole, BLIC,[g] aztreonam,[f] imipenem,[o] or TGCpo[e,n]
Providencia stuartii
TGC[e,k] or fluoroquinolone[b,r]
Trimethoprim-sulfamethoxazole, aztreonam,[f] imipenem,[o] or meropenem[o]
Pseudomonas aeruginosa
Cefepime, ceftazidime, piperacillin-tazobactam, or ticarcillin-clavulanate plus aminoglycoside[p]

(Continued)

TABLE 34–2. (Continued)

Ciprofloxacin,[b] levofloxacin,[b] aztreonam,[f] imipenem,[o] or meropenem[o]
UTI only: Aminoglycoside[p]
Ciprofloxacin,[b] levofloxacin,[b] or gatifloxacin[b]
Salmonella typhi
Ciprofloxacin,[b] levofloxacin,[b] ceftriaxone,[e] or cefotaxime[e]
Trimethoprim-sulfamethoxazole
Serratia marcescens
Piperacillin-tazobactam, ticarcillin-clavulanate, or TGC,[e,k] ± gentamicin
Trimethoprim-sulfamethoxazole, ciprofloxacin,[b] levofloxacin,[b] aztreonam,[f] imipenem,[g] meropenem,[a] or ertapenem
Stenotrophomonas (Xanthomonas) maltophilia
Trimethoprim-sulfamethoxazole
Generally very resistant to all antimicrobials; check sensitivities to ceftazidime,[e] ticarcillin-clavulanate, doxycycline,[a] and minocycline[a]

MISCELLANEOUS MICROORGANISMS

Chlamydia pneumoniae
Doxycycline[a]
Erythromycin, azithromycin, clarithromycin,[j] or fluoroquinolone[b,r]
C. trachomatis
Doxycycline[a] or azithromycin
Levofloxacin[b] or ofloxacin[b]
Mycoplasma pneumoniae
Erythromycin, azithromycin, clarithromycin[j]
Doxycycline[a] or fluoroquinolone[b,r]

VIII

SPIROCHETES

Treponema pallidum
Neurosyphilis
Penicillin G
Ceftriaxone[e]
Primary or secondary
Benzathine penicillin G
Doxycycline[a] or ceftriaxone[e]
Borrelia burgdorferi (choice depends on stage of disease)
Ceftriaxone[e] or cefuroxime axetil,[e] doxycycline,[a] amoxicillin
High-dose penicillin, cefotaxime,[e] azithromycin, or clarithromycin[j]

---

[a]Not for use in pregnant patients or children younger than 8 yr.
[b]Not for use in pregnant patients or children younger than 18 yr.
[c]Penicillinase-resistant penicillin: nafcillin or oxacillin.
[d]First-generation cephalosporins—IV: cefazolin; PO: cephalexin, cephradine, or cefadroxil.
[e]Some penicillin-allergic patients may react to cephalosporins.
[f]Not reliably bactericidal; should not be used for endocarditis.
[g]β-Lactamase inhibitor combination—IV: ampicillin-sulbactam, piperacillin-tazobactam, ticarcillin-clavulante; PO: amoxicillin-clavulanate.
[h]Either aqueous penicillin G or benzathine penicillin G (pharyngitis only).
[i]Only for soft tissue infections or upper respiratory infections (pharyngitis, otitis media).
[j]Do not use in pregnant patients.
[k]Third-generation cephalosporins—IV: cefotaxime, ceftriaxone.
[l]Gentamicin should be added if tolerance or moderately susceptible (MIC >0.1 g/mL) organisms are encountered; streptomycin is used but may be more toxic.
[m]Second-generation cephalosporins—IV: cefuroxime; PO: cefaclor, cefditoren, cefprozil, cefuroxime axetil, and loracarbef.
[n]Third-generation cephalosporins—PO: cefdinir, cefixime, cefetamet, cefpodoxime proxetil, and ceftibuten.
[o]Reserve for serious infection.
[p]Aminoglycosides: gentamicin, tobramycin, and amikacin; use per sensitivities.
[q]Cefoxitin, cefotetan.
[r]IV/PO: ciprofloxacin, ofloxacin, levofloxacin, gatifloxacin, and moxifloxacin.
[s]Reserve for serious infection when less toxic drugs are not effective.
[t]Generally reserved for patients with hypersensitivity reactions to penicillin.

- When selecting antimicrobial regimens, local susceptibility data should be considered whenever possible rather than information published by other institutions or national compilations.
- Empiric therapy is directed at organisms that are known to cause the infection in question.

HOST FACTORS

- In evaluating a patient for initial or empiric therapy, the following factors should be considered:
  - Allergy or history of adverse drug reactions
  - Age of patient
  - Pregnancy
  - Metabolic abnormalities
  - Renal and hepatic function
  - Concomitant drug therapy
  - Concomitant disease states
- Patients with diminished renal and/or hepatic function will accumulate certain drugs unless dosage is adjusted. Any concomitant therapy the patient is receiving may influence the selection of drug therapy, the dose, and monitoring.
- A list of selected drug interactions involving antimicrobials is provided in Table 34–3.

DRUG FACTORS

- Integration of both pharmacokinetic and pharmacodynamic properties of an agent is important when choosing antimicrobial therapy to ensure efficacy and prevent resistance.
- The importance of tissue penetration varies with the site of infection. The central nervous system (CNS) is one body site where the importance of antimicrobial penetration is relatively well defined and correlations with clinical outcomes are established. Drugs that do not reach significant concentrations in cerebrospinal fluid (CSF) should be avoided in treating meningitis.
- Apart from the bloodstream, other body fluids where drug concentration data are clinically relevant include urine, synovial fluid, and peritoneal fluid.
- Certain pharmacokinetic parameters such as area under the concentration-time curve (AUC) and maximal plasma concentration (C_{max}) can be predictive of treatment outcome when specific ratios of AUC or C_{max} to the minimum inhibitory concentration (MIC) are achieved. For some agents, the ratio of AUC to MIC, peak to MIC ratio, or the time that the drug concentration is above the MIC may predict efficacy.
- Antimicrobials that affect cell wall synthesis (e.g., β-lactams and vancomycin) display time-dependent bactericidal effects. Therefore, the most important pharmacodynamic relationship for these antimicrobials is the duration that drug concentrations exceed the MIC (T greater than MIC).
  - The costs of drug therapy are increasing dramatically, especially as new products derived from biotechnology are introduced. The total cost of antimicrobial therapy includes much more than just the acquisition cost of the drugs.

▶ COMBINATION ANTIMICROBIAL THERAPY

Combinations of antimicrobials are generally used to broaden the spectrum of coverage for empiric therapy, achieve synergistic activity against the infecting organism, and prevent the emergence of resistance.

VIII

TABLE 34–3. Major Drug Interactions with Antimicrobials

Antimicrobial	Other Agent(s)	Mechanism of Action/Effect	Clinical Management
Aminoglycosides	Neuromuscular blocking agents	Additive adverse effects	Avoid
	Nephrotoxins (N) or ototoxins (O) (e.g., amphotericn B (N) cisplatin (N/O), cyclosporine (N), furosemide (O), NSAIDs (N), radio contrast (N), vancomycin (N)	Additive adverse effects	Monitor aminoglycoside SDC and renal function
Amphotericin B	Nephrotoxins (e.g., aminoglycosides, cidofovir, cyclosporine, foscarnet, pentamidine)	Additive adverse effects	Monitor renal function
Azoles			
Chloramphenicol	Phenytoin, tolbutamide, ethanol	Decreased metabolism of other agents	Monitor phenytoin SDC, blood glucose
Foscarnet	Pentamidine IV	Increased risk of severe nephrotoxicity/ hypocalcemia	Monitor renal function/serum calcium
Isoniazid	Carbamazepine, phenytoin	Decreased metabolism of other agents (nausea, vomiting, nystagmus, ataxia)	Monitor drug SDC
Macrolides/azalides	Digoxin	Decreased digoxin bioavailability and metabolism	Monitor digoxin SDC; avoid if possible
	Theophylline	Decreased metabolism of theophylline	Monitor theophylline SDC
Metronidazole (also cefamandole, cefoperazone)	Ethanol (drugs containing ethanol)	Disulfiram-like reaction	Avoid
Penicillins and cephalosporins	Probenecid, aspirin	Blocked excretion of β-lactams	Use if prolonged high concentration of β-lactam desirable
Ciprofloxacin/ norfloxacin	Theophylline	Decreased metabolism of theophylline	Monitor theophylline
Quinolones	Class Ia and III Antiarrhythmics	Increased Q-T interval	Avoid
	Multivalent cations (antacids, iron, sucralfate, zinc, vitamins, dairy, citric acid) didanosine	Decreased absorption of quinolone	Separate by 2 h
Rifampin	Azoles, cyclosporine, methadone propranolol, protease inhibitors (PI), oral contraceptives, tacrolimus, warfarin	Increased metabolism of other agent	Avoid if possible
Sulfonamides	Sulfonylureas, phenytoin, warfarin	Decreased metabolism of other agent	Monitor blood glucose, SDC, PT
Tetracyclines	Antacids, iron, calcium, sucralfate	Decreased absorption of tetracycline	Separate by 2 h
	Digoxin	Decreased digoxin bioavailability and metabolism	Monitor digoxin SDC; avoid if possible

Azalides: azithromycin; azoles: fluconazole, itraconazole, ketoconazole, and voriconazole; macrolides: erythromycin, clarithromycin; protease inhibitors: aprenavir, indinavir, lopinavir/ritonavir, nelfinavir, ritonavir, and saquinavir; quinolones: ciprofloxacin, gatifloxacin, levofloxacin, moxifloxacin. SDC = serum drug concentrations.

BROADENING THE SPECTRUM OF COVERAGE

- Increasing the coverage of antimicrobial therapy is generally necessary in mixed infections where multiple organisms are likely to be present. This is the case in intraabdominal and female pelvic infections in which a variety of aerobic and anaerobic bacteria may produce disease.
- Another clinical situation in which increased spectrum of activity is desirable is with nosocomial infection. Hospital-acquired infections, except as previously noted, are generally caused by only one organism, but many different organisms may be possible.

Synergism

- The achievement of synergistic antimicrobial activity is advantageous for infections caused by gram-negative bacilli in immunosuppressed patients.
- Traditionally, combinations of aminoglycosides and β-lactams have been used since these drugs together generally act synergistically against a wide variety of bacteria. However, the data supporting superior efficacy of synergistic over nonsynergistic combinations are weak.
- Synergistic combinations may produce better results in infections caused by *Pseudomonas aeruginosa,* in certain infections caused by *Enterococcus* spp., and, perhaps, in patients with profound, persistent neutropenia.

VIII

PREVENTING RESISTANCE

The use of combinations to prevent the emergence of resistance is widely applied but not often realized. The only circumstance where this has been clearly effective is in the treatment of tuberculosis.

DISADVANTAGES OF COMBINATION THERAPY

- Although there are potentially beneficial effects from combining drugs, there are also potentially serious liabilities. Examples include additive nephrotoxicity from drugs such as aminoglycosides, amphotericin, and possibly vancomycin. Inactivation of aminoglycosides by penicillins may be clinically significant when excessive doses of penicillin are given to a patient in renal failure.
- Some combinations of antimicrobials are potentially antagonistic. Such combinations should probably be avoided whenever possible, unless the clinical situation warrants the use of both drugs for different pathogens. Agents that are capable of inducing β-lactamase production in bacteria may antagonize the effects of enzyme-labile drugs such as penicillins.

FAILURE OF ANTIMICROBIAL THERAPY

A variety of factors may be responsible for apparent lack of response to therapy. Factors include those directly related to the host, those related to the pathogen, and, although unlikely, laboratory error in identification and/or susceptibility testing. Factors directly related to the antimicrobial agents being utilized are only a small proportion of the possibilities.

Failures Caused by Drug Selection

- Factors directly related to the drug selection include an inappropriate selection of drug, dosage, or route of administration. Malabsorption of a drug product because of gastrointestinal disease (e.g., short-bowel syndrome) or a drug interaction (e.g., complexation of fluoroquinolones with multivalent cations resulting in reduced absorption) may lead to potentially subtherapeutic serum concentrations.

- Accelerated drug elimination is also a possible reason for failure and may occur in patients with cystic fibrosis or during pregnancy, when more rapid clearance or larger volumes of distribution may result in low serum concentrations, particularly for aminoglycosides.
- Finally, a common cause of failure of therapy is poor penetration into the site of infection. This is especially true for the so-called privileged sites such as the CNS, the eye, and the prostate gland.

Failures Caused by Host Factors

- Patients who are immunosuppressed (e.g., granulocytopenia from chemotherapy, AIDS) may respond poorly to therapy because their own defenses are inadequate to eradicate the infection despite seemingly adequate drug regimens.
- Other host factors are related to the necessity for surgical drainage of abscesses or removal of foreign bodies and/or necrotic tissue. If these situations are not corrected, they result in persistent infection and, occasionally, bacteremia, despite adequate antimicrobial therapy.

Failures Caused by Microorganisms

- Factors related to the pathogen include the development of drug resistance during therapy. Primary resistance refers to the intrinsic resistance of the pathogens producing the infection. However, acquisition of resistance during treatment has become a major problem as well.
- The increase in resistance among pathogenic organisms is believed to be due, in large part, to continued overuse of antimicrobials in the community, as well as in hospitals, and the increasing prevalence of immunosuppressed patients receiving long-term suppressive antimicrobials for the prevention of infections.

See Chapter 104, Antimicrobial Regimen Selection, authored by David S. Burgess and Betty J. Abate, for a more detailed discussion of this topic.

Chapter 35

▶ CENTRAL NERVOUS SYSTEM INFECTIONS

▶ DEFINITION

Central nervous system (CNS) infections include a wide variety of clinical conditions and etiologies: meningitis, meningoencephalitis, encephalitis, brain and meningeal abscesses, and shunt infections. The focus of this chapter is meningitis.

▶ PATHOPHYSIOLOGY

- Infections are the result of hematogenous spread from a primary infection site, seeding from a parameningeal focus, reactivation from a latent site, trauma, or congenital defects in the CNS.
- CNS infections may be caused by a variety of bacteria, fungi, viruses, and parasites. The most common causes of bacterial meningitis include *Streptococcus pneumoniae, Neisseria meningitides, Listeria monocytogenes,* and *Haemophilus influenzae.*
- The critical first step in the acquisition of acute bacterial meningitis is nasopharyngeal colonization of the host by the bacterial pathogen. The bacteria must first attach themselves to nasopharyngeal epithelial cells through structures called lectins. The bacteria are then phagocytized across nonciliated columnar nasopharyngeal cells into the host's bloodstream.
- A common characteristic of most CNS bacterial pathogens (e.g., *H. influenzae, Escherichia coli,* and *N. meningitidis*) is the presence of an extensive polysaccharide capsule that is resistant to neutrophil phagocytosis and complement opsonization.
- The exact site and mechanism of bacterial invasion into the CNS is unknown; however, studies suggest that invasion into the subarachnoid space occurs by continuous exposure of the CNS to large bacterial innocula.
- Bacterial cell death then causes the release of cell wall components such as lipopolysaccharide (LPS), lipid A (endotoxin), lipoteichoic acid, teichoic acid, and peptidoglycan depending on whether the pathogen is gram-positive or gram-negative. These cell wall components cause capillary endothelial cells and CNS macrophages to release cytokines (interleukin-1 [IL-1], tumor necrosis factor [TNF], and other inflammatory mediators). Products of the cyclooxygenase–arachidonic acid pathway (prostaglandins and thromboxanes) and platelet activating factor (PAF) are also released. PAF activates the coagulation cascade, and arachidonic acid metabolites stimulate vasodilatation. These lead to cerebral edema, elevated intracranial pressure, cerebrospinal fluid (CSF) pleocytosis, disseminated intravascular coagulation (DIC), syndrome of inappropriate antidiuretic hormone secretion (SIADH), decreased cerebral blood flow, cerebral ischemia, and death.

▶ CLINICAL PRESENTATION

- The clinical signs and symptoms of meningitis are variable (See Table 35-1).

GENERAL

- Clinical presentation varies with age, and generally, the younger the patient, the more atypical and the less pronounced is the clinical picture.

TABLE 35–1. Mean Values of the Components of Normal and Abnormal Cerebrospinal Fluid

Type	Normal	Bacterial	Viral	Fungal	Tuberculosis
WBC (cells/mm³)	<5	1000–5000	100–1000	40–400	100–500
Differential (%)	>90[a]	≥80 PMNs	50[b,c]	>50[b]	>80[b,c]
Protein (mg/dL)	<50	100–500	30–150	40–150	≤40–150
Glucose (mg/dL)	50–66% simultaneous serum value	<40 (<60% simultaneous serum value)	<30–70	<30–70	<30–70

[a]Monocytes.
[b]Lymphocytes.
[c]Initial Cerebrospinal fluid (CSF), while blood cell (WBC) count may reveal a predominance of polymorphonuclear neutrophils (PMNs).

- Up to 50% of patients may receive antibiotics before a diagnosis of meningitis is made, delaying presentation to the hospital. Prior antibiotic therapy may cause the Gram stain and CSF culture to be negative, but the antibiotic therapy rarely affects CSF protein or glucose.   VIII

SIGNS AND SYMPTOMS

- Classic signs and symptoms include fever, chills, vomiting, photophobia, severe headache, and nuchal rigidity associated with Kernig's and Brudzinski's signs. Kernig's and Brudzinski's signs are poorly sensitive and frequently are absent in children.
- Other signs and symptoms include irritability, delirium, drowsiness, lethargy, and coma.
- Clinical signs and symptoms in young children may include bulging fontanelle, apneas, purpuric rash, and convulsions in addition to those just mentioned.
- Seizures occur more commonly in children (20% to 30%) than in adults (0% to 12%).

DIFFERENTIAL SIGNS AND SYMPTOMS

- Purpuric and petechial skin lesions typically indicate meningococcal involvement, although the lesions may be present with *H. influenzae* meningitis. Rashes rarely occur with pneumococcal meningitis.
- Waterhouse-Friderichsen syndrome, a rapid eruption of multiple hemorrhagic lesions associated with a shocklike state, is associated with meningococcal meningitis.
- *H. influenza* meningitis and meningococcal meningitis both can cause involvement of the joints during the illness.
- A history of head trauma with or without skull fracture or presence of a chronically draining ear is associated with pneumococcal involvement.

LABORATORY TESTS

- Several tubes of CSF are collected via lumbar puncture for chemistry, microbiology, and hematology tests. Theoretically, the first tube has a higher likelihood of being contaminated with both blood and bacteria during the puncture, although the total volume is more important in practice than the tube cultured. CSF should not be refrigerated or stored on ice.

- Analysis of CSF chemistries typically includes measurement of glucose and total protein concentrations. An elevated CSF protein of 100 mg/dL or greater and a CSF glucose concentration of less than 50% of the simultaneously obtained peripheral value suggest bacterial meningitis (see Table 35–1).
- The values for CSF glucose, protein, and WBC concentrations found with bacterial meningitis overlap significantly with those for viral, tuberculous, and fungal meningitis (see Table 35–1) Therefore, CSF WBC counts and CSF glucose and protein concentrations cannot always distinguish the different etiologies of meningitis.

OTHER DIAGNOSTIC TESTS

- Blood and other specimens should be cultured according to clinical judgment because meningitis frequently can arise via hematogenous dissemination or can be associated with infections at other sites. A minimum of 20 mL of blood in each of two to three separate cultures per each 24-hour period is necessary for the detection of most bacteremias.
- Gram stain and culture of the CSF are the most important laboratory tests performed for bacterial meningitis. The Gram stain continues to be the most rapid and accurate method of presumptively diagnosing acute bacterial meningitis. When performed before antibiotic therapy is initiated, Gram stain is both rapid and sensitive and can confirm the diagnosis of bacterial meningitis in 75% to 90% of cases. The sensitivity of the Gram stain decreases to 40% to 60differentiate the various bacterial etiologies.
- Polymerase chain reaction (PCR) techniques can be used to diagnose meningitis caused by *N. meningitidis, S. pneumoniae,* and Hib. PCR is considered to be highly sensitive, but use of this diagnostic approach is limited owing to expense.
- Latex fixation, latex coagglutination, and enzyme immunoassay (EIA) tests provide for the rapid identification of several bacterial causes of meningitis, including *S. pneumoniae*, *N. meningitidis,* and Hib. Rapid-identification latex tests work by bringing potential capsular antigens of the pathogen causing meningitis in contact with a specific antibody, causing an antigen-antibody reaction. This capsular antigen-antibody reaction can be observed visually and quickly without waiting for culture results. The rapid antigen tests should be used in situations in which the Gram stain is negative. The sensitivity and specificity of latex fixation and coagglutination tests can vary with the manufacturer of the antibody, density of the antigen present in the CSF, and pathogen being tested.
- Diagnosis of tuberculosis meningitis employs acid-fast staining, culture, and PCR of the CSF.
- PCR testing of the CSF is the preferred method of diagnosing most viral meningitis infections.
- The standard diagnostic tests for fungal meningitis include culture, direct microscopic examination of stained and unstained specimens of CSF, antigen detection of cryptococcal or histoplasmal antigens, and antibody assay of serum and/or CSF.

▶ DESIRED OUTCOME

The goals of treatment include eradication of infection with amelioration of signs and symptoms, and prevention of neurologic sequelae, such as seizures, deafness, coma, and death.

VIII

► TREATMENT

GENERAL PRINCIPLES

- The administration of fluids, electrolytes, antipyretics, analgesia, and other supportive measures are particularly important for patients presenting with acute bacterial meningitis.
- Empiric antimicrobial therapy should be instituted as soon as possible to eradicate the causative organism. Antimicrobial therapy should last at least 48 to 72 hours or until the diagnosis of bacterial meningitis can be ruled out.
- Antibiotic dosages for treatment of CNS infections must be maximized to optimize penetration to the site of infection.
- Menigitis caused by *S. pneumoniae* and *H. influenzae* is successfully treated with 10 to 14 days of antibiotic therapy. Meningitis caused by *N. meningitides* usually can be treated with a 7-day course. A longer course, 14 to 21 days, is recommended for patients infected with *Listeria monocytogenes*, group B streptococcus, and enteric gram-negative bacilli. Therapy should be individualized, and some patients may require longer courses.

VIII

PHARMACOLOGIC TREATMENT

- Isolation and identification of the causative agent can direct the selection of the most appropriate antimicrobial therapy for the patient (Tables 35–2, 35–3, and 35–4).
- With increased meningeal inflammation, there will be greater antibiotic penetration (Table 35–5). Problems of CSF penetration may be overcome by direct instillation of antibiotics by intrathecal, intracisternal, or intraventricular routes of administration (Table 35–6).

Dexamethasone as an Adjunctive Treatment for Meningitis

- In addition to antibiotics, **dexamethasone** is a commonly used therapy for the treatment of pediatric meningitis. Dexamethasone may cause a significant improvement in CSF concentrations of glucose protein and lactate as well as a significantly lower incidence of neurologic sequela commonly associated with bacterial meningitis.
- The American Academy of Pediatrics suggests that the use of dexamethasone be considered for infants and children aged 2 months or older with pneumococcal meningitis and that it be given to those with *H. influenzae* meningitis. The commonly used intravenous (IV) dexamethasone dose is 0.15 mg/kg every 6 hours for 4 days. Alternatively, dexamethasone given 0.15 mg/kg every 6 hours for 2 days or 0.4 mg/kg every 12 hours for 2 days is equally effective and a potentially less toxic regimen.
- Dexamethasone should be administered prior to the first antibiotic dose, and serum hemoglobin and stool guaiac should be monitored for evidence of gastrointestinal (GI) bleeding.

Neisseria meningitidis (Meningococcus)

N. meningitidis meningitis is the leading cuase of bacterial meningitis in children and young adults in the United States. Most cases usually occur in the winter or spring, at a time when viral meningitis is relatively uncommon.

TABLE 35–2. Bacterial Meningitis: Most Likely and Empirical Therapy by Age Group

Age Commonly Affected	Most Likely Organisms	Empirical Therapy	Risk Factors for All Age Groups
Newborn–1 month	Gram-negative enterics[a] Group B *Streptococcus* *Listeria monocytogenes*	Ampicillin + cefotaxime or ceftriaxone or aminoglycoside	Respiratory tract infection Otitis media Mastoiditis Head trauma Alcoholism High-dose steroids
1 month–4 yr	*H. influenzea* *N. meningitidis* *S. pneumoniae*	Cefotaxime or ceftriaxone and vancomycin[b]	Splenectomy Sickle cell disease Immunoglobulin deficiency Immunosuppression
5–29 yr	*N. meningitidis* *S. pneumoniae* *H. influenzae*	Cefotaxime or ceftriaxone and vancomycin[b]	
30–60 yr	*S. pneumoniae* *N. meningitidis*	Cefotaxime or ceftriaxone and vancomycin[b]	
>60 yr	*S. pneumoniae* Gram-negative enterics *L. monocytogenes*	Ampicillin + cefotaxime or ceftriaxone or aminoglycoside and vancomycin[b]	

[a]*Escherichia coli, Klebsiella* spp., *Enterobacter* spp. common.
[b]Vancomycin use should be based on local incidence of penicillin-resistant *S. pneumoniae* and until cefotaxime or ceftriaxone minimum inhibitory concentration results are available.

Clinical Presentation

- Approximately 10 to 14 days after the onset of the disease and despite successful treatment, the patient develops a characteristic immunologic reaction of fever, arthritis (usually involving large joints), and pericarditis.
- The synovial fluid is characterized by a large number of polymorphonuclear cells, elevated protein concentrations, and sterile cultures.
- Deafness unilaterally, or more commonly bilaterally, may develop early or late in the disease course.
- Approximately 50% of patients with meningococcal meningitis have purpuric lesions, petechiae, or both. Patients may have an obvious or subclinical picture of DIC, which may progress to infarction of the adrenal glands and renal cortex and cause widespread thrombosis.

Treatment and Prevention

- Aggressive, early intervention with **high-dose IV crystalline penicillin G, 50,000 units/kg every 4 hours,** is usually recommended for treatment of *N. meningitidis* meningitis.
- **Chloramphenicol** may be used in place of penicillin G. Several third-generation cephalosporins (e.g., **cefotaxime, ceftizoxime, ceftriaxone, and cefuroxime**) approved for the treatment of meningitis are acceptable alternatives to penicillin G (see Table 35–4).
- Close contacts of patients contracting *N. meningitidis* meningitis are at an increased risk of developing meningitis. Prophylaxis of contacts should be started without delay and, therefore, without the aid of culture and sensitivity studies.

TABLE 35-3. Antimicrobial Agents of First Choice and Alternative Choice in the Treatment of Meningitis Caused by Gram-Positive Microorganisms

Organism	Antibiotic of First Choice[a]	Alternative Antibiotics[a]
Streptococcus pneumoniae		
Penicillin susceptible	Penicillin G 200,000–300,000 units/kg/day every 4 h IV; max: 4 million units every 4 h IV	Cefotaxime 200 mg/kg/day every 4–6 h IV; max: 2 g every 4 h Ceftriaxone 100 mg/kg/day every 12 h IV[b]; max: adults 2 g every 12 h Chloramphenicol[e] 100 mg/kg/day every 6 h; max: 1.5 g every 6 h
Penicillin resistant[c]	Cefotaxime or ceftriaxone and vancomycin[e] 30–40 mg/kg/day IV (60 mg/kg/day IV every 6 h[b])	Cefepime 50 mg/kg/dose every 12 h[b]; max: adult 2 g every 8 h IV Or meropenem 40 mg/kg every 8 h IV[b]; max: adults 1 g every 8 h IV with vancomycin[e] Linezolid 600 mg every 12 h IV[d]
Group B *streptococcus*	Penicillin ± gentamicin[e]	Ampicillin ± gentamicin[e] Cefotaxime Ceftriaxone Chloramphenicol[e]
Staphylococcus aureus		
Penicillin resistant	Nafcillin 200 mg/kg/day every 4 h IV; max: 2 g every 4 h IV	Vancomycin[e] Linezolid[d]
Methicillin resistant	Vancomycin[e]	
Staphylococcus epidermidis		
Penicillin resistant	Nafcillin	Vancomycin[e] Linezolid[d]
Methicillin resistant	Vancomycin[e]	
Listeria monocytogenes	Ampicillin 220–400 mg/kg/day, every 6 h IV or penicillin G max: 2 g every 4 h IV plus gentamicin[e]	Trimethoprim 10 mg/kg/day and sulfamethoxazole 50 mg/kg/day, every 6 h
Bacillus anthracis	A consensus regarding recommended agents for the treatment of CNS infections caused by anthrax or other biologic warfare agents has not been reached. Optimal treatment must be tailored to the particular pathogen and/or genetic variants of the pathogen	

[a]Recommended doses for adults and pediatric patients with normal renal and/or hepatic function.
[b]Pediatrics.
[c]Incidence of resistance is 20% to 45% worldwide.
[d]Clinical data are lacking, but linezolid may offer an alternative for the treatment of such infections.
[e]Monitor drug levels in serum.

TABLE 35–4. Antimicrobial Agents of First Choice and Alternative Choice in the Treatment of Meningitis Caused by Gram-Negative Microorganisms

Organism	Antibiotic of First Choice[a]	Alternative Antibiotics[a]
Neisseria meningitis (meningococcal)	Penicillin G 200,000–300,000 units/kg/day	Cefotaxime 200 mg/kg/day every 4 h; max: 2 g IV every 4 h Ceftriaxone 100 mg/kg/day every 24 h[b]; max: adults 2 g IV every 12 h Chloramphenicol[e] 100 mg/kg/day every 6 h; max: 1.5 g IV every 6 h
Escherichia coli	Cefotaxime or ceftriaxone	Cefepime 50 mg/kg/dose every 12 h[b]; max: adult 2 g every 8 h IV Meropenem 40 mg/kg every 8 h IV[b]; max: adults 1 g every 8 h IV
Hemophilus influenzae		
β-Lactamase positive	Cefotaxime	Ceftriaxone
β-Lactamase negative	Ampicillin 200–400 mg/kg/day every 6 h IV; max: 2 g every 4 h IV	Cefotaxime Ceftriaxone
Pseudomonas aeruginosa	Ceftazidime 85 mg/kg/day; max: 2 g IV every 6 h plus tobramycin[e] 5–7.5 mg/kg/day IV[c]	Meropenem Piperacillin 200–300 mg/kg/day; max: 3 g every 4 h IV plus tobramycin[e] Colistin sulfomethate[e] 5 mg/kg/day IV[d]
Enterobacteriaceae	Cefotaxime	Ceftriaxone Piperacillin plus aminoglycoside[e] Meropenem

[a]Recommended doses for adults and pediatric patients with normal renal and/or hepatic function.
[b]Pediatrics.
[c]Direct central nervous system administration may be added; see Table 35–6 for dosage.
[d]Should be reserved for multidrug-resistant pseudomonal or *Actinetobacter* infections for which all other therapeutic options have been exhausted.
[e]Monitor drug levels in serum.

- Adult patients should receive 600 mg of **rifampin** orally every 12 hours for 4 doses. Children 1 month to 12 years of age should receive 10 mg/kg of rifampin orally every 12 hours for 4 doses, and children younger than 1 month should receive 5 mg/kg orally every 12 hours for 4 doses.

Streptococcus pneumoniae (Pneumococcus or Diplococcus)

Pneumococcal meningitis occurs in the very young (less than 2 years of age) and the very old.

Treatment
See Table 35–3.

- The treatment of choice until susceptibility of the organism is known is the combination of **vancomycin** plus **ceftriaxone.** Penicillin may be used for drug-susceptible isolates with MICs of 0.06 mcg/mL or less. Treatment with IV **penicillin G** in adults with a penicillin-susceptible isolate and normal renal function usually results in a favorable outcome. However, a high percent of *S. pneumoniae* are either intermediately or highly resistant to penicillin.
- Vancomycin in combination with ceftriaxone is probably the most effective regimen for penicillin-resistant strains.

VIII

TABLE 35–5. Penetration of Antimicrobial Agents into the Cerebrospinal Fluid

Therapeutic Levels in CSF with or without Inflammation

Sulfonamides	Trimethoprim
Choramphenicol	Isoniazid
Rifampin	Pyrazinamide
Ethionamide	Cycloserine
Metronidazole	

Therapeutic Levels in CSF with Inflammation of Meninges

Penicillin G	Ampicillin ± sulbactam
Carbenicillin	Ticarcillin ± clavulanic acid
Nafcillin	Mezlocillin
Piperacillin	Cefuroxime
Cefotaxime	Ceftizoxime
Ceftriaxone	Ceftazidime
Imipenem	Aztreonam
Meropenem	Ofloxacin
Vancomycin	Ciprofloxacin
Vidarabine	Ethambutol
Flucytosine	Fluconazole
Pyrimethamine	Ganciclovir
Acyclovir	Foscarnet
Linezolid	Quinupristin/dalfopristin
Colistin	

Nontherapeutic Levels in CSF with or without Inflammation

Aminoglycosides	First-generation cephalosporins
Cefoperazone	Second-generation cephalosporins[a]
Clindamycin[b]	Ketoconazole
Amphotericin B	Itraconazole[c]

[a]Cefuroxime is an exception.
[b]Achieves therapeutic brain tissue concentrations.
[c]Achieves therapeutic concentrations for *Cryptococcus neoformans* therapy.
CSF, cerebrospinal fluid.

VIII

TABLE 35–6. Intraventricular and Intrathecal Antibiotic Dosage Recommendation

Antibiotic	Dose (mg)	Expected CSF Concentration[a] (mg/L)	Reference
Ampicillin	10–50	60–300	104–106
Methicillin	25–100	160–600	104–106
Nafcillin	75	500	105
Cephalothin	25–100	160–600	104–106
Chloramphenicol	25–100	160–600	104, 106, 107
Gentamicin	1–10	6–60	104–108
Quinupristin/dalfopristin	1–2	7–13	109
Tobramycin	1–10	6–60	108
Vancomycin	5	30	110–112
Amphotericin B	0.05–0.25 mg/day to 0.05–1 mg 1–3 times weekly	—	113

[a]Assumes adult CSF volume = 150 mL. CSF, cerebrospinal fluid.

- **Ceftriaxone** and **cefotaxime** may be used for penicillin-sensitive or intermediate-resistant isolates.
- Virtually all serotypes of *S. pneumoniae* exhibiting intermediate or complete resistance to penicillin are found in the current **23 serotype pneumococcal vaccine.** A heptavalent conjugate vaccine is available for use in infants between 2 months and 9 years of age. Current recommendations are for all healthy infants younger than 2 years of age to be immunized with the heptavalent vaccine at 2, 4, 6, and 12 to 15 months.

Gram-Negative Bacillary Meningitis
Currently, gram-negative bacteria are the fourth leading cause of meningitis.

Treatment
See Table 35–4.

- Optimal antibiotic therapies for gram-negative bacillary meningitis have not been fully defined. Meningitis caused by *Pseudomonas aeruginosa* is initially treated with **ceftazidime** or **piperacillin, cefepime** or **meropenem** plus an aminoglycoside, usually **tobramycin.**
- If the pseudomonad is suspected to be antibiotic resistant or becomes resistant during therapy, an intraventricular aminoglycoside (preservative-free) should be considered along with IV aminoglycoside. Intraventricular aminoglycoside dosages are adjusted to the estimated CSF volume (0.03 mg of tobramycin or **gentamicin** per mL of CSF and 0.1 mg of **amikacin** per mL of CSF every 24 hours). Ventricular levels of aminoglycoside are monitored every 2 or 3 days, just prior to the next intraventricular dose, and "trough levels" should approximate 2 to 10 mg/L.
- Gram-negative organisms, other than *P. aeruginosa,* that cause meningitis can also be treated with a third-generation cephalosporin such as **cefotaxime, ceftriaxone,** or **ceftazidime.** In adults, daily doses of 8 to 12 g/day of these third-generation cephalosporins or 2 g of ceftriaxone twice daily should produce CSF concentrations of 5 to 20 mg/L.
- Therapy for gram-negative meningitis is continued for a minimum of 21 days. CSF cultures may remain positive for several days or more on a regimen that will eventually be curative.

Haemophilus influenzae
In the past, *H. influenzae* was the most common cause of meningitis in children 6 months to 3 years of age, but this has declined dramatically since the introduction of effective vaccines. The disease is often a complication of primary infectious involvement of the middle ear, paranasal sinuses, or lungs.

Treatment
Approximately 30% to 40% of *H. influenzae* are ampicillin resistant. For this reason, many clinicians use a third-generation cephalosporin (**cefotaxime** or **ceftriaxone**) or **chloramphenicol with ampicillin** for initial antimicrobial therapy. Once bacterial susceptibilities are available, ampicillin may be used if the isolate proves ampicillin sensitive.

Prevention
- Secondary cases may occur within 30 days of the index case, and so treatment of close contacts (household members, individuals sharing sleeping quarters, crowded confined populations, day care attendees, and nursing home residents) of patients is usually recommended. The goal of prophylaxis is to eliminate nasopharyngeal and oropharyngeal carriage of *H. influenzae.*

VIII

- Prophylaxis of close contacts should be started only after consultation with the local health department. In general, children should receive 20 mg/kg (maximum 600 mg) and adults 600 mg daily in one dose for 4 days. Fully vaccinated individuals should not receive prophylaxis.
- Vaccination with *H. influenzae* type b (HIB) conjugate vaccines is usually begun in children at 2 months.
- The vaccine should be considered in patients older than 5 years with sickle cell disease, asplenia, or immunocompromising diseases.

Listeria monocytogenes

L. monocytogenes is a gram-positive diphtheroid-like organism and is responsible for 8% of all reported cases of meningitis. The disease affects primarily neonates, alcoholics, immunocompromised patients, and the elderly.

Treatment

- The combination of **penicillin G** or **ampicillin** with an aminoglycoside results in a bactericidal effect. Patients should be treated for 2 to 3 weeks after defervescence to prevent the possibility of relapse.
- **Trimethoprim-sulfamethoxazole** may be an effective alternative because adequate CSF penetration is achieved with these agents.

VIII

Mycobacterium tuberculosis

M. tuberculosis var. *hominis* is the primary cause of tuberculous meningitis. Tuberculous meningitis may exist in the absence of disease in the lung or extrapulmonary sites. Upon initial examination, CSF usually contains 100 to 1000 WBC/mm^3, which may be 75% to 80% polymorphonuclear cells. Over time, the pattern of WBCs in the CSF will shift to lymphocytes and monocytes.

Treatment

- **Isoniazid** is the mainstay in virtually any regimen to treat *M. tuberculosis.* In children, the usual dose of isoniazid is 10 to 20 mg/kg/day (maximum 300 mg/day). Adults usually receive 5 to 10 mg/kg/day or a daily dose of 300 mg.
- Supplemental doses of **pyridoxine hydrochloride (vitamin B$_6$)**, 50 mg/day, are recommended to prevent the peripheral neuropathy associated with isoniazid administration.
- The CDC recommends a regimen of four drugs for empiric treatment of *M. tuberculosis.* This regimen should consist of **isoniazid, rifampin, pyrazinamide,** and **ethambutol,** 15 to 20 mg/kg/day (maximum 1.6 g/day)for the first 2 months generally followed by isoniazid plus rifampin for the duration of therapy.
- Concurrent administration of rifampin is recommended at doses of 10 to 20 mg/kg/day (maximum 600 mg/day) for children and 600 mg/day for adults. The addition of pyrazinamide (children and adults, 15 to 30 mg/kg/day; maximum in both, 2 g/day) to the regimen of isoniazid and rifampin is now recommended. The duration of concomitant pyrazinamide therapy should be limited to 2 months to avoid hepatotoxicity.
- Patients with *M. tuberculosis* meningitis should be treated for a duration of 9 months or longer with multiple-drug therapy, and patients with rifampin-resistant strains should receive 18 to 24 months of therapy.
- The use of glucocorticoids for tuberculous meningitis remains controversial. The administration of steroids such as oral **prednisone,** 60 to 80 mg/day, or 0.2 mg/kg/day of IV **dexamethasone,** tapered over 4 to 8 weeks, improve neurologic suquelae and survival in adults and decrease mortality, long-term neurologic complications, and permanent sequelae in children.

Cryptococcus neoformans

- In the United States, cryptococcal meningitis is the most common form of fungal meningitis and is a major cause of morbidity and mortality in immuno-suppressed patients.
- Fever and a history of headaches are the most common symptoms of crypto-coccal meningitis, although altered mentation and evidence of focal neurologic deficits may be present. Diagnosis is based on the presence of a positive CSF, blood, sputum, or urine culture for *C. neoformans.*
- CSF cultures are positive in greater than 90% of cases.

Treatment

- **Amphotericin B** is the drug of choice for treatment of acute *C. neoformans* meningitis. Amphotericin B, 0.5 to 1 mg/kg/day, combined with **flucytosine,** 100 mg/kg/day, is more effective than amphotericin alone. In the AIDS popu-lation, flucytosine is often poorly tolerated, causing bone marrow suppression and GI distress.
- Due to the high relapse rate following acute therapy for *C. neoformans,* AIDS patients require lifelong maintenance or suppressive therapy. The standard of care for AIDS-associated cryptococcal meningitis is primary therapy, generally using amphotericin B with or without flucytosine followed by maintenance therapy with fluconazole for the life of the patient.

Viral Meningitis

- Meningitis is typically characterized as being either purulent or aseptic. While purulent meningitis refers to a bacterial etiology, aseptic meningitis historically was defined by diagnosis of exclusion.
- Common signs in adults include headache, mild fever (less than 40°C), nuchal rigidity, malaise, drowsiness, nausea, vomiting, and photophobia. Only fever and irritability may be evident in the infant, and meningitis must be ruled out as a cause of fever when no other localized findings are observed in a child.
- Laboratory examination of CSF usually reveals a pleocytosis with 100 to 1000 WBCs/mm^3, which are primarily lymphocytic; however, 20% to 75% of pa-tients with viral meningitis may have a predominance of polymorphonuclear cells on initial examination of the CSF, especially in enteroviral meningitis.

Treatment

- **Acyclovir** is the drug of choice for herpes simplex encephalitis. In patients with normal renal function, acyclovir is usually administered as 10 mg/kg every 8 hours for 2 to 3 weeks. Herpes virus resistance to acyclovir has been reported with increasing incidence, particularly from immunocompromised patients with prior or chronic exposures to acyclovir.
- The alternative treatment for acyclovir-resistant herpes simplex virus is **fos-carnet,** which must be individualized for renal function.

See Chapter 105, Central Nervous System Infections, authored by Elizabeth D. Hermsen and John C. Rotschafer, for a more detailed discussion of this topic.

Chapter 36

▶ ENDOCARDITIS

▶ DEFINITION

Endocarditis is an inflammation of the endocardium, the membrane lining the chambers of the heart and covering the cusps of the heart valves. Infective endocarditis (IE) refers to infection of the heart valves by microorganisms.

Endocarditis is often referred to as either acute or subacute depending on the clinical presentation. Acute bacterial endocarditis is a fulminating infection associated with high fevers, systemic toxicity, and death within a few days to weeks if untreated. Subacute infectious endocarditis is a more indolent infection, usually occurring in a setting of prior valvular heart disease.

▶ PATHOPHYSIOLOGY

- Most patients with IE have risk factors, such as preexisting cardiac valve abnormalities.
- Most types of structural heart disease resulting in turbulence of blood flow will increase the risk for IE. Some of the most important include the following:
  - Presence of a prosthetic valve (400-fold increased risk)
  - Previous endocarditis (400-fold increased risk)
  - Complex cyanotic congenital heart disease (e.g., single ventricle states)
  - Surgically constructed systemic pulmonary shunts or conduits
  - Acquired valvular dysfunction (e.g., rheumatic heart disease)
  - Hypertrophic cardiomyopathy
  - Mitral valve prolapse with regurgitation
  - Intravenous drug abuse
- Three groups of organisms cause most cases of IE: streptococci (55% to 62%), staphylococci (25% to 35%), and enterococci (5% to 18%) (Table 36–1).

▶ CLINICAL PRESENTATION

- The clinical presentation of patients with IE is highly variable and nonspecific (Table 36–2).

TABLE 36–1. Etiologic Organisms in Infective Endocarditis

Agent	Percentage of Cases
Streptococci	55–62
Viridans streptococci	30–40
Other streptococci	15–25
Staphylococci	20–35
Coagulase-positive	10–27
Coagulase-negative	1–3
Enterococci	5–18
Gram-negative aerobic bacilli	1.5–13
Fungi	2–4
Miscellaneous bacteria	<5
Mixed Infections	1–2
"Culture negative"	<5–24

TABLE 36–2. Clinical Presentation of Infective Endocarditis

General

The clinical presentation of IE is highly variable and nonspecific.

Symptoms

The patient may complain of fever, chills, weakness, dyspnea, night sweats, weight loss, and/or malaise.

Signs

Fever is common as well as a heart murmur (sometimes new or changing). The patient may or may not have embolic phenomenon, spleanomegaly, or skin manifestations (e.g., Osler nodes, Janeway lesions).

Laboratory Tests

The patient's WBC count may be normal or only slightly elevated. Nonspecific findings include anemia (normocytic, normochromic), thrombocytopenia, an elevated erythrocyte sedimentation rate or C-reactive protein, and altered urinary analysis (proteinuria/microscopic hematuria).

The hallmark laboratory finding is continuous bacteremia; three sets of blood cultures should be collected over 24 h.

Other Diagnostic Tests

An electrocardiogram, chest radiograph, and echocardiogram are commonly performed. Echocardiography to determine the presence of valvular vegetations plays a key role in the diagnosis of IE; it should be performed in all suspected cases.

- Important clinical signs, especially prevalent in subacute illness, may include the following peripheral manifestations ("stigmata") of endocarditis:
  - Osler nodes
  - Janeway lesions
  - Splinter hemorrhages
  - Petechiae
  - Clubbing of the fingers
  - Roth spots
  - Emboli
- Without appropriate antimicrobial therapy and surgery IE is usually fatal. With proper management, recovery can be expected in most patients.
- Factors associated with increased mortality include the following:
  - Congestive heart failure
  - Culture-negative endocarditis
  - Endocarditis caused by resistant organisms such as fungi and gram-negative bacteria
  - Left-sided endocarditis caused by *Staphylococcus aureus*
  - Prosthetic valve endocarditis

LABORATORY AND DIAGNOSTIC FINDINGS

- The hallmark of IE is a continuous bacteremia caused by shedding of bacteria from the vegetation into the bloodstream. More than 95% of patients with IE have a positive blood culture when three samples are obtained during a 24-hour period.
- Transesophageal echocardiography (TEE) is important in identifying and localizing valvular lesions in patients suspected of having IE. TEE is more sensitive for detecting vegetations (90% to 100%), compared to transthoracic echocardiography (TTE) (58% to 63%).
- The Modified Duke criteria, encompassing major findings of persistent bacteremia and echocardiographic findings and other minor findings, are used to categorize patients as "definite IE" or "possible IE."

▶ DESIRED OUTCOME

- Relieve the signs and symptoms of disease
- Decrease morbidity and mortality associated with infection
- Eradicate the causative organism with minimal drug exposure
- Provide cost-effective antimicrobial therapy
- Prevent IE in high-risk patients with appropriate antimicrobials

▶ TREATMENT

GENERAL PRINCIPLES

- The most important approach to treatment of IE includes isolation of the infecting pathogen and determination of antimicrobial susceptibilities, followed by high-dose, bactericidal antibiotics for an extended period.
- For most patients 4 to 6 weeks of therapy are required.
- Specific recommendations for treating IE caused by the most common organisms are discussed in this chapter.
- β-Lactam antimicrobials, such as penicillin G, nafcillin, and ampicillin, remain the drugs of choice for streptococcal, staphylococcal, and enterococcal VIII ◀ endocarditis, respectively.
- For some pathogens, such as enterococci, the use of synergistic antimicrobial combinations (including an aminoglycoside) is essential to obtain a bactericidal effect.

NONPHARMACOLOGIC THERAPY

- Surgery is an important adjunct to management of endocarditis in certain patients. In most cases, valvectomy and valve replacement are performed to remove infected tissues and restore hemodynamic function. The most important indications for surgical intervention in the past have been heart failure in left-sided IE and persistent infections in right-sided IE.

STREPTOCOCCAL ENDOCARDITIS

- Viridans streptococci (*Streptococcus mutans, S. sanguis,* and *S. mitis*) are common cause of IE, especially in cases involving native valves. *S. bovis* is not a viridans streptococcus but is included here because it is penicillin sensitive and treatment regimens are the same as for viridans streptococci.
- Most viridans streptococci are exquisitely sensitive to penicillin G with minimal inhibitory concentrations (MICs) less than or equal to 0.1 mcg/mL. The MIC should be determined for all viridans streptococci and the results used to guide therapy. Approximately 10% to 20% are moderately susceptible (MIC 0.1 to 0.5 mcg/mL).
- Recommended therapy in the uncomplicated case caused by fully susceptible strains is 4 weeks of either high-dose **penicillin G** or **ceftriaxone,** or 2 weeks of combined therapy with high-dose penicillin G plus an aminoglycoside (Table 36–3).
- The following conditions should all be present to consider a 2-week treatment regimen:
  - The isolate is penicillin sensitive (MIC less than or equal to 0.1 mcg/mL)
  - There are no cardiovascular risk factors such as heart failure, aortic insufficiency, or conduction abnormalities
  - No evidence of thrombotic disease
  - Native valve infection

TABLE 36-3. Suggested Regimens for Therapy of Native-Valve Endocarditis Due to Penicillin-Susceptible Viridans Streptococci and *Streptococcus bovis* (Minimum Inhibitory Concentration ≤0.1 mcg/mL)[a]

Antibiotic	Dosage and Route	Duration (wks)	Comments
Aqueous crystalline penicillin G sodium	12–18 million units/24 h IV either continuously or in six equally divided doses	4	Preferred in most patients older than 65 years and in those with impairment of the eighth nerve or renal function
or			
Ceftriaxone sodium	2 g once daily IV or IM[b]	4	
Aqueous crystalline penicillin G sodium	12–18 million units/24 h IV either continuously or in six equally divided doses	2	
With gentamicin sulfate[c]	1 mg/kg IM or IV every 8 h	2	When obtained 1 h after a 20–30 min IV infusion or IM injection, serum concentration of gentamicin of approximately 3 mcg/mL is desirable; trough concentration should be <1 mcg/mL.
Vancomycin hydrochloride[d]	30 mg/kg per 24 h IV in two equally divided doses, not to exceed 2 g/24 h unless serum levels are monitored	4	Vancomycin therapy is recommended for patients allergic to β-lactams (see text regarding drug levels); according to the guidelines, serum concentrations of vancomycin should be obtained 1 h after completion of the infusion and should be in the range of 30–45 mcg/mL for twice-daily dosing

[a]Dosages recommended are for patients with normal renal function. For nutritionally variant streptococci, see Table 36-7. IV = intravenous; IM = intramuscular.

[b]Patients should be informed that IM injection of ceftriaxone is painful.

[c]Dosing of gentamicin on a mg/kg basis will produce higher serum concentrations in obese patients than in lean patients. Therefore, in obese patients, dosing should be based on ideal body weight. (Ideal body weight for men is 50 kg + 2.3 kg/inch over 5 feet, and ideal body weight for women is 45.5 kg + 2.3 kg/inch over 5 feet.) Relative contraindications to the use of gentamicin are age > 65 yr, renal impairment, or impairment of the eighth nerve. Other potentially nephrotoxic agents (e.g., nonsteroidal anti-inflammatory drugs) should be used cautiously in patients receiving gentamicin.

[d]Vancomycin dosage should be reduced in patients with impaired renal function. Each dose of vancomycin should be infused over at least 1 h to reduce the risk of the histamine-release "red man" syndrome.

From Wilson WR, Karchmer AW, Dajani AS, et al. *Antibiotic treatment of adults with infective endocarditis due to streptococci, enterococci, and staphylococci, and HACEK microorganisms. JAMA* 1995;274:1706–1713, with permission. Copyright 1995–1997, American Medical Association.

- No vegetation greater than 5 mm diameter
- Clinical response is evident within 7 days.
- **Vancomycin** is effective and is the drug of choice for the patient with a history of immediate-type hypersensitivity reaction to penicillin.
- For patients with complicated infection or when the organism is relatively resistant (MIC = 0.1 to 0.5 μg/mL), combination therapy with penicillin and an aminoglycoside is recommended for 2 weeks followed by penicillin alone for an additional 2 weeks (Table 36–4).

STAPHYLOCOCCAL ENDOCARDITIS

- *Staphylococcus aureus* is the most common organism causing IE both among IV drug abusers and in persons with venous catheters. Coagulase-negative staphylococci (CNST, usually *S. epidermidis*) are prominent causes of prosthetic valve endocarditis (PVE).
- Management requires consideration of several factors:
  - Is the organism methicillin resistant?
  - Should combination therapy be used?
  - Is the infection on a native valve or a prosthetic valve?
  - Is the patient an intravenous drug abuser?
  - Is the infection on the left or right side of the heart?
- The recommended therapy for patients with left-sided IE caused by methicillin-sensitive *S. aureus* (MSSA) is 4 to 6 weeks of **nafcillin** or **oxacillin,** often combined with a short course of gentamicin (Table 36–5).
- If a patient has a mild, delayed allergy to penicillin, **first-generation cephalosporins** are effective alternatives but should be avoided in patients with an immediate-type hypersensitivity reaction.
- In a patient with appositive penicillin skin test or a history of immediate hypersensitivity to penicillin, **vancomycin** is the agent of choice. Vancomycin, however, kills *S. aureus* slowly and is generally regarded as inferior to penicillinase-resistant penicillins for MSSA.
- **Rifampin** may be added to vancomycin in refractory or complicated infections in patients with left-sided IE and, in some cases, addition of rifampin appeared to result in dramatic patient improvement.
- **Vancomycin** is the drug of choice for methicillin-resistant staphylococci since most methicillin-resistant *S. aureus* (MRSA) and most CNST are susceptible (see Table 36–5).

Treatment of Staphylococcus Endocarditis in Intravenous
Drug Abusers
- IE in IV drug abusers is most frequently (60% to 70%) caused by *S. aureus,* although other organisms may be more common in certain geographic locations.
- Standard treatment for MSSA consists of 4 weeks of therapy with a **penicillinase-resistant penicillin** (see Table 36–5).
- A 2-week course of **nafcillin** or **oxacillin** plus an aminoglycoside may be effective.
- Short-course vancomycin, in place of nafcillin or oxacillin appears to be ineffective.

PROSTHETIC VALVE ENDOCARDITIS

- PVE that occurs within 2 months of cardiac surgery is usually caused by staphylococci implanted at the time of surgery. Methicillin-resistant organisms are common. Vancomycin is the cornerstone of therapy.

VIII

TABLE 36-4. Therapy for Native-Valve Endocarditis Due to Strains of Viridans Streptococci and *Streptococcus bovis* Relatively Resistant to Penicillin G (Minimum Inhibitory Concentration >0.1 mcg/mL and <0.5 mcg/mL)[a]

Antibiotic	Dosage and Route	Duration (wks)	Comments
Aqueous crystalline penicillin G sodium	18 million units/24 h IV either continuously or in 6 equally divided doses	4	Cefazolin or other first-generation cephalosporins may be substituted for penicillin in patients whose penicillin hypersensitivity is not of the immediate type
With gentamicin sulfate[b]	1 mg/kg IM or IV every 8 h	2	
Vancomycin hydrochloride[c]	30 mg/kg per 24 h IV in two equally divided doses, not to exceed 2 g/24 h unless serum levels are monitored	4	Vancomycin therapy is recommended for patients allergic to β lactams

[a]Dosages recommended are for patients with normal renal function. IV = intravenous; IM = intramuscular.

[b]For specific dosing adjustment and issues concerning gentamicin, see Table 36–3 footnotes.

[c]For specific dosing adjustment and issues concerning vancomycin, see Table 36–3 footnotes.

From Wilson WR, Karchmer AW, Dajani AS, et al. Antibiotic treatment of adults with infective endocarditis due to streptococci, enterococci, and staphylococci, and HACEK microorganisms. JAMA 1995;274:1706–1713, with permission. Copyright 1995–1997, American Medical Association.

TABLE 36–5. Therapy for Endocarditis Due to Staphylococcus in the Absence of Prosthetic Material[a]

Antibiotic	Dosage and Route	Duration (wk)	Comments
Methicillin-Susceptible Staphylococci			
Regimens for non-β-lactam-allergic patients			
Nafcillin sodium or oxacillin sodium	2 g IV every 4 h	4–6	Benefit of additional aminoglycosides has not been established
With optional addition of gentamicin sulfate[†]	1 mg/kg IM or IV every 8 h	3–5 days	
Regimens for β-lactam-allergic patients Cefazolin (or other first-generation cephalosporins in equivalent dosages)	2 g IV every 8 h	4–6	Cephalosporins should be avoided in patients with immediate type hypersensitivity to penicillin
With optional addition of gentamicin[b]	1 mg/kg IM or IV every 8 h	3–5 days	
Vancomycin hydrochloride[c]	30 mg/kg per 24 h IV in two equally divided doses, not to exceed 2g/24 h unless serum levels are monitored	4–6	Recommended for patients allergic to penicillin
Methicillin-Resistant Staphylococci			
Vancomycin hydrochloride[c]	30 mg/kg per 24 h IV in two equally divided doses, not to exceed 2 g/24 h unless serum levels are monitored	4–6	

[a]For treatment of endocarditis due to penicillin-susceptible staphylococci (minimum inhibitory concentration ≤0.1 μg/mL), aqueous crystalline penicillin G sodium (Table 36–3, first regimen) can be used for 4 to 6 wk instead of nafcillin or oxacillin. Shorter antibiotic courses have been effective in some drug addicts with right-sided endocarditis due to Staphylococcus aureus (see text). See text for comments on use of rifampin. IV, intravenous; IM, intramuscular.

[b]For specific dosing adjustment and issues concerning gentamicin, see Table 36–3 footnotes.

[c]For specific dosing adjustment and issues concerning vancomycin, see Table 36–3 footnotes.

From Wilson WR, Karchmer AW, Dajani AS, et al. Antibiotic treatment of adults with infective endocarditis due to streptococci, enterococci, and staphylococci, and HACEK microorganisms. JAMA 1995;274:1706–1713, with permission. Copyright 1995–1997, American Medical Association.

- Because of the high morbidity and mortality associated with PVE and refractoriness to therapy, combinations of antimicrobials are usually recommended.
- For methicillin-resistant staphylococci (both MRSA and CNST), **vancomycin** is used with **rifampin** for 6 weeks or more (Table 36–6). An **aminoglycoside** is added for the first 2 weeks if the organism is susceptible.
- For methicillin-susceptible staphylococci, a **penicillinase-stable penicillin** is used in place of vancomycin.

ENTEROCOCCAL ENDOCARDITIS

- Enterococci cause 5% to 18% of endocarditis cases and are noteworthy for the following reasons: (1) no single antibiotic is bactericidal; (2) MICs to penicillin are relatively high (1 to 25 mcg/mL); (3) they are intrinsically resistant to all cephalosporins and relatively resistant to aminoglycosides (i.e., "low-level" aminoglycoside resistance); (4) combinations of a cell wall–active agent, such as a penicillin or vancomycin, plus an aminoglycoside are necessary for killing; (5) resistance to all available drugs is increasing.
- Enterococcal endocarditis ordinarily requires 4 to 6 weeks of high-dose **penicillin G** or **ampicillin,** plus an **aminoglycoside** for cure (Table 36–7). A 6-week course is recommended for patients with symptoms lasting longer than 3 months, recurrent cases, and patients with mitral valve involvement.
- In addition to isolates with high-level aminoglycoside resistance, β-lactamase-producing enterococci (especially *Enterococcus faecium*) are increasingly reported. If these organisms are discovered, use of vancomycin or ampicillin-sulbactam should be considered.
- Vancomycin-resistant enterococci, particularly *E. faecium*, are becoming more common.

GRAM-NEGATIVE BACILLI

- Endocarditis caused by gram-negative bacilli is relatively uncommon, although the incidence may be increasing. Patients at higher risk include IV drug abusers and those with prosthetic valves.
- The organism most commonly associated with gram-negative rod endocarditis in IV drug abusers is *Pseudomonas aeruginosa*. Other gram-negative bacilli causing IE include *Salmonella* spp., *Escherichia coli, Citrobacter* spp., *Klebsiella-Enterobacter* spp., *Serratia marcescens, Proteus* spp., and *Providencia* spp. Generally, these infections have a poor prognosis, with mortality rates as high as 60% to 80%.
- If medical management is implemented, large doses of a penicillin with activity against *Pseudomonas* (e.g. piperacillin 18 g/day) combined with an aminoglycosdie are necessary for an extended period (6 weeks).

▶ EVALUATION OF THERAPEUTIC OUTCOMES

- The evaluation of patients treated for IE includes assessment of signs and symptoms, blood cultures, microbiologic tests (e.g., MIC, minimum bactericidal concentration [MBC], or serum bactericidal titers), serum drug concentrations, and other tests to evaluate organ function.
- Persistence of fever may indicate ineffective antimicrobial therapy, emboli, infections of intravascular catheters, or a drug reaction. In some patients, low-grade fever may persist even with appropriate antimicrobial therapy.
- With effective therapy, blood cultures should be negative within a few days, although microbiological response to vancomycin may be unusually slower.

VIII

TABLE 36-6. Treatment of Staphylococcal Endocarditis in the Presence of a Prosthetic Valve or Other Prosthetic Material[a]

Antibiotic	Dosage and Route	Duration (wks)	Comments
Regimen for Methicillin-Resistant Staphylococci			
Vancomycin hydrochloride[b]	30 mg/kg/24 h IV in 2 or 4 equally divided doses, not to exceed 2 g/24 h unless serum levels are monitored	≥6	
With rifampin[c]	300 mg orally every 8 h	≥6	Rifampin increases the amount of warfarin sodium required for antithrombotic therapy.
And with gentamicin sulfate[d],[e]	1 mg/kg IM or IV every 8 h	2	
Regimen for Methicillin-Susceptible Staphylococci			
Nafcillin sodium or oxacillin sodium	2 g IV every 4 h	≥6	First-generation cephalosporins or vancomycin should be used in patients allergic to β lactam.
With rifampin[c]	300 mg orally every 8 h	≥6	Cephalosporins should be avoided in patients with immediate-type hypersensitivity to penicillin or with methicillin-resistant staphylococci.
And with gentamicin sulfate[d],[e]	1 mg/kg IM or IV every 8 h	2	

[a]Dosages recommended are for patients with normal renal function. IV = intravenous; IM = intramuscular.
[b]For specific dosing adjustment and issues concerning vancomycin, see Table 36–3 footnotes.
[c]Rifampin plays a unique role in the eradication of staphylococcal infection involving prosthetic material (see text); combination therapy is essential to prevent emergence of rifampin resistance.
[d]For specific dosing adjustment and issues concerning gentamicin, see Table 36–3 footnotes.
[e]Use during initial 2 wk.
From Wilson WR, Karchmer AW, Dajani AS, et al. Antibiotic treatment of adults with infective endocarditis due to streptococci, enterococci, and staphylococci, and HACEK microorganisms. JAMA 1995;274:1706–1713, with permission. Copyright 1995–1997, American Medical Association.

TABLE 36-7. Standard Therapy for Endocarditis Due to Enterococci[a]

Antibiotic	Dosage and Route	Duration (wks)	Comments
Aqueous crystalline penicillin G sodium	18–30 million units/24 h IV either continuously or in 6 equally divided doses	4–6	Four-week therapy recommended for patients with symptoms <3 months in duration; 6-wk therapy recommended for patients with symptoms >3 months in duration
With gentamicin sulfate[b]	1 mg/kg IM or IV every 8 h	4–6	
Ampicillin sodium	12 g/24 h IV either continuously or in six equally divided doses	4–6	
With gentamicin sulfate[b]	1 mg/kg IM or IV every 8 h	4–6	
Vancomycin hydrochloride[c]	30 mg/kg per 24 h in two equally divided doses, not to exceed 2 g/24 h unless serum levels are monitored	4–6	Vancomycin therapy is recommended for patients allergic to β lactams; cephalosporins are not acceptable alternatives for patients allergic to penicillin
With gentamicin sulfate[b]	1 mg/kg IM or IV every 8 h	4–6	

[a]All enterococci causing endocarditis must be tested for antimicrobial susceptibility in order to select optimal therapy (see text). This table is for endocarditis due to gentamicin- or vancomycin-susceptible enterococci; viridans streptococci with a minimum inhibitory concentration of >0.5 mcg/mL, nutritionally variant viridans streptococci, or prosthetic valve endocarditis caused by viridans streptococci or *Streptococcus bovis*. Antibiotic dosages are for patients with normal renal function. IV = intravenous; IM = intramuscular.

[b]For specific dosing adjustment and issues concerning gentamicin, see Table 36–3 footnotes.

[c]For specific dosing adjustment and issues concerning vancomycin, see Table 36–3 footnotes.

From Wilson WR, Karchmer AW, Dajani AS, et al. Antibiotic treatment of adults with infective endocarditis due to streptococci, enterococci, and staphylococci, and HACEK microorganisms. *JAMA 1995;274:1706–1713, with permission. Copyright 1995–1997, American Medical Association.*

TABLE 36–8. Cardiac Conditions Associated with Endocarditis

Endocarditis Prophylaxis Recommended
High-risk category
    Prosthetic cardiac valves, including biprosthetic and homograft valves
    Previous bacterial endocarditis
    Complex cyanotic congenital heart disease (e.g., single ventricle states, transposition of the great
        arteries, tetralogy of Fallot)
    Surgically constructed systemic pulmonary shunts or conduits
Moderate-risk category
    Most other congenital cardiac malformations (other than above and below)
    Acquired valvular dysfunction (e.g., rheumatic heart disease)
    Hypertrophic cardiomyopathy
    Mitral valve prolapse with valvar regurgitation and/or thickened leaflets
Endocarditis Prophylaxis Not Recommended
Negligible-risk category (no greater risk than the general population)
    Isolated secundum atrial septal defect
    Surgical repair of atrial septal defect, ventricular septal defect, or patent ductus arteriosus (without
        residua beyond 6 months)
    Previous coronary artery bypass graft surgery
    Mitral valve prolapse without valvar regurgitation
    Physiologic, functional, or innocent heart murmurs
    Previous Kawasaki disease without valvar dysfunction
    Previous rheumatic fever without valvar dysfunction
    Cardiac pacemakers (intravascular and epicardial) and implanted defibrillators

VIII

From Dajani AS, Taubert KA, Wilson W, et al. Prevention of bacterial endocarditis: Recommendations by the American Heart Association. JAMA 1997;277:1794–1801, with permission. Copyright 1995–1997, American Medical Association.

TABLE 36–9. Dental Procedures and Endocarditis Prophylaxis

Endocarditis Prophylaxis Recommended[a]
Dental extractions
Periodontal procedures including surgery, scaling and root planing, probing, and recall maintenance
Dental implant placement and reimplantation of avulsed teeth
Endodontic (root canal) instrumentation or surgery only beyond the apex
Subgingival placement of antibiotic fibers or strips
Initial placement of orthodontic bands but not brackets
Intraligamentary local anesthetic injections
Prophylactic cleaning of teeth or implants where bleeding is anticipated
Endocarditis Prophylaxis Not Recommended
Restorative dentistry[b] (operative and prosthodontic) with or without retraction cord[c]
Local anesthetic injections (nonintraligamentary)
Intracanal endodontic treatment; after placement and buildup
Placement of rubber dams
Postoperative suture removal
Placement of removable prosthodontic or orthodontic appliances
Taking of oral impressions
Fluoride treatments
Taking of oral radiographs
Orthodontic appliance adjustment
Shedding of primary teeth

[a]Prophylaxis is recommended for patients with high- and moderate-risk cardiac conditions.
[b]This includes restoration of decayed teeth (filling cavities) and replacement of missing teeth.
[c]Clinical judgment may indicate antibiotic use in selected circumstances that may create significant bleeding.
From Dajani AS, Taubert KA, Wilson W, et al. Prevention of bacterial endocarditis: Recommendations by the American Heart Association. JAMA 1997;277:1794–1801, with permission. Copyright 1995–1997, American Medical Association.

TABLE 36–10. Other Procedures and Endocarditis Prophylaxis

Endocarditis Prophylaxis Recommended
Respiratory tract
    Tonsillectomy and/or adenoidectomy
    Surgical operations that involve respiratory mucosa
    Bronchoscopy with a rigid bronchoscope
Gastrointestinal tract[a]
    Sclerotherapy for esophageal varices
    Esophageal stricture dilation
    Endoscopic retrograde cholangiography with biliary obstruction
    Biliary tract surgery
    Surgical operations that involve intestinal mucosa
Genitourinary tract
    Prostatic surgery
    Cystoscopy
    Urethral dilation

Endocarditis Prophylaxis Not Recommended
Respiratory tract
    Endotracheal intubation
    Bronchoscopy with a flesible bronchoscope, with or without biopsy[b]
    Tympanostomy tube insertion
Gastrointestinal tract
    Transesophageal echocardiography[b]
    Endoscopy with or without gastrointestinal biopsy[b]
Genitourinary tract
    Vaginal hysterectomy[b]
    Vaginal delivery[b]
    Cesarean section
    In uninfected tissue
        Urethral catheterization
        Uterine dilation and curettage
        Therapeutic abortion
        Sterilization procedures
        Insertion or removal of intrauterine devices
Other
    Cardiac catheterization, including balloon angioplasty
    Implanted cardiac pacemakers, implanted defibrillators, and coronary stents
    Incision or biopsy of surgically scrubbed skin
    Circumcision

[a]Prophylaxis is recommended for high-risk patients; optional for medium-risk patients.
[b]Prophylaxis is optional for high-risk patients.
From Dajani AS, Taubert KA, Wilson W, et al. *Prevention of bacterial endocarditis: Recommendations by the American Heart Association. JAMA 1997;277:1794–1801, with permission. Copyright 1995–1997, American Medical Association.*

VIII

- After the initiation of therapy, blood cultures should be rechecked until they are negative. During the remainder of the therapy, frequent blood culturing is not necessary.
- MICs should be determined for all isolates from blood cultures. MBCs are not routinely recommended.
- Serum bactericidal titers (SBTs) may be useful only when the causative organisms are moderately susceptible to antimicrobials, when less well-established regimens are used, or when response to therapy is suboptimal and dosage escalation is considered.

TABLE 36–11. Prophylactic Regimens for Dental, Oral, Respiratory Tract, or Esophageal Procedures

Situation	Agent	Regimen[a]
Standard general prophylaxis	Amoxicillin	Adults: 2 g; children: 50 mg/kg orally 1 h before procedure
Unable to take oral medications	Ampicillin	Adults: 2 g intramuscularly (IM) or intravenously (IV); children: 50 mg/kg IM or IV within 30 min before procedure
Allergic to penicillin	Clindamycin *or*	Adults: 600 mg; children: 20 mg/kg orally 1 h before procedure
	Cephalexin[b] or cefadroxil[b] *or*	Adults: 2 g; children: 50 mg/kg orally 1 h before procedure
	Azithromycin or chlarithromycin	Adults: 500 mg; children: 15 mg/kg orally 1 h before procedure
Allergic to penicillin and unable to take oral medications	Clidamycin *or*	Adults: 600 mg; children: 20 mg/kg IV within 30 min before procedure
	Cefazolin[b]	Adults 1 g; children: 25 mg/kg IM or IV within 30 min before procedure

[a]Total children's dose should not exceed adult dose.
[b]Cephalosporins should not be used in individuals with immediate-type hypersensitivity reaction (urticaria, angioedema, or anaphylaxis) to penicillins.
From Dajani AS, Taubert KA, Wilson W, et al. Prevention of bacterial endocarditis: Recommendations by the American Heart Association. JAMA 1997;277:1974–1801, with permission. Copyright 1995–1997, American Medical Association.

- Serum concentrations of the antimicrobial should generally exceed the MBC of the organism, however, in practice this principle is usually not helpful in monitoring patients with endocarditis.

▶ PREVENTION OF ENDOCARDITIS

- Antimicrobial prophylaxis is used to prevent IE in patients believed to be at high risk.
- The use of antimicrobials for this purpose requires consideration of the types of patients who are at risk; the procedures causing bacteremia; the organisms that are likely to cause endocarditis; and the pharmacokinetics, spectrum, cost, and ease of administration of available agents. The objective of prophylaxis is to diminish the likelihood of IE in high-risk individuals who are undergoing procedures that cause transient bacteremia.

PATIENTS AT RISK

- Patients with certain cardiac lesions, particularly those with a history of rheumatic heart disease and prosthetic heart valves, are at risk for developing endocarditis (Table 36–8). However, only 15% to 25% of patients who develop IE are in a definable high-risk category, and only a small proportion of high-risk patients will develop IE if prophylaxis is not given.

PROCEDURES CAUSING BACTEREMIA

See Tables 36–9 and 36–10.
For dental procedures of the gums and oral structures that cause bleeding, viridans streptococci frequently cause bacteremia, whereas instrumentation and surgery of

TABLE 36–12. Prophylactic Regimens for Genitourinary Gastrointestinal (Excluding Esophageal) Procedures

Situation	Agent[a]	Regimen[b]
High-risk patients	Ampicillin plus gentamicin	Adults: Ampicillin 2 g intramuscularly (IM) or intravenously (IV) plus gentamicin 1.5 mg/kg (not to exceed 120 mg) within 30 min of starting the procedure; 6 h later, ampicillin 1 g IM/IV or amoxicillin 1 g orally. Children: Ampicillin 50 mg/kg IM or IV (not to exceed 2 g) plus gentamicin 1.5 mg/kg within 30 min of starting the procedure; 6 h later, ampicillin 25 mg/kg IM/IV or amoxicillin 25 mg/kg orally.
High-risk patients allergic to ampicillin/amoxicillin	Vancomycin plus gentamicin	Adults: Vancomycin 1 g IV over 1–2 h plus gentamicin 1.5 mg/kg IV/IM (not to exceed 120 mg); complete injection/infusion within 30 min of starting the procedure. Children: Vancomycin 20 mg/kg IV over 1–2 h plus gentamicin 1.5 mg/kg IV/IM; complete injection or infusion within 30 min of starting the procedure.
Moderate-risk patients	Amoxicillin or Ampicillin	Adults: Amoxicillin 2 g orally 1 h before procedure, or ampicillin 2 g IM/IV within 30 min of starting the procedure. Children: Amoxicillin 50 mg/kg orally 1 h before procedure, or ampicillin 50 mg/kg IM/IV within 30 min of starting the procedure.
Moderate-risk patients allergic to ampicillin/amoxicillin	Vancomycin	Adults: Vancomycin 1 g IV over 1–2 h; complete infusion within 30 min of starting the procedure. Children: Vancomycin 20 mg/kg IV over 1–2 h; complete infusion within 30 min of starting the procedure.

[a]Total children's dose should not exceed adult dose.
[b]No second dose of vancomycin or gentamicin is recommended.

From Dajani AS, Taubert KA, Wilson W, et al. Prevention of bacterial endocarditis: Recommendations by the American Heart Association. JAMA 1997;277:1794–1801, with permission. Copyright 1995–1997, American Medical Association.

the gastrointestinal and genitourinary tracts more often result in enterococcal bacteremia.

ANTIBIOTIC REGIMENS

- A 2-g dose of amoxicillin is recommended for adult patients at risk, given 60 minutes prior to undergoing procedures associated with bacteremia (Table 36–11). For penicillin-allergic patients or those undergoing gastrointestinal surgery, alternative prophylaxis is recommended (Tables 36–11 and 36–12).

See Chapter 109, Infective Endocarditis, authored by Michael A. Crouch and Angie Veverka, for a more detailed discussion of this topic.

VIII ◄

Chapter 37

▶ FUNGAL INFECTIONS, INVASIVE

Systemic mycoses, such as histoplasmosis, coccidioidomycosis, cryptococcosis, blastomycosis, paracoccidioidomycosis, and sporotrichosis, are caused by primary or "pathogenic" fungi that can cause disease in both healthy and immunocompromised individuals. In contrast, mycoses caused by opportunistic fungi such as *Candida albicans, Aspergillus* spp., *Trichosporon, Torulopsis (Candida) glabrata, Fusarium, Alternaria,* and *Mucor* are generally found only in the immunocompromised host. Advances in medical technology, including organ and bone marrow transplantation, cytotoxic chemotherapy, the widespread use of indwelling intravenous (IV) catheters, and the increased use of potent, broad-spectrum antimicrobial agents, have all contributed to the dramatic increase in the incidence of fungal infections worldwide.

▶ SPECIFIC FUNGAL INFECTIONS

HISTOPLASMOSIS

- Histoplasmosis is caused by inhalation of dust-borne microconidia of the dimorphic fungus *Histoplasma capsulatum.*
- In the United States, most disease is localized along the Ohio and Mississippi river valleys.

Clinical Presentation

- In the vast majority of patients, low-inoculum exposure to *H. capsulatum* results in mild or asymptomatic pulmonary histoplasmosis. The course of disease is generally benign, and symptoms usually abate within a few weeks of onset. Patients exposed to a higher inoculum during a primary infection or reinfection may experience an acute, self-limited illness with flulike pulmonary symptoms, including fever, chills, headache, myalgia, and nonproductive cough.
- Chronic pulmonary histoplasmosis generally presents as an opportunistic infection imposed on a preexisting structural abnormality such as lesions resulting from emphysema. Patients demonstrate chronic pulmonary symptoms and apical lung lesions that progress with inflammation, calcified granulomas, and fibrosis. Progression of disease over a period of years, seen in 25% to 30% of patients, is associated with cavitation, bronchopleural fistulas, extension to the other lung, pulmonary insufficiency, and often death.
- In patients exposed to a large inoculum and in immunocompromised hosts, progressive illness, disseminated histoplasmosis, occurs. The clinical severity of the diverse forms of disseminated histoplasmosis (Table 37–1) generally parallels the degree of macrophage parasitization observed.
- Acute (infantile) disseminated histoplasmosis is seen in infants and young children and (rarely) in adults with Hodgkin's disease or other lymphoproliferative disorders. It is characterized by unrelenting fever; anemia; leukopenia or thrombocytopenia; enlargement of the liver, spleen, and visceral lymph nodes; and gastrointestinal (GI) symptoms, particularly nausea, vomiting, and diarrhea. Untreated disease is uniformly fatal in 1 to 2 months.
- Most adults with disseminated histoplasmosis demonstrate a mild, chronic form of the disease. Untreated patients are often ill for 10 to 20 years, with long asymptomatic periods interrupted by relapses.
- Adult patients with AIDS demonstrate an acute form of disseminated disease that resembles the syndrome seen in infants and children.

TABLE 37–1. Clinical Manifestations and Therapy of Histoplasmosis

Type of Disease and Common Clinical Manifestations	Approximate Frequency (%)[a]	Therapy/Comments
Nonimmunosuppressed Host		
Acute pulmonary histoplasmosis		
Asymptomatic or mild disease	50–99	*Asymptomatic, mild, or symptoms <4 wk:* No therapy generally required
		Symptoms >4 weeks: Itraconazole 200 mg once daily × 6–12 weeks[b]
Self-limited disease	1–50	*Self-limited disease:* Amphotericin B[c] 0.3–0.5 mg/kg/day × 2–4 weeks (total dose 500 mg) or ketoconazole 400 mg orally daily × 3–6 months may be beneficial in patients with severe hypoxia following inhalation of large inocula
		Antifungal therapy generally not useful for arthritis or pericarditis; NSAIDs[d] or corticosteroids may be useful in some cases
Mediastinal granulomas	1–50	Most lesions resolve spontaneously; surgery or antifungal therapy with amphotericin B 40–50 mg/day × 2–3 weeks or itraconazole 400 mg/day orally × 6–12 months may be beneficial in some severe cases; mild to moderate disease may be treated with itraconazole for 6–12 months
Severe diffuse pulmonary disease		Amphotericin B 0.7 mg/kg/day, for a total dose of ≤35 mg/kg (or 3 mg/kg/day of one of the lipid preparations) + prednisone 60 mg daily tapered over 2 weeks,[e] followed by itraconazole 200 mg twice daily for 6–12 weeks; in patients who do not require hospitalization, itraconazole 200 mg once or twice daily for 6–12 weeks can be used
Inflammatory/fibrotic disease	0.02	*Fibrosing mediastinitis:* The benefit of antifungal therapy (itraconazole 200 mg twice daily × 3 months) is controversial but should be considered, especially in patients with elevated ESR[f] or CF[g] titers ≥1:32; surgery may be of benefit if disease is detected early; late disease may not respond to therapy
		Sarcoid-like: NSAIDs or corticosteroids may be of benefit for some patients
		Pericarditis: Severe disease: corticosteroids 1 mg/kg/day or pericardial drainage procedure
Chronic pulmonary histoplasmosis	0.05	Antifungal therapy generally recommended for all patients to halt further lung destruction and reduce mortality
		Mild–moderate disease: Itraconazole 200–400 mg PO daily × 6–24 months is the treatment of choice
		Itraconazole and ketoconazole (200–800 mg/day orally for 1 year) are effective in 74% to 86% of cases, but relapses are common; fluconazole 200–400 mg daily is less effective (64%) than ketoconazole or itraconazole, and relapses are seen in 29% of responders

VIII

(Continued)

TABLE 37–1. Continued

Type of Disease and Common Clinical Manifestations	Approximate Frequency (%)[a]	Therapy/Comments
		Severe disease: Amphotericin B 0.7 mg/kg/day for a minimum total dose of 35 mg/kg is effective in 59% to 100% of cases and should be used in patients who require hospitalization or are unable to take itraconazole because of drug interactions, allergies, failure to absorb drug, or failure to improve clinically after a minimum of 12 weeks of itraconazole therapy
Immunosuppressed Host		
Disseminated histoplasmosis	0.02–0.05	*Disseminated histoplasmosis:* Untreated mortality 83% to 93%; relapse 5% to 23% in non-AIDS patients; therapy is recommended for all patients
Acute (Infantile)		*Nonimmunosuppressed patients:* Ketoconazole 400 mg/day orally × 6–12 months or amphotericin B 35 mg/kg IV
Subacute		*Immunosuppressed patients: (non-AIDS) or endocarditis or CNS disease:* Amphotericin B >35 mg/kg × 3 months followed by fluconazole or itraconazole 200 mg orally twice daily × 12 months
Progressive histoplasmosis (immunocompetent patients and immunosuppressed patients without AIDS)		*Life-threatening disease:* Amphotericin B 0.7–1 mg/kg/day IV for a total dosage of 35 mg/kg over 2–4 months; once the patient is afebrile, able to take oral medications, and no longer requires blood pressure or ventilatory support, therapy can be changed to itraconazole 200 mg orally twice daily for 6–18 months
		Non–life-threatening disease: Itraconazole 200–400 mg orally daily for 6–18 months; fluconazole therapy 400–800 mg daily) should be reserved for patients intolerant to itraconazole, and the development of resistance may lead to relapses
Progressive disease of AIDS	25–50[h]	Amphotericin B 15–30 mg/kg (1–2 g over 4–10 weeks)[i] or itraconazole 200 mg 3 times daily for 3 days then twice daily for 12 weeks, followed by lifelong suppressive therapy with itraconazole 200–400 mg orally daily; a study is in progress to determine whether itraconazole therapy can be discontinued after one year if CD4+ counts are >150 cells/mm3

VIII

[a]As a percentage of all patients presenting with histoplasmosis.
[b]Itraconazole plasma concentrations should be measured during the second week of therapy to ensure that detectable concentrations have been achieved. If the concentration is below 1 mcg/mL, the dose may be insufficient or drug interactions may be impairing absorption or accelerating metabolism, requiring a change in dosage. If plasma concentrations are greater than 10 mcg/mL, the dosage may be reduced.
[c]Desoxycholate amphotericin B.
[d]Nonsteroidal anti-inflammatory drugs.
[e]Effectiveness of corticosteroids is controversial.
[f]Erythrocyte sedimention rate.
[g]Complement fixation.
[h]As a percentage of AIDS patients presenting with histoplasmosis as the initial manifestation of their disease.
[i]Liposomal amphotericin B (AmBisome) may be more appropriate for disseminated disease.

Diagnosis

- Identification of mycelial isolates from clinical cultures can be made by conversion of the mycelium to the yeast form (requires 3 to 6 weeks) or by the more rapid (2-hour) and 100% sensitive DNA probe that recognizes ribosomal DNA.
- In most patients, serologic evidence remains the primary method in the diagnosis of histoplasmosis. Results obtained from complement fixation, immunodiffusion, and latex antigen agglutination antibody tests are used alone or in combination.
- In the AIDS patient with progressive disseminated histoplasmosis, the diagnosis is best established by bone marrow biopsy and culture, which yield positive cultures in 90% of patients.

Treatment

- Recommended therapy for the treatment of histoplasmosis is summarized in Table 37–1.
- Asymptomatic or mildly ill patients and patients with sarcoid-like disease generally do not benefit from antifungal therapy. Therapy may be helpful in symptomatic patients whose conditions have not improved during the first month of infection.
- Patients with mild, self-limited disease, chronic disseminated disease, or chronic pulmonary histoplasmosis who have no underlying immunosuppression can usually be treated with either oral ketoconazole or IV amphotericin B.
- In AIDS patients, intensive 12-week primary (induction and consolidation therapy) antifungal therapy is followed by lifelong suppressive (maintenance) therapy with **itraconazole**.
- In AIDS patients, **amphotericin B** should be administered in patients who require hospitalization. Itraconazole 200 mg twice daily may be used to complete a 12-week course.
- Response to therapy should be measured by resolution of radiologic, serologic, and microbiologic parameters and improvement in signs and symptoms of infection.
- Once the initial course of therapy for histoplasmosis is completed, lifelong suppressive therapy with oral azoles or **amphotericin B** (1 to 1.5 mg/kg weekly or biweekly) is recommended, because of the frequent recurrence of infection.
- Relapse rates in AIDS patients not receiving preventive maintenance are 50% to 90%.

BLASTOMYCOSIS

- North American blastomycosis is a systemic fungal infection caused by *Blastomyces dermatitidis*.
- Pulmonary disease probably occurs by inhalation conidia, which convert to the yeast forms in the lungs. It may be acute or chronic and can mimic infection with tuberculosis, pyogenic bacteria, other fungi, or malignancy.
- Blastomycosis can disseminate to virtually every other body organ including skin, bones and joints, or the genitourinary tract without any evidence of pulmonary disease.

Clinical Presentation

- Acute pulmonary blastomycosis is generally an asymptomatic or self-limited disease characterized by fever, shaking chills, and a productive, purulent cough.

- Pulmonary blastomycosis may present as a more chronic or subacute disease, with low-grade fever, night sweats, weight loss, and a productive cough resembling that of tuberculosis rather than bacterial pneumonia.
- Chronic pulmonary blastomycosis is characterized by fever, malaise, weight loss, night sweats, and cough.

Diagnosis
- The simplest and most successful method of diagnosing blastomycosis is by direct microscopic visualization of the large, multinucleated yeast with single, broad-based buds in sputum or other respiratory specimens, following digestion of cells and debris with 10% potassium hydroxide.
- Histopathologic examination of tissue biopsies and culture of secretions should be used to identify *B. dermatitidis*.

Treatment
- In patients with mild pulmonary blastomycosis, the clinical presentation of the patient, the immune competence of the patient, and the toxicity of the antifungal agents are the main determinants of whether or not to administer antifungal therapy. All immunocompromised patients and patients with progressive disease or with extrapulmonary disease should be treated (Table 37-2).
- Some authors recommend **ketoconazole** therapy for the treatment of self-limited pulmonary disease, with the hope of preventing late extrapulmonary disease.
- **Itraconazole**, 200 to 400 mg/day, is an effective as a first-line agent in the treatment of non–life-threatening non-CNS blastomycosis.
- All patients with disseminated blastomycosis and those with extrapulmonary disease require therapy (**ketoconazole**, 400 mg/day orally for 6 months). CNS disease should be treated with **amphotericin B** for a total cumulative dose greater than 1 g.
- Patients who fail or are unable to tolerate itraconazole therapy, or who develop CNS disease, should be treated with amphotericin B for a total cumulative dose of 1.5 to 2.5 g.
- HIV-infected patients should receive induction therapy with **amphotericin B** and chronic suppressive therapy with an oral azole antifungal. Itraconazole is the drug of choice for non–life-threatening histoplasmosis.

COCCIDIOIDOMYCOSIS

Coccidioidomycosis is caused by infection with *Coccidioides immitis*. The endemic regions encompass the semi-arid regions of the southwestern United States from California to Texas, known as the Lower Sonoran Zone.

Clinical Presentation
- Most of those infected are asymptomatic or have nonspecific symptoms that are often indistinguishable from those of ordinary upper respiratory infections, including fever, cough, headache, sore throat, myalgias, and fatigue. A fine, diffuse rash may be appear during the first few days of illness.
- "Valley fever" is a syndrome characterized by erythema nodosum and erythema multiforme of the upper trunk and extremities in association with diffuse joint aches or fever. Valley fever occurs in approximately 25% of infected persons, although, more commonly, a diffuse mild erythroderma or maculopapular rash is observed.
- Pulmonary coccidioidomycosis can also present as acute pneumonia or develop into a chronic, persistent pneumonia complicated by hemoptysis, pulmonary scarring, and the formation of cavities of bronchopleural fistulas.

VIII

TABLE 37–2. Therapy of Blastomycosis

Type of Disease	Preferred Treatment	Comments
Pulmonary[a]		
Life-threatening	Amphotericin B[b] IV 0.7–1 mg/kg/day IV (total dose 1.5–2.5 g)	Patients may be initiated on amphotericin B and changed to oral itraconazole 200–400 mg orally daily once patient is clinically stabilized and a minimum dose of 500 mg of amphotericin B has been administered
Mild to moderate	Itraconazole 200 mg orally twice daily x ≥6 months[c]	*Alternative therapy:* Ketoconazole 400–800 mg orally daily × ≥6 months or fluconazole 400–800 mg orally daily × ≥6 months[d]
		In patients intolerant of azoles or in whom disease progresses during azole therapy: Amphotericin B 0.5–0.7 mg/kg/day IV (total dose 1.5–2.5 g)
Disseminated or Extrapulmonary		
CNS[e]	Amphotericin B 0.7–1 mg/kg/day IV (total dose 1.5–2.5 g)	For patients unable to tolerate a full course of amphotericin B, consider lipid formulations of amphotericin B or fluconazole ≥ 800 mg orally daily
Non-CNS		
Life-threatening	Amphotericin B 0.7–1 mg/kg/day IV (total dose 1.5–2.5 g)	Patients may be initiated on amphotericin B and changed to oral itraconazole 200–400 mg orally daily once stabilized
Mild to moderate	Itraconazole 200–400 mg orally daily × ≥6 months	Ketoconazole 400–800 mg orally daily or fluconazole 400–800 mg orally daily × ≥6 months
		In patients intolerant of azoles or in whom disease progresses during azole therapy: Amphotericin B 0.5–0.7 mg/kg/day IV (total dose 1.5–2.5 g)
		Bone disease: Therapy with azoles should be continued for 12 months
Immunocompromised Host (Including Patients with AIDS, Transplants, or Receiving Chronic Glucocorticoid Therapy)		
Acute disease	Amphotericin B 0.7–1 mg/kg/day IV (total dose 1.5–2.5 g)	Patients without CNS infection may be switched to itraconazole once clinically stabilized and a minimum dose of 1 g of amphotericin B has been administered; long-term suppressive therapy with an azole is advised
Suppressive therapy	Itraconazole 200–400 mg orally daily	For patients with CNS disease or those intolerant of itraconazole, consider fluconazole 800 mg orally daily

[a]Some patients with acute pulmonary infection may have a spontaneous cure. Patients with progressive pulmonary disease should be treated.
[b]Desoxycholate amphotericin B.
[c]In patients not responding to 400 mg, dosage should be increased by 200 mg increments every 4 wk to a maximum of 800 mg daily.
[d]Therapy with ketoconazole is associated with relapses, and fluconazole therapy achieves a lower response rate than itraconazole.
[e]Central nervous system.

- Disseminated infection occurs in less than 1% of infected patients. Dissemination may occur to the skin, lymph nodes, bone, meninges, spleen, liver, kidney, and adrenal gland.

Diagnosis

- Most patients develop a positive skin test within 3 weeks of the onset of symptoms.

- Infection is characterized by the development of IgM to *C. immitis*, which peaks within 2 to 3 weeks of infection and then declines rapidly, and IgG, which peaks in 4 to 12 weeks and declines over months to years.
- Recovery of *C. immitis* from infected tissues or secretions for direct examination and culture provides an accurate and rapid method of diagnosis.

Treatment

- Only 5% of infected persons require therapy. Candidates for therapy include those with severe primary pulmonary infection or concurrent risk factors (e.g., HIV infection, organ transplant, or high doses of glucocorticoids), particularly patients with high complement fixation antibody titers in whom dissemination is likely.
- Specific antifungals (and their usual dosages) for the treatment of coccidioidomycosis include amphotericin B IV (0.5 to 0.7 mg/kg/day), ketoconazole (400 mg orally daily), IV or oral fluconazole (usually 400 to 800 mg daily, although dosages as high as 1200 mg/day have been utilized without complications), and itraconazole (200 to 300 mg orally twice daily as either capsules or solution). If itraconazole is used, measurement of serum concentrations may be helpful to ascertain whether oral bioavailability is adequate. Amphotericin B is generally preferred as initial therapy in patients with rapidly progressive disease, whereas azoles are generally preferred in patients with subacute or chronic presentations. Treatments for primary respiratory disease (mainly symptomatic patients) are 3- to 6-month courses of therapy.

CRYPTOCOCCOSIS

Cryptococcosis is a noncontagious, systemic mycotic infection caused by the ubiquitous encapsulated soil yeast *Cryptococcus neoformans*.

Clinical Presentation

- Primary cryptococcosis in humans almost always occurs in the lungs. Symptomatic infections are usually manifested by cough, rales, and shortness of breath that generally resolve spontaneously.
- Disease may remain localized in the lungs or disseminate to other tissues, particularly the CNS, although the skin can also be affected.
- In the non-AIDS patient, the symptoms of cryptococcal meningitis are nonspecific. Headache, fever, nausea, vomiting, mental status changes, and neck stiffness are generally observed.
- In AIDS patients, fever and headache are common, but meningismus and photophobia are much less common than in non-AIDS patients.

Diagnosis

- Examination of cerebrospinal fluid (CSF) in patients with cryptococcal meningitis generally reveals an elevated opening pressure, CSF pleocytosis (usually lymphocytes), leukocytosis, a decreased CSF glucose, an elevated CSF protein, and a positive cryptococcal antigen.
- Antigens to *C. neoformans* can be detected by latex agglutination.
- *C. neoformans* can be detected in approximately 60% of patients by india ink smear of CSF and cultured in more than 96% of patients.

Treatment

- Treatment of cryptococcosis is detailed in Table 37–3.
- For asymptomatic, immunocompetent persons with isolated pulmonary disease and no evidence of CNS disease, careful observation may be warranted. With symptomatic infection, **fluconazole** or **amphotericin B** is warranted.

TABLE 37–3. Therapy of Cryptococcosis[a,b]

Type of Disease and Common Clinical Manifestations	Therapy/Comments
Nonimmunocompromised Host	Comparative trials for amphotericin B[c] versus azoles not available
Isolated pulmonary disease (without evidence of CNS infection)	*Asymptomatic disease:* Durg therapy generally not required; observe carefully or fluconazole 400 mg orally daily × 3–6 months
	Mild to moderate symptoms: Fluconazole 200–400 mg orally daily × 3–6 months; *Severe disease or inability to take azoles:* Amphotericin B 0.4–0.7 mg/kg/day (total dose of 1–2 g)
Cryptococcemia with positive serum antigen titer (>1:8), cutaneous infection, a positive urine culture, or prostatic disease	Clinician must decide whether to follow the pulmonary therapeutic regimen or the CNS (disseminated) regimen
Recurrent or progressive disease not responsive to amphotericin B	Amphotericin B[d] IV 0.5–0.75 mg/kg/day ± IT amphotericin B 0.5 mg 2–3 times weekly
Isolated pulmonary disease (without evidence of CNS infection)	*Mild to moderate symptoms or asymptomatic with a positive pulmonary specimen:* Fluconazole 200–400 mg orally daily × lifelong *or*
	Itraconazole 200–400 mg orally daily × lifelong *or*
	Fluconazole 400 mg orally daily + flucytosine 100–150 mg/kg/day orally × 10 wk
	Severe disease: Amphotericin B until symptoms are controlled, followed by fluconazole
CNS disease	
Acute (induction/consolidation therapy) (follow all regimens with suppressive therapy)	Amphotericin B[d] IV 0.7–1 mg/kg/day + flucytosine 100 mg/kg/day orally × ≥2 weeks, then fluconazole 400 mg orally daily × ≥8 wk[e] *or*
	Amphotericin B[d] IV 0.7–1 mg/kg/day + flucytosine 100 mg/kg/day orally × 6–10 wk[e] *or*
	Amphotericin B[d] IV 0.7–1 mg/kg/day × 6–10 wk[e] *or*
	Fluconazole 400–800 mg orally daily × 10–12 wk *or*
	Itraconazole 400–800 mg orally daily × 10–12 wk *or*
	Fluconazole 400–800 mg orally daily + flucytosine 100–150 mg/kg/day orally × 6 wk[e] *or*
	Lipid formulation of amphotericin B IV 3–6 mg/kg/day × 6–10 wk
	Note: Induction therapy with azoles alone is discouraged.
CNS disease	Amphotericin B[d] IV 0.7–1 mg/kg/day + flucytosine 100 mg/kg/day orally × 2 wk, followed by fluconazole 400 mg orally daily for a minimum of 10 wk (in patients intolerant to fluconazole, substitute itraconazole 200–400 mg orally daily) *or*
	Amphotericin B[d] IV 0.7–1 mg/kg/day + 5-FC 100 mg/kg/day orally × 6–10 wk *or*
	Amphotericin B[d] IV 0.7–1 mg/kg/day × 10 wk
	Refractory disesase: Intrathecal or intraventricular amphotericin B

VIII ◄

TABLE 37–3. (Continued)

Type of Disease and Common Clinical Manifestations	Therapy/Comments
Immunocompromised Patients	
Non-CNS pulmonary and extrapulmonary disease	Same as nonimmunocompromised patients with CNS disease
CNS disease	Amphotericin B[d] IV 0.7–1 mg/kg/day × 2 wk, followed by fluconazole 400–800 mg orally daily 8–10 wk, followed by fluconazole 200 mg orally daily × 6–12 months (in patients intolerant to fluconazole, substitute itraconazole 200–400 mg orally daily)
	Refractory disesase: Intrathecal or intraventricular amphotericin B
HIV-Infected Patients	
Suppressive/maintenance therapy	Fluconazole 200–400 mg orally daily × lifelong
	or
	Itraconazole 200 mg orally twice daily × lifelong
	or
	Amphotericin B IV 1 mg/kg 1–3 times weekly × lifelong

[a]When more than one therapy is listed, they are listed in order of preference.
[b]See text for definitions of induction, consolidation, suppressive/maintenance therapy, and prophylactic therapy.
[c]Deoxycholate amphotericin B; IV, intravenous; IT, intrathecal; CNS, central nervous system.
[d]In patients with significant renal disease, lipid formulations of amphotericin B can be substituted for deoxycholate amphotericin B during the induction.
[e]Or until CSF cultures are negative

- The combination of **amphotericin B** with **flucytosine** for 6 weeks is often used for treatment of cryptococcal meningitis. An alternative is amphotericin B for 2 weeks followed by **fluconazole** for an additional 8 to 10 weeks.
- The use of intrathecal **amphotericin B** is not recommended for the treatment of cryptococcal meningitis except in very ill patients or in those with recurrent or progressive disease despite aggressive IV amphotericin B therapy. The dosage of amphotericin B employed is usually 0.5 mg administered via the lumbar, cisternal, or intraventricular (via an Ommaya reservoir) route 2 or 3 times weekly.
- **Amphotericin B** with **flucytosine** is the initial treatment of choice for acute therapy of cryptococcal meningitis in AIDS patients. Many clinicians will initiate therapy with amphotericin B, 0.7 mg/kg/ day IV (with flucytosine, 100 mg/kg/day). After 2 weeks, consolidation therapy with either itraconazole 400 mg/day orally or **fluconazole** 400 mg/day orally can be administered for 8 weeks or until CSF cultures are negative. Lifelong therapy with fluconazole is then recommended.
- Relapse of *C. neoformans* meningitis occurs in approximately 50% of AIDS patients after completion of primary therapy. **Fluconazole** (200 mg daily) is currently recommended for chronic suppressive therapy of cryptococcal meningitis in AIDS patients.

▶ *CANDIDA* INFECTIONS

Eight species of *Candida* are regarded as clinically important pathogens in human disease: *C. albicans, C. tropicalis, C. parapsilosis, C. krusei, C. stellatoidea, C. guilliermondi, C. lusitaniae*, and *C. glabrata*.

HEMATOGENOUS CANDIDIASIS

- Hematogenous candidiasis describes the clinical circumstances in which hematogenous seeding to deep organs such as the eye, brain, heart, and kidney occurs.
- *Candida* is generally acquired via the GI tract, although organisms may also enter the bloodstream via indwelling IV catheters. Immunosuppressed patients, including those with lymphoreticular or hematologic malignancies, diabetes, immunodeficiency diseases, or those receiving immunosuppressive therapy with high-dose corticosteroids, immunosuppressants, antineoplastic agents, or broad-spectrum antimicrobial agents are at high risk for invasive fungal infections. Major risk factors include the use of central venous catheters, total parenteral nutrition, receipt of multiple antibiotics, extensive surgery and burns, renal failure and hemodialysis, mechanical ventilation, and prior fungal colonization.
- Three distinct presentations of disseminated *C. albicans* have been recognized: (1) the acute onset of fever, tachycardia, tachypnea, and occasionally chills or hypotension (similar to bacterial sepsis); (2) intermittent fevers; (3) progressive deterioration with or without fever; and (4) hepatosplenic candidiasis manifested only as fever while the patient is neutropenic. VIII
- No test has demonstrated reliable accuracy in the clinical setting for diagnosis of disseminated *Candida* infection. Blood cultures are positive in only 25% to 45% of neutropenic patients.
- Treatment of candidiasis is presented in Table 37-4.
- In patients with an intact immune system, removal of all existing central venous catheters should be considered.
- Amphotericin B may be switched to fluconazole (IV or oral) for completion of therapy.
- Lipid-associated formulations of amphotericin B, liposomal amphotericin B (AmBisome) and amphotericin B lipid complex (Abelcet) have been approved for use in proven cases of candidiasis; however, patients with invasive candidiasis have also been treated successfully with amphotericin B colloid dispersion (Amphotec or Amphocil). The lipid-associated formulations are less toxic but as effective as amphotericin B deoxycholate.
- Many clinicians advocate early institution of empiric IV **amphotericin B** in patients with neutropenia and persistent fever (more than 5 to 7 days). Suggested criteria for the empiric use of amphotericin B include (1) fever of 5 to 7 days' duration that is unresponsive to antibacterial agents, (2) neutropenia of more than 7 days' duration, (3) no other obvious cause for fever, (4) progressive debilitation, (5) chronic adrenal corticosteroid therapy, and (6) indwelling intravascular catheters.

▶ *ASPERGILLUS* INFECTIONS

- Of more than 300 species of *Aspergillus*, three are most commonly pathogenic: *A. fumigatus*, *A. flavus*, and *A. niger*.
- Aspergillosis is generally acquired by inhalation of airborne conidia that are small enough (2.5 to 3 mm) to reach the alveoli or the paranasal sinuses.

SUPERFICIAL INFECTION

Superficial or locally invasive infections of the ear, skin, or appendages can often be managed with topical antifungal therapy.

TABLE 37–4. Therapy of Invasive Candidiasis

Type of Disease and Common Clinical Manifestations	Therapy/Comments
Prophylaxis of Candidemia	
Nonneutropenic patients[a]	Not recommended except for severely ill/high-risk patients in whom fluconazole IV/PO 400 mg daily should be used (see text)
Neutropenic patients[a]	The optimal duration of therapy is unclear but at a minimum should include the period at risk for neutropenia: Fluconazole IV/PO 400 mg daily *or* itraconazole solution 2.5 mg/kg q 12 h PO *or* micafungin (unlicensed in U.S.) 50 mg (1 mg/kg in patients under 50 kg) intravenously daily
Solid-organ transplantation	*Patients with two or more key risk factors[b]:*
Liver transplantation	Amphotericin B IV 10–20 mg daily or lipoosmal amphotericin B (AmBisome) 1 mg/kg/day or fluconazole 400 mg orally daily
Empirical Antifungal Therapy (Unknown *Candida* Species)	
Suspected disseminated candidiasis in febrile nonneutropenic patients	None recommended; data are lacking defining subsets of patients who are appropriate for therapy (see text)
Febrile neutropenic patients with prolonged fever despite 4–6 days of empirical antibacterial therapy	*Treatment duration:* Until resolution of neutropenia
	Amphotericin B IV 0.5–0.7 mg/kg/day *or* liposomal amphotericin B (AmBisome) IV 3 mg/kg/day *or* itraconazole 200 mg IV q 12 h x 2 days, then 200 mg/day x 12 days, then 400 mg PO (solution) daily *or* voriconazole 6 mg/kg IV loading dose q 12 h x day, then 3 mg/kg q 12 h (restrict to allogeneic bone marrow transplant and relapsed leukemia patients) *or* fluconazole 400 mg/day IV/PO (restrict to patients with a low risk for invasive aspergillosis *or* azole-resistant strains of *Candida* in patients with no previous azole exposure *or* signs and symptoms suggesting aspergillosis)
Treatment of Candidemia and Acute Hematogenously Disseminated Candidiasis	
Nonimmunocompromised host[c]	*Treatment duration:* 2 wk after the last positive blood culture and resolution of signs and symptoms of infection
	Remove existing central venous catheters when feasible, plus:
C. albicans, C. tropicalis, C. parapsilosis	Amphotericin B IV 0.6 mg/kg/day *or* fluconazole IV/PO 6 mg/kg/day *or* caspofungin 70 mg loading dose then 50 mg IV daily *or* amphotericin B IV 0.7 mg/kg/day plus fluconazole IV/PO 800 mg/day
	Patients intolerant or refractory to other therapy[d]:
	Amphotericin B lipid complex IV 5 mg/kg/day
	Liposomal amphotericin B IV 3–5 mg/kg/day
	Amphotericin B colloid dispersion IV 2–6 mg/kg/day
C. krusei	Amphotericin B IV $\geq$1 mg/kg/day *or* caspofungin 70 mg loading dose then 50 mg IV daily
C. lusitaniae	Fluconazole IV/PO 6 mg/kg/day
C. glabrata	Amphotericin B IV $\geq$0.7 mg/kg/day *or* fluconazole IV/PO 6–12 mg/kg/day (400–800 mg/day in a 70-kg patient) *or* Caspofungin 70 mg loading dose then 50 mg IV daily
Neutropenic host[e]	*Treatment duration:* Until resolution of neutropenia
	Remove existing central venous catheters when feasible, plus:
	Amphotericin B IV 0.7–1.0 mg/kg/day (total dosages 0.5–1 g) *or*
	Patients failing therapy with traditional amphotericin B: Lipid formulation of amphotericin B IV 3–5 mg/kg/day

VIII

(Continued)

TABLE 37–4. (Continued)

Type of Disease and Common Clinical Manifestations	Therapy/Comments
Chronic Disseminated Candidiasis (hepatosplenic candidiasis)	*Treatment duration:* Until calcification or resolution of lesions
	Stable patients: Fluconazole IV/PO 6 mg/kg/day
	Acutely ill or refractory patients: Amphotericin B IV 0.6–0.7 mg/kg/day
	Asymptomatic disease: Generally no therapy is required
Urinary Candidiasis	*Symptomatic or high-risk patients[f]:* Removal of urinary tract instruments, stents, and Foley catheters) plus 7–14 days therapy with fluconazole 200 mg orally daily or amphotericin B IV 0.3–1 mg/kg/day

[a]Patients at significant risk for invasive candidiasis include those receiving standard chemotherapy for acute myelogenous leukemia, allogeneic bone marrow transplants, or high-risk autologous bone marrow transplants. However, among these populations, chemotherapy or bone marrow transplant protocols do not all produce equivalent risk, and local experience should be used to determine the relevance of prophylaxis.

[b]Risk factors include retransplantation, creatinine of more than 2 mg/dL, choledochojejunostomy, intraoperative use of 40 units or more of blood products, fungal coonization detected within the first 3 days after transplantation.

[c]Therapy is generally the same for AIDS/non-AIDS patients except where indicated and should continued for 2 wk after the last positive blood culture and resolution of signs and symptoms of infection. All patients should receive an ophthalmologic examination. Amphotericin B may be switched to fluconazole (intravenous or oral) for the completion of therapy. Susceptibility testing of the infecting isolate is a useful adjunct to species identification during selection of a therapeutic approach because it can be used to identify isolates that are unlikely to respond to fluconazole or amphotericin B. However, this is not currently available at most institutions.

[d]Often defined as failure of $\geq$500 mg amphotericin B, initial renal insufficiency (creatinine $\geq$2.5 mg/dL or creatinine clearance <25 mL/min), a significant increase in creatinine (to 2.5 mg/dL for adults or 1.5 mg/dL for children) or severe acute administration-related toxicity.

[e]Patients who are neutropenic at the time of developing candidemia should receive a recombinant cytokine (granulocyte colony-stimulating factor or granulocyte-monocyte colony-stimulating factor) that accelerates recovery from neutropenia

[f]Patients at high risk for dissemination include neutropenic patients, low-birth-weight infants, patients with renal allografts, and patients who will undergo urologic manipulation.

VIII

ALLERGIC BRONCHOPULMONARY ASPERGILLOSIS

- Allergic manifestations of *Aspergillus* range in severity from mild asthma to allergic bronchopulmonary aspergillosis (BPA) characterized by severe asthma with wheezing, fever, malaise, weight loss, chest pain, and a cough productive of blood-streaked sputum.
- Therapy is aimed at minimizing the quantity of antigenic material released in the tracheobronchial tree.
- Antifungal therapy is generally not indicated in the management of allergic manifestations of aspergillosis, although some patients have demonstrated a decrease in their glucocorticoid dose following therapy with itraconazole.

ASPERGILLOMA

- In the nonimmunocompromised host, *Aspergillus* infections of the sinuses most commonly occur as saprophytic colonization (aspergillomas, or "fungus balls") of previously abnormal sinus tissue. Treatment consists of removal of the aspergilloma. Therapy with glucocorticoids and surgery is generally successful.
- Although IV amphotericin B is generally not useful in eradicating as-pergillomas, intracavitary instillation of amphotericin B has been employed

successfully in a limited number of patients. Hemoptysis generally ceases when the aspergilloma is eradicated.

INVASIVE ASPERGILLOSIS

Patients often present with classic signs and symptoms of acute pulmonary embolus: pleuritic chest pain, fever, hemoptysis, a friction rub, and a wedge-shaped infiltrate on chest radiographs.

Diagnosis

- Demonstration of *Aspergillus* by repeated culture and microscopic examination of tissue provides the most firm diagnosis. A rapid test to detect galactomannan antigen in blood was recently approved in the United States.
- In the immunocompromised host, aspergillosis is characterized by vascular invasion leading to thrombosis, infarction, and necrosis of tissue.

Treatment

- Antifungal therapy should be instituted in any of the following conditions: (1) persistent fever or progressive sinusitis unresponsive to antimicrobial therapy; (2) an eschar over the nose, sinuses, or palate; (3) the presence of characteristic radiographic findings, including wedge-shaped infarcts, nodular densities, or new cavitary lesions; or (4) any clinical manifestation suggestive of orbital or cavernous sinus disease or an acute vascular event associated with fever. Isolation of *Aspergillus* sp. from nasal or respiratory tract secretions should be considered confirmatory evidence in any of the previously mentioned clinical settings.
- IV **amphotericin B** remains the preferred therapy, at least initially, in acutely ill patients. Since *Aspergillus* is only moderately susceptible to amphotericin B, full doses (1 to 1.5 mg/kg/day) are generally recommended, with response measured by defervescence and radiographic clearing. The lipid-based formulations may be preferred as initial therapy in patients with marginal renal function or in patients receiving other nephrotoxic drugs.
- **Itraconazole** should be reserved as a second-line agent for patients intolerant of or not responding to high-dose amphotericin B. If itraconazole is used, a loading dose of 200 mg three times daily with food for 2 to 3 days should be employed, followed by itraconazole, 200 mg twice daily with food, for a minimum of 6 months.
- **Caspofungin** is indicated for treatment of invasive aspergillosis in patients who are refractory to or intolerant of other therapies such as amphotericin B and/or itraconazole.
- The use of prophylactic antifungal therapy to prevent primary infection or reactivation of aspergillosis during subsequent courses of chemotherapy is controversial.

See Chapter 119, Invasive Fungal Infections, authored by Peggy L. Carver, for a more detailed discussion of this topic.

VIII

Chapter 38

► GASTROINTESTINAL INFECTIONS

Gastrointestinal (GI) infections are among the more common causes of morbidity and mortality around the world. Most are caused by viruses and some are caused by bacteria or other organisms. In underdeveloped and developing countries, acute gastroenteritis involving diarrhea is the leading cause of mortality in infants and children younger than 5 years of age. In the United States, there are approximately 211 million episodes of acute gastroenteritis each year, causing over 900,000 hospitalizations and over 6000 deaths.

► REHYDRATION THERAPY

- Fluid replacement is the cornerstone of therapy for diarrhea regardless of etiology.
- Initial assessment of fluid loss is essential for rehydration. Weight loss is the most reliable means of determining the extent of water loss. Clinical signs such as changes in skin turgor, sunken eyes, dry mucous membranes, decreased tearing, decreased urine output, altered mentation, and changes in vital signs can be helpful in determining approximate deficits (Table 38–1).
- Weight loss of 9% to 10% is considered severe and requires intravenous (IV) fluid replacement with Ringer's lactate or 0.9% sodium chloride. Intravenous therapy is also indicated in patients with uncontrolled vomiting, the presence of paralytic ileus, stool output greater than 10 mL/kg/h, shock, or loss of consciousness.
- The necessary components of oral rehydration therapy (ORT) solutions include glucose, sodium, potassium, chloride, and water (Table 38–2).
- The maintenance phase should not exceed 100 to 150 mL/kg/day and is generally adjusted to equal stool.
- Early refeeding as tolerated is recommended. Age-appropriate diet may be resumed as soon as dehydration is corrected. Early initiation of feeding shortens the course of diarrhea. Initially, easily digested foods, such as bananas, applesauce, and cereal, may be added as tolerated. Foods high in fiber, sodium, and sugar should be avoided.

► BACTERIAL INFECTIONS

- The bacterial species most commonly associated with GI infection and infectious diarrhea in the United States are *Shigella* spp., *Salmonella* spp., *Campylobacter* spp., *Yersinia* spp., *Escherichia* spp., *Clostridium* spp., and *Staphylococcus* spp.
- Antibiotics are not essential in the treatment of most mild diarrheas, and empirical therapy for acute GI infections may result in unnecessary antibiotic courses. Antibiotic choices for bacterial infections are given in Table 38–3.

ENTEROTOXIGENIC (CHOLERA-LIKE) DIARRHEA

Cholera *(Vibrio cholerae)*
- *Vibrio cholerae* is the organisms that most often causes human epidemics and pandemics. Four mechanisms for transmission have been proposed: animal reservoirs, chronic carriers, asymptomatic or mild disease victims, or water reservoirs.

TABLE 38–1. Clinical Assessment of Degree of Dehydration in Children Based on Percentage of Body Weight Loss[a]

Variable	Mild, 3%–5%	Moderate, 6%–9%	Severe, ≥10%
Blood pressure	Normal	Normal	Normal to reduced
Quality of pulses	Normal	Normal or slightly decreased	Moderately decreased
Heart rate	Normal	Increased	Increased (bradycardia in severe cases)
Skin turgor	Normal	Decreased	Decreased
Fontanelle	Normal	Sunken	Sunken
Mucous membranes	Slightly dry	Dry	Dry
Eyes	Normal	Sunken orbits/decreased tears	Deeply sunken orbits/decreased tears
Extremities	Warm, normal capillary refill	Delayed capillary refill	Cool, mottled
Mental status	Normal	Normal to listless	Normal to lethargic or comatose
Urine output	Slightly decreased	<1 mL/kg/h	<1 mL/kg/h
Thirst	Slightly increased	Moderately increased	Very thirsty or too lethargic to indicate
Fluid replacement	ORT 50 mL/kg over 2–4 h	ORT 100 mL/kg over 2–4 h	Ringer lactate 40 mL/kg in 15–30 min, then 20–40 mL/kg if skin turgor, alertness, and pulse have not returned to normal *or* Ringer lactate or NS 20 mL/kg, repeat if necessary, and then replace water and electrolyte deficits over 1–2 days Followed by ORT 100 mL/kg over 4 hours. Replace ongoing losses with low-sodium ORT (40–60 mEq/L Na+) at 10 mL/kg per stool or emesis
	Replace ongoing losses with low-sodium ORT (40–60 mEq/L Na+) at 10 mL/kg per stool or emesis	Replace ongoing losses with low-sodium ORT (40–60 mEq/L Na+) at 10 mL/kg per stool or emesis	

[a]Percentages vary among authors for each dehydration category; hemodynamic and perfusion status is most important; when unsure of category, therapy for more severe category is recommended.
ORT, oral rehydration therapy.

TABLE 38–2. Comparison of Common Solutions Used in Oral Rehydration and Maintenance

Product	Na (mEq/L)	K (mEq/L)	Base (mEq/L)	Carbohydrate (mmol/L)	Osmolality (mOsm/L)
Naturalyte (unlimited beverage)	45	20	48	140	265
Pediatric electrolyte (NutraMax)	45	20	30	140	250
Pedialyte (Ross)	45	20	30	140	250
Infalyte (formerly Ricelyte; Mead Johnson)	50	25	30	70	200
Rehydralyte (Ross)	75	20	30	140	310
WHO/UNICEF oral rehydration salts	90	20	30	111	310
Cola	2	0	13	700	750
Apple juice	5	32	0	690	730
Chicken broth	250	8	0	0	500
Sports beverage	20	3	3	255	330

- Most pathology of cholera is thought to result from an enterotoxin that increases cyclic AMP–mediated secretion of chloride ion into the intestinal lumen, which results in isotonic secretion (primarily in the small intestine) exceeding the absorptive capacity of the intestinal tract (primarily the colon).
- The incubation period of *V. cholerae* is 1 to 3 days.
- Cholera is characterized by a spectrum from the asymptomatic state to the most severe typical cholera syndrome. In the most severe state, this disease can progress to death in a matter of 2 to 4 hours if not treated.

Treatment

- The mainstay of treatment for cholera consists of fluid and electrolyte replacement with ORT. Rice-based rehydration formulations are the preferred ORT for cholera patients. In patients who cannot tolerate ORT intravenous therapy with Ringer's lactate can be used.
- Antibiotics shorten the duration of diarrhea, decrease the volume of fluid lost, and shorten the duration of the carrier state (see Table 38–3). A single dose of oral doxycycline is the preferred agent. In children younger than 7 years of age, **trimethoprim-sulfamethoxazole, erythromycin, and furazolidone** are preferred.

ESCHERICHIA COLI

- *Escherichia coli* GI disease may be caused by enterotoxigenic *E. coli* (ETEC), enteroinvasive *E. coli* (EIEC), enteropathogenic *E. coli* (EPEC), enteroadhesive *E. coli* (EAEC), and enterohemorrhagic *E. coli* (EHEC). ETEC is now incriminated as being the most common cause of traveler's diarrhea.
- ETEC is capable of producing two plasmid-mediated enterotoxins: heat-labile toxin (HLT) and heat-stable toxin (HST). The net effect of either toxin on the mucosa is production of a cholera-like secretory diarrhea.
- Nausea and watery stools, with or without abdominal cramping, are characteristic of the disease caused by ETEC. Most ETEC diarrhea resolves within 24 to 48 hours without complication.
- Most cases respond readily to ORT, and although antibiotic therapy is seldom necessary, prophylaxis has been shown to effectively prevent the development of ETEC diarrhea.
- Fluid and electrolyte replacement should be initiated at the onset of diarrhea.
- Antibiotics used for treatment are found in Table 38–3.

TABLE 38–3. Recommendations for Antibiotic Therapy

Pathogen	First-Line Agents	Alternative Agents
Enterotoxigenic (Cholera-Like) Diarrhea		
Vibrio cholerae O1 or O139	Doxycycline 300 mg oral single dose; tetracycline 500 mg orally 4 times daily × 3 days; or trimethoprim-sulfamethoxazole DS tablet twice daily × 3 days; norfloxacin 400 mg orally twice daily × 3 days; or ciprofloxacin 500 mg orally twice daily × 3 days or 1 g orally single dose	Chloramphenicol 50 mg/kg IV every 6 h, erythromycin 250–500 mg PO every 6–8 h, and furazolidone
Enterotoxigenic E. coli	Norfloxacin 400 mg or ciprofloxacin 500 mg orally twice daily × 3 days	Trimethoprim-sulfamethoxazole DS tablet every 12 h
C. difficile	Metronidazole 250 4 times daily to 500 mg 3 times daily × 10 days	Vancomycin 125 mg orally four times daily × 10 days; bacitracin 20,000–25,000 units 4 times daily × 7–10 days
Invasive (Dysentery-Like) Diarrhea		
Shigella species[a]	Trimethoprim-sulfamethoxazole DS twice daily × 3–5 days	Ofloxacin 300 mg, norfloxacin 400 mg, or ciprofloxacin 500 mg twice daily × 3 days, or nalidixic acid 1 g/day × 5 days; azithromycin 500 mg orally × 1, then 250 mg orally daily × 4 days.
Salmonella		
Nontyphoidal[a]	Trimethoprim-sulfamethoxazole DS twice daily; ofloxacin 300 mg, norfloxacin 400 mg, or ciprofloxacin 500 mg twice daily × 5 days; or ceftriaxone 2 g IV daily or cefotaxime 2 g IV 3 times daily × 5 days	Azithromycin 1000 mg orally × 1 day, followed by 500 mg orally once daily × 6 days
Enteric fever	Ciprofloxacin 500 mg orally twice daily × 3–14 days (ofloxacin and perfloxacin equally efficacious)	Azithromycin 1000 mg orally × 1 day, followed by 500 mg daily × 5 days; or cefixime, cefotaxime, and cefuroxime; or chloramphenicol 500 mg 4 times daily orally or IV × 14 days
Campylobacter[a]	Erythromycin 500 mg orally twice daily × 5 days; azithromycin 1000 mg orally × 1 day, followed by 500 mg daily or clarithromycin 500 mg orally twice daily	Ciprofloxacin 500 mg or norfloxacin 400 mg orally twice daily × 5 days
Yersinia species[a]	A combination therapy with doxycycline, aminoglycosides, trimethoprim-sulfamethoxazole, or fluoroquinolones	
Traveler's Diarrhea		
Prophylaxis[a]	Norfloxacin 400 mg or ciprofloxacin 500 mg orally daily (in Asia, Africa, and South America); trimethoprim-sulfamethoxazole DS tablet orally daily (in Mexico)	
Treatment	Norfloxacin 400 mg or ciprofloxacin 500 mg orally twice daily × 3 days, or trimethoprim-sulfamethoxazole DS tablet orally twice daily × 3 days (in Mexico), or azithromycin 500 mg orally once daily × 3 days (only in areas of high prevalence of quiniolone-resistant Campylobacter species, such as Thailand)	

[a]For high-risk patients only.

- Effective prophylactic agents include **doxycycline, trimethoprim/ sulfamethoxazole, or a fluoroquinolone.**

PSEUDOMEMBRANOUS COLITIS *(CLOSTRIDIUM DIFFICILE)*

- Pseudomembranous colitis (PMC) results from toxins produced by *C. difficile*. It occurs most often in epidemic fashion and affects high-risk groups such as the elderly, debilitated patients, cancer patients, surgical patients, any patient receiving antibiotics, patients with nasogastric tubes, or those who frequently use laxatives.
- PMC has been associated most often with broad-spectrum antimicrobials, including clindamycin, ampicillin, or third-generation cephalosporins.
- PMC may result in a spectrum of disease from mild diarrhea to enterocolitis. In colitis without pseudomembranes, patients present with malaise, abdominal pain, nausea, anorexia, watery diarrhea, low-grade fever, and leukocytosis. With pseudomembranes, there is more severe illness with severe abdominal pain, perfuse diarrhea, high fever, and marked leukocytosis. Symptoms can start a few days after the start of antibiotic therapy to several weeks after antibiotics have been stopped.
- Diagnosis is made by colonoscopic visualization of pseudomembranes, finding VIII ◄ cytotoxins A or B in stools, or stool culture for *C. difficile*.
- Initial therapy of PMC should include discontinuation of the offending agent. The patient should be supported with fluid and electrolyte replacement.
- Both vancomycin and metronidazole are effective, but **metronidazole** 250 mg orally 4 times daily is the drug of choice. Oral **vancomycin,** 125 mg orally 4 times daily, is second-line therapy. It should be reserved for patients not responding to metronidazole, organisms resistant to metronidazole, patients allergic or intolerant to metronidazole, other treatments that include alcohol-containing solutions, patients who are pregnant or younger than 10 years, critically ill patients, or those with diarrhea that is caused by *Staphylococcus aureus*.
- Drugs that inhibit peristalsis, such as **diphenoxylate**, are contraindicated.
- Relapse can occur in 20% to 25% of patients and may be treated with metronidazole or vancomycin for 10 to 14 days.

► INVASIVE (DYSENTERY-LIKE) DIARRHEA

BACILLARY DYSENTERY (SHIGELLOSIS)

- Four species of *Shigella* are most often associated with disease: *S. dysenteriae* type I, *S. flexneri, S. bovdii,* and *S. sonnei.*
- Poor sanitation, poor personal hygiene, inadequate water supply, malnutrition, and increased population density are associated with increased risk of *Shigella* gastroenteritis epidemics, even in developed countries. The majority of cases are thought to result from fecal–oral transmission.
- *Shigella* spp. cause dysentery upon penetrating the epithelial cells lining the colon. Microabscesses may eventually coalesce, forming larger abscesses. Some *Shigella* species produce a cytotoxin, or shigatoxin, the pathogenic role of which is unclear although it is thought to damage endothelial cells of the lamina propria, resulting in microangiopathic changes that can progress to hemolytic uremic syndrome. Watery diarrhea commonly precedes the dysentery and may be a result of these toxins.
- Initial signs and symptoms include abdominal pain, cramping, and fever followed by frequent watery stools. Watery stools start within 48 hours of infection

and are followed by bloody diarrhea and other signs of dysentery within a few days.

- If untreated, bacillary dysentery usually lasts about 1 week (range 1 to 30 days).
- Shigellosis is usually a self-limiting disease. Most patients recover in 4 to 7 days. Treatment of bacillary dysentery generally includes correction of fluid and electrolyte disturbances and, occasionally, antimicrobials.
- Antimicrobials are indicated in the infirm, those who are immunocompromised, children in day care centers, the elderly, malnourished children, and health care workers. Antimicrobials may shorten the period of fecal shedding and attenuate the clinical illness.
- The agent of choice is **trimethoprim/sulfamethoxazole** for infections acquired in the United States. For infections acquired outside the United States, the agents of choice are **ciprofloxacin, norfloxacin,** and **azithromycin.** Fluoroquinolones are generally contraindicated in children and adolescents.
- Fluid and electrolyte losses can generally be replaced with oral therapy, as dysentery is generally not associated with significant fluid loss. Intravenous replacement is necessary only for children or the elderly.
- Antimotility agents such as diphenoxylate are not recommended because they can worsen dysentery.

SALMONELLOSIS

- Human disease caused by *Salmonella* generally falls into four categories: acute gastroenteritis (enterocolitis), bacteremia, extraintestinal localized infection, and enteric fever (typhoid and paratyphoid fever), and a chronic carrier state. *S. typhimurium* is the most common cause of salmonellosis.
- *Salmonella* enterocolitis occurs secondary to mucosal invasion of microorganisms, but it may involve enterotoxin production or local inflammatory exudates as possible mechanisms of pathology. Organisms may invade beyond the mucosa and enter the mesenteric lymphatics, which then carry bacteria to the general circulation via the thoracic duct. Bacteria not cleared by the reticuloendothelial system may cause metastatic infection in various organs.
- With enterocolitis, patients often complain of nausea and vomiting within 72 hours of ingestion followed by crampy abdominal pain, fever, and diarrhea, although the actual presentation is quite variable.
- Stool cultures inevitably yield the causative organism, if obtained early. However, recovery of organisms continues to decrease with time so that by 3 to 4 weeks, only 5% to 15% of adult patients are passing *Salmonella*.
- Some patients may continue to shed *Salmonella* for a year or longer. These "chronic carrier" states are rare for serotypes other than *S. typhi*.
- *Salmonella* can produce bacteremia without classic enterocolitis or enteric fever. The clinical syndrome is characterized by persistent bacteremia and prolonged intermittent fever with chills. Stool cultures are frequently negative.
- Extraluminal infection and/or abscess formation can occur at any site after any of the other syndromes or may be the primary presentation. Metastatic infections have been reported to involve bone, cysts, heart, kidney, liver, lungs, pericardium, spleen, and tumors.
- Enteric fever caused by *S. typhi* is called typhoid fever. If caused by any other serotype, it is referred to as paratyphoid fever. The onset of symptoms is gradual. Nonspecific symptoms of fever, dull headache, malaise, anorexia, and myalgias are most common. Initially, fever tends to be remittent but gradually progresses over the first week to temperatures that are often sustained over

104°F. Other frequently encountered symptoms include chills, nausea, vomiting, cough, weakness, and sore throat.

- About 80% of patients have positive blood cultures. Bacteremia persists in about one-third of patients for several weeks if not treated. Diagnostic tests other than culture are unreliable.

Treatment

- Most patients with enterocolitis require no therapeutic intervention. The most important part of therapy for *Salmonella* enterocolitis is fluid and electrolyte replacement. Antimotility drugs should be avoided since they increase the risk of mucosal invasion and complications.
- Antibiotics have no effect on the duration of fever or diarrhea and their frequent use increases the likelihood of resistance and the duration of fecal shedding. Antibiotics should be used in neonates or infants younger than 6 months, patients with primary or secondary immunodeficiency, severely symptomatic patients with fever and bloody diarrhea, and patients after splenectomy.
- Recommended antibiotics with adult doses include:
  - Fluoroquinolones
  - Trimethoprim/sulfamethoxazole
  - Ampicillin
  - Third-generation cephalosporins

VIII

- For bacteremia, life-threatening treatment should include the combination of a third-generation cephalosporin (ceftriaxone 2 g IV daily) and ciprofloxacin 500 mg orally twice daily. The duration of antibiotic therapy is dictated by the site.
- Fluoroquinolones such as **ciprofloxacin** (500 mg orally twice daily for 10 days in adults) are the drugs of choice for enteric fever, particularly in areas where multidrug resistance is common. A short course of 3 to 5 days is effective but a minimum of 10 days is recommended in severe cases.
- The drug of choice for chronic carriers of *Salmonella* is **norfloxacin,** 400 mg orally twice daily for 28 days.
- Vaccines are recommended for high-risk groups. Live oral attenuated vaccine Ty21a and parenteral polysaccharide vaccine have been shown to confer 42% to 77% efficacy for a duration of 3 to 5 years.

CAMPYLOBACTERIOSIS

- *Campylobacter* species are thought to be a major cause of diarrhea.
- Transmission of infection occurs primarily by ingestion of contaminated food or water.
- Incubation usually averages 2 to 4 days.
- The most common symptoms include diarrhea of varying consistency and severity, abdominal pain, and fever. Nausea, vomiting, headache, myalgias, and malaise may also occur. Bowel movements may be numerous, bloody (dysentery-like), foul smelling, and melenic and range from loose to watery (dysentery-like).
- The disease is self-limiting, and signs and symptoms usually resolve in about a week but may persist longer in 10% to 20% of patients.
- As with other acute diarrheal illnesses, fluid and electrolyte support is a mainstay of therapy, mainly with ORT.
- Antibiotics are not useful unless started within 4 days of the start of illness, as they do not shorten the duration or severity of diarrhea.

- Antibiotics are warranted in patients who present with high fevers, severe bloody diarrhea, prolonged illness (greater than 1 week), pregnancy, and immunocompromised states, including HIV infection.
- Erythromycin is considered the drug of choice for treatment. Clarithromycin or azithromycin are equally effective. Antimotility drugs are contraindicated.

YERSINIOSIS

- *Yersinia enterocolitica* and *Y. pseudotuberculosis* are associated with intestinal infection. The organisms have been isolated from a variety of food sources, including raw goat and cow milk.
- These bacteria cause a wide spectrum of clinical syndromes.
- The majority of cases present with enterocolitis that is mild and self-limiting. Symptoms, generally lasting 1 to 3 weeks, include vomiting, abdominal pain, diarrhea, and fever.
- A clinical syndrome seen in older children may resemble appendicitis.
- Many patients develop a reactive arthritis 1 to 2 weeks after recovery from enteritis.
- These diseases are generally self-limiting and are easily managed with oral rehydration solutions.
- Antibiotics should be used in high-risk patients who develop bacteremia (i.e. infants younger than 3 months and patients with cirrhosis or iron overload) or in patients with bone and joint infections.
- *Y. enterocolitica* is generally susceptible to **fluoroquinolones,** alone or in combination with **third-generation cephalosporins** or **aminoglycosides.** Alternative agents include **chloramphenicol, tetracycline,** and **trimethoprim/sulfamethoxazole.**
- Suggested antibiotics of choice are given in Table 38–3.

VIII

▶ ACUTE VIRAL GASTROENTERITIS

ROTAVIRUSES

- The highest frequency of rotavirus-associated diarrhea appears in children between the age of 2 to 3 years. The exact mechanism by which the rotaviruses cause diarrhea is not known.
- Clinical manifestations of rotavirus infections vary from asymptomatic (which is common in adults) to severe nausea, vomiting, and diarrhea with dehydration. Symptoms are characterized initially by nausea and vomiting. Diarrhea occurs in most patients and lasts for 1 to 9 days, but some patients experience only loose stool with no increase in frequency. Other signs and symptoms include fever, respiratory symptoms, irritability, lethargy, pharyngeal erythema, rhinitis, red tympanic membranes, and palpable cervical lymph nodes. Dehydration and electrolyte disturbances occur more frequently in children.
- Treatment of rotavirus-associated vomiting and/or diarrhea is directed at prevention or correction of dehydration.

NORWALK AND NORWALK-LIKE AGENTS

- Norwalk-like viral gastroenteritis is characterized by sudden onset of abdominal cramps with nausea and/or vomiting. Although adults frequently experience nonbloody diarrhea, children experience vomiting more often. Other frequent complaints are myalgias, headache, and malaise, which are accompanied by

fever in about 50% of cases. Signs and symptoms generally last only 12 to 48 hours.
- The disease is generally self-limiting and does not require therapy. On occasion, oral rehydration may be required. Rarely is parenteral hydration necessary.

See Chapter 111, Gastrointestinal Infections and Enterotoxigenic Poisonings, authored by Steven Martin and Rose Jung, for a more detailed discussion of this topic.

VIII ◄

Chapter 39

▶ HIV/AIDS

▶ DEFINITION

Table 39–1 and Table 39–2 present the revised classification systems for adult and child HIV infection.

▶ PATHOGENESIS

TRANSMISSION OF HIV

- Infection with HIV occurs through three primary modes: sexual, parenteral, and perinatal. Sexual intercourse, primarily receptive anal and vaginal intercourse, is the most common vehicle for transmission. The probability of HIV transmission from receptive anorectal intercourse is 0.1% to 3% per sexual contact and 0.1% to 0.2% per sexual contact for receptive vaginal intercourse. In general, the risk is increased when the index partner is in an advanced stage of disease. Persons at higher risk for heterosexual transmission include those with ulcerative sexually transmitted diseases, those with multiple sex partners, and sexual partners of intravenous drug users.
- The use of contaminated needles or other injection-related paraphernalia by drug abusers has been the main cause of parenteral transmissions and currently accounts for one-fourth of AIDS cases reported in the United States.
- Health care workers have a small risk of occupationally acquiring HIV, mostly through needlestick injury.
- Perinatal infection, or vertical transmission, is the most common cause (greater than 90%) of pediatric HIV infection. The risk of mother-to-child transmission is approximately 25% in the absence of breast feeding or antiretroviral therapy. Breast feeding can also transmit HIV.

▶ CLINICAL PRESENTATION

- Clinical presentations of primary HIV infection vary, but patients often have a viral syndrome or mononucleosis-like illness with fever, pharyngitis, and adenopathy (Table 39-3). Symptoms may last for 2 weeks.
- Probability of progression to AIDS is related to RNA viral load; in one study, 5-year progression rates to AIDS were 8%, 26%, 49%, and 62% for RNA copies per milliliter of less than 4530, 4531 to 13,020, 13,021 to 36,270, and greater than 36,270, respectively.
- The classification scheme of the Centers for Disease Control and Prevention (CDC) divides HIV infection into a matrix of nine categories based on the CD4 cell count (see "Diagnosis" below) and clinical conditions (see Table 39-1).
- Most children born with HIV are asymptomatic. On physical examination, they often present with unexplained physical signs such as lymphadenopathy, hepatomegaly, splenomegaly, failure to thrive and weight loss or unexplained low birth weight, and fever of unknown origin. Laboratory findings include anemia, hypergammaglobulinemia, altered mononuclear cell function, and altered T-cell subset ratios. The normal range for CD4 cell counts in children is much different than for adults (Table 39-2).
- Clinical presentations of the opportunistic infections are presented in "Infectious Complications of HIV," below.

TABLE 39–1. Centers for Disease Control and Prevention 1993 Revised Classification System for HIV Infection in Adults and AIDS Surveillance Case Definition

CD4 + T-Cell Categories (Absolute Number and Percentage)	(A) Asymptomatic, Acute (Primary) HIV or PGL[a]	(B) Symptomatic, not (A) or (C) Conditions	(C) AIDS-Indicator Conditions
≥500/μL or ≥29%	A1	B1	C1
200–499/μL or 14–28%	A2	B2	C2
<200/μL or <14%	A3	B3	C3

AIDS-Indicator Conditions

Candidiasis of bronchi, trachea, or lungs
Candidiasis, esophageal
Cervical cancer, invasive
Coccidioidomycosis, disseminated or extrapulmonary
Cryptococcosis, extrapulmonary
Cryptosporidiosis, chronic intestinal (duration >1 month)
Cytomegalovirus disease (other than liver, spleen or nodes)
Cytomegalovirus retinitis (with loss of vision)
Encephalopathy, HIV-related
Herpes simplex: chronic ulcer(s) (duration >1 month); or bronchitis, pneumonitis, or esophagitis
Histoplasmosis, disseminated or extrapulmonary
Isosporiasis, chronic intestinal (duration >1 month)
Kaposi's sarcoma
Lymphoma, Burkitt's
Lymphoma, immunoblastic
Lymphoma, primary, or brain
Mycobacterium avium complex or M. kansasii, disseminated or extrapulmonary
Mycobacterium tuberculosis, any site (pulmonary or extrapulmonary)
Mycobacterium, other species or unidentified species, disseminated or extrapulmonary
Pneumocystis carinii pneumonia
Pneumonia, recurrent
Progressive multifocal leukoencephalopathy
Salmonella septicemia, recurrent
Toxoplasmosis of brain
Wasting syndrome due to HIV

[a]PCL, persistent generalized lymphadenopathy.

TABLE 39–2. Centers for Disease Control and Prevention 1994 Revised Classification System for HIV Infection in Children Younger than 13 Years

Immunologic Categories	12 Months Cells/μL (%)[a]	1–5 Years Cells/μL (%)[a]	6–12 Years Cells/μL (%)[a]
1. No evidence of suppression	≥1500 (≥25%)	≥1000 (≥25%)	≥500 (≥25%)
2. Evidence of moderate suppression	750–1499 (15%–24%)	500–999 (15%–24%)	200–499 (15%–24%)
3. Severe suppression	<750 (<15%)	<500 (<15%)	<200 (<15%)

Immunologic Categories	N: No Signs/Symptoms	A: Mild Signs/Symptoms	B: Moderate Signs/Symptoms	C: Severe Signs/Symptoms
1. No evidence of suppression	N1	A1	B1	C1
2. Evidence of moderate suppression	N2	A2	B2	C2
3. Severe suppression	N3	A3	B3	C3

[a]Percentage of total lymphocytes.

TABLE 39–3. Clinical Presentation of Primary HIV Infection in Adults

Symptoms

Fever, sore throat, fatigue, weight loss, and myalgia

40%–80% of patients will also exhibit a morbilliform or maculopapular rash usually involving the trunk

Diarrhea, nausea, and vomiting

Lymphadenopathy, night sweats

Aseptic meningitis (fever, headache, photophobia, and stiff neck) may be present in a quarter of presenting cases

Other

High viral load (exceeding 50,000 copies/mL in the adult or 500,000 copies/mL in the child

Persistent decrease in CD4 lymphocytes

▶ DIAGNOSIS

- The most commonly used screening method for HIV is an enzyme-linked immunosorbent assay (ELISA), which detects antibodies against HIV-1 and is both highly sensitive and specific. False positives can occur in multiparous women; in recent recipients of hepatitis B, HIV, influenza, or rabies vaccine; following multiple blood transfusions; and in those with liver disease or renal failure, or undergoing chronic hemodialysis. False negatives may occur if the patient is newly infected and the test is performed before antibody production is adequate. The minimum time to develop antibodies is 3 to 4 weeks from initial exposure.
- Positive ELISAs are repeated in duplicate and if one or both tests are reactive, a confirmatory test is performed for final diagnosis. Western blot assay is the most commonly used confirmatory test.
- The viral load test quantifies viremia by measuring the amount of viral RNA. There are several methods used for determining the amount of HIV RNA: reverse transcriptase-coupled polymerase chain reaction (RT-PCR), branched DNA (bDNA), and transcription-mediated amplification. Each assay has its own lower limit of sensitivity, and results can vary from one assay method to the other; therefore, it is recommended that the same assay method be used consistently within patients.
- Viral load can be used as a prognostic factor to monitor disease progression and the effects of treatment.
- The number of CD4 lymphocytes in the blood is a surrogate marker of disease progression. The normal adult CD4 lymphocyte count ranges between 500 and 1600 cells/μL, or 40% to 70% of all lymphocytes.

▶ TREATMENT

GOALS OF TREATMENT

The goal of antiretroviral therapy is to achieve the maximum suppression of HIV replication (HIV RNA level that is less than the lower limit of quantitation). Secondary goals include an increase in CD4 lymphocytes and an improved quality of life. The ultimate goal is decreased morbidity and mortality.

GENERAL APPROACH TO TREATMENT OF HIV INFECTION

- Regular, periodic measurement of plasma HIV RNA levels and CD4 cell counts is necessary to determine the risk of disease progression in an HIV-infected individual and to determine when to initiate or modify antiretroviral treatment regimens.

- Treatment decisions should be individualized by level of risk indicated by plasma HIV RNA levels and CD4 counts.
- The use of potent combination antiretroviral therapy to suppress HIV replication to below the levels of detection of sensitive plasma HIV RNA assays limits the potential for selection of antiretroviral-resistant HIV variants, the major factor limiting the ability of antiretroviral drugs to inhibit virus replication and delay disease progression.
- The most effective means to accomplish durable suppression of HIV replication is the simultaneous initiation of combinations of effective anti-HIV drugs with which the patient has not been previously treated and that are not cross resistant with antiretroviral agents with which the patient has been treated previously.
- Each of the antiretroviral drugs used in combination therapy regimens should always be used according to optimum schedules and dosages.
- Women should receive optimal antiretroviral therapy regardless of pregnancy status.
- The same principles of antiretroviral therapy apply to both HIV-infected children and adults, although the treatment of HIV-infected children involves unique pharmacologic, virologic, and immunologic considerations.
- Persons with acute primary HIV infections should be treated with combination antiretroviral therapy to suppress virus replication to levels below the limit of detection of sensitive plasma HIV RNA assays.
- HIV-infected persons, even those with viral loads below detectable limits, should be considered infectious and should be counseled to avoid sexual and drug-use behaviors that are associated with transmission or acquisition of HIV and other infectious pathogens.
- An excellent source for information on treatment guidelines can be found at www.aidsinfo.nih.gov.
- Treatment is recommended for all HIV-infected persons with symptomatic disease or CD4 lymphocyte counts less than 350 cell/μL or plasma HIV RNA greater than 55,000 copies/mL regardless of CD4 count (Table 39–4).

VIII

PHARMACOLOGIC THERAPY

Antiretroviral Agents

- Inhibiting viral replication with combination of potent antiretroviral therapy has been the most clinically successful strategy in the treatment of HIV infection. There have been three primary groups of drugs used: **nucleoside and nonnucleoside reverse transcriptase inhibitors** and **protease inhibitors** (Table 39–5).
- Reverse transcriptase inhibitors are of two types: those that are derivatives of purine- and pyrimidine-based nucleosides and nucleotides (NRTIs) and those that are not nucleoside or nucleotide based (NNRTIs).
- Current recommendations for treating HIV infection advocate a minimum of three antiretroviral agents. The typical regimen consists of two nucleoside analogues with either a protease inhibitor (PI) or an NNRTI.
- Significant drug interactions can occur with many antiretroviral agents:

  - **Amprenavir**, **Efavirenz**, **tipranavir**, and **nevirapine** are inducers of drug metabolism, whereas **delavirdine** and protease inhibitors inhibit drug metabolism.
  - **Ritonavir** is a potent inhibitor of cytochrome P4503A and is used to reduce clearance of other protease inhibitors.

TABLE 39–4. Treatment of HIV Infection: Antiretroviral Regimens Recommended in Antiretroviral-Naive Persons

Nonnucleoside Reverse Transcriptase Inhibitor (NNRTI)–Based Regimens	
Preferred	Efavirenz + lamivudine + zidovudine (or tenofovir DF or stavudine) except for pregnant women or women with pregnancy potential
Alternatives	Efavirenz + emtricitabine + zidovudine (or tenofovir DF or stavudine) except for pregnant women or women with pregnancy potential
	or
	Efavirenz + (lamivudine or emtricitabine) + didanosine except for pregnant women or women with pregnancy potential
	or
	Nevirapine + (lamivudine or emtricitabine) + zidovudine (or stavudine or didanosine)
Protease Inhibitor (PI)–Based Regimens	
Preferred	Lopinavir/ritonavir + lamivudine + zidovudine (or stavudine)
Alternatives	Amprenavir/ritonavir + lamivudine (or emtricitabine) + zidovudine (or stavudine)
	Atazanavir + lamivudine (or emtricitabine) + zidovudine (or stavudine)
	Indinavir-ritonavir + lamivudine (or emtricitabine) + zidovudine (or stavudine)
	Lopinavir-ritonavir + emtricitabine + zidovudine (or stavudine)
	Nelfinavir + lamivudine (or emtricitabine) + zidovudine (or stavudine)
	Saquinavir-ritonavir + lamivudine (or emtricitabine) + zidovudine (or stavudine)
Triple Nucleoside Reverse Transcriptase Inhibitor–Based Regimen	
(Only as an alternative to NNRTI- or PI-based regimens when these cannot be used as preferred therapy)	
	Abacavir + lamivudine + zidovudine
	Abacavir + lamivudine + stavudine

VIII

NTRI, nucleoside reverse transcriptase inhibitor; NNRTI, nonnucleoside reverse transcriptase inhibitor; PI, protease inhibitor.
From Panel on Clinical Practice for Treatment of HIV Infection. Guidelines for the use of antiretroviral agents in HIV-infected adults and adolescents. November 3, 2003. http://AIDSinfo.NIH.gov; accessed, January 5, 2004.

- Two NRTIs, **zidovudine** and **stavudine**, antagonize each other's metabolism and should not be given together.
- Rifampin may substantially reduce the concentrations of PIs
- Saint John's wort is a potent inducer of metabolism and is contraindicated with PIs and NNRTIs.

TREATMENT DURING PREGNANCY

Therapy during pregnancy is warranted, particularly in light of the dramatic reduction in transmission seen with **zidovudine** monotherapy. In general, pregnant women should be treated similar to nonpregnant adults; if possible, zidovudine should be used for both mother and infant.

POSTEXPOSURE PROPHYLAXIS

- Postexposure prophylaxis (PEP) with a triple-drug regimen consisting of two NRTIS and a PI is recommended for percutaneous blood exposure involving significant risk (i.e., large volume of blood or blood from patients with advanced AIDS).
- Two NRTIs may be offered to health care workers with lower risk of exposure such as that involving either the mucous membrane or skin. Treatment is not necessary if the source of exposure is urine or saliva.
- Treatment should ideally be initiated within 1 to 2 hours. The optimal duration of treatment is unknown, but at least 4 weeks of therapy is advocated.

TABLE 39–5. Pharmacologic Parameters of Antiretroviral Compounds

Drug	In Vitro Susceptibility (μM IC$_{50}$ range)	F (%)	V_d (L/kg)	$t_{1/2}$ (h)	CL/F (L/h)	Adult Dose[a] (doses/day)	Plasma C_{max}/C_{min} (μM)	Ratio Fetal-Maternal Conc.	Ratio CSF-Plasma Conc.
Nucleoside Reverse Transcriptase Inhibitors									
Abacavir	0.07–5.8	83	0.86	1.5	49.8	300 mg (2)	10.7/0.04	?	0.3
Didanosine	0.01–10	40	0.83	1.4	26.9	200 mg (2) 400 mg(1)	4/0.02	0.3–0.5	0.22
Emtricitabine	0.0013–0.64	93	3	10	21	200 mg (1)	7.3/0.04	?	?
Lamivudine	0.002–15	86	1.3	5	23.1	150 mg (2) 300 mg (1)	7.5/0.22	>0.7	0.12
Stavudine	0.009–4	86	0.53	1.4	34	40 mg (2)	4/0.004	>0.7	0.02
Tenofovir	0.04–8.5	40	1.2	17	35.7	300 mg (1)	1.13/0.2[b]	?	?
Zalcitabine	0.03–0.5	85	0.53	2	12	0.75 mg (3)	0.05/0.001	0.3–0.5	0.2
Zidovudine	0.01–0.048	64	1.6	1.1	112	200 mg (3) 300 mg (2)	2/0.2	>0.7	0.6
Nonnucleoside Reverse Transcriptase Inhibitors									
Delavirdine	0.05–0.1[c]	85	0.48[d]	5.8	4	400 mg (3)	35/14	?	0.004
Efavirenz	0.0017–0.025[c]	43	10.2[d]	48	10.3	600 mg (1)	12.9/5.6	?	0.007
Nevirapine	0.010–0.1	50	1.21	25	2.6	200 mg (2)[c]	5.5/3.0	1	0.45

(Continued)

Protease Inhibitors

Amprenavir	0.012–0.41	?	6.1^d	9	64.9	1200 mg (2)	10.7/0.56	?	0.02
Atazanavir	0.002–0.005	68	3.6^d	7	25.2	400 mg (1)	3.26/0.17	?	0.0021–0.0226
Indinavir	$0.025–0.1^c$	60	1.2^d	1.5	43	800 mg (3)	13/0.25	?	0.07
Lopinavir[f]	0.004–0.027	?	0.74^d	5.5	6.5	400 mg (2)	15.4/8.8	?	?
Nelfinavir	0.009–0.06	?	2^b	2.6	37.4	750 mg (3)	5.6/0.7	?	IND
						1250 mg (2)			
Ritonavir	0.0038–0.154	60	0.41^d	3–5	8.8	600 mg $(2)^e$	16/5	?	IND
Saquinavir[g]	0.001–0.03	12	10	3	80	1200 mg (3)	0.4/0.15	?	IND

[a] Dose adjustment may be required for weight, renal or hepatic disease, and drug interactions.

[b] Using PMPA molecular weight, not prodrug.

[c] Range given is for IC_{90} or IC_{95}.

[d] V_d/F.

[e] Initial dose escalation recommended to minimize side effects.

[f] Available as coformulation 4:1 lopinavir to ritonavir.

[g] Soft-gel formulation.

IND, indeterminate with standard analytical techniques; F, bioavailability; V_d, distribution volume; $t_{1/2}$, elimination half-life; CL, total-body clearance; C_{max}, Maximum plasma concentration; C_{min}, minimum plasma concentration; CSF, cerebrospinal fluid; IC_{50-90}, concentration required to produce 50 or 90% inhibition of HIV strains in vitro.

▶ EVALUATION OF THERAPEUTIC OUTCOMES

- Following the initiation of therapy, patients are usually monitored at 3-month intervals with immunologic (i.e., CD4 count), virologic (HIV RNA), and clinical assessments.
- There are two general indications to change therapy: significant toxicity or treatment failure.
- Specific criteria to indicate treatment failure have not been established through controlled clinical trials. As a general guide, the following events should prompt consideration for changing therapy:
  - Less than a 1 $\log_{10}$ reduction in HIV RNA 1 month after the initiation of therapy, or a failure to achieve maximal suppression of HIV replications within 4 to 6 months.
  - A persistent decline in the CD4 cell count or a return to the pretreatment value or an increase in HIV RNA of 0.3 to 0.5 $\log_{10}$ copies/mL from nadir.
  - Clinical disease progression, usually the development of a new opportunistic infection.

▶ VIII THERAPEUTIC FAILURE

- Therapeutic failure may be the result of nonadherence to medication, development of drug resistance, intolerance to one or more medications, adverse drug-drug interactions, or pharmacokinetic-pharmacodynamic variability.
- In general, patients failing their first regimens should be treated with a drug representing a new class. Therapy should be changed to at least two new antiretroviral drugs that are not cross resistant with the agents the patient previously received.

▶ INFECTIOUS COMPLICATIONS OF HIV

- The development of certain opportunistic infections is directly or indirectly related to the level of CD4 lymphocytes.
- The most common opportunistic diseases and their frequencies found before death in patients with AIDS between 1990 and 1994 were *Pneumocystis carinii* pneumonia, *Mycobacterium avium* complex (MAC), and cytomegalovirus (CMV) disease.
- The spectrum of infectious diseases observed in HIV-infected individuals and recommended first-line therapies are shown in Table 39–6.

PNEUMOCYSTIS CARINII

P. carinii pneumonia (PCP) is the most common life-threatening opportunistic infection in patients with AIDS. The taxonomy of the organism is unclear, having been classified as both protozoan and fungal.

Clinical Presentation

- Characteristic symptoms include fever and dyspnea; clinical signs are tachypnea, with or without rales or rhonchi, and a nonproductive or mildly productive cough. Chest radiographs may show florid or subtle infiltrates or may occasionally be normal, although infiltrates are usually interstitial and bilateral. Arterial blood gases may show minimal hypoxia (PaO_2 80 to 95 mm Hg) but in more advanced disease may be markedly abnormal.
- The onset of PCP is often insidious, occurring over a period of weeks, although more fulminant presentations can occur.

TABLE 39–6. Therapies for Common Opportunistic Pathogens in HIV-Infected Individuals

Clinical Disease	Selected Initial Therapies for Acute Infection in Adults	Common Drug- or Dose-Limiting Adverse Reactions
Fungi		
Candidiasis, oral	Fluconazole 200 mg orally single dose or 100 mg orally for 5 days	Taste; patient acceptance
	or	
	Nystatin 500,000 units oral swish 4–6 times daily for 7–10 days,	
	or	
	Clotrimazole 10 mg (1 troche) orally 5 times daily for 7–10 days	
Candidiasis, esophageal	Fluconazole 200 mg orally or intravenously on the first day then 100 mg/day for 10–14 days	Elevated liver function tests, hepatotoxicity, nausea and vomiting
	or	
	Ketoconazole 400 mg/day orally for 10–14 days	Elevated liver function tests, hepatotoxicity, rash, nausea and vomiting
Pneumocystis carinii pneumonia	Trimethoprim–sulfamethoxazole intravenously or orally 12–20 mg/kg/day as trimethoprim component in 3–4 divided doses for 21 days[a]	Skin rash, fever, leukopenia Thrombocytopenia
	or	
	Mild episodes	
	Pentamidine intravenously 3–4 mg/kg/day for 21 days[a]	Azotemia, hypoglycemia, Hyperglycemia
	Atovaquone suspension 750 mg (5 mL) orally twice daily with meals for 21 days[a]	Rash, elevated liver enzymes, diarrhea
Cryptococcal meningitis	Amphotericin B 0.5–1 mg/kg/day intravenously for a minimum of 2 wk *with* or *without* flucytosine 100–150 mg/kg/day orally in 4 divided doses *followed by*	Nephrotoxicity, hypokalemia, anemia, fever, chills Bone marrow suppression, Elevated liver enzymes
	Fluconazole 100 to 200 mg/day, orally[a]	Same as above

(Continued)

TABLE 39–6. (Continued)

Clinical Disease	Selected Initial Therapies for Acute Infection in Adults	Common Drug- or Dose-Limiting Adverse Reactions
Histoplasmosis	Amphotericin B 0.5–1 mg/kg/day intravenously for 6–8 wk[a]	Same as above
	or	
	Itraconazole 200–400 mg/day orally for 3 months[a]	Elevated liver function tests, hepatotoxicity, nausea and vomiting, hypertension
Coccidioidomycosis	Amphotericin B 0.5–1 mg/kg/day intravenously for ≥6–8 wk[a]	Same as above
Protozoa		
Toxoplasmic encephalitis	Pyrimethamine 200 mg orally once then 50–100 mg/day	Bone marrow suppression
	+	
	Sulfadiazine 1–1.5 g orally 4 times daily	Allergy, rash, drug fever
	and	
	Folinic acid 10–20 mg orally daily for a minimum of 28 days[a]	Same as above
Isosporiasis	Trimethoprim and sulfamethoxazole 1–2 double-strength tablets (160 mg trimethoprim and 800 mg sulfamethoxazole) orally twice daily for 2–4 wk	
Bacteria		
Organisms associated with T-cell defects:		
Mycobacterium avium complex	Clarithromycin 500 mg orally twice daily, + ethambutol 15 mg/kg/day orally to a maximum of 1000 mg/day, and Rifabutin 300 mg/day[a]	Gastrointestinal intolerance; Optic neuritis, peripheral neuritis; Rash, gastrointestinal intolerance; Neutropenia, discolored urine, uveitis
Salmonella enterocolitis or bacteremia	Ciprofloxacin 500–750 mg orally twice daily for 14 days,	Gastrointestinal intolerance
	or	
	Trimethoprim (160 mg)-sulfamethoxazole (800 mg) 1 tablet orally twice daily for 14 days	Same as above

Organisms associated with B-cell defects:		
Campylobacter enterocolitis	Ciprofloxacin 500 mg orally twice daily for 7 days	Same as above
	or	
	Erythromycin 250–500 mg orally four times daily for 7 days	Gastrointestinal intolerance, colitis ototoxicity
Shigella enterocolitis	Ciprofloxacin 500 mg orally twice daily for 5 days	Same as above
Viruses		
Mucocutaneous herpes simplex	Acyclovir 1–2 g/day orally in 3–5 divided doses for 7–10 days	Gastrointestinal intolerance
	or	
	Valacyclovir 500 mg orally every 12 h for 7–10 days	Gastrointestinal intolerance
	Famciclovir 500 mg orally every 12 h for 7–10 days	Headache, gastrointestinal intolerance
Varicella-zoster	Acyclovir 30 mg/kg/day intravenously in 3 divided doses *or* 4 g/day orally for 7–10 days	Obstructive nephropathy, CNS symptomatology
	or	
	Valacyclovir, 1 g orally every 8 h for 7–10 days	Gastrointestinal intolerance
	or	
	Famciclovir 500 mg orally every 8 h for 7–10 days	
Cytomegalovirus	Ganciclovir 7.5–10 mg/kg/day in 2–3 divided doses intravenously for 14 days[a]	Neutropenia, thrombocytopenia
	or	
	Foscarnet 180 mg/kg/day in 2 or 3 divided doses intravenously for 14 days[a]	Nephrotoxicity, hypohypercalcemia, hypohyperphosphatemia, anemia
Cytomegalovirus retinitis	Ganciclovir intraocular implant	

[a]Maintenance therapy is recommended.

Treatment

- Treatment with **trimethoprim–sulfamethoxazole** or parenteral pentamidine is associated with a 60% to 100% response rate. Trimethoprim–sulfamethoxazole is the regimen of choice for treatment and subsequent prophylaxis of PCP in patients with and without HIV.
- Trimethoprim–sulfamethoxazole is given in doses of 15 to 20 mg/kg/day (based on the trimethoprim component) as three to four divided doses for the treatment of PCP.
- Trimethoprim–sulfamethoxazole is usually initiated by the intravenous route, although oral therapy (as oral absorption is high) may suffice in mildly ill and reliable patients or to complete a course of therapy after a response has been achieved with intravenous administration.
- For treatment of HIV-associated PCP, **pentamidine isethionate** is administered intravenously, usually in doses of 4 mg/kg /day.
- The optimum length of therapy for treatment of PCP with either agent is not known, but 21 days is commonly recommended.
- The more common adverse reactions seen with trimethoprim–sulfamethoxazole are rash, fever, leukopenia, elevated serum transaminases, and thrombocytopenia. The incidence of these adverse reactions is higher in HIV-infected individuals than in those not infected with HIV.
- For pentamidine, side effects include hypotension, tachycardia, nausea, vomiting, severe hypoglycemia or hyperglycemia, pancreatitis, irreversible diabetes mellitus, elevated transaminases, nephrotoxicity, leukopenia, and cardiac arrhythmias.
- The early addition of adjunctive glucocorticoid therapy to anti-PCP regimens has been shown to decrease the risk of respiratory failure and improve survival in patients with AIDS and moderate to severe PCP (PaO_2 less than or equal to ≤ 0 mm Hg or [A–a] gradient $\geq$ reater than or equal to 35 mm Hg). The regimen currently recommended is 40 mg of prednisone orally twice daily during days 1 through 5; 40 mg once daily on days 6 through 10; and 20 mg once daily on days 11 through 21, or for the duration of therapy. In general, adjunctive glucocorticoid therapy should be initiated when antipneumocystis therapy is started, as the data supporting the use of glucocorticoids are based on initiation within the first 24 to 72 hours of the start of antipneumocystis therapy.

Prophylaxis

- Currently, PCP prophylaxis is recommended for all HIV-infected individuals who have already had previous PCP. Prophylaxis is also recommended for all HIV-infected persons who have a CD4 lymphocyte count of less than 200 cells/μL (i.e. their CD4 cells are less than 20% of total lymphocytes), unexplained fever (greater than 100 °F) for more than 2 weeks, or a history of oropharyngeal candidiasis. Patients on PCP prophylaxis whose CD4 counts increase above 200 cells/μL antiretroviral therapy should not discontinue PCP prophylaxis at this point (Table 39-7).
- Trimethoprim–sulfamethoxazole is the preferred therapy for both primary and secondary prophylaxis of PCP in adults and adolescents. The recommended dose in adults and adolescents is one double-strength tablet daily.
- Trimethoprim–sulfamethoxazole is also the recommended drug of choice for PCP prophylaxis in children. The trimethoprim–sulfamethoxazole regimen recommended (although other acceptable alternatives exist) is 150 mg/m^2/day of trimethoprim and 750 mg/m^2/day of sulfamethoxazole given in divided doses twice daily, 3 times weekly on consecutive days (e.g., Monday, Tuesday, and Wednesday). The total daily dose of trimethoprim–sulfamethoxazole

in children should not exceed 320 mg of trimethoprim with 1600 mg of sulfamethoxazole.

TOXOPLASMA GONDII

T. gondii can infect any organ of the body and cause an acute infection; it has a predilection for the brain and the eye.

Clinical Presentation

- The clinical signs and symptoms of toxoplasmosis are most frequently associated with involvement of the central nervous system (CNS) and, less commonly, the lungs and eyes, although any organ can be affected. Clinical presentation often includes fever, headache, seizures (in approximately 10% to 25% of patients), focal neurologic abnormalities (in approximately 60% to 90%), and mental status changes.
- Brain biopsy is required to make a definitive diagnosis of toxoplasmic encephalitis, although presumptive diagnosis is commonly made in *T. gondii*–seropositive patients with typical CNS lesions.

Treatment

- The initial treatment of CNS toxoplasmosis is usually empiric. Antitoxoplasmosis therapy is usually initiated in patients with AIDS who are seropositive for *Toxoplasma*, have clinical symptoms suspicious for toxoplasmosis, and have characteristic findings on neuroradiographic studies.
- The combination of **pyrimethamine** and **sulfadiazine** is considered the most effective regimen for acute therapy of AIDS-related CNS toxoplasmosis.
- Pyrimethamine loading doses of 75 mg orally on the first day followed by 25 mg/day thereafter have been commonly used. Others have recommended larger loading doses of 100 to 200 mg followed by daily oral doses of 1 to 1.5 mg/kg/day (50 to 100 mg/day).
- The usual dose of sulfadiazine is 1 to 1.5 g every 6 hours (4 to 8 g/day).
- **Folinic acid**, in doses of 10 to 20 mg/day (although doses as high as 50 mg/day have been used) is usually added to the combination to reduce the pyrimethamine-induced bone marrow toxicity.
- Acute therapy with this combination should be continued for at least 3 weeks, but 6 weeks of treatment is recommended for more severely ill patients.
- The combination of pyrimethamine and **clindamycin** appears to be less toxic, but less effective, than that of pyrimethamine and sulfadiazine.
- The discontinuation of pyrimethamine and sulfadiazine after successful initial therapy may be considered in persons who have a sustained CD4 cell count of greater then 200 cells/μL, for at least 6 months and have completed initial therapy and are asymptomatic.
- A regimen of pyrimethamine (25 to 50 mg/day with leukovorin 10 to 25 mg orally once dialy) and sulfadiazine (500 to 1000 mg four times daily) is recommended for maintenance therapy.

CRYPTOCOCCUS NEOFORMANS

Cryptococcal infection is now uncommon and occurs primarily in those with limited access to health care.

Clinical Presentation

- The usual clinical presentation of cryptococcal infection is meningitis. The clinical features of cryptococcal meningitis may be subtle, nonspecific, and not localized to the CNS. Fever, headache, and malaise are the most frequent symptoms.

TABLE 39-7. Therapies for Prophylaxis of First Episode Opportunistic Diseases in Adults and Adolescents

Pathogen	Indication	First Choice
I. Standard of Care		
Pneumocystis Carinii	CD4 + count <200/μL or oropharyngeal candidiasis	Trimethoprim-sulfamethoxazole, 1 double-strength tablet orally once daily or 1 single-strength tablet orally once daily
Mycobacterium tuberculosis Isoniazid-sensitive	TST reaction ≥5 mm or prior positive TST result without treatment *or* contact with case of active tuberculosis	Isoniazid 300 mg orally + pyridoxine, 50 mg orally once daily for 9 months, *or* isoniazid 900 mg orally + pyridoxine 50 mg orally twice weekly × 12 months
Isoniazid-resistant	Same as isoniazid-sensitive; high probability of exposure to isoniazid-resistant tuberculosis	Rifampin 600 mg orally once daily + pyrazinamide 200 mg/kg orally once daily for 2 months
Toxoplasma gondii	IgG antibody to *Toxoplasma* and CD4 + count <100/μL	Trimethoprim-sulfamethoxazole 1 double-strength tablet orally once daily
Mycobacterium avium complex	CD4 + count <50 μL	Azithromycin, 1200 mg orally once weekly or clarithromycin, 500 mg orally twice daily
Varicella zoster virus (VZV)	Significant exposure to chickenpox or shingles for patients who have no history of either condition or, if available, negative antibody to VZV	Varicella zoster immune globulin (VZIG), 5 vials (1.25 mL each) intramuscularly administered ideally within 48 h of exposure but ≤96 h.
II. Usually Recommended		
Streptococcus pneumoniae	CD4 count of ≥200 cells μL	23-valent polysaccharide vaccine, 0.5 mL intramuscularly
Hepatitis B virus	All suseptible (antihepatitis B core antigen negative) patients	Hepatitis B vaccine, 3 doses
Influenza virus	All patients (annually, before influenza season)	Inactivated trivalent influenza virus vaccine: 0.5 mL intramuscularly

Hepatitis A virus — All susceptible (anti-HAV-negative) patients at increased risk for hepatitis A infection (e.g., illegal drug users, men who have sex with men, hemophiliacs) or Patients with chronic liver disease Including chronic hepatitis B or C — Hepatitis A vaccine: 2 doses

III. Indicated for Use Only in Selected Circumstances

Bacteria	Neutropenia	Granulocyte-colony-stimulating factor (G-CSF), 5–10 mcg/kg subcutaneously once daily for 2–4 wk; or granulocyte-macrophage colony-stimulating factor (GM-CSF), 250 mcg/m^2 subcutaneously for 2–4 wk.
Cryptococcus neoformans	CD4 + count <50/μL	Fluconazole, 100–200 mg orally once daily
Histoplasma capsulatum	CD4 + count < 100/μL, endemic Geographic area	Itraconazole capsule, 200 mg orally once daily
Cytomegalovirus	CD4 + count <50/μL and CMV antibody positivity	Oral ganciclovir, 1 g orally 3 times daily

From Centers for Disease Control and Prevention. Guidelines for Preventing Opportunistic Infections Among HIV-Infected Persons—2002 Recommendations of the USPHS/IDSA. MMWR 2002;51:1–52.

- Methods for diagnosis of cryptococcal infection include serum and cerebrospinal fluid (CSF) testing for cryptococcal antigen and fungal cultures. Detection of cryptococcal antigen in serum and CSF is the most sensitive and specific test; an antigen titer greater than 1:8 should be regarded as evidence of infection. t2

Treatment

- The standard therapeutic approach has been **amphotericin B** for both acute and maintenance therapy.
- **Fluconazole** is also effective for treatment of cryptococcal meningitis; however, the combination of amphotericin B and **flucytosine** was found to be superior.
- Most patients with cryptococcal meningitis should receive amphotericin B in an intravenous dose of at least 0.5 mg/kg/day for a minimum of 2 weeks as acute therapy. Flucytosine in doses of 100 to 150 mg/kg/day can be considered for combination with amphotericin B.
- Serum concentrations of flucytosine should be monitored, and peak levels kept below 100 mcg/mL to minimize hematologic adverse reactions.
- Maintenance therapy is necessary to prevent relapse. Fluconazole is the drug of choice to prevent relapse of cryptococcal meningitis.

VIII

MYCOBACTERIUM INFECTIONS

Clinical Presentation

- The clinical syndrome associated with *Mycobacterium avium* complex (MAC) includes high spiking fevers, diarrhea, night sweats, malaise, weight loss, anemia, and neutropenia. Persistent diarrhea and abdominal pain, a malabsorption syndrome, and extrahepatic biliary obstruction are manifestations associated with MAC gastrointestinal infection.
- Diagnosis of MAC infection is usually based on culture of the organisms from the blood, although biopsies of the liver, bone marrow, and lymph nodes are also highly sensitive and specific.

Treatment

- Treatment regimens should contain at least two antimycobacterial agents.
- Every regimen should contain either **clarithromycin** or **azithromycin**, with clarithromycin (500 mg twice daily) being the preferred agent. For the second agent, numerous choices are available, although **ethambutol** (15 mg/kg/day) is preferred by many experts. Many clinicians would add a third (such as rifabutin), and some, a fourth drug to this regimen.
- Clinical responses usually occur within 2 to 8 weeks of the start of therapy. If a clinical and microbiologic response is observed, therapy should continue for the duration of the patient's life.
- MAC prophylaxis is now strongly recommended for all HIV-infected adults and adolescents with a CD4 count less than 50 cells/μL. The first-line choices are either azithromycin (1200 mg once weekly) or clarithromycin (500 mg twice daily). **Rifabutin** is an alternative.

HERPES VIRUS INFECTIONS

Herpes Simplex Virus (HSV)

- The manifestations of HSV disease observed in persons with AIDS include orolabial, genital, and anorectal mucocutaneous disease; esophagitis; and less commonly, encephalitis. Ulcerative HSV lesions present for longer than 1 month in an individual with laboratory evidence of HIV infection, or no other apparent cause for immunodeficiency, are considered an AIDS-defining condition.

- Symptoms of anorectal lesions, the most common clinically evident HSV disease causing morbidity in homosexual men, include pain, itching, and painful defecation.

- **Acyclovir** is the drug of choice for treatment of HSV disease. For mild to moderate mucocutaneous disease, oral acyclovir in doses of 200 mg five times daily or 400 mg three times daily are used, although 400 mg five times daily may be necessary. Intravenous acyclovir (15 mg/kg/day) should be used in those settings where absorption of an oral drug is questionable, oral tolerance is unlikely (HSV esophagitis), or perhaps when severe mucocutaneous disease is present.

- Treatment of mucocutaneous disease should be continued until all lesions have crusted.

- Intravenous acyclovir (30 mg/kg/day) should also be used for viscerally disseminated disease and for HSV encephalitis.

- Recurrent HSV disease can often be managed with low-dose suppressive oral acyclovir therapy, 200 mg four times daily, 400 mg twice daily, or 800 mg once daily.

VIII ◄

Varicella-Zoster Virus (VZV)

- Zoster usually begins as radicular pain followed by localized erythematous rash and characteristic vesicles. Zoster will usually remain confined to a limited number of dermatomes, but complications such as widespread cutaneous involvement and disseminated visceral zoster may occur.

- **Acyclovir** is the drug of choice for VZV infections. While an oral acyclovir regimen of 4 g/day has been shown effective for the treatment of zoster in immunocompetent adults, the drug has not been fully evaluated in immunocompromised patients such as those with AIDS.

- AIDS patients with disseminated cutaneous or visceral zoster should receive treatment with intravenous acyclovir in doses of 30 mg/kg/day for at least 7 days or until all lesions are crusted.

Cytomegalovirus (CMV)

- Manifestations of CMV infection include retinitis, esophagitis, hepatitis, gastrointestinal involvement, and less commonly radiculopathy, encephalitis, and pneumonitis. CMV retinitis is usually associated with a painless progressive loss of vision. Patients may initially complain of blurry vision, loss of visual acuity, or "floaters."

- **Ganciclovir** therapy for CMV disease has traditionally been divided into two phases—induction and maintenance—because high relapse rates are found after discontinuation of the drug following successful completion of a 2- to 3-week course of initial therapy. Induction regimens are typically 7.5 to 10 mg/kg/day intravenously in two or three equally divided doses for 14 days, or longer if there is a slow clinical response. Maintenance therapy is usually 5 to 6 mg/kg once daily, although doses of 10 mg/kg have been used, 5 to 7 days/wk for an indefinite period of time.

- **Foscarnet** is an alternative to ganciclovir that appears less likely to cause neutropenia; however, it has a variety of potential adverse effects, including renal insufficiency and metabolic disturbances (both increases and decreases) in calcium and phosphorus.

- Prophylaxis with oral ganciclovir should be considered in HIV-infected adults and adolescents who have a CD4 cell count of less than 50 cells/μL; ganciclovir prophylaxis is not a recommended standard of care.

See Chapter 123, Human Immunodeficiency Virus Infection, authored by Courtney V. Fletcher and Thomas N. KaKuda for a more detailed discussion of this topic.

▶ VIII

Chapter 40

▶ INTRA-ABDOMINAL INFECTIONS

▶ DEFINITION

Intra-abdominal infections are those contained within the peritoneum or retroperitoneal space. Two general types of intra-abdominal infection are discussed throughout this chapter: peritonitis and abscess.

- Peritonitis is defined as the acute, inflammatory response of peritoneal lining to microorganisms, chemicals, irradiation, or foreign body injury. Peritonitis may be classified as either primary or secondary. With primary peritonitis, an intra-abdominal focus of disease may not be evident. In secondary peritonitis, a focal disease process is evident within the abdomen.
- An abscess is a purulent collection of fluid separated by a more or less well-defined wall from surrounding tissue. It usually contains necrotic debris, bacteria, and inflammatory cells.

▶ PATHOPHYSIOLOGY

- Table 40–1 summarizes many of the potential causes of bacterial peritonitis. The causes of intra-abdominal abscess somewhat overlap those of peritonitis

TABLE 40–1. Causes of Bacterial Peritonitis

Primary Bacterial Peritonitis
    Peritoneal dialysis
    Cirrhosis with ascites
    Nephrotic syndrome

Secondary Bacterial Peritonitis
    Miscellaneous causes
        Diverticulitis
        Appendicitis
        Inflammatory bowel diseases
        Salpingitis
        Biliary tract infections
        Necrotizing pancreatitis
    Neoplasms
        Intestinal obstruction
        Perforation
    Mechanical gastrointestinal problems
        Any cause of small bowel obstruction (adhesions, hernia)
    Vascular causes
        Mesenteric arterial or venous occlusion (atrial fibrillation)
        Mesenteric ischemia without occlusion
    Trauma
        Blunt abdominal trauma with rupture of intestine
        Penetrating abdominal trauma
    Iatrogenic intestinal perforation (endoscopy)
    Intraoperative events
    Peritoneal contamination during abdominal operation
    Leakage from gastrointestinal anastomosis

and, in fact, both may occur sequentially or simultaneously. Appendicitis is the most frequent cause of abscess.

- Intra-abdominal infection results from entry of bacteria into the peritoneal or retroperitoneal spaces or from bacterial collections within intra-abdominal organs. When peritonitis results from peritoneal dialysis, skin surface flora are introduced via the peritoneal catheter.
- In secondary peritonitis, bacteria most often enter the peritoneum or retroperitoneum as a result of disruption of the integrity of the gastrointestinal tract caused by diseases or traumatic injuries.
- When bacteria become dispersed throughout the peritoneum, the inflammatory process involves the majority of the peritoneal lining.
- Peritonitis often results in mortality because of the effects on multiple organ systems. Fluid shifts and endotoxins may cause hypotension and shock. Fluid loss from the vasculature with generalized peritonitis is similar to that which occurs after a 50% second-degree skin burn.
- An abscess begins by the combined action of inflammatory cells (such as neutrophils), bacteria, fibrin, and other inflammatory components. A mature abscess may have a fibrinous capsule that isolates bacteria and the liquid core from antimicrobials and immunologic defenses.

VIII

MICROBIOLOGY

- Primary bacterial peritonitis is often caused by a single organism. In children, the pathogen is usually *Streptococcus pneumoniae* or a group A streptococcus. When peritonitis occurs in association with cirrhotic ascites, enteric organisms (such as *Escherichia coli*) are usually responsible.
- Peritonitis in patients undergoing peritoneal dialysis is most often caused by common skin organisms: *Staphylococcus epidermidis, Staphylococcus aureus*, streptococci, and diphtheroids.
- Secondary intra-abdominal infections are often polymicrobial. The mean number of isolates of microorganisms from infected intra-abdominal sites has ranged from 2.9 to 3.7, including an average of 1.3 to 1.6 aerobes and 1.7 to 2.1 anaerobes. The frequencies with which specific bacteria were isolated in intra-abdominal infections are given in Table 40–2.
- The combination of aerobic and anaerobic organisms appears to greatly increase pathogenicity. In intra-abdominal infections, facultative bacteria may provide an environment conducive to the growth of anaerobic bacteria.

TABLE 40–2. Pathogens Isolated from Patients with Secondary Peritonitis

Gram-Negative Bacteria	
E. coli	32–61%
Enterobacter	8–26%
Klebsiella	6–26%
Proteus	4–23%
Gram-Positive Bacteria	
Enterococci	18–24%
Streptococci	6–55%
Staphylococci	6–16%
Anaerobic Bacteria	
Bacteroides	25–80%
Clostridium	5–18%
Fungi	2–5%

- Aerobic enteric bacteria and anaerobic bacteria are both pathogens in intra-abdominal infection. Aerobic bacteria, particularly *E. coli,* appear responsible for the early mortality from peritonitis, whereas anaerobic bacteria are major pathogens in abscesses, with *Bacteroides fragilis* predominating.
- The role of *Enterococcus* as a pathogen is not clear. Enterococcal infection occurs more commonly in postoperative peritonitis, in the presence of specific risk factors indicating failure of the host defenses, or with the use of broad-spectrum antibiotics.

▶ CLINICAL PRESENTATION

- Intra-abdominal infections have a wide spectrum of clinical features often depending on the specific disease process, the location and the magnitude of bacterial contamination, and concurrent host factors. Patients with primary and secondary peritonitis present quite differently (Table 40–3).
- If peritonitis continues untreated, the patient may go into hypovolemic shock from fluid loss into the peritoneum, bowel wall, and lumen. This may be accompanied by generalized sepsis.

VIII ◀

▶ DESIRED OUTCOME

- The goals of treatment are the correction of intra-abdominal disease processes or injuries that have caused infection and the drainage of collections of purulent material (e.g., abscess).
- A secondary objective is to achieve resolution of infection without major organ system complications or adverse treatment effects.

▶ TREATMENT

GENERAL PRINCIPLES

- The three major modalities for the treatment of intra-abdominal infection are prompt drainage, support of vital functions, and appropriate antimicrobial therapy to treat infection not removed by surgery.
- Antimicrobials are an important adjunct to surgical procedures in the treatment of intra-abdominal infections; however, the use of antimicrobial agents without surgical intervention is usually inadequate. For some specific situations (e.g., most cases of primary peritonitis), drainage procedures may not be required, and antimicrobial agents become the mainstay of therapy.
- With generalized peritonitis, large volumes of intravenous fluids are required to restore vascular volume and improve cardiovascular function.

NONPHARMACOLOGIC TREATMENT

- Secondary peritonitis requires surgical correction of the underlying pathology. Drainage of the purulent material, either by open surgical procedure or drained percutaneously, is the critical element in the management of an intra-abdominal abscess.
- Aggressive fluid repletion and management are required for the purposes of achieving or maintaining proper intravascular volumes and adequate urine output and correcting acidosis.
- In the initial hour of treatment, a large volume of intravenous solution (lactated Ringers) may need to be administered to restore intravascular volume. This may be followed by up to 1 L/h until fluid balance is restored in a few hours.

Infectious Diseases

TABLE 40–3. Clinical Presentation of Peritonitis

Primary Peritonitis	

General
The patient may not be in acute distress, particularly with peritoneal dialysis.

Signs and Symptoms
The patient may complain of nausea, vomiting (sometimes with diarrhea), and abdominal tenderness.
Temperature may be only mildly elevated or not elevated in patients undergoing peritoneal dialysis.
Bowel sounds are hypoactive.
The cirrhotic patient may have worsening encephalopathy.
Cloudy dialysate fluid with peritoneal dialysis.

Laboratory Tests
The patient's WBC count may be only mildly elevated.
Ascitic fluid usually contains >300 leukocytes/mm^3, and bacteria, may be evident on Gram stain of a centrifuged specimen.
In 60–80% of patients with cirrhotic ascites, the Gram stain is negative.

Other Diagnostic Tests
Culture of peritoneal dialysate or ascitic fluid should be positive.

Secondary Peritonitis	

Signs and Symptoms
Generalized abdominal pain.
Tachypnea.
Tachycardia.
Nausea and vomiting.
Temperature normal initially then increasing to 100–102°F (37.7–38.8°C) within the first few hours and may continue to rise for the next several hours.
Hypotension and shock if volume is not restored.
Decreased urine output due to dehydration.

Physical Examination
Voluntary abdominal guarding changing to involuntary guarding and a "board-like abdomen."
Abdominal tenderness and distension.
Faint bowel sounds that cease over time.

Laboratory Tests
Leukocytosis (15,000–20,000 WBC/mm^3, with neutrophils predominating and an elevated percentage of immature neutrophils (bands).
Elevated hematocrit and blood urea nitrogen because of dehydration.
Patient progresses from early alkalosis because of hyperventilation and vomiting to acidosis and lactic acidemia.

Other Diagnostic Tests
Abdominal radiographs may be useful because free air in the abdomen (indicating intestinal perforation) or distension of the small or large bowel is often evident.

VIII

- In patients with significant blood loss (hematocrit of 25%), blood should be given. This is generally in the form of packed red blood cells.

PHARMACOLOGIC THERAPY

- The goals of antimicrobial therapy are to control bacteremia and to establish the metastatic foci of infection, to reduce suppurative complications after bacterial contamination, and to prevent local spread of existing infection.

TABLE 40–4. Likely Intra-abdominal Pathogens

Type of Infection	Aerobes	Anaerobes
Primary Bacterial Peritonitis		
Children (spontaneous)	Pneumococci, group A Streptococcus	—
Cirrhosis	E. coli, Klebsiella, pneumococci (many others)	—
Peritoneal dialysis	Staphylococcus, Streptococcus	—
Secondary Bacterial Peritonitis		
Gastroduodenal	Streptococcus, E. coli	—
Biliary tract	E. coli, Klebsiella, enterococci	Clostridium or Bacteroides (infrequent)
Small or large bowel	E. coli, Klebsiella spp., Proteus spp.	Bacteroides fragilis and other Bacteroides, Clostridium
Appendicitis	E. coli, Pseudomonas	Bacteroides spp.
Abscesses	E. coli, Klebsiella, enterococci	B. fragilis and other Bacteroides, Clostridium, anaerobic cocci
Liver	E. coli, Klebsiella, enterococci staphylococci, amoeba	Bacteroides (infrequent)
Spleen	Staphylococcus, Streptococcus	

VIII

- An empiric antimicrobial regimen should be started as soon as the presence of intra-abdominal infection is suspected on the basis of likely pathogens.
- Likely pathogens, those against which antimicrobial agents should be directed, are listed in Table 40–4.
- Table 40–5 presents recommended and alternative regimens for selected situations. These are general guidelines, not rules, because there are many factors that cannot be incorporated into such a table.

Recommendations

- Most patients with severe intra-abdominal infections (where there is generalized peritonitis or sepsis should be placed on a β-lactam or β-lactamase inhibitor combination, or carbapenem (**imipenem**, **ertapenem** or **meropenem**). Combinations of an aminoglycoside with an antianaerobic agent such as clindamycin or metronidazole may be used, but some authorities consider such combinations to be obsolete.
- The selection of a specific agent or combination should be based on culture and susceptibility data for peritonitis that occurs from CPD. If microbiologic data are unavailable, empiric therapy should be initiated.
- For established intra-abdominal infections, most patients are adequately treated with 5 to 7 days of antimicrobial therapy.
- Patients with peritonitis who are undergoing CPD may receive parenteral as well as intraperitoneal antimicrobial agents. Intraperitoneal antimicrobial agents alone are often sufficient, unless severe infection is present. Recommended concentrations of antimicrobial agents for intraperitoneal irrigation solutions are 8 mg/L for **gentamicin** and **tobramycin**, 1 to 3 mg/L for **clindamycin**, 50,000 U/L for **penicillin G**, 125 mg/L for **cephalosporins**, 100 to 150 mg/L for **ticarcillin** or **carbenicillin**, 50 mg/L for **ampicillin**, 100 mg/L for **methicillin**, 30 mg/L for **vancomycin**, and 3 mg/L for **amphotericin B**.
- The usual duration of therapy for peritonitis associated with CPD is 10 to 14 days but may extend to 3 weeks. Antimicrobial therapy should be continued

TABLE 40–5. Guidelines for Initial Antimicrobial Agents for Intra-abdominal Infections

	Primary Agents	Alternatives
Primary Bacterial Peritonitis		
Cirrhosis	Cefotaxime	1. Add clindamycin or metronidazole if anaerobes are suspected 2. Other third-generation cephalosporins, extended-spectrum penicillins, aztreonam, and imipenem as alternatives 3. Aminoglycoside with antipseudomonal penicillin
Peritoneal dialysis	Regimen based on organism isolated 1. *Staphylococcus*: penicillinase-resistant penicillin or first-generation cephalosporin 2. *Streptococcus*: penicillin G 3. Aerobic gram-negative bacilli: cefotaxime, ceftazidime, or aminoglycoside plus an antipseudomonal penicillin 4. *Pseudomonas aeruginosa*: aminoglycoside plus antipseudomonal penicillin or ceftazidime	1. Alternative for resistant staphylococci is vancomycin 2. Alternative for *Streptococcus* is a first-generation cephalosporin 3. Alternatives for gram-negative bacilli are other third-generation cephalosporins, aztreonam, and extended-spectrum penicillins with β-lactamase inhibitors
Secondary Bacterial Peritonitis		
Perforated peptic ulcer	First-generation cephalosporins	1. Antianaerobic cephalosporins[a] 2. Possibly add aminoglycoside if patient condition is poor 3. Aminoglycoside with clindamycin or metronidazole; add ampicillin if patient is immunocompromised or if biliary tract origin of infection
Other	Imipenem/cilistatin, meropenem, ertapenem, or extended-spectrum penicillins with β-lactamase inhibitor	1. Ciprofloxacin with metronidazole 2. Aztreonam with clindamycin or metronidazole 3. Antianaerobic cephalosporins.[a]

Condition	Recommended	Alternative
Abscess		
General	Imipenem/cilastatin, meropenem, ertapenem, or extended-spectrum penicillins with β-lactamase inhibitor	1. Aztreonam with clindamycin or metronidazole 2. Ciprofloxacin with metronidazole 3. Aminoglycoside with clindamycin or metronidazole; Use metronidazole if amebic liver abscess is suspected
Liver	As above, but add a first-generation cephalosporin	Alternatives for penicillinase-resistant penicillin are first-generation
Spleen	Aminoglycoside plus penicillinase-resistant penicillin	cephalosporins or vancomycin
Appendicitis		
Normal or inflamed	Antianaerobic cephalosporins[a] (discontinued immediately postoperation)	1. Ampicillin–sulbactam
Gangrenous or perforated	Imipenem/cilastatin, meropenem, ertapenem, antianaerobic cephalosporins or extended-spectrum penicillins with β-lactamase inhibitor	1. Aztreonam with clindamycin or metronidazole 2. Ciprofloxacin with metronidazole 3. Aminoglycoside with clindamycin or metronidazole
Acute Cholecystitis	First-generation cephalosporin	Aminoglycoside plus ampicillin if severe infection
Cholangitis	Aminoglycoside with ampicillin with or without clindamycin or metronidazole	Use vancomycin instead of ampicillin if patient is allergic to penicillin
Acute Contamination from Abdominal Trauma	Antianaerobic cephalosporins[a] or ampicillin–sulbactam	1. A carbapenem 2. Ciprofloxacin plus metronidazole
Pelvic Inflammatory Disease	Cefotetan or cefoxitin with doxycycline	1. Clindamycin with gentamicin 2. Ampicillin–sulbactam with doxycycline 3. Ciprofloxacin with doxycycline and metronidazole

[a]Cefoxitin, cefotetan, and ceftizoxime.

until dialysate fluid is clear, cultures are negative for 2 to 3 days, and the patient is asymptomatic.

- Antianaerobic cephalosporins or extended-spectrum penicillins are effective in preventing most infectious complications after acute bacterial contamination, such as with abdominal trauma where gastrointestinal contents enter the peritoneum, and when the patient is seen soon after injury (within 2 hours) and surgical measures are instituted promptly.
- Acute intra-abdominal contamination, such as after a traumatic injury, may be treated with a short course (24 hours). For established infections (peritonitis or intra-abdominal abscess), an antimicrobial course of at least 7 days is justified.

▶ EVALUATION OF THERAPEUTIC OUTCOMES

- The patient should be continually reassessed to determine the success or failure of therapies.
- Unsatisfactory outcomes in patients with intra-abdominal infections may result from complications that arise in other organ systems. A complication commonly associated with mortality after intra-abdominal infection is pneumonia.
- Once antimicrobials are initiated and other important therapies described earlier are used, most patients should show improvement within 2 to 3 days. Usually, temperature will return to near normal, vital signs should stabilize, and the patient should not appear in distress, with the exception of recognized discomfort and pain from incisions, drains, and nasogastric tube.
- At 24 to 48 hours, aerobic bacterial culture results should return. If a suspected pathogen is not sensitive to the antimicrobial agents being given, the regimen should be changed if the patient has not shown sufficient progress.
- If the isolated pathogen is extremely sensitive to one antimicrobial, and the patient is progressing well, concurrent antimicrobial therapy may often be discontinued.
- With present anaerobic culturing techniques and the slow growth of these organisms, anaerobes are often not identified until 4 to 7 days after culture, and sensitivity information is difficult to obtain. For this reason, there are usually few data with which to alter the antianaerobic component of the antimicrobial regimen.
- Superinfection in patients being treated for intra-abdominal infection is often due to *Candida,* but enterococci or opportunistic gram-negative bacilli such as *Pseudomonas* or *Serratia* may be involved.
- Treatment regimens for intra-abdominal infection can be judged successful if the patient recovers from the infection without recurrent peritonitis or intra-abdominal abscess and without the need for additional antimicrobials. A regimen can be considered unsuccessful if a significant adverse drug reaction occurs, if reoperation is necessary, or if patient improvement is delayed beyond 1 or 2 weeks.

See Chapter 112, Intra-abdominal Infections, authored by Joseph T. DiPiro and Thomas R. Howdieshell, for a more detailed discussion of this topic.

VIII

Chapter 41

▶ RESPIRATORY TRACT INFECTIONS, LOWER

Lower respiratory tract infections include infectious processes of the lungs and bronchi, pneumonia, bronchitis, bronchiolitis, and lung abscess.

▶ BRONCHITIS

ACUTE BRONCHITIS

- Bronchitis refers to an inflammatory condition of the large elements of the tracheobronchial tree that is usually associated with a generalized respiratory infection. The inflammatory process does not extend to include the alveoli. The disease entity is frequently classified as either acute or chronic.
- Acute bronchitis most commonly occurs during the winter months. Cold, damp climates and/or the presence of high concentrations of irritating substances such as air pollution or cigarette smoke may precipitate attacks.

Pathophysiology

- Respiratory viruses are by far the most common infectious agents associated with acute bronchitis. The common cold viruses, rhinovirus and coronavirus, and lower respiratory tract pathogens, including influenza virus, adenovirus, and respiratory syncytial virus, account for the majority of cases. *Mycoplasma pneumoniae* also appears to be a frequent cause of acute bronchitis. Other bacterial causes include *Chlamydia pneumoniae* and *Bordetella pertussis.*
- Infection of the trachea and bronchi causes hyperemic and edematous mucous membranes and an increase in bronchial secretions. Destruction of respiratory epithelium can range from mild to extensive and may affect bronchial mucociliary function. In addition, the increase in bronchial secretions, which can become thick and tenacious, further impairs mucociliary activity. Recurrent acute respiratory infections may be associated with increased airway hyperreactivity and possibly the pathogenesis of chronic obstructive lung disease.

Clinical Presentation

- Bronchitis is primarily a self-limiting illness and rarely a cause of death. Acute bronchitis usually begins as an upper respiratory infection. The patient typically has nonspecific complaints such as malaise and headache, coryza, and sore throat.
- Cough is the hallmark of acute bronchitis. It occurs early and will persist despite the resolution of nasal or nasopharyngeal complaints. Frequently, the cough is initially nonproductive but progresses, yielding mucopurulent sputum.
- Chest examination may reveal rhonchi and coarse, moist rales bilaterally. Chest radiographs, when performed, are usually normal.
- Bacterial cultures of expectorated sputum are generally of limited utility because of the inability to avoid normal nasopharyngeal flora by the sampling technique. Viral antigen detection tests can be used when a specific diagnosis is necessary. Cultures or serologic diagnosis of *M. pneumoniae* and culture or direct fluorescent antibody detection for *B. pertussis* should be obtained in prolonged or severe cases when epidemiologic considerations would suggest their involvement.

Desired Outcome

The goals of therapy are to provide comfort to the patient and, in the unusually severe case, to treat associated dehydration and respiratory compromise.

Treatment

- The treatment of acute bronchitis is symptomatic and supportive in nature. Reassurance and antipyretics alone are often sufficient. Bedrest and mild analgesic-antipyretic therapy are often helpful in relieving the associated lethargy, malaise, and fever. **Aspirin** or **acetaminophen** (650 mg in adults or 10–15 mg/kg per dose in children with a maximum daily adult dose of 4 g and 60 mg/kg for children) or **ibuprofen** (200 to 800 mg in adults or 10 mg/kg per dose in children with a maximum daily dose of 3.2 g for adults and 40 mg/kg for children) is administered every 4 to 6 hours.
- Patients should be encouraged to drink fluids to prevent dehydration and possibly decrease the viscosity of respiratory secretions.
- In children, aspirin should be avoided and acetaminophen used as the preferred agent because of the possible association between aspirin use and the development of Reye's syndrome.
- Mist therapy and/or the use of a vaporizer may further promote the thinning and loosening of respiratory secretions.
- Persistent, mild cough, which may be bothersome, may be treated with **dextromethorphan;** more severe coughs may require intermittent **codeine** or other similar agents.
- Routine use of antibiotics in the treatment of acute bronchitis is discouraged; however, in patients who exhibit persistent fever or respiratory symptomatology for more than 4 to 6 days, the possibility of a concurrent bacterial infection should be suspected.
- When possible, antibiotic therapy is directed toward anticipated respiratory pathogen(s) (i.e., *Streptococcus pneumoniae, Haemophilus influenzae*) and/or those demonstrating a predominant growth upon throat culture.
- *M. pneumoniae,* if suspected by history or positive cold agglutinins (titers greater than or equal to 1:32) or if confirmed by culture or serology, may be treated with **erythromycin** or its analogs (e.g., **clarithromycin** or **azithromycin**). Also, a fluoroquinolone with activity against these pathogens (**gatifloxacin** or increased dose **levofloxacin**) may be used in adults.
- During known epidemics involving the influenza A virus, **amantadine** or **rimantadine** may be effective in minimizing associated symptomatology if administered early in the course of the disease.

CHRONIC BRONCHITIS

Chronic bronchitis is a nonspecific disease that primarily affects adults.

Pathophysiology

- Chronic bronchitis is a result of several contributing factors, including cigarette smoking; exposure to occupational dusts, fumes, and environmental pollution; and bacterial (and possibly viral) infection.
- In chronic bronchitis, the bronchial wall is thickened and the number of mucus-secreting goblet cells in the surface epithelium of both larger and smaller bronchi is markedly increased. Hypertrophy of the mucus glands and dilatation of the mucus gland ducts are also observed. As a result of these changes, patients with chronic bronchitis have substantially more mucus in their peripheral airways, further impairing normal lung defenses and causing mucus plugging of the smaller airways.

- Continued progression of this pathology can result in residual scarring of small bronchi, augmenting airway obstruction and the weakening of bronchial walls.

Clinical Presentation

- The hallmark of chronic bronchitis is cough that may range from a mild "smoker's" cough to severe incessant coughing productive of purulent sputum. Expectoration of the largest quantity of sputum usually occurs upon arising in the morning, although many patients expectorate sputum throughout the day. The expectorated sputum is usually tenacious and can vary in color from white to yellow-green.
- By definition, any patient who reports coughing up sputum on most days for at least three consecutive months each year for two consecutive years suffers from chronic bronchitis. Table 41–1 presents a classification and treatment scheme for chronic bronchitis.

TABLE 41–1. Classification System for Patients with Chronic Bronchitis and Initial Treatment Options   VIII

Baseline Status	Criteria or Risky Factors	Usual Pathogens	Initial Treatment Options
Class I			
Acute tracheobronchitis	No underlying structural disease	Usually a virus	1. None unless symptoms persist 2. Amoxicillin; amoxicillin-clavulanate; or a macrolide/azalide
Class II			
Chronic bronchitis	$FEV_1 > 50\%$ predicted value, increased sputum volume and purulence	*Hemophilus influenzae*, *Hemophilus* spp., *Moraxella catarrhalis*, *Streptococcus pneumoniae* (β-lactam resistance possible)	1. Amoxicillin, or fluoroquinolone if prevalence of *H. influenzae* resistance to amoxicillin is >20% 2. Fluoroquinolone, amoxicillin-clavulanate, azithromycin, tetracycline, or trimethoprim-sulfamethoxazole
Class III			
Chronic bronchitis with complications	$FEV_1 < 50\%$ predicted value, increased sputum volume and purulence, advanced age, at least four flares per year, or significant comorbidity	Same as class II; also *Klebsiella pneumoniae*, *Pseudomonas aeruginosa*, *K. pneumoniae*, and other gram-negative organisms (β-lactam resistance common)	1. Fluoroquinolone 2. Expanded spectrum cephalosporin, amoxicillin-clavulanate, or azithromycin
Class IV			
Chronic bronchial Infection	Same as for class III plus yearlong production of purulent sputum	Same as class III	1. Oral or parenteral fluoroquinolone, carbapenem or expanded spectrum cephalosporin

1, Preferred therapy; 2, alternative treatment options. Fluoroquinolone: ciprofloxacin, gatifloxacin, levofloxacin; tetracycline: tetracycline HCL, doxycycline; carbapenem: imipenem-cilastatin, meropenem; expanded-spectrum cephalosporin: ceftazidime, cefepime.

TABLE 41–2. Clinical Presentation of Chronic Bronchitis

Signs and Symptoms
Cyanosis (advanced disease)
Obesity
Physical Examination
Chest auscultation usually reveals inspiratory and expiratory rales, rhonchi, and mild wheezing
  with an expiratory phase that is frequently prolonged. There is hyperresonance on percussion
  with obliteration of the area of cardiac dullness
Normal vesicular breathing sounds are diminished
Clubbing of digits (advanced disease)
Chest Radiograph
Increase in the anteroposterior diameter of the thoracic cage (observed as a barrel chest)
Depressed diaphragm with limited mobility
Laboratory Tests
Erythrocytosis (advanced disease)
Pulmonary Function Tests
Decreased vital capacity
Prolonged expiratory flow

VIII

- With the exception of pulmonary findings, the physical examination of patients with mild to moderate chronic bronchitis is usually unremarkable (Table 41–2).
- An increased number of polymorphonuclear granulocytes in sputum often suggests continual bronchial irritation, whereas an increased number of eosinophils may suggest an allergic component. The most common bacterial isolates (expressed in percentages of total cultures) identified from sputum culture in patients experiencing an acute exacerbation of chronic bronchitis are as follows:

Haemophilus influenzae	24% to 26% (often β-lactamase +)
Haemophilus parainfluenzae	20%
Streptococcus pneumoniae	15%
Moraxella catarrhalis	15% (often β-lactamase +)
Klebsiella pneumoniae	4%
Serratia marcescens	2%
Neisseria meningitidis	2% (often β-lactamase +)
Pseudomonas aeruginosa	2%

Desired Outcome
The goals of therapy for chronic bronchitis are to reduce the severity of symptoms, to ameliorate acute exacerbations, and to achieve prolonged infection-free intervals.

Treatment
General Principles
- A complete occupational/environmental history for the determination of exposure to noxious, irritating gases, as well as cigarette smoking, must be assessed. Attempts must be made to reduce exposure to bronchial irritants.
- Humidification of inspired air may promote the hydration (liquefaction) of tenacious secretions, allowing for more effective sputum production. The use of mucolytic aerosols (e.g., *N*-acetylcysteine; deoxyribonuclease [DNase]) is of questionable therapeutic value.
- Postural drainage may assist in promoting clearance of pulmonary secretions.

Pharmacologic Therapy

- Oral or aerosolized bronchodilators (e.g., **albuterol** aerosol) may be of benefit to some patients during acute pulmonary exacerbations. For patients who consistently demonstrate limitations in airflow, a therapeutic change of bronchodilators should be considered.
- The use of antimicrobials has been controversial, although antibiotics are an important component of treatment. Agents should be selected that are effective against likely pathogens, have the lowest risk of drug interactions, and can be administered in a manner that promotes compliance (see Table 41–1).
- Selection of antibiotics should consider that up to 30% to 40% of *H. influenzae* and 95% of *M. pneumoniae* are β-lactamase producers, and up to 30% of *S. pneumoniae* are at least moderately penicillin resistant.
- Antibiotics commonly used in the treatment of these patients and their respective adult starting doses are outlined in Table 41–3. Duration of symptom-free periods may be enhanced by antibiotic regimens using the upper limit of the recommended daily dose for 10 to 14 days.
- **Ampicillin** is often considered the drug of choice for the treatment of acute exacerbations of chronic bronchitis. Unfortunately, the need for multiple repeat daily doses (4 times daily) and the increasing incidence of penicillin-resistant β-lactamase-producing strains of bacteria have limited the usefulness of this safe and cost-effective antibiotic. VIII
- The value of macrolides when *Mycoplasma* is involved is unquestioned. **Azithromycin** should be considered as the macrolide of choice for *Mycoplasma*.

TABLE 41–3. Oral Antibiotics Commonly Used for the Treatment of Acute Respiratory Exacerbations in Chronic Bronchitis

Antibiotic	Usual Adult Dose (g)	Dose Schedule (doses/day)
Preferred Drugs		
Ampicillin	0.25–0.5	4
Amoxicillin	0.5	3
Cefprozil	0.5	2
Cefuroxime	0.5	2
Ciprofloxacin	0.5–0.75	2
Gatifloxacin	0.4	1
Levofloxacin	0.5–0.75	1
Doxycycline	0.1	2
Minocycline	0.1	2
Tetracycline HCl	0.5	4
Amoxicillin-clavulanate	0.5	3
Trimethoprim-sulfamethoxazole	1 DS[a]	2
Supplemental Drugs		
Azithromycin	0.25–0.5	1
Erythromycin	0.5	4
Clarithromycin	0.25–0.5	2
Cefixime	0.4	1
Cephalexin	0.5	4
Cefaclor	0.25–0.5	3

[a]DS, double-strength tablet (160 mg trimethoprim/800 mg sulfamethoxazole).

- The fluoroquinolones are effective alternative agents for adults, particularly when gram-negative pathogens are involved, or for more severely ill patients. Many *S. pneumoniae* are resistant to older fluoroquinolones such as ciprofloxacin, necessitating the use of newer agents such as **gatifloxacin.**
- In patients whose history suggests recurrent exacerbations of their disease that might be attributable to certain specific events (i.e., seasonal, winter months), a trial of prophylactic antibiotics might be beneficial. If no clinical improvement is noted over an appropriate period (e.g., 2 to 3 months per year for 2 to 3 years), prophylactic therapy could be discontinued.

BRONCHIOLITIS

- Bronchiolitis is an acute viral infection of the lower respiratory tract of infants that shows a definite seasonal pattern (peaks during the winter months and persists through early spring). The disease most commonly affects infants between the ages of 2 and 10 months.
- Respiratory syncytial virus is the most common cause of bronchiolitis, accounting for 45% to 60% of all cases. Parainfluenza viruses are the second most common cause. Bacteria serve as secondary pathogens in only a small minority of cases.

VIII

Clinical Presentation
- The most common clinical signs of bronchiolitis are found in Table 41–4.
- As a result of limited oral intake due to coughing combined with fever, vomiting, and diarrhea, infants are frequently dehydrated.
- The diagnosis of bronchiolitis is based primarily on history and clinical findings. The isolation of a viral pathogen in the respiratory secretions of a wheezing child establishes a presumptive diagnosis of infectious bronchioloitis.

Treatment
- Bronchiolitis is a self-limiting illness and usually requires no therapy (other than reassurance and antipyretics) unless the infant is hypoxic or dehydrated.
- In severely affected children, the mainstays of therapy for bronchiolitis are oxygen therapy and intravenous fluids.
- Aerosolized β-adrenergic therapy appears to offer little benefit for the majority of patients but may be useful in the child with a predisposition toward bronchospasm.

TABLE 41–4. Clinical Presentation of Bronchiolitis

Signs and Symptoms
Prodrome with irritability, restlessness, and mild fever
Cough and coryza
Vomiting, diarrhea, noisy breathing, and an increase in respiratory rate as symptoms progress
Labored breathing with retractions of the chest wall, nasal flaring, and grunting
Physical Examination
Tachycardia and respiratory rate of 40–80/min in hospitalized infants
Wheezing and inspiratory rales
Mild conjunctivitis in one third of patients
Otitis media in 5–10% of patients
Laboratory Examinations
Peripheral white blood cell count normal or slightly elevated
Abnormal arterial blood gases (hypoxemia and, rarely, hypercarbia)

- Because bacteria do not represent primary pathogens in the etiology of bronchiolitis, antibiotics should not be routinely administered. However, many clinicians frequently administer antibiotics initially while awaiting culture results because the clinical and radiographic findings in bronchiolitis are often suggestive of a possible bacterial pneumonia.
- **Ribavirin** may be considered for bronchiolitis caused by respiratory syncytial virus in a subset of patients (those with underlying pulmonary or cardiac disease or with severe acute infection). Use of the drug requires special equipment (small-particle aerosol generator) and specifically trained personnel for administration via oxygen hood or mist tent.

▶ PNEUMONIA

Pneumonia is the most common infectious cause of death in the United States. It occurs in persons of all ages, although the clinical manifestations are most severe in the very young, the elderly, and the chronically ill.

PATHOPHYSIOLOGY

- Microorganisms gain access to the lower respiratory tract by three routes: VIII they may be inhaled as aerosolized particles; they may enter the lung via the bloodstream from an extrapulmonary site of infection; or aspiration of oropharyngeal contents may occur.
- Lung infections with viruses suppress the bacterial clearing activity of the lung by impairing alveolar macrophage function and mucociliary clearance, thus setting the stage for secondary bacterial pneumonia.
- The vast majority of pneumonia cases acquired in the community by otherwise healthy adults are due to *S. pneumoniae* (pneumococcus) or *M. pneumoniae* (up to 70% and 10% to 20% of all acute bacterial pneumonias in the United States, respectively). Other common bacterial causes include *Legionella* and *C. pneumoniae*. Community-acquired pneumonias caused by *Staphylococcus aureus* and gram-negative rods are observed primarily in the elderly, especially those residing in nursing homes, and in association with alcoholism and other debilitating conditions.
- Gram-negative aerobic bacilli and *S. aureus* are also the leading causative agents in hospital-acquired pneumonia.
- Anaerobic bacteria are the most common etiologic agents in pneumonia that follows the gross aspiration of gastric or oropharyngeal contents.
- In the pediatric age group, most pneumonias are due to viruses, especially respiratory syncytial virus, parainfluenza, and adenovirus. Pneumococcus is the most common bacterial cause.

CLINICAL PRESENTATION

Gram-Positive and Gram-Negative Bacterial Pneumonia
See Table 41–5.

- Infection with *Legionella pneumophila* is characterized by multisystem involvement, including rapidly progressive pneumonia. It has a gradual onset, with prominent constitutional symptoms such as malaise, lethargy, weakness, and anorexia occurring early in the course of the illness. A dry, nonproductive cough is initially present that over several days becomes productive of mucoid or purulent sputum. Fevers exceed 40°C and are typically unremitting and associated with a relative bradycardia. Pleuritic chest pain and progressive

TABLE 41–5. Clinical Presentation of Pneumonia

Signs and Symptoms
Abrupt onset of fever, chills, dyspnea, and productive cough
Rust-colored sputum or hemoptysis
Pleuritic chest pain
Physical Examination
Tachypnea and tachycardia
Dullness to percussion
Increased tactile fremitus, whisper pectoriloquy, and egophony
Chest wall retractions and grunting respirations
Diminished breath sounds over the affected area
Inspiratory crackles during lung expansion
Chest Radiograph
Dense lobar or segmental infiltrate
Laboratory Examination
Leukocytosis with a predominance of polymorphonuclear cells
Low oxygen saturation on arterial blood gas or pulse oximetry

VIII

dyspnea may be seen, and fine rales are found on lung examination, progressing to signs of frank consolidation later in the course of the illness. Extrapulmonary manifestations remain evident throughout the course of the illness and include diarrhea, nausea, vomiting, myalgias, and arthralgias.

- Substantial changes in a patient's mental status, often out of proportion to the degree of fever, are seen in approximately one fourth of patients. Obtundation, hallucinations, grand mal seizures, and focal neurologic findings have also been associated with this illness.
- Laboratory findings include leukocytosis with predominance of mature and immature granulocytes in 50% to 75% of patients. Because *L. pneumophila* stains poorly with commonly used stains, routine microscopic examination of sputum is of little diagnostic value. Fluorescent antibody testing can be performed to diagnose Legionnaires' disease.

Anaerobic Pneumonia

The course of anaerobic pneumonia is typically indolent with cough, low-grade fever, and weight loss, although an acute presentation may occur. Putrid sputum, when present, is highly suggestive of the diagnosis. Chest radiographs reveal infiltrates typically located in dependent lung segments, and lung abscesses develop in 20% of patients 1 to 2 weeks into the course of the illness.

Mycoplasma pneumoniae

- *M. pneumoniae* pneumonia presents with a gradual onset of fever, headache, and malaise, with the appearance 3 to 5 days after the onset of illness of a persistent, hacking cough that initially is nonproductive. Sore throat, ear pain, and rhinorrhea are often present. Lung findings are generally limited to rales and rhonchi; findings of consolidation are rarely present.
- Nonpulmonary manifestations are extremely common and include nausea, vomiting, diarrhea, myalgias, arthralgias, polyarticular arthritis, skin rashes, myocarditis and pericarditis, hemolytic anemia, meningoencephalitis, cranial neuropathies, and Guillain-Barré syndrome. Systemic symptoms generally clear in 1 to 2 weeks, while respiratory symptoms may persist up to 4 weeks.
- Radiographic findings include patchy or interstitial infiltrates, which are most commonly seen in the lower lobes.

- Sputum Gram stain may reveal mononuclear or polymorphonuclear leukocytes, with no predominant organism. While *M. pneumoniae* can be cultured from respiratory secretions using specialized medium, 2 to 3 weeks may be necessary for culture identification.

Viral Pneumonia

- The clinical pictures produced by respiratory viruses are sufficiently variable and overlap to such a degree that an etiologic diagnosis cannot confidently be made on clinical grounds alone. Serologic tests for virus-specific antibodies are often used in the diagnosis of viral infections. The diagnostic fourfold rise in titer between acute and convalescent phase sera may require 2 to 3 weeks to develop; however, same-day diagnosis of viral infections is now possible through the use of indirect immunofluorescence tests on exfoliated cells from the respiratory tract.
- Radiographic findings are nonspecific and include bronchial wall thickening and perihilar and diffuse interstitial infiltrates.

Nosocomial Pneumonia

- The strongest predisposing factor for nosocomial pneumonia is mechanical VIII◄ ventilation. Risk is increased by prior antibiotic use, use of H_2-receptor antagonists, and severe illness.

    The diagnosis of nosocomial pneumonia is usually established by presence of a new infiltrate on chest radiograph, fever, worsening respiratory status, and the appearance of thick, neutrophil-laden respiratory secretions.

DESIRED OUTCOME

- Eradication of the offending organism and complete clinical cure are the primary objectives.
- Associated morbidity should be minimized (e.g., renal, pulmonary, or hepatic dysfunction).

TREATMENT

- The first priority on assessing the patient with pneumonia is to evaluate the adequacy of respiratory function and to determine whether there are signs of systemic illness, specifically dehydration or sepsis with resulting circulatory collapse.
- The supportive care of the patient with pneumonia includes the use of humidified oxygen for hypoxemia, fluid resuscitation, administration of bronchodilators when bronchospasm is present, and chest physiotherapy with postural drainage if there is evidence of retained secretions.
- Important therapeutic adjuncts include adequate hydration (by intravenous route if necessary), optimal nutritional support, and fever control.
- The treatment of bacterial pneumonia initially involves the empiric use of a relatively broad-spectrum antibiotic (or antibiotics) effective against probable pathogens after appropriate cultures and specimens for laboratory evaluation have been obtained. Therapy should be narrowed to cover specific pathogens once the results of cultures are known.
- Appropriate empiric choices for the treatment of bacterial pneumonias relative to a patient's underlying disease are shown in Table 41–6 for adults and Table 41–7 for children. Dosages for antibiotics to treat pneumonia are provided in Table 41–8.

TABLE 41–6. Empirical Antimicrobial Therapy for Pneumonia in Adults[a]

Clinical Setting	Usual Pathogen(s)	Presumptive Therapy
Previously healthy, ambulatory patient	Pneumococcus, *Mycoplasma pneumoniae*	Macrolide/azalide,[b] tetracycline[c]
Elderly	Pneumococcus, gram-negative bacilli (such as *Klebsiella pneumoniae*); *Staphylococcus aureus, Hemophilus influenzae*	Piperacillin/tazobactam, cephalosporin[d]; carbapenem[e]
Chronic bronchitis	*Pneumococcus, H. influenzae, M. catarrhalis*	Amoxicillin, tetracycline,[c] TMP-SMZ,[f] cefuroxime, amoxicillin/clavulanate, macrolide-azalide,[b] fluoroquinolone
Alcoholism	Pneumococcus, *K. pneumoniae, S. aureus, H. influenzae*, possibly mouth anaerobes	Ticarcillin-clavulanate, piperacillin-tazobactam, plus aminoglycoside; carbapenem,[e] fluoroquinolone[g]
Aspiration		
Community	Mouth anaerobes	Penicillin or clindamycin
Hospital/residential care	Mouth anaerobes, *S. aureus*, gram-negative enterics	Clindamycin, ticarcillin-clavulanate, piperacillin-tazobactam, plus aminoglycoside
Nosocomial pneumonia	Gram-negative bacilli (such as *K. pneumoniae, Enterobacter* spp., *Pseudomonas aeruginosa*), *S. aureus*	Piperacillin-tazobactam, carbapenem,[e] or expanded spectrum cephalosporin[h] plus aminoglycoside, fluoroquinolone[g]

[a]See section on treatment of bacterial pneumonia.
[b]Macrolide/azalide: erythromycin, clarithromycin-azithromycin.
[c]Tetracycline: tetracycline HCl, doxycycline.
[d]Cephalosporin: cefuroxime, ceftriaxone, cefotaxime.
[e]Carbapenem: imipenem-cilastatin, meropenem.
[f]TMP-SMZ: trimethoprim-sulfamethoxazole.
[g]Fluroquinolone: ciprofloxacin, gatifloxacin, or levofloxacin.
[h]Expanded-spectrum cephalosporin: ceftazidime, cefepime.

- Antibiotic concentrations in respiratory secretions in excess of the pathogen minimum inhibitory concentration (MIC) are necessary for successful treatment of pulmonary infections.
- Drugs recommended for empiric treatment of community-acquired pneumonia are presented in Table 41–9.
- The benefit of antibiotic aerosols or direct endotracheal instillation has not been consistently demonstrated.
- Prevention of pneumonia is possible through the use of vaccines against *S. pneumoniae* and *H. influenzae* type b. In addition, **amantadine** may be administered for prevention of influenza A infection, beginning as soon as possible after exposure and continuing for at least 10 days.

▶ EVALUATION OF THERAPEUTIC OUTCOMES

- With community-acquired pneumonia, time for resolution of cough, sputum production, and presence of constitutional symptoms (e.g., malaise, nausea or

TABLE 41–7. Empirical Antimicrobial Therapy for Pneumonia in Pediatric Patients[a]

Age	Usual Pathogen(s)	Presumptive Therapy
1 month	Group B streptococcus, *Hemophilus influenzae* (nontypable), *Escherichia coli, Staphylococcus aureus, Listeria*, CMV, RSV, adenovirus	Ampicillin-sulbactam, cephalosporin[b] carbapenem[c]
		Ribavirin for RSV
1–3 months	*Chlamydia*, possibly *Ureaplasma*, CMV, *Pneumocystis carinii* (afebrile pneumonia syndrome)	Macrolide-azalide,[d] trimethoprim-sulfamethoxazole
	RSV	Ribavirin
	Pneumococcus, *S. aureus*	Semisynthetic penicillin[e] or cephalosporin[f]
3 months–6 yr	Pneumococcus, *H. influenzae*, RSV, adenovirus, Parainfluenza	Amoxicillin or cephalosporin[f] Ampicillin-sulbactam, amoxicillin-clavulanate
		Ribavirin for RSV
>6 yr	Pneumococcus, *Mycoplasma pneumoniae*, adenovirus	Macrolide/azalide[d] cephalosporin,[f] amoxicillin-clavulanate

CMV, cytomegalovirus; RSV, respiratory syncytial virus.
[a]See section on treatment of bacterial pneumonia.
[b]Third-generation cephalosporin: ceftriaxone, cefotaxime, cefepime. Note that cephalosporins are not active against *Listeria*.
[c]Carbapenem: imipenem-cilastatin, meropenem.
[d]Macrolide/azalide: erythromycin, clarithromycin-azithromycin.
[e]Semisynthetic penicillin: nafcillin, oxacillin.
[f]Second-generation cephalosporin: cefuroxime, cefprozil.
See text for details regarding ribavirin treatment for RSV infection.

VIII

TABLE 41–8. Antibiotic Doses for the Treatment of Bacterial Pneumonia

		Daily Antibiotic dose	
Antibiotic Class	Antibiotic	Pediatric (mg/kg/day)	Adult (total dose/day)
Macrolide	Clarithromycin	15	0.5–1 g
	Erythromycin	30–50	1–2 g
Azalide	Azithromycin	10 mg/kg × 1 day, then 5 mg/kg/day × 4 days	500 mg day 1, then 250 mg/day × 4 days
Tetracycline[a]	Tetracycline HCL	25–50	1–2 g
	Oxytetracycline	15–25	0.25–0.3 g
Penicillin	Ampicillin	100–200	2–6 g
	Amoxicillin/amoxicillin-clavulanate[b]	40–90	0.75–1 g
	Piperacillin-tazobactam	200–300	12 g
	Ampicillin-sulbactam	100–200	4–8 g
Extended-spectrum cephalosporins	Ceftriaxone	50–75	1–2 g
	Ceftazidime	150	2–6 g
	Cefepime	100–150	2–4 g
Fluoroquinolones	Gatifloxacin[c]	10–20	0.4 g
	Levofloxacin	10–15	0.5–0.75 g
	Ciprofloxacin	20–30	0.5–1.5 g
Aminoglycosides	Gentamicin	7.5	3–6 mg/kg
	Tobramycin	7.5	3–6 mg/kg

Note: Doses may be increased for more severe disease and may require modification in patients with organ dysfunction.
[a]Tetracyclines are rarely used in pediatric patients, particularly in those younger than 8 yr of age because of tetracycline-induced permanent tooth discoloration.
[b]Higher dose amoxicillin, amoxicillin-clavulanate (e.g., 90 mg/kg/day) is used for penicillin-resistant *S. pneumoniae*.
[c]Fluoroquinolones are avoided in pediatric patients because of the potential for cartilage damage; however, their use in pediatrics is emerging. Doses shown are extrapolated from adults and will require further study.

TABLE 41–9. Guidelines for the Empirical Treatment of Community-Acquired Pneumonia

Clinical Setting	Empirical Therapy
Outpatients	Macrolide/azalide, doxycycline, or fluoroquinolone
Inpatients, general medical ward	Extended-spectrum cephalosporin + macrolide/azalide or β-lactam/β-lactamase inhibitor + macrolide/azalide or fluoroquinolone
Inpatients, intensive care unit	Extended-spectrum cephalosporin or β-lactam/β-lactamase inhibitor + fluoroquinolone or macrolide/azalide

vomiting, lethargy) should be assessed. Progress should be noted in the first 2 days, with complete resolution in 5 to 7 days.

- With nosocomial pneumonia, the above parameters should be assessed along with WBC counts, chest radiograph, and blood gas determinations.

See Chapter 106, Lower Respiratory Tract Infections, authored by Mark L. Glover and Michael D. Reed, for a more detailed discussion of this topic.

VIII

Chapter 42

▶ RESPIRATORY TRACT INFECTIONS, UPPER

▶ OTITIS MEDIA

DEFINITION

- Otitis media is an inflammation of the middle ear. Acute otitis media involves the rapid onset of signs and symptoms of inflammation in the middle ear that manifests clinically as one or more of the following: otalgia (denoted by pulling of the ear in some infants), hearing loss, fever, or irritability. Otitis media with effusion (accumulation of liquid in the middle ear cavity) differs from acute otitis media in that signs and symptoms of an acute infection are absent.
- Otitis media is the most frequent diagnosis in infants and children.
- Risk factors contributing to increased incidence of otitis media include the winter season, attendance at a day care center, non–breast feeding in infants, native American or Inuit origin, early age at first infection, and nasopharyngeal colonization with middle ear pathogens.
- Eustachian tube anatomy is different in children compared with adults and may cause improper drainage of the middle ear.
- Abnormal function of the eustachian tube can cause reflux transudation of liquid in the middle ear and proliferation of bacteria, resulting in acute otitis media.

PATHOPHYSIOLOGY

- *Streptococcus pneumoniae* is the most common cause of acute otitis media (20% to 35%). Nontypable strains of *Haemophilus influenzae* and *Moxarella catarrhalis* are each responsible for 20% to 30% and 20% of cases, respectively. In 44% of cases, a viral etiology is found with or without concomitant bacteria.
- *S. pneumoniae* isolates are often intermediate resistant to penicillin (8% to 34%) and some are highly penicillin resistant (12% to 21%). Penicillin-resistant isolates are often resistant to multiple antibiotics. β-Lactam resistance occurs in about 23% to 35% of *H. influenzae* and in up to 100% of *M. catarrhalis*.

CLINICAL PRESENTATION

- Acute otitis media presents as an acute onset of signs and symptoms of middle ear infection such as otalgia, irritability, and tugging on the ear, following cold symptoms of runny nose, nasal congestion, or cough (Table 42–1).
- Resolution of acute otitis media occurs over 1 week. Pain and fever tend to resolve over 2 to 3 days.

DESIRED OUTCOME

The goals of treatment include reduction in signs and symptoms, eradication of infection, and prevention of complications. Avoidance of unnecessary antibiotic use is another goal in view of *S. pneumonia*.

TREATMENT

- Antimicrobial therapy is used to treat otitis media; however, a high percentage of children will be cured with symptomatic treatment alone.
- **Acetaminophen** or a nonsteroidal anti-inflammatory agent, such as **ibuprofen**, can be used to relieve pain and malaise in acute otitis media. Decongestants,

Infectious Diseases

TABLE 42–1. Clinical Presentation of Acute Otitis Media

General
The acute onset of signs and symptoms of middle ear infection following cold symptoms of runny nose, nasal congestion, or cough
Signs and Symptoms
Pain that can be severe (>75% of patients)
Children may be irritable, tug on the involved ear, and have difficulty sleeping
Fever is present in less than 25% of patients and, when present, is more often in younger children
Examination shows a discolored, thickened, bulging eardrum
Pneumatic otoscopy or tympanometry demonstrates an immobile eardrum; 50% of cases are bilateral
Draining middle ear fluid occurs (<3% of patients) that usually reveals a bacterial etiology
Laboratory Tests
Gram stain, culture, and sensitivities of draining fluid or aspirated fluid if tympanocentesis is performed

---

antihistamines, topical corticosteroids, or expectorants have not been proven effective for acute otitis media
- Surgical insertion of tympanostomy tubes (T tubes) is an effective method for the prevention of recurrent otitis media.
- VIII • Amoxicillin is the drug of choice for acute otitis media (40 to 45 mg/kg/day). High-dose amoxicillin (80 to 90mg/kg/day) is recommended if drug-resistant *S. pneumoniae* is suspected or a patient is at high risk for a resistant infection. Treatment recommendations for acute otitis media are found in Table 42–2.
- If treatment failure occurs with amoxicillin, an agent should be chosen with activity against β-lactamase-producing *H. influenzae* and *M. catarrhalis* as well as drug-resistant *S. pneumoniae* (such as amoxicillin-clavulanate, cefuroxime, or intramuscular ceftriaxone).
- Patients with penicillin allergy can be treated with a cephalosporin (some clinicians feel that the incidence of cross-reaction is sufficiently low in patients who have not experienced immediate pencillin-hypersensitivity reactions) or a macrolide such as azithromycin, or clarithromycin, erythromycin/sulfisoxazole, trimethoprim/sulfamethoxazole, or, if *S. pneumoniae* is documented, clindamycin.
- It is difficult to identify who will benefit from antimicrobial therapy. With or without treatment, about 60% of children who have acute otitis media are symptom-free within 24 hours. In almost 40% of the remaining children, antibiotic use reduces the duration of symptoms by about 1 day.
- A meta-analysis reported no difference in cure rates with short (less than 7 days) and usual durations (at least 7 days) of antibiotic therapy in children. Five days of therapy is effective in acute uncomplicated otitis media.

Antibiotic Prophylaxis of Recurrent Infections
- Recurrent otitis media is defined as at least 3 episodes in 6 months or at least 4 episodes in 12 months. Recurrent infections are of concern because patients under 3 years of age are at high risk for hearing loss and language and learning disabilities. Data from studies generally do not favor prophylaxis. A meta-analysis demonstrated that prophylaxis against these infections leads to one infection prevented each time one child is treated for 9 months.
- Vaccination against influenza and pneumococcus may decrease risk of acute otitis media, especially in those with recurrent episodes. Immunization with the influenza vaccine reduces the incidence of acute otitis media by 36%.
- Treatment failure is a lack of clinical improvement after 3 days in the signs and symptoms of infection including pain, fever and redness or bulging of the tympanic membrane.

TABLE 42–2. Acute Otitis Media Treatment Recommendations[a,b]

Antibiotic Therapy in Prior Month	Day 0	Clinically Defined Treatment Failure Day 3	Clinically Defined Treatment Failure Days 10 to 28
No	Amoxicillin usual dose 40–45 mg/kg/day	Amoxicillin-clavulanate high dose[c] Amoxicillin component 80–90 mg/kg/day clavulanate component 6.4 mg/kg/day	Same as day 3
	Amoxicillin high dose 80–90 mg/kg/day (high-risk patients)	Cefuroxime axetil Suspension: 30 mg/kg/day divided twice daily (max: 1 g) Tablets: 250 mg twice daily	
		Intramuscular ceftriaxone 1 g (50 mg/kg) daily for 3 days	
Yes	Amoxicillin high dose 80–90 mg/kg/day	Intramuscular ceftriaxone 1 g (50 mg/kg) daily for 3 days	Amoxicillin-clavulanate high dose[c] Amoxicillin component 80–90 mg/kg/day Clavulanate component 6.4 mg/kg/day
	Amoxicillin-clavulanate high dose[c] Amoxicillin component 80–90 mg/kg/day Clavulanate component 6.4 mg/kg/day	Clindamycin[d] 10–30 mg/kg/day divided every 6–8 h (max: 1.8 g/day)	Cefuroxime axetil Suspension: 30 mg/kg/day divided twice daily (max: 1g) Tablets: 250 mg twice daily
	Cefuroxime axetil Suspension: 30 mg/kg/day divided twice daily (max: 1 g) Tablets: 250 mg twice daily	Tympanocentesis	Intramuscular ceftriaxone 1 g (50mg/kg) daily for 3 days
			Tympanocentesis

[a]These recommendations are made by a group convened by the Centers for Disease Control.

[b]The recommended duration of treatment for oral therapy is 7–10 days.

[c]Higher doses of clavulanate produce a significant increase in diarrhea.

[d]Clindamycin is only recommended in cases of documented *S. pneumoniae*. It is not effective against *H. influenzae* or *M. catarrhalis*.

► PHARYNGITIS

Pharyngitis is an acute infection of the oropharynx or nasopharynx that results in 1% to 2% of all outpatient visits. While viral causes are most common, group A β-hemolytic streptococcus, or streptococcus pyogenes, *is the primary bacterial cause.*

- Viruses cause most of the cases of acute pharyngitis. Specific etiologic agents include rhinovirus (20%), coronavirus (at least 5%), adenovirus (5%), influenza (2%) parainfluenza (2%), and Epstein-Barr virus (less than 1%). A bacterial etiology for acute pharyngitis is far less likely. Out of all of the bacterial causes, group A streptococcus is the most common (15 to 30% of persons of all ages with pharyngitis), and it is the the only commonly occurring form of acute pharyngitis for which antimicrobial therapy is indicated.
- Nonsuppurative complications such as acute rheumatic fever, acute glomerulonephritis, and reactive arthritis may occur as a result of pharyngitis with group A streptococcus.

VIII CLINICAL PRESENTATION

- The incubation period is 2 to 5 days, and the illness often occurs in clusters. The clinical presentation of group A streptococcal pharyngitis is presented in Table 42–3.
- Guidelines from the Infectious Disease Society of America, American Academy of Pediatrics, and the American Heart Association suggest that testing for group A streptococcus be done in all patients with signs and symptoms. Only those with a positive test for group A Streptococcus require antibiotic treatment.
- There are several options to test for group A streptococcal pharyngitis. A throat swab can be sent for culture or used for rapid antigen detection testing.

TREATMENT

- The goals of treatment of pharyngitis are to improve clinical signs and symptoms, minimize adverse drug reactions, prevent transmission to close contacts,

TABLE 42–3. Clinical Presentation and Diagnosis of Group A streptococcal Pharyngitis

General
A sore throat of sudden onset that is mostly self-limited
Fever and constitutional symptoms resolving in about 3–5 days
Clinical signs and symptoms are similar for viral causes as well as nonstreptococcal bacterial causes
Signs and Symptoms
Sore throat
Pain on swallowing
Fever
Headache, nausea, vomiting, and abdominal pain (especially children)
Erythema/inflammation of the tonsils and pharynx with or without patchy exudates
Enlarged, tender lymph nodes
Red swollen uvula, petechiae on the soft palate, and a scarlatiniform rash
Several symptoms that are not suggestive of group A *Streptococcus* are cough, conjunctivitis, coryza, and diarrhea
Laboratory Tests
Throat swab and culture or rapid antigen detection testing.

and prevent acute rheumatic fever and suppurative complications such as peritonsillar abscess, cervical lymphadenitis, and mastoiditis.

- Antimicrobial therapy should be limited to those who have clinical and epidemiological features of Group A streptococcal pharyngitis with a positive laboratory test.

- As pain is often the primary reason for visiting a physician, emphasis on analgesics such as acetaminophen and nonsteroidal anti-inflammatory drugs (NSAIDs) to aid in pain relief is strongly recommended. However, acetaminophen is a better option because there is some concern that NSAIDs may increase the risk for necrotizing fasciitis or toxic shock syndrome. Either systemic or topical analgesics can be used, as well as antipyretics and other supportive care including rest, fluids, lozenges, and salt water gargles.

- Antimicrobial treatment should be limited to those who have clinical and epidemiological features of group A streptococcal pharyngitis with a positive laboratory test. **Penicillin** is the drug of choice in the treatment of group A streptococcal pharyngitis (Table 42–4). Table 42–5 presents dosing guidelines for recurrent infections.

- In patients allergic to penicillin, a macrolide such as **erythromycin** or a first-generation cephalosporin such as **cephalexin** (if the reaction is non IgE-mediated hypersensitivity with hives or anaphylaxis) can be used. Newer macrolides such as azithromycin and clarithromycin are as effective as erythromycin and cause fewer gastrointestinal adverse effects.

- If patients are unable to take oral medications, intramuscular **benzathine penicillin** can be given although it is painful and no longer available in Canada.

EVALUATION OF THERAPEUTIC OUTCOMES

- Most cases of pharyngitis are self-limited; however, antimicrobial therapy will hasten resolution when given early to proven cases of group A streptococcus. Fever generally resolves by 3 to 5 days, and most other acute symptoms by 1 week. Tonsils and lymph nodes may take a few weeks to return to baseline. Children should be kept home from daycare or school until afebrile and for the first 24 hours after antimicrobial treatment is initiated, after which time transmission is unlikely. Follow-up testing is generally not necessary for index cases or in asymptomatic contacts of the index patient.

▶ SINUSITIS

- Sinusitis is an inflammation and/or infection of the paranasal sinus mucosa. The term *rhinosinusitis* is used by some specialists, because sinusitis typically also involves the nasal mucosa. The majority of these infections are viral in origin. It is important to differentiate between viral and bacterial sinusitis to aid in optimizing treatment decisions.

- Bacterial sinusitis can be categorized into acute and chronic disease. Acute disease lasts less than 30 days with complete resolution of symptoms. Chronic sinusitis is defined as episodes of inflammation lasting more than 3 months with persistence of respiratory symptoms.

- Acute bacterial sinusitis is most often caused by the same bacteria implicated in acute otitis media: *Streptococcus pneumoniae* and *Haemophilus influenzae*. These organisms are responsible for about 70% of bacterial causes of acute sinusitis in both adults and children. Chronic sinusitis can be polymicrobial, with an increased prevalence of anaerobes as well as less common pathogens including gram-negative bacilli and fungi.

TABLE 42–4. Dosing Guidelines for Pharyngitis

Drug	Adult Dosage	Pediatric Dosage	Duration
Penicillin VK	250 mg 3 times daily or 500 mg twice daily	50 mg/kg/day divided in 3 doses	10 days
Penicillin benzathine	1.2 million units intramuscularly	0.6 million units for under 27 kg (50,000 units/kg)	1 dose
Penicillin G procaine and benzathine mixture	Not recommended in adolescents and adults	1.2 million units (benzathine 0.9 million units, procaine 0.3 million units)	1 dose
Amoxicillin	500 mg 3 times daily	40–50 mg/kg/day divided in 3 doses	10 days
Erythromycin			10 days
Estolate	20–40 mg/kg/day divided 2–4 times daily (max: 1 g/day)	Same as adults	
Stearate	1 g daily divided 2–4 times daily (adolescents, adults)	—	
Ethylsuccinate	40 mg/kg/day divided 2–4 times daily (max: 1 g/day)	Same as adults	
Cephalexin	250–500 mg orally 4 times daily	25–50 mg/kg/day divided in 4 doses	10 days

TABLE 42–5. Antibiotics and Dosing for Recurrent Episodes of Pharyngitis

Drug	Adult Dosage	Pediatric Dosage
Clindamycin	600 mg orally divided in 2–4 doses	20 mg/kg/day in 3 divided doses (max: 1.8 g/day)
Amoxicillin-clavulanate	500 mg twice daily	40 mg/kg/day in 3 divided doses
Penicillin benzathine	1.2 million units intramuscularly for 1 dose	0.6 million units for under 27 kg (50,000 units/kg)
Penicillin benzathine with rifampin	As above	As above
	20 mg/kg/day orally in 2 divided doses × last 4 days of treatment with penicillin	Rifampin dose same as adults

TABLE 42–6. Clinical Presentation and Diagnosis of Bacterial Sinusitis[42–44,46–49]

General

A nonspecific upper respiratory tract infection that persists beyond 7–14 days

VIII

Signs and Symptoms

Acute

Adults:

Nasal discharge/congestion

Maxillary tooth pain, facial or sinus pain that may radiate (unilateral in particular) as well as deterioration after initial improvement

Severe or persistent (beyond 7 days) signs and symptoms are most likely bacterial and should be treated with antimicrobials

Children:

Nasal discharge and cough for greater than 10–14 days or severe signs and symptoms such as temperature 39°C or facial swelling or pain are indications for antimicrobial therapy

Chronic

Symptoms are similar to those of acute sinusitis but more nonspecific

Rhinorrhea is associated with acute exacerbations

Chronic unproductive cough, laryngitis, and headache may occur

Chronic/recurrent infections occur 3–4 times a year and are unresponsive to steam and decongestants

TABLE 42–7. Approach to Treatment of Acute Bacterial Sinusitis

Uncomplicated sinusitis	Amoxicillin
Uncomplicated sinusitis, penicillin-allergic patient	Immediate-type hypersensitivity: Clarithromycin or azithromycin or trimethoprim-sulfamethoxazole Nonimmediate-type hypersensitivity: β-Lactamase-stable cephalosporin
Treatment failure or prior antibiotic therapy in past 4–6 wk	High-dose amoxicillin with clavulanate or β-lactamase-stable cephalosporin
High suspicion of penicillin-resistant *S. pneumoniae*	High-dose amoxicillin or clindamycin

TABLE 42–8. Dosing Guidelines for Acute Bacterial Sinusitis

Drug	Adult Dosage	Pediatric Dosage
Amoxicillin	500 mg 3 times daily	Low dose: 40–50 mg/kg/day divided in 3 doses
	High dose: 1 g 3 times daily	High dose: 80–100 mg/kg/day divided in 3 doses
Amoxicillin-clavulanate	500/125 mg 3 times daily	40–50 mg/kg/day divided in 3 doses
		High dose: Can add 40–50 mg/kg/day amoxicillin
Cefuroxime	250–500 mg twice daily	15 mg/kg/day divided in 2 doses
Cefaclor	250–500 mg 3 times daily	20 mg/kg/day divided in 3 doses
Cefixime	200–400 mg twice daily	8 mg/kg/day in 1 dose or divided in 2 doses
Cefdinir	600 mg daily or divided in 2 doses	14 mg/kg/day in 1 dose or divided in 2 doses
Cefpodoxime	200 mg twice daily	10 mg/kg/day in 2 divided doses (max: 400 mg daily)
Cefprozil	250–500 mg twice daily	15–30 mg/kg/day divided in 2 doses
Trimethoprim-sulfamethoxazole	160/800 mg every 12 h	6–8 mg/kg/day trimethoprim, 30–40 mg/kg/day sulfamethoxazole divided in 2 doses
Clindamycin	150–450 mg every 6 h	30–40 mg/kg/day divided in 3 doses
Clarithromycin	250–500 mg twice daily	15 mg/kg/day divided in 2 doses
Azithromycin	500 mg day 1, then 250 mg/day × 4 days	10 mg/kg day 1, then 5 mg/kg/day × 4 days
Levofloxacin	500 mg daily	N/A

N/A, not applicable.

CLINICAL PRESENTATION

The typical clinical presentation of bacterial sinusitis is presented in Table 42–6.

TREATMENT

- The goals of treatment of acute sinusitis are the reduction in signs and symptoms, achieving and maintaining patency of the ostia, limiting antimicrobial treatment to those who may benefit, eradication of bacterial infection with appropriate antimicrobial therapy, minimizing the duration of illness, prevention of complications, and prevention of progression from acute disease to chronic disease.
- Approximately 40% to 60% of patients with acute sinusitis will recover spontaneously (these are likely patients with viral sinusitis).
- Nasal decongestant sprays such as **phenylephrine** and **oxymetazoline** that reduce inflammation by vasoconstriction are often used in sinusitis. Use should be limited to the recommended duration of the product to prevent rebound congestion. Oral decongestants may also aid in nasal or sinus patency. To reduce mucociliary function, irrigation of the nasal cavity with saline and steam inhalation may be used to increase mucosal moisture, and mucolytics (e.g. guaifenesin) may be used to decrease the viscosity of nasal secretions. Antihistamines should not be used for acute bacterial sinusitis in view of their anticholineric effects that can dry mucosa and disturb clearance of mucosal secretions.
- Antimicrobial therapy is superior to placebo in reducing or eliminating symptoms, although the benefit is small.
- **Amoxicillin** is first-line treatment for acute bacterial sinusitis. It is cost effective in acute uncomplicated disease, and intial use of newer broad-spectrum agents

is not justified. The approach to treating acute bacterial sinusitis is given in Table 42–7. Dosing guidelines are given in Table 42–8.
• The current recommendations are 10 to 14 days, or at least 7 days, of antimicrobial therapy after signs and symptoms are under control.

See Chapter 107, Upper Respiratory Tract Infections, authored by Yasmin Khaliq, Sarah Forgie, and George Zhanel, for a more detailed discussion of this topic.

VIII

Chapter 43

► SEPSIS AND SEPTIC SHOCK

► DEFINITIONS

Definitions of terms related to sepsis are given in Table 43–1. Physiologically similar systemic inflammatory response syndrome (SIRS) can be seen even in the absence of identifiable infection.

► PATHOPHYSIOLOGY

- The sites of infections that most frequently led to sepsis were the respiratory tract (40%), urinary tract (18%), and intra-abdominal space (14%). Sepsis may be caused by gram-negative or gram-positive bacteria, as well as by fungi or other microorganisms.
- *Escherichia coli* is the common pathogen isolated in sepsis; other common gram-negative pathogens include *Klebsiella* spp., *Serratia* spp., *Enterobacter* spp., and *Proteus* spp. *Pseudomonas aeruginosa* is the most frequent cause of sepsis fatality. Common gram-positive pathogens include *Staphylococcus aureus, Staphylococcus epidermidis, Streptococcus pneumoniae,* coagulase-negative staphylococci, and enterococci.
- *Candida* species (particularly *Candida albicans*) are a common cause of sepsis in hospitalized patients.
- The pathophysiologic focus of gram-negative sepsis has been on the lipopolysaccharide (endotoxin) component of the gram-negative cell wall.

TABLE 43–1. Definitions Related to Sepsis

Condition	Definition
Bacteremia (fungemia)	Presence of viable bacteria (fungi) in the bloodstream.
Infection	Inflammatory response to invasion of normally sterile host tissue by the microorganisms.
Systemic inflammatory response syndrome (SIRS)	Systemic inflammatory response to a variety of clinical insults which can be infection, but can be noninfectious etiology. The response is manifested by 2 or more of the following conditions: T > 38°C (100.4°F) or < 36°C (96.8°F); HR > 90 beats/min; RR > 20 breaths/min or $Paco_2$ < 32 torr; WBC > 12,000 cells/mm^3, < 4000 cells/mm^3, or > 10% immature (band) forms.
Sepsis	The SIRS secondary to infection.
Severe sepsis	Sepsis associated with organ dysfunction, hypoperfusion, or hypotension. Hypoperfusion and perfusion abnormalities may include, but are not limited to, lactic acidosis, oliguria, or acute alteration in mental status.
Septic shock	Sepsis with hypotension, despite fluid resuscitation, along with the presence of perfusion abnormalities. Patients who are on inotropic or vasopressor agents may not be hypotensive at the time perfusion abnormalities are measured.
Multiple-organ dysfunction syndrome (MODS)	Presence of altered organ function requiring intervention to maintain homeostasis.
Compensatory anti-inflammatory response syndrome (CARS)	Compensatory physiologic response to systemic inflammatory response syndrome that is considered secondary to the actions of anti-inflammatory cytokine mediators.

HR, heart rate; RR, respiratory rate; T, temperature.

Lipid A is a part of the endotoxin molecule that is highly immunoreactive and is responsible for most of the toxic effects. Endotoxin first associates with a protein called lipopolysaccharide-binding protein in plasma. This complex then engages a specific receptor (CD14) on the surface of the macrophage, which activates it and causes release of inflammatory mediators.

- Sepsis involves a complex interaction of proinflammatory (e.g., tumor necrosis factor α [TNF-α]; interleukin [IL]-1, IL-6) and anti-inflammatory mediators (e.g., IL-1 receptor antagonist, IL-4, and IL-10). IL-8, platelet activating factor, and a variety of prostaglandins, leukotrienes, and thromboxanes are also important.
- TNF-α is considered the primary mediator of sepsis, and concentrations are elevated early in the inflammatory response during sepsis. TNF-α release leads to activation of other cytokines associated with cellular damage and it stimulates release of arachidonic acid metabolites that contribute to endothelial cell damage.
- The balance between pro- and anti-inflammatory mechanisms determines the degree of inflammation. After the initiation of sepsis there is often an imbalance of proinflammatory cytokines, which causes a systemic inflammatory response syndrome (SIRS), followed by a compensatory anti-inflammatory response syndrome (CARS). VIII
- Figure 43–1 shows a schematic representation of the cascades of sepsis that is the pathogenesis of sepsis and septic shock.

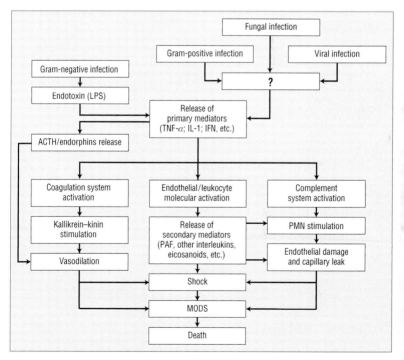

Figure 43–1. Cascades of sepsis. ACTH, adrenocorticotropic hormone.

- A primary mechanism of injury with sepsis is through endothelial cells. With inflammation, endothelial cells allow circulating cells (e.g., granulocytes) and plasma constituents to enter inflamed tissues, which may result in organ damage.
- Endotoxin activates complement, which then augments the inflammatory response through stimulation of leukocyte chemotaxis, phagocytosis and lysozomal enzyme release, increased platelet adhesion and aggregation, and production of toxic superoxide radicals.
- Proinflammatory mechanisms in sepsis are also procoagulant and antifibrinolytic. Levels of activated protein C, a fibrinolytic and anti-inflammatory substance, are decreased in sepsis.
- Shock is the most ominous complication associated with gram-negative sepsis and causes death in about one-half of patients. Other important complications of sepsis are disseminated intravascular coagulation (DIC), which occurs in 50% of patients with gram-negative sepsis. DIC causes activation of the coagulation cascade and inhibition of fibrinolysis, which can result in coagulopathy and microthrombosis. Acute respiratory distress syndrome (ARDS) is a common complication of sepsis, with mortality ranging from 19% to 90%.
- ►VIII The hallmark of the hemodynamic effect of sepsis is the hyperdynamic state characterized by high cardiac output and an abnormally low systemic vascular resistance (SVR).
- Sepsis results in distributive shock characterized by inappropriately increased blood flow to selected tissue at the expense of other tissue, independent of oxygen needs.

► CLINICAL PRESENTATION

- The signs and symptoms of early sepsis are quite variable and include fever, chills, and a change in mental status with lethargy and malaise. Hypothermia may occur instead of fever. Tachypnea and tachycardia are also evident. White blood cell count is usually elevated, as may be blood sugar. The patient may be hypoxic.
- Progression of uncontrolled sepsis leads to evidence of organ dysfunction, which may include oliguria, hemodynamic instability with hypotension or shock, lactic acidosis, hyperglycemia or hypoglycemia, possibly leukopenia, disseminated intravascular coagulation, thrombocytopenia, ARDS, gastrointestinal hemorrhage, or coma.

► DESIRED OUTCOME

► TREATMENT

The primary goals for treatment of sepsis are as follows:

1. Timely diagnosis and identification of the pathogen
2. Rapid elimination of the source of infection
3. Early initiation of aggressive antimicrobial therapy
4. Interruption of the pathogenic sequence leading to septic shock
5. Avoidance of organ failure

An important overall approach for treatment of sepsis is "goal-directed" therapy. Mortality can be reduced by early placement and use of a central venous catheter, increased fluid volume administration, dobutamine therapy if needed, and red blood cell transfusion, to achieve specific physiologic goals in the first 6 hours.

TABLE 43–2. Empirical Antimicrobial Regimens in Sepsis

Infection (Site or Type)	Antimicrobial Regimen		
	Community-Acquired	*Hospital-Acquired*	
Urinary tract	Ciprofloxacin *or* levofloxacin	Piperacillin *or* ceftazidime, ceftriaxone *or* ciprofloxacin, levofloxacin	± gentamicin
Respiratory tract	Newer fluoroquinolone[a] *or* ceftriaxone + clarithromycin-azithromycin	Piperacillin, ticarcillin *or* ceftazidime, cefipime	+ gentamicin or ciprofloxacin
Intra-abdominal	β-Lactamase inhibitor combo[b] *or* ciprofloxacin + metronidazole	Piperacillin-tazobactam *or* meropenem	
Skin/soft tissue	Nafcillin *or* cefazolin	Ceftriaxone +/− vancomycin	
Catheter-related		Vancomycin	
Unknown		Piperacillin *or* ceftazidime-cefipime *or* meropenem	+gentamicin +/− vancomycin

[a]Levofloxacin, gatifloxacin, moxifloxacin, gemifloxacin.
[b]Ampicillin-sulbactam, ticarcillin-clavulanic acid.

ANTIMICROBIAL THERAPY

- Aggressive, early antimicrobial therapy is critical in the management of septic patients. The regimen selected should be based on the suspected site of infection, likely pathogens and the local antibiotic susceptibility patterns, whether the organism was acquired from the community or a hospital, and the patient's immune status.
- The antibiotics that may be used for empiric treatment of sepsis are listed in Table 43–2.
- If *P. aeruginosa* is suspected, a dual regimen of **antipseudomonal penicillin** or **third-** or **fourth-generation cephalosporin** and an **aminoglycoside** is recommended. When an aminoglycoside is undesirable, an antipseudomonal fluoroquinolone such as ciprofloxacin or levofloxacin can be used.
- When aminoglycosides are used, single daily doses (4 to 7 mg/kg for gentamicin and tobramycin and 10 to 15 mg/kg for amikacin) may be preferred to achieve high peak concentrations early in treatment. Single daily dose administration should not be used in pediatric patients, burn victims, pregnant patients, patients with preexisting or progressive renal dysfunction, or patients requiring aminoglycosides for synergy against gram-positive pathogens.
- **Vancomycin** should be added whenever the risk of methicillin-resistant staphylococci is significant.
- The average duration of antimicrobial therapy in the normal host with sepsis is 10 to 14 days.

VIII

- Suspected systemic mycotic leading to sepsis is treated frequently with parenteral amphotericin B empirically, especially if the patient is clinically unstable. Alternative agents include fluconazole and caspofungin.

HEMODYNAMIC SUPPORT

- Maintenance of adequate tissue oxygenation is important in the treatment of sepsis and is dependent on adequate perfusion and adequate oxygenation of the blood.
- Rapid fluid resuscitation is the best initial therapeutic intervention for treatment of hypotension in sepsis. The goal is to restore tissue perfusion by maximizing cardiac output with increased left ventricular preload.
- Fluid administration should be titrated to clinical endpoints such as heart rate, urine output, blood pressure, and mental status. Isotonic crystalloids, such as 0.9% sodium chloride or lactated Ringer's solution, are commonly used for fluid resuscitation.
- Iso-oncotic colloid solutions (plasma and plasma protein fractions), such as 5% albumin and 6% hetastarch, offer the advantage of more rapid restoration of intravascular volume with less volume infused, but there is no significant clinical impact. Clinical outcome differences with the use of crystalloids or colloids have not been demonstrated, so crystalloids are generally recommended.

VIII

INOTROPE AND VASOACTIVE DRUG SUPPORT

When fluid resuscitation is insufficient to maintain tissue perfusion, the use of inotropes and vasoactive drugs is necessary. Selection and dosage are based on the pharmacologic properties of various catecholamines and how they influence hemodynamic parameters (Table 43–3).

Suggested Protocol for the Use of Inotropes and Vasoactive Agents

- **Dopamine** is widely used in low doses (1 to 5 μg/kg/min) to increase renal and mesenteric perfusion. Dopamine in moderate doses (greater than 5 μg/kg/min) may be used to support blood pressure.
- **Dobutamine** (in doses of 2 to 20 μg/kg/min) is a β-adrenergic inotropic agent that is the preferred drug for improving cardiac output and oxygen delivery. Dobutamine should be considered in severely septic patients with adequate filling pressures and blood pressure but low cardiac index.
- **Norepinephrine** is a potent α-adrenergic agent (0.01 to 3 μg/kg/min) useful in septic shock for vasoconstriction of peripheral beds. Phenylephrine may also be useful in patients with refractory hypotension.
- **Epinephrine,** in doses of 0.1 to 0.5 μg/kg/min, increases cardiac index and produces peripheral vasoconstriction. It is reserved for patients who fail to respond to traditional therapies.

TABLE 43–3. Receptor Activity of Cardiovascular Agents Commonly Used in Septic Shock

Agent	α_1	α_2	β_1	β_2	Dopaminergic
Dopamine	++/+++	?	++++	++	++++
Dobutamine	+	+	++++	++	0
Norepinephrine	+++	+++	+++	+/++	0
Phenylephrine	++/+++	+	?	0	0
Epinephrine	++++	++++	++++	+++	0

α_1, α_1-adrenergic receptor; α_2, α_2-adrenergic receptor; β_1, β_1-adrenergic receptor; β_2, β_2-adrenergic receptor; 0, no activity; ++++, maximal activity; ?, unknown activity.

- Prior to administering vasoactive agents, aggressive appropriate fluid resuscitation should occur. Vasoactive agents should not be considered an acceptable alternative to volume resuscitation.

ADJUNCTIVE THERAPIES

- **Glucocorticoids** may be useful for patients with ARDS and fibrotic disease when used 5 to 7 days after the onset of ARDS. Routine use of glucocorticoids in patients with sepsis or shock is not supported. It is now recognized that many critically ill patients have adrenal insufficiency and may require low doses of corticosteroids.
- Early enteral nutrition is recommended in patients with severe sepsis or septic shock.
- Administration of activated protein C (**drotrecogin**) to promote fibrinolysis and associated anti-inflammatory mechanisms may be beneficial in patients with APACHE II score greater than 25. This agent reduced mortality in severe sepsis but poses an increased risk of serious bleeding.

See Chapter 109, Sepsis and Septic Shock, authored by S. Lena Kang-Birken and Joseph T. DiPiro, for a more detailed discussion of this topic.   VIII

Chapter 44

▶ SEXUALLY TRANSMITTED DISEASES

▶ DEFINITION

The spectrum of sexually transmitted diseases (STDs) includes the classic venereal diseases—gonorrhea, syphilis, chancroid, lymphogranuloma venereum, and granuloma inguinale—as well as a variety of other pathogens known to be spread by sexual contact (Table 44–1). Common clinical syndromes associated with STDs are listed in Table 44–2. The most current information on epidemiology, diagnosis, and treatment of STDs provided by the Centers for Disease Control and Prevention (CDC) can be found at http://www.cdc.gov.

TABLE 44–1. Sexually Transmitted Diseases

Disease	Associated Pathogens
Bacterial	
Gonorrhea	*Neisseria gonorrhoeae*
Syphilis	*Treponema pallidum*
Chancroid	*Hemophilus ducreyi*
Granuloma inguinale	*Calymmatobacterium granulomatis*
Enteric disease	*Salmonella* spp., *Shigella* spp., *Campylobacter fetus*
Campylobacter infection	*Campylobacter jejuni*
Bacterial vaginosis	*Gardnerella vaginalis, Mycoplasma hominis, Bacteroides* spp., *Mobiluncus* spp.
Group B streptococcal infections	Group B *Streptococcus*
Chlamydial	
Nongonococcal urethritis	*Chlamydia trachomatis*
Lymphogranuloma venereum	*Chlamydia trachomatis*, type L
Viral	
Acquired immune-deficiency syndrome (AIDS)	Human immunodeficiency virus
Herpes genitalis	Herpes simplex virus, types I and II
Viral hepatitis	Hepatitis A, B, C, and D viruses
Condylomata acuminata	Human papillomavirus
Molluscum contagiosum	Poxvirus
Cytomegalovirus infection	Cytomegalovirus
Mycoplasmal	
Nongonococcal urethritis	*Ureaplasma urealyticum*
Protozoal	
Trichomoniasis	*Trichomonas vaginalis*
Amebiasis	*Entamoeba histolytica*
Giardiasis	*Giardia lamblia*
Fungal	
Vaginal candidiasis	*Candida albicans*
Parasitic	
Scabies	*Sarcoptes scabiei*
Pediculosis pubis	*Phthirus pubis*
Enterobiasis	*Enterobius vermicularis*

TABLE 44–2. Selected Syndromes Associated with Common Sexually Transmitted Pathogens

Syndrome	Commonly Implicated Pathogens	Common Clinical Manifestations[a]
Urethritis	*Chlamydia trachomatis*, herpes simplex virus, *Neisseria gonorrhoeae*, *Trichomonas vaginalis*, *Ureaplasma urealyticum*	Urethral discharge, dysuria
Epididymitis	*C. trachomatis*, *N. gonorrhoeae*	Scrotal pain, inguinal pain, flank pain, urethral discharge
Cervicitis/vulvovaginitis	*C. trachomatis*, *Gardnerella vaginalis*, herpes simplex virus, human papillomavirus, *N. gonorrhoeae*, *T. vaginalis*	Abnormal vaginal discharge, vulvar itching/irritation, dysuria, dyspareunia
Genital ulcers (painful)	*Hemophilus ducreyi*, herpes simplex virus	Usually multiple vesicular/pustular (herpes) or papular/pustular (*H. ducreyi*) lesions that may coalesce; painful, tender lymphadenopathy[b]
Genital ulcers (painless)	*Treponema pallidum*	Usually single papular lesion
Genital/anal warts	Human papillomavirus	Multiple lesions ranging in size from small papular warts to large exophytic condylomas
Pharyngitis	*C. trachomatis* (?), herpes simplex virus, *N. gonorrhoeae*	Symptoms of acute pharyngitis, cervical lymphadenopathy, fever[c]
Proctitis	*C. trachomatis*, herpes simplex virus, *N. gonorrhoeae*, *T. pallidum*	Constipation, anorectal discomfort, tenesmus, mucopurulent rectal discharge
Salpingitis	*C. trachomatis*, *N. gonorrhoeae*	Lower abdominal pain, purulent cervical or vaginal discharge, adnexal swelling, fever[d]

[a]For some syndromes, clinical manifestations may be minimal or absent.
[b]Recurrent herpes infection may manifest as a single lesion.
[c]Most cases of pharyngeal gonococcal infection are asymptomatic.
[d]Salpingitis increases the risk of subsequent ectopic pregnancy and infertility.

TABLE 44–3. Presentation of Gonorrhea Infections

	Males	Females
General	Incubation period 1–14 days Symptom onset in 2–8 days	Incubation period 1–14 days Symptom onset in 10 days
Site of infection	Most common—urethra Others—rectum (usually due to rectal intercourse in MSM), oropharynx, eye	Most common—endocervical canal Others—urethra, rectum (usually due to perineal contamination), oropharynx, eye
Symptoms	May be asymptomatic or minimally symptomatic Urethral infection—dysuria and urinary frequency Anorectal infection—asymptomatic to severe rectal pain Pharyngeal infection—asymptomatic to mild pharyngitis	May be asymptomatic or minimally symptomatic Endocervical infection—usually asymptomatic or mildly symptomatic Urethral infection—dysuria, urinary frequency Anorectal and pharyngeal infection—symptoms same as for men
Signs	Purulent urethral or rectal discharge can be scant to profuse Anorectal—pruritus, mucopurulent discharge, bleeding	Abnormal vaginal discharge or uterine bleeding; purulent urethral or rectal discharge can be scant to profuse
Complications	Rare (epididymitis, prostatitis, inguinal lymphadenopathy, urethral stricture) Disseminated gonorrhea	Pelvic inflammatory disease and associated complications (i.e., ectopic pregnancy, infertility) Disseminated gonorrhea (3 times more common than in men)

VIII

▶ GONORRHEA

- *Neisseria gonorrhoeae* is a gram-negative diplococcus estimated to cause up to 600,000 infections per year in the United States.

CLINICAL PRESENTATION

- Infected individuals may be symptomatic or asymptomatic, have complicated or uncomplicated infections, and have infections involving several anatomic sites.
- The most common clinical features of gonnococcal infections are presented in Table 44–3.
- Approximately 15% of women with gonorrhea develop pelvic inflammatory disease (PID). Left untreated, PID can be an indirect cause of infertility and ectopic pregnancies.
- In 0.5% to 3.0% of patients with gonorrhea, the gonococci invade the bloodstream and produce disseminated disease.
- The usual clinical manifestations of disseminated gonnococcal infection are tender necrotic skin lesions, tenosynovitis, and monoarticular arthritis.

DIAGNOSIS

- Diagnosis of gonococcal infections can be made by gram-stained smears, culture (the most reliable method), or newer methods based on the detection of cellular components of the gonococcus (e.g., enzymes, antigens, DNA, or lipopolysaccharide) in clinical specimens.

- Culture of exposed body areas is the most reliable means of diagnosing gonococcal infection.
- Alternative methods of diagnosis include enzyme immunoassay (EIA), DNA probes, and nucleic acid amplification techniques employing polymerase chain reaction and ligase chain reaction.

TREATMENT

- All currently recommended regimens are single-dose treatments with various oral or parenteral **cephalosporins** and **fluoroquinolones** (Table 44–4).
- **Ceftriaxone** (125 mg IM) is the only parenteral agent recommended by the CDC as a first-line agent for treatment of gonorrhea.
- Coexisting chlamydial infection, which is documented in up to 50% of women and 20% of men with gonorrhea, constitutes the major cause of postgonococcal urethritis, cervicitis, and salpingitis in patients treated for gonorrhea. As a result, concomitant treatment with **doxycycline** or **azithromycin** is recommended in all patients treated for gonorrhea. A single dose of azithromycin (2g) is highly effective against chlamydia.
- Pregnant women infected with *Neisseria gonorrhoeae* should be treated with either a **cephalosporin** or **spectinomycin,** because fluoroquinolones are contraindicated. **Erythromycin** or **amoxicillin** is the preferred treatment for presumed *Chlamydia trachomatis* infection.
- Treatment of gonorrhea during pregnancy is essential to prevent ophthalmia neonatorum. The American Academy of Pediatrics recommends that either **silver nitrate** (1%), **tetracycline** (1%), or **erythromycin** (0.5%) be instilled in each conjunctival sac immediately postpartum to prevent ophthalmia neonatorum.
- Infants born to infected mothers should also receive an intramuscular or intravenous injection of **ceftriaxone,** 50 mg/kg, for 7 days.

EVALUATION OF THERAPEUTIC OUTCOMES

- Combination gonorrhea/chlamydia therapy rarely results in treatment failures, and routine follow-up of patients treated with a regimen included in the CDC guidelines is not recommended.
- Persistence of symptoms following any treatment requires culture of the site(s) of gonorrheal infection, as well as susceptibility testing if gonococci are isolated.

▶ SYPHILIS

- The causative organism of syphilis is *Treponema pallidum,* a spirochete.
- Syphilis is usually acquired by sexual contact with infected mucous membranes or cutaneous lesions, although on rare occasions it can be acquired by nonsexual personal contact, accidental inoculation, or blood transfusion.

CLINICAL PRESENTATION

The clinical presentation of syphilis is varied, with progression through multiple stages possible in untreated or inadequately treat patients (Table 44–5).

Primary Syphilis

Primary syphilis is characterized by the appearance of a chancre on cutaneous or mucocutaneous tissue. Chancres persist only for 1 to 8 weeks before spontaneously disappearing.

VIII

TABLE 44-4. Treatment of Gonorrhea

Type of Infection	Recommended Regimens[a]	Alternative Regimens[b]
Uncomplicated infections of the cervix, urethra, and rectum in adults[c,d]	Ceftriaxone 125 mg IM once[e]; or ciprofloxacin 500 mg orally once[e]; or cefixime 400 mg orally once[f]; or ofloxacin 400 mg orally once[e] *plus* A treatment regimen for presumptive *C. trachomatis* coinfection (see Table 44–5)	Spectinomycin 2 g IM once; or cefitzoxime 500 mg IM once; or cefotaxime 500 mg IM once; or cefotetan 1 g IM once; or cefoxitin 2 g IM once with probenecid 1 g orally once; or lomefloxacin 400 mg orally once; or enoxacin 400 mg orally once; or norfloxacin 800 mg orally once *plus* A treatment regimen for presumptive *C. trachomatis* coinfection (see Table 44–5)
Gonococcal infections in pregnancy	Ceftriaxone 125 mg IM once[g,h] *plus* A recommended treatment regimen for presumptive *C. trachomatis* infection during pregnancy[h] (see Table 44–5)	Spectinomycin 2 g IM once *plus* a recommended treatment regimen for presumptive *C. trachomatis* infection during pregnancy[h] (see Table 44–5)
Disseminated gonococcal infection in adults (>45 kg)[h,i,j,k]	Ceftriaxone 1 g IM or IV every 24 h[l]	Cefitzoxime 1 g IV every 8 h[l] *or* Cefotaxime 1 g IV every 8 h[l]
Uncomplicated infections of the cervix, urethra, and rectum in children (<45 kg)	Ceftriaxone 125 mg IM once[m]	Spectinomycin 40 mg/kg IM once (not to exceed 2 g)

Gonococcal conjunctivitis in adults	Ceftriaxone 1 g IM once[n]
Ophthalmia neonatorum	Ceftriaxone 25–50 mg/kg IV or IM once (not to exceed 125 mg)
Infants born to mothers with gonococcal infection (prophylaxis)	Ceftriaxone 25–50 mg/kg IV or IM once (not to exceed 125 mg)

[a]Recommendations are those of the CDC.

[b]A number of other antimicrobials have demonstrated efficacy in treating uncomplicated gonorrhea but are not included in the CDC guidelines.

[c]Treatment failures are usually due to reinfection and necessitate patient education and sex-partner referral; additional treatment regimens for gonorrhea and chlamydia infections should be administered. Epididymitis should be treated for 10 days (see Table 44–8).

[d]Patients allergic to β-lactams should receive a quinolone. Persons unable to tolerate a β-lactam (penicillin or cephalosporin) or a quinolone should receive spectinomycin.

[e]Also recommended for the treatment of uncomplicated infections of the pharynx in combination with a treatment regimen for presumptive *C. trachomatis* infection; fluoroquinolones are *not* recommended for treating infections in MSM or infections acquired in Hawaii, California, or other parts of the world where high-level resistance to fluoroquinolones is reported.

[f]In July, 2002, Wyeth Pharmaceutical discontinued manufacturing cefixime; at the time of publication, there were no generic manufacturers of cefixime.

[g]Another recommendation IM or orally cephalosporin also may be used.

[h]The fluoroquinolones, doxycycline, and erythromycin ethylsuccinate are contraindicated during pregnancy.

[i]Patients treated with one of the recommended regimens should be treated with doxycycline or azithromycin for possible coexistent chlamydial infection.

[j]Patients with gonococcal meningitis should be treated for 10–14 days and those with endocarditis for at least 4 wk with ceftriaxone 1–2 g IV every 12 h.

[k]All treatment regimens should be continued for 24–48 h after improvement begins; at this time therapy can be switched to one of the following oral regimens to complete a 7-day course of treatment: cefixime 400 mg orally 2 times daily, or ciprofloxacin 500 mg orally 2 times daily, or ofloxacin 400 mg orally 2 time daily.

[l]All regimens should be continued for 24–48 h after improvement begins; at this time therapy can be switched to one of the following oral regimens to complete a 7-day course of treatment: cefixime 400 mg orally 2 times daily or ciprofloxacin 500 mg orally 2 times daily or ofloxacin 400 mg orally 2 times daily.

[m]Patients with bacteremia or arthritis should receive ceftriaxone 50 mg/kg (maximum 1 g) IM or IV once daily for 7 days.

[n]The eye should be lavaged 1 time with saline solution.

TABLE 44–5. Presentation of Syphilis Infections

General

Primary	Incubation period 10–90 days (mean 21 days)
Secondary	Develops 2–8 wk after initial infection in untreated or inadequately treated individuals
Latent	Develops 4–10 wk after secondary stage in untreated or inadequately treated individuals
Tertiary	Develops in approximately 30% of untreated or inadequately treated individuals 10–30 yr after initial infection

Site of Infection

Primary	External genitalia, perianal region, mouth, and throat
Secondary	Multisystem involvement secondary to hematogenous and lymphatic spread
Latent	Potentially multisystem involvement (dormant)
Tertiary	CNS, heart, eyes, bones, and joints

Signs and Symptoms

Primary	Single, painless, indurated lesion (chancre) that erodes, ulcerates, and eventually heals (typical); regional lymphadenopathy is common; multiple, painful, purulent lesions possible but uncommon
Secondary	Pruritic or nonpruritic rash, mucocutaneous lesions, flulike symptoms, lymphadenopathy
Latent	Asymptomatic
Tertiary	Cardiovascular syphilis (aoritits or aortic insufficiency), neurosyphilis (meningitis, general paresis, dementia, tabes dorsalis, eighth cranial nerve deafness, blindness), gummatous lesions involving any organ or tissue

► VIII

Secondary Syphilis

- The secondary stage of syphilis is characterized by a variety of mucocutaneous eruptions, resulting from widespread hematogenous and lymphatic spread of *T. pallidum*.
- Signs and symptoms of secondary syphilis disappear in 4 to 10 weeks; however, in untreated patients, lesions may recur at any time within 4 years.

Latent Syphilis

- Persons with a positive serologic test for syphilis but with no other evidence of disease have latent syphilis.
- Most untreated patients with latent syphilis have no further sequelae; however, approximately 25% to 30% progress to either neurosyphilis or late syphilis with clinical manifestations other than neurosyphilis.

Tertiary Syphilis and Neurosyphilis

Forty percent of patients with primary or secondary syphilis exhibit central nervous system (CNS) infection.

DIAGNOSIS

- Because *T. pallidum* is difficult to culture in vitro, diagnosis is based primarily on dark-field or direct fluorescent antibody microscopic examination of serous material from a suspected syphilitic lesion or on results from serologic testing.
- Serologic tests are the mainstay in the diagnosis of syphilis and are categorized as nontreponemal or treponemal. Commonly used nontreponemal tests include the Venereal Disease Research Laboratory (VDRL) slide test, the rapid plasma reagin (RPR) card test, the unheated serum regain (USR) test, and the tuluidine red unheated serum test (TRUST).

- Treponemal tests are more sensitive than nontreponemal tests and are used to confirm the diagnosis (i.e., the fluorescent treponemal antibody absorption [FTA-ABS]).

TREATMENT

- Treatment recommendations from the CDC for syphilis are presented in Table 44–6. Parenteral **penicillin G** is the treatment of choice for all stages of syphilis. Benzathine penicillin G is the only penicillin effective for single-dose therapy.
- Patients with abnormal CSF findings should be treated as having neurosyphilis.
- For pregnant patients, penicillin is the treatment of choice at the dosage recommended for that particular stage of syphilis. To ensure treatment success and prevent transmission to the fetus, some experts advocate an additional intramuscular dose of benzathine penicillin G, 2.4 million units, 1 week after completion of the recommended regimen.
- The majority of patients treated for primary and secondary syphilis experience the Jarisch–Herxheimer reaction after treatment, characterized by flulike symptoms such as transient headache, fever, chills, malaise, arthralgia, myalgia, tachypnea, peripheral vasodilation, and aggravation of syphilitic lesions.
- The Jarisch–Herxheimer reaction should not be confused with penicillin allergy. Most reactions can be managed symptomatically with analgesics, antipyretics, and rest.

VIII

EVALUATION OF THERAPEUTIC OUTCOMES

- CDC recommendations for serologic follow-up of patients treated for syphilis are given in Table 44–6. Quantitative nontreponemal tests should be performed at 6 and 12 months in all patients treated for primary and secondary syphilis and at 6, 12, and 24 months for early and late latent disease.
- For women treated during pregnancy, monthly quantitative nontreponemal tests are recommended in those at high risk of reinfection.

▶ CHLAMYDIA

Infections caused by *C. trachomatis* are believed to be the most common STD in the United States that has more than doubled in the past 10 years.

CLINICAL PRESENTATION

- In comparison with gonorrhea, chlamydial genital infections are more frequently asymptomatic, and when present, symptoms tend to be less noticeable. Table 44–7 summarizes the usual clinical presentation of chlamydial infections.
- Similar to gonorrhea, chlamydia may be transmitted to an infant during contact with infected cervicovaginal secretions. Nearly two thirds of infants acquire chlamydial infection after endocervical exposure, with the primary morbidity associated with seeding of the infant's eyes, nasopharynx, rectum, or vagina.

DIAGNOSIS

- Culture of endocervical or urethral epithelial cell scrapings is the most specific method for detection of chlamydia, but sensitivity is as low as 70%. Between 3 and 7 days are required for results.
- Tests that allow rapid identification of chlamydial antigens in genital secretions are the direct fluorescent antibody test, the enzyme immunoassay (requires just 30 minutes for results), and the DNA hybridization probe.

TABLE 44–6. Drug Therapy and Follow-up of Syphilis

Stage/Type of Syphilis	Recommended Regimens[a]	Follow-up Serology
Primary, secondary, or latent syphilis of less than 1-yr duration (early latent syphilis)	Benzathine penicillin G 2.4 million units IM in a single dose[b]	Quantitative nontreponemal tests at 6 and 12 months for primary and secondary syphilis; at 6, 12, and 24 months for early latent syphilis[c]
Latent syphilis of more than 1-yr duration (late latent syphilis) or syphilis of unknown duration	Benzathine penicillin G 2.4 million units IM once a week for 3 successive weeks (7.2 million units total)	Quantitative nontreponemal tests at 6, 12, and 24 months[d]
Neurosyphilis	Aqueous crystalline penicillin G 18–24 million units IV (3–4 million units every 4 h or by continuous infusion) for 10–14 days[e] *or* Aqueous procaine penicillin G 2.4 million units IM daily plus probenecid 500 mg orally four times daily, both for 10–14 days[e]	CSF[f] examination every 6 months until the cell count is normal; if it has not decreased at 6 months or is not normal by 2 yr, retreatment should be considered
Congenital syphilis	Aqueous crystalline penicillin G 50,000 units/kg IV every 12 h during the first 7 days of life and every 8 h thereafter for a total of 10 days *or* Procaine penicillin G 50,000 units/kg IM daily for 10 days	Quantitative nontreponemal tests every 2–3 months until nonreactive or titers have decreased 4-fold

Penicillin-allergic patients[a]

Primary, secondary, or early latent syphilis — Doxycycline 100 mg orally 2 times daily for 2 wk[h,i]

or

Tetracycline 500 mg orally 4 times daily for 2 wk[h,i]

Latent syphilis of more than 1 year's duration (late latent syphilis) or syphilis of unknown duration — Doxycycline 100 mg orally 2 times a day for 4 wk[i]

or

Tatracycline 500 mg orally 4 times daily for 4 wk[i]

Same as for non–penicillin-allergic patients

Same as for non–penicillin-allergic patients

---

[a]Recommendations are those of the CDC.

[b]Some experts recommend multiple doses of benzathine penicillin G or other supplemental antibiotics in addition to benzathine penicillin G in HIV-infected patients with primary or secondary syphilis; HIV-infected patients with early latent syphilis should be treated with the recommended regimen for latent syphilis of more than 1-yr duration.

[c]More frequent follow-up (i.e., 3, 6, 9, 12, and 24 months) recommended for HIV-infected patients.

[d]More frequent follow-up (i.e., 6, 12, 18, and 24 months) recommended for HIV-infected patients.

[e]Some experts administer benzathine penicillin G 2.4 million units IM once per week for up to 3 weeks after completion of the neurosyphilis regimens to provide a total duration of therapy comparable to that used for late syphilis in the absence of neurosyphilis.

[f]CSF, cerebrospinal fluid.

[g]For nonpregnant patients; pregnant patients should be treated with penicillin after desensitization.

[h]Although less effective than either the doxycycline or tetracycline regimen, erythromycin 500 mg orally 4 times daily can be considered as an alternative regimen for nonpregnant patients.

[i]Pregnant patients allergic to penicillin should be desensitized and treated with penicillin.

TABLE 44–7. Presentation of *Chlamydia* Infections

	Males	Females
General	Incubation period—35 days Symptom onset—7–21 days	Incubation period—7–35 days Usual symptom onset—7–21 days
Site of infection	Most common—urethra Others—rectum (receptive anal intercourse), oropharynx, eye	Most common—endocervical canal Others—urethra, rectum (usually due to perineal contamination), oropharynx, eye
Symptoms	Over 50% of urethral and rectal infections are asymptomatic Urethral infection—mild dysuria, discharge Pharyngeal infection—asymptomatic to mild pharyngitis	Over 66% of cervical infections are asymptomatic Urethral infection—usually subclinical; dysuria and frequency uncommon Rectal and pharyngeal infection—symptoms same as for men
Signs	Scant to profuse, mucoid to purulent urethral or rectal discharge Rectal infection—pain, discharge, bleeding	Abnormal vaginal discharge or uterine bleeding, purulent urethral, or rectal discharge can be scant to profuse
VIII Complications	Epididymitis, Reiter's syndrome (rare)	Pelvic inflammatory disease and associated complications (i.e., ectopic pregnancy, infertility) Reiter's syndrome (rare)

TREATMENT

- Recommended regimens for treatment of chlamydial infections are given in Table 44–8. Single-dose **azithromycin** and 7-day **doxycycline** are the agents of choice.
- For prophylaxis of ophthalmia neonatorum, various groups have proposed the use of **erythromycin** (0.5%) or **tetracycline** (1%) ophthalmic ointment in lieu

TABLE 44–8. Treatment of Chlamydial Infections

Infection	Recommended Regimens[a]	Alternative Regimen
Uncomplicated urethral, endocervical, or rectal infection in adults	Azithromycin 1 g orally once, or doxycycline 100 mg orally 2 times daily for 7 days	Ofloxacin 300 mg orally 2 times daily for 7 days, or levofloxacin 500 mg orally once daily for 7 days, or erythromycin base 500 mg orally 4 times daily for 7 days, or erythromycin ethyl succinate 800 mg orally 4 times daily for 7 days
Urogenital infections during pregnancy	Erythromycin base 500 mg orally 4 times daily for 7 days, or amoxicillin 500 mg orally 3 times daily for 7 days	Erythromycin base 250 mg orally 4 times daily for 14 days, or erythromycin ethyl succinate 800 mg orally 4 times daily for 7 days (or 400 mg orally 4 times daily for 14 days), or azithromycin 1 g orally as a single dose[b]
Conjunctivitis of the newborn or pneumonia in infants	Erythromycin base 50 mg/kg/day orally in 4 divided doses for 14 days[c]	

[a]Recommendations are those of the CDC.
[b]Data are insufficient to recommend routine use of azithromycin in pregnant women at this time.
[c]Topical therapy alone is inadequate and is unnecessary when systemic therapy is administered.

of silver nitrate. Although silver nitrate and antibiotic ointments are effective against gonococcal ophthalmia neonatorum, silver nitrate is not effective for chlamydial disease and may cause a chemical conjunctivitis.

- The only acceptable treatment for chlamydial ophthalmia neonatorum is systemic therapy with oral **erythromycin,** 50 mg/kg/day in four divided doses, for 10 to 14 days.

EVALUATION OF THERAPEUTIC OUTCOMES

- Treatment of chlamydial infections with the recommended regimens is highly effective; therefore, posttreatment cultures are not routinely recommended.
- Infants with pneumonitis should receive follow-up testing, because erythromycin is only 80% effective.

▶ GENITAL HERPES

The term *herpes* is used to describe two distinct but antigenically related serotypes of herpes simplex virus (HSV). Herpes simplex virus type 1 (HSV-1) is most commonly associated with oropharyngeal disease; type 2 (HSV-2) is most closely associated with genital disease.   VIII

CLINICAL PRESENTATION

A summary of the clinical presentation of genital herpes is provided in Table 44–9.

DIAGNOSIS

- A presumptive diagnosis of genital herpes commonly is made on the basis of the presence of dark-field-negative, vesicular, or ulcerative genital lesions. A history of similar lesions or recent sexual contact with an individual with similar lesions also is useful in making the diagnosis.
- Tissue culture is the most specific (100%) and sensitive method (80% to 90%) of confirming the diagnosis of first-episode genital herpes.

TREATMENT

- The goals of therapy in genital herpes infection are to shorten the clinical course, prevent complications, prevent the development of latency and/or subsequent recurrences, decrease disease transmission, and eliminate established latency.
- Palliative and supportive measures are the cornerstone of therapy for patients with genital herpes. Pain and discomfort usually respond to warm saline baths or the use of analgesics, antipyretics, or antipruritics.
- Specific chemotherapeutic approaches to treating genital herpes fall into six major areas: antiviral compounds, topical surfactants, photodynamic dyes, immune modulators, vaccines, and interferons.
- Specific recommendations are given in Table 44–10.
- Oral acyclovir, valacyclovir, and famciclovir are the treatments of choice for outpatients with first-episode genital herpes. Treatment does not prevent latency or alter the subsequent frequency and severity of recurrences.
- Continuous oral antiviral therapy reduces the frequency and the severity of recurrences in 70% to 90% of patients experiencing frequent recurrences.
- Acyclovir, valacyclovir, and famciclovir have been used to prevent reactivation of infection in patients seropositive for HSV who undergo transplantation procedures or induction chemotherapy for acute leukemia.

TABLE 44–9. Presentation of Genital Herpes Infections

General	Incubation period 2–14 days (mean - 4 days)
	Can be caused by either HSV-1 or HSV-2
Classification of Infection	
First-episode primary	Initial genital infection in individuals lacking antibody to either HSV-1 or HSV-2
First-episode nonprimary	Initial genital infection in individuals with clinical or serologic evidence of prior HSV (usually HSV-1) infection
Recurrent	Appearance of genital lesions at some time following healing of first-episode infection
Signs and Symptoms	
First-episode infections	Most primary infections are asymptomatic or minimally symptomatic
	Multiple painful pustular or ulcerative lesions on external genitalia developing over a period of 7–10 days; lesions heal in 2–4 wk (mean 21 days)
	Flulike symptoms (e.g., fever, headache, malaise) during first fews after appearance of lesions
	Others—local itching, pain or discomfort; vaginal or urethral discharge, tender inguinal adenopathy, paresthesias, urinary retention
	Severity of symptoms greater in females than in males
	Symptoms are less severe (e.g., fewer lesions, more rapid lesion healing, fewer or milder systemic symptoms) with nonprimary infections
	Symptoms more severe and prolonged in the immunocompromised
	On average viral shedding lasts approximately 11–12 days for primary infections and 7 days for nonprimary infections
Recurrent	Prodrome seen in approximately 50% of patients prior to appearance of recurrent lesions; mild burning, itching, or tingling are typical prodromal symptoms
	Compared to primary infections, recurrent infections associated with (1) fewer lesions that are more localized, (2) shorter duration of active infection (lesions heal within 7 days), and (3) milder symptoms
	Severity of symptoms greater in females than in males
	Symptoms more severe and prolonged in the immunocompromised
	On average viral shedding lasts approximately 4 days
Therapeutic implications of HSV-1 versus HSV-2 genital infection	Primary infections due to HSV-1 and HSV-2 virtually indistinguishable
	Recurrence rate is greater following primary infection with HSV-2
	Recurrent infections with HSV-2 tend to be more severe
Complications	Secondary infection of lesions; extragenital infection due to autoinoculation; disseminated infection (primarily in immuncompromised patients); meningitis or encephalitis; neonatal transmission

- The safety of acyclovir therapy during pregnancy is not established, although there is no evidence of teratogenic effects in humans.

▶ TRICHOMONIASIS

- Trichomoniasis is caused by *Trichomonas vaginalis,* a flagellated, motile protozoan that is responsible for 3 to 5 million cases per year in the United States.
- Coinfection with other STDs (such as gonorrhea) is common in patients diagnosed with trichomoniasis.

CLINICAL PRESENTATION

The typical presentation of trichomoniasis in males and females is presented in Table 44–11.

VIII

TABLE 44–10. Treatment of Genital Herpes

Type of Infection	Recommended Regimens[a,b]	Alternative Regimen
First clinical episode of genital herpes[c]	Acyclovir 400 mg orally 3 times daily for 7–10 days, *or* Acyclovir 200 mg orally 5 times daily for 7–10 days, *or* Famciclovir 250 mg orally 3 times daily for 7–10 days, *or* Valacyclovir 1 g orally 2 times daily for 7–10 days	Acyclovir 5–10 mg/kg IV every 8 h for 2–7 days until clinical improvement occurs, followed by oral therapy to complete at least 10 days of total therapy[d]
First clinical episode of herpes proctitis or oral infection including stomatitis or pharyngitis	Acyclovir 400 mg orally 5 times daily for 7–10 days[e]	Acyclovir 5–10 mg/kg IV every 8 h for 2–7 days until clinical improvement occurs, followed by oral therapy to complete at least 10 days of total therapy[d]
Recurrent infection		
Episodic therapy	Acyclovir 400 mg orally 3 times daily for 5 days,[f] *or* Acyclovir 800 mg orally 2 times daily for 5 days,[f] *or* Famciclovir 125 mg orally 2 times daily for 5 days,[f] *or* Valacyclovir 500 mg orally 2 times daily for 3–5 days,[f] *or* Valacyclovir 1 g orally once daily for 5 days[f] Acyclovir 400 mg orally twice daily,[g] *or*	
Suppressive therapy	Famciclovir 250 mg orally 2 times daily, or Valacyclovir 500 mg or 1000 mg orally once daily[h]	

VIII

[a]Recommendations are those of the CDC.
[b]HIV-infected patients may require more aggressive therapy.
[c]Primary or nonprimary first episode.
[d]Only for patients with severe symptoms or complications that necessitate hospitalization.
[e]Recommendations based on studies utilizing this dosage regimen rather than the lower dosage regimens recommended for first clinical episodes of genital herpes. It is not clear whether lower dosage regimens would have comparable efficacy. Famciclovir and valacyclovir are probably also effective for proctitis and oral infection, but clinical experience is limited.
[f]Requires initiation of therapy within 24 h of lesion onset or during the prodrome that precedes some outbreaks.
[g]Indicated only for patients with frequent and/or severe recurrences; although safety and efficacy are documented in patients receiving acyclovir daily therapy for as long as 6 yr and valacyclovir and famciclovir therapy for 1 yr, it is recommended that therapy be discontinued periodically (e.g., once a year) to reassess the need for continued suppressive therapy.
[h]Valacyclovir 500 mg appears less effective than valacyclovir 1000 mg in patients with approximately 10 recurrences per year.

DIAGNOSIS

- *T. vaginalis* produces nonspecific symptoms also consistent with bacterial vaginosis, and thus laboratory diagnosis is required.
- The simplest and most reliable means of diagnosis is a wet-mount examination of the vaginal discharge. Trichomoniasis is confirmed if characteristic pear-shaped, flagellating organisms are observed. Newer diagnostic tests such as monoclonal antibody or DNA probe techniques, as well as PCR tests are highly sensitive and specific.

TABLE 44–11. Presentation of Trichomonas Infections

	Males	Females
General	Incubation period 3–28 days Organism may be detectable within 48 hours after exposure to infected partner	Incubation period 3–28 days
Site of infection	Most common—urethra Others—rectum (usually due to rectal intercourse in MSM), oropharynx, eye	Most common—endocervical canal Others—urethra, rectum (usually due to perineal contamination), oropharynx, eye
Symptoms	May be asymptomatic (more common in males than females) or minimally symptomatic Urethral discharge (clear to mucopurulent) Dysuria, prurius	May be asymptomatic or minimally symptomatic Scant to copious, typically malodorous vaginal discharge (50–75%) and pruritus (worsen during menses) Dysuria, dyspareunia
Signs	Urethral discharge	Vaginal discharge Vaginal pH 4.5–6 Inflammation/erythema of vulva, vagina, and/or cervix Urethritis
Complications	Epididymitis and chronic prostatitis (uncommon) Male infertility (decreased sperm motility and viability)	Pelvic inflammatory disease and associated complications (i.e., ectopic pregnancy, infertility) Premature labor, premature rupture of membranes, and low-birth-weight infants (risk of neonatal infections is low) Cervical neoplasia

VIII

TABLE 44–12. Treatment of Trichomoniasis

Type	Recommended Regimen[a]	Alternative Regimen
Symptomatic and asymptomatic infections	Metronidazole 2 g orally in a single dose[b]	Metronidazole 500 mg orally 2 times daily for 7 days[c]
Treatment in pregnancy	Metronidazole 2 g orally in a single dose[d]	
Neonatal infections[e]	Metronidazole 10–30 mg/kg daily for 5–8 days	

Note: Tinidazole was approved by the FDA in 2004 for for the treatment of trichomonasis. The recommended dosage is 2 g orally in a single dose.

[a]Recommendations are those of the CDC.

[b]Treatment failures should be treated with metronidazole 500 mg orally 2 times daily for 7 days. Persistent failures should be managed in consultation with an expert. Metronidazole 2 g orally daily for 3–5 days has been effective in patients infected with *T. vaginalis* strains mildly resistant to metronidazole, but experience is limited; higher doses also have been used.

[c]Metronidazole labeling approved by the FDA does not include this regimen. Dosage regimens for treatment of trichomoniasis included in the product labeling are the single 2 g dose; 250 mg 3 times daily for 7 days; and 375 mg 2 times daily for 7 days. The 250 mg and 375 mg dosage regimens are currently not included in the CDC recommendations.

[d]Metronidazole is contraindicated in the first trimester of pregnancy. While the CDC recommends a single 2-g dose for treatment during pregnancy, a 7-day regimen is preferred by some since it produces lower peak serum drug concentrations.

[e]Only infants with symptomatic trichomoniasis or with urogenital trichomonal colonization that persists beyond the fourth week of life.

TABLE 44–13. Treatment Regimens for Miscellaneous Sexually Transmitted Diseases

Infection	Recommended Regimen[a]	Alternative Regimen
Chancroid (*Haemophilus ducreyi*)	Azithromycin 1 g orally in a single dose, *or* Ceftriaxone 250 mg IM in a single dose, *or* Ciprofloxacin 500 mg orally 2 times daily for 3 days, *b or* Erythromycin base 500 mg orally 4 times daily for 7 days	
Lymphogranuloma venereum	Doxycycline 100 mg orally 2 times daily for 21 days	Erythromycin base 500 mg orally 4 times daily for 21 days
Human Papillomavirus Infection: External genital warts	*Provider-Administered Therapies:* Cryotherapy (e.g., liquid nitrogen or cryoprobe), *or* Podophyllin 10–25% in compound tincture of benzoin applied to lesions; repeat weekly if necessary,[c,d] *or* Trichloroacetic acid (TCA) 80–90% or bichloroacetic acid (BCA) 80–90% applied to warts; repeat weekly if necessary, *or* Surgical removal (tangential scissor excision, tangential shave excision, curettage, or electrosurgery) *Patient-Applied Therapies:* Podofilox 0.5% solution or gel applied 2 times daily for 3 days, followed by 4 days of no therapy; cycle is repeated as necessary for a total of 4 cycles,[d] *or* Imiquimod 5% cream applied at bedtime 3 times weekly for up to 16 wk[d]	Intralesional interferon or laser surgery
Human Papillomavirus Infection: Vaginal, urethral meatus, and anal warts	Cryotherapy with liquid nitrogen, or TCA or BCA 80–90% as for external HPV warts; repeat weekly as necessary (*not* for urethral meatus warts), *or* Podophyllin 10–25% in compound tincture of benzoin applied at weekly intervals (*not* for vaginal or anal warts),[d] *or* Surgical removal (*not* for vaginal or urethral meatus warts)	

[a]Recommendations are those of the CDC.
[b]Ciprofloxacin is contraindicated for pregnant and lactating women and for persons aged <18 yr.
[c]Some experts recommended washing podophyllin off after 1–4 h to minimize local irritation.
[d]Safety during pregnancy is not established.

TREATMENT

- **Metronidazole** is the only antimicrobial agent available in the United States that is consistently effective in *T. vaginalis* infections.
- Treatment recommendations for *Trichomonas* infections are given in Table 44–12.
- Gastrointestinal complaints (e.g., anorexia, nausea, vomiting, diarrhea) are the most common adverse effects, with the single 2-g dose of metronidazole, occurring in 5% to 10% of treated patients. Some patients complain of a bitter metallic taste in the mouth.
- Patients intolerant of the single 2-g dose because of gastrointestinal adverse effects usually tolerate the multidose regimen.
- To achieve maximal cure rates and prevent relapse with the single 2-g dose of metronidazole, simultaneous treatment of infected sexual partners is necessary.
- Patients who fail to respond to an initial course usually respond to a second course of metronidazole therapy.
- Patients taking metronidazole should be instructed to avoid alcohol ingestion during therapy and for 1 to 2 days after completion of therapy because of a possible disulfiram-like effect.
- VIII • At present, no satisfactory treatment is available for pregnant women with *Trichomonas* infections.

EVALUATION OF THERAPEUTIC OUTCOMES

- Follow-up is considered unnecessary in patients who become asymptomatic after treatment with metronidazole.
- When patients remain symptomatic, it is important to determine if reinfection has occurred. In these cases, a repeat course of therapy, as well as identification and treatment or retreatment of infected sexual partners, is recommended.

▶ OTHER SEXUALLY TRANSMITTED DISEASES

Several STDs other than those previously discussed occur with varying frequency in the United States and throughout the world. While an in-depth discussion of these diseases is beyond the scope of this chapter, recommended treatment regimens are given in Table 44–13.

See Chapter 115, Sexually Transmitted Diseases, authored by Leroy C. Knodel, for a more detailed discussion of this topic.

Chapter 45

▶ SKIN AND SOFT TISSUE INFECTIONS

▶ DEFINITION

- Bacterial infections of the skin can be classified as primary (pyodermas or cellulitis) or secondary (invasion of the wound) (Table 45–1). Primary bacterial infections are usually caused by a single bacterial species and involve areas of generally healthy skin (e.g., impetigo, erysipelas). Secondary infections, however, develop in areas of previously damaged skin and are frequently polymicrobic in nature.
- The conditions that may predispose a patient to the development of skin and soft tissue infections (SSTIs) include (1) a high concentration of bacteria, (2) excessive moisture of the skin, (3) inadequate blood supply, (4) availability of bacterial nutrients, and (5) damage to the corneal layer allowing for bacterial penetration.
- The majority of SSTISs are caused by gram-positive organisms and, less commonly, gram-negative bacteria present on the skin surface. *Staphylococcus aureus* and *Streptococcus pyogenes* account for the majority of SSTIs.

▶ CELLULITIS

- Cellulitis is an acute, spreading infectious process that initially affects the epidermis and dermis and may subsequently spread within the superficial fascia. This process is characterized by inflammation but with little or no necrosis or suppuration of soft tissue.
- Cellulitis is most often caused by *S. pyogenes* or by *S. aureus* (see Table 45–1).

TABLE 45–1. Bacterial Classification of Important Skin and Soft Tissue Infections

Primary Infections	
Erysipelas	Group A streptococci
Impetigo	*Staphylococcus aureus*, group A streptococci
Lymphangitis	Group A streptococci; occasionally *S. aureus*
Cellulitis	Group A streptococci, *S. aureus*; occasionally other gram-positive cocci, gram-negative bacilli, and/or anaerobes
Necrotizing fasciitis	
Type I	Anaerobes (*Bacteroides* spp., *Peptostreptococcus* spp.) and facultative bacteria (streptococci, Enterobacteriaceae)
Type II	Group A streptococci
Secondary Infections	
Diabetic foot infections	*S. aureus*, streptococci, Enterobacteriaceae, *Bacteroides* spp., *Peptostreptococcus* spp., *Pseudomonas aeruginosa*
Pressure sores	*S. aureus*, streptococci, Enterobacteriaceae, *Bacteroides* spp., *Peptostreptococcus* spp., *Pseudomonas aeruginosa*
Bite wounds	
Animal	*Pasteurella multocida*, *S. aureus*, streptococci, *Bacteroides* spp.
Human	*Eikenella corrodens*, *S. aureus*, streptococci, *Corynebacterium* spp., *Bacteroides* spp., *Peptostreptococcus* spp.
Burn wounds	*Pseudomonas aeruginosa*, Enterobacteriaceae, *S. aureus*, streptococci

CLINICAL PRESENTATION

- Cellulitis is characterized by erythema and edema of the skin. The lesion, which may be extensive, is painful and nonelevated and has poorly defined margins. Tender lymphadenopathy associated with lymphatic involvement is common. Malaise, fever, and chills are also commonly present. There is usually a history of an antecedent wound from minor trauma, an ulcer, or surgery.
- A Gram stain of a smear obtained by injection and aspiration of 0.5 mL of saline (using a small-gauge needle) into the advancing edge of the erythematous lesion may help in making the microbiologic diagnosis but often yields negative results.
- Acute cellulitis with mixed aerobic-anaerobic flora generally occurs in diabetes, where the skin is near a traumatic site or surgical incision, at sites of surgical incisions to the abdomen or perineum, or when host defenses are compromised.

TREATMENT

- The goal of therapy of acute bacterial cellulitis is rapid eradication of the infection and prevention of further complications.
- Antimicrobial therapy of bacterial cellulitis is directed toward the type of bacteria either documented to be present or suspected.
- Local care of cellulitis includes elevation and immobilization of the involved area to decrease local swelling.
- As streptococcal cellulitis is indistinguishable clinically from staphylococcal cellulitis, administration of a semisynthetic penicillin (**nafcillin** or **oxacillin**) is recommended until a definitive diagnosis, by skin or blood cultures, can be made (Table 45–2). If documented to be a mild cellulitis secondary to streptococci, oral **penicillin VK,** 250 to 500 mg four times daily for 7 to 10 days, or intramuscular **procaine penicillin** may be administered. More severe streptococcal infections should be treated with intravenous antibiotics (such as **ceftriaxone** 50 to 100 mg/kg as a single dose). Mild to moderate staphylococcal infections may be treated orally with **dicloxacillin,** 250 to 500 mg four times daily.
- In penicillin-allergic patients, oral or parenteral **clindamycin** may be used. Alternatively, a first-generation cephalosporin such as **cefazolin** (1 to 2 g intravenously every 6 to 8 hours) may be used cautiously for patients who have not experienced immediate or anaphylactic penicillin reactions and are penicillin skin test negative. In mild cases where an oral cephalosporin can be used, **cefadroxil,** 500 mg twice daily, or **cephalexin,** 250 to 500 mg four times daily, is recommended. **Cefaclor, cefprozil**, and **cefpodoxime proxetil** are effective but more expensive.
- Alternative agents for documented infections with resistant gram-positive bacteria such as methicillin-resistant staphylococci and vancomycin-resistant enterococci include linezolid, quinupristin/dalfopristin, and daptomycin. In severe cases in which cephalosporins cannot be used because of documented methicillin resistance or severe allergic reactions to β-lactam antibiotics, intravenous **vancomycin** should be administered.
- For cellulitis caused by gram-negative bacilli or a mixture of microorganisms, immediate antimicrobial chemotherapy as determined by Gram stain is essential, along with appropriate surgical excision of necrotic tissue and drainage. Gram-negative cellulites may be treated appropriately with an aminoglycoside or first- or second-generation cephalosporin. If gram-positive aerobic bacteria

TABLE 45–2. Initial Treatment Regimens for Cellulitis Caused by Various Pathogens

Antibiotic	Adult Dose and Route	Pediatric Dose and Route
Staphylococcal or Unknown Gram-Positive Infection		
Mild infection	Dicloxacillin 0.25–0.5 g orally every 6 h[a,b]	Dicloxacillin 25–50 mg/kg/day orally in 4 divided doses[a,b]
Moderate to severe infection	Nafcillin or oxacillin 1–2 g IV every 4–6 h[a,b]	Nafcillin or oxacillin 150–200 mg/kg/day (not to exceed 12 g/24 h) IV in 4–6 equally divided doses[a,b]
Streptococcal (Documented)		
Mild infection	Penicillin VK 0.5 g orally every 6 h[a] or procaine penicillin G 600,000 units IM every 8–12 h[a]	Penicillin VK 125–250 mg orally every 6–8 h, or procaine penicillin G 25,000–50,000 units/kg (not to exceed 600,000 units) IM every 8–12 h[a]
Moderate to severe infection	Aqueous penicillin G 1–2 million units IV every 4–6 h[a,c]	Aqueous penicillin G 100,000–200,000 units/kg/day IV in four divided doses[a]
Gram-Negative Bacilli		
Mild infection	Cefaclor 0.5 g orally every 8 h[d] or cefuroxime axetil 0.5 g orally every 12 h[d]	Cefaclor 20–40 mg/kg/day (not to exceed 1 g) orally in 3 divided doses or cefuroxime axetil 0.125–0.25 g (tablets) orally every 12 h
Moderate to severe infection	Aminoglycoside[e] or IV cephalosporin (first- or second-generation depending on severity of infection or susceptibility pattern)[d]	Aminoglycoside[e] or intravenous cephalosporin (first- or second-generation depending on severity of infection or susceptibility pattern)
Polymicrobic Infection without Anaerobes		
	Aminoglycoside[e] + penicillin G 1–2 million units every 4–6 h or a semisynthetic penicillin (nafcillin 1–2 g every 4–6 h) depending on isolation of staphylococci or streptococci[b]	Aminoglycoside[e] + penicillin G 100,000 to 200,000 units/kg/day IV in 4 divided doses or a semisynthetic penicillin (nafcillin 150–200 mg/kg/day [not to exceed 12 g/24 h] IV in 4–6 equally divided doses) depending on isolation of staphylococci or streptococci[b]

Continued

TABLE 45-2. (Continued)

Antibiotic	Adult Dose and Route	Pediatric Dose and Route
Polymicrobic Infection with Anaerobes		
Mild infection	Amoxicillin/clavulanate 0.875 g orally every 12 h	Amoxicillin/clavulanic acid 20 mg/kg/day orally in 3 divided doses
	or	
	A fluoroquinolone (ciprofloxacin 0.4 g orally every 12 h or levofloxacin 0.5–0.75 g orally every 24 h) plus clindamycin 0.3–0.6 g orally every 8 h or metronidazole 0.5 g orally every 8 h	
Moderate to severe infection	Aminoglycoside[e,f] + clindamycin 0.6–0.9 g IV every 8 h or metronidazole 0.5 g IV every 8 h	Aminoglycoside[e] plus clindamycin 15 mg/kg/day IV in 3 divided doses or metronidazole 30–50 mg/kg/day IV in 3 divided doses
	or	
	Monotherapy with second- or third-generation cephalosporin (cefoxitin 1–2 g IV every 6 h or ceftizoxime 1–2 g IV every 8 h)	
	or	
	Monotherapy with imipenem 0.5 g IV every 6–8 h, meropenem 1 g IV every 8 h, or extended-spectrum penicillins with a β-lactamase inhibitor (piperacillin/tazobactam 4.5 g IV every 6 h)	

[a]For penicillin-allergic patients, use clindamycin 150–300 mg orally every 6–8 h (pediatric dosing: 10–30 mg/kg/day in 3–4 divided doses).

[b]For methicillin-resistant staphylococci, use vancomycin 0.5–1 g every 6–12 h (pediatric dosing 40 mg/kg/day in divided doses) with dosage adjustments made for renal dysfunction.

[c]For type II necrotizing fasciitis, use clindamycin 0.6–0.9 g IV every 8 h (in children, clindamycin 15 mg/kg/day IV in 3 divided doses) should be added.

[d]For penicillin-allergic adults, use a fluoroquinolone (ciprofloxacin 0.5–0.75 g orally every 12 h or 0.4 g IV every 12 h; levofloxacin 0.5–0.75 g orally or IV every 24 h; gatifloxacin 0.4 g orally or IV every 24 h; or moxifloxacin 0.4 g orally or IV every 24 h).

[e]Gentamicin or tobramycin, 2 mg/kg loading dose, then maintenance dose determined by serum concentrations.

[f]A fluoroquinolone or aztreonam 1 g IV every 6 h may be used in place of the aminoglycoside in patients with severe renal dysfunction or other relative contraindications to aminoglycoside use.

are also present, penicillin G or a semisynthetic penicillin should be added to the regimen. Therapy should be 10 to 14 days in duration.

▶ ERYSIPELAS

- Erysipelas (Saint Anthony's fire) is an infection of the superficial layers of the skin and cutaneous lymphatics. The infection is almost always caused by β-hemolytic streptococci, with *S. pyogenes* (group A streptococci) responsible for most infections.
- Erysipelas manifests as a bright red, edematous, indurated, and painful lesion sharply circumscribed by an elevated border. Leukocytosis is common. Patients often experience flulike symptoms (fever and malaise) prior to the appearance of the lesions.
- The lower extremities are the most common sites for erysipelas.
- Mild to moderate cases of erysipelas in adults are treated with **procaine penicillin G**, 600,000 units intramuscularly twice daily, or **penicillin VK**, 250 to 500 mg orally four times daily, for 7 to 10 days.
- Penicillin-allergic patients can be treated with clindamycin, 150 to 300 mg orally every 6 to 8 hours (10 to 30 mg/kg/day in three to four divided doses VIII ◀ for children). For more serious infections, aqueous penicillin G, 2 to 8 million units daily, should be administered intravenously.

▶ IMPETIGO

Impetigo is a superficial skin infection that is seen most commonly in children. It is highly communicable and spreads through close contact. Most cases are caused by *S. pyogenes*, but *S. aureus* either alone or in combination with *S. pyogenes* has emerged as a principal cause of impetigo.

CLINICAL PRESENTATION

- Exposed skin, especially the face, is the most common site for impetigo.
- Pruritus is common, and scratching of the lesions may further spread infection through excoriation of the skin.
- Other systemic signs of infection are minimal.
- Weakness, fever, and diarrhea are sometimes seen with bullous impetigo.
- Nonbullous impetigo manifests initially as small, fluid-filled vesicles. These lesions rapidly develop into pus-filled blisters that readily rupture. Purulent discharge from the lesions dries to form golden yellow crusts that are characteristic of impetigo.
- In the bullous form of impetigo, the lesions begin as vesicles and turn into bullae containing clear yellow fluid. Bullae soon rupture, forming thin, light brown crusts.
- Regional lymph nodes may be enlarged.

TREATMENT

- Penicillinase-resistant penicillins (such as **dicloxacillin** 12.5 mg/kg orally daily in for divided doses for children) are the agents of first choice because of the increased isolation of *S. aureus*. First-generation cephalosporins (such as cephalexin 25 to 50 mg/kg orally daily in two divided doses for children) are also effective. **Penicillin** may be used for impetigo caused by *S. pyogenes*. It may be administered as either a single intramuscular dose of benzathine

penicillin G (300,000 to 600,000 units in children, 1.2 million units in adults) or as oral penicillin VK given for 7 to 10 days.
- Penicillin-allergic patients can be treated with oral **clindamycin** (adults 150 to 300 mg orally every 6 to 8 hours; children 10 to 30 mg/kg per day in three to four divided doses)
- The duration of therapy is 7 to 10 days.
- **Mupirocin ointment** is as also effective.

▶ INFECTED PRESSURE ULCERS

- Many factors are thought to predispose patients to the formation of pressure ulcers: paralysis, paresis, immobilization, malnutrition, anemia, infection, and advanced age. Four factors thought to be most critical to their formation are pressure, shearing forces, friction, and moisture; however, there is still debate as to the exact pathophysiology of pressure sore formation. The areas of highest pressure are generated over the bony prominences.
- Pressure sores are routinely colonized by a wide variety of microorganisms; gram-negative aerobes and anaerobes are most often associated with the infections.
- Most pressure sores are colonized by bacteria; however, bacteria frequently infect healthy tissue. A large variety of aerobic gram-positive and gram-negative bacteria, as well as anaerobes, are frequently isolated.

CLINICAL PRESENTATION

- More than 95% of all pressure sores are located on the lower part of the body.
- Pressure sores can be classified in stages (Table 45–3).
- Pressure sores vary greatly in their severity, ranging from an abrasion to large lesions that can penetrate into the deep fascia involving both bone and muscle.
- Without treatment, an initial small localized area of ulceration can rapidly progress to 5 to 6 cm within days.

PREVENTION AND TREATMENT

- Prevention is the single most important aspect in the management of pressure sores. Friction and shearing forces can be minimized by proper positioning. Skin care and prevention of soilage are important, with the intent being to keep the surface relatively free from moisture. Relief of pressure (even for 5 minutes once every 2 hours) is probably the single most important factor in preventing pressure sore formation.

TABLE 45–3. Pressure Sore Classification

Stage 1	Pressure sore is generally reversible, is limited to the epidermis, and resembles an abrasion. It is best described as an irregularly shaped area of soft tissue swelling with induration and heat.
Stage 2	A stage 2 sore may also, be reversible; it extends through the dermis to the subcutaneous fat along with extensive undermining.
Stage 3	In this instance, the sore or ulcer extends further into subcutaneous fat along with extensive undermining.
Stage 4	The sore or ulcer is characterized by penetration into deep fascia involving both muscle and bone.

Note: Stage 3 and 4 lesions are unlikely to resolve on their own and often require surgical intervention.

MEDICAL MANAGEMENT

- Medical management is generally indicated for lesions that are of moderate size and of relatively shallow depth (stage 1 or 2 lesions) and are not located over a bony prominence.
- The main factors to be considered for successful topical therapy (local care) are the relief of pressure, debridement of necrotic tissue, wound cleansing, dressing selection, and prevention and treatment of infection.

Debridement

- Debridement can be accomplished by surgical or mechanical means (wet-to-dry dressing changes). Other effective therapies are hydrotherapy, wound irrigation, and dextranomers. Pressure sores should be cleaned with normal saline.
- A number of agents have been used to disinfect pressure sores (e.g., **acetic acid, sodium hypochlorite, hydrogen peroxide, mupirocin, bacitracin**) as well as other types of open wounds; however, these agents should be avoided as they impair healing.
- A short, 2-week trial of topical antibiotic (**silver sulfadiazine** or **triple antibiotic**) is recommended for a clean ulcer that is not healing or is producing a moderate amount of exudate despite appropriate care.

▶ INFECTED BITE WOUNDS

DOG BITES

- Patients at risk of acquiring an infection after a bite have had a puncture wound, have not sought medical attention within 12 hours of injury, and are older than 50 years of age.
- The infected dog bite is usually characterized by a localized cellulitis and pain at the site of injury. The cellulitis usually spreads proximally from the initial site of injury. If *Pasteurella multocida* is present, a rapidly progressing cellulitis with a gray malodorous discharge may be encountered.
- Most infections are polymicrobial, and the most frequently isolated organisms are *Pasteurella* spp., streptococci, staphylococci, *Moraxella,* and *Neisseria.* The most common anaerobes are *Fusobacterium* spp., *Bacteroides* spp., *Porphyromonas*, and *Prevotella.*
- Wounds should be thoroughly irrigated with a sterile saline solution. Proper irrigation will reduce the bacterial count in the wound.
- The role of antimicrobials for noninfected dog bite wounds remains controversial because only 20% of wounds become infected. Antibiotic recommendations for empiric treatment include a 3- to 5-day course of (1) a β-lactam antibiotic with β-lactamase inhibitor, (2) a second-generation cephalosprin with anaerobic activity, or (3) **penicillin** in combination with a first-generation **cephalosporin** or **clindamycin**.
- **Tetracycline** or **trimethoprim-sulfamethoxazole** is recommended as an alternative form of therapy for patients allergic to penicillins. **Erythromycin** may be considered an alternative for tetracycline in growing children or pregnant women.
- Prophylactic therapy should be given for 3 to 5 days. In addition to irrigation and antibiotics, when indicated, the injured area should be immobilized and elevated.
- Infections developing within the first 24 hours of a bite are most often caused by *P. multocida* and should be treated with **penicillin VK** or **amoxicillin/**

clavulanic acid (tetracycline is an alternative for nonpregnant adult penicillin-allergic patients). Treatment should be given for 10 to 14 days.

- For infections developing more than 36 to 48 hours after the bite, the risk of *P. multocida* being involved dramatically decreases in likelihood. Therapy in this instance includes a penicillinase-resistant penicillin (e.g., **dicloxacillin**) or a cephalosporin (e.g., **cefuroxime axetil**) and should be given for a full 10 to 14 days.
- If the immunization history of a patient with anything other than a clean minor wound is not known, tetanus/diphtheria toxoids (Td) and tetanus immune globulin (TIg) should be administered.
- If a patient has been exposed to rabies, the treatment objectives consist of thorough irrigation of the wound, tetanus prophylaxis, antibiotic prophylaxis (if indicated), and immunization. Postexposure prophylaxis immunization consists of both passive antibody administration and vaccine administration.

CAT BITES

- Approximately 30% to 50% of cat bites become infected. These infections are frequently caused by *P. multocida,* which has been isolated in the oropharynx of 50% to 70% of healthy cats.
- The management of cat bites is similar to that discussed for dog bites. Antibiotic therapy with **penicillin** is the mainstay, and therapy is as described for dog bites.

HUMAN BITES

- Infections can occur in up to 50% of patients with human bites.
- Infections caused by these injuries are most often caused by the normal oral flora, which includes both aerobic and anaerobic microorganisms. The most frequent aerobic organisms are streptococcal species, *S. aureus, Klebsiella pneumoniae*, and *Eikenella corrodens*. The most common anaerobic organisms are *Prevotella, Fusobacterium, Veillonella*, and *Peptostreptococcus* species. Anaerobic microorganisms have been isolated in the range of 40% of human bites and 55% of clenched-fist injuries.
- Management of bite wounds consists of aggressive irrigation, surgical debridement, and immobilization of the affected area. Primary closure for human bites is not generally recommended. If damage to a bone or joint is suspected, radiographic evaluation should be undertaken. Tetanus toxoid and antitoxin may be indicated.
- If the biter is HIV positive, the victim should have a baseline HIV status determined and then repeated in 3 and 6 months. The bite should be thoroughly irrigated with a virucidal agent such as povidone-iodine. Victims may be offered antiretroviral chemoprophylaxis.
- Patients with noninfected bite injuries should be given prophylactic antibiotic therapy. Initial therapy should consist of a penicillinase-resistant penicillin (e.g., **dicloxacillin**) in combination with **penicillin.** Prophylactic therapy should be given for 3 to 5 days as for dog bites. A first-generation cephalosporin or macrolide is not recommended, as the sensitivity to *E. corrodens* is variable.
- For infected bite wounds, penicillin and a **penicillinase-resistant penicillin** or **amoxicillin/clavulanic acid** should be empirically started and changed pending the culture results. Duration of therapy for infected bite injuries should be 7 to 14 days.

BACTERIAL DIABETIC FOOT INFECTIONS

- Three key factors are involved in the causation of diabetic foot problems: neuropathy, ischemia, and immunologic defects. Any of these disorders can occur in isolation; however, they frequently occur together.
- There are three major types of diabetic foot infections: deep abscesses, cellulitis of the dorsum, and mal perforans ulcers of the sole of the foot. Osteomyelitis may occur in 30% to 40% of infections.
- Diabetic foot infections are typically polymicrobic (an average of 4.1 to 5.8 isolates per culture). Staphylococci (especially *S. aureus*)and streptococci are the most common pathogens, although gram-negative bacilli and anaerobes are common. Other common isolates include *Escherichia coli, Klebsiella* spp., *Proteus* spp., *P. aeruginosa, B. fragilis*, and *Peptostreptococcus* spp.

TREATMENT

- The goal of therapy is preservation of as much normal limb function as possible while preventing infectious complications. Most infections can be successfully treated on an outpatient basis with wound care and antibiotics.
- Diabetic control should be maximized to ensure optimal healing.
- The patient should initially be restricted to bedrest, leg elevation, and control of edema, if present.
- After healing of the infected ulcer has occurred, a program for prevention should be designed.
- **Amoxicillin/clavulanate** is the agent of choice for oral outpatient treatment; however, this agent does not cover *P. aeruginosa*. Fluoroquinolones with metronidazole or clindamycin are reasonable alternatives.
- Serious polymicrobic infections may be treated with agents used for anaerobic cellulitis (Table 45–2).
- Monotherapy with broad-spectrum parenteral antimicrobials, along with appropriate medical and/or surgical management, is often effective in treating moderate to severe infections (including those in which osteomyelitis is present).
- Vancomycin is used frequently in severe infections with gram-positive pathogens. With increasing staphylococcal resistance, linezolid, quinupristin/dalfopristin, and daptomycin are alternatives.
- Treatment of soft tissue infections in diabetic patients should generally be at least 10 to 14 days in duration, and up to 21 days in severe infections. However, in cases of underlying osteomyelitis, treatment should continue for 6 to 12 weeks.

See Chapter 108, Skin and Soft Tissue Infections, authored by Susan L. Pendland, Douglas N. Fish, and Larry H. Danzinger, for a more detailed discussion of this topic.

Chapter 46

▶ SURGICAL PROPHYLAXIS

▶ DEFINITION

- Antibiotics administered prior to contamination of previously uninfected tissues or fluids are considered prophylactic. The goal for prophylactic antibiotics is to prevent a surgical-site infection (SSI) from developing. The prevention and management of non-SSI postoperative infections, such as catheter-related urinary tract infections, occasionally require antibiotics, but prevention of non-SSI infections is not the goal of surgical prophylaxis.
- Presumptive antibiotic therapy is administered when an infection is suspected but not yet proven. Therapeutic antibiotics are required for established infection.
- SSIs are classified as either incisional (such as cellulites of the incision site) or involving an organ or space (such as with meningitis). Incisional SSIs may be superficial (skin or subcutaneous tissue) or deep (fascial and muscle layers). Both types, by definition, occur by postoperative day 30. This period extends to 1 year in the case of deep infection associated with prosthesis implantation.

▶ RISK FACTORS FOR SURGICAL WOUND INFECTION

The traditional classification system developed by the National Research Council (NRC) stratifying surgical procedures by infection risk is reproduced in Table 46–1. The NRC wound classification for a specific procedure is determined intraoperatively.

INDIVIDUALIZING RISK FOR SURGICAL WOUND INFECTION

- The Study on the Efficacy of Nosocomial Infection Control (SENIC) analyzed more than 100,000 surgery cases and identified abdominal operations, operations lasting more than 2 hours, contaminated or dirty procedures, and more than three underlying medical diagnoses as factors associated with an increased incidence of SSI. When the NRC classification described in Table 46–1 was stratified by the number of SENIC risk factors present, the infection rates varied by as much as a factor of 15 within the same operative category.
- The SENIC risk assessment technique has been modified to include the American Society of Anesthesiologists (ASA) preoperative assessment score (Table 46–2). An ASA score of 3 or above was associated with increased SSI risk.

▶ MICROBIOLOGY

- Bacteria involved in SSI are either acquired from the patient's normal flora (endogenous) or from contamination during the surgical procedure (exogenous).
- Loss of protective flora via antibiotics can upset the balance and allow pathogenic bacteria to proliferate and increase infectious risk.
- Normal flora can become pathogenic when translocated to a normally sterile tissue site or fluid during surgical procedures.
- According to the National Nosocomial Infections Surveillance System (NNIS), the five most common pathogens encountered in surgical wounds are *Staphylococcus aureus*, coagulase-negative staphylococci, enterococci, *Escherichia coli*, and *Pseudomonas aeruginosa*.

TABLE 46–1. NRC[a] Wound Classification, Risk of SSI[b], and Indication for Antibiotics

Classification	SWI Rate (%)		Criteria	Antibiotics
	Preoperative Antibiotics	No Preoperative Antibiotics		
Clean	5.1	0.8	No acute inflammation or transection of gastrointestinal, oropharyngeal, genitourinary, biliary, or respiratory tracts. Elective case, no technique break.	Not indicated unless high-risk procedure[c]
Clean-contaminated	10.1	1.3	Controlled opening of aforementioned tracts with minimal spillage/minor technique break. Clean procedures performed emergently or with major technique breaks.	Prophylactic antibiotics indicated
Contaminated	21.9	10.2	Acute, nonpurulent inflammation present. Major spillage/technique break during clean-contaminated procedure.	Prophylactic antibiotics indicated
Dirty	N/A	N/A	Obvious preexisting infection present (abscess, pus, or necrotic tissue present).	Therapeutic antibiotics required

[a]National Research Council.
[b]surgical-site infection.
[c]High-risk procedures include implantation of prosthetic materials and other procedures where surgical-site infection is associated with high morbidity (see text).

TABLE 46–2. American Society of Anesthesiologists Physical Status Classification

Class	Description
1	Normal healthy patient
2	Mild systemic disease
3	Severe systemic disease that is not incapacitating
4	Incapacitating systemic disease that is a constant threat to life
5	Not expected to survive 24 h with or without operation

- Impaired host defenses, vascular occlusive states, traumatized tissues, or presence of a foreign body greatly decrease the number of bacteria required to cause a SSI.

▶ ANTIBIOTIC ISSUES

SCHEDULING ANTIBIOTIC ADMINISTRATION

The following principles must be considered when providing antimicrobial surgical prophylaxis.

- Antimicrobials should be delivered to the targeted tissue site prior to the initial incision. They should be administered with anesthesia, just prior to initial incision.
- Bactericidal antibiotic tissue concentrations should be maintained throughout the surgical procedure.

Strategies to ensure appropriate antimicrobial prophylaxis use are described in Table 46–3.

ANTIMICROBIAL SELECTION

- The choice of the prophylactic antimicrobial depends on the type of surgical procedure, most likely pathogenic organisms, safety and efficacy of the antimicrobial, track record for success based on published literature, and costs.

TABLE 46–3. Strategies for Implementing an Institutional Program to Ensure the Appropriate Use of Antimicrobial Prophylaxis in Surgery

1. Educate
Develop an educational program that enforces the importance and rationale of timely antimicrobial prophylaxis. Make this educational program available to all health care practitioners involved in the patient's care.

2. Standardize the Ordering Process
Establish a protocol (e.g., a preprinted order sheet) that standardizes antibiotic choice according to current published evidence, formulary availability, institutional resistance patterns, and cost.

3. Standardize the Delivery and Administration Process
Employ as system that ensures that antibiotics are prepared and delivered to the holding area in a timely fashion. Standardize the administration time to less than 1 hour preoperatively. Designate responsibility and accountability for antibiotic administration.
Provide visible reminders to prescribe or administer prophylactic antibiotics (e.g., checklists).
Develop a system to remind surgeons or nurses to readminister antibiotics intraoperatively during long procedures.

4. Provide Feedback
Follow up with regular reports of compliance and infection rates.

VIII

- Typically, gram-positive coverage is included in the choice of surgical prophylaxis, because organisms such as *S. aureus* and *Staphylococcus epidermidis* are common skin flora.
- Parenteral antibiotic administration is favored because of its reliability in achieving suitable tissue concentrations.
- First-generation cephalosporins (particularly cefazolin) are the preferred choice, particularly for clean surgical procedures.
- Vancomycin may be considered for prophylactic therapy in surgical procedures involving implantation of a prosthetic device in which the rate of methicillin resistant staphylococcus aureus (MRSA) is high.
- If the risk of MRSA is low and a β-lactam hypersensitivity exists, clindamycin can be used instead of cefazolin in order to limit vancomycin use.
- In cases where broader gram-negative and anaerobic coverage is desired, the antianaerobic cephalosporins such as cefoxitin, or cefotetan, are appropriate.

▶ RECOMMENDATIONS FOR SPECIFIC TYPES OF SURGERY

Specific recommendations are summarized in Table 46–4.

VIII ◀

GASTRODUODENAL SURGERY

- The risk of infection rises with conditions that increase gastric pH and subsequent bacterial overgrowth, such as obstruction, hemorrhage, malignancy, or acid-suppression therapy (clean-contaminated).
- A single dose of intravenous (IV) **cefazolin** will provide adequate prophylaxis for most cases.
- Postoperative therapeutic antibiotics may be indicated if perforation is detected during surgery, depending on whether an established infection is present.

BILIARY TRACT SURGERY

- Antibiotic prophylaxis has been proven beneficial for surgery involving the biliary tract.
- Most frequently encountered organisms include *E. coli, Klebsiella*, and enterococci. Single-dose prophylaxis with **cefazolin** is currently recommended.
- For low-risk patients undergoing elective laparoscopic cholecystectomy, antibiotic prophylaxis is of no benefit and is not recommended.
- Antibiotic prophylaxis is not currently recommended prior to endoscopic retrograde cholangiopancreatography.
- Some surgeons use presumptive antibiotics for cases of acute cholecystitis or cholangitis and defer surgery until the patient is afebrile, in an attempt to decrease infection rates further, but this practice is controversial.
- Detection of an active infection during surgery (gangrenous gallbladder, suppurative cholangitis) is an indication for therapeutic postoperative antibiotics.

COLORECTAL SURGERY

- Anaerobes and gram-negative aerobes predominate in SSIs (see Table 46–4), although gram-positive aerobes are also important. Therefore, the risk of SSI in the absence of an adequate prophylactic regimen is substantial.
- Reducing bacteria load with a thorough bowel preparation regimen (4 L of polyethylene glycol solution administered orally the day before surgery) is controversial, even though it is used by most surgeons.

TABLE 46–4. Most Likely Pathogens and Specific Recommendations for Surgical Prophylaxis

Type of Operation	Likely Pathogens	Recommended Prophylaxis Regimen[a]	Comments
Gastroduodenal	Enteric gram-negative bacilli, gram-positive cocci, oral anaerobes	Cefazolin 1 g x 1	High-risk patients only (obstruction, hemorrhage, malignancy, acid suppression therapy, morbid obesity)
Biliary tract	Enteric gram-negative bacilli, anaerobes	Cefazolin 1 g × 1 for high-risk patients Laparoscopic: None	High-risk patients only (acute cholecystitis, common duct stones, previous biliary surgery, jaundice, age >60 y, obesity, diabetes mellitus)
Colorectal	Enteric gram-negative bacilli, anaerobes	PO: Neomycin 1 g + erythromycin base 1 g at 1 PM, 2 PM, and 11 PM 1 day preop plus mechanical bowel prep. IV: Cefoxitin or cefotetan 1 g × 1	Benefits of oral plus IV is controversial except for colostomy reversal and rectal resection
Appendectomy	Enteric gram-negative bacilli, anaerobes	Cefoxitin or cefotetan 1 g × 1	A second intraoperative dose of cefoxitin may be required if procedure lasts longer than 3 h
Urologic	E. coli	Cefazolin 1 g × 1	Generally not recommended in patients with sterile preoperative urine cultures
Cesarean section	Enteric gram-negative bacilli, anaerobes, group B streptococci, enterococci	Cefazolin 2 g × 1	Give after cord is clamped
Hysterectomy	Enteric gram-negative bacilli, anaerobes, group B streptococci, enterococci	Vaginal: Cefazolin 1 g × 1 Abdominal: Cefotetan 1 g × 1 or Cefazolin 1 g × 1	Antibiotic prophylaxis should not exceed 24 h

Procedure	Organisms	Antibiotic regimen	Comments
Head and neck	*S. aureus*, streptococci oral anaerobes	Cefazolin 2 g or clindamycin 600 mg at induction and every 8h × 2 more doses	Addition of gentamicin to clindamycin is controversial
Cardiothoracic	*S. aureus*, *S. epidermidis*, *Corynebacterium*, enteric gram-negative bacilli	Cefazolin 1 g every 8h × 48 h	Second-generation cephalosporins also have been advocated In areas with high prevalence of *S. aureus* resistance, vancomycin should be considered
Vascular	*S. aureus*, *S. epidermidis*, enteric gram-negative bacilli	Cefazolin 1 g at induction and every 8h × 2 more doses	Abdominal and lower extremities have the highest infection rates
Orthopedic	*S. aureus*, *S. epidermidis*	Joint replacement: Cefazolin 1 g × 1 preop, then every 8h × 2 more doses Hip fracture repair: Same as above, except continue for 48 h	Open fractures assumed contaminated with gram-negative bacilli; aminoglycosides often used
Neurosurgery	*S. aureus*, *S. epidermidis*	CSF shunt procedures: Cefazolin 1 g × 1 or ceftriaxone 2 g × 1 Craniotomy: Cefazolin 1 g × 1 or cefotaxime 1 g × 1 or trimethoprim-sulfamethoxazole (160/800) IV × 1	No agents have been shown better than cefazolin in randomized control comparative trials.

[a]One-time doses are optimally infused at induction of anesthesia except as noted. Repeat doses may be required for long procedures.

- The combination of 1 g of **neomycin** and 1 g of **erythromycin base** given orally 19, 18, and 9 hours preoperatively is the most commonly used oral regimen in the United States.
- Whether perioperative parenteral antibiotics, in addition to the standard preoperative oral antibiotic regimen, will lower SSI rates further is controversial.
- Postoperative antibiotics are unnecessary in the absence of any untoward events or findings during surgery.

APPENDECTOMY

- A cephalosporin with antianaerobic activity such as **cefoxitin** or **cefotetan** is currently recommended as a first-line agent. Cefotetan may be superior for longer operations because of its longer duration of action.
- Single-dose therapy with cefotetan is adequate. Intraoperative dosing of cefoxitin may be required if the procedure extends beyond 3 hours.
- Established intra-abdominal infections require appropriate therapeutic postoperative antibiotics.

UROLOGIC PROCEDURES

- ►VIII As long as the urine is sterile preoperatively, the risk of SSI after urologic procedures is low and the benefit of prophylactic antibiotics in this setting is controversial. *E. coli* is the most frequently encountered organism.
- Antibiotic prophylaxis is warranted in high-risk patients (e.g., prolonged indwelling catheterization, positive urine cultures, and neutropenia) undergoing transurethral, perineal, or suprapubic resection of the prostate, resection of bladder tumors, or cystoscopy.
- Specific recommendations are listed in Table 46–4.
- Urologic procedures requiring an abdominal approach such as a nephrectomy or cystectomy require prophylaxis appropriate for a clean-contaminated abdominal procedure.

CESAREAN SECTION

- Antibiotics are efficacious to prevent SSIs for women undergoing cesarean section regardless of underlying risk factors.
- **Cefazolin,** 2 g IV, remains the drug of choice. Providing a broader spectrum by using cefoxitin against anaerobes or piperacillin for better coverage against *Pseudomonas* or enterococci, for example, does not lower postoperative infection rates any further in comparative studies.
- Antibiotics should be administered just after the umbilical cord is clamped, avoiding exposure of the infant to the drug.

HYSTERECTOMY

- Vaginal hysterectomies are associated with a high rate of postoperative infection when performed without the benefit of prophylactic antibiotics.
- **Cefazolin** is the drug of choice. Single-dose therapy should be adequate, but most reports used a 24-hour regimen.
- Abdominal hysterectomy SSI rates are correspondingly lower than vaginal hysterectomy rates. However, prophylactic antibiotics are still recommended regardless of underlying risk factors.
- Both cefazolin and antianaerobic cephalosporins (e.g., **cefoxitin, cefotetan**) have been studied extensively. Single-dose cefotetan is superior to single-dose cefazolin.
- The antibiotic course should not exceed 24 hours in duration.

HEAD AND NECK SURGERY

- Use of prophylactic antibiotics during head and neck surgery depends on the procedure type. Clean procedures, such as parotidectomy or a simple tooth extraction, are associated with low rates of SSI.
- Head and neck procedures involving an incision through a mucosal layer carry a high risk of SSI.
- Specific recommendations for prophylaxis are listed in Table 46–4.
- While typical doses of **cefazolin** are ineffective for anaerobic infections, the recommended 2-g dose produces concentrations high enough to be inhibitory to these organisms. A 24-hour duration has been used in most studies, but single-dose therapy may also be effective.
- For most head and neck cancer sections, 24 hours of clindamycin is appropriate.

CARDIAC SURGERY

- Although most cardiac surgeries are technically clean procedures, prophylactic antibiotics have been shown to lower rates of SSI.
- The usual pathogens are skin flora (see Table 46–4) and, rarely, gram-negative enteric organisms. VIII
- Risk factors for developing an SSI after cardiac surgery include obesity, renal insufficiency, connective tissue disease, reexploration for bleeding, and poorly timed administration of antibiotics.
- **Cefazolin** has been extensively studied and is currently considered the drug of choice. Patients weighing 80 kg should receive 2 g cefazolin rather than 1 g. Doses should be administered no earlier than 60 minutes before the first incision and no later than the beginning of induction of anesthesia.
- Extending antibiotic administration beyond 48 hours does not lower SSI rates. Single-dose cefazolin therapy may be sufficient.
- It may be necessary to use **vancomycin** in hospitals with a high incidence of SSI with MRSA or when sternal wounds are to be explored for possible mediastinitis.

NONCARDIAC VASCULAR SURGERY

- Prophylactic antibiotics are beneficial, especially in procedures involving the abdominal aorta and the lower extremities.
- Twenty-four hours of prophylaxis with IV **cefazolin** is adequate. For patients with β-lactam allergy, 24 hours of oral ciprofloxacin is effective.

ORTHOPEDIC SURGERY

- Prophylactic antibiotics are beneficial in cases involving implantation of prosthetic material (pins, plates, artificial joints).
- The most likely pathogens mirror those of other clean procedures and include staphylococci and, infrequently, gram-negative aerobes.
- **Cefazolin** is the best-studied antibiotic and is thus the drug of choice. For hip fracture repairs and joint replacements, it should be administered for 24 hours.

NEUROSURGERY

- The use of prophylactic antibiotics in neurosurgery is controversial.
- Single doses of **cefazolin** or, where required, **vancomycin** appear to lower SSI risk after craniotomy.

MINIMALLY INVASIVE AND LAPAROSCOPIC SURGERY

The role of prophylactic antimicrobials depends on the type of procedure performed and preexisting risk factors for infection. There are insufficient clinical trials to provide general recommendations.

See Chapter 121, Antimicrobial Prophylaxis in Surgery, authored by Salmaan Kanji and John W. Devlin, for a more detailed discussion of this topic.

◄ VIII

Chapter 47

▶ TUBERCULOSIS

- Tuberculosis (TB) is a communicable infectious disease caused by *Mycobacterium tuberculosis*. It can produce silent, latent infection as well as progressive, active disease.
- Globally, 2 billion people are infected and 2 to 3 million people die from tuberculosis each year.
- *M. tuberculosis* is transmitted from person to person by coughing or sneezing. Close contacts of TB patients are most likely to become infected.
- Fifty-one percent of TB patients in the United States are foreign born, most often from Mexico, the Philippines, Vietnam, India, China, Haiti, or South Korea. In the United States, TB disproportionately affects ethnic minorities (blacks and Hispanics).
- HIV is the most important risk factor for active TB, especially among people 25 to 44 years of age. An HIV-infected individual with tuberculous infection is over 100-fold more likely to develop active disease than an HIV-seronegative patient.

▶ PATHOPHYSIOLOGY

- Primary infection is initiated by the alveolar implantation of organisms in droplet nuclei that are small enough (1 to 5 mm) to escape the ciliary epithelial cells of the upper respiratory tract. Once implanted, the organisms multiply and are ingested by pulmonary macrophages, where they continue to multiply, albeit more slowly. Tissue necrosis and calcification of the originally infected site and regional lymph nodes may occur, resulting in the formation of a radiodense area referred to as a Ghon complex.
- Large numbers of activated macrophages surround the solid caseous (cheeselike) tuberculosis foci (the necrotic area) as a part of cell-mediated immunity. Delayed-type hypersensitivity also develops through activation and multiplication of T lymphocytes. Macrophages form granulomas to contain the organisms.
- Successful containment of *M. tuberculosis* requires activation of a subset of CD4 lymphocytes, referred to as Th-1 cells, which activate macrophages through secretion of interferon γ.
- Approximately 90% of patients who experience primary disease have no further clinical manifestations other than a positive skin test either alone or in combination with radiographic evidence of stable granulomas.
- Approximately 5% of patients (usually children, the elderly, or the immunocompromised) experience progressive primary disease at the site of the primary infection (usually the lower lobes) and frequently by dissemination, leading to meningitis and often to involvement of the upper lobes of the lung as well.
- Approximately 10% of patients develop reactivation disease, which arises subsequent to the hematogenous spread of the organism.
- Occasionally, a massive inoculum of organisms may be introduced into the bloodstream, causing widely disseminated disease and granuloma formation known as miliary tuberculosis.

TABLE 47–1. Clinical Presentation of Tuberculosis

Signs and Symptoms
- Patients typically present with weight loss, fatigue, a productive cough, fever, and night sweats
- Frank hemoptysis

Physical Examination
Dulness to chest percussion, rales, and increased vocal fremitus are observed frequently on ausculation

Laboratory Tests
Moderate elevations in the white blood cell (WBC) count with a lymphocyte predominance

Chest Radiograph
- Patchy or nodular infiltrates in the apical area of the upper lobes or the superior segment of the lower lobes
- Cavitation that may show air-fluid levels as the infection progresses

▶ CLINICAL PRESENTATION

NON–HIV-INFECTED PATIENTS

▶ VIII
- The clinical presentation of pulmonary TB is nonspecific, indicative only of a slowly evolving infectious process (Table 47–1).
- Physical examination is nonspecific, suggestive of progressive pulmonary disease.
- Clinical features associated with extrapulmonary TB vary depending on the organ system(s) involved but typically consist of slowly progressive compromise of organ function with low-grade fever and other constitutional symptoms.

HIV-INFECTED PATIENTS

- The clinical features of patients with HIV infection who develop TB may be markedly different from those classically observed in immunocompetent individuals. (In AIDS patients, TB is much more likely to present as the progressive primary form, to involve extrapulmonary sites, and to involve multiple lobes of the lung.
- TB in AIDS patients is less likely to involve cavitary disease, be associated with a positive skin test, or be associated with fever.

▶ DIAGNOSIS

TUBERCULIN SKIN TEST

- The most widely used screening method for tuberculous infection is the tuberculin skin test, which uses purified protein derivative (PPD). Populations most likely to benefit from skin testing are listed in Table 47–2.
- The Mantoux method of PPD administration, which is the most reliable technique, consists of the intradermal injection of PPD containing 5 TU. The test is read 48 to 72 hours after injection by measuring the diameter of the zone of induration.
- Some patients may exhibit a positive test after an initial negative test, and this is referred to as a booster effect.

SYMPTOMATIC DISEASE

Confirmatory diagnosis of a clinical suspicion of TB must be made via chest x-ray and microbiologic examination of sputum or other infected material to rule out active disease.

TABLE 47–2. Criteria for Tuberculin Positivity, by Risk Group

Reaction ≥5 mm of Induration	Reaction ≥10 mm of Induration	Reaction ≥15 mm of Induration
Human immunodeficiency virus (HIV)-positive persons	Recent immigrants (i.e., within the last 5 yr) from high prevalence countries	Persons with no risk factors for TB
Recent contacts of tuberculosis (TB) case patients	Injection drug users	
Fibrotic changes on chest radiograph consistent with prior TB	Residents and employees[a] of the following high-risk congregate settings: prisons and jails, nursing homes and other long-term facilities for the elderly, hospitals and other health care facilities, residential facilities for patients with acquired immunodeficiency syndrome (AIDS), and homeless shelters	
Patients with organ transplants and other immunosuppressed patients (receiving the equivalent of ≥15 mg/d of prednisone for 1 month or more)[b]	Mycobacteriology laboratory personnel	
	Persons with the following clinical conditions that place them at high risk: silicosis, diabetes mellitus, chronic renal failure, some hematologic disorders (e.g., leukemias and lymphomas), other specific malignancies (e.g., carcinoma of the head or neck and lung), weight loss of ≥10% of ideal body weight, gastrectomy, and jejunoileal bypass	
	Children younger than 4 yr of age or infants, children, and adolescents exposed to adults at high risk	

[a] For persons who are otherwise at low risk and are tested at the start of employment, a reaction of ≥15 mm induration is considered positive.
[b] Risk of TB in patients treated with corticosteroids increases with higher dose and longer duration.

Adapted from Centers for Disease Control and Prevention. Screening for tuberculosis and tuberculosis infection in high-risk populations: recommendations of the Advisory Council for the Elimination of Tuberculosis. MMWR 1995;44(No. RR-11):19–34.

▶ DESIRED OUTCOME

- Rapid identification of new cases of TB
- Isolation of the patient with active disease to prevent spread
- Collection of appropriate samples for smears and cultures
- Prompt resolution of signs and symptoms of disease after initiation of treatment
- Achievement of a noninfectious state, thus ending isolation
- Adherence to the treatment regimen
- Cure as quickly as possible (generally with at least 6 months of treatment)

▶ TREATMENT

GENERAL PRINCIPLES

- Drug treatment is the cornerstone of TB management. A minimum of two drugs, and generally three or four drugs, must be used simultaneously.
- Drug treatment is continued for at least 6 months and up to 2 to 3 years for some cases of multidrug-resistant TB (MDR-TB).
- Measures to assure adherence, such as directly observed therapy (DOT), are important.

PHARMACOLOGIC TREATMENT

Latent Infection

- As described in Table 47–3, Chemoprophylaxis should be initiated in patients to reduce the risk of progression to active disease.
- **Isoniazid** (INH), 300 mg daily in adults, is the primary treatment for latent TB in the United States, generally given for 9 months.
- Individuals likely to be noncompliant may be treated with a regimen of 15 mg/kg (to a maximum of 900 mg) twice weekly with observation.
- If the individual has been exposed to a patient with INH-resistant *M. tuberculosis* or a patient who has failed chemotherapy, chemoprophylaxis with **rifampin** (RIF) (for 4 months) should be initiated.
- Pregnant women, alcoholics, and patients with poor diets who are treated with isoniazid should receive pyridoxine, 10 to 50 mg daily, to reduce the incidence of central nervous system (CNS) effects or peripheral neuropathies.

Treating Active Disease

- Table 47–4 lists options for treatment of active TB. Doses of antituberculosis drugs are given in Table 47–5.
- Appropriate samples should be sent for culture and susceptibility testing prior to initiating therapy. Drug susceptibility testing should be done on the initial isolate for all patients with active TB, and this data should guide the initial drug selection for the new patient. If the source case cannot be identified, the drug resistance pattern in the area where the patient likely acquired TB should be used.
- If the patient is being evaluated for the retreatment of TB, it is imperative to know what drugs were used previously and for how long.
- Patients must complete 6 months or more of treatment. HIV-positive patients should be treated for an additional 3 months and at least 6 months from the time that they convert to smear and culture negativity. When isoniazid and rifampin cannot be used, treatment duration becomes 2 years or more, regardless of immune status.

VIII

TABLE 47–3. Recommended Drug Regimens for Treatment of Latent Tuberculosis (TB) Infection in Adults

Drug	Interval and Duration	Comments	Rating[a] (Evidence)[b]	
			HIV[−]	HIV[+]
Isoniazid	Daily for 9 months[c,d]	In human immunodeficiency virus (HIV)-infected patients, isoniazid may be administered concurrently with nucleoside reverse transcriptase inhibitors (NRTIs), protease inhibitors, or non-nucleoside reverse transcriptase inhibitors (NNRTIs)	A (II)	A (II)
	Twice weekly for 9 months[c,d]	Directly observed therapy (DOT) must be used with twice-weekly dosing	B (II)	B (II)
Isoniazid	Daily for 6 months[d]	Not indicated for HIV-infected persons, those with fibrotic lesions on chest radiographs, or children	B (I)	C (I)
	Twice weekly for 6 months[d]	DOT must be used with twice-weekly dosing	B (II)	C (I)
Rifampin	Daily for 4 months	For persons who cannot tolerate pyrazinamide	B (II)	B (III)
		For persons who are contacts of patients with isoniazid-resistant, rifampin-susceptible TB who cannot tolerate pyrazinamide		

[a]Strength of recommendation: A, preferred; B, acceptable alternative; C, offer when A and B cannot be given.

[b]Quality of evidence: I, randomized clinical trial data; II, data from clinical trials that are not randomized or were conducted in other populations; III, expert opinion.

[c]Recommended regimen for children younger than 18 yr of age.

[d]Recommended regimens for pregnant women. Some experts would use rifampin and pyrazinamide for 2 months as an alternative regimen in HIV-infected pregnant women, although pyrazinamide should be avoided during the first trimester.

Adapted from Centers for Disease Control and Prevention. Targeted tuberculin testing and treatment of latent tuberculosis infection. MMWR 2000;49(RR-6):31.

TABLE 47-4. Drug Regimens for Culture-Positive Pulmonary Tuberculosis Caused by Drug-Susceptible Organisms

	Initial Phase			Continuation Phase			Range of Total Doses (Minimal Duration)	Rating[a] [Evidence][b]	
Regimen	Drugs	Interval and Doses[c] (Minimal Duration)	Regimen	Drugs	Interval and Doses[c,d] (Minimal Duration)			HIV−	HIV+
1	INH RIF PZA EMB	7 days/wk for 56 doses (8 wk) or 5 days/wk for 40 doses (8 wk)[c]	1a	INH/RIF	7 days/wk for 126 doses (18 wk) or 5 days/wk for 90 doses (18 wk)[c]		182–130 (26 wk)	A (I)	A (II)
			1b	INH/RIF	Twice weekly for 36 doses (18 wk)		92–76 (26 wk)	A (I)	A (II)[g]
			1c[f]	INH/RPT	Once weekly for 18 doses (18 wk)		74–58 (26 wk)	B (I)	E (I)
2	INH RIF PZA EMB	7 days/wk for 14 doses (2 wk), then twice weekly for 12 doses (6 wk) or 5 days/wk for 10 doses (2 wk)[e] then twice weekly for 12 doses (6 wk)	2a	INH/RIF	Twice weekly for 36 doses (18 wk)		62–58 (26 wk)	A (II)	B (II)[g]
			2b[f]	INH/RPT	Once weekly for 18 doses (18 wk)		44–40 (26 wk)	B (I)	E (I)
3	INH RIF PZA EMB	3 times weekly for 24 doses (8 wk)	3a	INH/RIF	3 times weekly for 54 doses (18 wk)		78 (26 wk)	B (I)	B (II)
4	INH RIF EMB	7 days/wk for 56 doses (8 wk) or 5 days/wk for 40 doses (8 wk)[c]	4a	INH/RIF	7 days/wk for 217 doses (31 wk) or 5 days/wk for 155 doses (31 wk)[e]		273–195 (39 wk)	C (I)	C (II)
			4b	INH/RIF	Twice weekly for 62 doses (31 wk)		118–102 (39 wk)	C (I)	C (II)

Definition of abbreviations: EMB, Ethambutol; INH, isoniazid; PZA, pyrazinamide; RIF, rifampin; RPT, rifapentine.

[a] Definitions of evidence ratings: A, preferred; B, acceptable alternative; C, offer when A and B cannot be given; E, should never be given.

[b] Definitions of evidence ratings: I, randomized clinical trial; II, data from clinical trials that were not randomized or were conducted in other populations; III, expert opinion.

[c] When DOT is used, drugs may be given 5 days/wk and the necessary number of doses adjusted accordingly. Although there are no studies that compare 5 with 7 daily doses, extensive experience indicates this would be an effective practice.

[d] Patients with cavitation on initial chest radiograph and positive cultures at completion of 2 months of therapy should receive a 7-month (31 wk: either 217 doses [daily] or 62 doses [twice weekly]) continuation phase.

[e] Five-day-a-week administration is always given by DOT. Rating for 5 day/wk regimens is AIII.

[f] Options 1c and 2b should be used only in HIV-negative patients who have negative sputum smears at the time of completion of 2 months of therapy and who do not have cavitation on initial chest radiograph (see text). For patients started on this regimen and found to have a positive culture from the 2-month specimen, treatment should be extended an extra 3 months.

[g] Not recommended for HIV-infected patients with CD4+ cell counts <100 cells/μL.

[g] Options 1c and 2b should be used only in HIV-negative patients who have negative sputum smears at the time of completion of 2 months of therapy and who do not have cavitation on initial chest radiograph (see text). For patients started on this regimen and found to have a positive culture from the 2-month specimen, treatment should be extended an extra 3 months.

From Centers for Disease Control and Prevention. Treatment of tuberculosis. MMWR 2003;52 (RR-11).

TABLE 47–5. Doses[a] of Antituberculosis Drugs for Adults and Children[b]

Drug	Preparation	Adults/Children	Daily	1×/wk	2×/wk	3×/wk
First-Line Drugs						
Isoniazid	Tablets (50 mg, 100 mg, 300 mg); elixir (50 mg/5 ml); aqueous solution (100 mg/mL) for intravenous or intramuscular injection	Adults (max.)	5 mg/kg (300 mg)	15 mg/kg (900 mg)	15 mg/kg (900 mg)	15 mg/kg (900 mg)
		Children (max.)	10–15 mg/kg (300 mg)	—	20–30 mg/kg (900 mg)	—
Rifampin	Capsule (150 mg, 300 mg); powder may be suspended for oral administration; aqueous solution for intravenous injection	Adults[c] (max.)	10 mg/kg (600 mg)	—	10 mg/kg (600 mg)	10 mg/kg (600 mg)
		Children (max.)	10–20 mg/kg (600 mg)	—	10–20 mg/kg (600 mg)	—
Rifabutin	Capsule (150 mg)	Adults[c] (max.)	5 mg/kg (300 mg)	10 mg/kg (continuation phase) (600 mg)	5 mg/kg (300 mg)	5 mg/kg (300 mg)
		Children	Appropriate dosing for children is unknown	Appropriate dosing for children is unknown	Appropriate dosing for children is unknown	Appropriate dosing for children is unknown
Rifapentine	Tablet (150 mg, film coated)	Adults	The drug is not approved for use in children	The drug is not approved for use in children	The drug is not approved for use in children	The drug is not approved for use in children
		Children	The drug is not approved for use in children	The drug is not approved for use in children	The drug is not approved for use in children	The drug is not approved for use in children
Pyrazinamide	Tablet (500 mg, scored)	Adults	1000 mg (40–55 kg) 1500 mg (56–75 kg) 2000 mg (76–90 kg)[d]	—	2000 mg (40–55 kg) 3000 mg (56–75 kg) 4000 mg (76–90 kg)[d] 50 mg/kg (2 g)	1500 mg (40–55 kg) 2500 mg (56–75 kg) 3000 mg (76–90 kg)[d]
		Children (max.)	15–30 mg/kg (2 g)	—	—	—
Ethambutol	Tablet (100 mg, 400 mg)	Adults	800 mg (40–55 kg) 1200 mg (56–75 kg) 1600 mg (76–90 kg)[d]	—	2000 mg (40–55 kg) 2800 mg (56–75 kg) 4000 mg (76–90 kg)[d] 50 mg/kg (2.5 g)	1200 mg (40–55 kg) 2000 mg (56–75 kg) 2400 mg (76–90 kg)[d]
		Children[e] (max.)	15–20 mg/kg daily (1 g)	—	—	—

TABLE 47-5. (Continued)

Drug	Preparation	Adults/Children	Daily	11×/wk	2×/wk	3×/wk
					Doses	
Second-Line Drugs						
Cycloserine	Capsule (250 mg)	Adults (max.)	10–15 mg/kg/day (1 g in two doses), usually 500–750 mg/d in two doses^f	There are no data to support intermittent administration	There are no data to support intermittent administration	There are no data to support intermittent administration
		Children^g (max.)	10–15 mg/kg/day (1 g/day)			
Ethionamide	Tablet (250 mg)	Adults^g (max.)	15–20 mg/kg/day (1 g/day), usually 500–750 mg/day in a single daily dose or two divided doses^g	There are no data to support intermittent administration	There are no data to support intermittent administration	There are no data to support intermittent administration
		Children (max.)	15–20 mg/kg/day (1 g/day)			
Streptomycin	Aqueous solution (1-g vials) for intravenous or intramuscular administration	Adults (max.)	h	h	h	h
		Children (max.)	20–40 mg/kg/day (1 g)	—	20 mg/kg	—
Amikacin/ kanamycin	Aqueous solution (500-mg and 1-g vials) for intravenous or intramuscular administration	Adults (max.)	h	h	h	h
		Children (max.)	15–30 mg/kg/day (1 g) intravenous or intramuscular as a single daily dose	—	15–30 mg/kg	—
Capreomycin	Aqueous solution (1-g vials) for intravenous or intramuscular administration	Adults (max.)	h	h	h	h
		Children (max.)	15–30 mg/kg/day (1 g) as a single daily dose	—	15–30 mg/kg	—
p-Aminosalicylic acid (PAS)	Granules (4-g packets) can be mixed with food; tablets	Adults	8–12 g/day in 2–3 doses	There are no data to support intermittent administration	There are no data to support intermittent administration	There are no data to support intermittent administration

			Daily	2–3 times/wk	1 time/wk
	(500 mg) are still available in some countries, but not in the United States; a solution for intravenous administration is available in Europe	Children	200–300 mg/kg/day in 2–4 divided doses (10 g)	There are no data to support intermittent administration	There are no data to support intermittent administration
Levofloxacin	Tablets (250 mg, 500 mg, 750 mg); aqueous solution (500-mg vials) for intravenous injection	Adults	500–1000 mg daily	There are no data to support intermittent administration	There are no data to support intermittent administration
		Children	i	i	i
Moxifloxacin	Tablets (400 mg); aqueous solution (400 mg/250 mL) for intravenous injection	Adults	400 mg daily	There are no data to support intermittent administration	There are no data to support intermittent administration
		Children	j	j	j
Gatifloxacin	Tablets (400 mg); aqueous solution (200 mg/20 mL; 400 mg/40 mL) for intravenous injection	Adults	400 mg daily	There are no data to support intermittent administration	There are no data to support intermittent administration
		Children	k	k	k

aDose per weight is based on ideal body weight. Children weighing more than 40 kg should be dosed as adults.

bFor purposes of this document adult dosing begins at age 15 yr.

cDose may need to be adjusted because of weight.

dMaximum dose regardless of weight.

eThe drug can likely be used safely in older children but should be used with caution in children less than 5 yr of age, in whom visual acuity cannot be monitored. In younger children EMB at the dose of 15 mg/kg/day can be used if there is suspected or proven resistance to INH or RIF.

fIt should be noted that, although this is the dose recommended generally, most clinicians with experience using cycloserine indicate that it is unusual for patients to be able to tolerate this amount. Serum concentration measurements are often useful in determining the optimal dose for a given patient.

gThe single daily dose can be given at bedtime or with the main meal.

hDose: 15 mg/kg/day (1 g), and 10 mg/kg in persons more than 59 yr of age (750 mg). Usual dose: 750–1000 mg administered intramuscularly or intravenously, given as a single dose 5–7 days/wk and reduced to 2 or 3 times/wk after the first 2–4 months or after culture conversion, depending on the efficacy of the other drugs in the regimen.

iThe long-term (more than several weeks) use of levofloxacin in children and adolescents has not been approved because of concerns about effects on bone and cartilage growth. However, most experts agree that the drug should be considered for children with tuberculosis caused by organisms resistant to both INH and RIF. The optimal dose is not known.

jThe long-term (more than several weeks) use of moxifloxacin in children and adolescents has not been approved because of concerns about effects on bone and cartilage growth. The optimal dose is not known.

kThe long-term (more than several weeks) use of gatifloxacin in children and adolescents has not been approved because of concerns about effects on bone and cartilage growth. The optimal dose is not known.

- If the organism is drug resistant, the aim is to introduce two or more active agents that the patient has not received previously. With MDR-TB, no standard regimen can be proposed. It is critical to avoid monotherapy or adding only a single drug to a failing regimen.

Drug Resistance

Drug resistance should be suspected in the following situations:

- Patients who have received prior therapy for TB
- Patients from geographic areas with a high prevalence of resistance (New York City, Mexico, Southeast Asia, and the former Soviet states)
- Patients who are homeless, institutionalized, intravenous drug abusers, and/or infected with HIV
- Patients who still have acid-fast bacilli (AFB)-positive sputum smears after 2 months of therapy
- Patients who still have positive cultures after 3 to 4 months of therapy
- Patients who require retreatment

Special Populations

VIII *TUBERCULOUS MENINGITIS AND EXTRAPULMONARY DISEASE*

In general, **isoniazid, pyrazinamide, ethionamide**, and **cycloserine** penetrate the cerebrospinal fluid (CSF) readily. Patients with CNS tuberculosis are often treated for longer periods (9 to 12 months). Extrapulmonary TB of the soft tissues can be treated with conventional regimens. TB of the bone is typically treated for 9 months, occasionally with surgical debridement.

CHILDREN

Tuberculosis in children may be treated with regimens similar to those used in adults, although some physicians still prefer to extend treatment to 9 months.

PREGNANT WOMEN

- The usual treatment of pregnant women is isoniazid, rifampin, and ethambutol for 9 months.
- Women with TB should be cautioned against becoming pregnant, as the disease poses a risk to the fetus as well as to the mother. Isoniazid or ethambutol are relatively safe when used during pregnancy. Supplementation with B vitamins is particularly important during pregnancy. **Rifampin** has been rarely associated with birth defects, but those seen are occasionally severe, including limb reduction and CNS lesions. **Pyrazinamide** has not been studied in a large number of pregnant women, but anecdotal information suggests that it may be safe. **Ethionamide** may be associated with premature delivery, congenital deformities, and Down's syndrome when used during pregnancy. **Streptomycin** has been associated with hearing impairment in the newborn, including complete deafness.

IHIV-INFECTED PATIENTS

AIDS patients and other immunocompromised hosts may be managed with chemotherapeutic regimens similar to those used in immunocompetent individuals, although treatment is often extended to 9 months.

RENAL FAILURE

In nearly all patients, isoniazid and rifampin do not require dose modifications in renal failure. Pyrazinamide and ethambutol typically require a reduction in dosing frequency from daily to three times weekly (Table 47–6).

TABLE 47–6. Dosing Recommendations for Adults Patients with Reduced Renal Function and for Adult Patients Receiving Hemodialysis

Drug	Change in Frequency?	Recommended Dose and Frequency for Patients with Creatinine Clearance <30 mL/min or for Patients Receiving Hemodialysis
Isoniazid	No change	300 mg once daily, or 900 mg 3 times/wk
Rifampin	No change	600 mg once daily, or 600 mg 3 times/wk
Pyrazinamide	Yes	25–35 mg/kg per dose 3 times/wk (not daily)
Ethambutol	Yes	15–25 mg/kg per dose 3 times/wk (not daily)
Levofloxacin	Yes	750–1000 mg per dose 3 times/wk (not daily)
Cycloserine	Yes	250 mg once daily, or 500 mg/dose 3 times/week[a]
Ethionamide	No change	250–500 mg per dose daily
p-Aminosalicylic acid	No change	4 g per dose, twice daily
Streptomycin	Yes	12–15 mg/kg per dose 2 or 3 times/wk (not daily)
Capreomycin	Yes	12–15 mg/kg per dose 2 or 3 times/wk (not daily)
Kanamycin	Yes	12–15 mg/kg per dose 2 or 3 times/wk (not daily)
Amikacin	Yes	12–15 mg/kg per dose two or 3 times/wk (not daily)

Note: Standard doses are given unless there is intolerance.

The medications should be given after hemodialysis on the day of hemodialysis.

Monitoring of serum drug concentrations should be considered to ensure adequate drug absorption, without excessive accumulation, and to assist in avoiding toxicity.

Data currently are not available for patients receiving peritoneal dialysis. Until data become available, begin with doses recommended for patients receiving hemodialysis and verify adequacy of dosing, using serum concentration monitoring.

[a]The appropriateness of 250-mg daily doses has not been established. There should be careful monitoring for evidence of neurotoxicity.

VIII ◄

▶ EVALUATION OF THERAPEUTIC OUTCOMES AND PATIENT MONITORING

- Symptomatic patients should be isolated and have sputum samples sent for AFB stains every 1 to 2 weeks until two consecutive smears are negative.
- Once on maintenance therapy, patients should have sputum cultures performed monthly until negative, which generally occurs over 2 to 3 months. If sputum cultures continue to be positive after 2 months, drug susceptibility testing should be repeated and serum drug concentrations should be checked.
- Patients should have blood urea nitrogen, serum creatinine, aspartate transaminase or alanine transaminase, and a complete blood count determined at baseline and periodically, depending on the presence of other factors that may increase the likelihood of toxicity (advanced age, alcohol abuse, and possibly pregnancy). Hepatotoxicity should be suspected in patients whose transaminases exceed 5 times the upper limit of normal or whose total bilirubin exceeds 3 mg/dL. At this point, the offending agent(s) should be discontinued, and alternatives selected.
- Therapy with isoniazid results in a transient elevation in serum transaminases in 12% to 15% of patients and usually occurs within the first 8 to 12 weeks of therapy. Risk factors for hepatotoxicity include patient age, preexisting liver disease, and pregnancy or postpartum state. Isoniazid also may result in neurotoxicity, most frequently presenting as peripheral neuropathy or, in overdose, seizures and coma. Patients with pyridoxine deficiency, such as alcoholics, children, and the malnourished, are at increased risk, as are patients who are

slow acetylators of INH and those predisposed to neuropathy, such as those with diabetes.

- Elevations in hepatic enzymes have been attributed to rifampin in 10% to 15% of patients, with overt hepatotoxicity occurring in less than 1%. More frequent adverse effects of RIF include rash, fever, and gastrointestinal distress.
- Rifampin's induction of hepatic enzymes may enhance the elimination of a number of drugs, most notably protease inhibitors. Women who use oral contraceptives should be advised to use another form of contraception during therapy.
- The red colorizing effects of rifampin on urine, other secretions, and contact lenses should be discussed with the patient.
- Retrobulbar neuritis is the major adverse effect noted in patients treated with ethambutol. Patients usually complain of a change in visual acuity and/or inability to see the color green. Vision testing should be performed on all patients who must receive ethambutol for more than 2 months.
- Impairment of eighth cranial nerve function is the most important adverse effect of streptomycin. Vestibular function is most frequently affected, but hearing may also be impaired. Audiometric testing should be performed in patients who must receive streptomycin for more than 2 months. Streptomycin occasionally causes nephrotoxicity.
- The most serious problem with TB therapy is nonadherence to the prescribed regimen. The most effective way to ensure adherence is with DOT.

See Chapter 110, Tuberculosis, authored by Charles A. Peloquin, for a more detailed discussion of this topic.

VIII

Chapter 48

► URINARY TRACT INFECTIONS AND PROSTATITIS

► DEFINITION

- Infections of the urinary tract represent a wide variety of clinical syndromes including urethritis, cystitis, prostatitis, and pyelonephritis.
- A urinary tract infection (UTI) is defined as the presence of microorganisms in the urine that cannot be accounted for by contamination. The organisms have the potential to invade the tissues of the urinary tract and adjacent structures.
- Lower tract infections include cystitis (bladder), urethritis (urethra), prostatitis (prostate gland), and epididymitis. Upper tract infections involve the kidney and are referred to as pyelonephritis.
- Uncomplicated UTIs are not associated with structural or neurologic abnormalities that may interfere with the normal flow of urine or the voiding mechanism. Complicated UTIs are the result of a predisposing lesion of the urinary tract such as a congenital abnormality or distortion of the urinary tract, a stone, indwelling catheter, prostatic hypertrophy, obstruction, or neurologic deficit that interferes with the normal flow of urine and urinary tract defenses.
- Recurrent UTIs are characterized by multiple symptomatic episodes with asymptomatic periods occurring between these episodes. These infections are either due to reinfection or to relapse.
- Reinfections are caused by a new organism and account for the majority of recurrent UTIs.
- Relapse represents the development of repeated infections caused by the same initial organism.

► PATHOPHYSIOLOGY

- The bacteria causing UTIs usually originate from bowel flora of the host.
- UTIs can be acquired via three possible routes: the ascending, hematogenous, or lymphatic pathways.
- In females, the short length of the urethra and proximity to the perirectal area make colonization of the urethra likely. Bacteria are then believed to enter the bladder from the urethra. Once in the bladder, the organisms multiply quickly and can ascend the ureters to the kidney.
- Three factors determine the development of urinary tract infection: the size of the inoculum, virulence of the microorganism, and competency of the natural host defense mechanisms.
- Patients who are unable to void urine completely are at greater risk of developing urinary tract infections and frequently have recurrent infections.
- An important virulence factor of bacteria is their ability to adhere to urinary epithelial cells by fimbriae. Other virulence factors include hemolysin, a cytotoxic protein produced by bacteria that lyses a wide range of cells including erythrocytes, polymorphonuclear leukocytes, and monocytes; and aerobactin, which facilitates the binding and uptake of iron by *Escherichia coli*.

MICROBIOLOGY

- The most common cause of uncomplicated UTIs is *E. coli*, accounting for more than 85% of community-acquired infections, followed by *Staphylococcus saprophyticus* (coagulase-negative staphylococcus), accounting for 5% to 15%.

TABLE 48–1. Clinical Presentation of Urinary Tract Infections in Adults

Signs and Symptoms
Lower UTI: Dysuria, urgency, frequency, nocturia, suprapublic heaviness
Gross heamturia
Upper UTI: Flank pain, fever, nausea, vomiting malaise
Physical Examination
Upper UTI—costovertebral tenderness
Laboratory Tests
Bacteriuria
Pyuria (white blood cell count >10/mm^3
Nitrite-positive urine (with nitrite reducers)
Leukocyte esterase-positive urine
Antibody-coated bacteria (upper UTI)

- The urinary pathogens in complicated or nosocomial infections may include *E. coli*, which accounts for less than 50% of these infections, *Proteus* spp., *Klebsiella pneumoniae*, *Enterobacter* spp., *Pseudomonas aeruginosa*, staphylococci, and enterococci. *Candida* spp. have become common causes of urinary infection in the critically ill and chronically catheterized patient.

➤VIII

- The majority of UTIs are caused by a single organism; however, in patients with stones, indwelling urinary catheters, or chronic renal abscesses, multiple organisms may be isolated.

▶ CLINICAL PRESENTATION

- The typical symptoms of lower ad upper urinary tract infections are presented in Table 48–1.
- Symptoms alone are unreliable for the diagnosis of bacterial UTIs. The key to the diagnosis of UTI is the ability to demonstrate significant numbers of microorganisms present in an appropriate urine specimen to distinguish contamination from infection.
- A standard urinalysis should be obtained in the initial assessment of a patient. Microscopic examination of the urine should be performed by preparation of a Gram stain of unspun or centrifuged urine. The presence of at least one organism per oil-immersion field in a properly collected uncentrifuged specimen correlates with more than 100,000 bacteria/mL of urine.
- Criteria for defining significant bacteriuria are listed in Table 48–2.
- The presence of pyuria (more than 10 WBCs/mm^3) in a symptomatic patient correlates with significant bacteriuria.
- The nitrite test can be used to detect the presence of nitrate-reducing bacteria in the urine (such as *E. coli*). The leukocyte esterase test is a rapid dipstick test to detect pyuria.

TABLE 48–2. Diagnostic Criteria for Significant Bacteriuria

$\geq 10^2$ CFU coliforms/mL or $\geq 10^5$ CFU noncoliforms/mL in a symptomatic female
$\geq 10^3$ CFU bacteria/mL in a symptomatic male
$\geq 10^5$ CFU bacteria/mL in asymptomatic individuals on two consecutive specimens
Any growth of bacteria on suprapubic catheterization in a symptomatic patient
$\geq 10^2$ CFU bacteria/mL in a catheterized patient

- The most reliable method of diagnosing UTIs is by quantitative urine culture. Patients with infection usually have more than 10^5 bacteria/mL of urine, although as many as one-third of women with symptomatic infection have less than 10^5 bacteria/mL.
- A method to detect upper UTI is the antibody-coated bacteria (ACB) test, an immunofluorescent method that detects bacteria coated with immunoglobulin in freshly voided urine.

▶ DESIRED OUTCOME

The goals of treatment for UTIs are to prevent or to treat systemic consequences of infection, eradicate the invading organism, and prevent recurrence of infection.

▶ TREATMENT

GENERAL PRINCIPLES

- The management of a patient with a UTI includes initial evaluation, selection of an antibacterial agent and duration of therapy, and follow-up evaluation.
- The initial selection of an antimicrobial agent for the treatment of UTI is primarily based on the severity of the presenting signs and symptoms, the site of infection, and whether the infection is determined to be complicated or uncomplicated.

PHARMACOLOGIC TREATMENT

- The ability to eradicate bacteria from the urinary tract is directly related to the sensitivity of the organism and the achievable concentration of the antimicrobial agent in the urine.
- Table 48–3 lists the most common agents used in the treatment of UTIs, along with comments concerning their general use.
- Table 48–4 presents an overview of various therapeutic options for outpatient therapy for UTI.
- Table 48–5 describes empiric treatment regimens for selected clinical situations.

Acute Uncomplicated Cystitis

- These infections are predominantly caused by *E. coli*, and antimicrobial therapy should be directed against this organism initially. Other causes include *S. saprophyticus* and occasionally *K. pneumoniae* and *Proteus mirabilis*.
- Because the causative organisms and their susceptibilities are generally known, a cost-effective approach to management is recommended that includes a urinalysis and initiation of empiric therapy without a urine culture (Figure 48–1).
- Short-course therapy (3-day therapy) with **trimethoprim-sulfamethoxazole** or a **fluoroquinolone** (e.g., **ciprofloxacin, levofloxacin, norfloxacin, or gatifloxacin**) is superior to single-dose therapy for uncomplicated infection and should be the treatment of choice. Amoxicillin or sulfonamides are not recommended because of the high incidence of resistant *E. coli*. Follow-up urine cultures are not necessary in patients who respond.

Symptomatic Abacteriuria

- Single-dose or short-course therapy with **trimethoprim-sulfamethoxazole** has been used effectively, and prolonged courses of therapy are not necessary for the majority of patients.

TABLE 48–3. Commonly Used Antimicrobial Agents in the Treatment of Urinary Tract Infections

Agent	Comments
Oral Therapy	
Sulfonamides	These agents generally have been replaced by more agents due to resistance.
Trimethoprim-sulfamethoxazole (TMP-SMX)	This combination is highly effective against most aerobic enteric bacteria except *Pseudomonas aeruginosa*. High urinary tract tissue levels and urine levels are achieved, which may be important in complicated infection treatment. Also effective as prophylaxis for recurrent infections.
Penicillins Ampicillin Amoxicillin-clavulanic acid Carbenicillin indanyl	Ampicillin is the standard penicillin that has broad-spectrum activity. Increasing *E. coli* resistance has limited amoxicillin use in acute cystitis. Drug of choice for enterococci sensitive to penicillin. Amoxicillin-clavulanate is preferred for resistance problems. Carbenicillin indanyl is only indicated for the treatment of urinary tract infections.
Cephalosporins Cephalexin Cephradine Cefaclor Cefadroxil Cefuroxime Cefixime Cefzil Cefpodoxime	There are no major advantages of these agents over other agents in the treatment of urinary tract infections, and they are more expensive. They may be useful in cases of resistance to amoxicillin and trimethoprim-sulfamethoxazole. These agents are not active against enterococci.
Tetracyclines Tetracycline Doxycycline Minocycline	These agents have been effective for initial episodes of urinary tract infections; however, resistance develops rapidly, and their use is limited. These agents also lead to candidal overgrowth. The are useful primarily for chlamydial infections.
Fluoroquinolones Ciprofloxacin Norfloxacin Levofloxacin	The newer quinolones have a greater spectrum of activity, including *Pseudomonas aeruginosa*. These agents are effective for pyelonephritis and prostatitis. Avoid in pregnancy and children. Moxifloxacin should not be used owing to inadequate urinary concentrations.
Nitrofurantoin	This agent is effective as both a therapeutic and prophylactic agent in patients with recurrent UTIs. Main advantage is the lack of resistance even after long courses of therapy. Adverse effects may limit use (GI intolerance, neuropathies, pulmonary reactions).
Azithromycin	Single-dose therapy for chlamydial infections.
Methanamine hippurate-mandalate	These agents are reserved for prophylactic therapy or suppressive use between episodes of infection.
Fosfomycin	Single-dose therapy for uncomplicated infections.
Parenteral Therapy	
Aminoglycosides Centamicin Tobramycin Amikacin Netilmicin	Gentamicin and tobramycin are equally effective; gentamicin is less expensive. Tobramycin has better pseudomonal activity, which may be important in serious systemic infections. Amikacin generally is reserved for multiresistant bacteria.
Penicillins Ampicillin Ampicillin-sulbactam Ticarcillin-clavulanate Piperacillin Piperacillin-tazobactam	These agents generally are equally effective for susceptible bacteria. The extended-spectrum penicillins are more active against *P. aeruginosa* and enterococci and often are preferred over cephalosporins. They are very useful in renally impaired patients or when an aminoglycoside is to be avoided.

VIII

(Continued)

TABLE 48–3. (Continued)

Agent	Comments
Cephalosporins, first-, second-, and third-generation	Second- and third-generation cephalosporins have a broad spectrum of activity against gram-negative bacteria but are not active against enterococci and have limited activity against *P. aeruginosa*. Ceftazidime and cefepime are active against *P. aeruginosa*. They are useful for nosocomial infections and urosepsis due to susceptible pathogens.

Carbapenems
  Imipenem-cilastatin
  Meropenem
  Ertapenem
  Aztreonam
	These agents have broad spectrum of activity, including gram-positive, gram-negative, and anaerobic bacteria.
	Imipenem and meropenem are active against *P. aeruginosa* and enterococci, but ertapenem is not. All may be associated with candidal superinfections.
	A monobactam that is only active against gram-negative bacteria, including some strains of *P. aeruginosa*. Generally useful for nosocomial infections when aminoglycosides are to be avoided and in penicillin-sensitive patients.

Quinolones
  Ciprofloxacin
  Levofloxacin
  Gatifloxacin
	These agents have broad-spectrum activity against both gram-negative and gram-positive bacteria. They provide urine and high-tissue concentrations and are actively secreted in reduced renal function

VIII

- If single-dose or short-course therapy is ineffective, a culture should be obtained.
- If the patient reports recent sexual activity, therapy for *Chlamydia trachomatis* should be considered (azithromycin 1 g as a single dose or doxycycline 100 mg twice daily).

Asymptomatic Bacteriuria

- The management of asymptomatic bacteriuria depends on the age of the patient and, if female, whether she is pregnant. In children, treatment should consist of conventional courses of therapy, as described for symptomatic infections.
- In the nonpregnant female, therapy is controversial; however, it appears that treatment has little effect on the natural course of infections.
- Most clinicians feel that asymptomatic bacteriuria in the elderly is a benign disease and may not warrant treatment. The presence of bacteriuria can be confirmed by culture if treatment is considered.

Complicated Urinary Tract Infections
Acute Pyelonephritis

- The presentation of high-grade fever (greater than 38.3°C) and severe flank pain should be treated as acute pyelonephritis, and aggressive management is warranted. Severely ill patients with pyelonephritis should be hospitalized and intravenous drugs administered initially.
- At the time of presentation, a Gram stain of the urine should be performed, along with urinalysis, culture, and sensitivities.
- In the mild to moderately symptomatic patient for whom oral therapy is considered, an effective agent should be administered for at least a 2-week period, although use of highly active agents for 7 to 10 days may be sufficient. Oral antibiotics that have shown efficacy in this setting include **trimethoprim-sulfamethoxazole** or **fluoroquinolones.** If a Gram stain reveals gram-positive cocci, *S. faecalis* should be considered and treatment directed against this pathogen (**ampicillin**).

TABLE 48–4. Overview of Outpatient Antimicrobial Therapy for Lower Tract Infections in Adults

Indications	Antibiotic	Dose[a]	Interval	Duration
Lower tract Infections		2 DS tablets	Single dose	1 day
Uncomplicated	Trimethoprim-sulfamethoxazole	1 DS tablet	Twice a day	3 days
	Ciprofloxacin	250 mg	Twice a day	3 days
	Norfloxacin	400 mg	Twice a day	3 days
	Gatifloxacin	200–400 mg	Once a day	3 days
	Levofloxacin	250 mg	Once a day	3 days
	Lomefloxacin	400 mg	Once a day	3 days
	Enoxacin	200 mg	Once a day	3 days
	Amoxicillin	6 × 500 mg	Single dose	1 day
		500 mg	Twice a day	3 days
	Amoxicillin-clavulanate	500 mg	Every 8 h	3 days
	Trimethoprim	100 mg	Twice a day	3 days
	Nitrofurantoin	100 mg	Every 6 h	3 days
	Fosfomycin	3 g	Single dose	1 day
Complicated	Trimethoprim-sulfamethoxazole	1 DS tablet	Twice a day	7–10 days
	Trimethoprim	100 mg	Twice a day	7–10 days
	Norfloxacin	400 mg	Twice a day	7–10 days
	Ciprofloxacin	250–500 mg	Twice a day	7–10 days
	Gatifloxacin	400 mg	Once a day	7–10 days
	Moxifloxacin (PO only)	400 mg	Once a day	7–10 days
	Lomefloxacin	400 mg	Once a day	7–10 days
	Levofloxacin	250 mg	Once a day	7–10 days
	Amoxicillin-clavulanate	500 mg	Every 8 h	7–10 days
Recurrent Infections	Nitrofurantoin	50 mg	Once a day	6 months
	Trimethoprim	100 mg	Once a day	6 months
	Trimethoprim-sulfamethoxazole	1/2 ss tablet	Once a day	6 months
Acute urethral syndrome	Trimethoprim-sulfamethoxazole	1 DS	Twice a day	3 days
Failure of TMP-SMX	Azithromycin	1 g	Single dose	
	Doxycycline	100 mg	Twice a day	7 days
Acute pyelonephritis	Trimethoprim-sulfamethoxazole	1 DS tablet	Twice a day	14 days
	Ciprofloxacin	500 mg	Twice a day	14 days
	Gatifloxacin	400 mg	Once a day	14 days
	Norfloxacin	400 mg	Twice a day	14 days
	Levofloxacin	250 mg	Once a day	14 days
	Lomefloxacin	400 mg	Once a day	14 days
	Enoxacin	400 mg	Twice a day	14 days
	Amoxicillin-clavulanate	500 mg	Every 8 h	14 days

[a]Dosing intervals for normal renal function.

- In the seriously ill patient, the traditional initial therapy has included an intravenous **fluoroquinolone,** an **aminoglycoside** with or without **ampicillin,** or an extended-spectrum **cephalosporin** with or without an aminoglycoside.
- If the patient has been hospitalized in the last 6 months, has a urinary catheter, or is in a nursing home, the possibility of *P. aeruginosa* and *enterococci* infection, as well as multiply resistant organisms, should be considered. In this setting, **ceftazidime, ticarcillin–clavulanic acid, piperacillin, aztreonam, meropenem,** or **imipenem,** in combination with an **aminoglycoside,** is recommended. If the patient responds to initial combination therapy, the aminoglycoside may be discontinued after 3 days.
- Follow-up urine cultures should be obtained 2 weeks after the completion of therapy to ensure a satisfactory response and to detect possible relapse.

TABLE 48–5. Empirical Treatment of Urinary Tract Infections and Prostatitis

Diagnosis	Pathogens	Treatment	Comments
Acute uncomplicated cystitis	E. coli S. saprophyticus	1. Trimethoprim-sulfamethoxazole × 3 days 2. Quinolone × 3 days	Short-course therapy more effective than single dose
Pregnancy	As above	1. Amoxicillin-clavulanate × 7 days 2. Cephalosporin × 7 days 3. Trimethoprim-sulfamethoxazole × 7 days	Avoid trimethoprim-sulfamethoxazole durig third trimester
Acute pyelonephritis Uncomplicated	E. coli	1. Trimethoprim-sulfamethoxazole × 14 days 2. Quinolone × 14 days	Can be managed as outpatient
Complicated	E. coli, P. mirabilis K. pneumoniae Pseudomonas aeruginosa, E. fecalis	1. Quinolone × 14 days 2. Extended-spectrum penicillin Plus aminoglycoside	Severity of illness will determine duration of IV therapy; culture results should direct therapy Oral therapy may complete 14 days of therapy
Postatitis	E. coli, K. pneumoniae Proteus spp, Pseudomonas aeruginosa	1. Trimethoprim-sulfamethoxazole × 4–6 weeks 2. Quinolone × 4–6 weeks	Acute prostatitis may require IV therapy initially Chronic prostatitis may require longer treatment periods or surgery

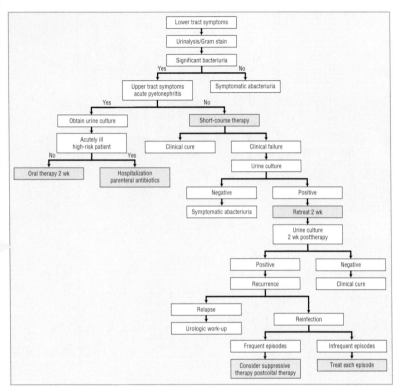

Figure 48–1. Management of UTIs in females.

Urinary Tract Infections in Males
- The conventional view is that therapy in males requires prolonged treatment (Figure 48–2).
- A urine culture should be obtained before treatment, because the cause of infection in men is not as predictable as in women.
- If gram-negative bacteria are presumed, **trimethoprim-sulfamethoxazole** or a **fluoroquinolone** is a preferred agent. Initial therapy is for 10 to 14 days. For recurrent infections in males, cure rates are much higher with a 6-week regimen of **trimethoprim-sulfamethoxazole**.

Recurrent Infections
- Recurrent episodes of urinary tract infection (reinfections and relapses) account for a significant portion of all UTIs.
- These patients are most commonly women and can be divided into two groups: those with fewer than two or three episodes per year and those who develop more frequent infections.
- In patients with infrequent infections (i.e., fewer than three infections per year), each episode should be treated as a separately occurring infection. Short-course therapy should be used in symptomatic female patients with lower tract infection.

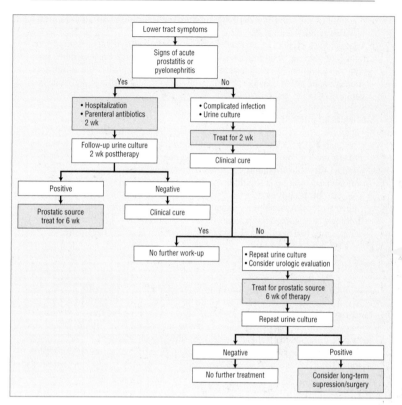

Figure 48–2. Management of UTIs in male.

- In patients who have frequent symptomatic infections, long-term prophylactic antimicrobial therapy may be instituted (see Table 48–4). Therapy is generally given for 6 months, with urine cultures followed periodically.
- In women who experience symptomatic reinfections in association with sexual activity, voiding after intercourse may help prevent infection. Also, self-administered, single-dose prophylactic therapy with **trimethoprim-sulfamethoxazole** taken after intercourse has been found to significantly reduce the incidence of recurrent infection in these patients.
- Women who relapse after short-course therapy should receive a 2-week course of therapy. In patients who relapse after 2 weeks, therapy should be continued for another 2 to 4 weeks. If relapse occurs after 6 weeks of treatment, therapy for 6 months or even longer may be considered.

SPECIAL CONDITIONS

Urinary Tract Infection in Pregnancy

- In patients with significant bacteriuria, symptomatic or asymptomatic, treatment is recommended in order to avoid possible complications during the pregnancy. Therapy should consist of an agent with a relatively low adverse-effect

501

potential (a **sulfonamide, cephalexin, amoxicillin, amoxicillin/clavulanate, nitrofurantoin**) administered for 7 days.

- Tetracyclines should be avoided because of teratogenic effects, and sulfonamides should not be administered during the third trimester because of the possible development of kernicterus and hyperbilirubinemia. Also, the quinolones should not be given because of their potential to inhibit cartilage and bone development in the newborn.

Catheterized Patients

- When bacteriuria occurs in the asymptomatic, short-term catheterized patient (less than 30 days), the use of systemic antibiotic therapy should be withheld and the catheter removed as soon as possible. If the patient becomes symptomatic, the catheter should again be removed and treatment as described for complicated infections should be started.
- The use of prophylactic systemic antibiotics in patients with short-term catheterization reduces the incidence of infection over the first 4 to 7 days. In long-term catheterized patients, however, antibiotics only postpone the development of bacteriuria and lead to emergence of resistant organisms.

VIII
▶ PROSTATITIS

Prostatitis is an inflammation of the prostate gland and surrounding tissue as a result of infection. It can be either acute or chronic. The acute form is characterized by a severe illness characterized by a sudden onset of fever and urinary and constitutional symptoms. Chronic bacterial prostatitis (CBP) represents a recurring infection with the same organism (relapse). Pathogenic bacteria and significant inflammatory cells must be present in prostatic secretions and urine to make the diagnosis of bacterial prostatitis.

PATHOGENESIS AND ETIOLOGY

- The exact mechanism of bacterial infection of the prostate is not well understood. The possible routes of infection include ascending infection of the urethra, reflux of infected urine into prostatic ducts, invasion by rectal bacteria through direct extension or lymphatic spread, and by hematogenous spread.
- Gram-negative enteric organisms are the most frequent pathogens in acute bacterial prostatitis (ABP). *E. coli* is the predominant organism, occurring in 75% of cases.
- CBP is most commonly caused by *E. coli*, with other gram-negative organisms isolated much less often.

CLINICAL PRESENTATION AND DIAGNOSIS

- The clinical presentation of bacterial prostatitis is presented in Table 48–6.
- Digital palpation of the prostate via the rectum may reveal a swollen, tender, warm, tense, or indurated prostate. Massage of the prostate will express a purulent discharge, which will readily grow the pathogenic organism. However, prostatic massage is contraindicated in ABP because of a risk of inducing bacteremia and associated pain.
- CBP is characterized by recurrent urinary tract infections with the same pathogen.
- Urinary tract localization studies are critical to the diagnosis of CBP.
- Both ABP and CBP are characterized by the presence of numerous white blood cells and lipid-containing macrophages (oval fat bodies) on microscopic examination of expressed prostatic secretions.

TABLE 48–6. Clinical Presentation of Bacterial Prostatitis

Signs and Symptoms
Acute bacterial prostatitis: High fever, chills, malaise, myalgia, localized pain (perineal, rectal, sacrococcygeal), frequency, urgency, dysuria, nocturia, and retention
Chronic bacterial prostatitis: Voiding difficulties (frequency, urgency, dysuria), low back pain, and perineal and suprapubic discomfort
Physical Examination
Acute bacterial prostatitis: Swollen, tender, tense, or indurated gland
Chronic bacterial prostatitis: Boggy, indurated (enlarged) prostate in most patients
Laboratory Tests
Bacteriuria
Bacteria in expressed prostatic secretions

TREATMENT

- The majority of patients can be managed with oral antimicrobial agents, such as **trimethoprim-sulfamethoxazole** or the fluoroquinolones (**ciprofloxacin, levofloxacin, gatifloxacin**). When intravenous treatment is necessary, intravenous to oral sequential therapy with **trimethoprim-sulfamethoxazole** or a fluoroquinolone, such as ciprofloxacin or **ofloxacin,** would be appropriate.
- The total course of therapy should be 4 weeks, which may be prolonged to 6 to 12 weeks with chronic prostatitis.
- Parenteral therapy should be maintained until the patient is afebrile and less symptomatic. The conversion to an oral antibiotic can be considered if the patient has been afebrile for 48 hours or after 3 to 5 days of intravenous therapy.
- The choice of antibiotics in CBP should include those agents that are capable of crossing the prostatic epithelium into the prostatic fluid in therapeutic concentrations and which also possess the spectrum of activity to be effective.
- Currently, the fluoroquinolones (given for 4 to 6 weeks) appear to provide the best therapeutic option in the management of CBP.

See Chapter 114, Urinary Tract Infections and Prostatitis, authored by Elizabeth A. Coyle and Randall A. Prince, for a more detailed discussion of this topic.

VIII

Chapter 49

▶ VACCINES, TOXOIDS, AND OTHER IMMUNOBIOLOGICS

▶ DEFINITIONS

- Immunization is the process of introducing an antigen into the body to induce protection against an infectious agent without causing disease.
- Vaccines are substances administered to generate a protective immune response.
- Toxoids are inactivated bacterial toxins. They retain the ability to stimulate the formation of antitoxin.
- Adjuvants are inert substances, such as aluminum salts (i.e., alum), which enhance vaccine antigenicity by prolonging antigen absorption.
- Immune sera are sterile solutions containing antibody derived from human (immune globulin) or equine (antitoxin) sources.
- Antitoxins contain antibodies that are made by immunizing animals with an antigen and then harvesting the antibodies from serum.

▶ VACCINE AND TOXOID RECOMMENDATIONS

- The recommended schedules for routine immunization of children and adults are shown in Tables 49–1 and 49–2, respectively.
- In general, inactivated vaccines can be administered simultaneously at separate sites. Killed and live antigens may be administered simultaneously or, if they cannot be administered simultaneously, at any interval between doses with the exception of cholera (killed) and yellow fever (live) vaccines, which should be given at least 3 weeks apart. If live vaccines are not administered simultaneously, their administration should be separated by at least 4 weeks.
- Vaccination of pregnant women generally is deferred until after delivery because of concern over potential risk to the fetus. Administration of live attenuated vaccines should not be done during pregnancy, and inactivated vaccines may be administered to pregnant women when the benefits outweigh the risks. Hepatitis A, hepatitis B, meningococcal, inactivated polio, and pneumococcal polysaccharide vaccines should be administered to pregnant women who are at risk for contracting these infections.
- Patients with chronic conditions that cause limited immune deficiency (e.g., renal disease, diabetes, liver disease, and asplenia) and who are not receiving immunosuppressants may receive live attenuated and killed vaccines, and toxoids.
- Patients with active malignant disease may receive killed vaccines or toxoids but should not be given live vaccines. Live virus vaccines may be administered to persons with leukemia who have not received chemotherapy for at least 3 months.
- If a person has been receiving high-dose corticosteroids or have had a course lasting longer than 2 weeks, then at least 1 month should pass before immunization with live virus vaccines.
- Responses to live and killed vaccines generally are suboptimal for HIV-infected patients and decrease as the disease progresses.
- General contraindications to vaccine administration include a history of anaphylactic reaction to a previous dose or an unexplained encephalopathy occurring within 7 days of a dose of pertussis vaccine. Immunosuppression and pregnancy are temporary contraindications to live vaccines.

TABLE 49–1. Childhood Immunization Schedule (2004)

Vaccine ▲ / Age ▲	Birth	1 months	2 months	4 months	6 months	12 months	15 months	18 months	24 months	4–6 yr	11–12 yr	13–18 yr
Hepatitis B[1]	HepB #1	only if mother HBsAg (–) — HepB #2			HepB #3						HepB series	
Diphtheria, Tetanus, Pertussis[2]			DTaP	DTaP	DTaP		DTaP			DTaP	Td	Td
Hemophilus Influenzae type b[3]			Hib	Hib	Hib[3]	Hib						
Inactivated poliovirus			IPV	IPV	IPV	IPV				IPV		
Measles, Mumps, Rubella[4]						MMR #1				MMR #2	MMR #2	
Varicella[5]						Varicella				Varicella		
Pneumococcal[6]			PCV	PCV	PCV	PCV			PCV	PPV		
Influenza[8]					Influenza (yearly)							

Vaccines below this line are for selected populations

| Hepatitis A[7] | | | | | | | | | Hepatitis A series | | | |

TABLE 49–1. (Continued)

This schedule indicates the recommended ages for routine administration of currently licensed childhood vaccines, as of December 1, 2003, for children through age 18 years. Any dose not given at the recommended age should be given at any subsequent visit when indicated and feasible. ☐ Indicates age groups that warrant special effort to administer those vaccines not previously given. Additional vaccines may be licensed and recommended during the year. Licensed combination vaccines may be used whenever any components of the combination are indicated and the vaccine's other components are not contraindicated. Providers should consult the manufacturers' package inserts for detailed recommendations. Clinically significant adverse events that follow immunization should be reported to the Vaccine Adverse Event Reporting System (VAERS). Guidance about how to obtain and complete a VAERS form can be found on the Internet: *http://www.vaers.org/* or by calling 1-800-822-7967.

1. Hepatitis B (HepB) vaccine. All infants should receive the first dose of hepatitis B vaccine soon after birth and before hospital discharge; the first dose may also be given by age 2 months if the infant's mother is hepatitis B surface antigen (HBsAg) negative. Only monovalent HepB can be used for the birth dose. Monovalent or combination vaccine containing HepB may be used to complete the series. Four doses of vaccine may be administered when a birth dose is given. The second dose should be given at least 4 weeks after the first dose, except for combination vaccines, which cannot be administered before age 6 weeks. The third dose should be given at least 16 weeks after the first dose and at least 8 weeks after the second dose. The last dose in the vaccination series (third of fourth dose) should not be administered before age 24 weeks.

Infants born to HBsAg-positive mothers should receive HepB and 0.5 mL of Hepatitis B Immune Globulin (HBIG) within 12 hours of birth at separate sites. The second dose is recommended at age 1 to 2 months. The last dose in the immunization series should not be administered before age 24 weeks. These infants should be tested for HBsAg and antibody to HBsAg (anti-HBs) at age 9 to 15 months.

Infants born to mothers whose HBsAg status is unknown should receive the first dose of the HepB series within 12 hours of birth. Maternal blood should be drawn as soon as possible to determine the mother's HBsAg status; if the HBsAg test is positive, the infant should receive HBIG as soon as possible (no later than age 1 week). The second dose is recommended at age 1 or 2 months. The last dose in the immunization series should not be administered before age 24 weeks.

2. Diphtheria and tetanus toxoids and acellular pertussis (DTaP) vaccine. The fourth dose of DTaP may be administered as early as age 12 months, provided 6 months have elapsed since the third dose and the child is unlikely to return at age 15 to 18 months. The final dose in the series should be given at age ≥4 years. **Tetanus and diphtheria toxoids (Td)** is recommended at age 11 to 12 years if at least 5 years have elapsed since the last dose of tetanus and diphtheria toxoid–containing vaccine. Subsequent routine Td boosters are recommended every 10 years.

3. *Haemophilus influenzae* type b (Hib) conjugate vaccine. Three Hib conjugate vaccines are licensed for infant use. If PRP-OMP (PedvaxHIB or ComVax [Merck]) is administered at ages 2 and 4 months, a dose at age 6 months is not required. DTaP/Hib combination products should not be used for primary immunization in infants at ages 2, 4, or 6 months but can be used as boosters following any Hib vaccine. The final dose in the series should be given at age ≥12 months.

4. Measles, mumps, and rubella vaccine (MMR). The second dose of MMR is recommended routinely at age 4 to 6 years but may be administered during any visit, provided at least 4 weeks have elapsed since the first dose and both doses are administered beginning at or after age 12 months. Those who have not previously received the second dose should complete the schedule by the 11- to 12-year-old visit.

5. Varicella vaccine. Varicella vaccine is recommended at any visit at or after age 12 months for susceptible children (i.e., those who lack a reliable history of chickenpox). Susceptible persons age ≥13 years should receive 2 doses, given at least 4 weeks apart.

6. Pneumococcal vaccine. The heptavalent **pneumococcal conjugate vaccine (PCV)** is recommended for all children age 2 to 23 months. It is also recommended for certain children age 24 to 59 months. The final dose in the series should be given at age ≥12 months.

Pneumococcal polysaccharide vaccine (PPV) is recommended in addition to PCV for certain high-risk groups. See *MMWR* 2000;49(RR-9):1–38.

7. Hepatitis A vaccine. Hepatitis A vaccine is recommended for children and adolescents in selected states and regions and for certain high-risk groups; consult your local public health authority. Children and adolescents in these states, regions, and high-risk groups who have not been immunized against hepatitis A can begin the hepatitis A immunization series during any visit. The 2 doses in the series should be administered at least 6 months apart. See *MMWR* 1999;48(RR-12):1–37.

8. Influenza vaccine. Influenza vaccine is recommended annually for children age ≥6 months with certain risk factors (including but not limited to children with asthma, cardiac disease, sickle cell disease, human immunodeficiency virus infection, and diabetes; and household members of persons in high-risk groups [see *MMWR* 2003;52(RR-8):1–36]) and can be administered to all others wishing to obtain immunity. In addition, healthy children age 6 to 23 months are encouraged to receive influenza vaccine if feasible, because children in this age group are at substantially increased risk of influenza-related hospitalizations. For healthy persons age 5 to 49 years, the intranasally administered live-attenuated influenza vaccine (LAIV) is an acceptable alternative to the intramuscular trivalent inactivated influenza vaccine (TIV). See *MMWR* 2003;52(RR-13):1–8. Children receiving TIV should be administered a dosage appropriate for their age (0.25 mL if age 6 to 35 months or 0.5 mL if age ≥3 years). Children age ≤8 years who are receiving influenza vaccine for the first time should receive 2 doses (separated by at least 4 weeks for TIV and at least 6 weeks for LAIV).

Adapted from material approved by the Advisory Committee on Immunization Practices (www.cdc.gov/nip/acip), the American Committee of Pediatrics (www.aap.org), and the American Academy of Family Physicians (www.aafp.org).

TABLE 49–2. Adult Immunization Schedual (2004)

	by Medical Conditions						
Vaccine ▶ **Medical Conditions ▼**	Tetanus-Diphtheria (Td)[a,1]	Influenza[2]	Pneumo-coccal (polysacch-aride)[3,4]	Hepatitis B[a,5]	Hepatitis A[6]	Measles, Mumps, Rubella (MMR)[a,7]	Varicella[a,8]
Pregnancy	A						
Diabetes, heart disease, chronic pulmonary disease, chronic liver disease, including chronic alcoholism	B	C			D		
Congenital Immunodeficiency, leukemia, lymphoma, generalized malignancy, therapy with alkylating agents, antimetabolites, radiation or large amounts of corticosteroids		E					F
Renal failure / end-stage renal disease, recipients of hemodialysis or clotting factor concentrates		E	G				
Asplenia including elective splenectomy and terminal complement component deficiencies	H	E, I, J					
HIV infection		E, K				L	

▨ For all persons in this group	▨ Catch-up on childhood vaccinations	▨ For persons with medical / exposure indications	▨ Contraindicated

Special Notes for Medical Conditions

A. For women, vaccinate if pregnancy will be during influenza season. For women with chronic deseases/conditions, vaccinate at any time during the pregnancy.

B. Although chronic liver disease and alcoholism are not indicator conditions for influenza vaccination, give 1 dose annually if the patient is ≥50 years, has other indications for influenza vaccine, or if the patient requests vaccination.

C. Asthma is an indicator condition for influenza but not for pneumococcal vaccination.

D. For all persons with chronic liver disease.

E. For persons <65 years, revaccinate once after 5 years or more have elapsed since initial vaccination.

F. Persons with impaired humoral immunity but intact cellular immunity may be vaccinated. *MMWR* 1999;48 (RR-06): 1–5.

G. Hemodialysis patients: Use special formulation of vaccine (40 ug/mL) or two 1-mL 20-ug doses given at one site. Vaccinate early in the course of renal disease. Assess antibody titers to hepatitis B surface antigen (anti-HBs) levels annually. Administer additional doses if anti-HBs levels decline to <10 milliinternational units (mIU)/ mL.

H. There are no data specifically on risk of severe or complicated influenza infections among persons with asplenia. However, influenza is a risk factor for secondary bacterial infections that may cause severe disease in asplenics.

I. Administer meningococcal vaccine and consider Hib vaccine.

J. Elective splenectomy: vaccinate at least 2 weeks before surgery.

K. Vaccinate as close to diagnosis as possible when CD4 cell counts are highest.

L. Withhold MMR or other measles containing vaccines from HIV-infected persons with evidence of severe immunosuppression. *MMWR* 1998;47 (RR-8):21–22; *MMWR* 2002;51 (RR-02): 22–24.

[a]Covered by the Vaccine Injury Compensation Program.

This schedule indicates the recommended age groups for routine administration of currently licensed vaccines for persons 19 years of age and older. Licensed combination vaccines may be used whenever any components of the combination are indicated and the vaccine's other components are not contraindicated. Providers should consult the manufacturers' package inserts for detailed recommendations.

(Continued)

TABLE 49–2. (Continued)

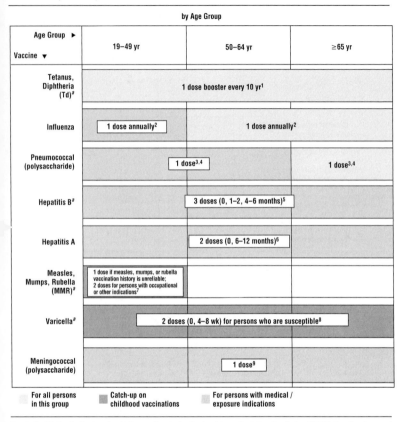

	by Age Group		
Age Group ▶ Vaccine ▼	19–49 yr	50–64 yr	≥65 yr
Tetanus, Diphtheria (Td)[a]	1 dose booster every 10 yr[1]		
Influenza	1 dose annually[2]	1 dose annually[2]	
Pneumococcal (polysaccharide)		1 dose[3,4]	1 dose[3,4]
Hepatitis B[a]	3 doses (0, 1–2, 4–6 months)[5]		
Hepatitis A	2 doses (0, 6–12 months)[6]		
Measles, Mumps, Rubella (MMR)[a]	1 dose if measles, mumps, or rubella vaccination history is unreliable; 2 doses for persons with occupational or other indications[7]		
Varicella[a]	2 doses (0, 4–8 wk) for persons who are susceptible[8]		
Meningococcal (polysaccharide)		1 dose[9]	

▨ For all persons in this group	▨ Catch-up on childhood vaccinations	▨ For persons with medical / exposure indications

Report all clinically significant postvaccination reactions to the Vaccine Adverse Event Reporting System (VAERS). Reporting forms and instructions on filing a VAERS report are available by calling 800-822-7967 or from the VAERS Web site at *www.vaers.org*.

For additional information about the vaccines listed above and contraindications for immunization, visit the National Immunization Program Web site at *www.cdc.gov/nip/* or call the National Immunization Hotline at 800-232-2522 (English) or 800-232-0233 (Spanish).

1. **Tetanus and diphtheria (Td)**. Adults including pregnant women with uncertain histories of a complete primary vaccination series should receive a primary series of Td. A primary series for adults is 3 doses: the first 2 doses given at least 4 weeks apart and the 3rd dose, 6–12 months after the second. Administer 1 dose if the person had received the primary series and the last vaccination was 10 years ago or longer. Consult *MMWR* 1991; 40 (RR-10): 1–21 for administering Td as prophylaxis in wound management. The ACP Task Force on Adult Immunization supports a second option for Td use in adults: a single Td booster at age 50 years for persons who have completed the full pediatric series, including the teenage/young adult booster. *Guide for Adult Immunization*. 3rd ed. ACP 1994: 20.

2. **Influenza vaccination**. Medical indications: chronic disorders of the cardiovascular or pulmonary systems including asthma; chronic metabolic diseases including diabetes mellitus, renal dysfunction, hemoglobinopathies, or immunosuppression (including immunosuppression caused by medications or by human immunodeficiency virus [HIV]), requiring regular medical follow-up or hospitalization during the preceding year; women who will be pregnant during the influenza season. Occupational indications: health care workers. Other indications: residents of nursing homes and other long-term care facilities; persons likely to transmit influenza to persons at high-risk (in-home care givers to persons with medical indications, household contacts and out-of-home caregivers of children birth to 23 months of age, or children with asthma or other indicator conditions for influenza vaccination, household members and care givers of elderly and adults with high-risk conditions); and anyone who wishes to be vaccinated. For healthy persons aged 5–49 years without high risk conditions, either the inactivated vaccine or the intranasally administered influenza vaccine (Flumist) may be given. *MMWR* 2003;52 (RR-8):1–36; *MMWR* 2003;53 (RR-13): 1–8.

(Continued)

TABLE 49–2. (Continued)

3. **Pneumococcal polysaccharide vaccination**. Medical indications: chronic disorders of the pulmonary system (excluding asthma), cardiovascular diseases, diabetes mellitus, chronic liver diseases including liver disease as a result of alcohol abuse (e.g., cirrhosis), chronic renal failure or nephrotic syndrome, functional or anatomic asplenia (e.g., sickle cell disease or splenectomy), immunosuppressive conditions (e.g., congenital immunodeficiency, HIV infection, leukemia, lymphoma, multiple myeloma, Hodgkins disease, generalized malignancy, organ or bone marrow transplantation), chemotherapy with alkylating agents, anti-metabolites, or long-term systemic corticosteroids. Geographic/other indications: Alaskan Natives and certain American Indian populations. Other indications: residents of nursing homes and other long-term care facilities. *MMWR* 1997;46 (RR-8):1–24.

4. **Revaccination with pneumococcal polysaccharide vaccine**. One-time revaccination after 5 years for persons with chronic renal failure or nephrotic syndrome, functional or anatomic asplenia (e.g., sickle cell disease or splenectomy), immunosuppressive conditions (e.g., congenital immunodeficiency, HIV infection, leukemia, lymphoma, multiple myeloma, Hodgkin's disease, generalized malignancy, organ or bone marrow transplantation), chemotherapy with alkylating agents, anti-metabolites, or long-term systemic corticosteroids. For persons 65 and older, one-time revaccination if they were vaccinated 5 or more years previously and were aged less than 65 years at the time of primary vaccination. *MMWR* 1997;46 (RR-8):1–24.

5. **Hepatitis B vaccination**. Medical indications: hemodialysis patients, patients who receive clotting-factor concentrates. Occupational indications: health care workers and public safety workers who have exposure to blood in the workplace, persons in training in schools of medicine, dentistry, nursing, laboratory technology, and other allied health professions. Behavioral indications: injecting drug users, persons with more than one sex partner in the previous 6 months, persons with a recently acquired sexually-transmitted disease (STD), all clients in STD clinics, men who have sex with men. Other indications: household contacts and sex partners of persons with chronic HBV infection, clients and staff of institutions for the developmentally disabled, international travelers who will be in countries with high or intermediate prevalence of chronic HBV infection for more than 6 months, inmates of correctional facilities. *MMWR* 1991;40 (RR-13):1–19.

6. **Hepatitis A vaccination**. For the combined HepA-HepB vaccine use 3 doses at 0, 1, and 6 months). Medical indications: persons with clotting-factor disorders or chronic liver disease. Behavioral indications: men who have sex with men, users of injecting and noninjecting illegal drugs. Occupational indications: persons working with HAV-infected primates or with HAV in a research laboratory setting. Other indications: persons traveling to or working in countries that have high or intermediate endemicity of hepatitis A. *MMWR* 1999;48 (RR-12):1–37.

7. **Measles, Mumps, and Rubella vaccination (MMR)**. Measles component: Adults born before 1957 may be considered immune to measles. Adults born in or after 1957 should receive at least dose of MMR unless they have a medical contraindication, documentation of at least one dose or other acceptable evidence of immunity. A second dose of MMR is recommended for adults who

- are recently exposed to measles or in an outbreak setting
- were previously vaccinated with killed measles vaccine
- were vaccinated with an unknown vaccine between 1963 and 1967
- are students in post-secondary educational institutions
- work in health care facilities
- plan to travel internationally

Mumps component: 1 dose of MMR should be adequate for protection. Rubella component: Give 1 dose of MMR to women whose rubella vaccination history is unreliable and counsel women to avoid becoming pregnant for 4 weeks after vaccination. For women of child-bearing age, regardless of birth year, routinely determine rubella immunity and counsel women regarding congenital rubella syndrome. Do not vaccinate pregnant women or those planning to become pregnant in the next 4 weeks. If pregnant and susceptible, vaccinate as early in postpartum period as possible. *MMWR* 1998;47 (RR-8): 1–57; *MMWR* 2001;50:1117.

8. **Varicella vaccination**. Recommended for all persons who do not have reliable clinical history of varicella infection, or serological evidence of varicella zoster virus (VZV) infection who may be at high risk for exposure or transmission. This includes, health-care workers and family contacts of immunocompromised persons, those who live or work in environments where transmission is likely (e.g., teachers of young children, day care employees, and residents and staff members in institutional settings), persons who live or work in environments where VZV transmission can occur (e.g., college students, inmates and staff members of correctional institutions, and military personnel), adolescents and adults living in households with children,women who are not pregnant but who may become pregnant in the future, international travelers who are not immune to infection. *Note:* Greater than 95% of U.S. born adults are immune to VZV. Do not vaccinate pregnant women or those planning to become pregnant in the next 4 weeks. If pregnant and susceptible, vaccinate as early in postpartum period as possible. *MMWR* 1996; 45 (RR-11): 1–36;*MMWR* 1999;48 (RR-6):1–5.

9. **Meningococcal vaccine (quadrivalent polysaccharide for serogroups A, C, Y, and W-135)**. Consider vaccination for persons with medical indications: adults with terminal complement component deficiencies, with anatomic or functional asplenia. Other indications: travelers to countries in which disease is hyperendemic or epidemic ("meningitis belt" of sub-Saharan Africa, Mecca, Saudi Arabia for Hajj). Revaccination at 3–5 years may be indicated for persons at high risk for infection (e.g., persons residing in areas in which disease is epidemic). Counsel college freshmen, especially those who live in dormitories, regarding meningococcal disease and the vaccine so that they can make an educated decision about receiving the vaccination. *MMWR* 2000;49 (RR-7): 1–20. *Note:* The AAFP recommends that colleges should take the lead on providing education on meningococcal infection and vaccination and offer it to those who are interested. Physicians need not initiate discussion of the meningococcal quadrivalent polysaccharide vaccine as part of routine medical care.

Adapted from material approved by the Advisory Committee on Immunization Practices (ACIP), and accepted by the American College of Obstetricians and Gynecologists (ACOG) and the American Academy of Family Physicians (AAFP)

▶ DIPHTHERIA TOXOID ADSORBED (DTA) AND DIPHTHERIA ANTITOXIN (DA)

- Two strengths of diphtheria toxoid are available (pediatric [D] and adult [d], which contains less antigen). Primary immunization with DTA is indicated for children less than 6 weeks of age. Generally, DTA is given along with acellular pertussis and tetanus vaccines (DTaP) at 2, 4, and 6 months of age, and then at 15 to 18 months and 4 to 6 years of age.
- For nonimmunized adults, a complete three-dose series of diphtheria toxoid should be administered, with the first two doses given at least 4 weeks apart and the third dose given 6 to 12 months after the second. The combined preparation, Td, is recommended in adults because it contains less diphtheria toxoid than DTaP, with fewer reactions seen from the diphtheria preparation. Booster doses are given every 10 years.
- DA is a sterile diphtheria antitoxin derived from hyperimmunized horses and is indicated for immediate use in patients with diphtheria. Sensitivity testing by performing an intradermal or scratch test and a conjunctival test should be performed before administration.
- The usual dose of DA is 20,000 to 40,000 units for pharyngeal disease, 40,000 to 60,000 units for nasopharyngeal lesions, and 80,000 to 120,000 units for extensive disease of 3 or more days.

VIII

▶ TETANUS TOXOID (TT), TETANUS TOXOID ADSORBED (TTA), AND TETANUS IMMUNE GLOBULIN (TIG)

- In children, primary immunization against tetanus is usually done in conjunction with diphtheria and pertussis vaccination using DTaP or a combination vaccine that includes hepatitis B and polio vaccines. A 0.5-mL dose is recommended at 2, 4, 6, and 15 to 18 months of age.
- Additional doses of tetanus toxoid are recommended as part of traumatic wound management if a patient has not received a dose of tetanus toxoid within the preceding 5 years (Table 49–3).
- In adults or children older than 7 years of age where primary immunization against tetanus alone is needed, a series of three doses of Td is administered intramuscularly; the initial dose is followed by a repeat dose in 1 to 2 months, then the third at 6 to 12 months after the first dose. Boosters are recommended every 10 years.
- Tetanus toxoid may be given to immunosuppressed patients if indicated.
- TIG is used to provide passive tetanus immunization following the occurrence of traumatic wounds in nonimmunized or suboptimally immunized persons (see Table 49–3). A dose of 250 to 500 units is administered intramuscularly. When administered with tetanus toxoid, separate sites for administration should be used.

TABLE 49–3. Tetanus Prophylaxis

	Clean, Minor		All Other	
Vaccination history	Td	TIG	Td	TIG
Unknown or <3 doses	Yes	No	Yes	Yes
≥3 doses	No[a]	No	No[b]	No

[a] Yes if >10 yr since last dose.
[b] Yes if >5 yr since last dose.

TABLE 49–4. *H. influenzae* Type b Conjugate Vaccine Products

Vaccine	Trade Name	Protein Carrier
HbOC	HibTITER (Wyeth Vaccines)	Mutant diphtheria toxin protein
PRP-T	ActHIB (Aventis Pasteur)	Tetanus toxoid
PRP-OMP	PedvaxHIB (Merck)	*Neisseria meningitides* serogroup B outer membrane protein

Note: The polysaccharide is polyribosyl-ribitol-phosphate (PRP).

- TIG is also used for the treatment of tetanus. In this setting, a single dose of 3000 to 6000 units is administered intramuscularly.

▶ HAEMOPHILUS INFLUENZAE TYPE b (HIB) VACCINES

- Hib vaccines currently in use are conjugate products, consisting of either a polysaccharide or oligosaccharide of polyribosylribitol phosphate (PRP) covalently linked to a protein carrier.
- Hib conjugate vaccines are indicated for routine use in all infants and children less than 5 years of age.
- The primary series of Hib vaccination consists of 0.5-mL IM doses at 2, 4, and 6 months of age (for HibTITER [HbOC] and ActHIB [PRP-T]) or doses at 2 and 4 months if PRP-OMP is used (Table 49–4). A booster dose is recommended at age 12 to 15 months.
- For infants aged 7 to 11 months who have not been vaccinated, three doses of HbOC, PRP-OMP, and PRP-T should be given: two doses, spaced 4 weeks apart, and then a booster dose at age 12 to 15 months (but at least 8 weeks since dose 2). For unvaccinated children aged 12 to 14 months, two doses should be given, with an interval of 2 months between them. In a child older than 15 months, a single dose of any of the four conjugate vaccines is indicated.

VIII

▶ HEPATITIS VACCINES

Information on hepatitis vaccines can be found in Chapter 24.

▶ INFLUENZA VIRUS VACCINE

- Annual influenza vaccination is strongly recommended for individuals over the age of 6 months with chronic medical conditions that make them at increased risk for the complications of influenza. Indications for annual influenza vaccination are as follows:
  - All individuals 50 years of age and older
  - Residents of nursing homes
  - Adults and children with chronic cardiovascular or pulmonary diseases including asthma
  - Adults and children with chronic metabolic disease, renal dysfunction, hemoglobinopathies, or immunosuppression (including immunosuppression from drugs or HIV)
  - Children and teenagers receiving chronic aspirin therapy
  - Pregnant women
  - Health care workers
  - Employees of residential care facilities for high-risk patients
  - Household members of persons in high-risk groups.

- Individuals who should not be vaccinated are those with anaphylactic hypersensitivity to eggs or other components of the vaccine or adults with febrile illness (until the fever abates).

▶ MEASLES VACCINE

- Measles vaccine is a live attenuated vaccine that is administered for primary immunization to persons 12 to 15 months of age or older, usually as a combination of measles, mumps, and rubella (MMR). A second dose is recommended at 4 to 6 years of age.
- The vaccine should not be given to immunosuppressed patients (except those infected with HIV) or pregnant women.
- The vaccine should not be given within 1 month of any other live vaccine unless the vaccine is given on the same day (as with the MMR vaccine).
- Measles vaccine is indicated in all persons born after 1956 or in those who lack documentation of wild virus infection either by history or antibody titers.
- For postexposure prophylaxis, the vaccine is effective if given within 72 hours of exposure. In addition, immune globulin may be administered intramuscularly at a dose of 0.25 mg/kg (maximum dose 15 mL), if given within 6 days of exposure.

▶ MENINGOCOCCAL POLYSACCHARIDE VACCINE (MPV)

- MPV is indicated in high-risk populations such as those exposed to the disease, those in the midst of uncontrolled outbreaks, travelers to an area with epidemic hyperendemic meningococcal disease, or individuals who have terminal complement deficiencies or asplenia.
- The vaccine should be made available to students starting college who wish to decrease their risk for meningococcal disease.
- The vaccine is administered subcutaneously as a single 0.5-mL dose.

▶ MUMPS VACCINE

- The vaccine (usually given in conjunction with measles and rubella, MMR) is given beginning at age 12 to 15 months, with a second dose prior to entry into elementary school. If the vaccine is given before 12 months of age, revaccination is necessary and should be given after reaching 1 year of age.
- The vaccine is also indicated in previously unvaccinated adults and in those in whom a poor history of wild virus infection or previous administration of killed mumps exists.
- Postexposure vaccination is of no benefit.
- Mumps vaccine should not be given to pregnant women or immunosuppressed patients. The vaccine should not be given within 6 weeks (preferably 3 months) of administration of immune globulin.

▶ PERTUSSIS VACCINE

- Acellular pertussis vaccine is usually administered in combination with diphtheria and tetanus toxoids (as DTaP).
- The primary immunization series for pertussis vaccine consists of four doses given at ages 2, 4, 6, and 15 to 18 months. A booster dose is recommended at age 4 to 6 years.

- Systemic reactions, such as moderate fever, occur in 3% to 5% of those receiving vaccines. Very rarely, high fever, febrile seizures, persistent crying spells, and hypotonic hyporesponsive episodes occur after vaccination.
- There are only two absolute contraindications to pertussis administration: an immediate anaphylactic reaction to a previous dose or encephalopathy within 7 days of a previous dose, with no evidence of other cause.

▶ PNEUMOCOCCAL VACCINE

- Pneumococcal vaccine is a mixture of capsular polysaccharides from 23 of the 83 most prevalent types of *Streptococcus pneumoniae* seen in the United States.
- Pneumococcal vaccine is recommended for the following immunocompetent persons:
  - Persons 65 or more years of age. If an individual received vaccine more than 5 years earlier and was under age 65 at the time of administration, revaccination should be given.
  - Persons aged 2 to 64 years with chronic illness.
  - Persons aged 2 to 64 years with functional or anatomic asplenia. When splenectomy is planned, pneumococcal vaccine should be given at least 2 weeks prior to surgery.
  - Persons aged 2 to 64 years living in environments where the risk of invasive pneumococcal disease or its complications is increased. This does not include daycare center employees and children.
- Pneumococcal vaccination is recommended for immunocompromised persons 2 years of age or older with
  - HIV infection
  - leukemia, lymphoma, Hodgkin's disease, or multiple myeloma
  - generalized malignancy
  - chronic renal failure of nephritic syndrome

and patients receiving

  - immunosuppressive therapy
  - organ or bone marrow transplant

- A single revaccination should be given if 5 or more years have passed since the first dose in persons older than 10 years. In those who are 10 years or younger, revaccination should be given 3 years after the previous dose.
- Because children less than 2 years of age do not respond adequately to the pneumococcal polysaccharide vaccine, a heptavalent pneumococcal conjugate vaccine was created that can be administered at 2, 4, and 6 months of age and between 12 and 15 months of age.

▶ POLIOVIRUS VACCINES

- Two types of trivalent poliovirus vaccines are currently licensed for distribution in the United States: an enhanced inactivated vaccine (IPV) and a live attenuated, oral vaccine (OPV). IPV is the recommended vaccine for the primary series and booster dose for children in the United States, whereas OPV is recommended in areas of the world that have circulating poliovirus.
- IPV is given to children aged 2, 4, and 6 to 18 months and 4 to 6 years. Primary poliomyelitis immunization is recommended for all children and young adults

VIII

up to age 18 years. Allergies to any component of IPV, including streptomycin, polymixin B, and neomycin, are contraindications to vaccine use.

- OPV is not recommended for persons who are immunodeficient or for normal individuals who reside in a household where another person is immunodeficient. OPV should not be given during pregnancy because of the small but theoretical risk to the fetus.

▶ RUBELLA VACCINE

- The vaccine is given with measles and mumps vaccines (MMR) at 12 to 15 months of age, then at 4 to 6 years.
- The vaccine should not be given to immunosuppressed individuals, although MMR vaccine should be administered to young children with HIV without severe immunosuppression as soon as possible after their first birthday. The vaccine should not be given to individuals with anaphylactic reaction to neomycin.
- Although the vaccine has not been associated with congenital rubella syndrome, its use in pregnancy is contraindicated. Women should be counseled not to become pregnant for 4 weeks following vaccination.

VIII

▶ VARICELLA VACCINE

- Varicella virus vaccine is recommended for all children 12 to 18 months of age and for persons above this age if they have not had chickenpox. Persons aged 13 years and older should receive two doses separated by 4 to 8 weeks.
- The vaccine is contraindicated in immunosuppressed or pregnant patients.
- Children with asymptomatic or mildly symptomatic HIV should receive two doses of varicella vaccine 3 months apart.

▶ VARICELLA-ZOSTER IMMUNE GLOBULIN

- Varicella-zoster immune globulin (VZIG) is used for passive immunization of susceptible immunodeficient patients exposed to varicella-zoster (VZ) infection.
- Use of VZIG should be considered in exposed children and certain adults who are immunocompromised and susceptible to VZ. Conditions warranting consideration of VZIG after VZ virus exposure are as follows:
  - Children with primary or acquired immunodeficiency, neoplastic disease, or who require immunosuppressive therapy
  - Neonates whose mothers develop varicella within 5 days before or 2 days after delivery
  - Preterm infants (less than 28 weeks' gestation or who weigh less than 1000 g) who are exposed to varicella while hospitalized
  - Susceptible pregnant women
  - Immunosuppressed adults and adolescents
- For maximum effectiveness, VZIG must be given within 48 hours and not more than 96 hours following exposure.
- Administration of VZIG is by the intramuscular route (never intravenously).

▶ IMMUNE GLOBULIN

- Immune globulin (IG) is available as both intramuscular (IGIM) and intravenous (IGIV) preparations.

TABLE 49–5. Indications and Dosage of Intramuscular Immune Globulin in Infectious Diseases

Primary immunodeficiency states	1.2 mL/kg IM, then 0.6 mL/kg every 2–4 wk
Hepatitis A exposure	0.02 mL/kg IM within 2 wk
Hepatitis A prophylaxis	0.02 mL/kg IM for exposure <3 months' duration
	0.06 mL/kg IM for exposure up to 5 months' duration
Hepatitis B exposure	0.06 mL/kg (HBIG preferred in known exposures)
Measles exposure	0.25 mL/kg (maximum dose 15 mL) as soon as possible
	0.5 mL/kg (maximum dose 15 mL) as soon as possible for immunocompromised individuals
Varicella exposure	0.6–1.2 mL/kg as soon as possible when VZIG not available

- Table 49–5 lists the suggested dosages for IGIM in various disease states.
- The uses for IVIG are as follows:
  - Primary immunodeficiency states including both antibody deficiencies and combined deficiencies
  - Idiopathic thrombocytopenic purpura (ITP)
  - Chronic lymphocytic leukemia (CLL) in patients who have had a serious bacterial infection   VIII ◄
  - Kawasaki disease (mucocutaneous lymph node syndrome)
  - Bone marrow transplant
  - Varicella-zoster

▶ Rho(D) IMMUNE GLOBULIN (RDIg)

- RDIg suppresses the antibody response and formation of anti-Rho(D) in Rho(D)-negative, D^u-negative women exposed to Rho(D)-positive blood and prevents the future chance of erythroblastosis fetalis in subsequent pregnancies with a Rho(D)-positive fetus.
- RDIg, when administered within 72 hours of delivery of a full-term infant, reduces active antibody formation from 12% to between 1 and 2%.
- RDIg is also used in the case of a premenopausal woman who is Rho(D) negative and has inadvertently received Rho(D)-positive blood or blood products.
- RDIg may be used after abortion, miscarriage, amniocentesis, or abdominal trauma.
- RDIg is administered intramuscularly only.

See Chapter 122, Vaccines, Toxoids, and Other Immunobiologics, authored by Mary S. Hayney, for a more detailed discussion of this topic.

Neurologic Disorders
Edited by Barbara G. Wells

Chapter 50 _____

▶ EPILEPSY

▶ DEFINITIONS

Epilepsy implies a periodic recurrence of seizures with or without convulsions. A seizure results from an excessive discharge of cortical neurons and is characterized by changes in electrical activity as measured by the electroencephalogram (EEG). A convulsion implies violent, involuntary contraction(s) of the voluntary muscles.

▶ PATHOPHYSIOLOGY

- A seizure is traceable to an unstable cell membrane or its surrounding cells. Excess excitability spreads either locally (focal seizure) or more widely (generalized seizure).
- An abnormality of potassium conductance, a defect in the voltage-sensitive calcium channels, or a deficiency in the membrane adenosine triphosphatase (ATPase) linked to ion transport may result in neuronal membrane instability and a seizure.
- Normal neuronal activity depends on normal functioning of excitatory (e.g., glutamate, aspartate, acetylcholine, norepinephrine, histamine, corticotropin-releasing factor, purines, peptides, cytokines, and steroid hormones) and inhibitory (e.g., dopamine, γ-aminobutyric acid [GABA]) neurotransmitters; an adequate supply of glucose, oxygen, sodium, potassium, chloride, calcium, and amino acids; normal pH; and normal receptor function.
- Prolonged seizures, continued exposure to glutamate, large numbers of generalized tonic-clonic (GTC) seizures (greater than 100), and multiple episodes of status epilepticus may be associated with neuronal damage.

▶ CLINICAL PRESENTATION

GENERAL

- In most cases, the health care provider will not be in a position to witness a seizure. Many patients (particularly those with complex partial or generalized tonic-clonic seizures) are amnestic to the actual seizure event. Obtaining an adequate history and description of the ictal event (including time course) from a third party (e.g., significant other, family member, or witness) is critically important.

SYMPTOMS

- Symptoms of a specific seizure will depend on seizure type. While seizures can vary between patients, they tend to be stereotyped within an individual.

  - Complex partial seizures may include somatosensory or focal motor features.
  - Complex partial seizures are associated with altered conciousness.
  - Absence seizures may appear relatively bland, with only very brief (seconds) periods of altered conciousness.

- Generalized tonic-clonic seizures are major convulsive episodes and are always associated with a loss of conciousness.

SIGNS

- Interictally (between seizure episodes), there are typically no objective, pathognomonic signs of epilepsy.

LABORATORY TESTS

- There are currently no diagnostic laboratory tests for epilepsy. In some cases, particularly following generalized tonic-clonic (or perhaps complex partial) seizures, serum prolactin levels may be transiently elevated. Laboratory tests may be done to rule out treatable causes of seizures (e.g., hypoglycemia, altered electrolyte concentrations, infections, etc.) that do not represent epilepsy.

OTHER DIAGNOSTIC TESTS

- EEG is very useful in the diagnosis of various seizure disorders.
- The EEG may be normal in some patients who still have the clinical diagnosis of epilepsy.
- While MRI is very useful (especially imaging of the temporal lobes), CT scan typically is not helpful except in the initial evaluation for a brain tumor or cerebral bleeding.
- The International Classification of Epileptic Seizures (Table 50–1) classifies epilepsy on the basis of clinical description and electrophysiologic findings.
- Partial seizures begin in one hemisphere of the brain and, unless they become secondarily generalized, result in an asymmetric seizure. Partial seizures manifest as alterations in motor functions, sensory or somatosensory symptoms, or automatisms. If there is no loss of consciousness, the seizures are called simple partial. If there is loss of consciousness, they are termed complex partial, and the patients may have automatisms, memory loss, or aberrations of behavior.

IX

TABLE 50–1. International Classification of Epileptic Seizures

I. Partial seizures (seizures begin locally)
   A. Simple (without impairment of consciousness)
      1. With motor symptoms
      2. With special sensory or somatosensory symptoms
      3. With psychic symptoms
   B. Complex (with impairment of consciousness)
      1. Simple partial onset followed by impairment of consciousness—with or without automatisms
      2. Impaired consciousness at onset—with or without automatisms
   C. Secondarily generalized (partial onset evolving to generalized tonic-clonic seizures)
II. Generalized seizures (bilaterally symmetrical and without local onset)
   A. Absence
   B. Myoclonic
   C. Clonic
   D. Tonic
   E. Tonic-clonic
   F. Atonic
   G. Infantile spasms
III. Unclassified seizures
IV. Status epilepticus

- Absence seizures generally occur in young children or adolescents and exhibit a sudden onset, interruption of ongoing activities, a blank stare, and possibly a brief upward rotation of the eyes. Absence seizures have a characteristic 2–4 cycle/second spike and slow-wave EEG pattern.
- In generalized seizures, motor symptoms are bilateral, and there is altered consciousness.
- Generalized tonic-clonic seizures may be preceded by premonitory symptoms (i.e., an aura). A tonic-clonic seizure that is preceded by an aura is likely a partial seizure that is secondarily generalized. Tonic-clonic seizures begin with a short tonic contraction of muscles followed by a period of rigidity. The patient may lose sphincter control, bite the tongue, or become cyanotic. The episode may be followed by unconsciousness, and frequently the patient goes into a deep sleep.
- Myoclonic jerks are brief shock-like muscular contractions of the face, trunk, and extremities. They may be isolated events or rapidly repetitive.
- In atonic seizures, there is a sudden loss of muscle tone that may be described as a head drop, dropping of a limb, or slumping to the ground.

▶ DIAGNOSIS

- The patient and family should be asked to characterize the seizure for frequency, duration, precipitating factors, time of occurrence, presence of an aura, ictal activity, and postictal state.
- Physical, neurologic, and laboratory examination (SMA-20, complete blood cell count [CBC], urinalysis, and special blood chemistries) may identify an etiology. A lumbar puncture may be indicated if there is fever.

▶ DESIRED OUTCOME

The goal of treatment is to control or reduce the frequency of seizures and ensure compliance, allowing the patient to live as normal a life as possible. Complete suppression of seizures must be balanced against tolerability of side effects, and the patient should be involved in defining the balance.

▶ TREATMENT

GENERAL APPROACH

- The treatment of choice depends on the type of epilepsy (Table 50–2) and on drug-specific adverse effects and patient preferences. Figure 50–1 is a suggested algorithm for treatment of epilepsy.
- Begin with monotherapy; about 50% to 70% of patients can be maintained on one antiepileptic drug (AED), but all are not seizure free.
- Up to 60% of patients with epilepsy are noncompliant, and this is the most common reason for treatment failure.
- Drug therapy may not be indicated in patients who have had only one seizure or those whose seizures have minimal impact on their lives. Patients who have had two or more seizures should generally be started on AEDs.
- Factors favoring successful withdrawal of AEDs include a seizure-free period of 2 to 4 years, complete seizure control within 1 year of onset, an onset of seizures after age 2 and before age 35 years, and a normal EEG. Poor prognostic factors include a history of a high frequency of seizures, repeated episodes of status epilepticus, a combination of seizure types, and development of abnormal

TABLE 50–2. Drugs of Choice for Specific-Seizure Disorders

Seizure Type	First-Line Drugs	Alternative Drugs
Partial seizures	Carbamazepine Phenytoin Lamotrigine Valproic acid Oxcarbazepine	Gabapentin Topiramate Levetiracetam Zonisamide Tiagabine Primidone, phenobarbital Felbamate
Generalized seizures		
Absence	Valproic acid, ethosuximide	Lamotrigine, levetiracetam
Myoclonic	Valproic acid, clonazepam	Lamotrigine, topiramate, felbamate, zonisamide, levetiracetam
Tonic-clonic	Phenytoin, carbamazepine, valproic acid	Lamotrigine, topiramate, phenobarbital, primidone, oxcarbazepine, levetiracetam

mental functioning. A 2-year seizure-free period is suggested for absence and rolandic epilepsy, while a 4-year seizure-free period is suggested for simple partial, complex partial, and absence associated with tonic-clonic seizures. According to the American Academy of Neurology guidelines, discontinuation of AEDs may be considered if the patient is seizure free for 2 to 5 years, if there is a single type of partial seizure or single type of primary generalized tonic-clonic seizure, if the neurologic examination and IQ are normal, and if the EEG normalized with treatment. AED withdrawal should always be done gradually.

- Patient knowledge of epilepsy and treatment correlates with an improved quality of life.

MECHANISM OF ACTION

The mechanism of action of most AEDs includes effects on ion channels (sodium and calcium), inhibitory neurotransmission (GABA), or excitatory neurotransmission (glutamate and aspartate). AEDs that are effective against generalized tonic-clonic and partial seizures probably reduce sustained repetitive firing of action potentials by delaying recovery of sodium channels from activation. Drugs that reduce corticothalamic T-type calcium currents are effective against generalized absence seizures.

SPECIAL CONSIDERATIONS IN THE FEMALE PATIENT

- Enzyme-inducing AEDs, including topiramate and oxcarbazepine, may cause treatment failures in females taking **oral contraceptives**; a supplemental form of birth control is advised if breakthrough bleeding occurs.
- For catamenial epilepsy (seizures just before or during menses) or seizures that occur at the time of ovulation, conventional AEDs should be tried first, but hormonal therapy (**progestational agents**) may also be effective. Intermittent acetazolamide has also been used.
- About 25% to 30% of women have increased seizure frequency during pregnancy, and a similar percentage have decreased frequency.
- AED monotherapy is preferred in pregnancy. Clearance of **phenytoin, carbamazepine, phenobarbital, ethosuximide, lamotrigine,** and **clorazepate** increases during pregnancy, and protein binding may be altered. There is a higher incidence of adverse pregnancy outcomes in women with epilepsy, and the risk of congenital malformations is 4% to 6% (twice as high as

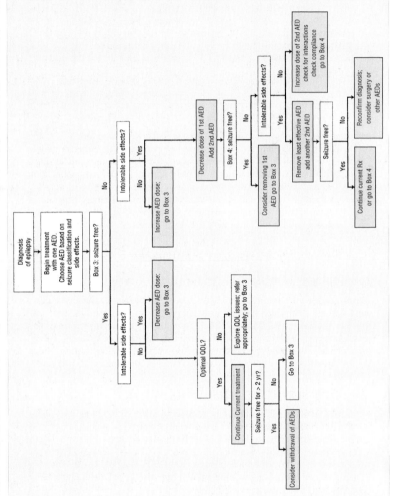

Figure 50-1 Algorithm for treatment of epilepsy. AED, antiepileptic drug; QOL, quality of life.

in nonepileptic women). Barbiturates and phenytoin are associated with congenital heart malformations and facial clefts. **Valproic acid** and **carbamazepine** are associated with spina bifida and hypospadias. Other adverse outcomes are growth, psychomotor, and mental retardation. Some of these events can be prevented by adequate **folate** intake; **prenatal vitamins with folic acid** (approximately 0.4 to 5 mg/day) should be given to women of childbearing potential who are taking AEDs. **Vitamin K**, 10 mg/day orally, given to the mother during the last month before delivery can prevent neonatal hemorrhagic disorder.

PHARMACOKINETICS

- AED pharmacokinetic data are summarized in Table 50–3. For populations known to have altered plasma protein binding, free rather than total serum concentrations should be measured if the AED is highly protein bound. Conditions altering AED protein binding include chronic renal failure, liver disease, hypoalbuminemia, burns, pregnancy, malnutrition, displacing drugs, and age (neonates and the elderly). Unbound concentration monitoring is especially useful for **phenytoin**.
- Neonates may metabolize drugs more slowly, and infants and children may metabolize drugs more rapidly than adults. Lower doses of AEDs are required in the elderly. Some elderly patients have increased receptor sensitivity to central nervous system (CNS) drugs, making the accepted therapeutic range invalid.

THE ROLE OF SERUM CONCENTRATION MONITORING

Seizure control may occur before the "minimum" of the accepted therapeutic serum range is reached, and some patients may need serum concentrations beyond the "maximum." The therapeutic range for AEDs may be different for different seizure types (e.g., higher for complex partial seizures than for tonic-clonic seizures).

EFFICACY

- The traditional treatment of tonic-clonic seizures is **phenytoin** or **phenobarbital**, but the use of **carbamazepine** and **valproic acid** is increasing, as efficacy is equal and side effects are more favorable.
- **Carbamazepine** and **valproic acid** had equal retention rates for tonic-clonic seizures, but carbamazepine was superior for partial seizures, and valproic acid caused more adverse effects.
- For a combination of absence and other generalized or partial seizures, **valproic acid** is preferred. If valproic acid is ineffective in treating a mixed seizure disorder that includes absence, **ethosuximide** should be used in combination with another AED.
- The newer AEDs were first approved as adjunctive therapy for patients with refractory partial seizures. To date, **lamotrigine** and **oxcarbazepine** have received Food and Drug Administration (FDA) approval for use in monotherapy in patients with partial seizures. **Felbamate** has monotherapy approval but causes some significant side effects.

ADVERSE EFFECTS

- Chronic and acute adverse effects of AEDs are listed in Table 50–4.
- When acute organ failure occurs, it usually happens within the first 6 months of AED therapy.

TABLE 50–3. Antiepileptic Drug Pharmacokinetic Data

AED	$t_{1/2}$ (h)[a]	Time to Steady State (days)	Unchanged (%)	V^D (l/kg)	Clinically Important Metabolite	Protein Binding (%)
Carbamazepine	12 M; 5–14 Co	21–28 for completion of auto-induction	<1	1–2	10,11-epoxide	40–90
Ethosuximide	A 60 C 30	6–12	10–20	0.67	No	0
Felbamate	16–22	5–7	50	0.73–0.82	No	~25
Gabapentin[b]	5–40[d]	1–2	100	0.65–1.04	No	0
Lamotrigine	25.4 M	3–15	0	1.28	No	40–50
Levetiracetam	7–10	2		0.7		<10%
Oxcarbazepine	3–13	2		0.7	10-Hydroxy-carbazepine	40%
Phenobarbital	A46–136 C37–73	14–21	20–40	0.6	No	50
Phenytoin	A10–34 C5–14	7–28	<5	0.6–8	No	90
Primidone	A3.3–19 C4.5–11	1–4	40	0.43–1.1	PB[c] PEMA[c]	80
Tiagabine	5–13		Negligible		No	95
Topiramate	18–21	4–5	50–70	0.55–0.8 (male) 0.23–0.4 (female)	No	15
Valproic acid	A8–20 C 7–14	1–3	<5	0.1–0.5	May contribute to toxicity	90–95 binding saturates
Zonisamide	24–60	5–15		0.8–1.6	No	40–60%

[a] A, adult; C, child; M, monotherapy; Co, combination therapy.
[b] The bioavailability of gabapentin is dose dependent.
[c] PB, phenobarbital; PEMA, phenylethylmalonamide.
[d] Half-life depends on renal function.

TABLE 50–4. Antiepileptic Drug Side Effects

AED	Acute Side Effects Concentration *Dependent*	*Idiosyncratic*	Chronic Side Effects
Carbamazepine	Diplopia Dizziness Drowsiness Nausea Unsteadiness Lethargy	Blood dyscrasias Rash	Hyponatremia
Ethosuximide	Ataxia Drowsiness GI distress Unsteadiness Hiccoughs	Blood dyscrasias Rash	Behavior changes Headache
Felbamate	Anorexia Nausea Vomiting Insomnia Headache	Aplastic anemia Acute hepatic failure	Not established
Gabapentin	Dizziness Fatigue Somnolence Ataxia	Pedal edema	Weight gain
Lamotrigine	Diplopia Dizziness Unsteadiness Headache	Rash	Not established
Levetiracetam	Sedation Behavioral disturbance	Not established	Not established
Oxcarbazepine	Sedation Dizziness Ataxia Nausea	Rash	Hyponatremia
Phenobarbital	Ataxia Hyperactivity Headache Unsteadiness Sedation Nausea	Blood dyscrasias Rash	Behavior changes Connective tissue disorders Intellectual blunting Metabolic bone disease Mood change Sedation
Phenytoin	Ataxia Nystagmus Behavior changes Dizziness Headache Incoordination Sedation Lethargy Cognitive impairment	Blood dyscrasias Rash Immunologic reaction	Behavior changes Cerebellar syndrome Connective tissue changes Skin thickening Folate deficiency Gingival hyperplasia Coarsening of facial features Acne

IX

Continued

TABLE 50–4. Continued

AED	Acute Side Effects Concentration *Dependent*	*Idiosyncratic*	Chronic Side Effects
	Fatigue		Cognitive impairment
	Visual blurring		Metabolic bone disease
			Sedation
Primidone	Behavior changes	Blood dyscrasias	Behavior change
	Headache	Rash	Connective tissue disorders
	Nausea		Cognitive impairment
	Sedation		Sedation
	Unsteadiness		
Tiagabine	Dizziness	Spike-wave stupor	Not established
	Fatigue		
	Difficulties concentrating		
	Nervousness		
	Tremor		
	Blurred vision		
	Depression		
	Weakness		
Topiramate	Difficulties concentrating	Metabolic acidosis	Kidney stones
	Psychomotor slowing	Acute angle glaucoma	Weight loss
	Speech or language problems	Oligohidrosis	
	Somnolence, fatigue		
	Dizziness		
	Headache		
Valproic acid	GI upset	Acute hepatic failure	Polycystic ovary-like syndrome(?)
	Sedation	Acute pancreatitis	Weight gain
	Unsteadiness	Alopecia	Hyperammonemia
	Tremor		
	Thrombocytopenia		
Zonisamide	Sedation		Kidney stones
	Dizziness	Rash	Weight loss
	Cognitive impairment	Oligohydrosis	
	Nausea		

- **Valproic acid** may cause less cognitive impairment than **phenytoin** and **phenobarbital**. Some of the newer agents (e.g., **gabapentin** and **lamotrigine**) have been shown to cause fewer cognitive impairments than the older agents (e.g., **carbamazepine**).

DRUG-DRUG INTERACTIONS

- Drug interactions involving AEDs are shown in Tables 50–5 and 50–6.
- **Phenobarbital**, **phenytoin**, **primidone**, and **carbamazepine** are potent inducers of cytochrome P450, epoxide hydrolase, and uridine diphosphate glucuronosyltransferase (UGT) enzyme systems. **Valproic acid** inhibits many hepatic enzyme systems and displaces some drugs from plasma albumin.

TABLE 50–5. Interactions Between Antiepileptic Drugs

AED	Added Drug	Effect[a]
Carbamazepine (CBZ)	Felbamate	Incr. 10, 11 epoxide
	Felbamate	Decr. CBZ
	Phenobarbital	Decr. CBZ
	Phenytoin	Decr. CBZ
Felbamate (FBM)	Carbamazepine	Decr. FBM
	Phenytoin	Decr. FBM
	Valproic acid	Incr. FBM
Gabapentin	No known interactions	
Lamotrigine (LTG)	Carbamazepine	Decr. LTG
	Phenobarbital	Decr. LTG
	Phenytoin	Decr. LTG
	Primidone	Decr. LTG
	Valproic acid	Incr. LTG
Levetiracetam	No known interactions	
Oxcarbazepine	Carbamazepine	Decrease MHD[b]
	Phenytoin	Decrease MHD[b]
	Phenobarbital	Decrease MHD[b]
Phenobarbital (PB)	Felbamate	Incr. PB
	Phenytoin	Incr. or decr. PB
	Valproic acid	Incr. PB
Phenytoin (PHT)	Carbamazepine	Decr. PHT
	Felbamate	Incr. PHT
	Methsuximide	Incr. PHT
	Phenobarbital	Incr. or decr. PHT
	Valproic acid	Decr. Total PHT
	Vigabatrin	Decr. PHT
Primidone (PRM)	Carbamazepine	Decr. PRM
		Incr. PB
	Phenytoin	Decr. PRM
		Incr. PB
	Valproic acid	Incr. PRM
		Incr. PB
Tiagabine (TGB)	Carbamazepine	Decr. TGB
	Phenytoin	Deer. TGB
Topiramate (TPM)	Carbamazepine	Decr. TPM
	Phenytoin	Decr. TPM
	Valproic acid	Decr. TPM
Valproic acid (VPA)	Carbamazepine	Decr. VPA
	Lamotrigine	Decr. VPA (slight)
	Phenobarbital	Decr. VPA
	Primidone	Decr. VPA
	Phenytoin	Decr. VPA
Zonisamide	Carbamazepine	Decrease zonisamide
	Phenytoin	Decrease zonisamide
	Phenobarbital	Decrease zonisamide

[a] Incr., increased; Decr., decreased.
[b] MHD, 10-monohydroxymetabolite.

IX

TABLE 50–6. Interactions with Other Medications

AED	Altered by	Result	Alters	Result
Carbamazepine	Cimetidine	Incr. CBZ	Oral contraceptives (OC)	Decr. efficacy of OC
	Erythromycin	Incr. CBZ	Doxycycline	Decr. doxycycline
	Fluoxetine	Incr. CBZ	Theophylline	Decr. theophylline
	Isoniazid	Incr. CBZ	Warfarin	Decr. warfarin
	Propoxyphene	Incr. CBZ		
Oxcarbazepine			OC	Decr. efficacy of OC
Phenobarbital	Acetazolamide	Incr. PB	OC	Decr. efficacy of OC
Phenytoin	Amiodarone	Incr. PHT		
	Antacids	Decr. absorption of PHT	Oral contraceptives	Decr. efficacy of oral contraceptives
	Cimetidine	Incr. PHT	Bishydroxycoumarin	Decr. anticoagulation
	Chloramphenicol	Incr. PHT	Folic acid	Decr. folic acid
	Disulfiram	Incr. PHT	Quinidine	Decr. quinidine
	Ethanol (acute)	Incr. PHT	Vitamin D	Decr. vitamin D
	Fluconazole	Incr. PHT		
	Fluoxetine	Incr. PHT		
	Isoniazid	Incr. PHT		
	Propoxyphene	Incr. PHT		
	Warfarin	Can both incr./decr. INR		
	Ethanol (chronic)	Decr. PHT		
Primidone	Isoniazid	Decr. metabolism of primidone	Chlorpromazine	Decr. chlorpromazine
	Nicotinamide	Decr. metabolism of primidone	Corticosteroids	Decr. corticosteroids
			Quinidine	Decr. quinidine
			Tricyclics	Decr. tricyclics
			Furosemide	Decr. renal sensitivity to furosemide
Topiramate			OC	Decr. efficacy of OC
Valproic acid	Cimetidine	Incr. VPA		
	Salicylates	Incr. free VPA		

Incr., increased; Decr., decreased.

Felbamate and **topiramate** can act as inducers with some isoforms and inhibitors with others.

- Except for **levetiracetam** and **gabapentin,** which are eliminated mostly unchanged by the renal route, AEDs are metabolized wholly or in part by hepatic enzymes.

DOSAGE AND ADMINISTRATION

Initial and maximal daily doses and target serum concentration ranges are shown in Table 50–7. Usually therapy is initiated at one fourth to one third of the anticipated maintenance dose, and gradually increased over 3 or 4 weeks to an effective dose. Serum concentrations may be useful, but the therapeutic range must be correlated with clinical outcome. Some patients need and tolerate concentrations above the range.

IX

SPECIFIC ANTIEPILEPTIC DRUGS

Carbamazepine

- **Carbamazepine** may act by inhibition of voltage-gated sodium channels.
- Food may enhance bioavailability.
- Controlled- and sustained-release preparations dosed every 12 hours are bioequivalent to immediate-release preparations dosed every 6 hours. These dosage forms, compared with immediate-release preparations, have lower peaks and higher troughs.
- The liver metabolizes 98% to 99% of a dose of carbamazepine (mostly by CYP3A4), and the major metabolite is carbamazepine-10,11-epoxide, which is active.
- Carbamazepine can induce its own metabolism (autoinduction); this effect begins within 3 to 5 days of dosing initiation and takes 21 to 28 days to become complete.
- Carbamazepine is considered an AED of first choice for newly diagnosed partial seizures. It is also useful for primary generalized convulsive seizures that are not considered an emergency.
- Neurosensory side effects (e.g., diplopia, blurred vision, nystagmus, ataxia, dizziness, and headache) are the most common, occurring in 35% to 50% of patients initially.
- Carbamazepine may induce hyponatremia, a condition similar to the syndrome of inappropriate antidiuretic hormone secretion. The incidence may increase with age.
- Thrombocytopenia and anemia are relatively rare events that respond to discontinuation of carbamazepine. Leukopenia is the most common hematologic side effect (up to 10%) but is usually transient. It may be persistent in 2% of patients. Carbamazepine may be continued unless the white cell count (WBC) drops to less than $2500/mm^3$ and the absolute neutrophil count drops to less than $1000/mm^3$.
- Rashes may occur in 10% of patients. Other side effects include hepatitis, osteomalacia, cardiac conduction defects, and lupus-like reactions.
- Carbamazepine may interact with other drugs by inducing their metabolism. **Valproic acid** increases concentrations of the 10,11-epoxide metabolite without affecting the concentration of carbamazepine. The interaction of **erythromycin** and **clarithromycin** (CYP3A4 inhibition) with carbamazepine is particularly significant.
- Loading doses are used only in critically ill patients.
- Although some patients, especially those on monotherapy, can be maintained on twice-a-day dosing, others may require more frequent administration, especially children. Larger doses can be given at bedtime. Dose increases can be made every 2 to 3 weeks.
- The sustained- and controlled-release dosage forms allow for twice-a-day dosing. The sustained-release capsule can be opened and sprinkled on food.

IX

Ethosuximide

- **Ethosuximide's** proposed mechanisms of action include inhibition of NADPH-linked aldehyde reductase, inhibition of sodium-potassium ATPase, a decrease in non-inactivating Na^+ currents, blocking of Ca^{2+}-dependent K^+ channels, and inhibition of T-type Ca^{2+} channel currents.
- It is a first-line treatment for absence seizures;
- There is some evidence for nonlinear metabolism at higher doses. Metabolites are believed to be inactive.

TABLE 50–7. AED Dosing and Target Serum Concentration Ranges

	Trade Name	Manufacturer	Year Introduced	Usual Initial Dose	Usual Maximum Daily Dose	Target Serum Concentration Range
Barbiturates						
Mephobarbital	Mebaral	Sanofi Winthrop	1935	50–100 mg/day	400–600 mg	Not defined
Phenobarbital	Various	Generic	1912	1–3 mg/kg/day (10–20 mg/kg LD)	180–300 mg	10–40 mcg/mL
Primidone	Mysoline	Wyeth-Ayerst	1954	100–125 mg/day	750–2000 mg	5–10 mcg/mL
Benzodiazepines						
Clonazepam	Klonopin	Roche	1975	1.5 mg/day	20 mg	20–80 ng/mL
Clorazepate	Tranxene	Abbott	1981	7.5–22.5 mg/day	90 mg	Not defined
Diazepam	Valium	Roche/generic	1968	PO: 4–40 mg IV:5–10 mg	PO: 4–40 mg IV: 5–30 mg	100–1000 ng/mL
Lorazepam	Ativan	Wyeth-Ayerst generic		PO: 2–6 mg	PO: 10 mg	10–30 mg/L
				IV: 0.05 mg/kg IM: 0.05 mg/kg		IV: 0.044 mg/kg
Hydantoins						
Ethotoin	Peganone	Abbott	1957	<1000 mg/day	2000–4000 mg with food	15–50 mcg/mL
Mephenytoin	Mesantoin	Sandoz	1947	50–100 mg/day	200–800 mg	25–40 mcg/mL
Phenytoin	Dilantin	Pfizer	1938	PO: 3–5 mg/kg (200–400 mg) (15–20 mg/kg LD)	PO: 500–600 mg	Total: 10–20 mcg/mL Unbound: 0.5–3 mcg/mL

Succinimides						
Ethosuximide	Zarontin	Pfizer	1960	500 mg/day	500–2000 mg	40–80 mcg/mL
Methsuximide	Celontin	Pfizer	1957	300 mg/day	300–1200 mg	N-desmethyl metabolite 10–40 mcg/mL
Other						
Carbamazepine	Tegretol	Novartis, generic	1974	400 mg/day	400–2400 mg	4–14 mcg/mL
Felbamate	Felbatol	MedPointe	1993	1200 mg/day	3600 mg	40–100 mcg/mL[a]
Gabapentin	Neurontin	Pfizer	1993	900 mg/day	4800 mg	4–16 mcg/mL[a]
Lamotrigine	Lamictal	Glaxo SmithKline	1994	25 mg qod if on VPA; 25–50 mg/day if not on VPA	100–150 mg if on VPA; 300–500 mg if not on VPA	4–20 mcg/mL[a]
Levetiracetam	Keppra	UCB-Pharma	2000	500–1000 mg/day	3000–4000 mg	Not defined
Oxcarbazepine	Trileptal	Novartis	2000	300–600 mg/day	2400–3000 mg	12–30 mcg/mL[a] (MHD)
Tiagabine	Gabitril	Abbott	1997	4–8 mg/day	80 mg	Not defined
Topiramate	Topamax	Ortho McNeil	1997	25–50 mg/day	200–1000 mg	Not defined.
Valproic acid	Depakene Depakote Depacon	Abbott	1978	15 mg/kg (500–1000 mg)	60 mg/kg (3000–5000 mg)	50–150 mcg/mL[a]
Zonisamide	Zonegran	Elan	2000	100–200 mg/day	600 mg	10–40 mcg/mL[a]

[a]Based on data from clinical trial—no established therapeutic ranges.

- A loading dose is not required. **Titration over 1 to 2 weeks to maintenance doses of 20 mg/kg/day (divided into two doses)** usually results in serum concentrations of 50 mcg/mL.

Felbamate

- **Felbamate** appears to act as a glycine receptor antagonist.
- It is approved for treating atonic seizures in patients with Lennox-Gastaut syndrome, and is effective for partial seizures as well.
- Because of the reports of aplastic anemia (1 in 3000 patients) and hepatitis (1 in 10,000 patients), it is now recommended only for patients refractory to other AEDs. Risk factors for aplastic anemia may be a history of cytopenia, AED allergy or toxicity, viral infection, and/or immunologic problems.
- It is recommended that the dose of **phenytoin**, **carbamazepine**, and **valproic acid** be decreased by about 30% when **felbamate** is added. Interactions with **warfarin** have also been reported.
- If felbamate is used as monotherapy, the dose is **initiated at 1200 mg/day (15 mg/kg in children) and then is increased by 600 mg every 2 weeks up to a maximum dose of 3600 mg/day (45 mg/kg in children).**

Gabapentin

- **Gabapentin** may modulate specific voltage-sensitive Ca^{2+} channels and elevates human brain GABA levels. It is a second-line agent for patients with partial seizures who have failed initial treatment. It may also have a role in patients with less severe seizure disorders, such as new-onset partial epilepsy, especially in elderly patients.
- Bioavailability decreases with increasing doses. It is eliminated exclusively renally, and dosage adjustment is necessary in patients with impaired renal function.
- Common side effects are fatigue, sleepiness, dizziness, and ataxia.
- **Dosing is initiated at 300 mg at bedtime and increased to 300 mg twice daily on the second day and 300 mg three times daily on the third day. Further titrations are then made. The manufacturer recommends maintenance doses up to 1800 to 2400 mg/day, but higher doses (5000 to 10,000 mg/day) have been used safely. Most clinicians use doses of 2400 to 4800 mg/day.**

Lamotrigine

- **Lamotrigine** blocks neuronal sodium channels, produces dose-dependent inhibition of high-voltage activation Ca^{2+} currents, and blocks release of excitatory amino acid neurotransmitters.
- It is useful as both adjunctive therapy and monotherapy in adults with partial epilepsy. It may also be useful in patients with primary generalized seizure types such as absence.
  It does not induce or inhibit the metabolism of other AEDs.
- The most frequent side effects are diplopia, drowsiness, ataxia, and headache. Rashes are usually mild to moderate, but Stevens-Johnson reaction has also occurred. The incidence of rash appears to be increased in patients who are also receiving **valproic acid** and who have rapid dosage titration.

Levetiracetam

- **Levetiracetam** has a unique chemical structure and mechanism of action.
- Renal elimination of unchanged drug accounts for 66% of drug clearance, and the dose should be adjusted for impaired renal function. The role of therapeutic drug monitoring is unknown. It has linear pharmacokinetics and is not metabolized by the cytochrome P450 (CYP) and UGT systems.

IX

- It is effective in the adjunctive treatment of partial seizures in adults who have failed initial therapy.
- Adverse effects include sedation, fatigue, and coordination difficulties. A slight decline in red and white blood cells was noted in clinical trials.
- It is believed to have a low potential for drug interactions.
- **The recommended initial dose is 500 mg orally twice daily, and this can be increased by 1000 mg/day every 2 weeks to a maximum recommended dose of 3000 mg/day (1500 mg b.i.d.).**

Oxcarbazepine

- **Oxcarbazepine** (a prodrug) is structurally related to **carbamazepine,** but it is converted to a monohydrate derivative (MHD), which is the active component.
- It blocks voltage-sensitive sodium channels, modulates the voltage-activated calcium currents, and increases potassium conductance.
- The MHD peaks within 4 to 6 hours after a dose. It undergoes glucuronide conjugation and is eliminated by the kidneys. Patients with significant renal impairment may require a dose adjustment. The half-life (9.3 ± 1.8 hours) is shorter in patients taking enzyme-inducing drugs. The relationship between dose and serum concentration is linear.
- It is indicated for use as monotherapy or adjunctive therapy for partial seizures in adults and as monotherapy and adjunctive therapy for partial seizures in patients as young as 4 years of age. It is also a potential first-line drug for patients with primary generalized convulsive seizures.
- The most frequently reported side effects are dizziness, nausea, headache, diarrhea, vomiting, upper respiratory tract infections, constipation, dyspepsia, ataxia, and nervousness. It generally has fewer side effects than **phenytoin**, **valproic acid**, or **carbamazepine**. Hyponatremia has been reported in up to 25% of patients and is more likely in the elderly. About 25% to 30% of patients who have had a rash with carbamazepine will have a cross-reaction with oxcarbazepine.
- Concurrent use of oxcarbazepine with **ethinyl estradiol**– and **levonorgestrel**-containing contraceptives may render these agents less effective. Oxcarbazepine may increase serum concentrations of **phenytoin** and decrease serum concentrations of **lamotrigine** (induction of UGT).
- **In adults, the starting dose of oxcarbazepine as monotherapy is 300 mg once or twice daily. This can be increased by 600 mg/day each week to a maximum dose of 2400 mg/day. For children aged 4 to 16 years, the starting dose is 8 to 10 mg/kg given twice daily, not to exceed 600 mg/day. This is titrated to the target dose over 2 weeks.** See manufacturer's recommendations for dosing by weight.
- **In patients converted from carbamazepine, the typical maintenance doses of oxcarbazepine are 1.5 times the carbamazepine dose.**

Phenobarbital and Primidone

- **Phenobarbital** decrease postsynaptic excitation, possibly through GABA mechanisms.
- Phenobarbital is the drug of choice for neonatal seizures, but in other situations it is reserved for patients who have failed other AEDs.
- Phenobarbital is a potent enzyme inducer.
- The amount of phenobarbital excreted renally can be increased by giving diuretics and urinary alkalinizers.

IX

- The most common side effects are fatigue, drowsiness, and depression. Phenobarbital impairs cognitive performance. In children, hyperactivity can occur (see Table 50–4).
- **Ethanol** increases phenobarbital metabolism, but **valproic acid**, **cimetidine**, phenytoin, felbamate, and **chloramphenicol** inhibit its metabolism.
- **Phenobarbital can usually be dosed once daily, and bedtime dosing may minimize daytime sedation.**

Phenytoin

- **Phenytoin** alters ion fluxes, thus altering depolarization, repolarization, and membrane stability.
- Phenytoin is a first-line AED for generalized seizures (except absence) and for partial seizures. Its place in therapy will be reevaluated as more experience is gained with the newer AEDs.
- Absorption may be saturable. Absorption is affected by particle size, and the brand should not be changed without careful monitoring. Food may slow absorption. The intramuscular route is best avoided, as absorption is erratic. Fosphenytoin can safely be administered intravenously and intramuscularly. Equations are available to normalize the phenytoin concentration in patients with hypoalbuminemia or renal failure.
- Phenytoin is metabolized in the liver mainly by CYP2C9, but CYP2C19 is also involved. Zero-order kinetics occurs within the usual dosage range, so any change in dose may produce disproportional changes in serum concentrations.
- **In nonacute situations, phenytoin may be initiated in adults at oral doses of 5 mg/kg/day and titrated upward. Subsequent dosage adjustments should be done cautiously because of nonlinearity in elimination. Most adult patients can be maintained on a single daily dose, but children often require more frequent administration. Only extended-release preparations should be used for single daily dosing.**
- One author suggested that if the phenytoin serum concentration is less than 7 mcg/mL, the daily dose should be increased by 100 mg; if the concentration is 7 to 12 mcg/mL, the daily dose can be increased by 50 mg; if the concentration is greater than 12 mcg/mL, the daily dose can be increased by 30 mg or less.
- Common but usually transient side effects are lethargy, incoordination, blurred vision, higher cortical dysfunction, and drowsiness. At concentrations greater than 50 mcg/mL, phenytoin can exacerbate seizures. Chronic side effects include gingival hyperplasia, impaired cognition, hirsutism, vitamin D deficiency, osteomalacia, folic acid deficiency, carbohydrate intolerance, hypothyroidism, and peripheral neuropathy.
- Phenytoin is prone to many drug interactions (see Tables 50–5 and 6). If protein-binding interactions are suspected, free rather than total phenytoin concentrations are a better therapeutic guide.
- Phenytoin decreases **folic acid** absorption, but folic acid replacement enhances phenytoin clearance and can result in loss of efficacy. Phenytoin tablets and suspension contain phenytoin acid, while the capsules and parenteral solution are phenytoin sodium, which is 92% phenytoin. Clinicians should remember that there are two different strengths of phenytoin suspension and capsules.

Tiagabine

- **Tiagabine** is a specific inhibitor of GABA reuptake into glial cells and other neurons.
- It is considered second-line therapy for patients with partial seizures who have failed initial therapy.

- The most frequently reported side effect is dizziness. Other side effects are asthenia, nervousness, tremor, and diarrhea. These side effects are usually transient.
- It is oxidized by CYP3A4 enzymes, and enzyme inducers increase its clearance.
- Tiagabine is displaced from protein by **naproxen**, **salicylates**, and **valproate**.
- **The minimal effective adult dose level is considered to be 30 mg/day. The initial dose is 4 mg/day, and this may be increased up to 56 mg/day in intervals of 4 to 8 mg/day added each week. The dosage typically employed is 32 to 56 mg daily.**

Topiramate

- **Topiramate** affects voltage-dependent sodium channels, GABA receptors, and antagonism of α-amino-3-hydroxy-5-methyl-4-isoxazole-4-propionic acid (AMPA) subtype glutamate receptors.
- It is a second-line AED for patients with partial seizures who have failed initial therapy.
- Approximately 50% of the dose is excreted renally, and tubular reabsorption may be prominently involved.
- The most common side effects are ataxia, impaired concentration, confusion, dizziness, fatigue, paresthesias, and somnolence. Nephrolithiasis occurs in 1.5% of patients. It has also been associated with acute narrow-angle glaucoma, oligohydrosis, and metabolic acidosis.
- Enzyme inducers may decrease topiramate serum levels.
- **Starting doses are 12.5 to 50 mg/day, increasing by 12.5 to 50 mg/day every week or two. The minimally effective dose is approximately 200 mg/day. For patients on other AEDs, doses greater than 600 mg/day do not appear to lead to improved efficacy and may increase side effects. Monotherapy doses of 1000 mg/day have been well tolerated and effective.**

Valproic Acid and Divalproex Sodium

- **Valproic acid** may increase synthesis or inhibit degradation of GABA. It may also potentiate postsynaptic GABA responses, have a direct membrane-stabilizing effect, and affect potassium channels.
- The free fraction may increase as the total concentration increases, and free concentrations may be a better monitoring parameter than total concentrations, especially at higher concentrations or in patients with hypoalbuminemia. Protein binding is decreased in patients with head trauma.
- At least 10 metabolites have been identified, and some may be active. One may account for hepatotoxicity (4-*en*-valproic acid), and it is increased by concurrent dosing with enzyme-inducing drugs. At least 67 cases have been reported, and most deaths were in mentally retarded children less than 2 years old who were receiving multiple drug therapy.
- The extended-release formulation (Depakote ER) is 15% less bioavailable than the enteric-coated preparation (Depakote).
- It is first-line therapy for primary generalized seizures, such as absence, myoclonic, and atonic seizures, and is approved for adjunctive and monotherapy treatment of partial seizures. It can also be useful in mixed seizure disorders.
- Side effects are usually mild and include gastrointestinal (GI) complaints, weight gain, drowsiness, ataxia, and tremor. GI complaints may be minimized with the enteric-coated formulation or by giving with food. Thrombocytopenia is common but is responsive to a decrease in dose. Other hematologic toxicities include leukopenia with transient neutropenia, transient erythroblastopenia, and bone marrow changes.

IX

- Polycystic ovary syndrome and menstrual irregularities have also been reported with valproic acid therapy.
- Although **carnitine** administration may partially ameliorate hyperammonemia, it is expensive, and there are only limited data to support routine supplemental use in patients taking valproic acid.
- Valproic acid is an enzyme inhibitor that increases serum concentrations of concurrently administered **phenobarbital** and may increase concentrations of **carbamazepine 10,11-epoxide** without affecting concentrations of the parent drug. It also inhibits the metabolism of **lamotrigine**.
- **Twice daily dosing is reasonable, but children and patients taking enzyme inducers may require 3 or 4 times daily dosing.**
- The enteric-coated tablet **divalproex sodium** causes fewer GI side effects. It is metabolized in the gut to valproic acid.

Zonisamide

- **Zonisamide** is a broad-spectrum **sulfonamide** AED that blocks voltage-sensitive sodium channels by reducing voltage-dependent T-type Ca^{2+} channels; it also facilitates dopaminergic and serotonergic neurotransmission, weakly inhibits carbonic anhydrase, and blocks K^+ evoked glutamate release.
- It is approved as adjunctive therapy with partial seizures, but it is potentially effective in a variety of partial and primary generalized seizure types.
- Zonisamide is 40% protein bound and has a half-life of 63 to 69 hours. It is metabolized by CYP3A4, and about 30% is excreted unchanged.
- The most common side effects include somnolence, dizziness, anorexia, headache, nausea, and irritability. Symptomatic kidney stones may occur in 2.6% of patients. Hypersensitivity reactions may occur in 0.02% of patients, and history of allergy to **sulfonamides** is a contraindication. Monitoring of renal function may be advisable in some patients.
- Enzyme inducers may reduce the half-life of zonisamide to 27 to 36 hours.
- **The initial dose in adults is 100 mg/day, and daily doses are increased by 100 mg every 2 weeks until a response is seen. The dosage range in adults 100 to 600 mg/day.**

▶ EVALUATION OF THERAPEUTIC OUTCOMES

- An individual therapeutic range should be established for each patient.
- Patients should be chronically monitored for seizure control, side effects, social adjustment, drug interactions, compliance, quality of life, and toxicity.
- Screening for neuropsychiatric disorders is also important. Clinical response is more important than serum drug concentrations.
- Patients should be asked to record severity and frequency of seizures in a seizure diary.

See Chapter 54, Epilepsy, authored by Barry E. Gidal and William R. Garnett, for a more detailed discussion of this topic.

Chapter 51

▶ HEADACHE: MIGRAINE AND TENSION-TYPE

▶ MIGRAINE HEADACHE

DEFINITION

Migraine is a recurring headache of moderate to severe intensity associated with gastrointestinal (GI), neurologic, and autonomic symptoms. In migraine with aura, a complex of focal neurologic symptoms precedes or accompanies the attack.

PATHOPHYSIOLOGY

- Neuronal dysfunction is now accepted as the primary basis of migraine pathophysiology. Symptoms of aura are thought to result from neuronal dysfunction characterized by a wave of depressed electrical activity that advances across the cerebral cortex. Aura is also associated with reduced cerebral blood flow.
- Migraine pain is believed to result from activity within the trigeminovascular system that results in release of vasoactive neuropeptides with subsequent vasodilation, dural plasma extravasation, and perivascular inflammation.
- The pathogenesis of migraine may be related to an imbalance in the activity of serotonin-containing neurons and/or noradrenergic pathways in brainstem nuclei that modulate cerebral vascular tone and nociception. This imbalance may result in vasodilation of intracranial blood vessels and activation of the trigeminovascular system.
- Serotonin (5-hydroxytryptamine, or 5-HT) is an important mediator of migraine. Acute antimigraine drugs such as ergot alkaloids and triptan derivatives are agonists of vascular and neuronal 5-HT_1 receptor subtypes, resulting in vasoconstriction and inhibition of vasoactive neuropeptide release and pain signal transmission. Drugs used for migraine prophylaxis stabilize serotonergic neurotransmission and raise the migraine threshold by antagonizing or down-regulating 5-HT_2 receptors, or by modulating serotonergic neuronal discharge.

▶ CLINICAL PRESENTATION

GENERAL

Migraine is a common, recurrent, severe headache that interferes with normal functioning. It is a primary headache disorder divided into two major subtypes, migraine without aura and migraine with aura.

SYMPTOMS

- Migraine is characterized by recurring episodes of throbbing head pain, frequently unilateral, that when untreated can last from 4 to 72 hours. Migraine headaches can be severe and associated with nausea, vomiting, and sensitivity to light, sound, and/or movement. Not all symptoms are present at every attack.
- In the headache evaluation, diagnostic alarms should be identified. These include: acute onset of the "first" or "worst" headache ever, accelerating pattern of headache following subacute onset, onset of headache after age 50, headache associated with systemic illness (e.g., fever, nausea, vomiting, stiff neck, and rash), headache with focal neurologic symptoms or papilledema, and new-onset

headache in a patient with cancer or human immunodeficiency virus (HIV) infection.

SIGNS

- A stable pattern, absence of daily headache, positive family history for migraine, normal neurologic examination, presence of food triggers, menstrual association, long-standing history, improvement with sleep, and subacute evolution are all signs of migraine headache. Aura may signal the migraine headache but is not required for diagnosis.
- Approximately 10% to 60% of migraineurs experience premonitory symptoms, or prodrome, in the hours or days before the onset of headache. Neurologic prodromal symptoms (phonophobia, photophobia, hyperosmia, difficulty concentrating) are most common, but psychologic (anxiety, depression, euphoria, irritability, drowsiness, hyperactivity, restlessness), autonomic (e.g., polyuria, diarrhea, constipation), and constitutional (e.g., stiff neck, yawning, thirst, food cravings, anorexia) symptoms may also occur.
- A migraine aura is experienced by approximately 31% of migraineurs. The aura typically evolves over 5 to 20 minutes and lasts less than 60 minutes. Headache usually occurs within 60 minutes of the end of the aura. Visual auras can include both positive features (e.g., scintillations, photopsia, teichopsia, fortification spectrum) and negative features (e.g., scotoma, hemianopsia). Sensory and motor symptoms such as paresthesias or numbness of the arms and face, dysphasia or aphasia, weakness, and hemiparesis may also occur.
- The actual migraine headache may occur at any time of day or night but usually occurs in the early morning hours on awakening. Pain is usually gradual in onset, peaking in intensity over minutes to hours, and lasting between 4 and 72 hours. Pain is typically reported as moderate to severe and most often involves the frontotemporal region. The headache is usually unilateral and throbbing or pulsating in nature. GI symptoms (e.g., nausea, vomiting) almost invariably accompany the headache. Other systemic symptoms include anorexia, constipation, diarrhea, abdominal cramps, nasal stuffiness, blurred vision, diaphoresis, facial pallor, and localized facial or periorbital edema. Sensory hyperacuity (photophobia, phonophobia, osmophobia) is frequently reported. Physical activity may aggravate the pain, and many patients seek a dark, quiet place for rest and relief.
- Once the headache pain wanes, a resolution phase characterized by exhaustion, malaise, and irritability ensues.

▶ DIAGNOSIS

LABORATORY TESTS

- In selected circumstances and secondary headache presentation, serum chemistries, urine toxicology profiles, thyroid function tests, lyme studies, and other blood tests such as a complete blood count, antinuclear antibody titer, erythrocyte sedimentation rate, and antiphospholipid antibody titer may be considered.

DIAGNOSTIC TESTS

- Perform a general medical and neurologic physical examination. Check for abnormalities: vital signs (fever, hypertension), funduscopy (papilledema, hemorrhage, and exudates), palpation and auscultation of the head and neck (sinus tenderness, hardened or tender temporal arteries, trigger points, temporomandibular joint tenderness, bruits, nuchal rigidity, and cervical spine tenderness), and neurologic examination (identify abnormalities or deficits in mental status, cranial nerves, deep tendon reflexes, motor strength, coordination, gait, and cerebellar function).

- Consider neuroimaging studies in patients with abnormal neurologic examination findings of unknown etiology and in those with additional risk factors warranting imaging.
- A comprehensive headache history is the most important element in establishing the clinical diagnosis of migraine.
- Diagnostic and laboratory testing may be warranted if there are suspicious headache features or abnormal examination findings. Neuroimaging (computed tomography or magnetic resonance imaging) should be considered in patients with unexplained neurologic physical findings or an atypical headache history.

DESIRED OUTCOME

- Acute therapy should provide consistent, rapid relief with minimal adverse effects and symptom recurrence, thereby enabling the patient to resume normal daily activities. Ideally, patients should be able to manage their headaches effectively without emergency department or physician office visits.
- Clinicians and migraineurs should collaborate to create a long-term management plan that reduces attack frequency and severity, minimizes disability and emotional distress, and improves quality of life.

TREATMENT

A treatment algorithm for acute migraine headache is shown in Figure 51–1.

Nonpharmacologic Treatment

- Application of ice to the head and periods of rest or sleep, usually in a dark, quiet environment, may be beneficial.
- Preventive management should begin with identification and avoidance of factors that provoke migraine attacks (Table 51–1).
- Behavioral interventions (relaxation therapy, biofeedback, cognitive therapy) are preventive options for patients who prefer nondrug therapy or when drug therapy is ineffective or not tolerated.

Pharmacologic Treatment of Acute Migraine

- Acute migraine therapies (Table 51–2) are most effective when administered at the onset of migraine.
- Pretreatment with antiemetics (e.g., **prochlorperazine, metoclopramide**) 15 to 30 minutes prior to administering abortive therapy or use of non-oral treatments (rectal suppositories, nasal spray, injections) may be advisable when nausea and vomiting are severe. In addition to its antiemetic effects, the prokinetic agent metoclopramide enhances absorption of oral medications.
- Acute migraine therapies should generally be limited to 2 days/wk to avoid the development of medication misuse (or rebound) headache.

Analgesics and Nonsteroidal Anti-inflammatory Drugs (NSAIDs)

- Simple analgesics and NSAIDs are effective treatment for mild to moderate migraine attacks. Aspirin, ibuprofen, naproxen sodium, tolfenamic acid, and the combination of acetaminophen plus aspirin and caffeine have shown most consistent evidence of efficacy.
- The COX-2 inhibitors and naproxen have been recently associated with cardiac events and stroke. The COX-2 inhibitors should not generally be chosen for this

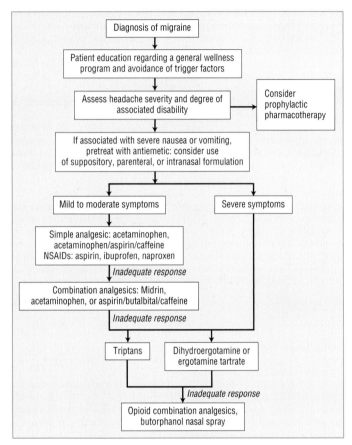

Figure 51–1. Treatment algorithm for migraine headaches.

indication. The Food and Drug Administration (FDA) urges that the naproxen product labeled dosing be carefully followed when it is used for any indication.

- NSAIDs appear to prevent neurogenically mediated inflammation in the trigeminovascular system by inhibiting prostaglandin synthesis.
- In general, NSAIDs with a long half-life that preclude their frequent use are preferred. Rectal suppositories and intramuscular **ketorolac** are options for patients with severe nausea and vomiting.
- The nonprescription combination of **acetaminophen, aspirin**, and **caffeine** is approved in the United States for relieving migraine pain and associated symptoms.
- Aspirin and acetaminophen are also available by prescription in combination with a short-acting barbiturate (**butalbital**) or an opioid (e.g., **codeine**). No randomized, placebo-controlled studies support the efficacy of butalbital-containing formulations for migraine.

TABLE 51–1. Precipitating Factors Associated with Migraine

Food Triggers
    Alcohol
    Caffeine/caffeine withdrawal
    Chocolate
    Citrus fruits, bananas, figs, raisins
    Dairy products
    Fermented and pickled foods
    Monosodium glutamate (e.g., in Chinese food, seasoned salt, and instant foods)
    Nitrate-containing foods (e.g., processed meats)
    Saccharin/aspartame (e.g., diet foods or diet sodas)
    Sulfites in shrimp
    Tyramine-containing foods
    Yeast products

Environmental Triggers
    Glare or flickering lights
    High altitude
    Loud noises
    Strong smells and fumes
    Tobacco smoke
    Weather changes

Behavioral-Physiologic Triggers
    Excess or insufficient sleep
    Fatigue
    Menstruation, menopause
    Skipped meals
    Strenuous physical activity (e.g., prolonged overexertion)
    Stress or post-stress

Medications
    Analgesic overuse
    Benzodiazepine withdrawal
    Cimetidine
    Decongestant overuse
    Ergotamine overuse
    Estrogen therapy
    Indomethacin
    Nifedipine
    Nitrates
    Oral contraceptives
    Reserpine
    Theophylline

IX

- **Midrin** is a proprietary combination of **acetaminophen**, **isometheptene mucate** (a sympathomimetic amine), and **dichloralphenazone** (a chloral hydrate derivative) that has shown modest benefits in placebo-controlled trials. It may be an alternative for patients with mild to moderate migraine attacks.

Ergot Alkaloids and Derivatives
- Ergot alkaloids are nonselective 5-HT$_1$ receptor agonists that constrict intracranial blood vessels and inhibit the development of neurogenic inflammation in the trigeminovascular system. They also have activity at α-adrenergic, β-adrenergic, and dopaminergic receptors.
- **Ergotamine tartrate** is available for oral, sublingual, and rectal administration. Oral and rectal preparations contain caffeine to enhance absorption and

TABLE 51–2. Acute Migraine Therapies[a]

Medication	Dosage	Comments
Analgesics		
Acetaminophen	1000 mg at onset; repeat every 4–6 h as needed	Maximum daily dose is 4 g
Acetaminophen 250 mg/aspirin 250 mg/caffeine 65 mg	2 tablets at onset and every 6 h	Available over-the-counter as Excedrin Migraine
Aspirin or acetaminophen with butalbital, caffeine	1–2 tablets every 4–6 h	Limit dose to 4 tablets/day and usage to 2 days/wk
Isometheptene 65 mg/dichloralphenazone 100 mg/acetaminophen 325 mg (Midrin)	2 capsules at onset; repeat 1 capsule every hour as needed	Maximum of 6 capsules/day and 20 capsules/month
Nonsteroidal Anti-inflammatory Drugs		
Aspirin	500–1000 mg every 4–6 h	Maximum daily dose is 4 g
Ibuprofen	200–800 mg every 6 h	Avoid doses >2.4 g/day
Naproxen sodium	550–825 mg at onset; may repeat 220 mg in 3–4 h	Avoid doses > 1.375 g/day
Diclofenac potassium	50–100 mg at onset; may repeat 50 mg in 8 h	Avoid doses > 150 mg/day
▶ IX **Ergotamine Tartrate**		
Oral tablet (1 mg) with caffeine 100 mg	2 mg at onset; then 1–2 mg every 30 min as needed	Maximum dose is 6 mg/day or 10 mg/wk; consider pretreatment with an antiemetic
Sublingual tablet (2 mg)		
Rectal suppository (2 mg) with caffeine 100 mg	Insert 1/2 to 1 suppository at onset; repeat after 1 h as needed	Maximum dose is 4 mg/day or 10 mg/wk; consider pretreatment with an antiemetic
Dihydroergotamine		
Injection 1 mg/mL	0.25–1 mg at onset IM or SQ; repeat every hour as needed	Maximum dose is 3 mg/day or 20 mg/wk
Nasal spray	One spray (0.5 mg) in each nostril at onset; repeat sequence 15 min later (total dose is 2 mg or 4 sprays)	Maximum dose is 3 mg/day; prime sprayer 4 times before using; do not tilt head back or inhale through nose while spraying; discard open ampules after 8 h
Serotonin Agonists (Triptans)		
Sumatriptan		
Injection	6 mg SC at onset; may repeat after 1 h if needed	Maximum daily dose is 12 mg
Oral tablets	25, 50, or 100 mg at onset; may repeat after 2 h if needed	Optimal dose is 50–100 mg; maximum daily dose is 200 mg
Nasal spray	5, 10, or 20 mg at onset; may repeat after 2 h if needed	Optimal dose is 20 mg; maximum daily dose is 40 mg; single-dose device delivering 5 or 20 mg; administer one spray in one nostril
Zolmitriptan	2.5 or 5 mg at onset as regular or orally disintegrating tablet; may repeat after 2 h if needed	Optimal dose is 2.5 mg; maximum dose is 10 mg/day. Do not divide ODT dosage form
Naratriptan	1 or 2.5 mg at onset; may repeat after 4 h if needed	Optimal dose is 2.5 mg; maximum daily dose is 5 mg

Continued

TABLE 51–2. (Continued)

Medication	Dosage	Comments
Rizatriptan	5 or 10 mg at onset as regular or orally disintegrating tablet; may repeat after 2 h if needed	Optimal dose is 10 mg; maximum daily dose is 30 mg; onset of effect is similar with standard and orally disintegrating tablets; use 5-mg dose (15 mg/day max) in patients receiving propranolol
Almotriptan	6.25 or 12.5 mg at onset; may repeat after 2 h if needed	Optimal dose is 12.5 mg; maximum daily dose is 25 mg
Frovatriptan	2.5 or 5 mg at onset; may repeat in 2 h if needed	Optimal dose 2.5–5 mg; maximum daily dose is 7.5 mg (3 tablets)
Eletriptan	20 or 40 mg at onset; may repeat after 2 h if needed	Maximum single dose is 40 mg; maximum daily dose is 80 mg
Miscellaneous		
Butorphanol nasal spray	1 spray in 1 nostril (1 mg) at onset; repeat in 1 h if needed	Limit to 4 sprays/day; consider use only when nonopioid therapies are ineffective or not tolerated
Metoclopramide	10 mg IV at onset	Useful for acute relief in the office or emergency department setting
Prochlorperazine	10 mg IV or IM at onset	Useful for acute relief in the office or emergency department setting

IX

[a]Limit use of symptomatic medications to 2 days/wk when possible to avoid medication misuse headache.

potentiate analgesia. Because oral ergotamine undergoes extensive first-pass hepatic metabolism, rectal administration is preferred. Dosage should be titrated to produce an effective but subnauseating dose.

- **Dihydroergotamine (DHE)** is available for intranasal and parenteral (intramuscular [IM], intravenous [IV], subcutaneous [SC]) administration. Patients can be trained to self-administer DHE by the IM or SC routes. The efficacy of intranasal DHE has been consistently demonstrated.
- Nausea and vomiting are common adverse effects of ergotamine derivatives. Ergotamine is 12 times more emetogenic than DHE; pretreatment with an antiemetic should be considered with ergotamine and IV DHE therapy. Other side effects include abdominal pain, weakness, fatigue, paresthesias, muscle pain, diarrhea, and chest tightness. Symptoms of severe peripheral ischemia (ergotism) include cold, numb, painful extremities; continuous paresthesias; diminished peripheral pulses; and claudication. Gangrenous extremities, myocardial infarction, hepatic necrosis, and bowel and brain ischemia have been reported rarely with ergotamine. Ergotamine derivatives and triptans should not be used within 24 hours of each other.
- Contraindications include renal and hepatic failure; coronary, cerebral, or peripheral vascular disease; uncontrolled hypertension; sepsis; and women who are pregnant or nursing.
- DHE does not appear to cause rebound headache, but dosage restrictions for ergotamine tartrate should be strictly observed to prevent this complication.

Serotonin Receptor Agonists (Triptans)
- **Sumatriptan**, **zolmitriptan**, **naratriptan**, **rizatriptan**, **almotriptan**, **frovatriptan**, and **eletriptan** are appropriate first-line therapy for patients with moderate to severe migraine or as rescue therapy when nonspecific medications are ineffective.

- These drugs are selective agonists of the 5-HT$_{1B}$ and 5-HT$_{1D}$ receptors. Relief of migraine headache results from (1) vasoconstriction of intracranial blood vessels through stimulation of vascular 5-HT$_{1B}$ receptors; (2) inhibition of vasoactive neuropeptide release from trigeminal perivascular nerves through stimulation of presynaptic 5-HT$_{1D}$ receptors; and (3) interruption of pain signal transmission within the brainstem through stimulation of 5-HT$_{1D}$ receptors. They also display varying affinity for 5-HT$_{1A}$, 5-HT$_{1E}$, and 5-HT$_{1F}$ receptors.
- **Sumatriptan** is available for oral, intranasal, and SC administration. The SC injection is packaged as an autoinjector device for self-administration by patients. The efficacies of 50-mg and 100-mg doses are comparable. When compared with the oral formulation, SC administration offers enhanced efficacy and a more rapid onset of action (10 vs. 30 minutes). Intranasal sumatriptan also has a faster onset of effect (15 minutes) than the oral formulation and produces similar rates of response. Approximately 30% to 40% of patients who respond to sumatriptan experience headache recurrence within 24 hours; a second dose given at the time of recurrence is usually effective. However, routine administration of a second oral or SC dose does not improve initial efficacy rates or prevent subsequent recurrence.
- Second-generation agents have higher oral bioavailability and longer half-lives than oral sumatriptan, which could theoretically improve within-patient treatment consistency and reduce headache recurrence. However, comparative clinical trials are necessary to determine their relative efficacy.
- Pharmacokinetic characteristics of the triptans are shown in Table 51–3.
- Clinical response to triptans varies among individual patients, and lack of response to one agent does not preclude effective therapy with another member of the class.
- Side effects of triptans include paresthesias, fatigue, dizziness, flushing, warm sensations, and somnolence. Minor injection site reactions are reported with SC use, and taste perversion and nasal discomfort may occur with intranasal

TABLE 51–3. Pharmacokinetic Characteristics of Triptans

Drug	Half-Life (h)	Time to Maximal Concentration (t_{max})	Bioavailability	Elimination
Almotriptan	3–4	1.4–3.8 h	70	MAO-A, CYP450 3A4 and 2D6
Eletriptan	5	1.4–2.8 h	50	CYP 3A4
Frovatriptan	25	2–4 h	24–30	CYP 1A2
Naratriptan	5–6	2–3 h	63–74	CYP450 (various isoenzymes)
Rizatriptan	2–3		40–45	MAO-A
Oral tablets		1–1.5 h		
Disintegrating		1.6–2.5 h		
Sumatriptan:	2			MAO-A
SC injection		12–15 min	97	
Oral tablets		2.5 h	14	
Nasal spray		1–2.5 h	17	
Zolmitriptan	3		40	CYP 1A2, MAO-A
Oral		1.5 h		
Disintegrating		3 h		
Nasal		4 h		

administration. Up to 15% of patients report chest tightness, pressure, heaviness, or pain in the chest, neck, or throat; although the mechanism of these symptoms is unknown, a cardiac source is unlikely in most patients. Isolated cases of myocardial infarction and coronary vasospasm with ischemia have been reported.

- Contraindications include ischemic heart disease, uncontrolled hypertension, cerebrovascular disease, and hemiplegic and basilar migraine. Triptans should not be given within 24 hours of ergotamine derivatives administration. Administration within 2 weeks of therapy with monoamine oxidase inhibitors is not recommended.

Opioids

- Opioids and derivatives (e.g., **meperidine, butorphanol, oxycodone, hydromorphone**) provide effective relief of intractable migraine but should be reserved for patients with moderate to severe infrequent headaches in whom conventional therapies are contraindicated or as rescue medication after failure to respond to conventional therapies.
- **Intranasal butorphanol** may provide an alternative to frequent office or emergency department visits for injectable migraine therapies. Onset of analgesia occurs within 15 minutes of administration. Adverse effects include dizziness, nausea, vomiting, drowsiness, and taste perversion. It is also a controlled substance that carries the potential for dependence and addiction.

IX◀

Glucocorticoids

- Short courses of oral or parenteral glucocorticoids (e.g., **prednisone, dexamethasone, hydrocortisone**) appear to be useful for refractory headache that has persisted for several days.
- Corticosteroids may be an effective rescue therapy for status migrainosus, which is a severe migraine that may last up to 1 week.

Pharmacologic Prophylaxis of Migraine

- Prophylactic therapies (Table 51–4) are administered on a daily basis to reduce the frequency, severity, and duration of attacks, as well as to increase responsiveness to acute symptomatic therapies. A treatment algorithm for prophylactic management of migraine headache is shown in Figure 51–2.
- Prophylaxis should be considered in the setting of recurring migraines that produce significant disability; frequent attacks requiring symptomatic medication more than twice per week; symptomatic therapies that are ineffective, contraindicated, or produce serious side effects; uncommon migraine variants that cause profound disruption and/or risk of neurologic injury; and patient preference to limit the number of attacks.
- Preventive therapy may also be administered intermittently when headaches recur in a predictable pattern (e.g., exercise-induced or menstrual migraine).
- Because efficacy of various prophylactic agents appears to be similar, drug selection is based on side-effect profiles and comorbid conditions of the patient. Individual response to a particular agent is unpredictable, and a trial of 2 to 3 months is necessary to judge the efficacy of each medication.
- Only propranolol, timolol, and valproic acid are approved by the FDA for this indication.
- Prophylaxis should be initiated with low doses and advanced slowly until a therapeutic effect is achieved or side effects become intolerable.
- Prophylaxis is usually continued for at least 3 to 6 months after headache frequency and severity have diminished, and then gradually tapered and discontinued, if possible.

β-Adrenergic Antagonists
- β Blockers (**propranolol, nadolol, timolol, atenolol**, and **metoprolol**) are the most widely used treatment for prevention of migraine. β Blockers with intrinsic sympathomimetic activity are ineffective.
- Side effects include drowsiness, fatigue, sleep disturbances, vivid dreams, memory disturbance, depression, GI intolerance, sexual dysfunction, bradycardia, and hypotension.
- β Blockers should be used with caution in patients with heart failure, peripheral vascular disease, atrioventricular conduction disturbances, asthma, depression, and diabetes.

Antidepressants
- **Amitriptyline** appears to be the tricyclic antidepressant (TCA) of choice, but **imipramine, doxepin, nortriptyline**, and **protriptyline** have also been used.
- Their beneficial effects in migraine prophylaxis are independent of antidepressant activity and may be related to down-regulation of central 5-HT$_2$ and adrenergic receptors.
- TCAs are usually well tolerated at the lower doses used for migraine prophylaxis, but anticholinergic effects may limit use, especially in patients with benign prostatic hyperplasia or glaucoma. Evening doses are preferred because of sedation.

➤ IX

TABLE 51–4. Prophylactic Migraine Therapies

Medication	Dose
β-Adrenergic Antagonists	
Atenolol	25–100 mg/day
Metoprotol[a]	50–300 mg/day in divided doses
Nadolol	80–240 mg/day
Propranolol[a,b]	80–240 mg/day in divided doses
Timolol[b]	20–60 mg/day in divided doses
Antidepressants	
Amitriptyline	25–150 mg at bedtime
Doxepin	10–200 mg at bedtime
Imipramine	10–200 mg at bedtime
Nortriptyline	10–150 mg at bedtime
Protriptyline	5–30 mg at bedtime
Fluoxetine	10–80 mg/day
Phenelzine[c]	15–60 mg/day in divided doses
Valproic Acid/Divalproex Sodium[b]	500–1500 mg/day in divided doses
Verapamil[a]	240–360 mg/day in divided doses
Methysergide,[b,c]	2–8 mg/day in divided doses with food
Nonsteroidal Anti-inflammatory Drugs[c]	
Aspirin	1300 mg/day in divided doses
Ketoprofen[a]	150 mg/day in divided doses
Naproxen sodium[a]	550–1100 mg/day in divided doses
Vitamin B$_2$	400 mg/day

[a]Sustained-release formulation available.
[b]FDA approved for prevention of migraine.
[c]Daily or prolonged use limited by potential toxicity.

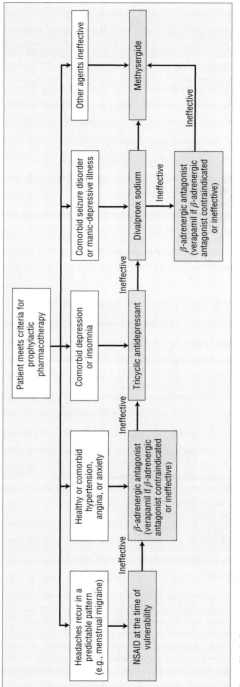

Figure 51–2. Treatment algorithm for prophylactic management of migraine headaches.

- Selective serotonin reuptake inhibitors (SSRIs) have not been extensively studied for migraine prophylaxis. There are inconsistent data for **fluoxetine**, and prospective data evaluating **sertraline, paroxetine, fluvoxamine,** and **citalopram** are lacking.
- SSRIs are considered to be less effective than TCAs for migraine prophylaxis and should not be considered first- or second-line therapy. However, they may be beneficial when depression is a significant contributor to headache.

Anticonvulsants

- **Valproic acid** and **divalproex sodium** (a 1:1 molar combination of valproate sodium and valproic acid) can reduce the frequency, severity, and duration of headaches by at least 50% in up to 65% of migraineurs.
- Efficacy of valproic acid may be due in part to inhibition of serotonergic neurons of the dorsal raphe nuclei.
- Side effects include nausea (less common with divalproex sodium and gradual dosing titration), tremor, somnolence, weight gain, hair loss, and hepatotoxicity (rare).
- Topiramate is undergoing FDA review for migraine prophylaxis. Gabapentin and other anticonvulsants may also have a role, but further study is required to establish their utility.

Methysergide

IX
- **Methysergide** is a semisynthetic ergot alkaloid that is a potent $5-HT_2$ receptor antagonist. It appears to stabilize serotonergic neurotransmission in the trigeminovascular system to block the development of neurogenic inflammation.
- Its use is limited by the occurrence of potentially serious retroperitoneal, endocardial, and pulmonary fibrotic complications that have occurred during long-term uninterrupted use. It is reserved for patients with refractory headaches that do not respond to other preventive therapies.
- Consequently, a 4-week medication-free period is recommended after each 6-month treatment period. Dosage should be tapered over 1 week to prevent rebound headaches.
- Monitoring for fibrotic complications should include periodic cardiac auscultation, chest x-ray, echocardiography, and abdominal imaging. Patients should report symptoms of flank pain, dysuria, chest pain, and shortness of breath.
- Methysergide is best tolerated when taken with meals. Side effects other than GI intolerance are many and include insomnia, vivid dreams, hallucinations, claudication, and muscle cramps. The labeling should be consulted for additional side effects and contraindications.

Calcium Channel Blockers

Verapamil provided only modest benefit in decreasing the frequency of attacks in two placebo-controlled studies. It has little effect on the severity of migraine attacks. It is generally considered a second- or third-line prophylactic agent.

Nonsteroidal Anti-inflammatory Drugs

- NSAIDs are modestly effective for reducing the frequency, severity, and duration of migraine attacks, but potential GI and renal toxicity limit daily or prolonged use.
- They may be used intermittently to prevent headaches that recur in a predictable pattern (e.g., menstrual migraine). Treatment should be initiated 1 to 2 days prior to the time of headache vulnerability and continued until vulnerability is passed.

▶ TENSION-TYPE HEADACHE

DEFINITION

Tension-type headache is the most common type of primary headache and is more common in women than men. Pain is usually mild to moderate and nonpulsatile. Episodic headaches may become chronic.

PATHOPHYSIOLOGY

- Pain is thought to originate from myofascial tissues.
- After activation of supraspinal pain perception structures, a headache occurs because of central modulation of incoming peripheral stimuli.

CLINICAL PRESENTATION

- Premonitory symptoms and aura are absent, and pain is usually mild to moderate, bilateral, and in the frontal and temporal areas, but occipital and parietal areas can also be affected.
- Mild photophobia or phonophobia may occur.
- Pericranial or cervical muscles may have tender spots or localized nodules in some patients.

TREATMENT

IX

- Simple analgesics (alone or in combination with caffeine) and NSAIDS are the mainstay of acute therapy.
- Nonpharmacologic therapies include reassurance and counseling, stress management, relaxation training, and biofeedback. physical therapeutic options (e.g., heat or cold packs, ultrasound, electrical nerve stimulation, massage, acupuncture, trigger point injections, occipital nerve blocks) have performed inconsistently.
- Acetaminophen, aspirin, ibuprofen, naproxen, ketoprofen, indomethacin, and ketorolac are effective.
- High-dose NSAIDS and the combination of aspirin or acetaminophen with butalbital or, rarely, codeine are effective options. The use of butalbital and codeine combinations should be avoided when possible.
- Acute medication for episodic headache should be taken no more often than 2 days/wk to prevent development of chronic tension-type headache.
- There is no evidence to support the efficacy of muscle relaxants for tension-type headache.
- Preventive treatment should be considered if headache frequency (more than 2 per week), duration (greater than 3 to 4 hours), or severity results in medication overuse or substantial disability.
- The TCAs are used most often for prophylaxis of tension headache. injection of botulinum toxin into pericranial muscles has demonstrated efficacy in prophylaxis of chronic tension-type headache in two studies.

▶ EVALUATION OF THERAPEUTIC OUTCOMES

- Patients should be monitored for frequency, intensity, and duration of headaches and for any change in the headache pattern.
- Patients taking abortive therapy should be monitored for frequency of use of prescription and over-the-counter medications and for side effects of medications.

- Patterns of abortive medication use can be documented to establish the need for prophylactic therapy. Prophylactic therapies should also be monitored closely for adverse reactions, abortive therapy needs, adequate dosing, and compliance.

See Chapter 59, Headache Disorders, authored by Deborah S. King and Katherine C. Herndon, for a more detailed discussion of this topic.

IX

Chapter 52

▶ PAIN MANAGEMENT

▶ DEFINITION

Pain is an unpleasant, subjective sensory and emotional experience associated with actual or potential tissue damage or described in terms of such damage.

▶ PATHOPHYSIOLOGY

NOCICEPTIVE PAIN

- Nociceptive (acute) pain is either somatic (arising from skin, bone, joint, muscle, or connective tissue) or visceral (arising from internal organs such as the large intestine or pancreas).
- Stimulation of free nerve endings known as nociceptors is the first step leading to the sensation of pain. These receptors are found in both somatic and visceral structures and are activated by mechanical, thermal, and chemical impulses. Release of bradykinins, K^+, prostaglandins, histamine, leukotrienes, serotonin, and substance P may sensitize and/or activate nociceptors. Receptor activation leads to action potentials that are transmitted along afferent nerve fibers to the spinal cord.
- Action potentials continue from the site of noxious stimuli to the dorsal horn of the spinal cord and then ascend to higher centers. The thalamus acts as a relay station and passes the impulses to central structures where pain is processed further.
- The body modulates pain through several processes. The endogenous opiate system consists of neurotransmitters (e.g., enkephalins, dynorphins, and β-endorphins) and receptors (e.g., μ, δ, κ) that are found throughout the central nervous system (CNS). Endogenous opioids bind to opioid receptors and inhibit the transmission of pain impulses.
- The CNS also contains a descending system for control of pain transmission. This system originates in the brain and can inhibit synaptic pain transmission at the dorsal horn. Important neurotransmitters here include endogenous opioids, serotonin, norepinephrine, γ-aminobutyric acid (GABA), and neurotensin.

NEUROPATHIC PAIN

- Neuropathic (chronic) pain is sustained by abnormal processing of sensory input by the peripheral or central nervous system. There are a large number of neuropathic pain syndromes that are often difficult to treat (e.g., low back pain, diabetic neuropathy, postherpetic neuralgia, cancer-related pain, spinal cord injury).
- Nerve damage or persistent stimulation may cause pain circuits to produce spontaneous nerve stimulation, autonomic neuronal pain stimulation, and a progressive increase in discharge of dorsal horn neurons.

▶ CLINICAL PRESENTATION

GENERAL

- Patients may be in obvious acute distress (trauma pain) or appear to have no noticeable suffering (chronic/persistent).

SYMPTOMS

- Pain can be described as sharp, dull, burning, shocklike, tingling, shooting, radiating, fluctuating in intensity, and varying in location.
- Over time, the same pain stimulus may cause symptoms that completely change (e.g., sharp to dull, obvious to vague).
- Nonspecific symptoms include anxiety, depression, fatigue, insomnia, anger, and fear.

SIGNS

- Acute pain can cause hypertension, tachycardia, diaphoresis, mydriasis, and pallor, but these signs are *not diagnostic*.
- In some acute cases and in most chronic/persistent pain, there may be no obvious signs.
- Pain is always subjective; thus pain is best diagnosed based on patient description and history.
- A comprehensive history and physical examination are required to evaluate underlying diseases and possible contributing factors. A baseline description of pain can be obtained by assessing PQRST characteristics (*p*alliative and *p*rovocative factors, *q*uality, *r*adiation, *s*everity, and *t*emporal factors). Attention should be given to mental factors that may lower the pain threshold (anxiety, depression, fatigue, anger, fear). Behavioral, cognitive, social, and cultural factors may also affect the pain experience.
- Nociceptive pain is often acute, localized, well described, and relieved with conventional analgesics. Somatic pain usually presents as throbbing and well-localized discomfort, but visceral pain can feel as if it were coming from other structures (referred) or present as a well-localized phenomenon.
- Neuropathic pain is often chronic, not well described, and not easily treated with conventional analgesics. Patients commonly present with pain described as burning, tingling, shock-like, or shooting; exaggerated painful responses to normally noxious stimuli (hyperalgesia); or painful responses to normally nonnoxious stimuli (allodynia).
- Ineffective pain treatment may result in hypoxia, hypercapnea, hypertension, excessive cardiac activity, and emotional difficulties.
- Chronic pain can be divided into four subtypes: (1) pain that persists beyond the normal healing time for an acute injury, (2) pain related to a chronic disease, (3) pain without an identifiable organic cause, and (4) pain involving both the chronic and acute pain associated with cancer.
- Patients with chronic pain may develop psychological problems, dependence on and tolerance to analgesics, trouble sleeping, and sensitivity to environmental changes that intensify pain.

▶ DESIRED OUTCOMES

The goals of therapy are to minimize pain and provide reasonable comfort at the lowest effective analgesic dose. With chronic pain, goals may include rehabilitation and resolution of psychosocial issues.

IX

TABLE 52–1. Pharmacokinetic and Pharmacodynamic Profiles of FDA-Approved Nonopioid Analgesics[a]

Agent	Time to Peak Concentration (h)	Elimination Half-Life (h)	Analgesic Onset (h)	Analgesic Duration (h)
Aspirin	0.25–2	0.25–0.33	0.5	3–6
Choline salicylate	1.5–2	—[b]	—[b]	4
Magnesium salicylate	1.5–2	—[b]	—[b]	4
Sodium salicylate	0.67	—[b]	—[b]	4
Diflunisal	2–3	8–12	1	8–12
Acetaminophen	0.5–2	1.25–3	0.5–1	3–6
Meclofenamate	0.5–2	0.8–5.3	—[b]	4–6
Mefenamic acid	2–4	2–4	—[b]	6
Etodolac	1	7	0.5–1	6–8
Diclofenac potassium	1	2	0.5	6–8
Ibuprofen	1–2	1–2.5	0.5	4–6
Fenoprofen	1–2	2–3	0.25–0.5	4–6
Ketoprofen	0.5–2	1.1–4	1	4–8
Naproxen	2–4	12–17	1	Up to 12
Naproxen sodium	1–2	12–13	0.5–1	Up to 12
Ketorolac (parenteral)	0.5–1	4–6	0.17	6
Ketorolac (oral)	0.5–1	4–6	0.5–1	4–6
Celecoxib	3	11	1	12–24
Valdecoxib	3	8–11	1	12–24

[a]Does not include agents approved only, for osteoarthritis or rheumatoid arthritis.
[b]Data not available to author.

▶ TREATMENT

ACUTE PAIN

The elderly and the young are at a higher risk for undertreatment of pain because of misunderstanding about the pathophysiology of their pain.

Nonopioid Agents

- Analgesia should be initiated with the most effective analgesic with the fewest side effects. Dosage, pharmacokinetic, pharmacodynamic, and side-effect profiles of Food and Drug Administration (FDA)-approved nonopioid analgesics are shown in Tables 52–1 to 52–3.
- These drugs (except acetaminophen) reduce prostaglandins produced by the arachidonic acid cascade, thereby decreasing the number of pain impulses received by the CNS.
- **Aspirin** given concurrently with other **nonsteroidal anti-inflammatory drugs** (NSAIDs) is more likely to cause gastrointestinal (GI) side effects. The **salicylate salts** cause fewer GI side effects than aspirin and do not inhibit platelet aggregation.
- Aspirin-like compounds should not be given to children or teenagers with influenza or chickenpox, as Reye's syndrome may result.
- **Acetaminophen** has analgesic and antipyretic activity but little anti-inflammatory action. It is highly hepatotoxic on overdose.

Opioid Agents

- With oral analgesics, the onset of action usually takes about 45 minutes, and peak effect usually is seen in about 1 to 2 hours.

TABLE 52–2. FDA-Approved Nonopioid Analgesics in Adults[a]

Class and Generic Name	Usual Dosage Range (mg)	Maximal Dose (mg/day)
Salicylates		
Acetylsalicylic acid[b] (aspirin)	325–650 every 4 h	4000
Choline[b]	870 every 3–4 h	5220
Magnesium[b]	650 every 4 h or 1090 three times daily	4800 in 3–4 divided doses
Sodium[b]	325–650 every 4 h	5400
Diflunisal	500–1000 initial	
	250–500 every 8–12 h	1500
para-Aminophenol		
Acetaminophen[b]	325–1000 every 4–6 h	4000
Fenamates		
Meclofenamate	50–100 every 4–6 h	400
Mefenamic acid	Initial 500	
	250 every 6 h (maximum of 7 days)	1000[c]
Pyranocarboxylic Acid		
Etodoloc	200–400 every 6–8 h (immediate release only)	1000
Acetic Acid		
Diclofenac potassium	In some patients, initial 100, 50 three times a day	150[d]
Propionic Acids		
Ibuprofen[b]	200–400 every 4–6 h	3200
		1200[e]
Fenoprofen	200 every 4–6 h	3200
Ketoprofen[b]	25–50 every 6–8 h	300
	12.5–25 every 4–6 h[d]	75[e]
Naproxen	500 initial	
	500 every 12 h or 250 every 6–8 h	1000[c]
Naproxen sodium[b]	In some patients, 440 initial[e]	
	220 every 8–12 h[e]	660[e]
Naproxen delayed-release[f]	500 every 12 h	1000
Naproxen controlled-release[f]	500–1000 every 24 h	1500
Pyrrolizine Carboxylic Acid		
Ketorolac (parenteral)	30–60 (single IM dose only)	30–60
	15–30 every 6 h (maximum of 5 days)	120
Ketorolac (oral) (indicated for continuation with parenteral only)	In some patients, initial oral dose 20 10 every 4–6 h (maximum of 5 days, which includes parenteral doses)	40
Cyclooxygenase-2 Inhibitors		
Celecoxib	Initial 400 followed by another 200 on first day then 200 twice daily[g]	400[g]
Valdecoxib	20 twice daily[h]	40[h]

[a]Does not include agents approved only for osteoarthritis or rheumatoid arthritis.
[b]Available both as an over-the-counter preparation and as a precription drug.
[c]Up to 1250 mg on the first day.
[d]Up to 200 mg on the first day.
[e]Over the counter.
[f]Not for the initial treatment of acute pain.
[g]For acute pain primary dysmenorrhea.
[h]For primary dysmenorrhea.

IX

TABLE 52–3. Relative Side Effects of FDA-Approved Nonopioid Analgesics[a]

Agent	GI Irritation	CNS Effects	Hepatic Toxicity	Renal Toxicity
Aspirin	+ + + + ++	+	++	++
Choline salicylate	+ + +	—[b]	—[b]	—[b]
Magnesium salicylate	+ + +	—[b]	—[b]	—[b]
Sodium salicylate	+ + +	—[b]	—[b]	—[b]
Diflunisal	++	+	+	+
Acetaminophen	+	+	++	+
Meclofenamate	++	+	+	++
Mefenamic acid	++	+	+	++
Etodolac	++	+	+	++
Diclofenac potassium	++	+	+	++
Ibuprofen	++	+	+	++
Fenoprofen	++	++	+	++
Ketoprofen	++	+	+	++
Ketorolac[c]	++	+	+	+
Naproxen	++	+	+	++
Celecoxib	+	+	+	++
Valdecoxib	+	+	+	++

[a] Does not include agents approved only for osteoarthritis or rheumatoid arthritis.
[b] No data available to author.
[c] Five-day use only.

IX

- Equianalgesic doses, dosing guidelines, major adverse effects, and pharmacokinetics of opioids are shown in Tables 52–4 to 52–7. The equianalgesic doses are only a guide, and doses must be individualized.
- Partial agonists and antagonists compete with agonists for opiate receptor sites and exhibit mixed agonist-antagonist activity. They may have selectivity for analgesic receptor sites and cause fewer side effects.
- In the initial stages of acute pain treatment, analgesics should be given around the clock. As the painful state subsides, as-needed schedules can be used.
- With patient-controlled analgesia (PCA), patients self-administer preset amounts of intravenous opioids via a syringe pump electronically interfaced with a timing device; thus, patients can balance pain control with sedation.
- Administration of opioids directly into the CNS (epidural and intrathecal/subarachnoid routes) is becoming prominent for acute pain. These methods require careful monitoring because of reports of marked sedation, respiratory depression, pruritus, nausea, vomiting, urinary retention, and hypotension. **Naloxone** is used to reverse respiratory depression, but continual infusion may be required. The analgesic effects of single doses of epidural opioids are given below:
  - **Morphine**, 1 to 6 mg (onset 30 minutes, duration 6 to 24 hours)
  - **Hydromorphone**, 1 to 2 mg (onset 15 minutes, duration 6 to 16 hours)
  - **Fentanyl**, 0.025 to 0.1 mg (onset 5 minutes, duration 1 to 4 hours)
- Intrathecal and epidural opioids are often administered by continuous infusion or PCA. They are safe and effective when given simultaneously with intrathecal or epidural local anesthetics such as **bupivacaine**. All agents administered directly into the CNS should be preservative free.
- Subarachnoid doses are smaller than epidural doses (e.g., morphine 0.1 to 0.3 mg, fentanyl 0.005 to 0.025 mg).

TABLE 52–4. Opioid Analgesics

Class and Generic Name	Route	Equianalgesic Dose (mg) (Adults)
Morphine-Like Agonists		
Morphine	IM	10
	PO	30
Hydromorphone	IM	1.5
	PO	7.5
Oxymorphone	IM	1
	R	5[a]
Levorphanol	IM (acute)	2
	PO (acute)	4
	IM (chronic)	1
	PO (chronic)	1
Codeine	IM	15–30[b]
	PO	15–30[b]
Hydrocodone	PO	5–10[b]
Oxycodone	PO	20–30[c]
Meperidine-Like Agonists		
Meperidine	IM	75
	PO	300[c] Not recommended
Fentanyl	IM	0.1–0.2
	Transdermal	25 mcg/h[d]
	Transmucosal for breakthrough pain only	
Methadone-Like Agonists		
Methadone	IM (acute)	Variable[e]
	PO (acute)	Variable[e]
	IM (chronic)	Variable[e]
	PO (chronic)	Variable[e]
Propoxyphene	PO	65[b]
Agonist-Antagonist Derivatives		
Pentazocine	IM	Not recommended
	PO	50[b]
Butorphanol	IM	2
	Intranasal	1[b]
		(one spray)
Nalbuphine	IM	10
Buprenorphine	IM	0.4
Dezocine	IM	10
Antagonists		
Naloxone	IV	0.4–1.2[f]
Central Analgesic		
Tramadol	PO	50–100[b]

[a] 5 mg rectal morphine = 5 mg rectal oxymorphone.
[b] Starting dose only (equianalgesia not shown).
[c] Starting doses lower (oxycodone, 5–10 mg).
[d] Equivalent IM morphine dose = 8–22 mg day.
[e] The equianalgesic dose of methadone when compared with other opioids will decrease progressively the higher the previous opioid dose has been.
[f] Starting doses to be used in cases of opioid overdose.

TABLE 52-5. Dosing Guidelines

Agent(s)	Doses (Titrate Up or Down Based on Patient Response)	Notes
NSAIDs/acetaminophen/aspirin	Dose to maximum before switching to another agent (see Table 52-2)	Used in mild to moderate pain May use in conjunction with opioid agents to decrease doses of each Regular alcohol use and high doses of acetaminophen may result in liver toxicity Care must be exercised to avoid overdose when combination products containing these agents are used
Morphine	PO 5–30 mg q 3–4 h[a] IM 5–10 mg q 3–4 h[a] IV 1–2.5 mg q 5 min prn[a] SR 15–30 mg q 12 h (may need to be q 8 h in some patients) Rectal 10–20 mg q 4 h[a]	Drug of choice in severe pain Use immediate-release product with SR product to control "breakthrough" pain in cancer patients Every 24-h product available
Hydromorphone	PO 2–4 mg q 3–6 h[a] IM 1–4 mg q 3–6 h[a] IV 0.1–0.5 mg q 5 min prn[a] Rectal 3 mg q 6–8 h[a]	Use in severe pain More potent than morphine; otherwise, no advantages Use immediate-release product with sustained-release product to control "breakthrough" pain in cancer patients Use sustained-release product only in those patients who have demonstrated opioid tolerance 12-mg, 16-mg, 24-mg, and 32-mg sustained-release capsules are available and should be dosed every 24 h
Oxymorphone	IM 1–1.5 mg q 4–6 h[a] IV 0.5 mg initially Rectal 5 mg q 4–6 h[a]	Use in severe pain No advantages over morphine
Levorphanol	PO 2–3 mg q 6–8 h[a] IM 1–2 mg q 6–8 h	Use in severe pain Extended half-life useful in cancer patients In chronic pain, wait 3 days between dosage adjustments
Codeine	PO 15–60 mg q 3–6 h[a] IM 15–60 mg q 3–6 h[a] IV 15–60 mg q 3–6 h[a] (max. 360 mg q day)	Use in moderate pain Weak analgesic; use with NSAIDs or aspirin or acetaminophen
Hydrocodone	PO 5–10 mg q 3–6 h[a]	Use in moderate/severe pain Most effective when used with NSAIDs or aspirin or acetaminophen
Oxycodone	PO 5–10 mg q 3–6 h[a] Controlled release, 10–20 mg q 12 h	Use in moderate/severe pain Most effective when used with NSAIDs or aspirin or acetaminophen Use immediate-release product with sustained-release product to control "breakthrough" pain in cancer patients
Meperidine	IM 50–150 mg q 3–4 h[a] IV 5–10 mg q 5 min prn[a]	Use in severe pain Oral not recommended

Continued

TABLE 52–5. (Continued)

Agent(s)	Doses (Titrate Up or Down Based on Patient Response)	Notes
Fentanyl	IV 25–50 mcg/h IM 0.05–0.1 mg q 1–2 h[a] Transdermal 25 mcg/h q 72 h Transmucosal 200 mcg may repeat × 1, 30 min after first dose is given then titrate	Do not use in renal failure May precipitate tremors, myoclonus, and seizures Monoamine oxidase inhibitors can induce hyperpyrexia and/or seizures or opioid overdose symptoms Used in severe pain Do not use transdermal in acute pain Transmucosal for "breakthrough" cancer pain
Methadone	PO 2.5–10 mg q 3–4 h (acute)[a] IM 2.5–10 mg q 3–4 h (acute)[a] PO 5–20 mg q 6–8 h (chronic)[a]	Effective in severe chronic pain Sedation can be major problem Some chronic pain patients can be dosed every 12 h The equianalgesic dose of methadone when compared with other opioids will decrease progressively the higher the previous opioid dose has been
Propoxyphene	PO 100 mg q 4 h[a] (napsylate) PO 65 mg q 4 h[a] (HCl) (max. q day 600 mg of napsylate, 390 mg HCl)	Use in moderate pain Weak analgesic; most effective when used with NSAIDs or aspirin or acetaminophen Will cause carbamazepine levels to increase 100 mg of napsylate salt = 65 mg of HCl salt
Pentazocine	PO 50–100 mg q 3–4 h[b] (max. 600 mg q day)	Third-line agent for moderate to severe pain May precipitate withdrawal in opiate-dependent patients Parenteral doses not recommended
Butorphanol	IM 1–4 mg q 3–4 h[b] IV 0.5–2 mg q 3–4 h[b] Intranasal 1 mg (1 spray) q 3–4 h[b] If inadequate relief after initial spray, may repeat in other nostril × 1 in 30–60 min Max 2 sprays (1 per nostril) q 3–4 h[b]	Second-line agent for moderate to severe pain May precipitate withdrawal in opiate-dependent patients
Nalbuphine	IM/IV 10 mg q 3–6 h[b] (max 20 mg dose, 160 mg q day)	Second-line agent for moderate to severe pain May precipitate withdrawal in opiate-dependent patients
Buprenorphine	IM 0.3 mg q 6 h[b] Slow IV 0.3 mg q 6 h[b] May repeat × 1, 30–60 min after initial dose	Second-line agent for moderate to severe pain May precipitate withdrawal in opiate-dependent patients
Dezocine	IM 5–20 mg q 3–6 h[b] IV 2.5–10 mg q 2–4 h[b]	Second-line agent for moderate to severe pain May precipitate withdrawal in opiate-dependent patients
Naloxone	IV 0.4–1.2 mg	When reversing opiate side effects in patients needing analgesia, dilute and titrate (0.1–0.2 mg q 2–3 min) so as not to reverse analgesia Maximum dose is 400 mg/24 h
Tramadol	PO 50–100 mg q 4–6 h[a] If rapid onset not required, start 25 mg/day and titrate over several days	Naloxone may not be effective in reversing respiratory depression Decrease dose in renal impairment and in the elderly

SR, sustained release; h, hour; q, every; mg, milligram; mcg, microgram; prn, as needed.

[b]May reach a ceiling analgesic effect.

TABLE 52–6. Major Adverse Effects of the Opioid Analgesics

Effects	Manifestation
Mood changes	Dysphoria, euphoria
Somnolence	Lethargy, drowsiness, apathy, inability to concentrate
Stimulation of chemoreceptor trigger zone	Nausea, vomiting
Respiratory depression	Decreased respiratory rate
Decreased gastrointestinal motility	Constipation
Increase in sphincter tone	Biliary spasm, urinary retention (varies among agents)
Histamine release	Urticaria, pruritus, rarely exacerbation of asthma (varies among agents)
Tolerance	Larger doses for same effect
Dependence	Withdrawal symptoms upon abrupt discontinuation

Morphine and Congeners

- **Morphine** is considered by many clinicians to be the first-line agent for moderate to severe pain. It can be given orally, parenterally, or rectally.
- Nausea and vomiting are more likely in ambulatory patients and with the initial dose.
- Respiratory depression increases progressively as doses are increased. It often manifests as a decrease in respiratory rate, and the cough reflex is also depressed. Patients with underlying pulmonary dysfunction are at risk for increased respiratory compromise. Respiratory depression can be reversed by naloxone.

IX

TABLE 52–7. Opioid Analgesic Pharmacokinetics[a]

Agent	Time to Peak (h)	Half-Life (h)	Analgesic Onset (min)	Analgesic Duration (h)
Morphine	0.5–1	2	10–20	3–5
Hydromorphone	0.5–1	2–3	10–20	3–5
Oxymorphone	0.5–1	2–3	10–20	4–6
Levorphanol	0.5–1	12–16	10–20	5–8
Hydrocodone (PO)	1	4	30–60	4–6
Codeine	0.5–1	3	10–20	4–6
Oxycodone (PO)	0.5–1	2–3	30–60	4–6
Meperidine	0.5–1	3–4	10–20	2–5
Fentanyl	0.17–0.33	3–4	7–15	1–2
Methadone	0.5–1	15–30	10–20	4–5 (acute) >8 (chronic)
Propoxyphene (PO)	2–2.5	6–12	30–60	4–6
Pentazocine	0.5–1	4–5	15–20	3–6
Butorphanol	0.5–1	2.5–3.5	10–20	4–6
Nalbuphine	0.5–1	2–5	<15	4–6
Buprenorphine	0.5–1	5	10–20	4–8
Dezocine	0.17–1.5 (IM)	0.6–5 (IV)	15–30 (IV)	2–4 (IV)
Naloxone[c] (IV/IM)	—[b]	1–1.5	1–2 (IV) 2–5 (IM)	0.5–2 (IV) IM may last longer
Tramadol (PO)	2–3	6–7	<60	4–6

[a]Based on intramuscular data unless otherwise indicated.
[b]No data available to author.
[c]Narcotic antagonist.

- The combination of opioid analgesics with alcohol or other CNS depressants amplifies CNS depression and is potentially harmful and possibly lethal.
- Morphine produces venous and arteriolar dilatation, which may result in orthostatic hypotension. Hypovolemic patients are more susceptible to morphine-induced hypotension. Morphine is often considered the opioid of choice when using opioids to treat pain associated with myocardial infarction, as it decreases myocardial oxygen demand.
- Morphine can cause constipation, spasms of the sphincter of Oddi, urinary retention, and pruritus (secondary to histamine release) (see Table 52–6). In head trauma patients who are not ventilated, morphine-induced respiratory depression can increase intracranial pressure and cloud the neurologic examination results.

Meperidine and Congeners (Phenylpiperidines)

- **Meperidine** is less potent and has a shorter duration of action than morphine. In most settings, it offers no advantages over morphine.
- With high doses or in patients with renal failure, the metabolite normeperidine accumulates, causing tremor, muscle twitching, and possibly seizures.
- Meperidine should not be combined with monoamine oxidase inhibitors because of the possibility of severe respiratory depression or excitation, delirium, hyperpyrexia, and convulsions.
- **Fentanyl** is a synthetic opioid structurally related to meperidine. It is often used in anesthesiology as an adjunct to general anesthesia. It is more potent and shorter acting than meperidine. Transdermal fentanyl can be used for treatment of chronic pain requiring opioid analgesics. After a patch is applied, it takes 12 to 24 hours to obtain optimal analgesic effect, and analgesic support may last 72 hours. It may take 6 days after increasing a dose before new steady-state levels are achieved. Thus, the fentanyl patch should not be used for acute pain. A fentanyl lozenge on a stick is available for treatment of breakthrough cancer pain.

Methadone and Congeners

Methadone has oral efficacy, extended duration of action, and ability to suppress withdrawal symptoms in heroin addicts. With repeated doses, the analgesic duration of action of methadone is prolonged, but excessive sedation may also result. Although effective for acute pain, it is usually used for chronic pain.

Opioid Agonist–Antagonist Derivatives

This class produces analgesia and has a ceiling effect on respiratory depression and lower abuse potential than morphine. However, psychotomimetic responses (e.g., hallucinations and dysphoria with **pentazocine**), a ceiling analgesic effect, and the propensity to initiate withdrawal in opioid-dependent patients have limited their widespread use.

Opioid Antagonists

Naloxone is a pure opioid antagonist that binds competitively to opioid receptors but does not produce an analgesic response. It is used to reverse the toxic effects of agonist and agonist-antagonist opioids.

Central Analgesic

- **Tramadol**, a centrally acting analgesic for moderate to moderately severe pain, binds to μ opiate receptors and weakly inhibits norepinephrine and serotonin reuptake.

TABLE 52–8. Local Anesthetics[a]

Agent	Onset (min)	Duration (h)
Esters		
Procaine	2–5	0.25–1
Chloroprocaine	6–12	0.5
Tetracaine	≤15	2–3
Amides		
Mepivacaine	3–5	0.75–1.5
Bupivacaine	5	2–4
Lidocaine	<2	0.5–1
Prilocaine	<2	≥1
Etidocaine	3–5	5–10
Ropivacaine[b]	11–26	1.7–3.2

[a]Unless otherwise indicated, values are for infiltrative anesthesia.
[b]Epidural administration in cesarean section.

- Although associated with less respiratory depression than morphine at recommended doses, tramadol has a side-effect profile similar to that of other opioid analgesics. It may also enhance the risk of seizures. It may be useful for treating chronic pain, especially that of neuropathic origin, but it has little advantage over other opioid analgesics for acute pain.

Combination Therapy
- The combination of an opioid and nonopioid oral analgesic often results in analgesia superior to monotherapy and may allow for lower doses of each agent. An NSAID with a scheduled opioid dose is often effective for painful bone metastases.

Regional Analgesia
- Regional analgesia with local anesthetics (Table 52–8) can provide relief of both acute and chronic pain. Anesthetics can be positioned by injection (i.e., in joints, in the epidural or intrathecal space, along nerve roots) or topically.
- High plasma concentrations can cause CNS excitation and depression (dizziness, tinnitus, drowsiness, disorientation, muscle twitching, seizures, respiratory arrest). Cardiovascular effects include myocardial depression and other effects. Skillful technical application, frequent administration, and specialized follow-up procedures are required.

CHRONIC PAIN
- An algorithm for pain management in oncology patients is shown in Figure 52–1.
- NSAIDs are especially effective for bone pain. **Strontium-89** and **samarium SM 153 lexidronam** are also effective.
- For cancer pain, round-the-clock schedules in conjunction with as-needed doses are employed when patients experience breakthrough pain.
- Methadone has regained prominence in treating cancer pain. It has a prolonged mechanism of action, *N*-methyl-d-aspartate (NMDA) receptor antagonist activity (d-isomer), and is inexpensive. However, it can be hard to titrate. Epidural

IX ◄

Mild pain

Agents: Nonpioid analgesics Nonsteroidal anti-inflammatory drugs (NSAIDs)	**Maximum daily dose:** Acetaminophen 4.0 g Ibuprofen 3.2 g Naproxen 1.0 g

Response

Good → Continue

Poor → Dose

Not tolerated →
GI: Take with food/milk/antacid
Switch to acetaminophen
Oral: Rectal acetaminophen

Principles of therapy

1. Assess the frequency/duration/occurrence/etiology of the pain on a routine basis.
2. If bone pain is present, use of an NSAID should be routine.
3. Always dose a medication to its maximum before reverting to the next step, unless pain is totally out of control.
4. If pain is constant or recurring, always dose round-the-clock (RTC).

Mild/moderate pain

Agents: Acetaminophen or NSAID combinations with opioids **Adjuncts:** Tricyclic antidepressants Anticonvulsants Steroids Radiopharmaceuticals (Bone pain)	**Maximum daily dose:** Acetaminophen 4.0 g Opioids Titrate Amitriptyline 10–50 mg Imipramine 10–50 mg Doxepin 10–50 mg Prednisone Titrate Dexamethasone Titrate NSAIDs (See above) Gabapentin (Neurontin) 3.6 g

Response

Good → Continue

Poor → Not tolerated →
GI: Take with food/milk/antacid
Delete NSAID
Oral: See below

Principles of therapy

1. Assess the frequency/duration/occurrence/etiology of the pain on a routine basis.
2. Whenever bone pain is present, use of an NSAID with opioid should be routine.
3. Pain management needs to take precedence over other therapies.
4. Fulminating sites of pain, especially in bone, need to be evaluated quickly for alternate therapy such as radiation/radiopharmaceuticals.
5. Accurate assessment and history of reported opiate allergies are important. A differentiation between allergy, sensitivity, and side effect needs to be made.
6. Always dose to the maximum of each agent when possible.
7. If pain is constant or recurring, always dose RTC.
8. Consider adjunct therapy when appropriate.
9. When using opioids, prevent constipation with a GI stimulant.

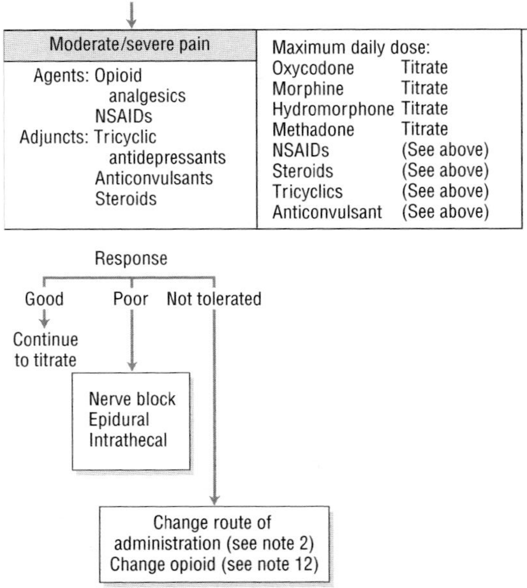

Moderate/severe pain		Maximum daily dose:		Principles of therapy

Agents: Opioid
analgesics
NSAIDs

Adjuncts: Tricyclic
antidepressants
Anticonvulsants
Steroids

Maximum daily dose:

Oxycodone	Titrate
Morphine	Titrate
Hydromorphone	Titrate
Methadone	Titrate
NSAIDs	(See above)
Steroids	(See above)
Tricyclics	(See above)
Anticonvulsant	(See above)

Principles of therapy

1. Assess the frequency/duration/occurrence/etiology of the pain on a routine basis.
2. Morphine is often the choice in this category: (1) multiple products available; (2) multiple route of administration options, such as oral, rectal, IM, SC, IV, epidural, and intrathecal; and (3) a known equipotency between these routes that allows a much easier transition.
3. No real practical dosage limits with opioids mentioned; can be titrated to patient response. If myoclonic jerking occurs, consider switching to alternative opioid.
4. Management should be RTC dosing, with sustained-release product and an immediate-release product as for breakthrough pain.
5. Utilize all possible adjuncts to minimize increases in dose.
6. Initial control may require doses higher than those needed in maintenance.
7. A fentanyl patch placed every 72 h may provide a more convenient dosing regimen when patients are on a stable oral dosing program.
8. Special situations of sudden-onset/sudden-resolution pain, especially along a nerve track, or neuralgias, may require an adjunct of an anticonvulsant and/or tricyclic antidepressant.
9. Any time nonpharmacologic options of radiation, chemotherapy, surgical debulking, or neurologic interventions are used, a total reevaluation of all drug treatment needs to be made.
10. When using opioids, prevent constipation with a GI stimulant.
11. Any new report of pain requires reevaluation.
12. If patient does not tolerate an opioid, consider switching to another opioid.

Response

Good — Continue to titrate

Poor / Not tolerated → Nerve block / Epidural / Intrathecal

Change route of administration (see note 2)
Change opioid (see note 12)

Figure 52–1. Algorithm for pain management in oncology patients. (*Adapted from the Kaiser Permanente Algorithm for Pain Management in Patients with Advanced Malignant Disease.*)

clonidine is also effective with epidurally administered opioid analgesics for treatment of refractory pain.

- The choice of opioid is controversial, but many clinicians prefer morphine for chronic cancer pain. The fentanyl patch may provide a more convenient dosing alternative in patients on stable regimens.
- Tricyclic antidepressants and anticonvulsants (e.g., **gabapentin**) can be effective for neuropathic pain.
- Meperidine is not recommended for long-term use because of its relatively short duration of action and CNS hyperirritability of normeperidine.

▶ EVALUATION OF THERAPEUTIC OUTCOMES

- Pain intensity, pain relief, and medication side effects must be assessed on a regular basis. The timing and regularity of assessment depend on the type of pain and the medications administered.
- Postoperative pain and acute exacerbations of cancer pain may require hourly assessment, whereas chronic nonmalignant pain may need only daily (or less frequent) monitoring.
- Quality of life must also be assessed on a regular basis in all patients.
- The best management of opioid-induced constipation is prevention. Patients should be counseled on proper intake of fluids and fiber, and a laxative may be added if needed.
- If acute pain does not subside within the anticipated time frame (usually 1 to 2 weeks), further investigation of the cause is warranted.

IX

See Chapter 58, Pain Management, authored by Terry J. Baumann, for a more detailed discussion of this topic.

Chapter 53

▶ PARKINSON'S DISEASE

▶ DEFINITION

Idiopathic Parkinson's disease (IPD) has highly characteristic neuropathologic findings and clinical presentation including motor deficits and, in some cases, mental deterioration.

▶ PATHOPHYSIOLOGY

- Loss of nigrostriatal dopamine neurons results in reduction of cortical activation; virtually all the motor deficits of IPD are attributable to the marked loss in dopaminergic neurons projecting to the putamen. There is a positive correlation between the degree of nigrostriatal dopamine loss and disease severity.
- Drugs enhancing dopaminergic or inhibiting acetylcholine or glutamate neurotransmission have been successful in IPD therapeutics. Recent findings suggest that adenosine A_{2A} receptor antagonists may also be promising.
- Activation of D_2 receptors appears to be of primary importance for mediating both clinical improvement and some adverse effects (e.g., hallucinations). D_1 receptors may be involved in producing dyskinesias.
- Degeneration of nigrostriatal dopamine neurons results in a relative increase of striatal cholinergic interneuron activity, which contributes to the tremor of IPD.

▶ CLINICAL PRESENTATION

- IPD develops insidiously and progresses slowly. Clinical features are summarized in Table 53–1. Initial symptoms may be sensory, but as the disease progresses, one or more classic primary features present (e.g., resting tremor, rigidity, bradykinesia, postural changes). Other characteristics include micrographia, decreased facial animation (hypomimia) and blink rate, shuffling gait, and decreased dexterity.
- Resting tremor is typical of IPD and often is the sole presenting complaint. However, only two-thirds of IPD patients have tremor on diagnosis, and some never develop this sign. Tremor is present most commonly in the hands, often begins unilaterally, and sometimes has a characteristic "pill-rolling" quality. The resting tremor is usually abolished by volitional movement and is absent during sleep.
- Muscular rigidity involves increased muscular resistance to passive range of motion and can be cogwheel in nature. Postural instability may lead to falls.
- Intellectual deterioration is not inevitable, but some patients deteriorate in a manner indistinguishable from Alzheimer's disease.

▶ DIAGNOSIS

- Diagnostic criteria specify that at least two of the following be present: (1) limb muscle rigidity, (2) resting tremor (at 3 to 6 Hz and abolished by movement), (3) bradykinesia, or (4) postural instability.
- A number of other conditions must also be excluded. Medication-induced parkinsonism must be ruled out (e.g., antipsychotics, antiemetics, or metoclopramide). Other diagnostic criteria include lack of other neurologic impairment and responsiveness to levodopa.

TABLE 53–1. Clinical Features

Cardinal Features	Diaphoresis
Bradykinesia	Orthostatic blood pressure changes
Postural instability	Paroxysmal flushing
Resting tremor (may have postural and action components)	Sexual disturbances
Rigidity	**Mental Status Changes**
Motor Symptoms	Bradyphrenia
Decreased dexterity	Confusional state
Dysarthria	Dementia
Dysphagia	Psychosis (paranoia, hallucinosis)
Festinating gait	Sleep disturbance
Flexed posture	**Other**
"Freezing" at initiation of movement	Fatiguability
Hypomimia	Oily skin
Hypophonia	Pedal edema
Micrographia	Seborrhea
Slow turning	Weight loss
Autonomic Symptoms	
Bladder and anal sphincter disturbances	
Constipation	

IX

▶ DESIRED OUTCOME

The goals of treatment are to minimize disability and side effects while maintaining quality of life. Families and patients should be involved in treatment decisions, and education of patients and caregivers is critical.

▶ TREATMENT

PHARMACOLOGIC THERAPY

- Treatment algorithms for early and late IPD are shown in Figures 53–1 and 53–2.
- A summary of available antiparkinsonian medications is listed in Table 53–2.
- In patients with mild symptoms, medications are often not needed if disabilities have not developed. Many patients have only mild slowness and resting tremor that can be managed effectively with anticholinergics or amantadine.
- The most effective treatment for IPD is replacement of the natural neurotransmitter dopamine by giving its immediate precursor, levodopa. Although levodopa is more effective than other available medications, concern for possible long-term risks causes some clinicians to limit its use.
- The decision to incorporate levodopa or dopamine agonist therapy is determined by advancing disability and ineffectiveness of alternative medications in providing adequate symptom control.
- L-dopa and dopaminergic agonists may cause psychiatric symptoms, including compulsive behaviors, delirium, agitation, paranoia, delusions, and hallucinations. These problems can be managed using the guidelines and antipsychotic medication as summarized in Table 53–3.

Anticholinergic Medications

- Anticholinergic drugs can be effective for tremor and dystonic features in some patients but rarely show substantial benefit for bradykinesia or other

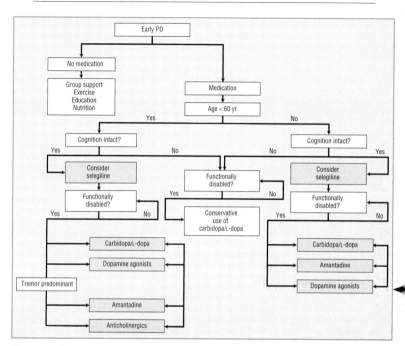

Figure 53–1. General algorithm for treating early idiopathic Parkinson's disease.

disabilities. They can be used as monotherapy or in conjunction with other antiparkinsonian drugs. They differ little from each other in therapeutic potential or adverse effects.

- Anticholinergic side effects include dry mouth, blurred vision, constipation, and urinary retention. More serious reactions include forgetfulness, sedation, depression, and anxiety. Patients with preexisting cognitive deficits and advanced age are at greater risk for central anticholinergic effects.

Amantadine

- **Amantadine** is often effective for mild symptoms, especially tremor. It may also decrease dyskinesia at relatively high doses (400 mg/day).
- Its precise mechanism of action is unknown but may involve dopaminergic or nondopaminergic mechanisms such as inhibition of *N*-methyl-*d*-aspartate receptors.
- Adverse effects include sedation, vivid dreams, dry mouth, depression, hallucinations, anxiety, dizziness, psychosis, and confusion. Livedo reticularis (a diffuse mottling of the skin) is a common but reversible side effect.
- Doses should be reduced in patients with renal dysfunction.

Levodopa and Carbidopa/Levodopa

- **Levodopa**, the most effective drug available, is the immediate precursor of dopamine. It crosses the blood-brain barrier, whereas dopamine does not.
- The decision to start L-dopa as soon as the diagnosis is made or only when symptoms compromise social, occupational, or psychological well-being has

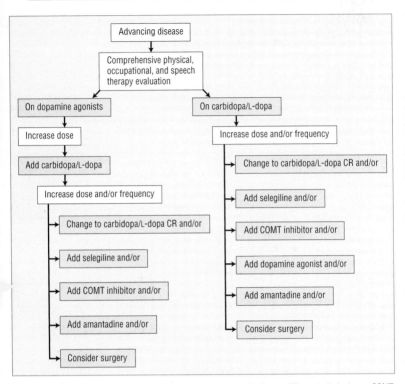

Figure 53–2. Algorithm for treating advanced idiopathic Parkinson's disease. CR, controlled release; COMT, catechol-*O*-methyltransferase.

generated controversy. A study is under way that should assist in making an informed decision.

- In the central nervous system (CNS) and elsewhere, levodopa is converted by l-amino acid decarboxylase (l-AAD) to dopamine. In the periphery, l-AAD can be blocked by administering **carbidopa**, which does not cross the blood–brain barrier. Carbidopa therefore increases the CNS penetration of exogenously administered levodopa and decreases adverse effects (e.g., nausea, vomiting, cardiac arrhythmias, postural hypotension, vivid dreams) from peripheral levodopa metabolism to dopamine.
- Starting levodopa at 200 to 300 mg/day in combination with carbidopa often achieves adequate relief of disability. The usual maximal dose of levodopa is 800 mg/day.
- About 75 mg of carbidopa is required to prevent peripheral adverse effects, but some patients may benefit from as much as 150 mg/day. Carbidopa/levodopa is most widely used in a 25-mg/100-mg tablet, but 25-mg/250-mg and 10-mg/100-mg dosage forms are also available. Controlled-release preparations of carbidopa/levodopa are available in 50-mg/200-mg and 25-mg/100-mg strengths. If peripheral adverse effects are prominent, 25-mg carbidopa (Lodosyn) tablets are available.

Generic Name	Trade Name	Manufacturer	Dosage Range (mg/day)	Dosage Forms (mg)	Cost Index[a]
Amantadine	Symmetrel	Endo Labs	200–300	100.50/5 mL	14, 13
		Generic brands, various			6, 7
Carbidopa/L-Dopa	Sinemet	Bristol-Meyers Squibb	[b]	10/100, 25/100,	8,9, 11
		Generic brands, various		25/250	7,8,10
Controlled-release Carbidopa/L-Dopa	Sinemet CR	Bristol-Meyers Squibb	[b]	25/100, 50/200	10, 19,
		Generic brands, various			9,18
Carbidopa/L-Dopa/entacapone	Stalevo	Novartis	[b]	12.5/50/200	21
				25/100/200	21
				37.5/150/200	21
Carbidopa	Lodosyn	Bristol-Meyers Squibb	[b]	25	6
Selegiline	Eldepryl	Somerset	10	5	27
		Generic brands, various			22
Tolcapone	Tasmar	Roche	300–600	100, 200	24, 26
Entacapone	Comtan	Novartis	200 with each dose of carbidopa/L-Dopa	200	19
Agonists					
Bromocriptine	Parlodel	Novartis	[b]	2.5, 5	30, 46
		Generic brands, various			23, 27
Pergolide	Permax	Amarin	[b]	0.05, 0.25, 1	12, 21, 45
		Generic brands, various			12, 19, 40
Pramipexole	Mirapex	Pfizer	1.5–4.5	0.125, 0.25, 0.5	10, 13, 22
				1, 1.5	22, 22
Ropinirole	Requip	GlaxoSmithKline	24	0.25, 0.5; 1	13, 13, 13
				2, 3, 4, 5	13, 23, 23, 23
Anticholinergic Drugs					
Benztropine	Cogentin	Merck and Co.	0.5–6	0.5, 1, 2	2, 2, 3
		Generic brands, various			1, 1, 1
Diphenhydramine	Benadryl	Parke-Davis	25–100	25, 50	2, 3
		Generic brands, various			1, 1
Trihexyphenidyl	Artane	Lederle	1–15	2, 5, 2/5 mL	2, 4, 4
		Generic brands, various			1, 3

[a]Cost index calculated from February 2004 average wholesale price per 100 (or per pint for solutions) equivalent to index × $10.00

[b]Dosage must be individualized.

TABLE 53–3. Stepwise Approach to Drug-Induced Psychosis in Parkinson's Disease

1. General measures such as evaluating for hypoxemia, infection (especially encephalitis, systemic sepsis, or urinary tract infection), or electrolyte disturbance (especially hypercalcemia or hyponatremia).
2. Simplify the antiparkinsonian regimen as much as possible by discontinuing the medications with the highest risk-benefit ratio first.
   a. Discontinue anticholinergics, including other nonparkinsonian medications with anticholinergic activity such as antidepressants, e.g., amitriptyline.
   b. Discontinue selegiline.
   c. Taper and discontinue dopamine agonists.
   d. Taper and discontinue amantadine, being aware that amantadine withdrawal delirium has been reported.
   e. Consider reduction of levodopa (especially at the end of day) and discontinuation of COMT inhibitors.
3. Consider atypical antipsychotic medication if psychosis persists.
   a. Quetiapine 12.5–50 mg at bedtime and gradually increased upward by 12.5–25 mg/wk until psychosis controlled, *or*
   b. Clozapine 12.5–50 mg at bedtime and gradually increased upward by 12.5 mg/wk until psychosis controlled (requires weekly monitoring for leukopenia).

- Between 5% and 10% of IPD patients develop involuntary movements or short-duration responses with each year of levodopa treatment. Movement complications associated with long-term use of carbidopa/levodopa and their suggested treatments are listed in Table 53–4.
- End-of-dose deterioration ("wearing off") has been related to increasing loss of neuronal storage capability for dopamine. Carbidopa/levodopa can be given more frequently or a controlled-release product can be tried. Some patients taking sustained-release forms require increased levodopa doses because of decreased bioavailability, and a conventional carbidopa/levodopa dose in the morning may be needed for more rapid absorption and response. Dopamine agonists also can be added to carbidopa/levodopa to treat wearing off.
- Monoamine oxidase B (MAO-B) inhibitors (**selegiline**) and the catechol-*O*-methyltransferase (COMT) inhibitors (**tolcapone** and **entacapone**) extend the action of levodopa, as discussed later in this chapter.
- Rapid fluctuations from "on" to "off" motor states can develop in patients taking levodopa chronically. Infusions of L-dopa or long-acting dopaminergic agonists tend to alleviate these fluctuations. The addition of MAO inhibitors or COMT inhibitors also may be beneficial. Drug-free periods (drug holidays) have not proven useful as therapeutic interventions because of the discomforts, risks, and limited gains observed in most patients.
- Dyskinesias and dystonias are usually associated with peak antiparkinsonian benefit. In this situation, the use of smaller, more frequent levodopa doses, sustained-release preparations, or addition of a dopamine agonist may be helpful.
- Psychiatric side effects of levodopa include delirium, agitation, paranoia, delusions, and hallucinations. These are especially likely in older patients and those with underlying confusion or dementia. **Clozapine** in low doses may improve psychotic symptoms while improving tremor and other motor symptoms. **Quetiapine** is also safe and effective (Table 53–3). **Olanzapine** and **risperidone** may improve psychotic symptoms but often worsen parkinsonian features.
- There is marked intra- and intersubject variability in the time to peak plasma concentrations after oral levodopa, and there may be more than one peak plasma concentration after a single dose because of erratic gastric emptying. Meals delay but antacids promote gastric emptying. Levodopa is primarily absorbed in the proximal duodenum by a saturable large neutral amino

IX

TABLE 53–4. Motor Fluctuations and Possible Interventions in IPD

Effect	Possible Treatments
End of dose deterioration ("wearing off")	Increase frequency of doses; controlled-release carbidopa/ʟ-dopa; consider dopamine agonists, selegiline, COMT inhibitors, or amantadine;duodenal or intravenous ʟ-dopa infusions; carbidopa/ʟ-dopa oral solution; subcutaneous apomorphine infusions; transdermal dopamine agonists
Delayed onset of response	Give on empty stomach before meals; crush or chew and take with a full glass of water; reduce dietary protein intake; antacids; morning standard-release carbidopa/ʟ-dopa if on sustained-release carbidopa/ʟ-dopa; infusions of ʟ-dopa; dopamine agonists
Drug-resistant "off" periods	Increase carbidopa/ʟ-dopa dose and/or frequency; give on empty stomach before meals; crush or chew and take with a full glass of water; infusions of ʟ-dopa or dopamine agonists; apomorphine subcutaneous injection; consider deep brain stimulation
Random oscillations ("on/off")	Dopamine agonists; controlled-release carbidopa/ʟ-dopa, selegiline; COMT inhibitors; infusions of ʟ-dopa or dopamine agonists; consider drug holiday and deep brain stimulation
Start hesitation ("freezing")	Increase carbidopa/ʟ-dopa dose; dopamine agonists; gait modifications (tapping, rhythmic commands, stepping over objects, rocking)
Peak-dose dyskinesia (I-D-I response[a])	Smaller more frequent doses of carbidopa/ʟ-dopa; controlled-release carbidopa/ʟ-dopa; dopamine agonist; consider amantadine, propranolol, fluoxetine, buspirone, clozapine, deep brain stimulation
Diphasic dyskinesias (D-I-D response[b])	Reduce anticholinergic medication
Dystonia	Baclofen; nighttime carbidopa/ʟ-dopa; morning standard-release carbidopa/ʟ-dopa if on sustained-release carbidopa/ʟ-dopa; dopamine agonists; anticholinergics; selective denervation with botulinum toxin
Myoclonus	Decrease nighttime ʟ-dopa doses; clonazepam
Akathisia	Benzodiazepines; propranolol; dopamine agonists; gabapentin

[a]I-D-1 is the improvement-dyskinesia/dystonia-improvement pattern of response.
[b]D-I-D is the dyskinesia-improvement-dyskinesia pattern of response.

IX ◀

acid (LNAA) transport system. Dietary LNAAs can compete for this site and compete with levodopa for transport into the brain. The elimination half-life of levodopa is about 1 hour and is extended to about 1.5 hours with carbidopa.

- Levodopa should not be administered with MAO-A inhibitors, because of a risk of hypertensive crisis, or with traditional antipsychotic agents, because of possible antagonism of levodopa efficacy.

Monoamine Oxidase B Inhibitors

- **Selegiline** (deprenyl; Eldepryl) is an irreversible MAO-B inhibitor that blocks dopamine breakdown and can modestly extend the duration of action of levodopa (up to 1 hour). It often permits reduction of levodopa dose by as much as one-half.
- Selegiline also increases the peak effects of levodopa and can worsen pre-existing dyskinesias or psychiatric symptoms such as delusions and hallucinations.
- Metabolites of selegiline are l-methamphetamine and l-amphetamine. Adverse effects are minimal and include insomnia and jitteriness.

- Studies evaluating its neuroprotective properties suggest that selegiline can delay the need for levodopa by about 9 months and has symptomatic effects, but there is no firm evidence that it can slow neurodegeneration.
- Rasagiline, another MAO-B inhibitor, has similar effects as selegiline in enhancing L-dopa effects and modest beneficial effect as monotherapy.

COMT Inhibitors

- **Tolcapone** (Tasmar) and **entacapone** (Comtan) are used only in conjunction with carbidopa/levodopa to prevent the peripheral conversion of levodopa to its metabolite 3-O-methyldopa (3OMD) and thus prolong the action of levodopa, that is, increas "on" time by about 1 hour. These agents significantly decrease "off" time and decrease levodopa requirements. Concomitant use of nonselective MAO inhibitors should be avoided to prevent inhibition of the pathways for normal catecholamine metabolism.
- COMT inhibition is more effective than controlled-release carbidopa-L-dopa in providing consistent extension of effect and avoids the delay in time to maximal effect seen with controlled-release L-dopa products. It is unclear whether use of these adjunctive agents will be more beneficial and cost effective than maximizing therapy with carbidopa/L-dopa alone.
- The starting and recommended dose of tolcapone is 100 mg three times daily as an adjunct to carbidopa/levodopa. Its use is limited by the potential for serious liver dysfunction; several deaths have been reported. Strict monitoring of liver function is required, and tolcapone should be discontinued if liver function tests are above the upper limit of normal or any signs or symptoms suggestive of hepatic failure exist.
- Because entacapone has a shorter half-life, 200 mg is given with each dose of carbidopa/levodopa up to 8 times a day. Dopaminergic adverse effects may occur and are managed easily by reducing the carbidopa/levodopa dose. Brownish-orange urine discoloration may occur (as with tolcapone), but there is no evidence of hepatotoxicity from entacapone.

Dopamine Agonists

- The ergot derivatives **pergolide** (Permax) and **bromocriptine** (Parlodel) and the nonergots **pramipexole** (Mirapex) and **ropinirole** (Requip) are beneficial adjuncts in patients with deteriorating response to levodopa, those experiencing fluctuation in response to levodopa, and those with limited clinical response to levodopa due to inability to tolerate higher doses. They decrease the frequency of "off" periods and provide a levodopa-sparing effect.
- The dose of dopamine agonists is best determined by slow titration to enhance tolerance and to find the least dose that provides optimal benefit.
- Pergolide with levodopa is similar or perhaps more efficacious with fewer side effects than bromocriptine with levodopa.
- When used as monotherapy, pergolide, pramipexole, and ropinirole seem to be more effective than bromocriptine as alternatives to levodopa, but only pramipexole and ropinirole are approved for monotherapy.
- Using the combination of levodopa with a dopamine agonist or dopamine agonist monotherapy as initial treatment revealed a decreased risk for the development of response fluctuations. This has raised the question of whether initial therapy of IPD should consist of dopamine agonist monotherapy. Because younger patients are more likely to develop motor fluctuations because of their longer life expectancy, dopamine agonists may be preferred in this population. Older patients are more likely to experience psychosis from dopamine agonists; therefore, carbidopa/levodopa may be the

best initial medication, particularly if cognitive problems or dementia is present.

- There is no rationale at present to choose one dopamine agonist over another on the basis of receptor specificity. A recommended initial dose of bromocriptine is 1.25 mg once or twice daily; the dose should be escalated slowly by 1.25 to 2.5 mg/day every week and maintained at the minimum effective dose. Average daily doses less than 30 mg may be effective for several years in many patients, but some patients require up to 120 mg/day.
- A recommended initial dose of pergolide is 0.05 mg/day for 2 days, gradually increasing by 0.1 to 0.15 mg/day every 3 days over a 12-day period. If higher doses are needed, the dose may be increased by 0.25 mg every 3 days until symptoms are eliminated or adverse effects occur. The mean therapeutic dose in most clinical trials was approximately 3 mg/day.
- Pramipexole is initiated at a dose of 0.125 mg three times daily and increased every 5 to 7 days as tolerated. In a fixed-dose study, doses greater than 3 mg/day were no more effective than 1.5 mg/day and were associated with more frequent adverse effects. It is primarily renally excreted, and the initial dose must be adjusted in renal insufficiency.
- Ropinirole is initiated at 0.25 mg three times daily and increased by 0.25 mg three times daily on a weekly basis to a maximum of 24 mg/day. It is metabolized by cytochrome P450 1A2; fluoroquinolones and smoking may alter ropinirole clearance.
- **Apomorphine** is a dopamine agonist that will soon be released in the United States as a subcutaneous injection. **Cabergoline** is a selective D_2 ergot agonist with a half-life of 70 hours that is available in the United States for treatment of hyperprolactinemia.
- Nausea is the most common side effect, followed by sedation, light-headedness, and vivid dreams. Asymptomatic postural hypotension is common but does not always require medication adjustment. CNS effects (e.g., confusion, hallucinations, and sedation) are often dose limiting. Pedal edema can also occur. The ergot dopamine agonists are associated rarely with pleuropulmonary fibrosis, and recently, cases of cardiac valvulopathy have been reported with pergolide.

▶ EVALUATION OF THERAPEUTIC OUTCOMES

- Patients and caregivers should be educated so that they can participate in treatment by recording medication administration times and duration of "on" and "off" periods.
- Symptoms, side effects, and activities of daily living must be scrupulously monitored and therapy individualized.

See Chapter 57, Parkinson's Disease, authored by Merlin V. Nelson, Richard C. Berchou, and Peter A. LeWitt, for a more detailed discussion of this topic.

Chapter 54

► STATUS EPILEPTICUS

► DEFINITION

Status epilepticus (SE) is recurrent seizures without an intervening period of consciousness before the next seizure or any seizure lasting longer than 30 minutes whether or not consciousness is impaired. Table 54–1 shows the classification of SE. The most common manifestation of SE is tonic-clonic or generalized convulsive SE (GCSE).

► PATHOPHYSIOLOGY

- An increase in excitatory (e.g., glutamate, acetylcholine) or a decrease in inhibitory (e.g., γ-aminobutyric acid [GABA]) neurotransmitters can cause sustained seizures with subsequent neuronal death.
- During SE, the GABA system does not function to inhibit seizures. There is evidence that $GABA_A$ receptors are modified during SE in a way that contributes

TABLE 54–1. International Classification of Status Epilepticus (SE)

Convulsive		Nonconvulsive	
International	*Traditional Terminology*	*International*	*Traditional Terminology*
Primary generalized SE • Tonic-clonic[a,b] • Tonic[a,c] • Clonic[c] • Myoclonic[b] • Erratic[d]	Grand mal, epilepticus convulsivus	Absence[c]	Petit mal, spike-and-wave stupor, spike-and-slow-wave or 3/s spike-and-wave, epileptic fugue, epilepsia minora continua, epileptic twilight, minor SE
Secondary generalized SE[a,b] • Tonic • Partial seizures with secondary generalization		Partial SE[a,b]	Focal motor, focal sensory, epilepsia partialis continuans, adversive SE

		Simple partial
		    Somatomotor
		    Dysphasic
		    Other types
			Elementary

		Complex partial	Temporal lobe, psychomotor, epileptic fugue state, prolonged epileptic stupor, prolonged epileptic confusional state, continuous epileptic twilight state

[a]Most common in older children.
[b]Most common in adolescents and adults.
[b]Most common in infants and young children.
[d]Most common in neonates.

to persistent seizures. However, it is unlikely that loss of GABA inhibition is the sole mechanism for SE.

- Two phases of GCSE have been identified. During phase I, each seizure produces marked increases in plasma epinephrine, norepinephrine, and steroid concentrations that may cause hypertension, tachycardia, and cardiac arrhythmias. Acidosis, hypotension, shock, rhabdomyolysis, secondary hyperkalemia, and acute tubular necrosis may ensue.

- Phase II begins 60 minutes into the seizure, and the patient begins to decompensate. The patient may become hypotensive and cerebral blood flow may be compromised. Glucose may be normal or decreased, and hyperthermia, respiratory deterioration, hypoxia, and ventilatory failure may develop.

- In prolonged seizures, motor activity may cease, but electrical seizures may persist.

► OUTCOMES OF GCSE

- Age, seizure duration, and severe preexisting brain disease are related to SE-induced morbidity. The younger the child, the greater is the risk for sequelea. Seizures exceeding 60 minutes can cause neuronal damage.

- Morbidity may be higher in patients with preexisting epilepsy.

- Mortality from GCSE depends on etiology, time from onset of SE to initiation of treatment, seizure duration, and patient age. More frequently, death is a result of the illness that precipitated the attack of SE, not the SE itself. The longer the duration of SE, the worse the prognosis. Recent estimates suggest a mortality rate up to 10% in children, up to 20% in adults, and up to 38% in the elderly.

► CLINICAL PRESENTATION AND DIAGNOSIS

GENERAL

Status epilepticus (SE) is a medical emergency that may be associated with significant morbidity and mortality.

SYMPTOMS

- Impaired consciousness (e.g., lethargy to coma)
- Disorientation once GCSE is controlled
- Pain associated with injuries (e.g., tongue lacerations, shoulder dislocations, head trauma, facial trauma)

EARLY SIGNS

- Acute injuries or CNS insults that cause extensor or flexor posturing
- Fever or intercurrent illnesses (signs of sepsis or meningitis)
- Evidence of head or other CNS injury (bradycardia, tachypnea, and hypertension; poor pupillary response; asymmetry on neurologic examination; abnormal posturing
- Generalized convulsions
- Hypothermia or fever suggestive of intercurrent illnesses
- Incontinence
- Muscle contractions, spasms
- Normal blood pressure or hypotension
- Respiratory compromise

LATE SIGNS

- Pulmonary edema with respiratory failure
- Cardiac failure (dysrhythmias, arrest, cardiogenic shock)
- Hyoptension/hypertension
- Disseminated intravascular coagulation, multi-organ failure
- Rhabdomyolysis
- Hyperpyremia

INITIAL LABORATORY TESTS

- Complete blood count (CBC) with differential
- Serum chemistry profile (e.g., electrolytes, calcium, magnesium, glucose, serum creatinine, ALT, AST)
- Urine drug/alcohol screen
- Blood cultures
- Arterial blood gas to assess for metabolic and respiratory acidosis
- Serum drug concentration if previous anticonvulsant suspected or known

OTHER DIAGNOSTIC TESTS

- Lumbar puncture if CNS infection suspected
- EEG—should be obtained on presentation and once clinical seizures are controlled
- CT with and without contrast (to assess for bleeding, infection, arteriovenous malformations, neoplasm)
- MRI later
- X-ray if indicated to diagnose fractures
- ECG, especially if ingestion confirmed

ALT, alanine aminotransferase; AST, aspartate aminotransferase; CBC, complete blood count; CNS, central nervous system; CT, computed tomography; ECG, electrocardiogram; EEG, electroencephalograph; GCSE, generalized convulsive status epilepticus; MRI, magnetic resonance imaging; SE, status epilepticus

- Most patients have altered consciousness ranging from obtunded to marked lethargy and somnolence with pronounced eyes-open unresponsiveness and waxy rigidity.
- After seizures have stopped, it is important to determine if the patient is febrile or has a systemic or central nervous system (CNS) infection.

▶ DESIRED OUTCOME

The goals of treatment are (1) patient stabilization (e.g., adequate oxygenation, preservation of cardiorespiratory function, and management of systemic complications), (2) correct diagnosis of the subtype and identification of precipitating factors, (3) stopping clinical and electrical activity as soon as possible, and (4) preventing seizure recurrence.

▶ TREATMENT

- For any tonic-clonic seizure that does not stop automatically or when doubt exists regarding the diagnosis, treatment should begin during the diagnostic workup. An algorithm for treatment of GCSE is shown in Figure 54–1.
- Concurrent with initiation of anticonvulsants, vital signs should be assessed and an adequate airway with ventilation should be established and maintained.

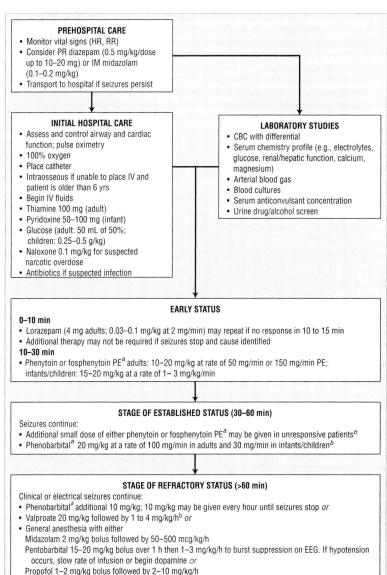

PREHOSPITAL CARE
- Monitor vital signs (HR, RR)
- Consider PR diazepam (0.5 mg/kg/dose up to 10–20 mg) or IM midazolam (0.1–0.2 mg/kg)
- Transport to hospital if seizures persist

INITIAL HOSPITAL CARE
- Assess and control airway and cardiac function; pulse oximetry
- 100% oxygen
- Place catheter
- Intraosseous if unable to place IV and patient is older than 6 yrs
- Begin IV fluids
- Thiamine 100 mg (adult)
- Pyridoxine 50–100 mg (infant)
- Glucose (adult: 50 mL of 50%; children: 0.25–0.5 g/kg)
- Naloxone 0.1 mg/kg for suspected narcotic overdose
- Antibiotics if suspected infection

LABORATORY STUDIES
- CBC with differential
- Serum chemistry profile (e.g., electrolytes, glucose, renal/hepatic function, calcium, magnesium)
- Arterial blood gas
- Blood cultures
- Serum anticonvulsant concentration
- Urine drug/alcohol screen

EARLY STATUS

0–10 min
- Lorazepam (4 mg adults; 0.03–0.1 mg/kg at 2 mg/min) may repeat if no response in 10 to 15 min
- Additional therapy may not be required if seizures stop and cause identified

10–30 min
- Phenytoin or fosphenytoin PE[a] adults: 10–20 mg/kg at rate of 50 mg/min or 150 mg/min PE; infants/children: 15–20 mg/kg at a rate of 1– 3 mg/kg/min

STAGE OF ESTABLISHED STATUS (30–60 min)

Seizures continue:
- Additional small dose of either phenytoin or fosphenytoin PE[a] may be given in unresponsive patients[b]
- Phenobarbital[a] 20 mg/kg at a rate of 100 mg/min in adults and 30 mg/min in infants/children[b]

STAGE OF REFRACTORY STATUS (>60 min)

Clinical or electrical seizures continue:
- Phenobarbital[a] additional 10 mg/kg; 10 mg/kg may be given every hour until seizures stop *or*
- Valproate 20 mg/kg followed by 1 to 4 mg/kg/h[b] *or*
- General anesthesia with either
  Midazolam 2 mg/kg bolus followed by 50–500 mcg/kg/h
  Pentobarbital 15–20 mg/kg bolus over 1 h then 1–3 mg/kg/h to burst suppression on EEG. If hypotension occurs, slow rate of infusion or begin dopamine *or*
  Propofol 1–2 mg/kg bolus followed by 2–10 mg/kg/h
Once seizures controlled, taper midazolam, pentobarbital, propofol over 12 h. If seizures recur restart infusion and titrate to effective dose over 12 h.

[a]Because variability exists in dosing, monitor serum concentration.
[b]If seizure is controlled, begin maintenance dose and optimize using serum concentration monitoring.

Figure 54–1. Algorithm for the management of generalized convulsive status epilepticus (GCSE). RR, respiratory rate; HR, heart rate; BP, blood pressure; PE, phenytoin sodium equivalents; IVIG, intravenous immunoglobulin.

Oxygen should be administered. If there is poor air exchange, the patient should be intubated and ventilated mechanically. Temperature should be monitored frequently.

- Normal to high blood pressure should be maintained.
- All patients should receive glucose, and thiamine (100 mg) should be given prior to glucose in adults.
- Metabolic and/or respiratory acidosis should be assessed by arterial blood gas measurements to determine pH, Pao_2, $Paco_2$, and HCO_3. If pH is less than 7.2, secondary to metabolic acidosis, sodium bicarbonate should be given.

BENZODIAZEPINES

- A **benzodiazepine** (BZ) should be administered as soon as possible if the patient is actively seizing. If seizures have stopped, a longer-acting anticonvulsant should be given.
- **Diazepam** is extremely lipophilic and quickly distributed into the brain but redistributes rapidly into body fat, causing a very short duration of effect (0.25 to 0.5 hours). Therefore, a longer-acting anticonvulsant (e.g., **phenytoin, phenobarbital**) should be given immediately after the diazepam.
- The recommended initial diazepam dose in children and adults is shown in Table 54–2. The maximum total dose is 5 mg in children under age of 5 years, 10 mg in children 5 years and older, and 40 mg in adults.
- ▶ IX **Lorazepam** is currently considered the BZ of choice. It takes slightly longer to reach peak brain levels than diazepam but has a longer duration of action (greater than 12 to 24 hours); thus, fewer patients require additional anticonvulsants for seizure termination. One dose provides seizure protection for 24 hours. The initial dosing of lorazepam is shown in Table 54–2. If the seizure continues after 5 minutes, a second dose may be given. If there is no response in another 5 minutes, a third (final) dose can be given. Patients chronically on BZs may require larger doses. The administration of diazepam and lorazepam should not exceed 5 and 2 mg/min, respectively.
- **Midazolam** is water soluble and diffuses rapidly into the central nervous system (CNS) but has a very short half-life (0.8 hours). It must be given by continuous infusion when given chronically. There is increasing interest in using it buccally, intranasally, and intramuscularly when intravenous access cannot be obtained readily.
- With BZ administration, a brief period of cardiorespiratory depression (less than 1 minute) may occur and can necessitate assisted ventilation or require intubation, especially if BZs are used with a barbiturate. Hypotension may occur with high doses of BZs.

PHENYTOIN

- **Phenytoin** has a long half-life (20 to 36 hours), but it cannot be delivered fast enough to be considered a first-line agent. It takes longer to control seizures than do the BZs because it enters the brain more slowly. It is also associated with administration-related cardiovascular toxicity and is ineffective in some forms of nonconvulsive SE (NCSE).
- See Table 54–2 for dosing guidelines.
- If the patient has been on phenytoin prior to admission and the phenytoin concentration is known, this should be considered in determining a loading dose.
- A reduction in the loading dose is recommended for elderly patients, and a larger loading dose is required in obese patients.

TABLE 54-2. Medications Used in the Initial Treatment of GCSE

Anticonvulsant (Route)	Loading Dose (Maximum Dose)		Rate of Infusion		Maintenance Dose	
	Adult	Pediatric	Adult	Pediatric	Adult	Pediatric
Diazepam (IV bolus)	0.25 mg/kg[a,b,c] (40 mg)	0.25–0.5 mg/kg[a,c] (0.75 mg/kg)	<5 mg/min	<5 mg/min	Not used	Not used
Fosphenytoin IV	15–20 mg PE/kg	15–20 mg PE/kg	150 mg PE/min	3 mg PE/kg/min	4–5 mg PE/kg/day	5–10 mg PE/kg/day
Lorazepam (IV bolus)	4 mg[a,b,c] (8 mg)	0.1 mg/kg[a,c] (4 mg)	2 mg/min	Over 2–5 min	Not used	Not used
Midazolam IV	200 mcg/kg[a,d]	150 mcg/kg[a,d]	0.5–1 mg/min	2–3 min	50–500 mcg/kg/h[e]	60–120 mcg/kg/h[e]
Phenobarbital IV	10–20 mg/kg[e]	15–20 mg/kg[e]	100 mg/min	30 mg/min	1–4 mg/kg/day[e]	3–5 mg/kg/day[e]
Phenytoin IV	15–20 mg/kg[f]	15–20 mg/kg[f]	50 mg/min	1 mg/kg/min	4–5 mg/kg/day[e]	5–10 mg/kg/day[e]

[a]Doses may be repeated every 10 to 15 min until the maximum dosage is given.
[b]Initial doses in the elderly are 2 to 5 mg.
[c]Larger doses may be required if patients chronically on a benzodiazepine (e.g., clonazepam).
[d]May be given by the intramuscular, rectal, or buccal routes.
[e]Titrate dose as needed.
[f]Administer additional loading dose based on serum concentration.

- For seizures continuing after the initial loading dose, some practitioners have recommended an additional loading dose of 5 mg/kg (after waiting 60 minutes for response), but additional phenytoin may result in toxicity and exacerbation of seizures. There is no evidence that a total loading dose greater than 20 mg/kg will be of benefit in these patients.
- Maintenance dosing should be started within 12 to 24 hours of the loading dose.
- The propylene glycol vehicle may cause hypotension and arrhythmias, especially in older patients with heart disease and critically ill patients with marginal blood pressures. The maximum rate of infusion is 50 mg/min in adults, 25 mg/min in the elderly and those with atherosclerotic heart disease, and 1 mg/kg/min in children weighing less than 50 kg. Vital signs and an electrocardiogram (ECG) should be obtained during administration.
- Phenytoin is associated with pain and burning during infusion. Phlebitis may occur with chronic infusion, and tissue necrosis is likely on infiltration. Intramuscular administration is not recommended.

FOSPHENYTOIN

- **Fosphenytoin,** the water-soluble phosphate ester of phenytoin, is a phenytoin prodrug.
- The dose of fosphenytoin sodium is expressed as phenytoin sodium equivalents (PE).
- Adverse reactions include nystagmus, dizziness, pruritus, paresthesias, headache, somnolence, and ataxia.
- Dosing guidelines are given in Table 54–2. In adults, the rate of administration should be 100 to 150 mg PE/min. Pediatric patients should receive fosphenytoin at a rate of 1 to 3 mg PE/kg/min.
- Continuous ECG, blood pressure, and respiratory status monitoring is required for all loading doses of fosphenytoin. Serum phenytoin concentrations should not be obtained for at least 2 hours or more following fosphenytoin dosing.

PHENOBARBITAL

- The Working Group on Status Epilepticus recommends that **phenobarbital** be given after a benzodiazepine plus phenytoin has failed. Most practitioners agree that phenobarbital is the long-acting anticonvulsant of choice in patients with hypersensitivity to the hydantoins or in those with cardiac conduction abnormalities. Some clinicians, especially in pediatric institutions feel that phenobarbital should be the drug of choice after the benzodiazepines have been administered.
- There is no maximum dose beyond which further doses are likely to be ineffective.
- The dosing guidelines are given in Table 54–2. In order to avoid overdosing, estimated lean body mass should be used in obese patients.
- Peak brain concentrations occur 12 to 60 minutes after intravenous dosing. On average, seizures are controlled within minutes of the loading dose.
- If the initial loading dose does not stop the seizures within 20 to 30 minutes, an additional 10- to 20-mg/kg dose may be given. If seizures continue, a third 10-mg/kg load may be given. Once seizures are controlled, the maintenance dose should be started within 12 to 24 hours.
- Medical personnel should be ready to provide respiratory support whenever phenobarbital and the BZs are used together. If significant hypotension develops, the infusion should be slowed or stopped.

IX

REFRACTORY GCSE

- When adequate doses of a **BZ, phenytoin**, and **phenobarbital** have failed, the condition is termed refractory. Failure to aggressively treat early increases the likelihood of nonresponse. Doses of agents used to treat refractory GCSE are given in Table 54–3.

Benzodiazepines

- **Midazolam** has been suggested as the first-line treatment for refractory GCSE and as the third-line agent in patients unresponsive to lorazepam plus phenytoin. The infusion rate should be increased every 15 minutes until seizures are controlled. Most patients respond within 65 minutes.
- Once SE is terminated, dosages can be decreased by 1 mcg/kg/min every 2 hours. Successful discontinuation is enhanced by maintaining serum phenytoin serum concentrations near 20 mg/L and phenobarbital concentrations above 40 mg/L.
- Dosing should be guided by electroencephalogram (EEG) response.
- Hypotension and poikilothermia can occur and may require supportive therapies.
- Refractory GCSE has also been treated with large-dose continuous infusion **lorazepam** or **diazepam**. Lorazepam contains propylene glycol, which can accumulate and cause marked osmolar gap, metabolic acidosis, and renal toxicity.

Medically Induced Coma

- If there is inadequate response to high doses of midazolam, anesthetizing is recommended. Intubation and respiratory support are mandatory during **barbiturate** coma, and continuous monitoring of vital signs is essential. A short-acting barbiturate (e.g., **pentobarbital** or **thiopental**) is generally preferred (see Figure 54–1).
- **Pentobarbital** should be initiated with a loading dose in accordance with the guidelines given in Table 54–3. If hypotension occurs, the rate of administration should be slowed or dopamine should be administered. The loading dose should be followed immediately by an infusion according to Table 54–3, increasing gradually until there is burst suppression on the EEG or adverse effects occur. Twelve hours after a burst suppression pattern is obtained, the rate of pentobarbital infusion should be titrated downward every 2 to 4 hours to determine if GCSE is in remission.

Valproate

- Refer to Table 54–3 for dosing guidelines for adults and children. The manufacturer recommends that intravenous **valproate** be given no faster than 3 mg/kg/min.
- Some have suggested that the maintenance infusion rate should be adjusted as follows: (1) if no inducers are present, the continuous infusion rate is 1 mg/kg/h; (2) if one or more inducers are present (e.g., phenobarbital, phenytoin), the rate is 2 mg/kg/h; and (3) if inducers and pentobarbital coma are present, the rate is 4 mg/kg/h.

Propofol

- **Propofol** is very lipid soluble, has a large volume of distribution, and has a rapid onset of action. It appears to be effective for GCSE, and the dosing guidelines

TABLE 54-3. Medications Used to Traet Refractory GCSE

Anticonvulsant (Route)	Loading Dose		Rate of Infusion		Maintenance Dose	
	Adult	Pediatric	Adult	Pediatric	Adult	Pediatric
Lidocaine	50–100 mg	1 mg/kg (maximum dose = 3–5 mg/kg in first hour)		≤2 min	1.5–3.5 mg/kg/h	1.2–3 mg/kg/h
Midazolam IV	200 mcg/kg[a]	150 mcg/kg[a]	0.5–1 mg/min	2–3 min	50–500 mcg/kg/h[b]	60–120 mcg/kg/h[b]
Pentobarbital (IV)	10–20 mg/kg	15–20 mg/kg	1–2 h	1–2 h	1–5 mg/kg/h[b]	1–5 mg/kg/h[b]
Propofol IV	2 mg/kg	3 mg/kg	10 seconds	20–30 seconds	5–10 mg/kg/h	2–18 mg/kg/h[b]
Valproate	15–20 mg/kg	20–25 mg/kg	3 mg/kg/min	3 mg/kg/min	1–4 mg/kg/h[b]	1–4 mg/kg/h[b]

[a]Doses may be repeated twice every 10–15 min until the maximum dosage is given.
[b]Titrate dose as needed.

are given in Table 54–3. It may cause respiratory and cerebral depression, and bradycardia. Metabolic acidosis has also been reported but is controversial.

- An adult dose can provide more than 1000 cal/day as lipid and cost over $1000/day.

Lidocaine

- **Lidocaine** is not recommended unless other agents have failed. Table 54–3 shows the recommended dosing guidelines. It has a rapid onset of action. Fasiculations, visual disturbances, and tinnitus may occur at serum concentrations between 6 and 8 mg/L. Seizures and obtundation may develop when serum concentrations exceed 8 mg/L.

▶ EVALUATION OF THERAPEUTIC OUTCOMES

An EEG is a very important tool that allows practitioners to determine when abnormal electrical activity has been aborted and may assist in determining which anticonvulsant was effective. Vital signs must be monitored during the infusion. It may also be necessary to monitor the ECG in some patients. The infusion site must be assessed for any evidence of infiltration before and during administration of **phenytoin.**

See Chapter 55, Status Epilepticus, authored by Stephanie J. Phelps, Collin A. Hovinga, and Bradley A. Boucher, for a more detailed discussion of this topic. IX◄

Chapter 55

► ASSESSMENT AND NUTRITION REQUIREMENTS

► DEFINITION

- Nutrition assessment allows identification of individuals at risk for under- and overnutrition.
- Undernutrition is the result of inadequate nutrition intake or inappropriate use of ingested nutrients. Changes in subcellular, cellular, and/or organ function can occur and increase the risk of morbidity and mortality.

► CLASSIFICATION OF NUTRITIONAL DISEASES

- Undernutrition can result from a deficiency in protein and calories or from a single nutrient (e.g., vitamins, trace elements).
- The types of protein-energy malnutrition are marasmus (deficiency in total intake or nutrient utilization), kwashiorkor (relative protein deficiency), and mixed marasmus-kwashiorkor.
- Single-nutrient deficiencies can occur, usually in combination with any protein-energy malnutrition.
- For information on overnutrition or obesity, see Chapter 57.

► NUTRITION SCREENING

- Nutrition screening provides a systematic way to identify individuals at risk for undernutrition.
- Risk factors for undernutrition include any disease state, complicating condition, treatment, or socioeconomic condition that result in decreased nutrient intake, altered metabolism, and/or malabsorption. The presence of three to four risk factors puts a person at risk for undernutrition.
- The Joint Commission on Accreditation of Healthcare Organizations standards require a nutrition screening typically within 24 to 72 hours of hospital admission. Patients determined not to be at risk for malnutrition should be reevaluated every 7 to 14 days. Patients determined to be at risk for malnutrition need a nutrition assessment and care plan.

► DESIRED OUTCOME

The goals of nutrition assessment are to identify the presence (or risk) of developing undernutrition and complications, estimate nutrition needs, and establish baseline parameters for assessing the outcome of therapy.

► NUTRITION ASSESSMENT

Nutrition assessment is the first step in developing a nutrition care plan and includes a clinical evaluation, anthropometric measurements, and biochemical and immune function studies.

TABLE 55–1. Evaluation of Actual Body Weight (ABW)

ABW Compared With Ideal Body Weight (IBW)

Undernutrition

ABW <69% IBW	Severe malnutrition
ABW 70–79% IBW	Moderate malnutrition
ABW 80–90% IBW	Mild malnutrition

Normal

ABW 90–120% IBW	Normal

Overnutrition

ABW > 120% IBW	Overweight
ABW ≥ 150% IBW	Obese
ABW ≥ 200% IBW	Morbidly obese

ABW Compared with Usual Body Weight (UBW)

ABW 85–95% UBW	Mild malnutrition
ABW 75–84% UBW	Moderate malnutrition
ABW <74% UBW	Severe malnutrition

CLINICAL EVALUATION

- Clinical evaluation remains the oldest, simplest, and most widely used method of evaluating nutrition status.
- The medical and dietary history should include weight changes within 6 months, dietary intake changes, gastrointestinal symptoms, functional capacity, and disease states. X
- Physical examination should focus on assessment of lean body mass (LBM) and physical findings of vitamin, trace element, and essential fatty acid deficiencies.

ANTHROPOMETRIC MEASUREMENTS

- Anthropometric measurements are gross measurements of body cell mass used to evaluate LBM and fat stores. The most common measurements are weight, height, limb size (e.g., skinfold thickness and midarm muscle, wrist, and waist circumferences), and bioelectrical impedance analysis (BIA).
- Interpretation of actual body weight (ABW) should consider ideal weight for height, usual body weight (UBW), fluid status, and age. Change over time can be calculated as percentage of UBW or ideal body weight (IBW). Unintentional weight loss of more than 10% in less than 6 months correlates with poor clinical outcome in adults.
- IBW provides a population reference standard against which the ABW can be compared to detect both under- and overnutrition (Table 55–1). Although calculation of IBW is based on gender and height (Table 55–2), it can lead to misclassification of nutrition status in some individuals.

TABLE 55–2. Body Weight Equations

Ideal Body Weight (IBW)

Adult males:	IBW (kg) $= 50 + 123 \times$ height in inches >5 ft)
Adult females:	IBW (kg) $= 45.5 + (2.3 \times$ height in inches >5 ft)
Children (1–18 yr):	IBW (kg) $= ([\text{height in cm}]^2 \times 1.65)/1000$

Adjusted Body Weight for Obesity

Adjusted body weight $=\{[\text{Actual body weight (kg)} - \text{IBW (kg)}] \times 0.25\} + \text{IBW}$

TABLE 55–3. Expected Grown Velocities in Children

Age	Weight (g/day)	Height (cm/mo)
0–3 months	24–35	2.8–3.4
3–5 months	15–21	1.7–2.4
6–12 months	10–13	1.3–1.6
1–3 yr	5–9	0.6–1.0
4–6 yr	5–6	0.5–0.6
7–10 yr	7–11	0.4–0.5

- The best indicator of adequate nutrition in children is appropriate growth. Weight and height should be plotted on the appropriate growth curve and compared with usual growth velocities (Table 55–3). Additionally, the average weight gain for infants is 20 to 30 g/day for term infants and 10 to 25 g/day for preterm infants.
- Body mass index (BMI) appears to be a better indicator than IBW and is becoming the standard for defining obesity. Interpretation of BMI should include consideration of gender and frame size. BMI values greater than 25 kg/m^2 are indicative of overweight, and values less than 18.5 kg/m^2 are indicative of malnutrition. BMI is calculated as follows:

X

$$\text{Body weight (kg)/[height (m)]}^2$$

- Measurements of skinfold thickness estimate subcutaneous fat, midarm muscle circumference estimate skeletal muscle mass, and waist circumference estimate abdominal fat content.
- BIA is a simple, noninvasive, and relatively inexpensive way to measure LBW. It is based on differences between fat tissue and lean tissue's resistance to conductivity. Fluid status should be considered in interpretation of BIA results.

BIOCHEMICAL AND IMMUNE FUNCTION STUDIES

- LBM can be assessed by measuring serum visceral proteins (Table 55–4). They are best for assessing uncomplicated semistarvation and recovery, and poor for assessing status during acute stress. Visceral proteins must be interpreted relative to overall clinical status because they are affected by factors other than nutrition.
- Immune function tests have the advantage of being simple, readily available, and inexpensive markers of nutrition status. Immune function tests have the disadvantage of being nonspecific, but they might be useful for monitoring response to a nutrition regimen including immunotherapy.
- Total lymphocyte count is obtained from a complete blood count with differential. Values less than 1500 cells/mm^3 are associated with moderate nutrition depletion, and values greater than 900 cells/mm^3 denote severe depletion.
- Delayed cutaneous hypersensitivity is commonly assessed using antigens to which the patient has been previously sensitized. The recall antigens used most frequently are mumps, *Candida albicans*, streptokinase-streptodornase, *Trichophyton*, coccidioidin, and purified protein derivative. Anergy is associated with malnutrition.

TABLE 55–4. Summary of Visceral Proteins Used for Assessment of Lean Body Mass

Serum Protein	Half-life (days)	Function	Factors Resulting in Increased Values	Factors Resulting in Decreased Values
Albumin	18–20	Maintains plasma oncotic pressure; transports small molecules	Dehydration, anabolic steroids, insulin, infection	Overhydration, edema, renal insufficiency, nephrotic syndrome, poor dietary intake impaired digestion, burns, congestive heart failure, cirrhosis, thyroid/adrenal/pituitary hormones, trauma, sepsis
Transferrin	8	Binds iron in plasma and transports to bone	Iron deficiency, pregnancy, hypoxia, chronic blood loss, estrogens	Chronic infection, cirrhosis, enteropathies, nephrotic syndrome, cortisone, testosterone
Prealbumin (transthyretin)	1–2	Binds T_3 and to a lesser extent T_4; carrier for retinol-binding protein	Renal dysfunction	Cirrhosis, hepatitis, stress, inflammation, surgery, hyperthyroidism, cystic fibrosis, renal dysfunction, zinc deficiency

X

► SPECIFIC NUTRIENT DEFICIENCIES

- Biochemical assessment of trace element, vitamin, and essential fatty acid deficiencies should be based on the nutrient's function, but few practical methods are available. Therefore, most assays measure serum concentrations of the individual nutrient.
- Deficiency states have been described for the following trace elements: zinc, copper, manganese, selenium, chromium, iodine, fluoride, molybdenum, and iron.
- Single vitamin deficiencies are uncommon; multiple vitamin deficiencies more commonly occur with undernutrition. For information on iron-deficiency and other anemias, see Chapter 32.
- Essential fatty acid deficiency is rare but can occur with prolonged lipid-free parenteral nutrition, very low fat enteral formulas, severe fat malabsorption, or severe malnutrition. The body can synthesize most fatty acids except for linoleic and linolenic acid, which should constitute approximately 2% to 4% of total calorie intake. Diagnosis of essential fatty acid deficiency is based on a triene-to-tetraene ratio of greater than 0.4.
- Carnitine can be synthesized from lysine and methionine, but synthesis is decreased in premature infants. Low carnitine levels can occur in premature infants receiving parenteral nutrition or carnitine-free diets.

► ASSESSMENT OF NUTRIENT REQUIREMENTS

- Assessment of nutrient requirements must be made in the context of patient-specific factors (e.g., age, gender, size, disease state, clinical condition, nutrition status, physical activity).
- To replace recommended dietary allowances (RDAs), the Food and Nutrition Board created a new family of nutrition reference values, the dietary reference intakes (DRIs) and seven nutrient groups (refer to http://www.nal.usda.gov\fnic\etext\000105.html#q3).

ENERGY REQUIREMENTS

- Adults should consume 45% to 65% of total calories from carbohydrates, 20% to 35% from fat, and 10% to 35% from protein. Recommendations are similar for children, except that infants and younger children should consume 40% to 50% of total calories from fat.
- Daily energy requirements are 20 to 25 kcal/kg for healthy adults, 25 to 30 kcal/kg for malnourished or mildly metabolically stressed adults, 30 to 35 kcal/kg for critically ill or hypermetabolic adults, and 35 to 40 kcal/kg for adults with major burns. Unfortunately, this simple approach fails to consider age- and gender-related differences in energy metabolism.
- Daily energy requirements for children are approximately 150% of basal metabolic rate (BMR) with additional calories to support activity and growth (Table 55–5). Requirements increase with fever, sepsis, major surgery, trauma, burns, long-term growth failure, and chronic conditions (e.g., bronchopulmonary dysplasia, congenital heart disease, and cystic fibrosis).
- Equations are available to estimate resting energy expenditure (Table 55–6). The result should be multiplied by a factor to correct for stress, which ranges from 1.2 for no stress (i.e., confined to bed) up to 2.0 for severe stress (e.g., severe trauma or burns).

TABLE 55–5. Dietary Reference Intakes for Energy and Protein in Healthy Children

Age (Reference age/weight)	Estimated Energy Requirement (kcal/day)		Protein RDA (g/kg/day)
	Male	**Female**	
0–6 months (3 months/6 kg)	570	520	1.52[a]
7–12 months (9 months/9 kg)	743	676	1.5
1–2 yr (24 months/12 kg)	1046	992	
1–3 yr (24 months/12 kg)			1.1
3–8 yr (6 yr/20 kg)	1742	1642	
4–8 yr (6 yr/20 kg)			0.95
9–13 yr (11 yr/M: 36 kg; F: 37 kg)	2279	2071	0.95
14–18 yr (16 yr/M: 61 kg; F: 54 kg)	3152	2368	0.85

F, female; M, male; RDA, recommended dietary allowance.
[a]Adequate intake.

- Each equation for estimating energy requirements has advantages and disadvantages, but none has been shown to be superior to another. The most popular is the Harris-Benedict equation.
- The most accurate clinical tool for estimating energy requirements is indirect calorimetry or metabolic gas monitoring. This noninvasive procedure determines oxygen consumption (Vo_2, mL/minute) and carbon dioxide production

X

TABLE 55–6. Equations to Estimate Basal Energy Expenditure in Adults and Children

Harris-Benedict (kcal/day)
Males: BEE = 66 + [13.7W] + [5H (cm)] – (6.8A)
Females: BEE = 655 + [9.6W] + [1.8H (cm)] – (4.7A)

Modified Harris-Benedict (kcal/day)
Males: BEE = [8.8W] + [1128H (m)] – 1071
Females: BEE – [9.2W] + [637H (m)] – 302

Caldwell-Kennedy (kcal/day)
Infants (<3 yr of age): BEE = 22 + (31W) + [1.2H (cm)]

Schofield (MJ/day) (to convert to kcal/day multiply by 239.2)
3–10 yr of age
Males: BMR – (0.08W) + [0.55H (m)] + 1.74
Females: BMR = (0.07W) + [0.68H (m)] + 1.55
10–18 yr of age
Males: BMR = (0.07W) + [0.57H (m)] + 2.16
Females: BMR = (0.04W) + [1.95H (m)] + 0.84

FAO/WHO/UNU (kcal day)
3–10 yr of age
Males: BMR = 22.7W + 495
Females: BMR = 22.5W + 499
10–18 yr of age
Males: BMR = 17.5W + 651
Females: BMR = 12.2W + 746

A, age in years; BEE, basal energy expenditure; BMR, basal metabolic rate; FAO/WHO/UNU, Food and Agriculture Organization/World Health Organization/United Nations University; H, height in centimeters (cm) or meters (m), as indicated; MJ, megajoules; W, weight in kilograms.

(Vco$_2$, mL/minute). Resting energy expenditure (REE, kcal/day) is then calculated using the abbreviated Weir equation:

$$REE = (3.9\ Vo_2 + 1.1\ Vco_2) \times 1.44$$

- Data from indirect calorimetry can also be used to determine a respiratory quotient. Values greater than 1.0 suggest overfeeding, whereas values less than 0.7 suggest a ketogenic diet, fat gluconeogenesis, or ethanol oxidation. Respiratory quotient (RQ) is calculated as follows:

$$RQ = Vco_2/Vo_2$$

- Limitations of indirect calorimetry include limited availability, calibration errors, and other errors.

PROTEIN, FLUID, AND MICRONUTRIENT REQUIREMENTS

Protein

- Protein requirements are based on age, nutrition status, disease state, and clinical condition. The usual recommended daily protein allowances are 0.8 g/kg for adults, 1.5 to 2.0 g/kg for patients with metabolic stress (e.g., infection, trauma, and surgery), and 2.5 to 3.0 g/kg for patients with burns. See Table 55–5 for recommendations for children.
- Daily protein requirements can be individualized by measuring the nitrogen in a 24-hour urine collection (UUN), because nitrogen is found only in protein and at a relatively constant ratio of 1 g/6.25 g protein. Nitrogen output is then compared with nitrogen intake. Nitrogen output is approximated by the following:

$$\text{Nitrogen output (g/day)} = UUN + 4$$

Fluid

- Daily adult fluid requirements are approximately 30 to 35 mL/kg, 1 mL/kcal, or 1500 mL/m^2.
- Daily fluid requirements for children and preterm infants who weigh less than 10 kg are at least 100 mL/kg. An additional 50 mL/kg should be provided for each kilogram of body weight between 11 and 20 kg, and 20 mL/kg for each kilogram above 20 kg.
- Fluid requirements increase with increased insensible or gastrointestinal losses, fever, sweating, and increased metabolism. Fluid requirements decrease with renal failure, expanded extracellular fluid volume (e.g., cardiac failure), or hypoalbuminemia with starvation.
- Fluid status is assessed by monitoring urine output and specific gravity, serum electrolytes, and weight changes. An hourly urine output of at least 1.0 mL/kg for children and 50 mL for adults is needed to ensure tissue perfusion.

Micronutrients

- Requirements for micronutrients (i.e., electrolytes, trace elements, and vitamins) vary with age, gender, route of administration, and underlying clinical conditions.
- In patients with renal failure, sodium, potassium, magnesium, and phosphorus requirements are typically decreased, whereas and calcium requirements are increased (see chapters 74 and 76).

DRUG-NUTRIENT INTERACTIONS

- Concomitant drug therapy can alter serum concentrations of vitamins (Table 55–7), minerals, and electrolytes.

TABLE 55–7. Drug Effects on Vitamin Status

Drug	Possible Vitamin Effect
Antacids	Thiamine deficiency
Antibiotics	Vitamin K deficiency
Anticonvulsants	Vitamin D and folic acid impaired absorption
Antineoplastics	Folic acid antagonism and malabsorption
Antipsychotics	Decreased riboflavin
Cathartics	Increased requirements for vitamins D, C, and B_6
Cholestyramine	Vitamins A, D, E, and K, β-carotene malabsorption
Colestipol	Vitamins A, D, E, and K, β-carotene malabsorption
Corticosteroids	Decreased vitamins A and C
Diuretics (loop)	Thiamine deficiency
Histamine$_2$-antagonists	Vitamin B_{12} deficiency
Isoniazid	Vitamin B_6 deficiency
Mineral oil	Vitamins A, D, E, and K malabsorption
Orlistat	Vitamins A, D, E, and K malabsorption
Pentamidine	Folic acid deficiency
Proton pump inhibitors	Vitamin B_{12} deficiency

- Some drug delivery systems contain nutrients. For example, the vehicle for propofol is 10% lipid emulsion and most intravenous therapies include dextrose or sodium.

X

▶ EVALUATION OF THERAPEUTIC OUTCOMES

- Most markers of nutrition status are not ideal. They were first used in epidemiologic studies of large populations and, when applied to individuals, lack specificity and sensitivity.
- Weight and serum albumin concentration have the best correlation with clinical outcome; the cost-effectiveness of other biochemical parameters is not known.
- Other anthropometric measures are probably most useful with long-term nutrition support.
- Continuous reassessment is required because nutrition requirements are dynamic.

See Chapter 135, Assessment of Nutrition Status and Nutrition Requirements, authored by Katherine Hammond Chessman and Vanessa J. Kumpf, for a more detailed discussion of this topic.

Chapter 56

▶ ENTERAL NUTRITION

▶ DEFINITION

Enteral nutrition (EN) is the delivery of nutrients by tube or mouth into the gastrointestinal (GI) tract. This chapter focuses on delivery through a feeding tube.

▶ PATHOPHYSIOLOGY

- Digestion and absorption are the GI processes that generate usable fuels for the body. Understanding the mechanisms of these processes can enhance rational use of EN support.
- Digestion is the stepwise conversion of complex chemical and physical nutrients via mechanical, enzymatic, and physicochemical processes into molecular forms that can be absorbed from the GI tract.
- Nutrients are absorbed across the brush border membrane of intestinal cells and reach the systemic circulation through the portal venous or splanchnic lymphatic systems, provided the GI or biliary tract does not excrete them.
- Many factors can alter these stepwise processes and interfere with digestion and absorption, such as functional immaturity of the neonatal gut.

▶ CLINICAL PRESENTATION AND INDICATIONS

- Clinical presentation of protein-energy malnutrition and nutrition assessment are discussed in Chapter 55.
- EN is indicated for the patient who cannot or will not eat enough to meet nutritional requirements and who has a functioning GI tract. Additionally, a method of enteral access must be possible. Potential indications include neoplastic disease, organ failure, hypermetabolic states, GI disease, and neurologic impairment.
- The only absolute contraindications are mechanical obstruction and necrotizing enterocolitis. Conditions that challenge the success of EN include severe diarrhea, protracted vomiting, enteric fistulae, severe GI hemorrhage, and intestinal dysmotility.
- EN has replaced parenteral nutrition (PN) (see Chapter 58) as the preferred method of specialized nutrition support. Advantages of EN over PN include maintaining GI tract structure and function; fewer metabolic, infectious, and technical complications; and lower costs.
- The optimal time to initiate EN is controversial. Early initiation within 24 to 48 hours of hospitalization is recommended for critically ill patients because this approach appears to decrease infectious complications and reduce mortality. If patients are only mildly to moderately stressed and well nourished, initiation can be delayed until oral intake is (or expected to be) inadequate for 7 to 14 days.

▶ DESIRED OUTCOME

The goals of EN are to reverse protein-calorie malnutrition, maintain adequate nutritional state, promote growth and development of infants and children, and reduce disease-related morbidity and mortality.

▶ TREATMENT

ENTERAL ACCESS

- EN can be administered through four routes, which have different indications, tube placement options, advantages, and disadvantages (Table 56–1). The choice depends on the anticipated duration of use and the feeding site (i.e., stomach versus small bowel).
- Short-term access is generally easier, less invasive, and less costly than long-term access. Feeding tubes used for short-term access are not suitable for long-term use owing to patient discomfort, long-term complications, and mechanical failure.
- The most frequently used short-term routes are accessed by inserting a tube through the nose and threading it into the stomach (nasogastric), duodenum (nasoduodenal), or jejunum (nasojejunal).
- The stomach is generally the least expensive and least labor-intensive access site; however, patients who have impaired gastric emptying are at risk for aspiration and pneumonia.
- Greater skill is required to place the feeding tube beyond the pylorus. Techniques to facilitate manual placement include using a stylet or weighted tube, or administering **metoclopramide** or **erythromycin**.
- Long-term access should be considered when EN is anticipated for more than 4 to 6 weeks. The most popular option is gastrostomy followed by jejunostomy.
- The gastrostomy exit site requires general stoma care to prevent inflammation and infection. The gastrostomy tube is easily removed after it is no longer needed. If the fistula does not close spontaneously, histamine$_2$-antagonist therapy and silver nitrate cautery usually prevent further leaking.

ADMINISTRATION METHODS

- EN can be administered by continuous, continuous cyclic, bolus, and intermittent methods. The choice depends on the feeding tube location, patient's clinical condition, intestinal function, residence environment, and tolerance to tube feeding.
- Continuous EN is preferred for initiation, for critically ill patients, and for patients with limited absorption capacity because of rapid GI transit time or severely impaired digestion. Continuous EN has the advantage of being well tolerated. It has the disadvantages of cost and inconvenience owing to pump and administration sets.
- Cyclic EN has the advantage of allowing breaks from the infusion system, thereby facilitating activities of daily living, especially if EN is administered nocturnally.
- Bolus EN is most commonly used in long-term care residents who have a gastrostomy. This method has the advantage of requiring little administration time (e.g., 5 to 10 minutes) and minimal equipment (e.g., a syringe). Bolus EN has the potential disadvantages of causing cramping, nausea, vomiting, aspiration, and diarrhea.
- Intermittent EN is similar to bolus EN except that the feeding is administered over 20 to 60 minutes, which improves tolerability but requires more equipment (e.g., reservoir bag and infusion pump). Like bolus EN, intermittent EN mimics normal eating patterns and is suitable only for the patient with a gastrostomy.

TABLE 56–1. Options and Considerations in the Selection of Enteral Access

Access	Indications	Tube Placement Options	Advantages	Disadvantages
Nasogastric or orogastric	Short-term Intact gag reflex Normal gastric emptying	Manually at bedside	Ease of placement Allows for all methods of administration Inexpensive Many available tubes and sizes	Potential tube displacement Potential increased aspiration risk
Nasoduodenal or nasojejunal	Short-term Impaired gastric motility or emptying High risk of GER or aspiration	Manually at bedside Fluoroscopically Endoscopically	Potential reduced aspiration risk Allows for early postinjury or postoperative feeding Many available tubes and sizes	Manual transpyloric passage requires greater skill Potential tube displacement of clogging Bolus or intermittent feeding not tolerated
Gastrostomy	Long-term Normal gastric emptying	Surgically Endoscopically Radiologically Laparoscopically	Allows for all methods of administration Large-bore tubes less likely to clog Many available tubes and sizes Low-profile buttons available	Attendant risk associated with each type of procedure Potential increased aspiration risk Requires stoma site care
Jejunostomy	Long-term Impaired gastric motility or gastric emptying High risk of GER or aspiration	Surgically Endoscopically Radiologically Laparoscopically	Allows for early postinjury or postoperative feeding Potential reduced aspiration risk Many available tubes and sizes	Attendant risks associated with each type of procedure Bolus or intermittent feeding not tolerated Requires stoma site care

GER, gastroesophageal reflux.

FORMULATIONS

- Historically, EN formulations were created to provide essential nutrients including macronutrients (e.g., carbohydrates, fats, and proteins) and micronutrients (e.g., electrolytes, trace elements, and vitamins).
- Over time, formulations have been enhanced to improve tolerance and meet specific patient needs. For example, nutraceuticals or pharmaconutrients are added to modify the disease process or improve clinical outcome; however, these health claims are not regulated by the Food and Drug Administration (FDA).
- Fiber, in the form of soy polysaccharides, has been added to several EN formulations. In addition to providing an excellent energy source, potential benefits include trophic effects on colonic mucosa, promotion of sodium and water absorption, and regulation of bowel function.
- Osmolality is a function of the size and quantity of ionic and molecular particles primarily related to protein, carbohydrate, electrolyte, and mineral content. Osmolality is commonly thought to affect GI tolerability, but there is a lack of supporting evidence.
- EN formulations are classified by their composition and intended patient population (Table 56–2). Most formularies should contain no more than one product per category. Some categories can be omitted depending on the patient population.
- Most EN products are ready-to-use prepackaged liquids, which have the advantages of convenience and lower susceptibility to microbiologic contamination. The major disadvantage is storage space. Closed-system containers provide a prefilled, sterile 1- to 1.5-L supply of EN formula; they can be cost effective when water, electrolytes, or drugs must be added. X
- Polymeric formulations contain intact macronutrients and are similar to table food.
- Standard polymeric formulations have a well-proportioned mix of macronutrients, with or without fiber. These formulations are best suited for tube feeding because, to maintain isotonicity (300 mOsm/L), they are not sweetened and not palatable. Standard formulations have a nonprotein calorie–nitrogen ratio of 125 : 1 to 150 : 1.
- High-protein formulations have a nonprotein calorie–nitrogen ratio of less than 125:1. Candidates for these formulations require more than 1.5 g of protein/kg/day and are generally critically ill because of trauma, burns, pressure sores, surgical wounds, or high fistula output.
- High caloric density formulations are indicated for patients requiring restriction of fluids, electrolytes, or both, such as patients with renal insufficiency or congestive heart failure.
- Elemental or peptide-based formulations have partially hydrolyzed protein or fat components. Peptide-based formulations replace some of the protein with dipeptides and tripeptides, thereby optimizing absorption. Although indications are not clearly established, they probably include patients who do not tolerate standard formulations because of malabsorption and patients who benefit from medium-chain triglycerides (e.g., patients with pancreatic insufficiency).
- Disease state-specific formulations are designed to meet specific nutrient requirements and to manage metabolic abnormalities. Unfortunately, scientific and clinical research supporting their efficacy is minimal, except for low carbohydrate formulations supplemented with specific fatty acids for patients with acute respiratory distress syndrome (ARDS).

TABLE 56–2. Adult Enteral Feeding Formulation Classification System

Category	Features[a]	Product Examples[b]
Standard polymeric	Isotonic 1–1.2 kcal/mL NPC:NB 125:1 to 150:1 May contain fiber	Osmolite 1 Cal, Isocal (MJ), Isocal HN (MJ) Osmolite 1 Cal (R), Jevity 1 Cal (R), Ultracal (MJ), Jevity 1.2 Cal (R), Nutren 1.0 (N), Isosource (No), Nutren w/Fiber (N), Fibersource (No)
High protein	NPC:N < 125:1 May contain fiber	Promote (R), Replete (N), Promote w/Fiber (R), Replete w/Fiber (N), TraumaCal (MJ), Isosource VHN (No)
High caloric density	1.5–2 kcal/mL Lower electrolyte content per calorie Hypertonic	Nutren 1.5 (N), Deliver 2.0 (MJ), Two-Cal HN (R), Nutren 2.0 (N), Novasource 2.0 (No)
Elemental	High proportion of free amino acids Low in fat	Tolerex (No), Criticare HN (MJ), Vital HN (R), Vivonex TEN (No)
Peptide-based	Contains dipeptides and tripeptides Contain MCTs	Peptamen (N), Subdue (MJ), Peptamen VHP (N), Subdue Plus (MJ), Perative (R), Crucial (N), Peptinex DT (No)
Disease-specific		
Renal	Caloric dense Protein content varies Low electrolyte content	Suplena (R), Magnacal Renal (MJ), Nepro (R), Novasource Renal (No), Renalcal (N), NutriRenal (N)
Hepatic	Increased branched-chain and decreased aromatic amino acids	Nutri-Hep (N)
Pulmonary	High fat, low carbohydrate	Pulmocare (R), Oxepa (R), Respalor (MJ), Novasource Pulmonary (No), NutriVent (N)
Diabetic	High fat, low carbohydrate	Glucerna (R), Resource Diabetic (No), Choice DM (MJ), Glytrol (N), Diabetisource AC (No)

Metabolic stress	Supplemented with glutamine,
	  arginine, nucleotides, and/or
	  omega-3 fatty acids
		Impact varieties (No), Perative (R),
		Crucial (N), AlitraQ (R),

Oral supplement	Sweetened for taste Hypertonic	Ensure varieties (R), Boost (MJ), Resource varieties (No), ProSure (R), NuBasic varieties (N)

X

[a]MCT, medium-chain triglyceride; NPC: N. nonprotein calorie-nitrogen ratio.
[b]Manufacturers: MJ, Mead Johnson Nutritionals; R, Ross Products Division, Abbott Laboratories; N. Nestlé, Clinical Nutrition; NO, Novartis.

- Oral supplements are not intended for tube feeding. They are sweetened to improve taste and are therefore hypertonic.
- A module is a powder or liquid that can be added to a commercially available product (Table 56–3). Alternatively, a modular product can be mixed to concentrate nutrients in less volume.
- Hydration formulations are used to maintain hydration or treat dehydration. They can be administered by mouth or feeding tube. The glucose content of these formulations can decrease fecal water loss and generate a positive electrolyte balance.
- Conditionally essential amino acids (e.g., glutamine and arginine) are added to some formulations for critically ill patients, but their benefit is questionable.

TABLE 56–3. Modular Enteral Products

Primary Nutrient Supplied	Example Products (M)[a]
Carbohydrate	Moducal (MJ), Polycose (R)
Protein	ProMod (R), Casec (MJ)
Fat	MCT Oil (MJ), Microlipid (MJ)
Human milk fortifier	Enfamil Human Milk Fortifier (MJ), Similac Human Milk Fortifier (R)
Pectin/carbohydrate/potassium	Benana Flakes (K)
Carbohydrate and fat	Duocal (SHS)

[a]Manufacturers: R, Ross Products Division, Abbott Laboratories; MJ, Mead Johnson Nutritionals; K, Kanana; SHS, SHS International, Ltd.

INITIATION AND TITRATION OF ENTERAL NUTRITION REGIMENS

- Schedules for progression from initial to target rates should be individualized. The need to reach nutrient goal should be balanced with the need for tolerance.
- In adults, continuous EN feedings are typically started at 20 to 50 mL/h and advanced by 10 to 25 mL/h every 4 to 8 hours until the goal is achieved. Intermittent EN feedings are started at 120 mL every 4 hours and advanced by 30 to 60 mL/h every 8 to 12 hours.
- In children, EN feedings are typically started at 1 to 2 mL/kg/h for continuous feeding or 20 to 25 mL/kg per bolus and advanced by similar volumes every 4 to 12 hours.
- In premature infants, feedings are started at lower rates or volumes, usually 10 to 20 mL/kg/day.
- The practice of diluting hyperosmolar EN formulations should be avoided unless necessary to increase fluid intake.

COMPLICATIONS

- Patients should be monitored for metabolic, GI, and mechanical complications (Table 56–4).
- Metabolic complications associated with EN are analogous to those of PN (see Chapter 58), but the occurrence is lower.
- Gastric residual volume is thought to increase the risk of vomiting and aspiration. Residual volume is measured by aspirating the stomach contents into a syringe attached to the open end of the feeding tube. Although the definition is controversial, residual is probably excessive if it is greater than 200 to 500 mL in adults, or if it is twice the bolus volume or hourly infusion rate in children. The determination should be based on a trend rather than an isolated finding and should be made in conjunction with the presence of symptoms.
- The stepwise approach for managing excessive gastric residual volume with GI symptoms is slowing, not stopping, the tube feeding; initiating metoclopramide; considering a transpyloric feeding tube; trying a proton pump inhibitor or histamine$_2$-receptor antagonist; and minimizing use of narcotics, sedatives, and other agents that delay gastric emptying.
- In addition to avoiding excessive gastric residuals, methods for preventing aspiration pneumonia include keeping the head of the bed at 30° to 45° during feeding and for 30 to 60 minutes after intermittent infusions, changing from bolus to intermittent or continuous administration, providing good oral care, and monitoring tube placement for proper positioning.

TABLE 56–4. Monitoring for Complications

Parameter	Initiation of Enteral Nutrition	Frequency
Vital signs	Every 4–6 h	As needed
Clinical assessment		
Weight	Daily	Weekly
Length/height (children)	Weekly–monthly	Monthly
Head circumference (<3 yr of age)	Weekly–monthly	Monthly
Total intake/output	Daily	As needed
Tube feeding intake	Daily	Daily
Enterostomy tube site assessment	Daily	Daily
GI tolerance		
Stool frequency/volume	Daily	Daily
Abdomen assessment	Daily	Daily
Nausea or vomiting	Daily	Daily
Gastric residual volumes	Every 4–8 h (varies)	As needed
Tube placement	Prior to starting, then ongoing	Ongoing
Laboratory		
Electrolytes, BUN/S_{cr}, glucose	Daily	As needed
Calcium, magnesium, phosphorus	3–7 times/wk	As needed
Liver function tests	Weekly	As needed
Trace elements, vitamins	Patient-specific	Patient-specific

BUN, blood urea nitrogen; S_{cr}, serum creatinine.

X

- Management of diarrhea should be directed at identifying and correcting the cause. The most common causes are sorbitol, drug therapy, infection, malabsorption, and factors related to tube feeding (e.g., rapid delivery or advancement, intolerance to composition, large volume administered into small bowel, and formula contamination). Switching to a fiber-containing, lower fat, peptide-based, or lactose-free formulation can be beneficial. As a last resort, pharmacologic intervention (e.g., opiates, **diphenoxylate,** or **loperamide**) can be used to control severe diarrhea.
- Techniques for clearing occluded tubes include pancreatic enzymes in sodium bicarbonate and using a declogging device. Techniques for maintaining patency include flushing with at least 30 mL of water before and after medication administration, at least every 8 hours during continuous feeding, and after each intermittent feed.

DRUG DELIVERY VIA FEEDING TUBE

- Administering drugs via tube feeding is a common practice, but drug dissolution or therapeutic effect can be altered if the tube tip is placed in the small bowel. If the drug is a solid that can be crushed (e.g., *not* a sublingual, sustained-release, or enteric-coated formulation) or is a capsule, the powder can be mixed with 15 to 30 mL of solvent and administered. Otherwise, a liquid dosage preparation should be used. Multiple medications should be administered separately, each followed by flushing the tube with 5 mL or more of water.
- Mixing of liquid medications with EN formulations can cause physical incompatibilities that inhibit drug absorption and clog small-bore feeding tubes. Incompatibility is more common with formulations containing intact (versus

TABLE 56–5. Medications with Special Considerations for Enteral Feeding Tube Administration

Drug	Interaction	Comments
Phenytoin	Reduced bioavailability in the presence of EN	Holding tube feeding 1–2 h before and after phenytoin has no proven benefit Adjust tube feeding rate for time held for phenytoin administration Monitor phenytoin serum concentrations and clinical response and, if necessary switch to IV phenytoin route
Antibiotics (selected)	Potential for reduced bioavailability due to complexation of drug with divalent and trivalent cations found in enteral feeding	May influence quinolone antibiotics, penicillin, tetracycline, isoniazid, and rifampin Consider holding tube feeding before and after administration Avoid jejunal administration of ciprofloxacin Monitor clinical response
Warfarin	Decreased absorption of warfarin due to enteral feeding; therapeutic effect antagonized by vitamin K content of enteral formulations	Adjust warfarin dose based on INR Anticipate need to increase warfarin dose when enteral feedings are started, and decrease dose when enteral feedings are stopped
Antacids	Altered pharmacologic effect of antacid if administered into the small bowel	Administer antacids only into a feeding tube with the tip placed in the stomach
Omeprazole	Rapid degradation in acid environment of stomach when omeprazole granules are crushed	Mix omeprazole granules with acidic juice, not water, to avoid clumping; give via large-, not small-, bore tube to avoid occlusion. Prepare oral liquid suspension for administration via a feeding tube

EN, enteral nutrition; INR, International Normalized Ratio.

TABLE 56–6. Parameters Used to Monitor Enteral Nutrition Efficacy

Parameter	Comments
Anthropometrics	Weight at least weekly; daily in neonates and infants Serial measurement of triceps skinfold and midarm muscle circumference in patients on long-term enteral nutrition
Muscle function	Physical endurance Grip strength
Metabolic	Visceral proteins (albumin and transferrin) at least monthly 24-h urine urea nitrogen weekly to monthly Indirect calorimetry tailored to patient-specific situations
Nutrition intake	Calories, portein, fluid, electrolytes, trace elements, and vitamins
Skin integrity	Wound healing Pressure sores

hydrolyzed) protein and medications formulated as acidic syrups. Mixing of liquid medications and EN formulations should be avoided whenever possible.
- The most significant drug-nutrient interactions result in reduced bioavailability and suboptimal pharmacologic effect (Table 56–5).

▶ EVALUATION OF THERAPEUTIC OUTCOMES

- Assessing the outcome of EN includes monitoring objective measures of body composition, protein and energy balance, and subjective outcome for physiologic muscle function and wound healing (Table 56–6).
- Measures of disease-related morbidity include length of hospital stay, infectious complications, and patient's sense of well-being.

See Chapter 138, Enteral Nutrition, authored by Vanessa J. Kumpf and Katherine Hammond Chessman, for a more detailed discussion of this topic.

X

Chapter 57

▶ OBESITY

▶ DEFINITION

Obesity is the state of excess body fat stores, which should be distinguished from overweight (i.e., excess body weight relative to a person's height).

▶ PATHOPHYSIOLOGY

ETIOLOGY

- The etiology of obesity is usually unknown, but it is likely multifactorial and related to varying contributions from genetic, environmental, and physiologic factors.
- Genetic factors appear to be the primary determinants of obesity in some individuals, whereas environmental factors are more important in others. The specific gene that codes for obesity is unknown; there is probably more than one gene.
- Environmental factors include reduced physical activity or work; abundant and readily available food supply; increased fat intake; increased consumption of refined simple sugars; and decreased ingestion of vegetables, fruits, and complex carbohydrates.
- Excess caloric intake is a prerequisite to weight gain and obesity, but whether the primary consideration is total calorie intake or macronutrient composition is debatable.
- Many neurotransmitters, receptors, and peptides stimulate or decrease food intake in humans and animals (Table 57–1). An understanding of the relationships among these factors is still evolving.
- Activity is thought to play a role in obesity, but studies designed to test the benefit of increased physical activity yield inconsistent results.
- Weight gain can be caused by medical conditions (e.g., hypothyroidism, Cushing's syndrome, hypothalamic lesion) or genetic syndromes (e.g., Prader-Willi syndrome), but these are unusual to rare causes of obesity.

TABLE 57–1. Effects of Various Neurotransmitters, Receptors, and Peptides on Food Intake

Neurotransmitter/ Receptor/Peptide	Action	Food Intake
Norepinephrine	⇑ Concentration	⇓
α_1 and β_1	Stimulates receptor	⇓
α_2	Stimulates receptor	⇑
Serotonin	⇑ Concentration	⇓
5-HT$_{1A}$	Stimulates receptor	⇑
5-HT$_{1B}$ and 5-HT$_{2C}$	Stimulates receptor	⇓
Histamine H$_1$ and H$_3$	Stimulates receptor	⇓
Dopamine D$_1$ and D$_2$	Stimulates receptor	⇓
Leptin	⇑ Concentration	⇓
Neuropeptide Y	⇑ Concentration	⇑
Galanin	⇑ Concentration	⇑

Nutritional Disorders

PHYSIOLOGY AND COMORBIDITIES

- The degree of obesity is determined by the net balance of energy ingested relative to energy expended over time. The single largest determinant of energy expenditure is metabolic rate, which is expressed as resting energy expenditure (REE) or basal metabolic rate (BMR). The two terms are frequently used interchangeably because they differ by less than 10%.
- The major types of adipose tissue are (1) white adipose tissue, which manufactures, stores, and releases lipid; and (2) brown adipose tissue, which dissipates energy via uncoupled mitochondrial respiration. Obesity research includes evaluation of the activity of adrenergic receptors and their effect on adipose tissue with respect to energy storage and expenditure or thermogenesis.
- Obesity, especially excessive central adiposity, is associated with serious health risks and increased mortality. Hypertension, hyperlipidemia, insulin resistance, and glucose intolerance are known cardiac risk factors that cluster in obese individuals.

▶ CLINICAL PRESENTATION AND DIAGNOSIS

- Excess body fat can be determined by skinfold thickness, body density using underwater body weight, bioelectrical impedance and conductivity, dual-energy x-ray absorptiometry (DEXA), computed axial tomography (CT) scan, and magnetic resonance imaging (MRI). Unfortunately, many of these methods are too expensive and time consuming for routine use.
- Body mass index (BMI) and waist circumference (WC) are recognized, acceptable markers of excess body fat, which independently predict disease risk (Table 57–2).
- BMI is calculated as weight (kg) divided by the square of the height (m^2).
- WC, the most practical method of characterizing central adiposity, is the narrowest circumference between the last rib and top of the iliac crest.

▶ DESIRED OUTCOME

The goal of therapy should be reasonable and should consider initial body weight, patient motivation and desire, comorbidities, and patient age. If, for example, the

TABLE 57–2. Classification of Overweight and Obesity by BMI, Waist Circumference, and Associated Disease Risk

	BMI (kg/m²)	Obesity Class	Disease Risk[a] (Relative to Normal Weight and Waist Circumference)	
			Men ≤40 in. (≤102 cm) Women ≤35 in. (≤88 cm)	>40 in. (>102 cm) >35 in. (>88 cm)
Underweight	<18.5		—	—
Normal[b]	18.5–24.9		—	—
Overweight	25.0–29.9		Increased	High
Obesity	30.0–34.9	I	High	Very high
	35.0–39.9	II	Very high	Very high
Extreme obesity	≥ 40	III	Extremely high	Extremely high

[a] Disease risk for type 2 diabetes, hypertension, and cardiovascular disease.

[b] Increased waist circumference can also be a marker for increased risk even in persons of normal weight.

primary goal is improved blood glucose, blood cholesterol, or hypertension, then the endpoint should be target levels of glycosylated hemoglobin, low-density lipoprotein cholesterol, or blood pressure; weight loss goals may be as little as 5%. If the primary goal is relief of osteoarthritis or sleep apnea, then weight loss of 10% or 20% may be more appropriate.

▶ TREATMENT

- Successful obesity treatment plans incorporate diet, exercise, behavior modification with or without pharmacologic therapy, and/or surgery (Figure 57–1).
- The primary aim of behavior modification is to help patients choose lifestyles conducive to safe and sustained weight loss. Behavioral therapy is based on principles of human learning, which use stimulus control and reinforcement to substitute desirable for learned, undesirable behavior.
- Many diets exist to aid weight loss. Regardless of the program, energy consumption must be less than energy expenditure. Highly restrictive diets often yield rapid short-term, but disappointing long-term, results.
- Surgery, which reduces the stomach volume or absorptive surface of the alimentary tract, remains the most effective intervention for obesity. Although modern techniques are safer than older procedures and have an operative mortality of 1%, there are still many potential complications. Therefore, surgery should be reserved for those with BMI greater than 35 or 40 kg/m^2.

PHARMACOLOGIC THERAPY

See Table 57–3.   X◀

- The debate regarding the role of pharmacotherapy remains heated, fueled by the need to treat a growing epidemic and by the fallout from the removal of agents from the market. Reasons for withdrawal were cardiac valvular insufficiency and structural abnormalities for **fenfluramine**, potential cardiac valve problems for **dexfenfluramine**, and hemorrhagic stroke for **phenylpropanolamine**. **Mazindol** was also removed from the market.
- The National Task Force on the Prevention and Treatment of Obesity concluded that short-term use of anorectic agents is difficult to justify because of the predictable weight regain that occurs upon discontinuation. Long-term use may have a role for patients who have no contraindications, but further study is needed before widespread, routine use is implemented.
- **Orlistat** induces weight loss by lowering dietary fat absorption and improves lipid profiles, glucose control, and other metabolic markers. Soft stools, abdominal pain or colic, flatulence, fecal urgency, and/or incontinence occur in 80% of individuals, are mild to moderate in severity, and improve after 1 to 2 months of therapy. Orlistat interferes with the absorption of fat-soluble vitamins and **cyclosporine**.
- **Sibutramine** is more effective than placebo, but patients tended to regain weight after 6 months of treatment. Dry mouth, anorexia, insomnia, constipation, increased appetite, dizziness, and nausea occur 2 to 3 times more often than with placebo. Sibutramine should not be used in patients with coronary artery disease, stroke, congestive heart failure, arrhythmias, or monoamine oxidase inhibitor (MAOI) use.
- **Phentermine** (30 mg in the morning or 8 mg before meals) has less powerful stimulant activity and lower abuse potential than amphetamines and was an effective adjunct in placebo-controlled studies. Adverse effects (e.g., increased blood pressure, palpitations, arrhythmias, mydriasis, altered insulin or

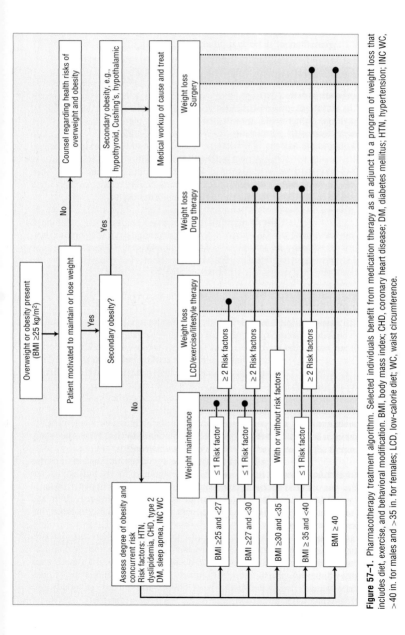

Figure 57-1. Pharmacotherapy treatment algorithm. Selected individuals benefit from medication therapy as an adjunct to a program of weight loss that includes diet, exercise, and behavioral modification. BMI, body mass index; CHD, coronary heart disease; DM, diabetes mellitus; HTN, hypertension; INC WC, >40 in. for males and >35 in. for females; LCD, low-calorie diet; WC, waist circumference.

TABLE 57–3. Pharmacotherapeutic Agents for Weight Loss

Class	Status	Daily Dosages (mg)
Gastrointestinal lipase inhibitor		
Orlistat (Xenical)	Long-term use	360
Noradrenergic/serotonergic agent		
Sibutramine (Meridia)	Long-term use	5–15
Noradrenergic agents		
Phendimetrazine (Prelu-2, Bontril, Plegine, X-Trazine)	Short-term use	70–105
Phentermine (Fastin, Oby-trim, Adipex-P, Ionamin)	Short-term use	15–37.5
Diethylpropion (Tenuate, Tenuate Dospan)	Short-term use	75
Methamphetamine HCl (desoxyephedrine HCl)[a]	Not recommended	5–15
Amphetamine sulfate[a]	Not recommended	5–30
Dextroamphetamine sulfate (Dexedrine)[a]	Not recommended	5–30
Amphetamine/dextroamphetamine mixtures (Adderall)[a]	Not recommended	5–30
Benzphetamine (Didrex)[a]	Not recommended	25–150
Ephedrine (various)[b]	Unlabeled use	20–60
Serotonergic agents		
Fluoxetine (Prozac)	Unlabeled use	60
Sertraline (Zoloft)	Unlabeled use	200

[a] High abuse potential.
[b] Available without a prescription; other agents require prescriptions.

oral hypoglycemic requirements) and interactions with MAO inhibitors have implications for patient selection.

- **Diethylpropion** (25 mg before meals or 75 mg of extended-release formulation every morning) is more effective than placebo in achieving short-term weight loss. Diethylpropion is one of the safest noradrenergic appetite suppressants and can be used in patients with mild to moderate hypertension or angina, but it should not be used in patients with severe hypertension or significant cardiovascular disease.
- **Amphetamines** should generally be avoided because of their powerful stimulant and addictive potential.
- **Ephedrine** (20 mg with or without caffeine 200 mg, up to 3 times daily) had better appetite-suppressive and thermogenic activity than placebo in trials lasting up to 6 months. The most common side effects are tremor, agitation, nervousness, increased sweating, and insomnia. Palpitations and tachycardia have also been reported.
- Serotonergic agents lack the central stimulant effects and abuse potential associated with noradrenergic compounds, but serotonergic agents can alter sleep patterns and change affect. Patients receiving **fluoxetine** (60 mg daily) had an initial weight loss of 2 to 4 kg in placebo-controlled trials, but there were no differences between groups over periods of up to 1 year. Similar findings have been noted with **sertraline** (200 mg daily).
- Peptides (e.g., leptin, neuropeptide Y, galanin) are being investigated because exogenous manipulation may provide future therapeutic approaches to the management of obesity.
- Herbal, natural, and food-supplement products are often used to promote weight loss (Table 57–4). The Food and Drug Administration (FDA) does not strictly regulate these products, so the ingredients may be inactive and present in variable concentrations. In contrast with popular belief, these products are not inherently safer than prescription drugs. For example, more than

TABLE 57–4. Herbal/Natural Products and Food Supplements Used for Weight Loss[a]

Herbal/Natural/ Food, Supplements	Active Moiety	Proposed Mechanism
Chromium picolinate	Chromium	Unclear
St. John's wort	Hypericin	Serotonergic/monoamine oxidase inhibition
Hoodia	P57	Unclear
White willow bark	Salicylate	Inhibit norepinephrine breakdown
Calcium pyruvate	Pyruvate	Unclear
Guarana extract	Caffeine	Noradrenergic
Various tea extracts	Caffeine	Noradrenergic
Garcinia gambogia extract (citrin)	Hydroxycitric acid	Unclear
Chitosan	Cationic polysaccharide	Block fat absorption

[a]Safety and efficacy not documented.

800 reports of serious adverse events (e.g., seizures, stroke, and death) were attributed to ephedrine alkaloids, which led the FDA to exclude them from dietary supplements.

► EVALUATION OF THERAPEUTIC OUTCOMES

- Specific weight goals that are consistent with medical needs and patient desire should be established. Loss of 5% to 30% of initial weight at a rate of 1 pound per week is reasonable.
- Evaluation requires careful clinical, biochemical, and, if necessary, psychological evaluation. Progress should be assessed in a health care setting once or twice monthly for the first 1 to 2 months, then monthly. Each encounter should document weight, WC, BMI, blood pressure, medical history, and tolerability of drug therapy.
- Diabetic patients require more intense medical monitoring and self-monitoring of blood glucose. Some anorectic agents have direct effects that improve glucose tolerance.
- Patients with hyperlipidemia or hypertension should be monitored to assess the effects of weight loss on appropriate endpoints.

See Chapter 140, Obesity, authored by John V. St. Peter and Mehmood A. Khan, for a more detailed discussion of this topic.

Chapter 58

▶ PARENTERAL NUTRITION

▶ DEFINITION

Parenteral nutrition (PN) provides macro- and micronutrients by central or peripheral venous access to meet specific nutritional requirements of the patient, promote positive clinical outcomes, and improve quality of life. PN is also referred to as total parenteral nutrition (TPN) or hyperalimentation.

▶ INDICATIONS

- Identifying candidates and deciding when to initiate PN are difficult because data are conflicting and published guidelines are not consistent.
- In general, PN should be considered when a patient cannot meet nutritional requirements through use of the gastrointestinal tract. Consensus guidelines are based on clinical experience and investigations in specific populations (Table 58–1).
- PN should be considered after suboptimal nutritional intake for 1 day in preterm infants, 2 to 3 days in term infants, 5 to 7 days in well-nourished children, and 7 to 14 days in older children and adults. The route and type of PN depend on the patient's clinical state and expected length of PN therapy (Figure 58–1).
- Peripheral PN (PPN) is a relatively safe and simple method of nutritional support. PPN candidates do not have large nutritional requirements, are not fluid restricted, and are expected to begin enteral intake within 7 to 10 days. Thrombophlebitis is a common complication; this risk is greater with solution osmolaritites greater than 600 to 900 mOsm/L (Table 58–2).
- Central PN is useful in patients who require PN for more than 7 to 10 days and who have large nutrient requirements, poor peripheral venous access, or fluctuating fluid requirements.

▶ DESIRED OUTCOME

- Optimal nutrition therapy requires defining the patient's nutrition goals, determining the nutrient requirements to achieve those goals, delivering the required nutrients, and assessing the nutrition regimen.
- Goals of nutrition support include correcting caloric and nitrogen imbalances, fluid or electrolyte abnormalities, and vitamin or trace element abnormalities, without causing or worsening other metabolic complications.
- Specific caloric goals include adequate energy intake to promote growth and development in children, energy equilibrium and preservation of fat stores in well-nourished adults, and positive energy balance in malnourished patients with depleted fat stores.
- Specific nitrogen goals are positive nitrogen balance or nitrogen equilibrium and improvement in serum concentration of protein markers (e.g., transferrin or prealbumin).

▶ TREATMENT

PARENTERAL NUTRITION COMPONENTS

Both macronutrients (i.e., water, protein, dextrose, and intravenous lipid emulsion [IVLE]) and micronutrients (i.e., vitamins, trace elements, and electrolytes) are necessary to maintain normal metabolism.

TABLE 58–1. Indications for Parenteral Nutrition (PN)

1. Inability to absorb nutrients via the gastrointestinal tract because of one or more of the following:
   a. Massive small bowel resection.
   b. Intractable vomiting when adequate enteral intake is not expected for 7–14 days.
   c. Severe diarrhea especially in infants younger than 3 months who have persistent diarrhea for >2 wk and who have failed enteral nutrition support.
   d. Inflammatory bowel disease (Crohn's disease or ulcerative colitis during acute exacerbations of ulcerative colitis when preservation of lean body mass and functional capacity with enteral nutrition is impossible and for children who have near-complete bowel obstruction, high-output fistulae, GI bleeding, and progressive surgical resection resulting in short bowel syndrome.
   e. Bowel obstruction in patients with prolonged dysmotility of the gastrointestinal tract distal to the pylorus, or in patients who cannot grow and gain weight with enteral nutrition alone.
   f. GI fistulae when enteral intake must be restricted >7 days.
2. Cancer: Antineoplastic therapy, radiation therapy, or hematopoietic stem cell transplantation.
   a. Severely malnourished cancer patients or those in whom GI or other toxicities are anticipated to preclude adequate oral nutritional intake for a prolonged period.
   b. Not for well-nourished or mildly malnourished patients.
   c. Not for patients with advanced cancer unresponsive to chemotherapy or radiation therapy.
3. Pancreatitis when adequate enteral intake is not expected for 5–7 days or when enteral feeding exacerbates abdominal pain, ascites, or fistula output in patients with limited oral intake.
4. Critical care:
   a. Patients in whom enteral nutrition is contraindicated or is unlikely to provide adequate nutrition within 5–10 days.
   b. Organ failure (liver, renal, or respiratory) and moderate to severe catabolism, when enteral feeding is contraindicated.
   c. Burn patients in whom enteral nutrition is contraindicated or is unlikely to provide adequate nutritional requirements within 4–5 days.
5. Perioperative PN:
   a. Preoperative: When the gastrointestinal tract is not functional and surgery is not expected for at least 7 days.
   b. Postoperative: When enteral nutrition is contraindicated or is unlikely to provide adequate nutritional requirements within 7–10 days.
6. Hyperemesis gravidarum: When enteral tube feeding is not tolerated.
7. Eating disorders: Patients with anorexia nervosa and severe malnutrition who require nonvolitional feeding, but who cannot tolerate enteral support.
8. Low-birth-weight (premature) infants: Within the first day of life in selected low-birth-weight infants such as those diagnosed with necrotizing enterocolitis or bronchopulmonary dysplasia, before enteral nutrition is initiated and as a supplement while enteral nutrition is being advanced.
9. Inborn errors of metabolism: Children who are unable to tolerate specialized formulas enterally because of disease-induced nausea and vomiting and poor palatability of the formulas.

GI, gastrointestinal.

Macronutrients

Macronutrients are used for energy (dextrose, fat) and as structural substrates (protein, fats).

Amino Acids

- Protein is provided as crystalline amino acids (CAAs).
- When oxidized, 1 g of protein yields 4 kcal. Including the caloric contribution from protein in calorie calculations is controversial; therefore, calories can be calculated as either total or nonprotein calories.
- Standard CAA products contain a balanced profile of essential, semiessential, and nonessential L-amino acids and are designed for patients with "normal"

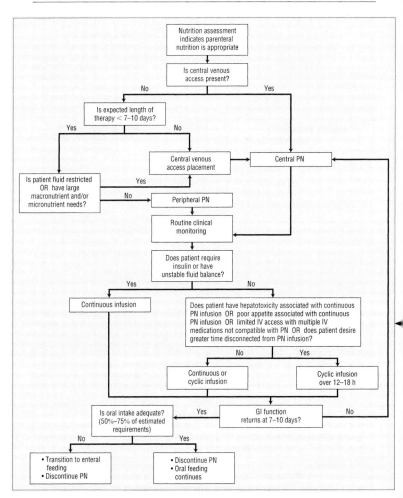

Figure 58–1. Algorithm for parenteral nutrition (PN) route and infusion pattern.

organ function and nutritional requirements. Standard CAA products differ in amino acid, total nitrogen, and electrolyte content but have similar effects on protein markers.

- Conditionally essential amino acids (CEAAs) such as taurine, aspartic acid, and glutamic acid are available in some commercially available CAA solutions (**Aminosyn PF**, **Trophamine**). Other CEAAs such as cysteine, carnitine, and glutamine are not included because they are unstable or insoluble.
- Higher concentrated CAA solutions (i.e., 10% and 15%) are attractive for patients who have large protein needs, such as the critically ill, but are fluid restricted.
- Modified amino acid solutions are designed for patients with altered protein requirements owing to hepatic encephalopathy (**Aminosyn HF**, **Hepatasol**,

607

TABLE 58–2. Osmolarities of Selected Parenteral Nutrients

Nutrient	Osmolarity
Amino acid	100 mOsm/%
Dextrose	50 mOsm/%
Lipid emulsion	1.7 mOsm/%
Sodium (acetate, chloride, phosphate)	2 mOsm/mEq
Potassium (acetate, chloride, phosphate)	2 mOsm/mEq
Magnesium sulfate	1 mOsm/mEq
Calcium gluconate	1.4 mOsm/mEq

Hepatamine), renal failure (**Aminosyn RF, RenAmine, Aminess, Nephr-Amine**), metabolic stress or trauma (**Aminosyn HBC, BranchAmin, FreAmine HBC**), or young age (**Aminosyn PF, Trophamine, Premasol**). However, these solutions are expensive and their role in disease-specific PN regimens is controversial.

Dextrose
- The primary energy source in PN solutions is carbohydrate, usually as dextrose monohydrate. Available concentrations range from 5% to 70%. When oxidized, 1 g of hydrated dextrose provides 3.4 kcal.
- Recommended doses for routine clinical care rarely exceed 5 mg/kg/min in older children and adults. Higher infusion rates contribute to the development of hyperglycemia, excess carbon dioxide production, and increased biochemical markers for liver function. Doses in infants and young children can exceed 5 mg/kg/min.
- Glycerol is a non–insulin-dependent source of carbohydrate that can be used to avoid stress-related hyperglycemia in critically ill patients. A major disadvantage of the available glycerol solution is the dilute concentration of carbohydrate and amino acids (3% of each). Most patients require 3 to 4 L of glycerol solution (**ProcalAmine**) and supplemental IVLE to meet minimal energy requirements.

Lipid Emulsion
- Commercially available IVLEs provide calories and essential fatty acids (EFAs). These products differ in triglyceride source, fatty acid content, and EFA concentration.
- When oxidized, 1 g of fat yields 9 kcal. Because of the caloric contribution from egg phospholipid and glycerol, caloric content of IVLE is 1.1 kcal/mL for the 10%, 2 kcal/mL for the 20%, and 3 kcal/mL for the 30% emulsions.
- Essential fatty acid deficiency (EFAD) can be prevented by giving IVLE, 0.5 to 1 g/kg/day for neonates and infants and 100 g/wk for adults.
- IVLE 10% and 20% products can be administered by a central or peripheral vein, added directly to PN solution as a total nutrient admixture (TNA) or three-in-one system (lipids, protein, glucose, and additives), or piggybacked with a CAA and dextrose solution. IVLE 30% is approved only for TNA preparation.
- IVLE is contraindicated in patients with an impaired ability to clear lipid emulsion and should be administered cautiously to patients with egg allergy.
- The caloric contribution from **propofol** infusions can require adjustment of a patient's nutrition regimen. The caloric contribution from **amphotericin** liposomal and lipid complex formulations is not clinically relevant.

Micronutrients: Vitamins, Trace Elements, and Electrolytes

- Micronutrients are required to support metabolic activities for cellular homeostasis such as enzyme reactions, fluid balance, and regulation of electrophysiologic processes.
- Multivitamin products have been formulated to comply with guidelines for adults, children, and infants. These products contain 13 essential vitamins including vitamin K.
- Requirements for trace elements depend on the patient's age and clinical condition (e.g., higher doses of zinc in patients with high-output ostomies or diarrhea).
- Zinc, copper, chromium, manganese, and possibly selenium and molybdenum are the only trace elements that require supplementation during PN.
- Requirements for trace elements during organ failure are not clearly defined. Manganese and copper should be restricted or withheld in patients with cholestatic liver disease. Chromium, molybdenum, and selenium should be restricted or withheld in patients with renal failure.
- Sodium, potassium, calcium, magnesium, phosphorus, chloride, and acetate are necessary components of PN for maintenance of cellular functions such as acid-base balance and cellular growth.
- Patients with normal organ function and serum electrolyte concentrations should receive daily maintenance doses of electrolytes during PN.
- Electrolyte requirements depend on the patient's disease state, organ function, drug therapy, nutrition status, and extrarenal losses.

ORDERING, COMPOUNDING, AND STORING PN SOLUTIONS

- PN regimens for adults can be based on formulas (Figure 58–2), computer programs, or standardized order forms. Order forms are popular because they help educate practitioners and foster cost-efficient nutrition support by minimizing errors in ordering, compounding, and administering.
- PN regimens for infants and children typically require an individualized approach, which is highly variable among institutions.
- The two most common types of PN solutions are CAA and dextrose combination, with or without IVLE piggybacked into the PN line, and TNAs. A CAA and dextrose combination with separate IVLE administration is recommended for neonates and infants.
- Methods for compounding PN solutions vary among institutions and often involve automated compounders. Sterility should be assured during compounding, storage, and administration.
- CAA and dextrose solutions are generally stable for 1 to 2 months if refrigerated at 4°C and if protected from light, but TNA formulations are inherently unstable.
- Appropriate resources should be consulted for compatibility and stability information before mixing components (e.g., manufacturer's information, *Trissel's Handbook on Injectable Drugs*, and *King Guide to Parenteral Admixtures*).
- Precipitation of calcium and phosphorus is a common interaction that is potentially life-threatening.
- Bicarbonate should not be added to acidic PN solutions; a bicarbonate precursor salt (e.g., acetate) is preferred.
- Vitamins can be adversely affected by changes in solution pH, other additives, storage time, solution temperature, and exposure to light. Vitamins should be added to the PN solution near the time of administration and should not be in the PN solution for more than 24 hours.

Patient Case: A 53-year-old patient's estimated nutritional requirements are 95–105 g protein/day and 1800–2100 total kcal/day. The patient has a central venous access and no history of hyperlipidemia or allergy to eggs. The patient is not fluid restricted. The PN solution will be compounded as an individualized regimen utilizing a single-bag, 24-h infusion of a crystalline amino acid (CAA)/dextrose combination with intravenous lipid emulsion (IVLE) piggy-backed into the PN infusion line. The stock solutions used to compound this regimen are 10% CAA and 70% dextrose.

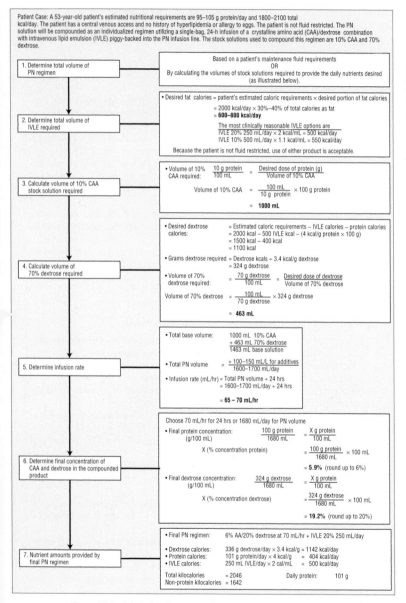

1. Determine total volume of PN regimen

Based on a patient's maintenance fluid requirements
OR
By calculating the volumes of stock solutions required to provide the daily nutrients desired (as illustrated below).

2. Determine total volume of IVLE required

- Desired fat calories = patient's estimated caloric requirements × desired portion of fat calories

  = 2000 kcal/day × 30%–40% of total calories as fat

  = 600–800 kcal/day

  The most clinically reasonable IVLE options are
  IVLE 20% 250 mL/day × 2 kcal/mL = 500 kcal/day
  IVLE 10% 500 mL/day × 1.1 kcal/mL = 550 kcal/day

  Because the patient is not fluid restricted, use of either product is acceptable.

3. Calculate volume of 10% CAA stock solution required

- Volume of 10% CAA required: $\dfrac{10 \text{ g protein}}{100 \text{ mL}} = \dfrac{\text{Desired dose of protein (g)}}{\text{Volume of 10\% CAA}}$

  Volume of 10% CAA $= \dfrac{100 \text{ mL}}{10 \text{ g protein}} \times 100 \text{ g protein}$

  = 1000 mL

4. Calculate volume of 70% dextrose required

- Desired dextrose calories: = Estimated caloric requirements – IVLE calories – protein calories
  = 2000 kcal – 500 IVLE kcal – (4 kcal/g protein × 100 g)
  = 1500 kcal – 400 kcal
  = 1100 kcal

- Grams dextrose required = Dextrose kcals ÷ 3.4 kcal/g dextrose
  = 324 g dextrose

- Volume of 70% dextrose required: $\dfrac{70 \text{ g dextrose}}{100 \text{ mL}} = \dfrac{\text{Desired dose of dextrose}}{\text{Volume of 70\% dextrose}}$

  Volume of 70% dextrose $= \dfrac{100 \text{ mL}}{70 \text{ g dextrose}} \times 324 \text{ g dextrose}$

  = 463 mL

5. Determine infusion rate

- Total base volume:
  1000 mL 10% CAA
  + 463 mL 70% dextrose
  1463 mL base solution

- Total PN volume = $\dfrac{+ 100\text{–}150 \text{ mL/L for additives}}{1600\text{–}1700 \text{ mL/day}}$

- Infusion rate (mL/hr) = Total PN volume ÷ 24 hrs
  = 1600–1700 mL/day ÷ 24 hrs

  = 65 – 70 mL/hr

6. Determine final concentration of CAA and dextrose in the compounded product

Choose 70 mL/hr for 24 hrs or 1680 mL/day for PN volume

- Final protein concentration: $\dfrac{100 \text{ g protein}}{1680 \text{ mL}} = \dfrac{X \text{ g protein}}{100 \text{ mL}}$
  (g/100 mL)

  X (% concentration protein) $= \dfrac{100 \text{ g protein}}{1680 \text{ mL}} \times 100 \text{ mL}$

  = 5.9% (round up to 6%)

- Final dextrose concentration: $\dfrac{324 \text{ g dextrose}}{1680 \text{ mL}} = \dfrac{X \text{ g protein}}{100 \text{ mL}}$
  (g/100 mL)

  X (% concentration dextrose) $= \dfrac{324 \text{ g dextrose}}{1680 \text{ mL}} \times 100 \text{ mL}$

  = 19.2% (round up to 20%)

7. Nutrient amounts provided by final PN regimen

- Final PN regimen: 6% AA/20% dextrose at 70 mL/hr + IVLE 20% 250 mL/day

- Dextrose calories: 336 g dextrose/day × 3.4 kcal/g = 1142 kcal/day
- Protein calories: 101 g protein/day × 4 kcal/g = 404 kcal/day
- IVLE calories: 250 mL IVLE/day × 2 cal/mL = 500 kcal/day

Total kilocalories = 2046   Daily protein: 101 g
Non-protein kilocalories = 1642

Figure 58–2. Calculation of a parenteral nutrition (PN) compounding plan.

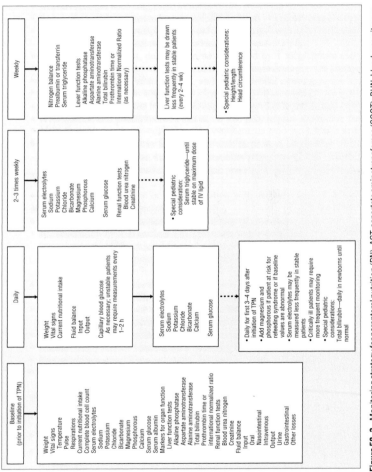

Figure 58–3. Monitoring strategy for parenteral nutrition (PN). AST, aspartate aminotransferase (SGOT); BUN, blood urea nitrogen; CBC, complete blood count; TPN, total PN.

TABLE 58–3. Substrate Intolerance in Parenteral Nutrition (PN)

Complication	Possible Causes	Intervention
Hyperglycemia	Stress, infection, corticosteroids, pancreatitis, diabetes mellitus, peritoneal dialysis, excessive dextrose administration	Decrease dextrose load by decreasing infusion rate or dextrose concentration (may substitute fat calories); administer insulin
Hypoglycemia	Abrupt withdrawal of dextrose, insulin overdose	Increase dextrose intake: decrease exogenous insulin Taper infusion rate down prior to discontinuing PN
Excess carbon dioxide production	Excess dextrose intake	Decrease dextrose intake; balance calories from fat and dextrose
Hypertriglyceridemia	Stress, familial hyperlipidemia, pancreatitis; excess IVLE dose; rapid IVLE infusion rate	Decrease IVLE dose; decrease rate of IVLE infusion; discontinue IVLE if indicated
Abnormal liver function tests (elevated AST, alkaline phosphatase, and bilirubin)	Stress, infection, cancer, excess carbohydrate intake, excess caloric intake, essential fatty acid deficiency	Decrease dextrose load (substitute fat); decrease total calories; provide essential fatty acids; cycle PN infusion; transition to enteral nutrition regimen

AST, aspartate aminotransferase (SGOT); IVLE, intravenous lipid emulsion.

- Using the PN admixture as a drug vehicle consolidates dosage units and has other advantages; however, compatibility and stability data are not available for many PN solutions. Medications frequently added to PN solutions include albumin, regular insulin, and histamine$_2$ antagonists.

ADMINISTERING PN SOLUTIONS

- PN solutions should be administered with an infusion pump.
- A 0.22-μm filter is recommended for CAA and dextrose solutions to remove particulate matter, air, and microorganisms. Because IVLE particles measure approximately 0.5 μm, IVLE should be administered separately and piggy-backed into the PN line beyond the in-line filter.
- Routine use of in-line filters with TNA solutions is controversial. A 1.2-μm filter can be used to prevent catheter occlusion caused by precipitates or lipid aggregates, and to remove *Candida albicans*.
- Although protocols for initiating PN differ, the rate is typically increased gradually over 12 to 24 hours to prevent hyperglycemia. When discontinuing PN, the infusion rate is gradually decreased to prevent hypoglycemia.
- The starting dose of IVLE is 0.5 g/kg/day in neonates and 0.5 to 1 g/kg/day in older children. This dose is increased by 0.5 to 1 g/kg/day to a maximum of 3 to 4 g/kg/day. The dose of IVLE in adults ranges from 1 to 2.5 g/kg/day, not to exceed 30% to 60% of total calories.
- Administering IVLE over 16 to 24 hours in adults and 20 to 24 hours (0.15 g/kg/h) in neonates appears to be the best strategy for promoting IVLE clearance and minimizing negative immune function effects.
- Cyclic PN (e.g., 12 to 18 h/day) is useful in hospitalized patients who have limited venous access and require other medications necessitating interruption of PN infusion, to prevent or treat hepatotoxicities associated with continuous PN therapy, and to allow home patients to resume normal lifestyles. Cyclic PN may be poorly tolerated by patients with severe glucose intolerance or unstable fluid balance.

COMPLICATIONS

PN can cause mechanical or technical (e.g., malfunctions in delivery system and catheter-related complications), infectious (e.g., colonization of the catheter or direct microbial invasion of the skin), metabolic (e.g., substrate intolerance [Table 58–3] and fluid, electrolyte, and acid-base disorders), and nutritional (e.g., hypertriglyceridemia, refeeding syndrome, EFAD, and metabolic bone disease) complications.

▶ EVALUATION OF THERAPEUTIC OUTCOMES

- Routine evaluation should include assessment of the clinical condition of the patient, with a focus on nutritional and metabolic effects of the PN regimen.
- Biochemical and clinical parameters should be monitored routinely in patients receiving PN (Figure 58–3).

See Chapter 137, Parenteral Nutrition, authored by Todd W. Mattox and Pamela D. Reiter, for a more detailed discussion of this topic.

Chapter 59

▶ BREAST CANCER

▶ DEFINITION

Breast cancer is a malignancy originating from breast tissue. This chapter distinguishes between early stages, which are potentially curable, and metastatic breast cancer, which is usually incurable.

▶ PATHOPHYSIOLOGY

- The development of malignancy is a multistep process with preinvasive (or noninvasive) and invasive phases.
- The strongest risk factors are female gender and increasing age. Additional risk factors include endocrine factors (e.g., early menarche, nulliparity, late age at first birth, estrogen therapy), genetics (e.g., personal and family history, mutations of tumor suppresser genes [*BRCA1* and *BRCA2*]), and environment (e.g., radiation exposure).
- Breast cancer spreads via the bloodstream early in the course of the disease, resulting in relapse and metastatic disease after local therapy. The most common metastatic sites are lymph nodes, skin, bone, liver, lungs, and brain.
- The likelihood of developing metastatic disease is related to prognostic factors as described below.

▶ CLINICAL PRESENTATION

- The initial sign in more than 90% of women with breast cancer is a painless lump that is typically solitary, unilateral, solid, hard, irregular, and nonmobile. Less common initial signs are pain and nipple changes. More advanced cases present with prominent skin edema, redness, warmth, and induration.
- Symptoms of metastatic breast cancer include bone pain, difficulty breathing, abdominal enlargement, jaundice, and mental status changes.
- Approximately 80% of women first detect some breast abnormalities themselves.
- It is increasingly common for breast cancer to be detected during routine screening mammography in asymptomatic women.

▶ DIAGNOSIS

- Initial workup for a woman presenting with a localized lesion or suggestive symptoms should include a careful history, physical examination of the breast, three-dimensional mammography, and possibly other breast imaging techniques such as ultrasound.
- Breast biopsy is indicated for a mammographic abnormality that suggests malignancy or a mass that is palpable on physical examination.

STAGING

- Stage is based on the size of the primary tumor (T_{1-4}), presence and extent of lymph node involvement (N_{1-3}), and presence or absence of distant metastases (M). Simplistically stated, these stages may be represented as follows:

  Early Breast Cancer
  Stage 0: Carcinoma in situ or disease that has not invaded the basement membrane.
  Stage I: Small primary tumor without lymph node involvement.
  Stage II: Metastasis to ipsilateral axillary lymph nodes.
  Locally Advanced Breast Cancer
  Stage III: Usually a large tumor with extensive nodal involvement in which node or tumor is fixed to the chest wall; also includes inflammatory breast cancer, which is rapidly progressive.
  Advanced or Metastatic Breast Cancer
  Stage IV: Metastases to organs distant from the primary tumor.

PATHOLOGIC EVALUATION

- The pathologic evaluation of breast lesions establishes the histologic diagnosis and presence or absence of prognostic factors.
- Most breast carcinomas are adenocarcinomas and are classified as ductal or lobular.
- Carcinoma in situ may be a preinvasive cancer or a marker of unstable epithelium that represents an increased risk for developing aggressive cancer.

PROGNOSTIC FACTORS

- Tumor size and the presence and number of involved axillary lymph nodes are primary factors in assessing the risk for breast cancer recurrence and subsequent metastatic disease. XI
- Hormone receptors are used as indicators of prognosis and to predict response to hormone therapy.
- The rate of tumor cell proliferation, nuclear grade, and tumor (histologic) differentiation are also independent prognostic research factors.
- Additional potential prognostic factors include overexpression of *erb*-B2 oncogene (or HER-2/*neu*), cathepsin-D, angiogenic growth factors, and mutations in the tumor suppressor p53 gene. HER-2/*neu* status is of interest because targeted therapy is available; however, the testing method is controversial. The widely used method, immunohistochemistry (IHC), can yield false-positive results at the 2+ level, which should be confirmed by fluorescence in situ hybridization (FISH) testing.

▶ DESIRED OUTCOME

The goal of therapy with early and locally advanced breast cancer is cure. The goals of therapy with metastatic breast cancer are to improve symptoms, improve quality of life, and prolong survival.

▶ TREATMENT

The treatment of breast cancer is rapidly evolving. Specific information regarding the most promising interventions can be found only in the primary literature.

Treatment can cause substantial toxicity, which differs depending on the individual agent, administration method, and combination regimen. Because a comprehensive review of toxicities is beyond the scope of this chapter, appropriate references should be consulted.

EARLY BREAST CANCER

Local-Regional Therapy

- Surgery alone can cure most patients with in situ cancers and approximately half of those with stage II cancers.
- Breast conservation is appropriate primary therapy for most women with stages I and II disease; it is preferable to modified radical mastectomy because it produces equivalent survival rates with cosmetically superior results. Breast conservation consists of lumpectomy (i.e., excision of the primary tumor and adjacent breast tissue) followed by radiation therapy to prevent local recurrence.
- Primary systemic or neoadjuvant therapy, which is administered before surgery, is gaining favor. Advantages include shrinking the tumor, making inoperable tumors resectable, assessing in vivo response to chemotherapy, and, in patients with complete pathologic response, prolonging disease-free survival.
- Simple or total mastectomy involves removal of the entire breast without dissection of underlying muscle or axillary nodes. This procedure is used for carcinoma in situ where the incidence of axillary node involvement is only 1%, for local recurrence following breast conservation therapy, or to avoid the inconvenience of radiation therapy and preserve the option for future breast reconstruction.
- Axillary lymph nodes should be sampled for staging and prognostic information. Lymphatic mapping with sentinel lymph node biopsy is a new, less invasive alternative to axillary dissection; however, the procedure is controversial because of the lack of long-term data.

Systemic Adjuvant Therapy

- Systemic adjuvant therapy is the administration of systemic therapy following surgery, radiation, or both. There is no evidence of metastatic disease but a high likelihood of recurrence because of undetectable micrometastases. The goal of such therapy is cure.
- The choice between chemotherapy and endocrine therapy, or both, as adjuvant therapy is evolving.
- Essentially all women with stage I and stage II breast cancer derive some benefit from chemotherapy, but the absolute benefit is greater in premenopausal women.
- The National Comprehensive Cancer Network (NCCN) practice guidelines reflect the trend toward the use of chemotherapy in all women regardless of menopausal status, and the addition of endocrine therapy in all women with receptor-positive disease regardless of menopausal status.

Adjuvant Chemotherapy

- Many combination regimens are used in the adjuvant setting (Table 59–1), which are typically derived from those that produce the highest response rate in advanced disease.
- **Doxorubicin**-containing regimens are popular because they are superior to **cyclophosphamide**, **methotrexate**, and **fluorouracil** (CMF) and require only four cycles.

XI

TABLE 59–1. Adjuvant Chemotherapy of Breast Cancer

AC
Doxorubicin 60 mg/m^2 IV, day 1
Cyclophosphamide 400–600 mg/m^2 IV, day 1
Repeat cycle every 21 days

CAF (or FAC)
Cyclophosphamide 600 (or 500) mg/m^2 IV, day 1
Doxorubicin 60 (or 50) mg/m^2 IV, day 1 (over 72 h)
Fluorouracil 600 mg/m^2 IV, day 1 (or 500 mg/m^2 days 1, 4)
Repeat cycle every 21–28 days

CEF (or FEC)
Cyclophosphamide 75 mg/m^2 PO, days 1–14 (or 500 mg/m^2 IV, day 1)
Epirubicin 60 (or 100) mg/m^2 IV, days 1, 8 (or day 1 only)
Fluorouracil 600 (or 500) mg/m^2 IV, days 1, 8 (or day 1 only)
Repeat cycle every 21 days and, for CEF, with prophylactic antibiotics or growth factor support

CMF
Cyclophosphamide 100 mg/m^2 PO, days 1–14 (or 600 mg/m^2 IV, day 1)
Methotrexate 40 mg/m^2 IV, days 1, 8 (or day 1 only)
Fluorouracil 600 mg/m^2 IV, days 1, 8
Repeat cycle every 28 days

TAC
Docetaxel[a] 75 mg/m^2 IV, day 1
Doxorubicin 50 mg/m^2 IV, day 1
Cyclophosphamide 600 mg/m^2 IV, day 1
Repeat cycle every 21–28 days

[a] Premedicate with dexamethasone.

- Taxanes, **docetaxel** and **paclitaxel,** are a newer class with activity against metastatic breast cancer rivaling that of anthracyclines. When used in combination regimens or given sequentially (e.g., doxorubicin and cyclophosphamide followed by paclitaxel [AC → T]), taxanes increase disease-free survival in women with node-positive breast cancer. Follow-up, however, is insufficient to assess impact on the decisive endpoint, overall survival.
- Clinical trials are being conducted to evaluate newer agents (e.g., **trastuzumab**).
- Chemotherapy should be initiated within 3 weeks of surgical removal of the primary tumor. The optimal duration of treatment is about 12 to 24 weeks.
- Dose intensity refers to the amount of drug administered per unit of time, which can be increased by increasing dose, decreasing time, or both. Dose density is equivalent to dose intensity except that it is increased only by decreasing time. Dose intensity, but not density, is an important determinant of outcome in adjuvant therapy. Therefore, the dose of standard regimens should *not* be reduced unless necessitated by severe toxicity.
- The short-term toxicities of chemotherapy are generally well tolerated in the adjuvant setting, especially with the availability of serotonin-antagonist antiemetics and colony-stimulating factors.

Adjuvant Endocrine Therapy
- **Tamoxifen** is the gold standard for adjuvant endocrine therapy because of extensive trial experience showing decreased recurrence and mortality. Additional benefits include estrogenic effects on lipids and bone density.
- The optimal daily dose of tamoxifen is 20 mg, beginning soon after completing chemotherapy and continuing for five years.

- Tamoxifen is usually well tolerated. Symptoms of estrogen withdrawal (hot flashes and vaginal bleeding) may occur but decrease in frequency and intensity over time. Tamoxifen increases the risks of stroke, pulmonary embolism, deep vein thrombosis, and endometrial cancer, especially in women older than 50 years of age.
- Other endocrine therapies show promise, but trials have insufficient follow-up to assess impact on survival. Such options included **toremifene** as an alternative to tamoxifen; the luteinizing hormone-releasing hormone (LHRH), **goserelin**, for premenopausal women; and aromatase inhibitors, either in place of or after tamoxifen, for postmenopausal women.

LOCALLY ADVANCED BREAST CANCER (STAGE III)

- Local-regional therapy with surgery, radiation, or both does not cure locally advanced breast cancer.
- Primary or neoadjuvant or chemotherapy is the initial treatment of choice. Benefits include rendering inoperable tumors resectable and increasing the rate of breast-conserving surgery.
- Combination regimens used as primary chemotherapy are similar to those used as adjuvant therapy and generally include an anthracycline and taxane.

METASTATIC BREAST CANCER (STAGE IV)

The choice of therapy for metastatic disease is based on the site of disease involvement and presence or absence of certain characteristics, as described below.

Endocrine Therapy

- Endocrine therapy is the treatment of choice for patients who have hormone receptor-positive metastases in soft tissue; bone; pleura; or, if asymptomatic, viscera. Compared with chemotherapy, endocrine therapy has an equal probability of response and a better safety profile.
- Patients are sequentially treated with endocrine therapy until they have rapidly growing metastatic disease, at which time chemotherapy can be given.
- Because most endocrine therapies are equally effective, the choice is based primarily on toxicity (Table 59–2).
- **Tamoxifen** is usually the agent of choice in both premenopausal and post-menopausal women whose tumors are hormone-receptor positive, unless metastases occur within a year of adjuvant tamoxifen. Maximal beneficial effects do not occur for 2 months or more. In addition to the side effects described for adjuvant therapy, tumor flare or hypercalcemia occurs in approximately 5% of patients with metastatic breast cancer. This may be a positive indication that the patient will have a response to endocrine therapy.
- New antiestrogens are being developed to maintain tamoxifen's beneficial effects on breast cells, bone, and lipids and avoid its effects on the endometrium. The new antiestrogen, **toremifene**, appears to have efficacy and safety similar to that of tamoxifen, but it is not suitable for tamoxifen-refractory disease because of cross-resistance.
- Ovarian ablation (oophorectomy) is considered by some to be the endocrine therapy of choice in *premenopausal* women and produces similar overall response rates as tamoxifen. Medical castration with an LHRH analogue, **goserelin, leuprolide,** or **triptorelin,** is a reversible alternative to ovarian ablation.
- Aromatase inhibitors reduce circulating estrogens by blocking peripheral conversion from an androgenic precursor, the primary source of estrogens in *postmenopausal* women. Newer agents are more selective and better toler-

XI

ated than the prototype, **aminoglutethimide**. As second-line therapy, **anastrozole** and **exemestane** improve overall survival and tolerability compared with progestins. As first-line therapy, anastrozole and **letrozole** improve time to progression and tolerability compared with tamoxifen.

- Progestins are generally reserved for third-line therapy. They cause weight gain, fluid retention, and thromboembolic events.

Chemotherapy

- Chemotherapy is preferred to endocrine therapy for women with hormone receptor-negative tumors; rapidly progressive lung, liver, or bone marrow involvement; or failure of endocrine therapy.
- The choice of treatment depends on the individual. Agents used as adjuvant therapy can be repeated unless the cancer recurred within a year. Sequential single-agent regimens are less toxic than combination regimens, but the latter are used to induce rapid response for symptomatic bulky metastases.
- Combinations produce objective responses in approximately 40% of patients previously unexposed to chemotherapy, but complete responses occur in less than 10% of patients. The median duration of response is 5 to 12 months; the median survival is 14 to 33 months.
- Single agents are associated with lower response rates, but time to progression and overall survival are similar. Single agents are better tolerated, an important consideration in the metastatic setting.
- **Anthracyclines** produce response rates of 50% to 60% when used as first-line therapy for metastatic breast cancer.
- Newer single agents, such as **paclitaxel** (50% to 60%), **docetaxel** (54% to 68%), **capecitabine** (25%), **vinorelbine** (30% to 50%), and **gemcitabine** (13% to 42%), produce impressive response rates in previously untreated patients. Although response rates are lower in previously treated patients, these agents are useful alternatives for anthracycline-refractory breast cancer. Furthermore, some of these agents are moving to first-line regimens, often in combination with anthracyclines.

TABLE 59–2. Endocrine Therapies Used for Metastatic Breast Cancer

Class	Drug	Dose	Side Effects
Aromatase inhibitors Nonsteroidal Steroidal	Anastrozole Letrozole Exemestane	1 mg PO daily 2.5 mg PO daily 25 mg PO daily	Hot flashes, arthralgias, myalgias, headaches, diarrhea, mild nausea
Antiestrogens SERMs	Tamoxifen Toremifene	20 mg PO daily 60 mg PO daily	Hot flahses, vaginal discharge, mild nausea, thromboembolism, endometrial cancer
SERDs	Fulvestrant	250 mg IM every 28 days	Hot flashes, injection site reactions, possibly thromboembolism.
LHRH analogues	Goserelin Leuprolide Triptorelin	3.6 mg SC every 28 days 7.5 mg IM every 28 days 3.75 mg Im every 28 days	Hot flashes, amenorrhea, menopausal symptoms, injection site reactions
Progestins	Megestrol acetate Medroxyprogesterone	40 mg PO 4 times a day 400–1000 mg IM every week	Weight gain, hot flashes, vaginal bleeding, edema, thromboembolsim

LHRH, luteinizing hormone-releasing hormone; SERD, selective estrogen receptor downregulator; SERM, selective estrogen receptor modulator.

TABLE 59–3. Single-Agent Chemotherapy for Metastatic Breast Cancer

Paclitaxel	**Vinorelbine**
175 mg/m^2 IV over 3 h every 21 days	Vinorelbine 30 mg/m^2 IV, days 1, 8 every 21 days
or	*or*
80 mg/m^2 IV over 1 h every 7 days	Vinorelbine 25–30 mg/m^2 IV every 7 days (adjust dose based on absolute neutrophil count; see product infomation)
Docetaxel	**Gemcitabine**
60–100 mg/m^2 IV over 1 h every 21 days	Gemcitabine 600–1000 mg/m^2 IV, days 1, 8, and 15,
or	every 28 days (may need to hold day-15 dose based on blood
30–35 mg/m^2 IV over 30 min every 7 days	counts)
Capecitabine	**Liposomal doxorubicin**
2000–2500 mg/m^2 PO divided twice daily for 14 days, every 21 days	30–50 mg/m^2 IV over 90 min every 21–28 days

- Different doses are available for single-agent therapy of metastatic breast cancer (Table 59-3). Weekly paclitaxel administration causes less myelosuppression and delayed onset of peripheral neuropathy compared with paclitaxel given every 21 days. The 100-mg/m^2 dose of docetaxel is indicated for symptomatic patients requiring rapid onset of activity, whereas 60 or 75 mg/m^2 is equally effective and appropriate for asymptomatic patients. Capecitabine is usually initiated at 2,000 mg/m^2 daily because the 2,500-mg/m^2 dose is poorly tolerated and does not improve efficacy.
- **Trastuzumab,** a monoclonal antibody that binds to HER-2/*neu* protein, produces responses rates of 15% to 20% when used as a single agent and prolongs survival when combined with chemotherapy. Trastuzumab is well tolerated, but it may increase the risk of doxorubicin-related cardiotoxicity. Non-anthracycline-containing combinations are being evaluated.

PREVENTION OF BREAST CANCER

- **Tamoxifen,** 20 mg daily, reduced the incidence of estrogen-receptor-positive breast cancer by 48% in a meta-analysis of women at risk for developing breast cancer. Because adverse effects may be unacceptable when tamoxifen is used as preventive therapy, candidates should be informed of potential benefits and risks.

▶ EVALUATION OF THERAPEUTIC OUTCOMES

EARLY BREAST CANCER

- The goal of adjuvant therapy in early-stage disease is cure. Because there is no clinical evidence of disease when adjuvant therapy is administered, assessment of this goal cannot be fully evaluated for years after initial diagnosis and treatment.
- Adjuvant chemotherapy can cause substantial toxicity. Because maintaining dose intensity is important in cure of disease, supportive care should be optimized with measures such as antiemetics and growth factors.

LOCALLY ADVANCED BREAST CANCER

- The goal of primary systemic therapy in locally advanced breast cancer is cure. Complete pathologic response, determined at the time of surgery, is the desired end point.

METASTATIC BREAST CANCER

- Optimizing quality of life is the therapeutic end point in the treatment of patients with metastatic breast cancer. Many valid and reliable tools are available for objective assessment of quality of life.
- The least toxic therapies are used initially, with increasingly aggressive therapies applied in a sequential manner that does not significantly compromise quality of life.
- Tumor response is measured by clinical chemistry (e.g., liver enzyme elevation in patients with hepatic metastases) or imaging techniques (e.g., bone scans or chest x-rays).
- Assessment of the clinical status and symptom control of the patient is often adequate to evaluate response to therapy.

See Chapter 125, Breast Cancer, authored by Celeste Lindley and Laura Boehnke Michaud, for a more detailed discussion of this topic.

XI

Chapter 60

► COLORECTAL CANCER

► DEFINITION

Colorectal cancer is a malignant neoplasm involving the colon, rectum, and anal canal.

► PATHOPHYSIOLOGY

- Development of a colorectal neoplasm is a multistep process of genetic and phenotypic alterations of normal bowel epithelium structure and function leading to unregulated cell growth, proliferation, and tumor development.
- Sequential mutations within colonic epithelium result in cellular replication or enhanced invasiveness. Genetic changes include mutational activation of oncogenes and inactivation of tumor suppressor genes.
- Adenocarcinomas account for more than 90% of tumors of the large intestine.

► CLINICAL MANIFESTATIONS

- Signs and symptoms of colorectal cancer can be extremely varied, subtle, and nonspecific. Patients with early-stage colorectal cancer are often asymptomatic, and lesions are usually detected by screening procedures.
- Blood in the stool is the most common sign; however, any change in bowel habits, vague abdominal discomfort, or abdominal distention may be a warning sign.
- Less common signs and symptoms include nausea, vomiting, and, if anemia is severe, fatigue.
- Approximately 20% of patients with colorectal cancer present with metastatic disease. The most common site of metastasis is the liver, followed by the lungs and then bones.

PREVENTION AND SCREENING

- Primary prevention is aimed at preventing colorectal cancer in an at-risk population. To date, the only strategy shown to reduce the risk is chemoprevention with celecoxib in people with familial adenomatous polyposis (FAP).
- Secondary prevention is aimed at preventing malignancy in a population that has already manifested an initial disease process. Secondary prevention includes procedures ranging from colonoscopic removal of precancerous polyps to total colectomy for high-risk individuals (e.g., FAP).
- American Cancer Society guidelines for average-risk individuals include annual occult fecal blood testing starting at age 50 years and examination of the colon every 5 or 10 years depending on the procedure. Digital rectal examination is not effective alone and should be performed with other screening examinations.

► DIAGNOSIS

- When colorectal carcinoma is suspected, a careful history and physical examination should be performed to identify risk factors and clinical manifestations.
- The entire large bowel should be evaluated by colonoscopy or proctosigmoidoscopy with double-contrast barium enema.

- Baseline laboratory tests should include complete blood cell count, prothrombin time (PT), activated partial thromboplastin time (aPTT), liver and renal function tests, and serum carcinoembryonic antigen (CEA). Serum CEA can serve as a marker for colorectal cancer and for monitoring response to treatment, but it is too insensitive and nonspecific to be used as a screening test for early-stage colorectal cancer.
- Radiographic imaging studies include chest x-ray, bone scan, abdominal computed tomography (CT) scan or ultrasound, positron emission tomography (PET), ultrasonography, and magnetic resonance imaging (MRI).
- Immunodetection of tumors using tumor-directed antibodies is an imaging technique for early detection of colorectal cancers. These tests might also be useful for identifying metastatic or recurrent disease in patients with rising CEA levels.
- Stage of colorectal cancer should be determined at diagnosis to predict prognosis and to develop treatment options. Stage is based on the size of the primary tumor (T_{1-4}), presence and extent of lymph node involvement (N_{1-2}), and presence or absence of distant metastases (M).

▶ DESIRED OUTCOME

The goal of treatment depends on the stage of disease. Stages I, II, and III are potentially curable; the goals are to eradicate micrometastatic disease and to prevent recurrence. Stage IV is incurable; the goals are to alleviate symptoms, avoid disease-related complications, and prolong survival. In all stages, treatment decisions require careful assessment of relative risks and benefits.

▶ TREATMENT

XI

GENERAL PRINCIPLES

- Treatment modalities are surgery, radiation therapy (XRT), and chemotherapy and biomodulators. This section on treatment begins with an overview of each modality and associated toxicities. Next, this section addresses separately adjuvant therapy and treatment of metastatic disease.
- Adjuvant therapy is administered after complete tumor resection to eliminate residual local or metastatic microscopic disease.
- Adjuvant therapy differs for colon and rectal cancer because their natural history and recurrence patterns differ. Rectal cancer is more difficult to resect with wide margins, so local recurrences are more frequent than with colon cancer. Adjuvant XRT plus chemotherapy is considered standard for stage II or III rectal cancer. Adjuvant chemotherapy is standard for stage III colon cancer and can be considered for high-risk stage II colon cancer. Adjuvant therapy is not indicated for stage I colorectal cancer because most patients are cured by surgical resection alone.
- Neoadjuvant therapy is administered before surgery to shrink the tumor, thereby making it resectable. Neoadjuvant XRT may also prevent local recurrence.
- Chemotherapy is the primary treatment modality for metastatic colorectal cancer. Treatment options are generally similar for metastatic cancer of the colon and rectum.

SURGERY

- Surgical removal of the primary tumor is the treatment of choice for most patients with operable disease.

- Surgery for *colon* cancer generally involves complete tumor resection with an appropriate margin of tumor-free bowel and a regional lymphadenectomy.
- Surgery for *rectal* cancer depends on the area involved. Although less than 33% of these patients require permanent colostomy, frequent complications include urinary retention, incontinence, impotence, and local-regional recurrence.
- Common complications of surgery for both colon and rectal caner include infection, anastomotic leakage, obstruction, adhesions, and malabsorption syndromes.
- Surgery is rarely indicated for metastatic colorectal cancer, except for discrete hepatic and possibly other metastases that can be resected.

RADIATION THERAPY

- XRT can be administered with curative surgical resection to prevent local recurrence of rectal cancer, before surgery to shrink a rectal tumor and make it operable, or in advanced or metastatic disease to alleviate symptoms. Adjuvant XRT, however, does not have a definitive role in colon cancer because recurrences are usually extrapelvic.
- Acute adverse effects associated with XRT include hematologic depression, dysuria, diarrhea, abdominal cramping, and proctitis. Chronic symptoms may persist for months after XRT and may involve diarrhea, proctitis, enteritis, small-bowel obstruction, perineal tenderness, and impaired wound healing.

CHEMOTHERAPY AND BIOMODULATORS

Fluoropyrimidines

- **Fluorouracil** (5-FU) is the most widely used chemotherapeutic agent for colorectal cancer. Biomodulators are usually added to 5-FU to modify its activity and improve response rates, unless it is administered by continuous intravenous (IV) infusion.
- Administration method affects clinical activity and toxicity. 5-FU is administered by IV bolus once weekly or daily for 5 days each month, or by continuous IV infusion over 5 days. Continuous infusion appears to have better clinical activity, but bolus administration is more popular in the United States because of ease of administration and lower cost.
- Continuous IV infusion of 5-FU is generally well tolerated but is associated with palmar-plantar erythrodysesthesia or hand-foot syndrome. This distinct skin toxicity can be acutely disabling, but it is reversible and not life-threatening. IV bolus administration is associated with leukopenia, which is dose limiting and can be life-threatening. Both methods are associated with a similar incidence of mucositis, diarrhea, nausea and vomiting, and alopecia.
- Oral cryotherapy reduces the incidence and severity of stomatitis. Patients should chew and hold ice chips in the mouth for 5 minutes before, during, and for 30 minutes after bolus administration of 5-FU.
- **Capecitabine** is an oral fluoropyrimidine, which has efficacy and safety profiles similar to those of IV infusion of 5-FU.
- Combined 5-FU and XRT results in severe hematologic toxicity, enteritis, and diarrhea compared with either chemotherapy or XRT alone.

Biomodulators

- **Leucovorin** improves 5-FU cytotoxicity. Toxicity depends on the regimen. High-dose leucovorin is associated with dose-limiting diarrhea, whereas low-dose leucovorin is associated with neutropenia and stomatitis.
- **Levamisole** is a synthetic, oral anthelmintic drug with immunomodulatory properties. Toxicities are generally minimal and reversible. Toxicities include

metallic taste, arthralgias, central nervous system (CNS) toxicities (e.g., mood changes, sleep disorders, or cerebellar ataxia), and hepatic toxicity.

Irinotecan

- **Irinotecan** is a topoisomerase I inhibitor. Irinotecan is associated with two distinct patterns of diarrhea that require appropriate intervention.
- Early-onset diarrhea occurs 2 to 6 hours after administration and is characterized by lacrimation, diaphoresis, abdominal cramping, flushing, and/or diarrhea. These cholinergic symptoms respond to atropine 0.25 to 1.0 mg IV or SC.
- Late-onset diarrhea occurs 1 to 12 days after administration, lasts 3 to 5 days, and can be fatal. Late-onset diarrhea requires aggressive, high-dose **loperamide** beginning with 4 mg after the first soft or watery stool, followed by 2 mg every 2 hours until symptom free for 12 hours.

Oxaliplatin

- **Oxaliplatin** has a mechanism similar to that of cisplatin and might have better activity against colorectal cancer.
- Unlike other platinums, oxaliplatin is associated with minimal renal toxicity, hematologic toxicity, and nausea and vomiting.
- Oxaliplatin is associated with neuropathies. Acute neuropathy is reversible within 2 weeks, usually occurs peripherally, and is precipitated by exposure to cold. Persistent neuropathy is cumulative and is characterized by paresthesias, dysesthesias, and hypoesthesias.

Monoclonal Antibodies

- **Bevacizumab** is a humanized monoclonal antibody directed against vascular endothelial growth factor (VEGF).
- Bevacizumab does not increase the frequency of typical adverse events when added to chemotherapy.
- Bevacizumab is associated with hypertension, which is easily managed with oral antihypertensive agents.
- Bevacizumab is also associated with gastrointestinal perforation. This rare, but potentially fatal, complication necessitates prompt evaluation of abdominal pain associated with vomiting or constipation.
- **Cetuximab** is a chimeric monoclonal antibody directed against epidermal growth factor receptor (EGFR).
- Cetuximab is generally well tolerated. The most common adverse events are acne-like skin rash, asthenia, lethargy, malaise, and fatigue.

ADJUVANT THERAPY FOR COLON CANCER

- 5-FU combined with leucovorin or levamisole significantly reduces the risk of relapse and death in patients with stage III colon cancer. 5-FU and leucovorin has become the standard (Table 60–1) because a 6-month course is as effective as 12 months of 5-FU and levamisole.
- The value of adjuvant therapy for stage II colon cancer is less clear, but high-risk individuals will probably benefit and should be offered adjuvant therapy in a clinical trial.
- None of the administration methods for 5-FU and leucovorin (Table 60–2) is considered standard. The regimens have similar efficacy but different toxicity profiles, treatment costs, and compliance issues. Many practitioners prefer the weekly, high-dose regimen (i.e., Roswell Park regimen) because of less toxicity, except for diarrhea.

XI

TABLE 60–1. National Comprehensive Cancer Network Recommendations for Adjuvant Therapy for Colon Cancer

Pathologic Stage	Treatment Options
$T_{1-2}N_0M_0$	None
$T_3N_0M_0$	Clinical trial *or* observation
T_3 high risk	Consider 5-FU and leucovorin *or* clinical trial *or* observation
$T_4N_0M_0$	Consider 5-FU and leucovorin $\pm$ XRT[a] *or* clinical trial *or* observation
$T_{1-3}N_{1-2}M_0$	5-FU and leucovorin *or* FOLFOX
$T_4N_{1-2}M_0$	5-FU and leucovorin $\pm$ XRT[a] *or* FOLFOX

5-FU, fluorouracil; FOLFOX, 5-FU, leucovorin, oxaliplatin; XRT, radiation therapy.
[a]Catogary 2B, defined as nonuniform consensus, based on lower-level evidence including clinical experience.

- New adjuvant regimens are being evaluated such as the addition of a newer agent to 5-FU and leucovorin.

ADJUVANT AND NEOADJUVANT THERAPY FOR RECTAL CANCER

- The goal of adjuvant XRT for rectal cancer is to decrease local tumor recurrence after surgery, preserve the sphincter, and, with preoperative radiotherapy, improve resectability.
- 5-FU enhances the cytotoxic effects of XRT. Compared with XRT alone, the combination reduces local tumor recurrence and improves survival in high-risk patients.
- Continuous infusions of 5-FU, which may provide more effective radiosensitization, significantly improve disease-free and overall survival compared with IV bolus injections. Unlike adjuvant therapy for colon cancer, leucovorin and other biomodulators have not yet been shown to improve the efficacy of adjuvant 5-FU in rectal cancer.
- More research is needed to determine the best way to combine surgery, XRT, and chemotherapy. Available findings indicate that the extent of tumor involvement is important. For resectable T2 or larger lesions, postoperative 5-FU-based chemotherapy and XRT is appropriate. For unresectable tumors, neoadjuvant

TABLE 60–2. Adjuvant Fluorouracil and Leucovorin for Colon Cancer

	Regimen	Major Dose-Limiting Toxicities
Weekly, high-dose leucovorin; Roswell Park regimen	Fluorouracil 600 mg/m^2 IV + lecovorin 500 mg/m^2 IV weekly $\times$ 6 of 8 wk	Diarrhea, mucositis
Consecutive day, low-dose leucovorin; Mayo Clinic regimen	Fluorouracil 425 mg/m^2/day IV + leucovorin 20 mg/m^2/day IV days 1–5, for 5 consecutive days, repeated every 4–5 wk	Mucositis, neutropenia
Bolus plus infusional fluorouracil; de Gramont regimen	Leucovorin 200 mg/m^2/day IV over 2 h followed by fluorouracil 400 mg/m^2/day IV bolus, then followed by fluorouracil 600 mg/m^2/day continuous IV infusion over 22 h, days 1 and 2 for 2 consecutive days; repeat every 2 wk	Neutropenia, mucositis

XI

chemoradiation followed by surgery followed by postoperative 5-FU, with or without postoperative XRT, should be considered.

TREATMENT OF METASTATIC COLORECTAL CANCER

- 5-FU is incorporated into first-line regimens for metastatic colorectal cancer, usually in combination with leucovorin (Table 60–3).
- The optimal combination of 5-FU with leucovorin regimen is controversial. Historically, 5-FU plus low-dose leucovorin (i.e., Mayo Clinic regimen) was the most popular regimen for metastatic colorectal cancer based on response

TABLE 60–3. First-Line Chemotherapeutic Regimens for Metastatic Colorectal Cancer

	Regimen	Major Dose-Limiting Toxicities
Pyrimidine only		
Roswell Park; Mayo Clinic, or de Gramont regimen	Fluorouracil + leucovorin (See Table 60-2)	Diarrhea, mucositis, neutropenia
Capecitabine	1250 mg/m^2 orally twice daily for 14 days, repeated every 3 wk	Diarrhea, hand-foot syndrome
Oxaliplatin + fluorouracil + leucovorin		
Oxaliplatin + bimonthly infusional fluorouracil; FOLFOX4	Oxaliplatin 85 mg/m^2 IV day 1 + bolus fluorouracil 400 mg/m^2 IV + leucovorin 200 mg/m^2 IV followed by fluorouracil 600 mg/m^2 IV in 22-h infusion on days 1 and 2, every 2 wk	Sensory neuropathy, neutropenia
High-dose oxaliplatin + bimonthly infusional fluorouracil; FOLFOX7	Oxaliplatin 130 mg/m^2 IV with leucovorin 400 mg/m^2 IV day 1, followed by fluorouracil 400 mg/m^2 IV bolus and 2400 mg/m^2 continuous IV infusion over 46 h started on day 1, repeated every 2 wk	Sensory neuropathy, diarrhea, myelosuppression
Irinotecan + fluorouracil + leucovorin		
Irinotecan + bolus fluorouracil; IFL; Saltz regimen	Irinotecan 125 mg/m^2 IV + fluorouracil 500 mg/m^2 IV + leucovorin 20 mg/m^2 IV weekly for 4 of 6 wk	Diarrhea, neutropenia
Irinotecan + infusional fluorouracil; FOLFIRI	Irinotecan 180 mg/m^2 IV + leucovorin 400 mg/m^2 IV + bolus fluorouracil 400 mg/m^2 IV, followed by fluorouracil 2400 mg/m^2 continuous IV infusion over 46 h on day 1, repeated every 2 wk	Nausea, diarrhea, mucositis neutropenia
Biweekly irinotecan + infusional fluorouracil	Irinotecan 180 mg/m^2 IV + leucovorin 200 mg/m^2 + fluorouracil 400 mg/m^2 IV, followed by fluorouracil 600 mg/m^2 continuous IV infusion over 22 h, day 1, repeated every 2 wk	Neutropenia, diarrhea
Weekly irinotecan + infusional fluorouracil	Irinotecan 80 mg/m^2 IV + leucovorin 500 mg/m^2 IV + fluorouracil 2300 mg/m^2 continuous IV infusion over 24 h day 1, repeated weekly	Neutropenia, diarrhea
Bevacizumab		
Bevacizumab + bolus; IFL	Irinotecan 125 mg/m^2 IV + fluorouracil 500 mg/m^2 IV + leucovorin 20 mg/m^2 IV weekly for 4 of 6 wk with bevacizumab 5 mg/m^2 IV day 1, repeated every 2 wk	Diarrhea, hypertension, asthenia, thrombosis, vomiting, proteinuria

XI

rates, toxicity, and drug costs. A weekly schedule of 5-FU (bolus or continuous IV) combined with leucovorin is more convenient for the patient.

- Adding a newer agent (i.e., triple-drug therapy) prolongs survival and is the standard first-line approach for patients who can tolerate the additional toxicity, which can be substantial. The optimal triple-drug regimen is unknown.
- Adding irinotecan to 5-FU and leucovorin prolonged survival by 2 to 3 months in previously untreated patients ($p < .05$ in two studies).
- Adding oxaliplatin to 5-FU and leucovorin improved response rates ($p < .05$ in two studies) and survival ($p < .05$ in one study) in previously untreated patients.
- Adding bevacizumab to 5-FU and leucovorin improved response rates and survival ($p < .05$ in two studies) in previously untreated patients. Bevacizumab is being evaluated in combination with other agents as first-line or salvage therapy.
- Capecitabine monotherapy is suitable for first-line therapy in patients not likely to tolerate triple-drug therapy. Capecitabine produced superior response rates and comparable survival compared with 5-FU and leucovorin in a pooled analysis. Capecitabine is being evaluated in combination with irinotecan or oxaliplatin.
- Second-line or salvage therapy is based on type of and response to previous treatment, site and extent of disease, and patient factors and treatment preferences (Table 60–4). The optimal sequence of regimens has not been established.
- A different regimen is generally used as salvage therapy, unless first-line therapy induced disease stabilization or a better response. Preliminary evidence supports reinstitution of previously active first-line therapy. Therefore, 5-FU can be included in salvage regimens, either in combination with an agent not previously used or by a different route (e.g., continuous IV infusion or capecitabine).

XI

TABLE 60–4. Salvage Chemotherapeutic Regimens for Metastatic Colorectal Cancer

	Regimen	Major Dose-Limiting Toxicities
Irinotecan		
Weekly irinotecan	Irinotecan 125 mg/m^2 IV every week for 4 out of 6 wk	Neutropenia, diarrhea
Every 3-weekly irinotecan	Irinotecan 350 mg/m^2 IV every 3 wk	Neutropenia, diarrhea
Oxaliplatin + fluorouracil + leucovorin		
FOLFOX4 or FOLFOX7	(See Table 60–3)	Sensory neuropathy, neutropenia
Cetuximab[a]		
Cetuximab + irinotecan	Continue irinotecan as previously dosed, + cetuximab 400 mg/m^2 IV loading dose, then cetuximab 250 mg/m^2 IV weekly thereafter	Asthenia, diarrhea, nausea acne-like rash, vomiting
Cetuximab	Cetuximab 400 mg/m^2 IV loading dose, then cetuximab 250 mg/m^2 IV weekly thereafter	Acne-like rash, asthenia, constipation, diarrhea
Fluorouracil		
Protracted continuous infusion	Fluorouracil 250–300 mg/m^2 per day continuous IV infusion until disease progression	Mucositis, hand-foot syndrome

[a] If irinotecan-refractory disease.

- After failure of first-line therapy, patients should be encouraged to participate in clinical trials, which are being conducted to evaluate sequencing and many new treatments.
- After failure of 5-FU, irinotecan monotherapy prolonged survival by 2 to 3 months compared with best supportive care (p <.05) and with 5-FU by continuous infusion (p not significant).
- The combination of oxaliplatin, 5-FU, and leucovorin is effective as salvage therapy. Unlike irinotecan, oxaliplatin does not have substantial activity as monotherapy.
- Cetuximab produced encouraging response rates in patients with irinotecan-refractory disease, especially when it was combined with irinotecan. Cetuximab is also suitable as salvage therapy for patients with oxaliplatin-refractory disease, and ongoing studies are evaluating cetuximab combined with oxaliplatin.

▶ EVALUATION OF THERAPEUTIC OUTCOMES

- The goals of monitoring are to evaluate the benefit of treatment and to detect recurrence.
- Patients who undergo curative surgical resection, with or without adjuvant therapy, require routine follow-up.
- Patients should be evaluated for anticipated side effects such as loose stools or diarrhea, nausea or vomiting, mouth sores, fatigue, and fever.
- Patients should be closely monitored for side effects that require aggressive intervention such as irinotecan-induced diarrhea and bevacizumab-induced gastrointestinal perforation. Patients should be evaluated for other treatment-specific side effects such as oxaliplatin-induced neuropathy, cetuximab-induced skin rash, and bevacizumab-induced hypertension.
- Less than half of patients develop symptoms of recurrence such as pain syndromes, changes in bowel habits, rectal or vaginal bleeding, pelvic masses, anorexia, and weight loss. CEA levels may help detect recurrences in asymptomatic patients.
- Quality of life indices should be monitored, especially in patients with metastatic disease.

XI

See Chapter 127, Colorectal Cancer, authored by Patrick J. Medina and Lisa E. Davis, for a more detailed discussion of this topic.

Chapter 61

▶ LUNG CANCER

▶ DEFINITION

Lung cancer is a solid tumor originating from bronchial epithelial cells. This chapter distinguishes between non-small cell lung cancer (NSCLC) and small cell lung cancer (SCLC) because they have different natural histories and responses to therapy.

▶ PATHOPHYSIOLOGY

- Lung carcinomas arise from pluripotent epithelial cells after exposure to carcinogens, which cause chronic inflammation that leads to genetic and cytologic changes and ultimately to carcinoma.
- Activation of protooncogenes, inhibition or mutation of tumor suppressor genes, and production of autocrine growth factors contribute to cellular proliferation and malignant transformation. Molecular changes, such as P53 mutations and overexpression of epidermal growth factor receptor (EGFR), also affect disease prognosis and response to therapy.
- Cigarette smoking is responsible for about 83% of lung cancer cases. Exposure to asbestos, chloromethyl ethers, heavy metals, polycyclic aromatic hydrocarbons, and radon has also been implicated.
- The major cell types are SCLC (20% of all lung cancers), adenocarcinoma (40%), squamous cell carcinoma (less than 30%), and large cell carcinoma (15%). The last three types are grouped together and referred to as NSCLC.

▶ CLINICAL PRESENTATION

- The most common initial signs and symptoms include cough, dyspnea, chest pain, sputum production, and hemoptysis. Many patients also exhibit systemic symptoms such as anorexia, weight loss, and fatigue.
- Disseminated disease can cause neurologic deficits from CNS metastases, bone pain or pathologic fractures secondary to bone metastases, or liver dysfunction from hepatic involvement.
- Paraneoplastic syndromes commonly associated with lung cancers include cachexia, hypercalcemia, syndrome of inappropriate antidiuretic hormone secretion, and Cushing's syndrome.

▶ DIAGNOSIS

- In a patient with signs and symptoms of lung cancer, chest x-ray, computed tomography (CT) scan, and positron emission tomography (PET) scan are the most valuable diagnostic tests. Integrated CT-PET technology appears to improve diagnostic accuracy in staging NSCLC over CT or PET alone.
- Pathologic confirmation of lung cancer is established by examination of sputum cytology and/or tumor biopsy by fiberoptic bronchoscopy, percutaneous needle biopsy, or open-lung biopsy.
- All patients must have a thorough history and physical examination to detect signs and symptoms of the primary tumor, regional spread of the tumor, distant metastases, paraneoplastic syndromes, and ability to withstand aggressive surgery or chemotherapy.

STAGING

- The American Joint Committee on Cancer has established a TNM staging classification for lung cancer based on the primary tumor size and extent (T), regional lymph node involvement (N), and the presence or absence of distant metastases (M).
- A simpler system is commonly used to compare treatments. Stage I includes tumors confined to the lung without lymphatic spread, stage II includes large tumors with ipsilateral peribronchial or hilar lymph node involvement, stage IIIA includes locally advanced disease, stage IIIB includes bulky regional disease, and stage IV includes any tumor with distant metastases.
- A two-stage classification is widely used for SCLC. Limited disease is confined to one hemithorax and the regional lymph nodes. All other disease is classified as extensive.

▶ TREATMENT

NON-SMALL CELL LUNG CANCER

Desired Outcome

The goal of treating NSCLC depends on the disease stage. Stages I, II, and possibly III disease can be cured with appropriate therapy. In contrast, stage IV disease is not curable, but chemotherapy can decrease symptoms and prolong survival.

General Principles

- Surgery is the treatment of choice for localized disease (stage I or IIA).
- Radiation therapy is used as adjuvant therapy after surgery, as primary therapy if the tumor is not operable or the patient is not a good surgical candidate, and as palliative therapy for advanced disease.
- Historically, NSCLC has been considered to be insensitive to chemotherapy. New drugs and new combination regimens are yielding promising results. For example, a 3-drug regimen was recently shown to prolong survival when used as adjuvant therapy after surgery for stages I, II, and III disease.
- Management of locally advanced NSCLC (stages IIB, IIIA, and IIIB) is controversial. Postoperative adjuvant and preoperative neoadjuvant chemotherapy, with or without concurrent radiation therapy, have been used.
- New combinations improve response and survival rates in patients with stage IV disease. Patients most likely to benefit from chemotherapy have a good performance status, no or minimal weight loss, and less extensive disease.
- No single regimen is considered standard, so selection should be based on the patient's ability to tolerate expected toxicities and likelihood of radiation therapy (and impact on chemotherapy-induced toxicities).

Chemotherapy

- The most widely used and recommended regimens include **cisplatin** or **carboplatin** combined with another agent (Table 61–1). Historically, cisplatin combined with **etoposide** was considered to be the most active regimen for advanced NSCLC. Addition of a third drug does not appear to provide benefit and can increase toxicity.
- **Vinorelbine** and cisplatin improves survival compared with either agent alone. Vinorelbine has the advantage of minimal toxicity and is easily administered in the outpatient setting over 6 to 10 minutes followed by a 75- to 100-mL IV flush.

XI

TABLE 61–1. Combination Regimens Using Newer Agents for Stage III and IV Non–Small Cell Lung Cancer

Regimen	Overall Response Rates (%)	Median Survival Duration
Paclitaxel + cisplatin versus etoposide + cisplatin		
Etoposide 100 mg/m² IV days 1,2, and 3; cisplatin 75 mg/m² IV day 1; cycle; every 21 days	12	7.6 months
Paclitaxel 250 mg/m² IV over 24 hours day 1; cisplatin 75 mg/m² IV day 2; filgrastim 5 mcg/kg SC from day 3 until granulocytes ≥ 10,000/mcL; cycle: every 21 days	27.7	10 months
Paclitaxel 135 mg/m² IV over 24 hours day 1; cisplatin 75 mg/m² IV day 2; cycle: every 21 days	25.3	9.5 months
Cisplatin + paclitaxel or gemcitabine or docetaxel versus carboplatin + paclitaxel		
Cisplatin 75 mg/m² IV day 1; paclitaxel 175 mg/m² per 24 h IV day 1; cycle: every 21 days	21	7.8 months
Gemcitabine 1000 mg/m² IV days 1, 8, 15; cisplatin 100 mg/m² IV day 1; cycle: every 28 days	22	8.1 months
Docetaxel 75 mg/m² IV day 1; cisplatin 75 mg/m² IV day 1; cycle: every 21 days	17	7.4 months
Paclitaxel 225 mg/m² every 3 h IV day 1; carboplatin AUC 6 IV day 1; cycle: every 21 days	17	8.1 months
Paclitaxel + carboplatin versus vinorelbine + cisplatin		
Paclitaxel 225 mg/m² every 3 h IV day 1; carboplatin AUC 6 IV day 1; cycle: every 21 days	PR 27	8.0 months
Vinorelbine 25 mg/m² IV weekly; cisplatin 100 mg/m² IV day 1; cycle: every 28 days	PR 27	8.0 months
Cisplatin + vinorelbine or vindesine versus vinorelbine		
Vinorelbine 30 mg/m² IV weekly; cisplatin 120 mg/m² day 1 and 29, then every 6 weeks	30	9.2 months
Vindesine 3 mg/m² every week for 6 wk then every 2 weeks thereafter; cisplatin 120 mg/m² days 1 and 29, then every 6 weeks	19	7.4 months
Vinorelbine 30 mg/m² weekly	14	7.2 months
Cisplatin + gemcitabine or etoposide		
Gemcitabine 1250 mg/m² IV weekly on days 1 and 8; cisplatin 100 mg/m² IV day 1; cycle: every 21 days	40.6 (p=.02)	8.7 months
Etoposide 100 mg/m² IV days 1, 2, 3; cisplatin 100 mg/m² IV day 1; cycle: every 21 days	21.9	7.2 months
Irinotecan + cisplatin		
Irinotecan 60 mg/m² IV days 1, 8, 15; cisplatin 80 mg/m² IV day 1; cycle: every 28 days	43	50.3 weeks
Cisplatin 80 mg/m² IV day 1; vindesine 3 mg/m² IV days 1, 8, 15; cycle: every 28 days	31	47.7 weeks
Irinotecan 100 mg/m² IV days 1, 8, 15	21	46.1 weeks

ANC, absolute neutrophil count; AUC, area under the curve; PR, partial response.

XI

- More studies are needed to clarify how **paclitaxel** should be combined with other agents, whether the dose should be high or low, and whether the dose should be infused over 1 or 3 hours or given as a continuous 24-hour infusion. The 1-hour infusion is easy to administer in the outpatient setting and causes minimal myelosuppression, but it increases the rate of peripheral sensory neuropathy. Studies are being conducted to determine whether continuous infusion or high doses are more effective; these approaches are more myelosuppressive and require granulocyte colony-stimulating factor (G-CSF) support.
- **Docetaxel**, a taxane without the schedule-dependent efficacy and toxicity issues of paclitaxel, is given IV over 1 hour every 3 weeks. Docetaxel is approved as a single agent after failure of first-line therapy and in combination with platinum as first-line therapy. The dose-limiting toxicity is neutropenia.
- **Gemcitabine** is approved as first-line therapy when combined with cisplatin based on studies showing prolonged survival compared with cisplatin with or without etoposide. In a 4-way comparison of combination regimens, gemcitabine combined with cisplatin was associated with the least neutropenia but the most thrombocytopenia and renal dysfunction.
- **Irinotecan** is being evaluated in many combination regimens. Irinotecan is also being evaluated with chest radiotherapy at a dose selected to avoid the esophagitis, diarrhea, and unexpected severe pneumonitis seen at higher doses.
- Two oral EGFR inhibitors are indicated as single-agent therapy after failure of first-line therapy. Although not compared in a head-to-head study, **erlotinib** appears to be more active because it significantly prolonged survival whereas **gefitinib** did not.

SMALL CELL LUNG CANCER

Desired Outcome
The goal of treatment is cure or prolonged survival, which requires aggressive combination chemotherapy.

Surgery and Radiation Therapy
- Surgery is almost never indicated because SCLC disseminates early in the disease.
- SCLC is very radiosensitive. Radiotherapy has been combined with chemotherapy to treat tumors limited to the thoracic cavity. This combined-modality therapy prevents local tumor recurrences but only modestly improves survival over chemotherapy alone.
- Radiotherapy is utilized to prevent and treat brain metastases, a frequent occurrence with SCLC. Prophylactic cranial irradiation is controversial because of neurologic and cognitive impairment and should be limited to patients with limited disease and complete response to chemotherapy.

Chemotherapy
- Aggressive combination chemotherapy produces a four to fivefold increase in median survival for patients with SCLC.
- Combination chemotherapy is clearly superior to single-agent therapy. The most frequently used regimen is a platinum combined with **etoposide** or, less frequently, **irinotecan**.
- **Cisplatin**-containing regimens yielded improved survival and less life-threatening myelosuppression than regimens without cisplatin. **Carboplatin** is frequently used in place of cisplatin because it has similar efficacy and is less toxic.

- Alternating non–cross-resistant regimens and dose intensity are theoretically attractive, but neither provided substantial benefit in clinical studies. Dose-intensive regimens significantly increase toxicity such as granulocytopenia, febrile neutropenia, mucositis, and weight loss.
- Recurrent SCLC is usually less sensitive to chemotherapy. If recurrence is more than 6 months after induction chemotherapy, that regimen can be repeated. If recurrence is less than 6 months, another regimen should be used such as **ifosfamide**, **taxane**, **gemcitabine**, **topotecan**, CAV (**cyclophosphamide**, **doxorubicin**, and **vincristine**), **gemcitabine**, oral etoposide, **methotrexate**, or **vinorelbine**.

▶ EVALUATION OF THERAPEUTIC OUTCOMES

- The efficacy of induction therapy should be determined after two to three cycles of chemotherapy. If there is no response or progressive disease, a non–cross-resistant or investigational regimen should be considered.
- The optimal duration of chemotherapy after induction of response is contro-versial. Guidelines for NSCLC recommend a maximum of six or eight cycles of chemotherapy, but some experts recommend only three or four cycles. In-duction therapy for SCLC is administered for four to six cycles, but more than four cycles have not demonstrated a survival advantage and may reduce quality of life.
- Intensive therapeutic monitoring is required because of underlying medical problems in patients with lung cancer and because of drug- and radiotherapy-related toxicity.
- Patients receiving radiation therapy may experience esophagitis, fatigue, radi-ation pneumonitis, and cardiac toxicity.
- The aggressive chemotherapy regimens used for lung cancer cause many tox-icities. Although a comprehensive review is beyond the scope of this chap-ter, cisplatin-induced acute and delayed emesis merits consideration because the problem is common and severe, requiring aggressive management with **serotonin antagonists** and **dexamethasone**. Appropriate references should be consulted for management of other common toxicities such as dose-limiting myelosuppression, mucositis, nephrotoxicity, peripheral neuropathy, and oto-toxicity.

XI

See Chapter 126, Lung Cancer, authored by Rebecca S. Finley and Jeannine S. McCune, for a more detailed discussion of this topic.

Chapter 62

▶ LYMPHOMAS

▶ DEFINITION

Lymphomas are a heterogenous group of malignancies that arise from immune cells residing predominantly in lymphoid tissues. Differences in histology have led to classification as Hodgkin's and non-Hodgkin's lymphoma, which are addressed separately in this chapter.

▶ HODGKIN'S DISEASE

PATHOPHYSIOLOGY

- Current hypotheses indicate that B-cell transcriptional processes are disrupted, which prevent expression of B-cell surface markers and production of immunoglobulin mRNA. Alterations in the normal apoptotic pathways favor cell survival and proliferation.
- Malignant Reed-Sternberg cells overexpress nuclear factor-κB, which is associated with cell proliferation and anti-apoptotic signals. Infections with viral and bacterial pathogens upregulate nuclear factor-κB. Epstein-Barr virus (EBV) is found in many, but not all, Hodgkin's lymphoma tumors.

CLINICAL PRESENTATION

- Most patients with lymphomas present with adenopathy, which waxes and wanes and which is painless and rubbery. Adenopathy is usually localized to the cervical region but can also occur in the mediastinal, hilar, and retroperitoneal regions.
- Up to 40% of patients with Hodgkin's disease present with constitutional, or "B," symptoms (e.g., fever, night sweats, weight loss, and pruritus).

DIAGNOSIS AND STAGING

- Diagnosis requires the presence of Reed-Sternberg cells.
- Staging is performed to provide prognostic information and to guide therapy. Staging has evolved from previous classifications, and it continues to evolve.
- Approximately half of the patients have early-stage disease (stages I, II, and II$_E$). The other half have advanced disease, of which 10% to 15% is stage IV.
- Clinical staging is based on noninvasive procedures such as history, physical examination, laboratory tests, and radiography. Pathologic staging is based on biopsy findings of strategic sites (e.g., muscle, bone, skin, spleen, abdominal nodes) using an invasive procedure (e.g., laparoscopy).
- Prognostic factors that predict poor treatment outcome include advanced stage, advanced age, male gender, B symptoms, high number of involved nodal regions, large mediastinal mass, extranodal disease, elevated erythrocyte sedimentation rate (ESR), anemia, leukocytosis, lymphocytopenia, and low serum albumin.

DESIRED OUTCOME

The treatment goal for Hodgkin's disease is to maximize curability while minimizing treatment-related complications.

Oncologic Disorders

Oncologic Disorders

TREATMENT

- Treatment options include radiation therapy, chemotherapy, or both (combined-modality therapy). The choice depends on the stage of disease and presence of risk factors (Table 62–1).
- Studies are being conducted to identify how to maximize efficacy and minimize toxicity such as by limiting the volume of radiation therapy or the number of chemotherapy cycles.
- Surgery is rarely indicated unless pathologic staging would affect treatment. The use of laparotomy and splenectomy is diminishing because of associated morbidity and mortality.

Radiation Therapy

- Radiation therapy is an integral part of treatment and can be used alone for selected patients with early-stage disease. *Involved-field* radiation therapy targets a single field of Hodgkin's lymphoma. *Extended-field* or subtotal nodal radiation targets the involved field and an uninvolved area. *Total nodal* radiation therapy targets all areas.
- Low-dose consolidative radiation therapy can be beneficial for advanced-stage Hodgkin's disease if chemotherapy induces a partial response.
- The major concern with radiation therapy is long-term effects such as cardiovascular disease and secondary solid malignancies.

Initial Chemotherapy

- Combination regimens produce more rapid and durable remissions than single-agent therapy.

XI

TABLE 62–1. General Treatment Recommendations for Hodgkin's Disease[a,b]

Early-Stage Disease	
Favorable prognosis (CS I or II with no risk factors)	Extended-field radiation or 2–4 cycles of ABVD plus involved-field radiation
Unfavorable prognosis (CS I or II with risk factors)	4–6 cycles of ABVD plus involved-field radiation
Advanced-Stage Disease (CS III or IV)	6–8 cycles of ABVD, or MOPP/ABV, or ChIVPP, or MOPP plus radiation to residual lymphoma or sites of bulky disease
Relapsed Disease	
Relapse after radiation	6–8 cycles of chemotherapy with or without radiation (treat as if this were primary advanced disease)
Relapse after primary chemotherapy[c,d]	Salvage chemotherapy at conventional doses or high-dose chemotherapy and autologous hematopoietic stem cell transplantation

ABVD, doxorubicin, bleomycin, vinblastine, dacarbazine; CS, clinical stage.
[a]Patients should be considered for clinical trials when possible.
[b]In general, patients with large mediastinal adenopathy should be treated with chemotherapy followed by radiation to the mediastinum.
[c]A standard regimen or approach does not exist.
[d]Highly selected patients may be treated with radiation alone.

- Two to 8 cycles of chemotherapy should be administered, depending on the stage of disease and presence of risk factors (see Table 62-1). Maintenance therapy does not increase survival and can contribute to long-term complications.
- MOPP (**m**echlorethamine, **v**incristine [Oncovin], **p**rocarbazine, **p**rednisone) used to be the mainstay of treatment for advanced Hodgkin's disease (stages IIIB and IV) (Table 62–2). MOPP produces complete remissions in 84% of patients and has a 10-year cure rate of 54%.
- ABVD (**d**oxorubicin [Adriamycin], **b**leomycin, **v**inblastine, **d**acarbazine) has become the standard because it offers equal or improved efficacy and less toxicity compared with MOPP.
- None of the alternating (e.g., MOPP and ABVD), hybrid (MOPP and ABV), or sequential regimens provide clear advantages over fully dosed four-drug regimens.
- New regimens are being evaluated for advanced-stage Hodgkin's lymphoma, such as Stanford V and BEACOPP (see Table 62-2).

Salvage Chemotherapy

- Response to salvage therapy depends on the extent and site of recurrence, previous therapy, and duration of first remission. Choice of salvage therapy should be guided by response to initial therapy and patient's ability to tolerate therapy.
- Patients who relapse after an initial complete response can be treated with the same regimen, a non–cross-resistant regimen, radiation therapy, or high-dose chemotherapy and autologous hematopoietic stem cell transplantation (HSCT).
- Lack of complete remission after initial therapy or relapse within a year after completing initial therapy is associated with poor prognosis. Patients with these prognostic factors are candidates for high-dose chemotherapy and HSCT.

XI

Complications of Chemotherapy

- Myelosuppression is the major dose-limiting toxicity of most combination regimens. Hematopoietic growth factors can decrease neutropenia and allow delivery of optimal doses on schedule.
- Nausea and vomiting are frequently seen with dacarbazine, doxorubicin, and mechlorethamine. The severity has diminished with the use of the 5-HT3 antagonists.
- Neurotoxicity is frequently seen with vincristine.
- Other acute toxic effects include alopecia, dermatitis, mucositis, phlebitis, malaise and fatigue, pulmonary reactions, and renal dysfunction.
- Long-term complications include gonadal dysfunction, secondary malignancies, and cardiac disease. The risk of developing acute leukemia is highest after chemotherapy, with or without radiation therapy. The risk is higher with MOPP than with ABVD.

▶ NON-HODGKIN'S LYMPHOMA

PATHOPHYSIOLOGY

- Chromosomal translocations have become a hallmark of many lymphomas.
- Non-Hodgkin's lymphomas are derived from monoclonal proliferation of B or, less commonly, T lymphocytes and their precursors.
- There are many histologic subtypes of non-Hodgkin's lymphoma, and new entities are still being recognized.

TABLE 62–2. Combination Chemotherapy for Hodgkin's Lymphoma

Drug	Dosage (mg/m^2)	Rate	Days
MOPP (repeat every 21 days)			
Mechlorethamine	6	IV	1, 8
Vincristine	1.4	IV	1, 8
Procarbazine	100	Oral	1–14
Prednisone	40	Oral	1–14
ABVD (repeat every 28 days)			
Adriamycin (doxorubicin)	25	IV	1, 15
Bleomycin	10	IV	1, 15
Vinblastine	6	IV	1, 15
Dacarbazine	375	IV	1, 15
Stanford V (one course over 12 weeks)			
Doxorubicin	25	IV	Weeks 1, 3, 5, 7, 9, 11
Vinblastine	6	IV	Weeks 1, 3, 5, 7, 9, 11
Mechlorethamine	6	IV	Weeks 1, 5, 9
Etoposide	60	IV	Weeks 3, 7, 11
Vincristine	1.4[a]	IV	Weeks 2, 4, 6, 8, 10, 12
Bleomycin	5	IV	Weeks 2, 4, 6, 8
Prednisone	40	Oral	Every other day for 12 wk; begin tapering at week 10
BEACOPP (repeat every 21 days)			
Bleomycin	10	IV	8
Etoposide	100	IV	1–3
Adriamycin (doxorubicin)	25	IV	1
Cyclophosphamide	650	IV	1
Oncovin (vincristine)	1.4[a]	IV	8
Procarbazine	100	Oral	1–7
Prednisone	40	Oral	1–14
BEACOPP escalated (repeat every 21 days)			
Bleomycin	10	IV	8
Etoposide	200	IV	1–3
Adriamycin (doxorubicin)	35	IV	1
Cyclophosphamide	1250	IV	1
Oncovin (vincristine)	1.4[a]	IV	8
Procarbazine	100	Oral	1–7
Prednisone	40	Oral	1–14
Granulocyte colony-stimulating factor		SC	8+

[a]Vincristine dose capped at 2 mg.

CLINICAL PRESENTATION

- Patients present with a variety of symptoms, which depend on the site of involvement and whether it is nodal or extranodal.
- Adenopathy can be localized or generalized. Involved nodes are painless, rubbery, and discrete and are usually located in the cervical and supraclavicular regions. Mesenteric or gastrointestinal involvement can cause nausea, vomiting, obstruction, abdominal pain, palpable abdominal mass, or gastrointestinal bleeding. Bone marrow involvement can cause symptoms related to anemia, neutropenia, or thrombocytopenia.

- Lymphomas can be classified by degree of aggressiveness. Slow-growing or indolent lymphomas are favorable (untreated survival measured in years), whereas rapid-growing or aggressive lymphomas are unfavorable (untreated survival measured in months).
- Indolent lymphomas usually arise in middle-aged or older adults (median age 55 years). Most patients present with advanced disease, often the result of bone marrow involvement. These lymphomas have an indolent course with adenopathy waxing and waning for months to years before diagnosis.
- Aggressive lymphomas occur over a broader age range. Patients present at various stages of disease. Lymphoma tends to disseminate rapidly and often involves extranodal and privileged sites.
- Only 20% of patients with non-Hodgkin's lymphoma have constitutional, or B, symptoms.

DIAGNOSIS AND STAGING

- Diagnosis is established by biopsy of an involved lymph node.
- Diagnostic workup of non-Hodgkin's lymphoma is generally similar to that of Hodgkin's disease.
- There are many systems for classifying non-Hodgkin's lymphomas, which continue to evolve.
- Prognosis depends on histologic subtype and clinical risk factors (e.g., age more than 60 years, performance status of 2 or more, elevated lactic dehydrogenase, extranodal involvement, and stage III or IV disease). These risk factors are used to calculate the International Prognostic Index (IPI). A newer prognostic index uses similar risk factors except that low performance status is replaced with low hemoglobin (less than 12 g/dL).

XI

DESIRED OUTCOME

The primary treatment goals for non-Hodgkin's lymphoma are to relieve symptoms and, whenever possible, cure the patient of disease without causing unacceptable toxicity.

TREATMENT

General Principles

- Appropriate therapy for non-Hodgkin's lymphoma depends on many factors including patient age; disease type, stage, and site; and patient preference.
- Treatment options include radiation therapy, chemotherapy, and biologic agents.
- Radiation therapy is rarely suitable for remission induction because non-Hodgkin's lymphoma is rarely localized at diagnosis. Radiation therapy is used more commonly in advanced disease, mainly as a palliative measure.
- Effective chemotherapy ranges from single-agent therapy for indolent lymphomas to aggressive, complex combination regimens for aggressive lymphomas. Paradoxically, indolent or favorable lymphomas are rarely curable, whereas aggressive or unfavorable lymphomas are potentially curable.
- Treatment strategies are summarized for the most common non-Hodgkin's lymphomas as examples of how to treat indolent (i.e., follicular) and aggressive (i.e., diffuse large B-cell) lymphomas. Strategies are also summarized for AIDS-related lymphoma.

Follicular Lymphoma, an Indolent Lymphoma
Localized Follicular Lymphoma

- Options for stage I and II follicular lymphoma include locoregional radiation therapy, chemotherapy followed by radiation therapy, and extended-field radiation therapy.
- Radiation therapy is the standard treatment and is usually curative. Chemotherapy is not recommended, unless the patient has high-risk stage II disease.

Advanced Follicular Lymphoma

- Management of stages III and IV indolent lymphoma is controversial because standard approaches are not curative. Complete response can be induced in 50% to 80% of patients, but the median duration of remission is only 18 to 36 months. After relapse, response can be re-induced; however, response rates and durations decrease with each retreatment.
- Therapeutic options are diverse and include watchful waiting, single-agent therapy, combination chemotherapy, biologic therapy, and combined-modality therapy. Immediate aggressive therapy does not improve survival compared with conservative therapy (i.e., watchful waiting followed, only when needed, by single-agent chemotherapy).
- Oral alkylating agents, **chlorambucil**, 0.1 to 0.2 mg/kg, or **cyclophosphamide**, 1.5 to 2.5 mg/kg (adjusted to white blood cell and platelet counts), are the mainstay of treatment. These single agents are as effective as combination regimens and produce minimal toxicity, but secondary acute myelogenous leukemia (AML) is a concern. **Fludarabine** and **cladribine** produce high response rates without secondary AML, but they are more myelosuppressive.
- **Rituximab,** a chimeric monoclonal antibody directed at the CD20 molecule on B cells, has become one of the most widely used therapies for follicular lymphoma. Rituximab was initially used as salvage therapy and is also being used as first-line therapy, either alone or combined with CHOP (cyclophosphamide, doxorubicin [*h*ydroxydaunomycin], vincristine (*O*ncovin), *p*rednisone). Rituximab has the advantage of being suitable for retreatment therapy and, interestingly, produces a longer duration of remission after the second course than after the first course.
- The rituximab dosage is 375 mg/m^2 weekly for 4 weeks. Other dosages are being studied. For example, maintenance therapy every 6 months appears to improve the initial response rate and to prolong the duration of response.
- Adverse effects are usually infusion related, especially after the first infusion of rituximab. Adverse effects include fever, chills, respiratory symptoms, fatigue, headache, pruritus, and angioedema. Patients should receive **acetaminophen**, 650 mg, and **diphenhydramine**, 50 mg, 30 minutes before the infusion.
- Anti-CD20 radioimmunoconjugates are mouse antibodies linked to radioisotopes (e.g., ^{131}I-tositumomab and ^{90}Y-ibritumomab tiuxetan). They have the advantage of delivering radiation to tumor cells expressing the CD20 antigen and to adjacent tumor cells that do not express it. They have the disadvantage of damaging adjacent normal tissue (e.g., bone marrow).
- Radioimmunotherapy was initially used as salvage therapy and is being evaluated as first-line therapy in combination with CHOP.
- Radioimmunotherapy is generally well tolerated. Toxicities include infusion-related reactions, myelosuppression, and possibly myelodysplactic syndrome or AML. ^{131}I-tositumomab can cause thyroid dysfunction.
- The decision to use radioimmunotherapy requires consideration of the complexity, risks, and cost. The ideal candidate has limited bone marrow involvement and adequate blood cell counts.

XI

TABLE 62–3. Combination Chemotherapy for Non-Hodgkin's Lymphoma (CHOP)[a]

Drug	Dose (mg/m^2)	Route	Days
Cyclophosphamide	750	IV	1
Doxorubicin	50	IV	1
Vincristine	1.4	IV	1
Prednisone	100	PO	1–5

[a]Cycle should be repeated every 21 days.

- High-dose chemotherapy followed by HSCT is an option for relapsed follicular lymphoma. The recurrence rate is lower after allogeneic than after autologous HSCT, but the benefit is offset by increased treatment-related mortality. The ideal candidate is young and does not have serious comorbidities.

Diffuse Large B-Cell Lymphoma, an Aggressive Lymphoma
Early-Stage Diffuse Large B-Cell Lymphoma
- Stage I and nonbulky stage II should be treated with 3 cycles of CHOP (Table 62–3) followed by locoregional radiation therapy.
- If a poor prognostic factor is present, the patient should receive additional cycles of CHOP (e.g., total of six to eight cycles).

Advanced Diffuse Large B-Cell Lymphoma Disease
- Bulky stage II and stages III and IV lymphoma should be treated with intensive combination chemotherapy and continued for 2 cycles after inducing complete response. Maintenance therapy does not improve survival.
- Rapid response (i.e., complete response in first three treatment cycles) produces a more durable remission than responses requiring more prolonged treatment.
- CHOP remains the treatment of choice, but it is not ideal. Only half of patients have complete remissions, and only one-third are cured. Many institutions recommend adding rituximab to CHOP (R-CHOP) for treatment of all aggressive lymphomas.
- Elderly adults have lower complete response and survival rates than do younger patients, possibly because elderly adults do not tolerate intensive chemotherapy and therefore receive less aggressive chemotherapy.
- R-CHOP is becoming the standard for elderly adults with aggressive non-Hodgkin's lymphomas. Full-dose CHOP should be used whenever possible.
- Attempts to improve on CHOP include adding single agents, such as bleomycin (CHOP-Bleo, BACOP) or **methotrexate** (M-BACOD), and administering as many agents as possible. These strategies do not significantly affect treatment outcome and are more difficult to administer, more toxic, and more expensive.
- Patients with high-intermediate- or high-risk IPI scores are candidates for more aggressive regimens such as high-dose chemotherapy with autologous HSCT. A study is being conducted to determine whether high-dose chemotherapy with autologous HSCT should be administered early (as consolidation after first complete remission) or late (after relapse).

Salvage Therapy for Aggressive Lymphoma
- Salvage therapy is more likely to induce response if the response to initial chemotherapy was complete (chemosensitivity) than if it was less than complete (chemoresistance).

Oncologic Disorders

- High-dose chemotherapy with autologous HSCT is the therapy of choice for younger patients with chemosensitive relapse.
- Salvage regimens incorporate drugs not used as initial therapy. Commonly used regimens include DHAP (**dexamethasone**, *h*igh-dose **cytarabine** [*A*ra-C]**,** and **cisplatin** [*P*latinol]), ESHAP (**etoposide**, **methylprednisolone** [*S*olumedrol]**,** *h*igh-dose cytarabine [*A*ra-C], and cisplatin [*P*latinol]), and MINE (**mesna, ifosfamide, mitoxantrone** [*N*ovantrone], and **etoposide**). None is clearly superior to the others.
- ICE (*i*fosfamide, **carboplatin,** and *e*toposide) appears to be better tolerated than cisplatin-containing regimens, especially in elderly adults.
- Rituximab is being evaluated in combination with many salvage regimens.

Non-Hodgkin's Lymphoma in AIDS

- Patients with AIDS have a 150- to 250-fold increased risk of developing non-Hodgkin's lymphoma, which is usually aggressive.
- Treatment of AIDS-related lymphoma is difficult because underlying immunodeficiency increases the risk of treatment-related myelosuppression.
- Standard combination regimens (e.g., CHOP) yield disappointing results. The new approach, dose-adjusted EPOCH (*e*toposide, *p*rednisone, vincristine [*O*ncovin], *c*yclophosphamide, and doxorubicin [*h*ydroxydaunomycin]), is promising.
- Antiretroviral therapy and prophylactic antibiotics should be continued during chemotherapy.

▶ EVALUATION OF THERAPEUTIC OUTCOMES

- The primary outcome to be identified is tumor response, which is based on physical examination, radiologic evidence, and other baseline findings. Complete response is desirable because it yields the only chance for cure.
- Patients are evaluated for response at the end of 4 cycles or, if treatment is shorter, at the end of treatment.
- Optimal outcomes for most types of lymphoma require delivery of full doses on time. Hematopoietic growth factors and other supportive care measures are often needed to achieve this goal.
- To optimize chemotherapy administration, the clinician must identify, monitor, treat, and prevent or minimize treatment-related toxicity. Pertinent laboratory data and other procedures should be reviewed to establish a baseline for monitoring purposes. Major organ and system toxicities to be monitored include hematologic, neurologic, skin, pulmonary, gastrointestinal, renal, and cardiac.
- Myelosuppression and neutropenic fever with infection are constant concerns with aggressive chemotherapy. Appropriate patient education and monitoring are critical.

See Chapter 129, Lymphomas, authored by Val R. Adams and Gary C. Yee, for a more detailed discussion of this topic.

XI

Chapter 63

▶ PROSTATE CANCER

▶ DEFINITION

Prostate cancer is a malignant neoplasm that arises from the prostate gland.

▶ PATHOPHYSIOLOGY

- Genetic mutations involving, for example, E-cahedrin, p53, and the androgen receptor appear to contribute to the development of prostate cancer.
- The normal prostate is composed of acinar secretory cells that are altered when invaded by cancer. The major pathologic cell type is adenocarcinoma (more than 95% of cases).
- Prostate cancer can be graded. Well differentiated tumors grow slowly, whereas poorly differentiated tumors grow rapidly and have a poor prognosis.
- Metastatic spread can occur by local extension, lymphatic drainage, or hematogenous dissemination. Skeletal metastases from hematogenous spread are the most common sites of distant spread. The lung, liver, brain, and adrenal glands are the most common sites of visceral involvement, but these organs are not usually involved initially.

▶ CLINICAL PRESENTATION

- Localized prostate cancer is usually asymptomatic.
- Locally invasive prostate cancer is associated with ureteral dysfunction or impingement, such as alterations in micturition (e.g., urinary frequency, hesitancy, dribbling).
- Patients with advanced disease commonly present with back pain and stiffness due to osseous metastases. Untreated spinal cord lesions can lead to cord compression. Lower extremity edema can occur as a result of lymphatic obstruction. Anemia and weight loss are nonspecific signs of advanced disease.

▶ SCREENING AND DIAGNOSIS

- Digital rectal exam (DRE) is commonly employed for screening of prostate cancer. It has the advantages of specificity, low cost, safety, and ease of performance. DRE has the disadvantages of not being very sensitive and of interobserver variability.
- Prostate-specific antigen (PSA), a glycoprotein produced only in the cytoplasm of benign and malignant prostate cells, is more sensitive than DRE and is simple to perform. PSA has the disadvantage of low specificity.
- Screening for prostate cancer is controversial. The American Cancer Society recommends annual PSA and DRE for men who are 50 years or older.
- On DRE, prostate cancer is characterized by a rock-hard nodule or mass, whereas in benign prostatic hypertrophy (BPH) the gland is smooth and rubbery.
- The diagnosis must be confirmed by biopsy (e.g., transperianal or transrectal needle biopsy). Biopsy also yields a Gleason score of 1 through 10. Lower Gleason scores are assigned to well differentiated, slowly growing cells, and higher scores are assigned to poorly differentiated, rapidly dividing cells.
- Initial laboratory tests should include a complete blood chemistry, liver function tests, and serum phosphatases.

- Bone scan, excretory urogram, and chest x-ray are performed for staging purposes. Depending on the results, skeletal films, lymph node evaluation (e.g., pelvic computed tomography [CT], indium-111-labeled capromab pendetide scan, bipedal lymphangiogram), and transrectal magnetic resonance imaging (MRI) may also be needed.

▶ DESIRED OUTCOME

The goal of treatment for early-stage prostate cancer is to minimize morbidity and mortality. Advanced prostate cancer (stage D) is not curable, and the goal is to provide symptom relief and maintain quality of life.

▶ TREATMENT

GENERAL APPROACH TO TREATMENT

- The initial treatment for prostate cancer depends on the disease stage, Gleason score, presence of symptoms, and patient's life expectancy.
- The most appropriate therapy for early-stage prostate cancer is unknown.
- Radical prostatectomy and radiation therapy are generally considered equivalent for localized prostate cancer, and neither has been shown to be superior to observation alone.
- Men with no symptoms, Gleason score of 2 to 6, or PSA of less than 10 ng/mL are at low risk for recurrence and have a high 10-year survival rate. If life expectancy is less than 10 years, options are observation or radiation therapy. If life expectancy is more than 20 years, options are more aggressive (e.g., prostatectomy or radiation therapy).
- Men with T_{2b-c} disease, Gleason score of 7, or PSA of 10 to 20 ng/mL are at intermediate risk for recurrence. If life expectancy is less than 10 years, options are observation, radiation therapy, or radical prostatectomy. If life expectancy is more than 10 years, options are prostatectomy or radiation therapy.
- Men with T_{3a-b} disease, Gleason score of 8 to 10, or PSA of more than 20 ng/mL are at high risk for recurrence. If life expectancy is less than or equal to 5 years, options are observation or hormonal therapy. If life expectancy is more than 5 years, radiation therapy should be combined with hormonal therapy.
- Men with T_{3c} or T_4 disease are at very high risk for recurrence. Options are androgen ablation with or without radiation therapy. Hormonal therapy should be initiated at diagnosis instead of waiting for the onset of symptoms.
- The major initial treatment modality for advanced prostate cancer (stage D_2) is androgen ablation (e.g., orchiectomy or luteinizing hormone-releasing hormone [LH-RH] agonists with or without antiandrogens). After disease progression, secondary hormonal manipulations, cytotoxic chemotherapy, and supportive care are used.

RATIONALE FOR HORMONAL THERAPY

- The rationale for hormonal therapy is based on the effect of androgens on the growth and differentiation of the normal prostate (Figure 63–1).
- The testes and the adrenal glands are the major sources of androgens, specifically dihydrotestosterone (DHT).
- LH-RH from the hypothalamus stimulates the release of luteinizing hormone (LH) and follicle-stimulating hormone (FSH) from the anterior pituitary gland.

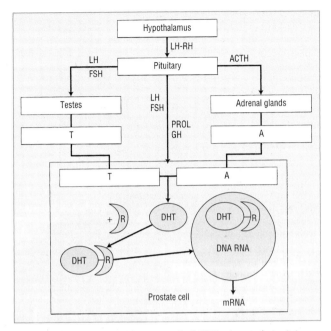

Figure 63–1. Hormonal regulation of the prostate gland. ACTH, adrenocorticotropic hormone; A, androgens; DHT, dihydrotestosterone; FSH, follicle-stimulating hormone; GH, growth hormone; LH, luteinizing hormone; LH-RH, luteinizing hormone-releasing hormone; PROL, prolactin; R, receptor; T, testosterone.

XI ◄

- LH complexes with receptors on the Leydig cell testicular membrane and stimulates the production of testosterone and small amounts of estrogen.
- FSH acts on testicular Sertoli cells to promote maturation of LH receptors and produce an androgen-binding protein.
- Circulating testosterone and estradiol influence the synthesis of LH-RH, LH, and FSH by a negative-feedback loop at the hypothalamic and pituitary level.
- Only 2% of total plasma testosterone is present in the active unbound state that penetrates the prostate cell, where it is converted to DHT by 5 α-reductase. DHT subsequently binds with a cytoplasmic receptor and is transported to the cell nucleus where transcription and translation of stored genetic material occur.

SURGERY AND RADIATION THERAPY

- Prostatectomy and radiation therapy are associated with complications that must be weighed against expected benefit. Consequently, many patients postpone therapy until the onset of symptoms.
- Complications of radical prostatectomy include blood loss, stricture formation, incontinence, lymphocele, fistula formation, anesthetic risk, and impotence. Nerve-sparing techniques facilitate return of potency after prostatectomy.
- Acute complications of radiation therapy include cystitis, proctitis, hematuria, urinary retention, penoscrotal edema, and impotence.
- Chronic complications of radiation therapy include proctitis, diarrhea, cystitis, enteritis, impotence, urethral stricture, and incontinence.

TABLE 63–1. Comparative Costs of Hormonal Therapy for Advanced Prostate Cancer

Drug	Dose	Average Wholesale Price/Month of Therapy
Leuprolide depot	7.5 mg/mo	$566.85
Leuprolide depot	22.5 mg/12 wk	$1700.63
Leuprolide depot	30 mg/16 wk	$2267.50
Goserelin implant	3.6 mg q 28 days	$439.24
Goserelin implant	10.8 mg/12 wk	$1317.74
Flutamide	750 mg/day	$315.70
Bicalutamide	50 mg/day	$319.74
Nilulamide	300 mg/day for 1st mo, then 150 mg/day	$467.16, then $233.58

- Bilateral orchiectomy rapidly reduces circulating androgen levels. Many patients are not surgical candidates owing to advanced age or perceived unacceptableness. Nonetheless, orchiectomy is the preferred initial treatment for patients with impending spinal cord compression or ureteral obstruction.

LH-RH AGONISTS

- LH-RH agonists provide response rates of approximately 80%, which is similar to that of orchiectomy, and have the advantage of being reversible.
- There are no comparative trials of LH-RH agonists, so the choice is usually based on cost (Table 63–1) and on patient and physician preference. **Leuprolide acetate** is administered daily. **Leuprolide depot** and **goserelin acetate implant** can be administered monthly, or every 12 or 16 weeks.
- The most common adverse effects of LH-RH agonists are disease flare-up during the first week of therapy (e.g., increased bone pain, urinary symptoms), hot flashes, erectile impotence, decreased libido, and injection-site reactions.

ANTIANDROGENS

- Monotherapy with **flutamide** (50% to 87%), **bicalutamide** (54% to 70%), and **nilutamide** (40%) produces objective response rates lower than those of LH-RH agonists. Antiandrogens are indicated for advanced prostate cancer only when combined with an LH-RH agonist (flutamide and bicalutamide) or orchiectomy (nilutamide). In combination, antiandrogens can reduce the LH-RH agonist-induced flare.
- The daily doses are flutamide, 750 mg; bicalutamide, 50 mg; and nilutamide, 300 mg for 1 month, followed by 150 mg.
- The adverse effects of antiandrogens are gynecomastia, hot flashes, gastrointestinal (GI) disturbances, liver function test abnormalities, and breast tenderness. GI disturbances consist of diarrhea for flutamide and bicalutamide and nausea or constipation for nilutamide. Flutamide is also associated with methemoglobinemia, whereas nilutamide causes visual disturbances (impaired dark adaptation), alcohol intolerance, and interstitial pneumonitis.

COMBINED HORMONAL BLOCKADE

- The role of combined hormonal therapy, also referred to as maximal androgen deprivation or total androgen blockade, continues to be evaluated.
- Randomized trial results are mixed when candidates for second-line therapy are treated with combinations of antiandrogens plus either LH-RH agonists or orchiectomy. The most recent meta-analysis showed only a slight survival benefit

at 5 years for maximal androgen blockade with flutamide or nilutamide (27.6%) compared with conventional medical or surgical castration alone (24.7%; $p = .0005$).

- Some investigators consider combination androgen ablation to be the initial hormonal therapy of choice for newly diagnosed patients because the major benefit is seen in patients with minimal disease. Some argue that treatment should not be delayed because combined androgen deprivation trials demonstrate a survival advantage for young patients with good performance status and minimal disease who were initially treated with hormonal therapy.
- Studies are needed to answer questions regarding the selection of modalities used as combined hormonal therapy, with careful consideration of effects on survival, time to progression, quality of life, patient preference, and economics.

ESTROGENS

Historically, estrogens were an important method of androgen ablation. The major agent, **diethylstilbestrol** (DES), was removed from the market in 1997. Alternatives (e.g., **ethinyl estradiol**, **conjugated estrogens**, **chlorotrianisene**, and **polyestradiol phosphate**) have not been as extensively studied and cost more than DES.

SALVAGE THERAPY

- The selection of salvage therapy depends on what was used as initial therapy. Radiotherapy can be used after radical prostatectomy. Androgen ablation can be used after radiation therapy or radical prostatectomy.
- If testosterone levels are not suppressed (i.e., greater than 20 ng/dL) after initial LH-RH agonist therapy, an antiandrogen or orchiectomy may be indicated. If testosterone levels are suppressed, the disease is considered to be androgen independent and should be treated with palliative therapy.
- If initial therapy consisted of an LH-RH agonist and antiandrogen, then androgen withdrawal should be attempted. Mutations of the androgen receptor may allow antiandrogens to become agonists. Withdrawal produces responses lasting 3 to 14 months in up to 35% of patients.
- Androgen synthesis inhibitors provide symptomatic, but brief, relief in approximately 50% of patients. **Aminoglutethimide** causes adverse effects in 50% of patients, such as lethargy, ataxia, dizziness, and self-limiting rash. The adverse effects of **ketoconazole** are GI intolerance, transient increases in liver and renal function tests, and hypoadrenalism.
- Bisphosphonates prevent hormone-induced bone loss when used early during androgen deprivation therapy and, in some studies, prevent skeletal morbidity when used for hormone-refractory prostate cancer. Usual dosages are **pamidronate**, 90 mg every month, and **zoledronic acid**, 4 mg every 3 to 4 weeks.
- After hormonal options are exhausted, palliation can be achieved with **strontium-89** or **samarium-153 lexidronam** for bone-related pain, analgesics, glucocorticoids, local radiotherapy, or chemotherapy.

CHEMOTHERAPY

- **Docetaxel**, 75 mg/m^2 every 3 weeks, combined with **prednisone**, 5 mg twice daily, is becoming the standard for hormone-refractory metastatic prostate cancer because it is the first chemotherapy regimen to show a survival benefit. In the randomized study, the most common adverse events were nausea, alopecia, and myelosuppression. Docetaxel can also cause fluid retention and peripheral neuropathy.

XI

- Single agents with modest activity include **cyclophosphamide, estramustine, fluorouracil, methotrexate, dacarbazine, mitoxantrone, doxorubicin, paclitaxel, gemcitabine, vinorelbine,** and **cisplatin**.
- Active combinations include estramustine and **vinblastine** or mitoxantrone, and mitoxantrone and prednisone. Other possible combinations are ketoconazole and doxorubicin, and estramustine and **etoposide** or paclitaxel.

▶ EVALUATION OF THERAPEUTIC OUTCOMES

- Monitoring depends on the stage of prostate cancer.
- For definitive, curative therapy, objective parameters include primary tumor size, involved lymph nodes, and tumor markers such as PSA.
- For treatment of metastatic disease, clinical benefit can be documented by evaluating performance status, weight, quality of life, analgesic requirements, and PSA or DRE.
- Patients should be monitored for treatment-related adverse events, especially events that are amenable to intervention.

See Chapter 128, Prostate Cancer, authored by Jill M. Kolesar, for a more detailed discussion of this topic.

▶XI

Chapter 64

▶ GLAUCOMA

▶ DEFINITION

Glaucomas are ocular disorders characterized by changes in the optic nerve head (optic disk) and by loss of visual sensitivity and field.

▶ PATHOPHYSIOLOGY

- There are two major types of glaucoma: open-angle glaucoma, which accounts for most cases and is therefore the focus of this chapter, and closed-angle glaucoma.
- In open-angle glaucoma, the specific cause of optic neuropathy is unknown. Increased intraocular pressure (IOP) was historically considered to be the sole cause. Additional contributing factors include increased susceptibility of the optic nerve to ischemia, reduced or dysregulated blood flow, excitotoxicity, autoimmune reactions, and other abnormal physiologic processes.
- Although IOP is a poor predictor of which patients will have visual field loss, the risk of visual field loss increases with increasing IOP.
- IOP is determined by the balance between the inflow and outflow of aqueous humor. Inflow is increased by β-adrenergic agents and decreased by α_2-, α-, and β-adrenergic blockers; dopamine blockers; carbonic anhydrase inhibitors; and adenylate cyclase stimulators. Outflow is increased by cholinergic agents, which contract the ciliary muscle and open the trabecular meshwork, and by prostaglandin analogs and α_2-adrenergic agonists, which affect uveoscleral outflow.
- Secondary open-angle glaucoma has many causes including systemic diseases, trauma, surgery, rubeosis, lens changes, ocular inflammatory diseases, and drugs. Secondary glaucoma can be classified as pretrabecular (normal meshwork is covered and prevents outflow of aqueous humor), trabecular (meshwork is altered or material accumulates the intertravecular spaces), or posttrabecular (episcleral venous blood pressure is increased).
- Many drugs can increase IOP (Table 64–1). The potential to induce or worsen glaucoma depends on the type of glaucoma and on whether it is adequately controlled.
- Closed-angle glaucoma occurs when the iris mechanically blocks the trabecular meshwork, resulting in increased IOP.

▶ CLINICAL PRESENTATION

- Open-angle glaucoma is slowly progressive and is usually asymptomatic until the onset of substantial visual field loss. Visual field defects include general peripheral visual field constriction, isolated scotomas or blind spots, nasal visual field depression or nasal step, enlargement of the blind spot, large arc-like scotomas, reduced contrast sensitivity, reduced peripheral acuity, and altered color vision.
- In closed-angle glaucoma, patients typically experience intermittent prodromal symptoms (e.g., blurred or hazy vision with halos around lights and,

TABLE 64–1. Drugs That May Induce or Potentiate Increased Intraocular Pressure

Open-angle glaucoma
Ophthalmic corticosteroids (high risk)
Systemic corticosteroids
Nasal/inhaled corticosteroids
Fenoldopam
Ophthalmic anticholinergics
Succinylcholine
Vasodilators (low risk)
Cimetidine (low risk)

Closed-angle glaucoma
Topical anticholinergics
Topical sympathomimetics
Systemic anticholinergics
Heterocyclic antidepressants
Low-potency phenothiazines
Antihistamines
Ipratropium
Benzodiazepines (low risk)
Theophylline (low risk)
Vasodilators (low risk)
Systemic sympathomimetics (low risk)
Central nervous system stimulants (low risk)
Serotonin selective reuptake inhibitors
Imipramine
Venlafaxine
Topiramate
Tetracyclines (low risk)
Carbonic anhydrase inhibitors (low risk)
Monoamine oxidase inhibitors (low risk)
Topical cholinergics (low risk)

occasionally, headache). Acute episodes produce symptoms associated with a cloudy, edematous cornea; ocular pain; nausea, vomiting, and abdominal pain; and diaphoresis.

▶ DIAGNOSIS

- The diagnosis of *open-angle glaucoma* is confirmed by the presence of characteristic optic disk changes and visual field loss, with or without increased IOP. *Normal tension glaucoma* refers to disk changes, visual field loss, and IOP of less than 21 mm Hg. *Ocular hypertension* refers to IOP of more than 21 mm Hg without disk changes or visual field loss.
- Optic disk findings associated with open-angle glaucoma include cup-disk ratio of more than 0.5, progressive increase in cup size, cup-disk ratio asymmetry more than 0.2, vertical elongation of the cup, excavation of the cup, increased exposure of lamina cribrosa, pallor of the cup, splinter hemorrhages, cupping to the edge of the disk, notching of the cup, and nerve fiber defects.
- For *closed-angle glaucoma*, the presence of a narrow angle is usually visualized by gonioscopy. IOP is generally markedly elevated (e.g., 40 to 90 mm Hg) when symptoms are present. Additional signs include hyperemic conjunctiva, cloudy cornea, shallow anterior chamber, and occasionally edematous and hyperemic optic disk.

▶ DESIRED OUTCOME

The goal of drug therapy in patients with glaucoma is to preserve visual function by reducing the IOP to a level at which no further optic nerve damage occurs.

▶ TREATMENT OF OCULAR HYPERTENSION AND OPEN-ANGLE

GLAUCOMA

- Treatment is indicated for ocular hypertension if the patient has a significant risk factor such as IOP greater than 25 mm Hg, vertical cup-disk ratio greater than 0.5, or central corneal thickness less than 555 μm. Additional risk factors to be considered include family history of glaucoma, black race, severe myopia, and presence of only one eye.
- Treatment is indicated for all patients with elevated IOP and characteristic optic disk changes or visual field defects.
- Drug therapy is the most common initial treatment and is initiated in a stepwise manner, starting with a single well tolerated topical agent (Table 64–2). Historically, β blockers were the treatment of choice and continue to be used if there are no contraindications to potential β blockade caused by systemic absorption. β blockers have the advantage of low cost owing to generic formulations.
- Newer agents are also suitable for first-line therapy. Prostaglandin analogues have the advantage of strong potency, unique mechanism suitable for combination therapy, good safety profile, and once-a-day dosing. **Brimonidine** has the theoretical advantage of neuroprotection, which has not yet been demonstrated in humans. Topical carbonic anhydrase inhibitors (CAIs) are also suitable for first-line therapy.
- **Pilocarpine** and **epinephrine** (or **dipivefrin**) are used as third-line therapies because of adverse events or reduced efficacy.
- **Carbachol**, topical cholinesterase inhibitors, and oral CAIs (Table 64–3) are used as last-resort options after failure of less toxic options.
- The optimal timing of argon laser or surgical trabeculectomy is controversial, ranging from initial therapy to after failure of third- or fourth-line drug therapy. Antiproliferative agents such as **fluorouracil** and **mitomycin C** are used to modify the healing process and maintain patency.

XII

▶ TREATMENT OF CLOSED-ANGLE GLAUCOMA

- Acute closed-angle glaucoma with high IOP requires rapid reduction of IOP. Iridectomy is the definitive treatment, which produces a hole in the iris that permits aqueous flow to move directly from the posterior to the anterior chamber.
- Drug therapy of an acute attack typically consists of an osmotic agent and secretory inhibitor (e.g., β blocker, α_2 agonist, **latanoprost**, or CAI), with or without pilocarpine.
- Osmotic agents are used because they rapidly decrease IOP. Examples include **glycerin**, 1 to 2 g/kg orally, and **mannitol**, 1 to 2 g/kg intravenously.
- Although traditionally the drug of choice, pilocarpine use is controversial as initial therapy. Once IOP is controlled, pilocarpine should be given every 6 hours until iridectomy is performed.
- Topical corticosteroids can be used to reduce ocular inflammation and synechiae.
- Epinephrine should be used with caution because it can precipitate acute closed-angle glaucoma, especially when used with a β blocker.

XII

TABLE 64-2. Topical Drugs Used in the Treatment of Glaucoma

Drug	Common Brand Names	Dose Form	Strength(%)	Usual Dose[a]	Mechanism of Action
β-Adrenergic blocking agents					
Betaxolol	Generic	Solution	0.5	1 drop b.i.d.	Reduce aqueous production by the ciliary body
	Betoptic-S	Suspension	0.25	1 drop b.i.d.	
Carteolol	Generic	Solution	1	1 drop b.i.d.	
Levobunolol	Betagan	Solution	0.25, 0.5	1 drop b.i.d.	
Metipranolol	OptiPranolol	Solution	0.3	1 drop b.i.d.	
Timolol	Timoptic, Betimol	Solution	0.25, 0.5	1 drop q.d. or b.i.d.	
	Timoptic-XE	Gelling solution	0.25, 0.5	1 drop q.d.	
Nonspecific adrenergic agonists					
Dipivefrin	Propine	Solution	0.1	1 drop b.i.d.	Increase aqueous humor outflow
α₂-Adrenergic agonists					
Apraclonidine	Iopidine	Solution	0.5, 1	1 drop b.i.d. or t.i.d.	Reduce aqueous humor production; brimonidine also increases uveoscleral outflow
Brimonidine	Alphagan P	Solution	0.15	1 drop b.i.d. or t.i.d.	
Cholinergic agonists					
Direct-acting					
Carbachol	Carboptic, Isopto Carbachol	Solution	0.75, 1.5, 2.25, 3	1 drop b.i.d. or t.i.d.	Increase aqueous humor outflow through trabecular meshwork
Pilocarpine	Isopto Carpine, Pilocar	Solution	0.25, 0.5, 1, 2, 4, 6, 8, 10	1 drop b.i.d. or t.i.d.	
	Pilopine HS	Gel	4	Every q.h.s.	

Cholinesterase inhibitors					
Echothiophate	Phospholine iodide	Solution	0.125	q.d. or b.i.d.	
Carbonic anhydrase inhibitors					
Brinzolamide	Azopt	Suspension	1	b.i.d. or t.i.d.	Reduce aqueous humor production by the ciliary body
Dorzolamide	Trusopt	Solution	2	b.i.d. or t.i.d.	
Prostaglandin analogues					
Latanoprost	Xalatan	Solution	0.005	1 drop q.h.s.	Increase aqueous uveoscleral outflow and, to a lesser extent, trabecular outflow
Bimatoprost	Lumigan	Solution	0.03	1 drop q.h.s.	
Travoprost	Travatan	Solution	0.004	1 drop q.h.s.	
Combinations					
Timolol-dorzolamide	Cosopt	Solution	Timolol 0.5% Dorzolamide 2%	1 drop b.i.d.	

[a]Use of nasolacrimal occlusion will increase number of patients successfully treated with longer dosage intervals.

XII

TABLE 64–3. Systemic Carbonic Anhydrase Inhibitors Used in the Treatment of Glaucoma

Drug	Common Brand Names	Dose Form	Strength (%)	Usual Dose
Acetazolamide	Generic	Tablet	125 mg, 250 mg	125–250 mg 2–4 times a day
		Injection	500 mg/vial	250–500 mg
	Diamox Sequels	Capsule	500 mg	500 mg twice a day
Dichlorphenamide	Daranide	Tablet	50 mg	25–50 mg 1–3 times a day
Methazolamide	Generic	Tablet	25 mg, 50 mg	25–50 mg 2–3 times a day

▶ EVALUATION OF THERAPEUTIC OUTCOMES

- Successful outcomes require identifying an effective, well tolerated regimen; closely monitoring therapy; and patient adherence. Whenever possible, therapy for open-angle glaucoma should be started as a single agent in one eye to facilitate evaluation of drug efficacy and tolerance. Many drugs or combinations may need to be tried before the optimal regimen is identified.
- Monitoring therapy for open-angle glaucoma should be individualized. IOP response is assessed every 4 to 6 weeks initially, every 3 to 4 months after IOPs become acceptable, and more frequently after therapy is changed. The visual field and disk changes are monitored annually, unless glaucoma is unstable or worsening.
- Patients should be monitored for tachyphylaxis, especially with β blockers or **apraclonidine**. Treatment can be temporarily discontinued to monitor its benefit.
- There is no specific target IOP because the correlation between IOP and optic nerve damage is poor. Typically, a 25% to 30% reduction is desired.
- The target IOP also depends on disease severity and is generally less than 21 mm Hg for early visual field loss or optic disk changes, with progressively lower targets for greater damage. Targets as low as less than 10 mm Hg are desired for very advanced disease, continued damage at higher IOPs, normal tension glaucoma, and pretreatment pressures in the low- to mid-teens.
- Using more than one drop per dose increases the risk of adverse events and cost, but not efficacy.
- Patients should be educated about possible adverse effects and methods for preventing them.
- Patients should be taught how to administer topical therapy. With a forefinger pulling down the lower eyelid to form a pocket, the patient should place the dropper over the eye, look at the tip of the bottle, and then look up and place a single drop in the eye. To maximize topical activity and minimize systemic absorption, the patient should close the lid for 1 to 3 minutes after instillation and place the index finger over the nasolacrimal drainage system in the inner corner of the eye.
- If more than one topical drug is required, instillation should be separated by 5 to 10 minutes to provide optimal ocular contact.
- Adherence to drug therapy should be monitored because it is commonly inadequate and a cause of therapy failure.

See Chapter 92, Glaucoma, authored by Timothy S. Lesar, Richard G. Fiscella, and Deepak Edward, for a more detailed discussion of this topic.

Chapter 65

▶ ALZHEIMER'S DISEASE

▶ DEFINITION

Alzheimer's disease (AD) is a progressive dementia affecting both cognition and behavior with no known cause or cure. Patients eventually lose all cognitive, analytical, and physical functioning, and the disease is ultimately fatal.

▶ PATHOPHYSIOLOGY

- AD destroys neurons in the cortex and limbic structures of the brain responsible for higher learning, memory, reasoning, behavior, and emotional control.
- The presence of neurofibrillary tangles (NFTs) and neuritic plaques (NPs) is necessary for AD to occur. Intracellular NFTs are composed of paired helical filaments formed from tau protein that aggregate in dense bundles. Abnormal phosphorylation of tau filaments results in microtubular collapse and eventual cell death.
- NPs (also called amyloid or senile plaques) are extracellular and are composed of beta amyloid protein (βAP) and an entwined mass of broken neurites. βAP deposition may initiate the process of NP formation. Proteases cleave the amyloid precursor protein to form the βAP.
- Inflammatory mediators and other immune system constituents are present near areas of plaque formation, suggesting that the immune system plays an active role in the pathogenesis.
- Cholinergic pathways, especially a large system of neurons located at the base of the forebrain in the nucleus basalis of Mynert, are profoundly damaged. Cholinergic cell loss appears to be a result of the disease pathology rather than the disease-producing event.
- Serotonergic neurons of the raphe nuclei and noradrenergic cells of the locus ceruleus are also lost, whereas monoamine oxidase type B (MAO-B) activity is increased.
- Glutamate and other excitatory amino acid neurotransmitters have been implicated as potential neurotoxins in AD.
- Elevated cholesterol levels in brain neurons may alter cell membrane functioning and result in the cascade leading to plaque formation.
- Estrogen interacts with nerve growth factor, which may explain its ability to promote synaptic growth. Estrogen also acts as an antioxidant and may help maintain normal cholinergic transmission.

▶ CLINICAL PRESENTATION

The onset of AD is almost imperceptible, but deficits progress over time.

GENERAL

The patient may have vague memory complaints initially, or the patient's significant other may report that the patient is "forgetful." Cognitive decline is gradual over the course of illness. Behavioral disturbances may be present in moderate stages. Loss of daily function is common in advanced stages.

Psychiatric Disorders

SYMPTOMS

- *Cognitive:* Memory loss (poor recall and losing items); aphasia (circumlocution and anomia); apraxia; agnosia; disorientation (impaired perception of time and unable to recognize familiar people); impaired executive function
- *Noncognitive:* Depression, psychotic symptoms (hallucinations and delusions), behavioral disturbances (physical and verbal aggression, motor hyperactivity, uncooperativeness, wandering, repetitive mannerisms and activities, and combativeness)
- *Functional:* Inability to care for self (dressing, bathing, toileting, and eating)

▶ DIAGNOSIS

- AD is currently a diagnosis of exclusion. The National Institute of Neurological and Communicative Disorders and Stroke (NINCDS) and the Alzheimer's disease and Related Disorders Association (ADRDA) developed criteria for diagnosing AD that reduce erroneous diagnoses to less than 10% (Table 65–1). The *Diagnostic and Statistical Manual of Mental Disorders, 4th ed., Text Revision* (DSM-IV-TR) criteria are also considered appropriate for making the diagnosis.
- Patients with suspected AD should have a history and physical examination with appropriate laboratory and other diagnostic tests, neurologic and psychiatric examinations, standardized rating assessments, functional evaluation, and a caregiver interview.
- Rule out vitamin B_{12} and folate deficiency, and rule out hypothyroidism with thyroid function tests. CT or MRI scans may aid diagnosis.
- Information about prescription drug use; alcohol or other substance use; family medical history; and history of trauma, depression, or head injury should be obtained. It is important to rule out medication use (e.g., anticholinergics, sedatives) as contributors to dementia symptoms.

XIII **TABLE 65–1.** NINCDS-ADRDA Criteria and Diagnostic Workup for Probable Alzheimer's Disease

I. History of progressive cognitive decline of insidious onset
- In-depth interview of patient and caregivers
II. Deficits in at least two or more areas of functioning
III. No disturbance of consciousness
- Confirmation with use of dementia rating scale (e.g., Mini-Mental Status Examination [MMSE] or Blessed Dementia Scale)
IV. Age between 40 and 90 yr (usually >65 yr)
V. No other explainable cause of symptoms
- Normal laboratory tests including hematology, full chemistries, B_{12} and folate, thyroid function tests, Veneral Disease Research Lab test (to rule out venereal disease or syphilis)
- Normal electrocardiogram and electroencephalogram
- Normal physical exam, including thorough neurologic exam
- Neuroimaging, CT or MRI scanning: No focal lesions signifying other possible causes of dementia are present. Abnormalities which are common, but not diagnostic for AD include general cerebral wasting, widening of sulci, widening of the ventricles, and lesions of white matter surrounding the ventricle deep in the brain

The Mini-Mental Status Examination is a commonly used scale that measures orientation, recall, short-term memory, concentration, constructional praxis, and language. The MMSE is scored from 0 to 30, with a score of 10–26 typical of mild to moderate Alzheimer's disease.

TABLE 65–2. Stages of Cognitive Decline: The Global Deterioration Scale (GDS)

Stage 1	Normal	No subjective or objective change in intellectual functioning.
Stage 2	Forgetfulness	Complaints of losing things or forgetting names of acquaintances. Does not interfere with job or social functioning. Generally a component of normal aging.
Stage 3	Early confusion	Cognitive decline causes interference with work and social functioning. Anomia, difficulty remembering right word in conversation, and recall difficulties are present and noticed by family members. Memory loss may cause anxiety for patient.
Stage 4	Late confusion (early AD)	Patient can no longer manage finances or homemaking activities. Difficulty remembering recent events. Begins to withdraw from difficult tasks and to give up hobbies. May deny memory problems.
Stage 5	Early dementia (moderate AD)	Patient can no longer survive without assistance. Frequently disoriented with regard to time (date, year, season). Difficulty selecting clothing. Recall for recent events is severely impaired; may forget some details of past life (e.g., school attended or occupation). Functioning may fluctuate from day to day. Patient generally denies problems. May become suspicious or tearful. Loses ability to drive safely.
Stage 6	Middle dementia (moderately severe AD)	Patients need assistance with activities of daily living (e.g., bathing, dressing, and toileting). Patients experience difficulty interpreting their surroundings; may forget names of family and caregivers; forget most details of past life; have difficulty counting backward from 10. Agitation, paranoia, and delusions are common.
Stage 7	Late dementia	Patient loses ability to speak (may only grunt or scream), walk, and feed self. Incontinent of urine and feces. Consciousness reduced to stupor or coma.

- The Folstein Mini-Mental Status Examination (MMSE) can help to establish a history of deficits in two or more areas of cognition and establish a baseline against which to evaluate change in severity. The average expected decline in an untreated patient is 2 to 4 points per year.
- After diagnosis, AD is staged using a scale such as the Global Deterioration Scale (GDS) (Table 65–2). This 7-point system correlates with psychometric measures and changes in computed tomography or positron emission tomography scans and is useful to monitor global changes in AD patients.

▶ DESIRED OUTCOME

The primary goal of treatment in AD is to maintain patient functioning as long as possible. Secondary goals are to treat the psychiatric and behavioral sequelea.

▶ TREATMENT

A proposed treatment algorithm for both cognitive and psychiatric/behavioral symptoms of AD is shown in Figure 65–1.

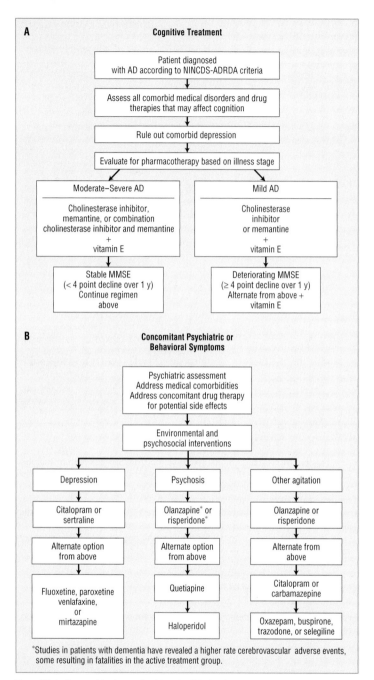

Figure 65–1. Proposed treatment algorithms for Alzheimer's disease: (A) cognitive treatment and (B) concomitant psychiatric or behavioral symptoms. NINCDS, National Institute of Neurological and Communicative Disorders and Stroke; ADRDA, Alzheimer's disease and Related Disorders Association; MMSE, Mini-Mental Status Examination; SSRI, selective serotonin reuptake inhibitor.

NONPHARMACOLOGIC THERAPY

On initial diagnosis, the patient and caregiver should be educated on the course of illness, available treatments, legal decisions, changes in lifestyle that will be necessary with disease progression, and other quality of life issues.

PHARMACOTHERAPY OF COGNITIVE SYMPTOMS

- Current pharmacotherapeutic interventions are primarily symptomatic attempts to improve or maintain cognition. There is evidence that some interventions (e.g., cholinesterase inhibitors, vitamin E) may prolong the time to critical functional end points. There are presently no medications that change the course of illness or cure AD.
- Change in disease severity may be assessed using the MMSE. Successful treatment reflects a decline of less than 2 points each year on the MMSE score.

Cholinesterase Inhibitors

- No direct comparative trials have been conducted to assess the effectiveness of one agent over another.
- If the decline in MMSE score is more than 2 to 4 points after treatment for 1 year with the initial agent, it is reasonable to change to a different cholinesterase inhibitor. Otherwise, treatment should be continued with the initial medication throughout the course of the illness.

Donepezil

- **Donepezil** (Acricept) is a piperidine derivative with specificity for inhibition of acetylcholinesterase rather than butyrylcholinesterase. This is purported to result in fewer peripheral side effects (e.g., nausea, vomiting, diarrhea) than with nonspecific cholinesterase inhibitors such as tacrine.
- It is approved for treatment of cognitive impairment in mild to moderately severe AD (MMSE score 10 to 26). Patients taking donepezil had improved cognition for the first 6 to 9 months, followed by a gradual decline. It may also be effective for patients with moderate to severe AD.
- Dosing strategies for donepezil are shown in Table 65–3.
- Donepezil is well tolerated by most patients. The most common side effects are nausea, vomiting, diarrhea, headache, and insomnia.   XIII

Rivastigmine

- **Rivastigmine** (Exelon) has central activity at acetylcholinesterase and butyrylcholinesterase sites, but low activity at these sites in the periphery. Theoretically, this should result in fewer peripheral side effects.
- One study indicated that treatment with rivastigmine improves or stabilizes cognition for about 6 to 12 months longer than in untreated patients. It has not been evaluated for severe dementia or for treatment of behavior symptoms.
- The initial dose is 1.5 mg twice daily, titrated upward at intervals of at least 2 weeks to a maximum dose of 6 mg twice daily. Tolerability and absorption are improved when it is given with food.

TABLE 65–3. Recommended Dosing Strategies for Cholinesterase Inhibitors

	Tacrine	Donepezil	Rivastigmine	Galantamine
Starting dose	10 mg 4 times a day	5 mg daily	1.5 mg twice a day	4 mg twice a day
Maintenance dose	20–40 mg 4 times a day	5–10 mg daily	3–6 mg twice a day	8–12 mg twice a day
Time between dose adjustment	4–6 wk	4–6 wk	2 wk	4 wk

Galantamine
- **Galantamine** (Reminyl) is a cholinesterase inhibitor that also has activity as a nicotinic receptor agonist.
- Galantamine causes modest cognitive improvement, which lasts about 9 months.
- Table 65–3 shows dosing strategies.
- Adverse effects of galantamine include nausea, vomiting, diarrhea, headache, and dizziness.

Tacrine
- **Tacrine** (Cognex) was the first cholinesterase inhibitor approved for the treatment of AD, but it has been replaced by safer, more tolerable agents.

Other Drugs
- **Memantine** (Namenda) is an antagonist of the *N*-methyl-D-aspartate (NMDA) receptor, which is indicated for treatment of moderate to severe AD. It is usually well tolerated, and side effects include constipation, confusion, dizziness, headache, coughing, and hypertension. It is used as monotherapy and in combination with cholinesterase inhibitors. It is initiated at 5 mg/day and increased weekly by 5 mg/day to the effective dose of 10 mg twice daily. Dosing must be adjusted in patients with renal impairment.
- **Vitamin E** is an antioxidant that has been studied in AD on the basis of pathophysiologic theories involving free radicals. Vitamin E may be used adjunctively with cholinesterase inhibitors throughout treatment.
- Current data do not support a role for **Estrogen** in treating or preventing dementia. It should be used only in women who have another medical reason for estrogen therapy.
- Nonsteroidal anti-inflammatory drug (NSAID) use on a regular basis has been associated with a lower incidence of AD in epidemiologic studies. These drugs have not been shown effective in treatment of cognitive symptoms in AD. However, because of limited prospective data and the potential for side effects, NSAIDs are not recommended for general use in prevention or treatment of AD.
- Recent interest has focused on the use of lipid lowering agents, especially the HMG-CoA-reductase inhibitors, to prevent AD. **Pravastatin** and **lovastatin**, but not **simvastatin**, were associated with a lower prevalence of AD. Further study is needed before these agents can be recommended for this use.
- **Egb 761**, an extract of **ginkgo biloba**, has been evaluated in many studies, but a recent meta-analysis determined that only 4 of 57 studies met minimal scientific standards for clinical trials. The results of the meta-analysis indicated that ginkgo biloba, 120 to 240 mg/day, may have some therapeutic effect, but the clinical relevance was minimal. Because of limited efficacy data, the potential for adverse effects (e.g., hemorrhage), and the poor standardization of herbal products, it is recommended that ginkgo biloba be used only with caution.

PHARMACOTHERAPY OF NONCOGNITIVE SYMPTOMS
- Secondary pharmacotherapeutic interventions are aimed at treating psychotic symptoms, inappropriate or disruptive behavior, and depression. Medications and recommended doses for noncognitive symptoms are shown in Table 65–4.
- General guidelines are as follows: (1) use reduced doses, (2) monitor closely, (3) titrate dosage slowly, (4) document carefully, and (5) periodically attempt to reduce medication (at least every 3 months).
- Psychotropic medications with anticholinergic effects should be avoided because they may worsen cognition. Other side effects from traditional

XIII

TABLE 65–4. Medications Used in Treating Noncognitive Symptoms of Dementia

Drugs	Suggested Dosage in Dementia (mg/day)	Indications
Antipsychotics		Psychosis: hallucinations, delusions, suspiciousness
Haloperidol	0.5–4 mg	Disruptive behaviors: agitation, aggression
Olanzapine	2.5–10 mg	
Quetiapine	12.5–200 mg	
Risperidone	0.25–2 mg	
Antidepressants		Depression: poor appetite, insomnia, hopelessness,
Citalopram	10–20 mg	anhedonia, withdrawal, suicidal thoughts, agitation
Fluoxetine	5–20 mg	
Mirtazapine	15–45 mg	
Paroxetine	10–40 mg	
Sertraline	50–200 mg	
Trazodone	75–400 mg[a]	
Venlafaxine	37.5–150 mg	
Anticonvulsants		Agitation or aggression
Carbamazepine	100–1,000 mg[a,b]	
Others		
Buspirone	10–45 mg	Disruptive behaviors
Oxazepam	10–60 mg[a]	Disruptive behaviors
Selegiline	10 mg	Disruptive behaviors, agitation, anxiety, depression

[a] Administer in divided doses.
[b] Dosage adjustment should be guided by drug serum concentrations.

psychotropic agents in the elderly include sedation, postural instability, and extrapyramidal side effects.

Antipsychotics

- Antipsychotic medications have traditionally been used to treat disruptive behaviors and psychosis in AD patients. Symptoms responding include assaultiveness, extreme agitation and hyperexcitability, hallucinations, delusions, suspiciousness, hostility, and uncooperativeness. Symptoms not responding include withdrawal, apathy, cognitive deficits, wandering, and incontinence.
- Placebo-controlled studies suggest that traditional (typical) antipsychotics are moderately effective at best. Newer atypical antipsychotics have been shown to be effective with fewer side effects. Consequently, atypical antipsychotics are preferred for treatment of psychosis or aggression in AD.
- Effective doses are much lower than those typically used to treat schizophrenia (see Table 65–4).
- **Risperidone** (Risperdal) has been studied in clinical trials and used in practice for psychotic symptoms or behavioral disturbances associated with dementia. The recommended initial dose is 0.25 mg daily, titrated in 0.25- to 0.5-mg increments up to 1 mg daily. If response is inadequate, further titration to 2 mg daily may be attempted if tolerated.
- **Olanzapine** (Zyprexa) has been shown to be beneficial in controlled trials. However, it has anticholinergic effects, raising concern about its utility for the treatment of AD.
- **Quetiapine** (Seroquel) has been evaluated only in open-label studies. It may be a reasonable alternative for patients who respond inadequately to or cannot tolerate risperidone or olanzapine.

XIII

- **Aripiprazole** (Abilify) and **ziprasidone** (Geodon) require further study before they can be recommended in this population.

Antidepressants

- Depression and dementia have many symptoms in common, and the diagnosis of depression can be difficult, especially later in the course of AD.
- There appears to be significant placebo response when treating depression in AD patients. Also, antidepressant response may not be as dramatic as in depressed nondemented patients. Up to 12 weeks of treatment may be required to achieve an antidepressant response.
- Symptoms of depression should be documented for several weeks prior to initiating antidepressant therapy. If nonspecific treatments fail (e.g., visiting with a clinician or increasing activity level), a trial of an antidepressant may be warranted. Pharmacotherapy should be initiated with an agent possessing a favorable side-effect profile.
- The selective serotonin reuptake inhibitors (SSRIs) **citalopram** and **sertraline** have been recommended as first-line agents because of demonstrated efficacy in placebo-controlled trials. **Fluoxetine** and **paroxetine**, as well as the serotonin/norepinephrine reuptake inhibitors venlafaxine and mirtazepine may be alternatives.

Miscellaneous Therapies

- **Carbamazepine**, mean dose 300 mg/day, and citalopram, 10 to 20 mg/day, have been shown to improve psychosis and behavioral disturbance in AD patients.
- **Oxazepam** and other benzodiazepines have been used to treat anxiety, agitation, and aggression, but they generally show inferior efficacy compared with antipsychotics.
- **Buspirone** has shown benefit in treating agitation and aggression in small studies with minimal adverse effects.
- **Selegiline** may decrease anxiety, depression, and agitation.

▶ EVALUATION OF THERAPEUTIC OUTCOMES

XIII
- A thorough assessment at baseline should define therapeutic goals and document cognitive status, physical status, functional performance, mood, thought processes, and behavior. Both the patient and caregiver should be interviewed.
- Objective assessments, such as the MMSE for cognition and the Functional Activities Questionnaire for activities of daily living, should be used to quantify changes in symptoms and function.
- Because target symptoms of psychiatric disorders may respond differently in demented patients, a detailed list of symptoms to be treated should be documented to aid in monitoring.
- The patient should be observed carefully for potential side effects of drug therapy. The specific side effects to be monitored and the method and frequency of monitoring should be documented.
- Assessments for drug effectiveness, side effects, compliance, need for dosage adjustment, or change in treatment should occur at least monthly.
- A treatment period of 6 months to 1 year may be required to determine whether therapy is beneficial.

See Chapter 63, Alzheimer's Disease, authored by Jennifer D. Faulkner, Jody Bartlett, and Paul Hicks, for a more detailed discussion of this topic.

Chapter 66

▶ ANXIETY DISORDERS

▶ DEFINITION

Anxiety disorders include a constellation of disorders in which anxiety and associated symptoms are irrational or experienced at a level of severity that impairs functioning. The characteristic features are anxiety and avoidance.

▶ PATHOPHYSIOLOGY

- *Noradrenergic model.* This model suggests that the autonomic nervous system of anxious patients is hypersensitive and overreacts to various stimuli. The locus ceruleus may have a role in regulating anxiety, as it activates norepinephrine (NE) release and stimulates the sympathetic and parasympathetic nervous systems. Chronic noradrenergic overactivity downregulates α_2 adrenoreceptors in patients with generalized anxiety disorder (GAD) and post-traumatic stress disorder (PTSD). Patients with social anxiety disorder (SAD) appear to have a hyperresponsive adrenocortical response to psychological stress.
- *γ-aminobutyric acid (GABA) receptor model.* GABA is the major inhibitory neurotransmitter in the central nervous system (CNS). Many antianxiety drugs target the GABA$_A$ receptor. **Benzodiazepines** (BZs) enhance or diminish the inhibitory effects of GABA, which has a strong regulatory or inhibitory effect on serotonin (5-HT), NE, and dopamine (DA) systems. Anxiety symptoms may be linked to underactivity of GABA systems or downregulated central BZ receptors. In patients with GAD, BZ binding in the left temporal lobe is reduced. Abnormal sensitivity to antagonism of the BZ binding site and decreased binding was demonstrated in panic disorder. Growth hormone response to baclofen in patients with generalized SAD suggests an abnormality of central GABA$_B$ receptor function. Abnormalities of GABA inhibition may lead to increased response to stress in PTSD patients.
- *Serotonin (5-HT) model.* GAD symptoms may reflect excessive 5-HT transmission or overactivity of the stimulatory 5-HT pathways. Patients with SAD have greater prolactin response to **buspirone** challenge, indicating an enhanced central serotonergic response. The role of 5-HT in panic disorder is unclear, but it may have a role in development of anticipatory anxiety. Preliminary data suggest that the 5-HT and 5-HT$_2$ antagonist *meta*-chlorophenylpiperazine (*m*-CPP) causes increased anxiety in PTSD patients.
- Patients with PTSD have a hypersecretion of corticotropin-releasing factor but demonstrate subnormal levels of cortisol at the time of trauma and chronically. Dysregulation of the hypothalamic-pituitary-adrenal axis may be a risk factor for eventual development of PTSD.
- Functional neuroimaging studies suggest that frontal and occipital brain areas are integral to the anxiety response. Patients with panic disorder may have abnormal activation of the parahippocampal region and prefrontal cortex at rest. Panic anxiety is associated with activation of brain stem and basal ganglia regions. GAD patients have an abnormal increase in cortical activity and a decrease in basal ganglia activity. In patients with SAD, there may be abnormalities in the amygdala, hippocampus, and various cortical regions. Lower hippocampal volumes in patients with PTSD may be a precursor for subsequent development of PTSD.

TABLE 66–1. Presentation of Generalized Anxiety Disorder

Psychological and cognitive symptoms
- Excessive anxiety
- Worries that are difficult to control
- Feeling keyed up or on edge
- Poor concentration or mind going blank

Physical symptoms
- Restlessness
- Fatigue
- Muscle tension
- Sleep disturbance
- Irritability

Impairment
- Social, occupational, or other important functional areas
- Poor coping abilities

Screening questions
- What is going on in your life?
- How do you feel about it?
- What troubles you the most?
- How are you handling that?

▶ CLINICAL PRESENTATION

GENERALIZED ANXIETY DISORDER

- The clinical presentation of GAD is shown in Table 66–1. The diagnostic criteria require persistent symptoms most days for at least 6 months. The anxiety or worry must be about a number of matters and is accompanied by at least three psychological or physiological symptoms. The illness has a gradual onset at an average age of 21 years. The course of illness is chronic, with multiple spontaneous exacerbations and remissions. There is a high percentage of relapse and a low rate of recovery.

XIII

PANIC DISORDER

- Symptoms usually begin as a series of unexpected panic attacks. These are followed by at least 1 month of persistent concern about having another panic attack.
- Symptoms of a panic attack are shown in Table 66–2. During an attack, there must be at least four physical symptoms in addition to psychological symptoms. Symptoms reach a peak within 10 minutes and usually last no more than 20 or 30 minutes.
- Many patients eventually develop agoraphobia, which is avoidance of specific situations (e.g., crowded places, bridges) where they fear a panic attack might occur. Patients may become homebound.

SOCIAL ANXIETY DISORDER (SAD)

- The essential feature of SAD is an intense, irrational, and persistent fear of being negatively evaluated in a social or performance situation. Exposure to the feared situation usually provokes a panic attack. Symptoms of social anxiety disorder are shown in Table 66–3. The fear and avoidance of the situation must interfere with daily routine or social/occupational functioning. It is a chronic disorder with a mean age of onset in the teens.

TABLE 66–2. Symptoms of a Panic Attack

Psychological symptoms
- Depersonalization
- Derealization
- Fear of losing control
- Fear of going crazy
- Fear of dying

Physical symptoms
- Abdominal distress
- Chest pain or discomfort
- Chills
- Dizziness or lightheadedness
- Feeling of choking
- Hot flushes
- Palpitations
- Nausea
- Paresthesias
- Shortness of breath
- Sweating
- Tachycardia
- Trembling or shaking

TABLE 66–3. Presentation of Social Anxiety Disorder

Fears
- Being scrutinized by others
- Being embarrassed
- Being humiliated

Some feared situations
- Addressing a group of people
- Eating or writing in front of others
- Interacting with authority figures
- Speaking in public
- Talking with strangers
- Use of public toilets

Physical symptoms
- Blushing
- "Butterflies in the stomach"
- Diarrhea
- Sweating
- Tachycardia
- Trembling

Types
- Generalized type: fear and avoidance extend to a wide range of social situations
- Nongeneralized type: fear is limited to one or two situations

Screening questions
- Are you uncomfortable or embarrassed at being the center of attention?
- Do you find it hard to interact with people?

XIII

- In the generalized subtype, fear is of many social situations where embarrassment may occur. In the discrete subtype, fear is limited to one or two situations (e.g., performing, public speaking).

SPECIFIC PHOBIA

- The primary characteristic is a marked and persistent fear of a specific object or situation such as thunderstorms, animals, or heights. These patients are not seriously impaired, as they simply avoid the feared object. Specific phobia is considered unresponsive to drug therapy but highly responsive to behavioral therapy.

POSTTRAUMATIC STRESS DISORDER

- In PTSD, exposure to a traumatic event causes immediate intense fear, helplessness, or horror.
- The clinical presentation of PTSD is shown in Table 66–4. Patients must have at least one reexperiencing symptom, three signs or symptoms of persistent avoidance of stimuli, and at least two symptoms of increased arousal. Symptoms from each category must be present longer than 1 month and cause significant distress or impairment. PTSD can occur at any age, and the course is variable.
- One-third of patients with PTSD have a poor prognosis, and about 80% have a concurrent depression or anxiety disorder. Over half of men with PTSD have comorbid alcohol abuse or dependence, and about 20% of patients attempt suicide.

TABLE 66–4. Presentation of Posttraumatic Stress Disorder

Reexperiencing symptoms
- Recurrent, intrusive distressing memories of the trauma
- Recurrent, disturbing dreams of the event
- Feeling that the traumatic event is recurring (e.g., dissociative flashbacks)
- Physiologic reaction to reminders of the trauma

Avoidance symptoms
- Avoidance of conversations about the trauma
- Avoidance of thoughts or feelings about the trauma
- Avoidance of activities that are reminders of the event
- Avoidance of people or places that arouse recollections of the trauma
- Inability to recall an important aspect of the trauma
- Anhedonia
- Estrangement from others
- Restricted affect
- Sense of a foreshortened future (e.g., does not expect to have a career, marriage)

Hyperarousal symptoms
- Decreased concentration
- Easily startled
- Hypervigilance
- Insomnia
- Irritability or angry outbursts

Subtypes
- Acute: duration of symptoms is less than 3 months
- Chronic: symptoms last for longer than 3 months
- With delayed onset: onset of symptoms is at least 6 months posttrauma

Screening questions
- Have you ever experienced a significant trauma in your life?
- Did this experience have a lasting negative impact or change your life?

XIII

TABLE 66–5. Common Medical Illnesses Associated with Anxiety Symptoms

Cardiovascular
Angina, arrhythmias, congestive heart failure, ischemic heart disease, myocardial infarction

Endocrine and metabolic
Cushing's disease, hyperparathyroidism, hyperthyroidism, hypothyroidism, hypoglycemia, hyponatremia, hyperkalemia, pheochromocytoma, vitamin B_{12} or folate deficiencies

Neurologic
Dementia, migraine, Parkinson's disease, seizures, stroke, neoplasms, poor pain control

Respiratory system
Asthma, chronic obstructive pulmonary disease, pulmonary embolus, pneumonia

Others
Anemias, systemic lupus erythematosus, vestibular dysfunction

▶ DIAGNOSIS

- Evaluation of the anxious patient requires a complete physical and mental status examination; appropriate laboratory tests; and a medical, psychiatric, and drug history.
- Anxiety symptoms may be associated with medical illnesses (Table 66–5) or drug therapy (Table 66–6). About 50% of patients with GAD have irritable bowel syndrome.
- Anxiety symptoms may be present in several major psychiatric illnesses (e.g., mood disorders, schizophrenia, organic mental syndromes, substance withdrawal).

▶ DESIRED OUTCOME

- The desired outcomes of treatment of GAD are to reduce severity, duration, and frequency of the symptoms and to improve overall functioning.
- The goals of therapy of panic disorder include a complete resolution of panic attacks (not always achievable), marked reduction in anticipatory anxiety and phobic fears, and resumption of normal activities.

TABLE 66–6. Drugs Associated with Anxiety Symptoms

Anticonvulsants: carbamazepine
Antidepressants: selective serotonin reuptake inhibitors, tricyclic antidepressants
Antihypertensives: felodipine
Antibiotics: quinolones, isoniazid
Bronchodilators: albuterol, theophylline
Corticosteroids: prednisone
Dopa agonists: levodopa
Herbals: ma huang, ginseng, ephedra
Nonsteroidal anti-inflammatory drugs: ibuprofen
Stimulants: amphetamines, methylphenidate, caffeine, cocaine
Sympathomimetics: pseudoephedrine
Thyroid hormones: levothyroxine
Toxicity: anticholinergics, antihistamines, digoxin
Withdrawal: alcohol, sedatives

- The goals of treatment of SAD are to reduce the physiologic symptoms and phobic avoidance and increase participation in desired social activities.
- The goals of therapy of PTSD are to decrease core symptoms, disability, and comorbidity and improve quality of life and resilience to stress.
- The goals of treatment of PTSD are to eliminate core symptoms and improve disability, comorbid conditions, and quality of life.

▶ TREATMENT

GENERALIZED ANXIETY DISOSRDER (GAD)

- For patients with GAD, nonpharmacologic modalities include short-term counseling, stress management, cognitive therapy, meditation, supportive therapy, and exercise. GAD patients should be educated to avoid caffeine, stimulants, excessive alcohol, and diet pills. Cognitive behavioral therapy is the most effective psychological therapy for GAD patients, and most patients with GAD require psychological therapy, alone or in combination with antianxiety drugs.
- An algorithm for the pharmacologic management of GAD is shown in Figure 66–1.

XIII

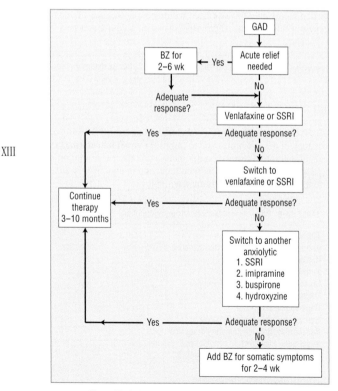

Figure 66–1. Algorithm for the pharmacotherapy of GAD.

TABLE 66–7. Drug Choices for Anxiety Disorders

Anxiety Disorders	First-Line Drugs	Second-Line Drugs	Alternatives
Generalized anxiety	Venlafaxine XR Paroxetine Escitalopram	Benzodiazepines Imipramine Buspirone	Hydroxyzine
Panic disorder	SSRIs	Imipramine Clomipramine Alprazolam Clonazepam	Phenelzine
Social anxiety disorder	Paroxetine Sertraline Venlafaxine XR	Citalopram Escitalopram Fluvoxamine Clonazepam	Buspirone Gabapentin Phenelzine

SSRI, selective serotonin reuptake inhibitor; XR, extended-release.

- Drug choices for anxiety disorders are shown in Table 66–7, and non-BZ antianxiety agents for GAD are shown in Table 66–8. Kava kava is not recommended as an anxiolytic because of reports of hepatotoxicity.
- The Food and Drug Administration (FDA) recently placed a black box warning on the use of all antidepressants in children and adolescents, and monitoring parameters were defined. The official approved labeling and/or the FDA should be consulted for additional information (see chapter 68).

Antidepressants

- **Antidepressants** are considered the treatment of choice for long-term management of chronic anxiety. Antianxiety response requires 2 to 4 weeks.
- **Venlafaxine** extended release alleviates anxiety in patients with or without comorbid depression, and it can be dosed once daily. **Paroxetine** and **escitalopram** are also more effective than placebo. In a four-parallel-group study, **imipramine** was more effective than **diazepam, trazodone,** or placebo; trazodone and diazepam were more effective than placebo.

XIII ◄

TABLE 66–8. Nonbenzodiazepine Antianxiety Agents for Generalized Anxiety Disorder

Generic Name	Trade Name	Starting Dose	Dosage Range (mg/day)[a]
Antidepressants			
Escitalopram[b]	Lexapro	10 mg/day	10–20
Imipramine	Tofranil	50 mg/day	75–200
Paroxetine[b,c]	Paxil	20 mg/day	20–50
Venlafaxine[b]	Effexor XR	37.5 or 75 mg/day	75–225[d]
Azapirones			
Buspirone[b,c]	BuSpar	7.5 mg twice per day	15–60[d]
Diphenylmethane			
Hydroxyzine[b,c,e]	Vistaril, Atarax	25 or 50 mg 4 times daily	200–400

[a]Elderly patients are usually treated with approximately one-half of the dose listed.
[b]FDA-approved for generalized anxiety disorder.
[c]Available generically.
[d]No dosage adjustment is required in elderly patients.
[e]FDA-approved for anxiety and tension in children in divided daily doses of 50–100 mg.

TABLE 66–9. Benzodiazepine Antianxiety Agents

Generic Name	Brand Name	Approved Dosage Range (mg/day)[a]	Approximate Equivalent Dose (mg)
Alprazolam[b]	Xanax	0.75–4	0.5
	Xanax XR	1–10c	
Chlordiazepoxide[b]	Librium	25–100	25
Clonazepam[b]	Klonopin	1–4c	0.25
Clorazepate[b]	Tranxene	7.5–60	7.5
Diazepam[b]	Valium	2–40	5
Lorazepam[b]	Ativan	0.5–10	0.75–1
Oxazepam[b]	Serax	30–120	15

[a]Elderly patients are usually treated with approximately one-half of the dose listed.
[b]Available generically.
[c]Panic disorder dose.

- Common side effects of venlafaxine are nausea, somnolence, and dry mouth. Common paroxetine side effects include somnolence, nausea, abnormal ejaculation, dry mouth, decreased libido, and asthenia. Escitalopram causes nausea, insomnia, fatigue, decreased libido, and ejaculation disorders. **Tricyclic antidepressants** (TCAs) commonly cause sedation, orthostatic hypotension, anticholinergic effects, and weight gain. TCAs are very toxic on overdose.

Evaluation of Therapeutic Outcomes
- Initially, anxious patients should be monitored once to twice weekly for reduction in anxiety symptoms, improvement in functioning, and side effects. The Visual Analog Scale may assist in the evaluation of drug response.

Benzodiazepine (BZ) Therapy
- The **BZs** are the most effective and safe medications for the treatment of acute anxiety symptoms (Table 66–9). All BZs are equally effective anxiolytics, and most of the improvement occurs in the first 2 weeks of therapy. They are considered to be more effective for somatic and autonomic symptoms of GAD, while antidepressants are considered more effective for the psychic symptoms (e.g., apprehension and worry).
- It is theorized that BZs ameliorate anxiety through potentiation of GABA activity.
- The dose must be individualized, and duration of therapy usually should not exceed 4 months. Some patients require longer treatment.
- The elderly have an enhanced sensitivity to BZs and may experience falls when on BZ therapy.

Pharmacokinetics
- BZ pharmacokinetic properties are shown in Table 66–10.
- **Diazepam** and **clorazepate** have high lipophilicity and are rapidly absorbed and distributed into the CNS. They have a shorter duration of effect after a single dose than would be predicted on the basis of half-life, as they are rapidly distributed to the periphery.
- **Lorazepam** and **oxazepam** are less lipophilic and have a slower onset but a longer duration of action. They are not recommended for immediate relief of anxiety.

TABLE 66–10. Pharmacokinetics of Benzodiazepine Antianxiety Agents

Generic Name	Time to Peak Plasma Level (h)	Elimination Half-Life, Parent (h)	Metabolic Pathway	Clinically Significant Metabolites	Protein Binding (%)
Alprazolam	1–2	12–15	Oxidation		80
Chlordiazepoxide	1–4	5–30	N-Dealkylation Oxidation	Desmethylchloridazepoxide Demoxepam DMDZ[a]	96
Clonazepam	1–4	30–40	Nitroreduction		85
Clorazepate	1–2	Prodrug	Oxidation	DMDZ	97
Diazepam	0.5–2	20–80	Oxidation	DMDZ Oxazepam	98
Lorazepam	2–4	10–20	Conjugation		85
Oxazepam	2–4	5–20	Conjugation		97

[a]Desmethyldiazepam (DMDZ) half-life 50–100 h.

XIII

- **IM diazepam** and **chlordiazepoxide** should be avoided because of variability in rate and extent of absorption. **IM lorazepam** provides rapid and complete absorption.
- **Clorazepate**, a prodrug, is converted to DMDZ in the stomach through a pH-dependent process that may be impaired by concurrent antacid use. Several other BZs are also converted to DMDZ, which has a long half-life.
- Intermediate- or short-acting BZs are preferred for chronic use in the elderly and those with liver disorders because of minimal accumulation and achievement of steady state within 1 to 3 days.

Adverse Events
- The most common side effect of BZs is CNS depression. Tolerance usually develops to this effect. Other side effects are disorientation, psychomotor impairment, confusion, aggression, excitement, and anterograde amnesia.

Abuse, Dependence, Withdrawal, and Tolerance
- Those with a history of drug abuse are at the greatest risk for becoming BZ abusers.
- BZ dependence is defined by the appearance of a predictable withdrawal syndrome (i.e., anxiety, insomnia, agitation, muscle tension, irritability, nausea, malaise, diaphoresis, nightmares, depression, hyperreflexia, tinnitus, delusions, hallucinations, and seizures) upon abrupt discontinuation.

Benzodiazepine Discontinuation
- After BZs are abruptly discontinued, three events can occur:
  - Rebound symptoms are an immediate, but transient, return of original symptoms with an increased intensity compared with baseline.
  - Recurrence or relapse is the return of original symptoms at the same intensity as before treatment.
  - Withdrawal is the emergence of new symptoms and a worsening of preexisting symptoms.
- The onset of withdrawal symptoms is 24 to 48 hours after discontinuation of short-$_{1/2}$ and 3 to 8 days after discontinuation of long-$_{1/2}$ drugs.
- Discontinuation strategies include the following:
  - A 25% per week reduction in dosage until 50% of the dose is reached, then dosage reduction by one-eighth every 4 to 7 days.
  - A BZ with a long-$t_{1/2}$ (e.g., **diazepam, clonazepam**) may be substituted for a drug with a short-$t_{1/2}$ (e.g., **lorazepam, oxazepam, alprazolam**). The substituted drug should be given for several weeks before gradual tapering begins.
  - Adjunctive use of **imipramine, valproic acid,** or **buspirone** can help to reduce withdrawal symptoms during the BZ taper.

Drug Interactions
- Drug interactions with the BZs are generally pharmacodynamic or pharmacokinetic (Table 66–11). The combination of **BZs** with **alcohol** or other **CNS depressants** may be fatal.
- **Alprazolam** dose should be reduced by 50% if **nefazodone** (Serzone) or **fluvoxamine** is added.

Dosing and Administration
- Initial doses should be low, and dosage adjustments can be made weekly. (see Table 66–9)
- Treatment of acute anxiety generally should not exceed 4 weeks. BZs can be given as needed, and if several acute courses are necessary, a BZ-free period

XIII

TABLE 66–11. Pharmacokinetic Drug Interactions with the Benzodiazepines

Drug	Effect
Alcohol (chroni)	Increased Cl of BZs
Carbamazepine	Decreased Cl of alprazolam
Cimetidine	Decreased Cl of alprazolam, diazepam, chlordiazepoxide, and clorazepate and increased $t_{1/2}$
Disulfiram	Decreased Cl of alprazolam and diazepam
Erythromycin	Decreased Cl of alprazolam
Fluoxetine	Decreased Cl of alprazolam and diazepam
Fluvoxamine	Decreased Cl of alprazolam and prolonged $t_{1/2}$
Itraconazole	Potentially decreased Cl of alprazolam and diazepam
Ketaconazole	Potentially decreased Cl of alprazolam
Nefazodone	Decreased Cl of alprazolam, AUC doubled, and $t_{1/2}$ prolonged
Omeprazole	Decreased Cl of diazepam
Oral contraceptives	Increased free concentration of chlordiazepoxide and slightly decreased Cl; decreased Cl and increased $_{1/2}$ of diazepam and alprazolam
Paroxetine	Decreased Cl of alprazolam
Phenobarbital	Increased Cl of clonazepam and reduced $t_{1/2}$
Phenytoin	Increased Cl of clonazepam and reduced $t_{1/2}$
Probenecid	Decreased Cl of lorazepam and prolonged $t_{1/2}$
Propranolol	Decreased Cl of diazepam and prolonged $t_{1/2}$
Ranitidine	Decreased absorption of diazepam
Rifampin	Increased metabolism of diazepam
Theophylline	Decreased alprazolam concentrations
Valproate	Decreased Cl of lorazepam

AUC, area under the plasma concentration curve; BZ, benzodiazepine; Cl, clearance; $t_{1/2}$, elimination half-life.

of 2 to 4 weeks should be implemented between courses. Persistent symptoms should be managed with **antidepressants** or **buspirone**.

- BZs with a long $t_{1/2}$ may be dosed once daily at bedtime and may provide nighttime hypnotic and anxiolytic effects the next day.
- In the elderly, doses should be low, and short-elimination half-life agents prescribed.

XIII

Buspirone Therapy

- **Buspirone** is a 5-HT_{1A} partial agonist that lacks anticonvulsant, muscle relaxant, sedative-hypnotic, motor impairment, and dependence properties.
- It is considered a second-line agent for GAD because of inconsistent reports of efficacy, delayed onset of effect, and lack of efficacy for comorbid depressive and anxiety disorders (e.g., panic disorder or SAD).
- It has a mean $t_{1/2}$ of 2.5 hours, and it is dosed 2 to 3 times daily.
- Side effects include dizziness, nausea, and headaches.

Drug Interactions

- **Buspirone** may increase **cyclosporine** and **haloperidol** levels and elevate blood pressure in patients taking a **monoamine oxidase inhibitor** (MAOI).
- **Verapamil, diltiazem, itraconazole, fluvoxamine, nefazodone,** and **erythromycin** increase and **rifampin** reduces buspirone blood levels.

Dosing and Administration
- The initial dose of buspirone is 7.5 mg two times daily, with increments of 5 mg/day every 2 or 3 days as needed. The usual therapeutic dose is 30 to 60 mg/day.
- The onset of anxiolytic effects requires 2 weeks or more; maximum benefit may require 4 to 6 weeks.
- It is not useful for situations requiring rapid antianxiety effects or as-needed therapy.
- When switching from a BZ to buspirone, the BZ should be tapered slowly.

PANIC DISORDER

General Therapeutic Principles
- Antipanic drugs are shown in Table 66–12. An algorithm for drug therapy of panic disorder is shown in Figure 66–2.
- Most patients without agoraphobia improve with pharmacotherapy alone, but if agoraphobia is present, cognitive-behavioral therapy (CBT) typically is initiated concurrently.
- Patients treated with CBT are less likely to relapse than those treated with imipramine alone. For patients who cannot or will not take medications, CBT alone is certainly indicated, as it is associated with improvement in 80% to 90% of patients short-term and 75% of patients at 6-month follow-up.
- Patients must be educated to avoid caffeine, drugs of abuse, and stimulants.
- **Antidepressants**, especially the selective serotonin reuptake inhibitors (**SSRIs**) are preferred in elderly patients and youth. The **BZs** are second line in these patients because of potential problems with disinhibition.

TABLE 66–12. Drugs Used in the Treatment of Panic Disorder

Class/Generic Name	Brand Name	Starting Dose	Antipanic Dosage[a] Range (mg)
Selective serotonin reuptake inhibitors			
Citalopram	Celexa	10 mg/day	20–60
Escitalopram	Lexapro	5 mg/day	10–20
Fluoxetine[b]	Prozac	5 mg/day	10–20
Fluvoxamine[b]	Luvox	25 mg/day	100–300
Paroxetine[b]	Paxil	10 mg/day	20–60[c]
Sertraline	Zoloft	25 mg/day	50–200[c]
Benzodiazepines			
Alprazolam[b]	Xanax	0.25 mg 3 times a day	4–10[c]
	Xanax XR	0.5–1 mg/day	1–10[c]
Clonazepam[b]	Klonopin	0.25 mg once or twice per day	1–4[c]
Diazepam[b]	Valium	2–5 mg 3 times a day	5–20
Lorazepam[b]	Ativan	0.5–1 mg 3 times a day	2–8
Tricyclic antidepressants			
Clomipramine[b]	Anafranil	25 mg twice a day	75–250
Imipramine[b]	Tofranil	10–25 mg/day	75–250
Monoamine oxidase inhibitor			
Phenelzine	Nardil	15 mg/day	45–90

[a]Dosage used in clinical trials but not FDA-approved.
[b]Available generically.
[c]Dosage is FDA-approved.

XIII

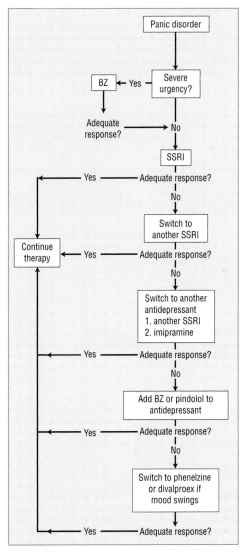

Figure 66–2. Algorithm for the pharmacotherapy of panic disorder.

Antidepressants

- Stimulatory side effects (e.g., anxiety, insomnia, jitteriness, irritability) can occur in TCA- and SSRI-treated patients. This may affect compliance and hinder dose increases. Low initial doses and gradual dose titration may eliminate these effects (Table 66–12).
- Imipramine blocks panic attacks within 4 weeks, but maximal improvement, including reduced anticipatory anxiety and antiphobic response, requires 8 to 12 weeks.

- About 25% of panic patients discontinue TCAs because of side effects.
- All SSRIs eliminate panic attacks in 60% to 80% of patients. The antipanic effect requires 4 weeks, and some patients do not respond until 8 to 12 weeks.
- Low initial doses of **SSRIs**, with gradual titration to the antipanic dose, are required to avoid stimulatory side effects.
- **MAOIs** are reserved for the most difficult or refractory panic disorder patients. Side effects and dietary and drug restrictions affect patient acceptance (see chapter 68 for food and drug restrictions).
  Fluoxetine must be stopped 5 weeks before **phenelzine** (or another MAOI) is started. Other antidepressants should be stopped 2 weeks before phenelzine is started.

Benzodiazepines

- **BZs** are second-line agents except when rapid response is essential. They should not be used as monotherapy in panic disorder patients with a history of depression or **alcohol** or drug abuse. BZs are often used concomitantly with antidepressants in the first weeks to offset the delay in onset of anti-panic effects.
- About 60% to 80% of panic patients respond to BZs, but relapse rates of 50% or higher are common despite slow drug tapering.
- **Alprazolam** and **clonazepam** are the most frequently used of the BZs and are well accepted by patients. Therapeutic response occurs in 1 to 2 weeks. With alprazolam, the duration of action may be as little as 4 to 6 hours with break-through symptoms between dosing. The use of extended-release alprazolam or clonazepam avoids this problem.

Dosing and Administration

- Initial doses should be low. **Imipramine** should be initiated at 10 mg/day at bedtime and slowly increased by 10 mg every 2 to 4 days as tolerated to 75 to 100 mg/day, then increased by 25 mg every 2 to 4 days. Most patients require at least 150 mg/day of imipramine or a combined imipramine-desipramine plasma level of 100 to 150 ng/mL.
- **Paroxetine** is started at 10 mg, with dose increases of 10 mg weekly; the target dose is 40 mg. The starting dose of **fluoxetine** is 5 mg/day, with dosage increases every 2 or 3 days to 10 to 20 mg/day within 2 weeks.
- **Phenelzine** is initiated at 15 mg/day after the evening meal and increased by 15 mg/day every 3 to 4 days until a minimum of 45 mg/day is reached (in divided doses). If improvement is not achieved after 8 to 12 weeks, further titration to as high as 90 mg/day can be undertaken.
- The starting dose of **clonazepam** is 0.25 mg twice daily, with a dose increase to 1 mg by the third day. Increases by 0.25 to 0.5 mg every 3 days to 4 mg/day can be made if needed.
- The starting dose of **alprazolam** is 0.25 to 0.5 mg three times daily (or 0.5 mg once daily of alprazolam extended release), slowly increased over several weeks to an ideal dose. Most patients require 3 to 6 mg/day.
- Usually patients are treated for 12 to 24 months before discontinuation (over 4 to 6 months) is attempted. Many patients require long-term therapy. Successful maintenance with single weekly doses of **fluoxetine** has been described.

Evaluation of Therapeutic Outcomes

- Patients with panic disorder should be seen weekly during the first few weeks to adjust medication doses based on symptom improvement and to monitor side effects. Once stabilized, they can be seen monthly. The Hamilton Rating Scale for Anxiety (score less than or equal to 7 to 10) can be used to measure anxiety, and the Sheehan Disability Scale (with a goal of less than or equal to 1 on each item) can be used to measure for disability. During drug discontinuation the frequency of appointments should be increased.

SOCIAL ANXIETY DISORDER

- SAD patients often respond more slowly and less completely than patients with other anxiety disorders. Treatment can be guided by symptoms, prior treatments, comorbid conditions, and history of substance abuse.
- After improvement, at least 1 year of maintenance treatment is recommended to maintain improvement and decrease the rate of relapse. Long-term treatment may be needed for patients with unresolved symptoms, comorbidity, an early onset of disease, or a prior history of relapse.
- CBT (exposure therapy, cognitive restructuring, relaxation training, and social skills training) and pharmacotherapy are considered equally effective in SAD, but CBT can lead to a greater likelihood of maintaining response after treatment termination.
- CBT and social skills training are effective in children with SAD, but evidence for effectiveness of pharmacotherapy (**fluoxetine, fluvoxamine, sertraline,** and **paroxetine**) is limited to case studies and open-label trials.
- Drugs used in treatment of SAD are shown in Table 66–13, and an algorithm for treatment of SAD is shown in Figure 66–3.
- Venlafaxine and paroxetine were equivalent in efficacy for SAD over a 12-week acute treatment period.
- Response rates of **SSRIs** in SAD ranged from 50% in controlled trials to 80% in open trials. Anxiety, avoidance, and disability are improved.
- With SSRI treatment, the onset of effect is delayed 4 to 8 weeks, and maximum benefit is often not observed until 12 weeks or longer.

TABLE 66–13. Drugs Used in the Treatment of Social Anxiety Disorder

Class/Generic Name	Brand Name	Starting Dose	Dosage Range[a] (mg/day)
Selective serotonin reuptake inhibitors			
Citalopram[b]	Celexa	20 mg/day	20–40
Escitalopram	Lexapro	10 mg/day	10–20
Fluvoxamine[b]	Luvox	50 mg/day	150–300
Paroxetine[b]	Paxil	10–20 mg/day	20–60[c]
Sertraline	Zoloft	25–50 mg/day	50–200[c]
Serotonin-norepinephrine reuptake inhibitor			
Venlafaxine	Effexor XR	75 mg/day	75–225[c]
Benzodiazepine			
Clonazepam[b]	Klonopin	0.25 mg/day	1–3
Monoamine oxidase inhibitor			
Phenelzine[b]	Nardil	15 mg q pm	60–90
Alternate agents			
Buspirone[b,d]	Buspar	10 mg twice per day	45–60
Gabapentin[b]	Neurontin	100 mg 3 times a day	900–3600

XIII

[a]Dosage used in clinical trials but not FDA-approved.
[b]Available generically.
[c]Dosage is FDA-approved.
[d]Used as augmenting agent.

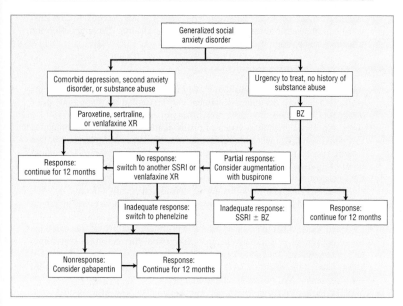

Figure 66–3. Algorithm for the pharmacotherapy of social anxiety disorder (SAD).

- Limited data suggest that **citalopram, escitalopram,** and **fluvoxamine** are also effective for SAD, but that **fluoxetine** is not effective.
- SSRIs are initiated at doses similar to those used for depression. If there is comorbid panic disorder, the SSRI dose should be started at one-fourth to one-half the usual starting dose of antidepressants. The dose should be tapered slowly during discontinuation to decrease the risk of relapse.
- Some patients unresponsive to SSRIs have improved with **venlafaxine.** Response has been reported by week 3.
- **BZs** should be reserved for patients at low risk of substance abuse, those who require rapid relief, or those who have not responded to other therapies.
- **Clonazepam** is the most extensively studied BZ for treatment of generalized SAD. It is effective within 1 to 2 weeks. It improved fear and phobic avoidance, interpersonal sensitivity, fears of negative evaluation, and disability measures. Adverse effects include sexual dysfunction, unsteadiness, dizziness, and poor concentration. It is often given with antidepressants or psychotherapy or both for initial relief.
- BZs must be tapered slowly on discontinuation.
- **Gabapentin** (900 to 3600 mg/day in three divided doses) was effective for SAD, and onset of effect was 2 to 4 weeks.
- β Blockers blunt the peripheral autonomic symptoms of arousal (e.g., rapid heart rate, sweating, blushing, and tremor) and are often used to decrease anxiety in performance-related situations. For specific SAD, 10 to 80 mg of **propranolol** or 25 to 100 mg of **atenolol** can be taken 1 hour before the performance. A test dose should be taken at home on a day before the performance to be sure adverse effects will not be problematic.
- Although effective, **MAOIs** are reserved for treatment-resistant patients because of dietary restrictions, potential drug interactions, and adverse effects.

XIII

- Patients should be monitored for symptom response, adverse effects, and over-all functionality and quality of life. Patients should be seen weekly during dosage titration, and monthly once stabilized. Patients should be asked to keep a diary, and the Liebowitz Social Anxiety Scale can be used to monitor severity of symptoms and symptom change.

POSTTRAUMATIC STRESS DISORDER (PTSD)

- Immediately after the trauma, patients should receive treatment individualized to their presenting symptoms (e.g., non-BZ hypnotic, short courses of CBT). Brief courses of CBT in close proximity to the trauma resulted in lower rates of PTSD 3 and 6 months later.
- If symptoms (e.g., hyperarousal, avoidance, dissociation, insomnia, depression) persist for 3 to 4 weeks and there is social or occupational impairment, patients should receive pharmacotherapy or psychotherapy, or both.
- Psychotherapies for PTSD include anxiety management (e.g., stress-inoculation training, relaxation training, biofeedback, distraction techniques), CBT, insight-oriented therapies, and psychoeducation.
- Table 66–14 shows antidepressants used in the treatment of PTSD, and Figure 66–4 shows an algorithm for the pharmacotherapy of PTSD.
- The **SSRIs** are first-line pharmacotherapy for PTSD. The TCAs and **MAOIs** may also be effective, but they have less favorable side-effect profiles.
- The **SSRIs** are believed to be more effective for numbing symptoms than other drugs. About 60% of **sertraline**-treated patients showed improvement in arousal and avoidance/numbing symptoms, but not reexperiencing symptoms. Similar numbers of patients have been shown to improve on **paroxetine**. **Fluoxetine** was effective in a placebo-controlled trial, and **fluvoxamine** was effective in an open trial. Citalopram may also be effective.
- **Amitriptyline** and **imipramine**, and the MAOI **phenelzine**, can be considered second- or third-line drugs for PTSD after SSRIs have failed. **Trazodone, mirtazapine,** and **venlafaxine** may also be effective.

XIII ◄

TABLE 66–14. Antidepressants Used in the Treatment of Posttraumatic Stress Disorder

Class/Generic Name	Brand Name	Starting Dose	Dosage Range[a] (mg/day)
Selective serotonin reuptake inhibitors			
Citalopram[c,b]	Celexa	20 mg/day	20–40
Escitalopram	Lexapro	10 mg/day	10–20
Fluoxetine[c,b]	Prozac	10–20 mg/day	10–60
Fluvoxamine[c,b]	Luvox	50 mg/day	100–250
Paroxetine[c,b]	Paxil	10–20 mg/day	20–60[c,b]
Sertraline	Zoloft	25–50 mg/day	50–200[c,b]
Other agents			
Amitriptyline	Elavil	25–50 mg/day	75–200
Imipramine	Tofranil	25–50 mg/day	75–200
Lamotrigine	Lamictal	25 mg/day	50–500
Phenelzine	Nardil	15 mg every night	45–75

[a]Dosage used in clinical trials but not FDA-approved.
[b]Available generically.
[c]Dosage is FDA-approved.

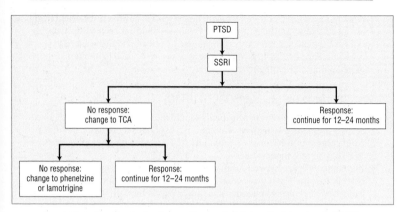

Figure 66–4. Algorithm for the pharmacotherapy of posttraumatic stress disorder (PTSD).

- If there is no improvement in the acute stress response 3 to 4 weeks post trauma, **SSRIs** should be started in a low dose with slow titration upward toward antidepressant doses. Eight to 12 weeks is an adequate duration of treatment to determine response. Clinical response after 3 months of treatment is considered a predictor of long-term outcome.
- Responders to drug therapy should continue treatment for at least 12 months (24 months if residual symptoms persist). When discontinued, drug therapy should be tapered slowly over a period of 1 month or more to reduce the likelihood of relapse.
- Anticonvulsants (**topiramate** and **divalproex sodium**), antiadrenergics drugs (**prazosin**), and antipsychotics (**risperidone, quetiapine**, and **olanzapine**) may be used as augmenting agents in partial responders.
- Patients should be seen weekly for the first month, then biweekly through the second month. During months 3 to 6, patients can be seen monthly, then every 1 to 2 months from months 6 to 12. Responders after 1 year of pharmacotherapy can be seen every 3 months. Patients should be monitored for symptom response, side effects, and treatment adherence.
- A symptom reduction of 75% is a good response, reduction of 25% to 75% is a partial response, and less than 25% symptom response is considered a nonresponse. Remission could be monitored with the Treatment Outcome PTSD Scale (score less than or equal to 5 and the Sheehan Disability Scale (score less than or equal to 1 on each item).

See Chapter 69, Anxiety Disorders I, authored by Cynthia K. Kirkwood and Sarah T. Melton, and Chapter 70, Anxiety Disorders II, authored by Cynthia K. Kirkwood, Eugene H. Makela, and Barbara G. Wells, for a more detailed discussion of this topic.

XIII

Chapter 67

▶ BIPOLAR DISORDER

▶ DEFINITION

Bipolar disorder, previously known as manic-depressive illness, is a cyclical disorder with recurrent extreme fluctuations in mood, energy, and behavior. Diagnosis requires the occurrence of a manic, hypomanic, or mixed episode during the course of the illness.

▶ PATHOPHYSIOLOGY

- Medical conditions, medications, and somatic treatments that may induce mania are shown in Table 67–1.
- Proposed pathophysiologic theories for bipolar disorder are as follows.
  - The kindling and behavioral sensitization model postulates that psychosocial stressors may result in manic or depressive episodes because brain networks are sensitized for exaggerated responses secondary to neurotransmitter imbalances, dysregulation, and voltage-gated ion channel abnormalities.
  - The monoamine hypothesis suggests a functional deficit of norepinephrine (NE), dopamine (DA), and/or serotonin (5-HT) in depression and an excess of catecholamines (NE and DA) in mania.

TABLE 67–1. Secondary Causes of Mania

Medical conditions that induce mania
- CNS disorders (brain tumor, strokes, head injuries, subdural hematoma, multiple sclerosis, systemic lupus erythematosus, temporal lobe seizures, Huntington's disease)
- Infections (encephalitis, neurosyphilis, sepsis, human immunodeficiency virus)
- Electrolyte or metabolic abnormalities (calcium or sodium fluctuations, hyper- or hypoglycemia)
- Endocrine or hormonal dysregulation (Addison's disease, Cushing's disease, hyper- or hypothyroidism, menstrual-related or pregnancy-related or perimenopausal mood disorders)
- Vitamin and nutritional deficiencies (essential amino acids, essential fatty acids, vitamin B_{12})

Medications or drugs that induce mania
- Alcohol intoxication
- Drug withdrawal states (alcohol, α_2-adrenergic agonists, antidepressants, barbiturates, benzodiazepines, opiates)
- Antidepressants (MAOIs, TCAs, 5-HT and/or NE and/or DA reuptake inhibitors, 5-HT antagonists)
- DA-augmenting agents (CNS stimulants: amphetamines, cocaine, sympathomimetics; DA agonists, releasers, and reuptake inhibitors)
- Hallucinogens (LSD, PCP)
- Marijuana intoxication precipitates psychosis, paranoid thoughts, anxiety, and restlessness
- NE-augmenting agents (α_2-adrenergic antagonists, β agonists, NE reuptake inhibitors)
- Steroids (anabolic, adrenocorticotropic hormone, corticosteroids)
- Thyroid preparations
- Xanthines (caffeine, theophylline)
- Over-the-counter weight loss agents and decongestants (ephedra, pseudoephedrine)
- Herbal products (St. John's wort)

Somatic therapies that induce mania
- Bright light therapy
- Sleep deprivation

CNS, central nervous system; DA, dopamine; 5-HT, serotonin; LSD, lysergic acid diethylamide; MAOI, monoamine oxidase inhibitor; NE, norepinephrine; PCP, phencyclidine; TCA, tricyclic antidepressant.

- The permissive hypothesis posits that central nervous system (CNS) 5-HT is low in both mania and depression, and superimposed low NE causes depression and high NE causes mania.
- The dysregulation hypothesis states that mood disorders may be caused by a dysregulation between neurotransmitter systems, neuropeptides, hormones, and secondary messenger systems.
- A γ-aminobutyric acid (GABA) deficiency hypothesis is proposed for mania since it inhibits NE and DA activity.
- Glutamate and aspartate, excitatory amino acid neurotransmitters, may be overactive and thus cause manic episodes.
- Cholinergic underactivity has been proposed to cause mania and overactivity of acetylcholine to cause depression. Acetylcholine is an antagonist of the catecholamine system and contributes to the interaction between phosphatidylinositol and phosphatidylcholine second messenger systems.
- Abnormal calcium, potassium, and sodium homeostasis may alter neurotransmitter release and the second messenger system.
- Hormonal changes during the menstrual cycle, postpartum period, and perimenopausal phase may contribute to mood dysregulation.
- L-tryptophan or 5-HT deficiency and changes in the light-dark cycle may result in reduced melatonin secretion from the pineal gland, which disrupts the sleep-wake cycle, alters circadian rhythms, and causes seasonal affective changes. Circadian rhythm desynchronization may cause diurnal variations in mood and seasonal recurrences of episodes.

▶ CLINICAL PRESENTATION AND DIAGNOSIS

The Diagnostic and Statistical Manual of Mental Disorders, 4th ed., text revision (DSM-IV-TR) classifies bipolar disorders as (1) bipolar I, (2) bipolar II, (3) cyclothymic disorder, and (4) bipolar disorder not otherwise specified (NOS). Table 67–2 defines mood disorders by type of episode. Table 67–3 describes the evaluation and diagnostic criteria for mood disorders.

▶ XIII MAJOR DEPRESSIVE EPISODE

In bipolar depression patients have an increased suicide risk and often have mood lability, hypersomnia, low energy, psychomotor retardation, cognitive impairments, anhedonia, decreased sexual activity, slowed speech, carbohydrate craving, and weight gain.

MANIC EPISODE

- Acute mania usually begins abruptly and symptoms increase over several days. The severe stages may include bizarre behavior, hallucinations, and paranoid or grandiose delusions. There is marked impairment in functioning or the need for hospitalization.
- Manic episodes may be precipitated by stressors, sleep deprivation, antidepressants, CNS stimulants, or bright light.

HYPOMANIC EPISODE

- Hypomanic episodes are described in Table 67–3. There is no marked impairment in social or occupational functioning, no delusions, and no hallucinations.
- During a hypomanic episode, some patients may be more productive and creative than usual, but 5% to 15% of patients may rapidly switch to a manic episode.

TABLE 67–2. Mood Disorders Defined by Episodes

Disorder Subtype	Episode(s)[a]
Major depressive disorder, single episode	Major depressive episode
Major depressive disorder, recurrent	Two or more major depressive episodes
Bipolar disorder, type I[b]	Major depressive episode + manic or mixed episode
Bipolar disorder, type II[c]	Major depressive episode + hypomanic episode
Dysthymic disorder	Chronic subsyndromal depressive episodes
Cyclothymic disorder[d]	Chronic fluctuations between subsyndromal depressive and hypomanic episodes (2 yr for adults and 1 yr for children and adolescents)
Mood disorder due to a general medical condition	Disturbance in mood that is secondary to a general medical condition (see Table 67–1)
Substance-induced mood disorder	Disturbance in mood that is secondary to the effects of a substance (e.g., medication, toxin, drug abuse, somatic treatments; see Table 67–1)
Bipolar disorder not otherwise specified	Mood states do not meet criteria for any specific bipolar disorder

[a]The length and severity of a mood episode and the interval between episodes varies from patient to patient. Manic episodes are usually briefer and end more abruptly than major depressive episodes. The average length of untreated manic episodes ranges from 4 to 13 months. Episodes may occur regularly (at the same time or season of the year) and often cluster at 12-month intervals. Women have more depressive episodes than manic episodes, whereas men have a more even distribution of episodes.
[b]For bipolar I disorder, 90% of individuals who experience a manic episode later have multiple recurrent major depressive, manic, hypomanic, or mixed episodes alternating with a normal mood state.
[c]Approximately 5–15% of patients with bipolar II disorder will develop a manic episode over a 5-year period. If a manic or mixed episode develops in a patient with bipolar II disorder, the diagnosis is changed to bipolar I disorder.
[d]Patients with cyclothymic disorder have a 15 to 50% risk of later developing a bipolar I or II disorder.

MIXED EPISODE

- Mixed episodes occur in up to 40% of all episodes, are often difficult to diagnose and treat, and are more common in younger and older patients and females.
- Patients with mixed states often have comorbid alcohol and substance abuse, severe anxiety symptoms, a higher suicide rate, and a poorer prognosis.

XIII

▶ COURSE OF ILLNESS

- The average age of onset of a first manic episode is 21 years. More than 80% of patients have more than four episodes during their lifetime, and the interval between episodes decreases with age. Usually there is normal functioning between episodes.
- Rapid cyclers (10% to 20% of bipolar patients) have four or more episodes per year (major depressive, manic, mixed, or hypomanic). Rapid-cycling and mixed states are associated with a poorer prognosis and nonresponse to anti-manic agents. Risk factors for rapid cycling include biologic rhythm dysregu-lation, antidepressant or stimulant use, hypothyroidism, and premenstrual and postpartum states.
- Women have more depressive than manic episodes, but men have an equal number of each.
- Suicide attempts occur in up to 50% of patients with bipolar disorder, and ap-proximately 10% to 19% of individuals with bipolar I disorder commit suicide. Bipolar II patients may be more likely than bipolar I patients to attempt suicide.
- Approximately 10% to 15% of adolescents with recurrent major depressive episodes subsequently have an episode of mania or hypomania.

TABLE 67–3. Evaluation and Diagnostic Criteria of Mood Episodes

Diagnostic work-up depends on clinical presentation and findings	• Mental status examination • Psychiatric, medical, and medication history • Physical and neurological examination • Basic laboratory tests: complete blood count, blood chemistry screen, thyroid function, urinalysis, urine drug screen • Psychological testing • Brain imaging: magnetic resonance imaging and functional scan; alternative: computed tomography scan, positron emission tomography scan • Lumbar puncture • Electroencephalogram

Diagnosis

Episode	Impairment of Functioning or Need for Hospitalization[a]	DSM-IV-TR Criteria[b]
Major depressive	Yes	>2-wk period of either depressed mood or loss of interest or pleasure in normal activities, associated with at least five of the following symptoms: • Depressed, sad mood (adults); may be irritable mood in children • Decreased interest and pleasure in normal activities • Decreased appetite, weight loss • Insomnia or hypersomnia • Psychomotor retardation or agitation • Decreased energy or fatigue • Feelings of guilt or worthlessness • Impaired concentration and decision making • Suicidal thoughts or attempts
Manic	Yes	>1-wk period of abnormal and persistent elevated mood (expansive or irritable), associated with at least three of the following symptoms (four if the mood is only irritable): • Inflated self-esteem (grandiosity) • Decreased need for sleep • Increased talking (pressure of speech) • Racing thoughts (flight of ideas) • Distractible (poor attention) • Increased activity (either socially, at work, or sexually) or increased motor activity or agitation • Excessive involvement in activities that are pleasurable but have a high risk for serious consequences (buying sprees, sexual indiscretions, poor judgment in business ventures)

XIII

Continued

TABLE 67–3. (Continued)

Hypomanic	No	At least 4 days of abnormal and persistent elevated mood (expansive or irritable); associated with at least three of the following symptoms (four if the mood is only irritable):
		• Inflated self-esteem (grandiosity)
		• Decreased need for sleep
		• Increased talking (pressure of speech)
		• Racing thoughts (flight of ideas)
		• Increased activity (either socially, at work, or sexually) or increased motor activity or agitation
		• Excessive involvement in activities that are pleasurable but have a high risk for serious consequences (buying sprees, sexual indiscretions, poor judgment in business ventures)
Mixed	Yes	Criteria for both a major depressive episode and manic episode (except for duration) occur nearly every day for at least a 1-wk period
Rapid cycling	Yes	>4 Major depressive or manic episodes (manic, mixed, or hypomanic) in 12 months

[a]Impairment in social or occupational functioning; need for hospitalization due to potential self-harm, harm to others, or psychotic symptoms.

[b]The disorder is not due to a medical condition (e.g., hypothyroidism) or substance-induced disorder (e.g., antidepressant treatment, medications, electroconvulsive therapy).

- Alcohol and drug abuse or dependence may occur in 46% and 41% of bipolar patients, respectively.

▶ DIAGNOSIS

The diagnosis of mood episodes is guided by the criteria shown in Table 67–3.

XIII

▶ DESIRED OUTCOME

The goals of treatment include resolution of symptoms, prevention of future episodes, minimization of adverse drug effects, good compliance with treatment, patient education about the disorder and treatment approaches, and avoidance of stressors that may precipitate an acute episode.

▶ TREATMENT

GENERAL APPROACH

An example treatment algorithm for the acute treatment of mood episodes in patients with bipolar I disorder is shown in Table 67–4.

NONPHARMACOLOGIC THERAPY

- Psychoeducation about bipolar disorder, treatment, and monitoring for the patient and family

TABLE 67–4. Algorithm and Guidelines for the Acute Treatment of Mood Episodes in Patients with Bipolar I Disorder

Acute Manic or Mixed Episode	Acute Depressive Episode
General guidelines • Assess for secondary causes of mania or mixed states (e.g., alcohol or drug use) • Taper off antidepressants, stimulants, and caffeine if possible • Treat substance abuse • Encourage good nutrition (with regular protein and essential fatty acid intake), exercise, adequate sleep, stress reduction, and psychosocial therapy • Optimize the dose of mood stabilizing medication(s) before adding on benzodiazepines; if psychotic features are present, add on antipsychotic; ECT used for severe or treatment-resistant manic/mixed episodes or psychotic features	**General guidelines** • Assess for secondary causes of depression (e.g., alcohol or drug use) • Taper off antipsychotics, benzodiazepines or sedative-hypnotic agents if possible • Treat substance abuse • Encourage good nutrition (with regular protein and essential fatty acid intake), exercise, adequate sleep, stress reduction, and psychosocial therapy • Optimize the dose of mood stabilizing medication(s) before adding on lithium, lamotrigine or antidepressant (e.g., bupropion or an SSRI); if psychotic features are present, add on an antipsychotic; ECT used for severe or treatment-resistant depressive episodes or for psychosis or catatonia
Mild to moderate symptoms of mania or mixed episode First, initiate and/or optimize mood-stabilizing medication: lithium[a] or valproate[a] or atypical antipsychotic (e.g., olanzapine, quetiapine, risperidone) Alternative anticonvulsants: carbamazepine, lamotrigine,[b] or oxcarbazepine Second, if response is inadequate, consider adding a benzodiazepine (lorazepam or clonazepam) for short-term adjunctive treatment of agitation or insomnia if needed	**Mild to moderate symptoms of depressive episode** First, initiate and/or optimize mood-stabilizing medication: lithium[a] or lamotrigine[b] Alternative anticonvulsants: carbamazepine, oxcarbazepine, or valproate
Moderate to severe symptoms of mania or mixed episode First, two-drug combinations: lithium[a] or valproate[a] **plus** an atypical antipsychotic (e.g., olanzapine, quetiapine, risperidone) for short-term adjunctive treatment of psychotic features (e.g., delusions or hallucinations) Alternative anticonvulsants: carbamazepine, lamotrigine,[b] or oxcarbazepine Second, if response is inadequate, consider adding a benzodiazepine (lorazepam or clonazepam) for short-term adjunctive treatment of agitation or insomnia if needed; lorazepam is recommended for catatonia	**Moderate to severe symptoms of depressive episode** First, two-drug combinations: lithium[a] or lamotrigine[a] **plus** an antidepressant[c]; lithium **plus** lamotrigine Alternative anticonvulsants: carbamazepine, oxcarbazepine, or valproate Second, if response is inadequate, consider adding an atypical antipsychotic for short-term adjunctive treatment of psychotic features (e.g., delusions or hallucinations) if needed

Third, if response is inadequate, consider a two-drug combination:

- Lithium **plus** an anticonvulsant or an atypical antipsychotic
- Anticonvulsant **plus** an anticonvulsant or atypical antipsychotic

Third, if response is inadequate, consider a three-drug combination:

- Lithium **plus** an anticonvulsant **plus** an atypical antipsychotic
- Anticonvulsant **plus** an anticonvulsant **plus** an atypical antipsychotic

Fourth, if response is inadequate, consider ECT for mania with psychosis or catatonia,[d] or add clozapine for treatment-refractory illness

Fifth, if response is inadequate, consider adding adjunctive therapies[e]

Third, if response is inadequate, consider a three-drug combination:

- Lithium **plus** an anticonvulsant **plus** an antidepressant
- Lamotrigine[b] **plus** an anticonvulsant **plus** an antidepressant

Fourth, if response is inadequate, consider ECT for treatment-refractory illness and depression with psychosis or catatonia[d]

Fifth, if response is inadequate, consider adding adjunctive therapies[e]

---

[a] Utilize standard therapeutic serum concentration ranges; if partial response or breakthrough episode, adjust dose to achieve higher serum concentrations without causing intolerable adverse effects; valproate is preferred over lithium for mixed episodes and rapid cycling; lithium and/or lamotrigine is preferred over valproate for bipolar depression.

[b] Lamotrigine is not approved for the acute treatment of depression, and the dose must be started low and slowly titrated up to decrease adverse effects if used for maintenance therapy of bipolar I disorder. A drug interaction and a severe dermatologic rash may occur when lamotrigine is combined with valproate (i.e., lamotrigine doses must be halved from standard dosing titration).

[c] Antidepressant monotherapy is not recommended for bipolar depression. Bupropion, selective serotonin reuptake inhibitors (SSRIs; e.g., citalopram, escitalopram, or sertraline), and serotonin–norepinephrine reuptake inhibitors (SNRIs; e.g., venlafaxine) have shown good efficacy and fewer adverse effects in the treatment of unipolar depression; monoamine oxidase inhibitors (MAOIs) and tricyclic antidepressants (TCAs) have more adverse effects (e.g., weight gain) and may have a higher risk of causing antidepressant-induced mania; fluoxetine, fluvoxamine, nefazodone, and paroxetine inhibit liver metabolism and should be used with caution in patients on concomitant medications that require cytochrome P450 clearance; paroxetine and venlafaxine have a higher risk for causing a discontinuation syndrome.

[d] Electroconvulsive therapy (ECT) is used for severe mania or depression during pregnancy and for mixed episodes; prior to treatment, anticonvulsants, lithium, and benzodiazepines should be tapered off to maximize therapy and minimize adverse effects.

[e] There are minimal or no efficacy data for some adjunctive (add-on) therapies; α2-adrenergic agonists, calcium channel blockers, gabapentin, tiagabine, topiramate, and zonisamide; topiramate may have efficacy as an adjunctive agent with standard agents for maintenance therapy, based on initial trials.

- Early signs and symptoms of mania and depression and charting mood changes
- Importance of compliance with therapy
- Psychosocial or physical stressors that may precipitate an episode
- Limiting substances and drugs that can trigger mood episodes
- Strategies for coping with stressful life events
- Development of a crisis intervention plan
- Psychotherapy (e.g., individual, group, and family), interpersonal therapy, and/or cognitive behavioral therapy
- Stress reduction techniques, relaxation therapy, massage, yoga, etc.
- Sleep (regular bedtime and awake schedule; avoid alcohol or caffeine intake prior to bedtime)
- Nutrition (regular intake of protein-rich foods or drinks and essential fatty acids; supplemental vitamins and minerals)
- Exercise (regular aerobic and weight training at least 3 times a week)
- The use of bilateral electroconvulsive therapy (ECT) for severe mania or mixed episodes, psychotic depression, or rapid cycling is still considered the best acute treatment approach (approximately 80% response rate) for those patients who do not respond to first-line mood stabilizers such as lithium and valproate.

PHARMACOLOGIC THERAPY

- Use an established mood stabilizer for the treatment of an acute mood episode and for continuation therapy. (see Table 68–9 for efficacy ratings and recommendations based on clinical trials, guidelines, and algorithms).
  - If a patient responded well to a specific pharmacologic agent in the past and it was well tolerated, then use the same treatment again.
  - If a patient had intolerance or adverse reactions to a specific pharmacologic agent in the past or has a strong preference against an agent, then do not use it.
  - It is preferable to slowly taper off a medication than to abruptly discontinue it.
- There are no specific guidelines for when to switch therapies or when combination approaches should be started.
  - In general, if a patient with mania or mixed states has not responded within 2 to 4 weeks with an established mood stabilizer (e.g., lithium, lamotrigine, or valproate), a second first-line agent can be added to the regimen for augmentation; alternative treatment options include adding carbamazepine, oxcarbazepine, or an atypical antipsychotic in lieu of a first-line agent.
  - Patients who are nonresponsive or intolerant to adverse effects of first-line pharmacologic approaches should be switched to another agent; when necessary, electroconvulsive therapy may be used to rapidly reduce manic or depressive symptoms and may be used for maintenance treatment.
  - Changes in medication therapies and doses should be based on treatment response (or change in symptoms), tolerability of side effects, serum drug levels when applicable, and avoidance of drug interactions.
- For patients with rapid cycling (more than 4 mood episodes per year):
  - Evaluate and treat underlying hypothyroidism, hormonal imbalance, or drug or alcohol abuse.
  - For antidepressant-induced rapid cycling, taper off antidepressant and other agents that increase norepinephrine or dopamine activity (e.g., central nervous system stimulants, sympathomimetics, and caffeine).
- Use combination therapies for patients who are partially responsive or unresponsive to monotherapy with an established mood stabilizer.

XIII

- Combination therapies may be needed for the treatment of acute mania or mixed episodes, breakthrough depression, and rapid cycling
- Reassessment of combination and adjunctive therapies should be done routinely and unnecessary medications should be tapered off gradually and discontinued.
- Use antidepressants or stimulants cautiously in patients with rapid cycling or with a history of antidepressant-induced mania; patients with recurrent depressive episodes may need long-term antidepressant therapy to minimize relapses.
- Some mood stabilizers have an increased teratogenic risk during the first trimester (e.g., carbamazepine, lithium, oxcarbazepine, and valproate); this risk is greater if the patient is on multiple agents.
  - Prenatal monitoring suggested: maternal serum α -fetoprotein screening for neural tube defects before the twentieth week of gestation and high-resolution ultrasound at 16 to 18 weeks' gestation to detect cardiac abnormalities; fetal echocardiography is recommended if lithium is used during the first trimester.
  - Routine serum level monitoring of medications (when applicable) is recommended during pregnancy, with dosage adjustments if indicated.
- Electroconvulsive therapy may be considered for patients with severe or treatment-resistant mania or depression and in pregnant women; maintenance drug therapy may be considered for patients whose acute episodes responded to electroconvulsive therapy.
- After the resolution of the mood episodes, maintenance treatment is generally recommended for both bipolar I and II disorder: lithium or valproate (first choices) and carbamazepine, lamotrigine, and oxcarbazepine (alternative choices).
  - Patients should be maintained on a 6-month continuation phase of the mood stabilizer while the adjunctive treatment(s) are tapered and discontinued if possible.
  - Patients who have had only one manic episode and who have responded to treatment should be continued on a mood stabilizer for 12 months, then gradually tapered off over several months (usually after 6 months of complete remission).
- Lifetime prophylaxis with a mood stabilizer is recommended for: XIII ◄
  - Bipolar I: after two manic episodes, after one severe manic episode, in the presence of a strong family history of bipolar disorder or major depressive disorder, with frequent episodes (more than one per year), or with rapid onset of manic episodes.
  - Bipolar II: after three hypomanic episodes or if the patient becomes hypomanic with antidepressant therapy.

Treatments of First Choice

- **Lithium**, **Divalproex sodium** (**valproate**), and **olanzapine** are currently approved by the Food and Drug Administration (FDA) for treatment of acute mania in bipolar I. Lithium and **lamotrigine** are approved for maintenance treatment of bipolar I disorder.
- Lithium is the drug of choice for classic bipolar disorder, whereas valproate has better efficacy for mixed states and rapid cycling compared with lithium.
- **Aripiprazole**, **quetiapine**, **risperidone**, and **ziprasidone** have been approved by the FDA for acute mania (monotherapy and adjunctive to lithium or valproate).
- Combination therapies (e.g., lithium plus valproate or **carbamazepine**; lithium or valproate plus an atypical antipsychotic) may provide better acute response

and prevention of relapse than monotherapy in some patients with mixes states or rapid cycling.
- Useful guidelines include the following: Practice Guideline for the Treatment of Patients with Bipolar Disorder (Revision) published by the American Psychiatric Association; Texas Medication Algorithm Project; World Federation of Societies of Biological Psychiatry; Practice Parameters for the Assessment and Treatment of Children and Adolescents with Bipolar Disorder by the American Academy of Child and Adolescent Psychiatry.
- Divalproex is now the most prescribed mood stabilizer in the United States.

Alternative Treatments
- High potency benzodiazepines (e.g., **clonazepam** and **lorazepam**) are common alternatives to antipsychotics for agitation, anxiety, panic, and insomnia. A relative contraindication for long-term benzodiazepines is drug and alcohol abuse or dependency.
- Tricyclic antidepressants are associated with an increased risk of inducing mania in bipolar I disorder and possibly cause rapid cycling. Some guidelines recommend avoiding antidepressants in the treatment of bipolar depression or limiting their use to brief intervals, but evidence suggests that coadministration of therapeutic doses of mood stabilizers can reduce the risk of antidepressant-induced switching. Generally the antidepressant should be withdrawn 2 to 6 months after remission and the patients maintained on a mood stabilizer.
- High doses of levothyroxine sodium (0.15 to 0.4 mcg/day) have been reported to have mood stabilizing properties in rapid-cycling bipolar patients when combined with mood-stabilizing agents.

Special Populations
- Table 67–5 shows treatment approaches in special populations of bipolar patients.
- Approximately 20% to 50% of women with bipolar disorder relapse postpartum; prophylaxis with mood stabilizers is recommended immediately postpartum to decrease the risk of relapse.

XIII Drug Class Information
- Product information, dosing and administration, clinical use, and proposed mechanisms of action for agents used for bipolar disorder are shown in Table 67–6.
- Pharmacokinetics and recommended therapeutic serum concentrations of lithium and selected anticonvulsants are shown in Table 67–7.
- Guidelines for baseline and routine laboratory testing and monitoring for patients receiving lithium and selected anticonvulsants are shown in Table 67–8.
- Efficacy ratings of drugs used in treating bipolar I disorder are shown in Table 67–9.

Adverse Drug Effects
Monitoring and management of adverse effects is an essential component of treatment to ensure tolerability and treatment adherence.

ANTIPSYCHOTICS
For a summary of antipsychotic adverse effects refer to Chapter 69.

CARBAMAZEPINE
For a summary of carbamazepine adverse effects refer to Chapter 50.

TABLE 67–5. Approaches to Treating Bipolar Disorder in Special Populations and with Comorbidities

Population Type or Comorbid Condition	First-Line Therapies	Second-Line Therapies
Aggression/violence/homicidal	Hospitalization: optimize dose and/or serum concentrations of lithium or valproate, then lithium or valproate ± atypical antipsychotic[a] Alternative: carbamazepine or oxcarbazepine ± atypical antipsychotic[a]	Lithium ± valproate ± atypical antipsychotic[a] ± benzodiazepines Alternative: carbamazepine or oxcarbazepine ± atypical antipsychotic[a] ± benzodiazepines
Anxiety disorders (panic or obsessive-compulsive disorder)	Valproate or add antidepressant (e.g., 5-HT reuptake inhibitor)	Adjunctive: benzodiazepine (short-term)
Attention deficit hyperactivity disorder	Add bupropion or atomoxetine; DA or NE augmenting agents may exacerbate mood changes and make it difficult to monitor bipolar disorder	CNS stimulants (use cautiously): amphetamine, dextroamphetamine, methylphenidate
Breast-feeding	All medications used in the treatment of bipolar disorder are secreted in breast milk, thus the risks versus benefits must be weighed.	There are no recommendations or treatment guidelines at this time. Valproate or carbamazepine are compatible with breast-feeding, but potential risks should be considered.
Cardiac disease/heart failure	Valproate: monitor for hypertension, tachycardia, peripheral edema	Calcium channel blocker: monitor for bradycardia, hypotension, peripheral edema ECT for acute treatment
Catatonia (mutism, motor excitement, and stereotypic movements)	Benzodiazepines (lorazepam) for acute treatment	
Children and adolescents	Lithium or valproate: maintenance treatment should continue for a minimum of 18 months after stabilization to decrease risk of relapse	Carbamazepine or oxcarbazepine. Alternative: atypical antipsychotics (for psychosis) or combination therapies

Continued

TABLE 67–5. (Continued)

Population Type or Comorbid Condition	First-Line Therapies	Second-Line Therapies
Geriatric patients (>65 yr of age and in good health)	Rule out general medical conditions, medications, or substance use that may cause a manic syndrome; valproate and lithium require lower doses, regular laboratory and serum concentration monitoring; concomitant medications and medical conditions may alter the metabolism and excretion of medications	Carbamazepine or oxcarbazepine induce liver enzymes and may affect the metabolism and blood levels of concomitant medications; lithium, antipsychotics, and benzodiazepines increase the risk of adverse effects and cognitive impairment
Liver disease	Lithium: not metabolized by the liver Alternative: gabapentin (no efficacy data)	All anticonvulsants (except gabapentin), atypical antipsychotics, benzodiazepines, and calcium channel blockers require liver metabolism, and dosage adjustments may be needed (e.g., 25–50% reduction of normal doses)
Neurologic disorders (migraine, seizures)	Valproate	Carbamazepine or oxcarbazepine Alternative: lamotrigine
Pregnancy[a]	Pregnancy should be planned in consultation with a psychiatrist and obstetrician to weigh risks versus benefits of treatment options (e.g., discontinuing medications before conception or at the beginning of pregnancy, discontinuing medications only for the first trimester, or continuing medications throughout pregnancy). Medications should be tapered off slowly to avoid recurrent mood episodes. Prophylactic medications such as lithium or valproate may prevent postpartum mood episodes. Alternative: ECT used for patients with severe mania, mixed states, depression, or psychosis.	Acute mania or mixed episode: first choice: lithium After first trimester: carbamazepine, lamotrigine, oxcarbazepine, or valproate Second choice: benzodiazepine (lorazepam) Third choice: calcium channel blocker With psychosis: first choice: adjunctive high-potency typical antipsychotic (haloperidol, perphenazine, thiothixene, or trifluoperazine) Second choice: adjunctive atypical antipsychotic[b] Acute depression: First choice: adjunctive 5-HT or 5-HT/NE reuptake inhibitors Second choice: adjunctive bupropion

Psychosis (delusions, hallucinations)	Optimize dose and/or serum concentrations of lithium or anticonvulsant Alternative: add atypical or typical antipsychotic for short-term adjunctive therapy	ECT
Renal disease or impairment	Carbamazepine and valproate: if creatinine clearance is <10 mL/min, administer 75% of standard dose; combining medications in patients with renal impairment should be done cautiously; use agents that have a therapeutic serum concentration range for blood level monitoring	Oxcarbazepine: initiate dosing at one-half the usually starting dose (300 mg/day) and increase slowly
Substance use disorders (e.g., alcohol, cocaine, methamphetamine)	Dual-diagnosis treatment program: substance abuse plus standard pharmacologic/nonpharmacologic treatments for bipolar disorder; hepatic dysfunction from chronic alcohol abuse or from hepatitis may alter the metabolism of some agents	Lithium or valproate Alternative: carbamazepine or oxcarbazepine or topiramate (alcohol dependence)
Suicidal behavior or attempts	Lithium: long-term treatment associated with reduction of suicide risk and mortality	

[a] Olanzapine, quetiapine, and risperidone are preferred; alternative atypicals: aripiprazole and ziprasidone are newer agents and may initially cause akathisia-like reactions; clozapine is usually reserved for treatment-resistant mania or mixed states.

[b] Teratogenic ratings: gabapentin, lamotrigine, olanzapine, oxcarbazepine, quetiapine, risperidone, topiramate, and verapamil are category C; carbamazepine, clonazepam, lithium, lorazepam, and valproate are category D. Lithium may have fewer teratogenic effects than previously thought and may be considered during the first trimester. Carbamazepine, oxcarbazepine, and topiramate increase the metabolism of oral contraceptives and may make them ineffective.

DA, dopamine; ECT, electroconvulsive therapy; 5-HT, serotonin; NE, norepinephrine.

TABLE 67–6. Product Formulations, Dosage and Administration, Clinical Use, and Proposed Mechanism of Action of Agents Used in the Treatment of Bipolar Disorder.

Generic Name	Trade Name	Formulations	Dosage and Administration	Clinical Use	Proposed Mechanism of Action
Lithium salts: FDA-approved for bipolar disorder					
Lithium carbonate	Eskalith	Capsule: 300 mg	900–2400 mg/day in 2–4 divided doses, preferably with meals. There is wide variation in the dosage needed to achieve therapeutic response and trough serum lithium concentration (i.e., 0.6–1.2 mEq/L for maintenance therapy and 1.0–1.2 mEq/L for acute mood episodes taken 8–12 h after the last dose).	Use alone or in combination with other drugs (e.g., valproate, carbamazepine, antipsychotics) for the acute treatment of mania and for maintenance treatment.	• Normalizes or inhibits secondary messenger systems (e.g., inhibits phosphoinositide and adenylate cyclase signaling; normalizes guanine nucleotide-binding protein [G protein] signal transduction system)
	Eskalith CR	Extended-release tablet: 450 mg			• Decreases 5-HT reuptake and increases postsynaptic 5-HT receptor sensitivity
	Lithobid	Extended-release tablet: 300 mg			• Inhibits the synthesis of DA, decreases the number of β-adrenergic receptors and inhibits DA_2 and β-adrenergic receptor supersensitivity
	Generic	Tablet: 300 mg (scored) Capsule: 150, 300, 600 mg			• Enhances GABAergic activity and normalizes GABA levels
Lithium citrate	Cibalith-S	8 mEq/5 mL			• Reduces glutaminergic activity (e.g., increases glutamate uptake) with chronic therapy
					• Decreases Ca^+ transport into cells, interferes with Ca^+-Na^+ active transport system, increases renal tubular reabsorption of Ca^+ and increases serum Ca^+ and parathyroid concentrations
					• Increases choline in red blood cells and potentiates the cholinergic secondary messenger system

Anticonvulsants: FDA-approved for bipolar disorder

Divalproex sodium	Depakote	Enteric-coated, delayed-release tablet: 125, 250, 500 mg Sprinkle capsule: 125 mg	750–3000 mg/day (20–60 mg/kg/day) in 2–3 divided doses for delayed-release divalproex or valproic acid.	Use alone or in combination with other drugs (e.g., lithium, carbamazepine, antipsychotics) for the acute treatment of mania and for maintenance treatment.	• Increases GABA levels in plasma and CNS; inhibits GABA catabolism, increases synthesis, and release; may prevent GABA reuptake; enhances the action of GABA at the GABA^a receptor
	Depakote ER	Enteric-coated extended release tablet: 250, 500 mg	Extended-release divalproex may be given once daily at bedtime after stabilization.	Use caution when combining with lamotrigine due to potential drug interaction.	• Normalizes Na$^+$ and Ca$^+$ channels • Reduces intracellular inositol and protein kinase C isozymes
Valproic acid	Depakene	Capsule: 250 mg	A loading dose of divalproex (20–30 mg/kg/day) can be given, then 20 mg/kg/day and titrated to a serum concentration of 50–125 mcg/mL.		• May modulate gene expression • Antikindling properties may decrease rapid cycling and mixed states
Valproate sodium	Depakene	Syrup: 250 mg/5 mL			• Blocks voltage-sensitive Na$^+$ and Ca$^+$ channels
Lamotrigine	Lamictal	Tablet: 25, 100, 150, 200 mg	50–400 mg/day in divided doses.	Use alone or in combination with other drugs (e.g., lithium, carbamazepine) for long-term maintenance treatment for bipolar I disorder.	• Modulates or decreases presynaptic aspartate and glutamate release
		Chewable tablet: 2, 5, 25 mg	Dosage should be slowly increased (e.g., 25 mg/day for 2 wk, then 50 mg/day for weeks 3 and 4, then 50-mg/day increments at weekly intervals up to 200 mg/day). When combined with valproate, initial and titration dosing should be decreased by 50% to minimize the risk of a serious rash.	Lamotrigine may have efficacy for prevention of bipolar depression.	• Antikindling properties may decrease rapid cycling and mixed states

Continued

TABLE 67–6. (Continued)

Generic Generic Name	Trade Name	Formulations	Dosage and Dosage and Administration	Clinical Use	Proposed Mechanism Proposed Mechanism of Action
Anticonvulsants: Not FDA-approved for bipolar disorder					

Carbamazepine	Tegretol, Epitol
	Tegretol
	
	Tegretol-XR
	
	Carbatrol
		Tablet: 200 mg
		Chewable tablet: 100 mg
		Suspension: 100 mg/5 mL
		Extended-release tablet:
		100, 200, 400 mg
		Extended-release capsule:
		200, 300 mg
			200–1800 mg/day in 2–4 divided doses.
			Dosage should be slowly increased
			according to response and adverse
			effects (e.g., 100–200 mg twice daily
			and increase by 200 mg/day at weekly
			intervals).
			Administer conventional tablets and
			suspension with meals.
			Extended-release tablets should be
			swallowed whole and not be broken or
			chewed.
			Carbatrol capsules may be opened and
			contents sprinkled over food.
				Use alone or in combination with other
				drugs (e.g., lithium, valproate,
				antipsychotics) for the acute and
				long-term maintenance treatment of
				mania or mixed episodes for bipolar I
				disorder. APA guidelines recommend
				reserving it for patients unable to
				tolerate or who have inadequate
				response to lithium or valproate.
					• Blocks voltage-sensitive Na^+
					  channels
					• Stimulates the release of antidiuretic
					  hormone and decreases Na^+ serum
					  concentrations
					• Blocks Ca^+ influx through the NMDA
					  glutamate receptor and decreases
					  Ca^+ serum concentrations
					• Modulates presynaptic aspartate and
					  glutamate release
					• Antikindling properties may decrease
					  rapid cycling and mixed states

Oxcarbazepine	Trileptal	Tablet: 150, 300, 600 mg
		Suspension: 300 mg/5 mL
			300–1200 mg/day in two divided doses.
			Dosage should be slowly adjusted up and
			down according to response and
			adverse effects (e.g., 150–300 mg twice
			daily and increase by 300–600 mg/day
			at weekly intervals).
				May have fewer adverse effects and be
				better tolerated than carbamazepine
					• Oxcarbazepine and its monohydroxy
					  metabolite increase K^+ conductance;
					  modulates the activity of high-voltage
					  activated Ca^+ channels; and blocks
					  Na^+ channels

Clonazepam	Klonopin	Tablet: 0.5, 1, 2 mg	0.5–20 mg/day in divided doses or one
			dose at bedtime.
			Dosage should be slowly adjusted up and
			down according to response and
			adverse effects.
				Use in combination with other drugs
				(e.g., antipsychotics, lithium,
				valproate) for the acute treatment of
				mania or mixed episodes. Use as a
				short-term adjunctive
				sedative-hypnotic agent.
					• Binds to the benzodiazepine site and
					  augments the action of $GABA^A$ by
					  increasing the frequency of Cl^-
					  channel opening, which causes
					  hyperpolarization (a less excitable
					  state) and inhibits neuronal firing

Lorazepam	Ativan	Tablet: 0.5, 1, 2 mg Oral solution: 2 mg/mL Injection: 2, 4 mg/mL	2–40 mg/day in divided doses or one dose at bedtime. Dosage should be slowly adjusted up and down according to response and adverse effects.	
Gabapentin	Neurontin	Capsule: 100, 300, 400 Solution: 250 mg/5 mL Tablets: 600, 800 mg	900–3600 mg/day in 3–4 divided doses. Dosage should be slowly increased to minimize adverse effects (e.g., 300 mg 3 times daily, and increase by 300 mg/day every 3–7 days up to 1800 mg/day).	Not recommended for the acute treatment of mania or mixed episodes for bipolar I disorder due to lack of efficacy. Used as an adjunctive agent for comorbid anxiety states and insomnia.	• Exact mechanism is unknown; although gabapentin is structurally related to GABA, it does not interact with GABA receptors • May modulate the action of the GABA synthetic enzyme (glutamic acid decarboxylase) and the glutamate synthetic enzyme; alters the synthesis and release of GABA; increases GABA levels
Topiramate	Topamax	Tablet: 25, 100, 200 mg Sprinkle capsule: 15, 25 mg	50–200 mg/day in divided doses. Dosage should be slowly increased to minimize adverse effects (e.g., 25 mg at bedtime for 1 wk, then 25–50 mg/day increments at weekly intervals).	Not recommended for the acute treatment of mania or mixed episodes due to lack of efficacy; used as an adjunctive agent with established mood stabilizers	• Modulates voltage-sensitive Na^+ channels • Inhibits Ca^+ channels • Blocks glutamate activity • Potentiates GABAergic activity and levels • Inhibits protein kinases A and C • Weak carbonic anhydrase inhibitor

Continued

TABLE 67-6. (Continued)

Generic Generic Name	Trade Name	Formulations	Dosage and Dosage and Administration	Clinical Use	Proposed Mechanism Proposed Mechanism of Action
Atypical antipsychotics: FDA-approved for bipolar disorder					
Aripiprazole	Abilify	Tablet: 5, 10, 15, 20, 30 mg	10–30 mg/day once daily	Use in combination with lithium or valproate for the acute treatment of mania or mixed states (primarily with psychotic features) for bipolar I disorder. Only olanzapine is FDA-approved at this time.	• Antagonist of postsynaptic DA_2 receptors; atypical agents also block $5-HT_{2A}$ receptors that increase the presynaptic release of DA, thus lowering the risk of extrapyramidal symptoms and prolactin release
Olanzapine	Zyprexa	Tablet: 2.5, 5, 7.5, 10, 15, 20 mg	5–20 mg/day in 1 or 2 doses		
	Zyprexa Zydis	Tablet, orally disintegrating: 5, 10, 15, 20 mg			• Receptors blockade varies by agent: DA_{1-4}, $5-HT_{2A-2C}$, α_{1-2}-adrenergic, muscarinic, and histamine$_1$
Quetiapine	Seroquel	Tablet: 25, 100, 200, 300 mg	50–800 mg/day in divided doses or once daily when stabilized		
Risperidone	Risperdal	Tablet: 0.25, 0.5, 1, 2, 3, 4 mg Oral solution: 1 mg/mL	0.5–6 mg/day in 1 or 2 doses		
Ziprasidone	Geodon	Capsule: 20, 40, 60, 80 mg	40–160 mg/day in divided doses		
Calcium channel blockers: Not FDA-approved for bipolar disorder					
Nimodipine	Nimotop	Capsule: 30 mg	30–120 mg/day	Use as third-line agent for combination with other drugs (e.g. carbamazepine, valproate, antipsychotics).	• Blocks Ca^+ influx through L-type Ca^+ channels
Verapamil	Verelan	Capsule: 120, 180, 240, 360 mg	80–480 mg/day		• Alters Ca^+-Na^+ exchange
	Calan, Isoptin	Film-coated tablet: 40, 80, 120 mg Extended-release tablet: 120, 180, 240 mg			• Decreases 5-HT, DA, and endorphin activity

APA, American Psychiatric Association; Ca^+, calcium; Cl^-, chloride; DA, dopamine; FDA, Food and Drug Administration; GABA, γ-aminobutyric acid; 5-HT, serotonin; K^+, potassium; Na^+, sodium; NMDA, N-methyl-D-aspartate; NE, norepinephrine.

TABLE 67–7. Pharmacokinetics and Therapeutic Serum Concentrations of Lithium and Anticonvulsants Used in the Treatment of Bipolar Disorder

	Lithium	Carbamazepine	Oxcarbazepine	Divalproex (DVPX) Sodium/ Valproic Acid (VPA)	Lamotrigine
Gastrointestinal absorption					
Regular release	Rapid: 95–100% within 1–6 h	Slow and erratic: 85–90%	Slow and complete: 100%	Rapid and complete (VPA)	Rapid: 98%
Syrup/suspension/ solution	Faster rate of absorption: 100%	Faster rate of absorption	Unknown	Faster rate of absorption than tablets	NA
Extended-release/ enteric-coated tablets	Delayed absorption: 60–90%	Delayed absorption: 89% of the suspension; and less than regular-release tablets	NA	Extended release: 90% of intravenous dose Delayed release: 81–90% of intravenous dose Delayed absorption with delayed-release tablets; valproate is rapidly converted to VPA in the stomach, then is rapidly and almost completely absorbed from the GI tract	NA
Delay in absorption by food	Yes	No; reports of increased rate of absorption with fatty meals (extended-release capsule)	Unknown	Yes; food slows the rate of absorption but not the extent for DVPX	Bioavailability not affected by food
Time to reach peak serum concentrations	0.5–3 h (regular-release) 4–12 h (extended-release) 0.25–1 h (oral solution)	4.5 h (regular-release); 1.5 h (suspension); 3–12 h (extended-release tablets); 4.1–7.7 h (extended-release capsules); higher peak concentrations with chewable tablets	4.5 h (range of 3–13 h)	1–4 h (VPA) 3–5 h (DVPX single dose) 7–14 h (DVPX extended-release multiple dosing)	1–4 h

Continued

TABLE 67–7. (Continued)

	Lithium	Carbamazepine	Oxcarbazepine	Divalproex (DVPX) Sodium/ Valproic Acid (VPA)	Lamotrigine
Distribution					
Volume of distribution	Initial: 0.3–0.4 L/kg Steady-state: 0.7–1 L/kg	0.6–2 L/kg (adults)	10-monohydroxy carbazepine (metabolite): 49 L/kg	11 L/1.73 m² (total valproate); 92 L/1.73 m² (free valproate)	0.9–1.3 L/kg
Crosses the placenta	Yes; pregnancy risk category: D Risk of cardiac defects: 0.1–0.5%	Yes; pregnancy risk category: D	Yes; pregnancy risk category: C	Yes; pregnancy risk category: D Risk of neural tube defects: 1–5%	Yes; pregnancy risk category: C
Crosses into breast milk	Yes: 35–50% of mother's serum concentration; breast-feeding not recommended	Yes: ratio of concentration in breast milk to plasma is 0.4 for drug and 0.5 for epoxide metabolite; considered compatible with breast-feeding	Yes: both drug and active metabolite; breast-feeding not recommended	Yes: considered compatible with breast-feeding	Yes: breast-feeding not recommended
Protein binding	No	75–90%	40% of active metabolite	80%–90% (dose dependent)	55%
Renal clearance	Yes: 10–40 mL/min with 90–98% of dose excreted in urine; 80% of lithium that is filtered by the renal glomeruli is reabsorbed	Yes: 1–3% excreted unchanged in urine	Yes: 95% excreted in the urine; less than 1% excreted unchanged	Yes: 30–50% excreted as glucuronide conjugate; less than 3% excreted unchanged	Yes: 94% excreted as glucuronide conjugate
Metabolism					
Hepatic metabolism	No	Yes: oxidation and hydroxylation Induces liver enzymes to increase its metabolism and other drugs	Yes: oxidation and conjugation	Yes: oxidation and glucuronide conjugation	Yes: glucuronic acid conjugation Induces its own metabolism in normal volunteers

Metabolites	No	Yes: 10, 11-epoxide (active)	Yes: 10-monohydroxy carbazepine (active)	Yes (not active)	No
Kinetics	First-order	First-order after initial enzyme induction phase	First-order	First-order	First-order
Half-life ($t_{1/2}$)	18–27 h (adult); greater than 36 h (elderly or patients with renal impairment)	$t_{1/2}$ decreases over time due to autoinduction: 25–65 h (initial) 12–17 h (adult multiple dosing) 8–14 h (children multiple dosing)	2 h (parent) 9 h (metabolite)	5–20 h (adult)	25 h; increases to 59 h with concomitant valproic acid therapy
Cytochrome P450 (CYP450) isoenzyme					
CYP450 substrate	No	2C8 and 3A3/4	Unknown	2C19	Unknown
CYP450 inhibitor	No	No	2C19	2C9, 2D6, and 3A3/4	Unknown
CYP450 inducer	No	1A2, 2C9/10, and 3A3/4	3A3/4	No	Unknown
Therapeutic serum/plasma concentrations					
Obtain blood level 10–12 hours postdose	1–1.5 mEq/L: for adult, acute mania 0.4–0.6 mEq/L: for elderly or medically ill 0.6–1.2 mEq/L: for adult, maintenance	4–12 mcg/mL: for adult, acute mania and maintenance 4–8 mcg/mL: for elderly or medically ill	No established therapeutic range; 12–30 mcg/mL for 10-hydroxy carbazepine based on epilepsy trials	50–125 mcg/mL: adult, acute mania and maintenance 40–75 mcg/mL: elderly or medically ill	No established therapeutic range; 4–20 mcg/mL based on epilepsy trials

NA, not applicable.

TABLE 67-8. Guidelines for Baseline and Routine Laboratory Tests and Monitoring for Agents Used in the Treatment of Bipolar Disorder

	Baseline: Physical Exam and General Chemistry[a]	Hematologic Tests[b]		Metabolic Tests[c]		Liver Function Tests[d]		Renal Function Tests[e]		Thyroid Function Tests[f]		Serum Electrolytes[g]		Dermatologic[h]	
	Baseline	Baseline	6–12 months	Baseline	6–12 months	Baseline	6–12 months	Baseline	6–12 months	Baseline	6–12 months	Baseline	6–12 months	Baseline	3–6 months
Atypical antipsychotics[i]	X			X	X										
Carbamazepine[j]	X	X	X			X	X	X					X	X	X
Lamotrigine[k]	X													X	X
Lithium[l]	X	X	X	X	X			X	X	X	X	X	X		
Oxcarbazepine[m]	X			X								X	X		
Valproate[n]	X	X	X	X	X	X	X							X	X

[a]Screen for drug abuse and serum pregnancy.

[b]Complete blood cell count (CBC) with differential and platelets.

[c]Fasting glucose, serum lipids, weight.

[d]Lactase dehydrogenase, aspartate aminotransferase, alanine aminotransferase, total bilirubin, alkaline phosphatase.

[e]Serum creatinine, blood urea nitrogen, urinalysis, urine osmolality, specific gravity.

[f]Triiodothyronine, total thyroxine, thyroxine uptake, and thyroid-stimulating hormone.

[g]Serum sodium.

[h]Rashes, hair thinning, alopecia.

[i]Atypical antipsychotics: Monitor for increased appetite with weight gain (primarily in patients with initial low or normal body mass index); monitor closely if rapid or significant weight gain occurs during early therapy; cases of hyperlipidemia and diabetes reported.

[j]Carbamazepine: Manufacturer recommends CBC and platelets (and possibly reticulocyte counts and serum iron) at baseline, and that subsequent monitoring be individualized by the clinician (e.g., CBC, platelet counts, and liver function tests every 2 wk during the first 2 months of treatment, then every 3 months if normal). Monitor more closely if the patient exhibits hematologic or hepatic abnormalities or if the patient is receiving a myelotoxic drug; discontinue if platelets are <100,000/mm³, if white blood cell (WBC) count is <3000/mm³ or if there is evidence of bone marrow suppression or liver dysfunction. Serum electrolyte levels should be monitored in the elderly or those at risk for hyponatremia. Carbamazepine interferes with some pregnancy tests.

[k]Lamotrigine: Serious dermatologic reactions have occurred within 2–8 wk of initiating treatment and are more likely to occur in patients receiving concomitant valproate, with rapid dosage escalation, or using doses exceeding the recommended titration schedule.

[l]Lithium: Obtain baseline electrocardiogram for patients over age 40 or if preexisting cardiac disease (benign, reversible T-wave depression may occur). Renal function tests should be obtained every 2–3 months during the first 6 months, then every 6–12 months; if impaired renal function, monitor 24-h urine volume and creatinine every 3 months; if urine volume >3L/d, monitor urinalysis, osmolality, and specific gravity every 3 months. Thyroid function tests should be obtained once or twice during the first 6 months, then every 6–12 months; monitor for signs and symptoms of hypothyroidism; if supplemental thyroid therapy is required, monitor thyroid function tests and adjust thyroid dose every 1–2 months until thyroid function indices are within normal range, then monitor every 3–6 months.

[m]Oxcarbazepine: Hyponatremia (serum sodium concentrations <125 mEq/L) has been reported and occurs more frequently during the first 3 months of therapy; serum sodium concentrations should be monitored in patients receiving drugs that lower serum sodium concentrations (e.g., diuretics or drugs that cause inappropriate antidiuretic hormone secretion) or in patients with symptoms of hyponatremia (e.g., contusion, headache, lethargy, and malaise). Hypersensitivity reactions have occurred in approximately 25–30% of patients with a history of carbamazepine hypersensitivity and requires immediate discontinuation.

[n]Valproate: Weight gain reported in patients with low or normal body mass index. Monitor platelets and liver function during first 3–6 months if evidence of increased bruising or bleeding. Monitor closely if patients exhibit hematologic or hepatic abnormalities or in patients receiving drugs that affect coagulation, such as aspirin or warfarin; discontinue if platelets are <100,000/mm³/L or if prolonged bleeding time. Pancreatitis, hyperammonemic encephalopathy, polycystic ovary syndrome, increased testosterone, and menstrual irregularities have been reported; not recommended during first trimester of pregnancy due to risk of neural tube defects.

TABLE 67–9. Efficacy Ratings of Pharmacological Treatments Used in Bipolar I Disorder

Drug	Acute Mania or Mixed States	Acute Bipolar Depression	Maintenance Therapy
Lithium			
Lithium carbonate	A+: monotherapy	A	A+
Anticonvulsants			
Carbamazepine	A: monotherapy	B	B
Divalproex	A+: monotherapy	C	A
Gabapentin	X: monotherapy and adjunctive	D	D
Lamotrigine	C: monotherapy / B: rapid cycling	A	A+
Levetiracetam	D	D	D
Oxcarbazepine	B: monotherapy	D	B
Tiagabine	X: monotherapy / D: adjunctive	D	D
Topiramate	C: monotherapy or adjunctive	C: adjunctive	C: adjunctive
Zonisamide	C: monotherapy	D	D
Antipsychotics			
Aripiprazole	A+: monotherapy	D	D
Clozapine	A: monotherapy for treatment-resistant patients	D	D
Haloperidol	A: monotherapy or adjunctive	D	D
Olanzapine	A+: monotherapy or adjunctive	B: adjunctive with fluoxetine	D
Risperidone	A+: monotherapy or adjunctive	B: adjunctive	D
Quetiapine	A+: monotherapy or adjunctive	D	D
Ziprasidone	A+: monotherapy	D	D

Definition of Ratings:

A, Efficacy established by two or more randomized, double-blind, placebo-controlled or comparator trials and/or recommended as a first-line agent by APA Practice Guidelines for the Treatment of Patients with Bipolar Disorder (Revision) or Texas Consensus Panel on Medication Treatment of Bipolar Disorder; +, approved by the FDA.

B, Efficacy suggested by one randomized, double-blind, placebo-controlled or comparator trial; recommended as a second-line (alternative) agent by APA Practice Guidelines for the Treatment of Patients with Bipolar Disorder (Revision) or Texas Consensus Panel on Medication Treatment of Bipolar Disorder; not approved by the FDA.

C, Efficacy suggested by two or more open-label and/or non–placebo-controlled trials; not approved by the FDA.

D, No controlled clinical trials and/or efficacy not established for monotherapy in bipolar disorder.

X, Not recommended due to negative results or no significant difference from placebo on a randomized, placebo-controlled or comparator trial.

APA, American Psychiatric Association, FDA, Food and Drug Administration.

Lamotrigine

For a summary of lamotrigine adverse effects refer to Chapter 50.

Lithium

- Initial side effects are often dose related and are worse at peak serum concentrations (1 to 2 hours postdose). Lowering the dose, taking smaller doses with food, extended-release products, and once-daily dosing at bedtime may help.
- Gastrointestinal distress may be minimized by standard approaches or by adding antacids or antidiarrheals.
- Muscle weakness and lethargy (transient) occur in about 30% of patients. Polydipsia with polyuria and nocturia occurs in up to 70% of patients, and is managed by changing to once-daily dosing at bedtime.
- Up to 40% of patients complain of headache, memory impairment, confusion, poor concentration, and impaired motor performance. A fine hand tremor may occur in up to 50% of patients. The hand tremor may be treated with propranolol 20 to 120 mg/day, atenolol 50 mg/day, or metoprolol 20 to 80 mg/day.
- Lithium reduces the kidney's ability to concentrate urine and may cause a nephrogenic diabetes insipidus with low urine specific gravity and low osmolality polyuria (urine volume greater than 3 L/day). This may be treated with loop diuretics, thiazide diuretics, or triamterene. If thiazide diuretics are used, lithium doses should be decreased by 50% and lithium and potassium levels monitored.
- Long-term lithium therapy is associated with a 10% to 20% risk of morphological renal changes (e.g., glomerular sclerosis, tubular atrophy, and interstitial nephritis).
- Lithium-induced nephrotoxicity is rare if patients are maintained on the lowest effective dose, if once-daily dosing is used, if good hydration is maintained, and if toxicity is avoided.
- Up to 30% of patients on maintenance lithium therapy develop transiently elevated thyroid-stimulating hormone serum concentrations, and 5% to 35% of patients develop a goiter and/or hypothyroidism, which is dose-related and more likely to occur in women. This is managed by adding levothyroxine to the regimen.
- Lithium may cause cardiac effects including T-wave flattening or inversion (up to 30% of patients), atrioventricular block, and bradycardia. If a patient has preexisting cardiac disease, a cardiologist should be consulted and an electrocardiogram obtained at baseline and regularly during therapy.
- Other late-appearing lithium side effects include benign reversible leukocytosis, acne, alopecia, exacerbation of psoriasis, pruritic dermatitis, maculopapular rash, folliculitis, and weight gain.
- Lithium toxicity can occur with serum levels greater than 1.5 mEq/L, but the elderly may have symptoms at therapeutic levels. Severe lithium intoxication may occur with serum concentrations above 2 mEq/L and include vomiting, diarrhea, incontinence, incoordination, impaired cognition, arrhythmias, and seizures. Permanent neurologic impairment and kidney damage may occur as a result of toxicity.
- Several factors predispose to lithium toxicity, including sodium restriction, dehydration, vomiting, diarrhea, drug interactions that decrease lithium clearance, heavy exercise, sauna baths, hot weather, and fever. Patients should be told to maintain adequate sodium and fluid intake and to avoid excessive coffee, tea, cola, and other caffeine-containing beverages and alcohol.
- If lithium toxicity is suspected, the patient should discontinue lithium and go immediately to the emergency room. Hemodialysis is generally required when

XIII

serum lithium levels are above 4 mEq/L for patients on long-term treatment, or greater than 6 to 8 mEq/L after acute poisoning.

Oxcarbazepine
- For a summary of oxcarbazepine adverse effects refer to Chapter 50.

Valproate Sodium and Valproic Acid
- For a summary of valproate and valproic acid adverse effects refer to Chapter 50.

▶ EVALUATION OF THERAPEUTIC OUTCOMES

- Patients with bipolar disorder should be seen regularly (every 1 to 2 weeks for acute or frequent episodes or 1 to 3 months for stable patients with infrequent episodes) and monitored for response of target symptoms, and presence of side effects.
- Patients should receive regular laboratory monitoring and compliance monitoring.
- Patients who have a partial response of nonresponse to therapy should be reassessed for an accurate diagnosis, concomitant medical or psychiatric conditions, and medications or substances that exacerbate mood symptoms.
- Patients and family members should be actively involved in treatment to monitor target symptoms, response, and side effects.

See Chapter 68, Bipolar Disorder, authored by Martha P. Fankhauser and Marlene P. Freeman, for a more detailed discussion of this topic.

XIII

Chapter 68

▶ DEPRESSIVE DISORDERS

▶ DEFINITION

Major depressive disorder and dysthymic disorder are two types of depressive disorders listed in *The Diagnostic and Statistical Manual of Mental Disorders*, 4th ed., text revision (DSM-IV-TR). The essential feature of major depressive disorder is a clinical course that is characterized by one or more major depressive episodes without a history of manic, mixed, or hypomanic episodes. Dysthymic disorder is a chronic disturbance of mood involving depressed mood and at least two other symptoms, and it is generally less severe than major depressive disorder. This chapter focuses exclusively on the diagnosis and treatment of major depressive disorder.

▶ PATHOPHYSIOLOGY

- *Biogenic amine hypothesis.* Depression may be caused by decreased brain levels of the neurotransmitters norepinephrine (NE), serotonin (5-HT), and dopamine (DA).
- *Postsynaptic changes in receptor sensitivity.* Changes in sensitivity of NE or 5-HT$_2$ receptors may relate to onset of depression.
- *Dysregulation hypothesis.* This theory emphasizes a failure of homeostatic regulation of neurotransmitter systems, rather than absolute increases or decreases in their activities.
- Both serotonergic and noradrenergic systems need to be functional for an antidepressant effect to be exerted.
- *The role of dopamine (DA).* Several reviews suggest that increased DA neurotransmission in the nucleus accumbens may be related to the mechanism of action of antidepressants.

▶ CLINICAL PRESENTATION

- Emotional symptoms may include diminished ability to experience pleasure, loss of interest in usual activities, sadness, pessimistic outlook, crying spells, hopelessness, anxiety (present in almost 90% of depressed outpatients), feelings of guilt, and psychotic features (e.g., auditory hallucinations, delusions).
- Physical symptoms may include fatigue, pain (especially headache), sleep disturbance, appetite disturbance (decreased or increased), loss of sexual interest, and gastrointestinal and cardiovascular complaints (especially palpitations).
- Intellectual or cognitive symptoms may include decreased ability to concentrate or slowed thinking, poor memory for recent events, confusion, and indecisiveness.
- Psychomotor disturbances may include psychomotor retardation (slowed physical movements, thought processes, and speech) or psychomotor agitation.

▶ DIAGNOSIS

- Major depression is characterized by one or more episodes of major depression, as defined by the DSM-IV-TR (Table 68–1).
- When a patient presents with depressive symptoms, it is necessary to investigate the possibility of a medical, psychiatric, and/or drug-induced cause (Table 68–2).

TABLE 68–1. DSM-IV-TR Criteria for Major Depressive Episode

A. Five (or more) of the following symptoms have been present during the same 2-wk period and represent a change from previous functioning; at least one of the symptoms is either (1) depressed mood or (2) loss of interest or pleasure.

Note: Do not include symptoms that are clearly due to a general medical condition or mood-incongruent delusions or hallucinations.

  1. Depressed mood most of the day nearly every day
  2. Markedly diminished interest or pleasure in all, or almost all, activities most of the day nearly every day
  3. Significant weight loss when not dieting or weight gain (e.g., a change of more than 5% of body weight in a month), or decrease or increase in appetite nearly every day
  4. Insomnia or hypersomnia nearly every day
  5. Psychomotor agitation or retardation nearly every day (observable by others, not merely subjective feelings of restlessness or being slowed down)
  6. Fatigue or loss of energy nearly every day
  7. Feelings of worthlessness or excessive or inappropriate guilt (which may be delusional) nearly every day
  8. Diminished ability to think or concentrate, or indecisiveness, nearly every day
  9. Recurrent thoughts of death (not just fear of dying), recurrent suicidal ideation without a specific plan, or a suicide attempt or a specific plan for committing suicide

B. The symptoms cause clinically significant distress or impairment in social, occupational, or other important areas of functioning.

C. The symptoms are not due to the direct physiological effects of a substance (e.g., a drug of abuse, a medication) or a general medical condition (e.g., hypothyroidism).

D. The symptoms are not better accounted for by bereavement (i.e., after the loss of a loved one), the symptoms persist for longer than 2 months or are characterized by marked functional impairment, morbid preoccupation with worthlessness, suicidal ideation, psychotic symptoms, or psychomotor retardation.

Modified and reprinted with permission from the Diagnostic and Statistical Manual of Mental Disorders, 4th ed., Text Revision. Washington, American Psychiatric Association, 2000.

TABLE 68–2. Common Medical Disorders, Psychiatric Disorders, and Drug Therapy Associated With Depression

Medical disorders		Psychiatric disorders
Medical disorders	Metabolic disorders	**Psychiatric disorders**
Endocrine diseases	Electrolyte imbalance	Alcoholism
Hypothyroidism	Hypokalemia	Anxiety disorders
Addison's disease	Hyponatremia	Eating disorders
Cushing's disease	Hepatic encephalopathy	Schizophrenia
Deficiency states	Cardiovascular disease	**Drug therapy**
Pernicious anemia	Coronary artery disease	Antihypertensives
Wernicke's encephalopathy	Congestive heart failure	Clonidine
Severe anemia	Myocardial infarction	Diuretics
Infections	Neurologic disorders	Guanethidine sulfate
AIDS	Alzheimer's disease	Hydralazine hydrochloride
Encephalitis	Epilepsy	Methyldopa
Influenza	Huntington's disease	Propranolol
Mononucleosis	Multiple sclerosis	Reserpine
Sexually transmitted diseases	Pain	**Hormonal therapy**
Tuberculosis	Parkinson's disease	Oral contraceptives
Collagen disorder	Poststroke	Steroids/adrenocorticotropic hormone
Systemic lupus erythematosus	Malignant disease	**Acne therapy**
		Isotretinoin
		Other
		Interferon-beta-1a

XIII

- Depressed patients should have a medication review, physical examination, mental status examination, a complete blood count with differential, thyroid function tests, and electrolyte determinations.

▶ DESIRED OUTCOME

The goals of treatment of the acute depressive episode are to eliminate or reduce the symptoms of depression, minimize adverse effects, ensure compliance with the therapeutic regimen, facilitate a return to a premorbid level of functioning, and prevent further episodes of depression.

▶ TREATMENT

NONDRUG TREATMENT

- The efficacy of psychotherapy and antidepressants is considered to be additive. Psychotherapy alone is not recommended for the acute treatment of patients with severe and/or psychotic major depressive disorders. For uncomplicated nonchronic major depressive disorder, combined treatment may provide no unique advantage. Cognitive therapy, behavioral therapy, and interpersonal psychotherapy appear to be equal in efficacy.
- Electroconvulsive therapy (ECT) is a safe and effective treatment for all sub-types of major depressive disorder. It is considered when a rapid response is needed, risks of other treatments outweigh potential benefits, there has been a poor response to drugs, and the patient expresses a preference for ECT. A rapid therapeutic response (10 to 14 days) has been reported. Relative con-traindications include increased intracranial pressure, cerebral lesions, recent myocardial infarction, recent intracerebral hemorrhage, bleeding, and other-wise unstable vascular conditions. Adverse effects of ECT include confusion, memory impairment, prolonged apnea, treatment emergent mania, headache, nausea, and muscle aches. Relapse rates during the year following ECT are high unless maintenance antidepressants are prescribed.
- ▶ XIII • Bright light therapy (i.e., the patient looking into a light box) may be used for patients with seasonal affective disorder.

GENERAL THERAPEUTIC PRINCIPLES

- In general, antidepressants are equal in efficacy when administered in compa-rable doses.
- Factors that influence the choice of antidepressant include the patient's history of response, history of familial response, subtype of depression, concurrent medical history, potential for drug-drug interactions, side-effect profile of var-ious drugs, and drug cost.
- Between 65% and 70% of patients with major depression improve with drug therapy.
- Melancholic depression appears to respond well to tricyclic antidepressants (**TCAs**), selective 5-HT reuptake inhibitors (**SSRIs**), and ECT.
- A preferential response to monoamine oxidase inhibitors (**MAOIs**) has been reported in patients with atypical depression.
- Patients who fail to respond to a TCA may well respond to an SSRI, and vice versa.
- Psychotically depressed individuals generally require either ECT or combina-tion therapy with an antidepressant and an antipsychotic agent.

DRUG CLASSIFICATION

- Table 68–3 shows the commonly accepted classification of available antidepressants, suggested therapeutic plasma concentration ranges, initial doses, and usual dosage ranges.
- Table 68–4 shows the relative potency and selectivity of the antidepressants for inhibition of NE and 5-HT reuptake and relative side-effect profiles.
- The SSRIs inhibit the reuptake of 5-HT into the presynaptic neuron.
- TCAs are effective in treating all depressive subtypes, especially the severe melancholic subtype.

TABLE 68–3. Adult Dosages for Currently Available Antidepressant Medications[a]

Generic Name	Trade Name	Suggested Therapeutic Plasma Concentration (ng/mL)	Initial Dose (mg/day)	Usual Dosage Range (mg/day)
Selective serotonin reuptake inhibitors				
Citalopram	Celexa		20	20–60
Escitalopram	Lexapro		10	10–20
Fluoxetine	Prozac		10–20	10–80
Fluvoxamine	Luvox		50	50–300
Paroxetine	Paxil		20	20–50
Sertraline	Zoloft		50	100–200
Serotonin/norepinephrine reuptake inhibitor				
Venlafaxine	Effexor		75	75–375
Aminoketone				
Bupropion	Wellbutrin		200	300–450
Triazolopyridines				
Nefazodone	Serzone		200	300–600
Trazodone	Desyrel		50–150	150–400
Tetracyclics				
Maprotiline	Ludiomil	200–300[b]	50–75	100–225
Mirtazapine	Remeron		15	15–45
Tricyclic antidepressants				
Tertiary amines				
Amitriptyline	Elavil	120–250[b]	50–75	100–300
Clomipramine	Anafranil		25	100–250
Doxepin	Sinequan	110–250[b]	50–75	100–300
Imipramine	Tofranil	200–300[b]	50–75	100–300
Trimipramine	Surmontil		50–75	100–300
Secondary amines				
Desipramine	Norpramin	125–300	50–75	100–300
Nortriptyline	Pamelor	50–150	25–50	50–150
Protriptyline	Vivactil	70–240	10–20	15–60
Dibenzoxazepine				
Amoxapine	Asendin	200–400[c]	50–150	100–400
Monoamine oxidase inhibitors				
Phenelzine	Nardil		15	15–90
Tranylcypromine	Parnate		20	20–60

XIII

[a]Doses listed are total daily doses; elderly patients are usually treated with approximately one-half of the dose listed.
[b]Parent durg plus demethylated metabolite.
[c]Parent drug plus hydroxymetabolite.

TABLE 68–4. Relative Potencies of Norepinephrine and Serotonin Reuptake Blockade and Side-Effect Profile of Antidepressant Drugs

	Reuptake Antagonism		Anticholinergic Effects	Sedation	Orthostatic Hypotension	Seizures	Conduction Abnormalities
	Norepinephreine	Serotonin					
Selective serotonin reuptake inhibitors							
Citalopram	0	+ + + +	0	+	0	+ +	0
Escitalopram	0	+ + + +	0	0	0	0	0
Fluoxetine	0	+ + +	0	0	0	+ +	0
Fluvoxamine	0	+ + + +	0	0	0	+ +	0
Paroxetine	0	+ + + +	+	+	0	+ +	0
Sertraline	0	+ + + +	0	0	0	+ +	0
Serotonin/norepinephrine reuptake inhibitor							
Venlafaxine	+ + + +	+ + + +	+	+	0	+ +	+
Aminoketone							
Bupropion	+	+	+	0	0	+ + + +	+
Triazolopyridines							
Nefazodone	0	+ +	0	+ + +	+ + +	+ +	+ +
Trazodone	0	+ +	0	+ + + +	+ + +	+ +	+ +
Tetracyclics							
Maprotiline	+ + +	+	+ + +	+ + +	+ +	+ + + +	+ + +
Mirtazapine	0	0	+	+ +	+ +	+	+

Tricyclic antidepressants

Tertiary amines

Amitriptyline	++	++++	++++	+++	+++	+++
Clomipramine	++	+++	++++	++	++++	+++
Doxepin	++	++	+++	++	+++	++
Imipramine	+++	+++	++++	+++	+++	+++
Trimipramine	++	++	++++	+++	+++	+++

Secondary amines

Desipramine	++++	+	++	++	++	++
Nortriptyline	+++	++	++	+	++	++
Protriptyline	+++	++	+	++	++	+++

Dibenzoxazepine

Amoxapine[a]	+++	++	+++	++	+++	++

Monoamine oxidase inhibitors

Phenelzine	++	+	++	++	+	
Tranylcypromine	++	+	+	++	+	+

++++, high; +++, moderate; ++, low; +, very low; 0, absent.

[a]Also blocks dopamine receptors.

- The MAOIs **phenelzine** and **tranylcypromine** increase the concentrations of NE, 5-HT, and DA within the neuronal synapse through inhibition of the monoamine oxidase enzyme system.
- The triazolopyridines **trazodone** and **nefazodone** are antagonists at the 5-HT$_2$ receptor and inhibit the reuptake of 5-HT. They have negligible affinity for cholinergic and histaminergic receptors.
- **Bupropion's** most potent neurochemical action is blockade of DA reuptake.
- **Venlafaxine** is a potent inhibitor of NE reuptake and a weak inhibitor of DA reuptake.
- **Maprotiline** and **Amoxapine** are inhibitors of NE reuptake, with less effect on 5-HT reuptake.
- **Mirtazapine** enhances central noradrenergic and serotonergic activity through the antagonism of central presynaptic α_2-adrenergic autoreceptors and heteroreceptors.
- **St John's Wort**, an herbal over-the-counter medication, may be effective for mild to moderate depression, but it is associated with several drug interactions. Its potency, purity, and manufacture are not regulated by the Food and Drug Administration (FDA). As depression is a potential life-threatening disease, all antidepressant treatments should be overseen by a trained health care professional.

ADVERSE EFFECTS

Adverse-effect profiles of the various antidepressants are summarized in Table 68–4.

Tricyclic Antidepressants and Other Heterocyclics

- Anticholinergic side effects (e.g., dry mouth, blurred vision, constipation, urinary retention, tachycardia, and memory impairment) and sedation are more likely to occur with the tertiary amine **TCAs** than with the secondary amine TCAs.
- Orthostatic hypotension and resultant syncope, a common and potentially serious adverse effect of the TCAs, occurs as a result of α_1-adrenergic antagonism.
- XIII • Additional side effects include cardiac conduction delays and heart block, especially in patients with preexisting conduction disease.
- Other side effects that may lead to noncompliance include weight gain, excessive perspiration, and sexual dysfunction.
- Abrupt withdrawal of TCAs (especially high doses) may result in symptoms of cholinergic rebound (e.g., dizziness, nausea, diarrhea, insomnia, restlessness).
- **Amoxapine** is a demethylated metabolite of loxapine and, as a result of its postsynaptic receptor DA-blocking effects, may be associated with extrapyramidal side effects (EPS).
- **Maprotiline,** a tetracyclic drug, causes seizures at a higher incidence than do standard TCAs and is contraindicated in patients with a history of seizure disorder. The ceiling dose is considered to be 225 mg/day.

Venlafaxine

Venlafaxine may cause a dose-related increase in diastolic blood pressure. Dosage reduction or discontinuation may be necessary if sustained hypertension occurs.

Selective Serotonin Reuptake Inhibitors

The **SSRIs** produce fewer sedative, anticholinergic, and cardiovascular adverse effects than the **TCAs** and are not associated with weight gain. The primary adverse effects include nausea, vomiting, diarrhea, and sexual dysfunction. Headache, insomnia, and fatigue are also reported commonly.

Triazolopyridines

- **Trazodone** and **nefazodone** cause minimal anticholinergic and gastrointestinal effects. Sedation, dizziness, and orthostatic hypotension are the most frequent dose-limiting side effects.
- Priapism occurs rarely with **trazodone** use (1 in 6000 male patients).
- A black box warning for life-threatening liver failure was recently added to the prescribing information for **nefazodone**. Treatment with nefazodone should not be initiated in individuals with active liver disease or with elevated baseline serum transaminases.

Aminoketone

The occurrence of seizures with **bupropion** is dose-related and may be increased by predisposing factors (e.g., history of head trauma or CNS tumor). At the ceiling dose (450 mg/day), the incidence of seizures is 0.4%.

Mixed Serotonin-Norepinephrine Effects

Mirtazapine's most common adverse effects are somnolence, weight gain, dry mouth, and constipation. In preclinical trials, liver function tests were elevated 1.6 times more frequently in the mirtazapine group than in the placebo group.

Monoamine Oxidase Inhibitors

- The most common adverse effect of MAOIs is postural hypotension (more likely with **phenelzine** than **tranylcypromine**), which can be minimized by divided-daily dosing. Anticholinergic side effects are common but less severe than with the TCAs. Phenelzine causes mild to moderate sedating effects, but tranylcypromine is often stimulating, and the last dose of the day is administered in early afternoon. Sexual dysfunction in both genders is common. **Phenelzine** has been associated with hepatocellular damage and weight gain.
- Hypertensive crisis is a potentially fatal adverse reaction that can occur when MAOIs are taken concurrently with certain foods, especially those high in tyramine (Table 68–5), and with certain drugs (Table 68–6). Symptoms of hypertensive crisis include occipital headache, stiff neck, nausea, vomiting, sweating, and sharply elevated blood pressure. In the past, hypertensive crisis was treated with 10 to 20 mg of nifedipine sublingually or swallowed, but a sharp fall in blood pressure and rebound catecholamine release has been reported. Alternative agents, such as captopril, should be considered. Education of patients taking MAOIs regarding dietary and medication restrictions is critical.

PHARMACOKINETICS

- The pharmacokinetics of the antidepressants is summarized in Table 68–7.
- The major metabolic pathways of the **TCAs** are demethylation, hydroxylation, and glucuronide conjugation. Metabolism of the TCAs appears to be linear within the usual dosage range, but dose-related kinetics cannot be ruled out in the elderly.
- The SSRIs, with the possible exception of **citalopram**, may have a nonlinear pattern of drug accumulation with chronic dosing.
- Factors reported to influence TCA plasma concentrations include disease states (e.g., renal or hepatic dysfunction), genetics, age, cigarette smoking, and concurrent drug administration. Similarly, hepatic impairment, renal impairment, and age have been reported to influence the pharmacokinetics of SSRIs.

TABLE 68–5. Dietary Restrictions for Patients Taking Monoamine Oxidase Inhibitors

Aged cheeses[a]
Sour cream[b]
Yogurt[b]
Cottage cheese[b]
American cheese[b]
Mild Swiss cheese[b]
Wine[c] (especially Chianti and sherry)
Beer
Herring[a] (pickled, salted, dry)
Sardines
Snails
Anchovies
Canned, aged, or processed meats
Monosodium glutamate
Liver (chicken or beef, more than 2 days old)
Fermented foods
Canned figs
Raisins
Pods of broad beans[a] (fava beans)
Yeast extract[a] and other yeast products
Meat extract (marmite)
Soy sauce
Chocolate[d]
Coffee[d]
Ripe avocado
Sauerkraut
Licorice

[a]Clearly warrants absolute prohibition (e.g., English Stilton, blue, Camembert, cheddar).
[b]Up to 2 oz daily is acceptable.
[c]3 oz white wine or a single cocktail is acceptable.
[d]Up to 2 oz daily is acceptable; larger amounts of decaffeinated coffee are acceptable.

XIII

TABLE 68–6. Medication Restrictions for Patients Taking Monoamine Oxidase Inhibitors

Amphetamines	Levodopa
Appetite suppressants	Local anesthetics containing sympathomimetic vasoconstrictors
Asthma inhalants	Meperidine
Buspirone	Methyldopa
Carbamazepine	Methylphenidate
Cocaine	Other antidepressants[a]
Cyclobenzaprine	Other MAOIs
Decongestants (topical and systemic)	Reserpine
Dextromethorphan	Rizatriptan
Dopamine	Stimulants
Ephedrine	Sumatriptan
Epinephrine	Sympathomimetics
Guanethidine	Tryptophan

[a]Tricyclic antidepressants may be used with caution by experienced clinicians in treatment-resistant populations.

TABLE 68–7. Pharmacokinetic Properties of Antidepressants

Generic Name	Elimination Half-Life (h)[a]	Time of Peak Plasma Concentration (h)	Plasma Protein Binding (%)	Percentage Bioavailable	Clinically Important Metabolites
Selective serotonin reuptake inhibitors					
Citalopram	33	2–4	80	≥80	Desmethyl- and didemethylcitalopram
Escitalopram	27–32	5	56	80	None
Fluoxetine	4–6 days[b]	4–8	94	95	Norfluoxetine
Fluvoxamine	15–26	2–8	77	53	None
Paroxetine	24–31	5–7	95	36[c]	None
Sertraline	27	6–8	99		N-Desmethylsertraline
Serotonin/norepinephrine reuptake inhibitor					
Venlafaxine	5	2	27–30		O-Desmethylvenlafaxine
Aminoketone					
Bupropion	10–21	3	82–88	[d]	Bupropion threoamino alcohol; bupropion morpholinol
Triazolopyridines					
Nefazodone	2–4	1	99	20	Meta-chlorophenylpiperazine hydroxynefazodone; triazoledione
Trazodone	6–11	1–2	92	[d]	Meta-chlorophenyl piperazine
Tetracyclic					
Maprotiline	28–105	4–24	88	79–87	Desmethylmaprotiline
Mirtazapine	20–40	2	85	50	None known

Continued

TABLE 68–7. (Continued)

Generic Name	Elimination Half-Life (h)[a]	Time of Peak Plasma Concentration (h)	Plasma Protein Binding (%)	Percentage Bioavailable	Clinically Important Metabolites
Tricyclic antidepressants					
Tertiary amines					
Amitriptyline	9–46	1–5	90–97	30–60	Nortriptyline; 10-hydroxynortriptyline
Clomipramine	20–24	2–6	97	36–62	
Doxepin	8–36	1–4	68–82	13–45	Desmethyldoxepin
Imipramine	6–34	1.5–3	63–96	22–77	2-Hydroxyimipramine; desipramine 2-hydroxydesipramine
Trimipramine	7–40	3	94–96	18–63	None
Secondary amines					
Desipramine	11–46	3–6	73–92	33–51	2-Hydroxydesipramine
Nortriptyline	16–88	3–12	87–95	46–70	10-Hydroxynortriptyline
Protriptyline	54–198	6–12	90–94	75–90	None
Dibezoxazepine					
Amoxapine	8–30[e]	1–2	90	[d]	8-Hydroxyamoxapine
Monoamine oxidase inhibitors					
Phenelzine	1.5–4	[d]	[d]	[d]	
Tranylcypromine	1.5–3	[d]	[d]	[d]	

[a]Biologic half-life in slowest phase of elimination.
[b]4–6 days with chronic dosing; norfluoxetine, 4–16 days.
[c]Increases 30–40% when taken with food.
[d]No data available.
[e]Amoxapine, 8 h; 8-hydroxyamoxapine, 30 h.

- In acutely depressed patients, there is a correlation between antidepressant effect and plasma concentrations for some TCAs. Table 68–3 shows suggested therapeutic plasma concentration ranges. The best-established therapeutic range is for **nortriptyline**, and data suggest a therapeutic window.
- Some indications for plasma level monitoring include inadequate response, relapse, serious or persistent adverse effects, use of higher than standard doses, suspected toxicity, elderly patients, children and adolescents, pregnant patients, patients of African or Asian descent (because of slower metabolism), cardiac disease, suspected noncompliance, suspected pharmacokinetic drug interactions, and changing brands.
- Plasma concentrations should be obtained at steady state, usually after a minimum of 1 week at constant dosage. Sampling should be done during the elimination phase, usually in the morning, 12 hours after the last dose. Samples collected in this manner are comparable for patients on once-daily, twice-daily, or thrice-daily regimens.

DRUG-DRUG INTERACTIONS

- Drug interactions of the **TCAs** are summarized in Tables 68–8 and 68–9. Table 68–10 summarizes the drug interactions of non-TCAs.
- The very slow elimination of fluoxetine and norfluoxetine makes it critical to ensure a 5-week washout after **fluoxetine** discontinuation before starting an **MAOI**. Potentially fatal reactions may occur when any **SSRI** or TCA is coadministered with an MAOI.
- Increased plasma concentrations of TCAs and symptoms of toxicity may occur when **fluoxetine**, **sertraline**, and **paroxetine** are added to a TCA regimen.
- Data to date suggest that citalopram may cause only moderate or no pharmacokinetic interactions when coadministered with the TCAs. **Fluvoxamine** may cause an increase in the plasma concentration of citalopram. **Escitalopram** is considered unlikely at present to cause many clinically important pharmacokinetic interactions, but it may cause a doubling of the area under the curve for **desipramine**.
- The drug interaction literature should be consulted for detailed information concerning any real or potential drug interaction involving any psychotherapeutic agent.
- Table 68–11 compares second- and third-generation antidepressants for their effects on the enzymes of the cytochrome P450 system.

XIII

SPECIAL POPULATIONS

Elderly Patients

- The **SSRIs** are often selected as first-choice antidepressants in elderly patients, and they may enable one to avoid adverse effects commonly associated with the **TCAs**.
- In healthy elderly patients, cautious use of a secondary amine TCA (**desipramine** or **nortriptyline**) may be appropriate because of their defined therapeutic plasma concentration ranges, well-established efficacy, and well-known adverse-effect profiles.
- **Nefazodone, bupropion,** and **venlafaxine** may also be chosen because of their milder anticholinergic and less frequent cardiovascular side effects.

Children and Adolescents

- Data supporting efficacy of antidepressants in children and adolescents are sparse. Fluoxetine is the only antidepressant that is FDA approved for treatment of depression in patients less than 18 years of age.

TABLE 68–8. Pharmacokinetic Drug Interactions Involving Tricyclic Antidepressants

Elevates plasma concentrations of TCAs
Cimetidine
Diltiazem
Ethanol, acute ingestion
SSRIs
Haloperidol
Labetalol
Methylphenidate
Oral contraceptives
Phenothiazines
Propoxyphene
Quinidine
Verapamil

Lowers plasma concentrations of TCAs
Barbiturates
Carbamazepine
Ethanol, chronic ingestion
Phenytoin

Elevates plasma concentrations of interacting drug
Hydantoins
Oral anticoagulants

Lowers plasma concentrations of interacting drug
Levodopa

TABLE 68–9. Pharmacodynamic Drug Interactions Involving Tricyclic Antidepressants

Interacting Drug	Effect
Alcohol	Increased CNS depressant effects
Amphetamines	Increased effect of amphetamines
Androgens	Delusions, hostility
Anticholinergic agents	Excessive anticholinergic effects
Bepredil	Increased antiarrhythmic effect
Clonidine	Decreased antihypertensive efficacy
Disulfiram	Acute organic brain syndrome
Estrogens	Increased or decreased antidepressant response; increased toxicity
Guanadrel	Decreased antihypertensive efficacy
Guanethidine	Decreased antihypertensive efficacy
Insulin	Increased hypoglycemic effects
Lithium	Possible additive lowering of seizure threshold
Methyldopa	Decreased antihypertensive efficacy; tachycardia; CNS stimulation
Monoamine oxidase inhibitors	Increased therapeutic and possibly toxic effects of both drugs; hypertensive crisis; delirium; seizures; hyperpyrexia; serotonin syndrome
Oral hypoglycemics	Increased hypoglycemic effects
Phenytoin	Possible lowering of seizure threshold and reduced antidepressant response
Sedatives	Increased CNS depressant effects
Sympathomimetics	Increased pharmacologic effects of direct-acting sympathomimetics; decreased effects of indirect-acting sympathomimetics
Thyroid hormones	Increased therapeutic and possibly toxic effects of both drugs; CNS stimulation; tachycardia

XIII

TABLE 68–10. Drug Interactions of Non-TCA Antidepressants

Non-TCA	Interacting Drug/Drug Class	Effect
Dibenzoxazepine		
Amoxapine	Many of the drugs that interact with the TCAs	Similar response to that seen with TCA interaction
Tetracyclic		
Maprotiline	Many of the drugs that interact with the TCAs	Similar response to that seen with TCA interaction
Mirtazapine	MAOIs	Theoretically central serotonin syndrome could occur
Triazolopyridines		
Nefazodone	Alprazolam	Increased plasma concentrations of alprazolam
	Astemizole	Theoretically increased plasma concentrations of astemizole with potentially serious cardiovascular adverse effects
	Digoxin	Increased C_{max}, C_{min}, and AUC of digoxin by 29%, 27%, and 15%, respectively
	Haloperidol	Decreased clearance of haloperidol by 35%
	MAOIs	Hypertensive crisis; serotonin syndrome; delirium; coma; seizures; hyperpyrexia
	Propranolol	Decreased C_{max} and AUC of propranolol; increased C_{max}, C_{min}, and AUC of m-CCP metabolite of nefazodone
	Ritonavir	Increased AUC of ritonavir with potential for increased adverse events: headaches, dry mouth, nausea, somnolence, dizziness
	Terfenadine	Theoretically increased plasma concentrations of terfenadine with potentially serious cardiovascular adverse effects
	Triazolam	Increased plasma concentrations of triazolam; increased psychomotor impairment
Trazodone	CNS depressants	Increased CNS depression
	Digoxin	Increased serum concentrations of digoxin
	Ethanol	Additive impairment in motor skills
	Fluoxetine	Increased plasma concentrations of trazodone
	MAOIs	Theoretically central serotonin syndrome could occur
	Neuroleptics	Increased hypotension
	Phenytoin	Increased serum concentrations of phenytoin
	Tryptophan	Agitation, restlessness, poor concentration, nausea
	Warfarin	Decreased hypoprothrombinemic response
Aminoketone		
Bupropion	MAOIs	Increased toxicity of bupropion
	Medications that lower seizure threshold	Increased incidence of seizures
	Levodopa	Increased incidence of adverse experiences
	Ritonavir	Increased blood level of bupropion with increased risk of seizures
Selective serotonin reuptake inhibitors		
Citalopram	Cimetidine	Reduced oral clearance of citalopram
	Fluvoxamine	Increased plasma concentrations of citalopram
	TCAs	Possible increased AUC of TCA

XIII

Continued

TABLE 68–10. (Continued)

Fluoxetine	Alprazolam	Increased plasma concentrations and half-life of alprazolam; increased psychomotor impairment
	Anticoagulants	Possible increased risk of bleeding
	β-Adrenergic blockers	Increased metoprolol serum concentrations and bradycardia; possible heart block
	Buspirone	Decreased therapeutic response to buspirone
	Carbamazepine	Increased plasma concentrations of carbamazepine with symptoms of carbamazepine toxicity
	Dextromethorphan	Visual hallucinations (one patient only)
	Haloperidol	Increased haloperidol concentrations and increased extrapyramidal side effects
	Lithium	Neurotoxicity—confusion, ataxia, dizziness, tremor, absence, seizures
	MAOIs	Severe or fatal reactions—confusion, nausea, double vision, hypomania, hypertension, tremor, serotonin syndrome
	Phenytoin	Increased plasma concentrations of phenytoin and symptoms of phenytoin toxicity
	TCAs	Markedly increased TCA plasma concentration with symptoms of TCA toxicity
	Terfenadine	Arrhythmias, shortness of breath, and orthostasis
	Trazodone	Headaches, dizziness, sedation
	Tryptophan	Agitation, restlessness, poor concentration, nausea
	Valproate	Increased valproate serum concentrations
Fluvoxamine	Alprazolam	Increased AUC of alprazolam by 96%, increased alprazolam half-life by 71%, and increased psychomotor impairment
	Astemizole	Theoretically increased plasma concentrations of astemizole with potentially serious cardiovascular effects
	β-Adrenergic blockers	Fivefold increase in propranolol serum concentration; bradycardia and hypotension with combined fluvoxamine and metoprolol
	Carbamazepine	Possible carbamazepine toxicity, although a controlled study did not support this
	Clozapine	Increased clozapine serum concentrations and increased risk for seizures and orthostatic hypotension
	Diazepam	Decreased clearance of diazepam and its active metabolite
	Diltiazem	Bradycardia
	Haloperidol	Increased haloperidol plasma concentrations
	Lithium	Increased serotonergic effects; seizures, nausea, tremor
	MAOIs	Potential for hypertensive crisis, serotonin syndrome, seizures, delirium
	Methadone	Increased methadone plasma concentrations with symptoms of methadone toxicity
	TCAs	Increased TCA plasma concentration

TABLE 68–10. (Continued)

Non-TCA	Interacting Drug/Drug Class	Effect
	Terfenadine	Theoretically increased plasma concentrations of terfenadine with potentially serious cardiovascular effects
	Theophylline	Increased serum concentrations of theophylline with symptoms of theophylline toxicity
	Tryptophan	Increased serotonergic effects and severe vomiting
	Warfarin	Increased hypoprothrombinemic response to warfarin
Paroxetine	Cimetidine	Increased paroxetine serum concentrations
	Desipramine	Increased plasma concentrations and half-life of desipramine
	MAOIs	Potential for hypertensive crisis, serotonin syndrome, seizures, delirium
	Warfarin	Possible increased risk for bleeding
Sertraline	Carbamazepine	Increased plasma concentrations of carbamazepine
	Diazepam	Small decrease in clearance of diazepam
	MAOIs	Serotonin syndrome, myoclonus, violent shaking
	TCAs	Increased plasma concentrations of secondary amine TCAs (desipramine, nortriptyline)
	Tolbutamide	Decreased clearance of tolbutamide (16%)
	Warfarin	Increased prothrombin time
Serotonin/norepinephrine reuptake inhibitor		
Venlafaxine	Cimetidine	Reduced clearance of venlafaxine by 43%
		AUC and peak serum concentration of venlafaxine increased by 60%
	MAOIs	Potential for hypertensive crisis, serotonin syndrome, seizures, delirium

AUC, area under the curve; C_{max}, maximum concentration; C_{min}, minimum concentration; MAOI, monoamine oxidase inhibitor.

TABLE 68–11. Second- and Third-Generation Antidepressants and Cytochrome (CYP) P450 Enzyme Inhibitory Potential

Drug	CYP Enzyme			
	1A2	2C	2D6	3A4
Buproprion	0	0	0	0
Citalopram	0	0	0	+++
Escitalopram	0	0	0	0
Fluoxetine	0	++	++++	++
Fluvoxamine	++++	++	0	++
Mirtazapine	0	0	0	0
Nefazodone	0	0	0	++++
Paroxetine	0	0	++++	0
Sertraline	0	+++	++	+
Venlafaxine	0	0	0	0

++++, high; +++, moderate; ++, low; +, very low; 0, absent.

- The FDA has established a link between antidepressant use and suicidality in children and adolescents. The FDA now requires that all antidepressants carry a black box warning providing cautions in the use of all antidepressants in this population, and the FDA also recommends specific monitoring parameters. The clinician should consult the FDA approved labeling or the FDA Web site for additional information.
- Several cases of sudden death have been reported in children and adolescents taking **desipramine**. A baseline electrocardiogram (ECG) is recommended before initiating a TCA in children and adolescents, and an additional ECG is advised when steady-state plasma concentrations are achieved. TCA plasma concentration monitoring is critical to ensure safety, and plasma concentrations above 450 ng/mL are associated with increased risk of serious adverse effects.

Pregnancy

- As a general rule, if effective, nondrug approaches are preferred when treating depressed pregnant patients.
- No major teratogenic effects have been identified with the **SSRIs** or **TCAs**. However, evaluations to date suggest a possible association of **fluoxetine** with premature birth and decreased fetal growth rate.
- When TCAs are withdrawn during pregnancy, they should be tapered gradually to avoid withdrawal symptoms. If possible, drug tapering is usually begun 5 to 10 days before the estimated day of confinement.

REFRACTORY PATIENTS

- Most "treatment-resistant" depressed patients have received inadequate therapy. Issues to be considered in patients who have not responded to treatment include the following: (1) Is the diagnosis correct? (2) Does the patient have a psychotic depression? (3) Has the patient received an adequate dose and duration of treatment? (4) Do adverse effects preclude adequate dosing? (5) Has the patient been compliant with the prescribed regimen? (6) Was treatment outcome measured adequately? (7) Is there a coexisting or preexisting medical or psychiatric disorder?
- XIII • The current antidepressant may be stopped, and a trial initiated with an agent of unrelated chemical structure.
- Alternatively, the current antidepressant may be augmented (potentiated) by the addition of **lithium, liothyronine**, or an atypical antipsychotic.
- A third approach is to use two different classes of antidepressants concurrently. The combination of an **SSRI** and **MAOI** should not be used. Two drugs should not be used when one drug will suffice. An algorithm for treatment of depression including refractory patients is shown in Figure 68–1.

DOSING

- The usual initial adult dose of most TCAs is 50 mg at bedtime, and the dose may be increased by 25 to 50 mg every third day (see Table 68–3).
- **Bupropion** is usually initiated at 100 mg twice daily, and this dose may be increased to 100 mg three times daily after 3 days. An increase to 450 mg/day (the ceiling dose), given as 150 mg three times daily, may be considered in patients with no clinical response after several weeks at 300 mg/day.
- A 6-week antidepressant trial at a maximum dosage is considered an adequate trial. Patients must be told about the expected lag time of 2 to 4 weeks before the onset of antidepressant effect.

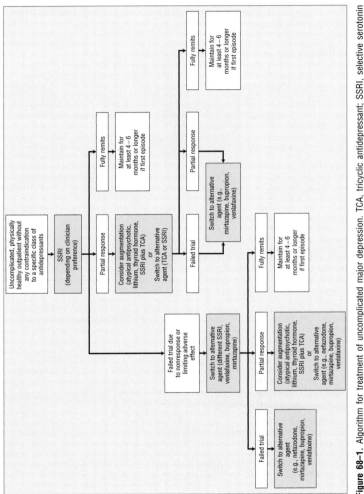

Figure 68–1. Algorithm for treatment of uncomplicated major depression. TCA, tricyclic antidepressant; SSRI, selective serotonin reuptake inhibitor.

- Elderly patients should receive half the initial dose given to younger adults, and the dose is increased at a slower rate. The elderly may require 6 to 12 weeks of treatment to achieve the desired antidepressant response.
- To prevent relapse, antidepressants should be continued at full therapeutic doses for 4 to 9 months after remission. Some investigators recommend lifelong maintenance therapy for persons at greatest risk for recurrence (e.g., persons greater than 50 years of age at onset of the first episode, persons greater than 40 years of age and with two or more prior episodes, and persons of any age with three or more prior episodes).

▶ PHARMACOECONOMIC CONSIDERATIONS

- Drug costs account for about 10% to 12% of the direct costs of treating depression. When evaluating the costs of treatment, more must be considered than the cost of medications alone. Several studies have shown that the **SSRIs** are a more economical approach to treatment of depression (compared with **TCAs**) when all treatment costs are considered.
- A recent evaluation found that both **nefazodone** and **fluoxetine** were cost effective when compared with **imipramine**, with **nefazodone** being slightly more cost effective than **fluoxetine**. Additional, longer-term studies in more diverse populations are needed before judgments can be made regarding which of the newer antidepressants offers a cost-effectiveness advantage.

▶ EVALUATION OF THERAPEUTIC OUTCOMES

- Several monitoring parameters, in addition to plasma concentrations, are useful in managing patients. Patients must be monitored for adverse effects, remission of previously documented target symptoms, and changes in social or occupational functioning. Regular monitoring should be assured for several months after antidepressant therapy is discontinued.
- Patients given **venlafaxine** and those given **TCAs** concurrently with adrenergic neuronal blocking antihypertensives should have blood pressure monitored regularly.
- Patients older than age 40 years should receive a pretreatment ECG before starting TCA therapy, and follow-up ECGs should be performed periodically.
- Patients should be monitored for emergence of suicidal ideation after initiation of any antidepressant.
- In addition to the clinical interview, psychometric rating instruments allow for rapid and reliable measurement of the nature and severity of depressive and associated symptoms.
- Patients should be monitored closely for relapse or recurrence if the brand of antidepressant is changed.

See Chapter 67, Depressive Disorders, authored by Judith C. Kando, Barbara G. Wells, and Peggy E. Hayes, for a more detailed discussion of this topic.

XIII

Chapter 69

▶ SCHIZOPHRENIA

▶ DEFINITION

Schizophrenia is a chronic heterogeneous syndrome of disorganized and bizarre thoughts, delusions, hallucinations, inappropriate affect, and impaired psychosocial functioning.

▶ PATHOPHYSIOLOGY

- Increased ventricular size, decreased brain size, and brain asymmetry have been reported. Lower hippocampal volume may correspond to impairment in neuropsychological testing and poorer response to first-generation antipsychotics (FGAs).
- *Dopaminergic hypothesis.* Psychosis may result from hyper- or hypoactivity of dopaminergic processes in specific brain regions. This may include the presence of a dopamine (DA) receptor defect.
- *Glutamatergic dysfunction.* Glutamatergic tracts interact with dopaminergic tracts. A deficiency of glutamatergic activity produces symptoms similar to those of dopaminergic hyperactivity and possibly those seen in schizophrenia.
- *Serotonin (5-HT) abnormalities.* Schizophrenic patients with abnormal brain scans have higher whole blood 5-HT concentrations.
- The primary abnormality may occur in one neurotransmitter with secondary changes in other neurotransmitters.
- Molecular research involving subtle changes in G-proteins, protein metabolism, and other subcellular processes may well identify the biologic disturbances in schizophrenia.

▶ CLINICAL PRESENTATION

- Symptoms of the acute episode may include the following: being out of touch with reality; hallucinations (especially hearing voices); delusions (fixed false beliefs); ideas of influence (actions controlled by external influences); disconnected thought processes (loose associations); ambivalence (contradictory thoughts); flat, inappropriate, or labile affect; autism (withdrawn and inwardly directed thinking); uncooperativeness, hostility, and verbal or physical aggression; impaired self-care skills; and disturbed sleep and appetite.
- After the acute psychotic episode, the patient typically has residual features (e.g., anxiety, suspiciousness, lack of volition, lack of motivation, poor insight, impaired judgment, social withdrawal, difficulty in learning from experience, and poor self-care skills).

▶ DIAGNOSIS

- *The Diagnostic and Statistical Manual of Mental Disorders,* 4th ed., text revision (DSM-IV-TR), specifies the following criteria for the diagnosis of schizophrenia:
  - Persistent dysfunction lasting longer than 6 months
  - Two or more symptoms (present for at least 1 month) including hallucinations, delusions, disorganized speech, grossly disorganized or catatonic behavior, and negative symptoms
  - Significantly impaired functioning (work, interpersonal, or self-care)

- DSM-IV-TR classifies symptoms as positive or negative.
  - Positive symptoms (the ones most affected by antipsychotic drugs) include delusions, disorganized speech (association disturbance), hallucinations, behavior disturbance (disorganized or catatonic), and illusions.
  - Negative symptoms include alogia (poverty of speech), avolition, affective flattening, anhedonia, and social isolation.
- Cognitive dysfunction is another symptom category that includes impaired attention, working memory, and executive function.

▶ DESIRED OUTCOME

The goals of treatment include the following: alleviation of target symptoms, avoidance of side effects, improvement in psychosocial functioning and productivity, compliance with the prescribed regimen, and involvement of the patient in treatment planning.

▶ TREATMENT

A thorough mental status examination (MSE), physical and neurologic examination, a complete family and social history, and laboratory workup (complete blood count, electrolytes, hepatic function, renal function, electrocardiogram, fasting serum glucose, serum lipids, thyroid function, and urine drug screen) must be performed prior to treatment.

GENERAL THERAPEUTIC PRINCIPLES

- Second-generation antipsychotics (SGAs) (also known as atypical antipsychotics), except **clozapine**, are the agents of first choice in treatment of schizophrenia. Growing, but still controversial, evidence supports that the SGAs (e.g., **clozapine**, **olanzapine**, **risperidone**, **quetiapine**, **ziprasidone**, and **aripiprazole**) have superior efficacy for treatment of negative symptoms, cognition, mood, and general psychopathology. They also generally have better tolerability than the FGAs.
- SGAs have few or no acutely occurring extrapyramidal side effects (EPSs). Other attributes ascribed include minimal or no propensity to cause tardive dyskinesia and less effect on serum prolactin than the FGAs. **Clozapine** is the only SGA that fulfills all these criteria.
- Figure 69–1 outlines a suggested algorithm for treatment of schizophrenia. Clozapine has superior efficacy in decreasing suicidal behavior, and is considered a higher (see algorithm) treatment option in suicidal patients.
- Selection of an antipsychotic should be based on (1) the need to avoid certain side effects, (2) concurrent medical or psychiatric disorders, and (3) patient or family history of response.
- All FGAs are equal in efficacy in groups of patients when used in equipotent doses. High-potency drugs (e.g., **haloperidol**) are as effective in treating acute agitation as low-potency, highly sedating FGAs (e.g., **chlorpromazine**).
- Dosage equivalents (expressed as CPZ-equivalent dosages—the equipotent dosage of an FGA compared with 100 mg of CPZ) may be useful when switching from one FGA to another FGA drug (Table 69–1).
- Predictors of good antipsychotic response include a prior good response to the drug selected, absence of alcohol or drug abuse, acute onset and short duration of illness, acute stressors or precipitating factors, later age of onset, affective

XIII

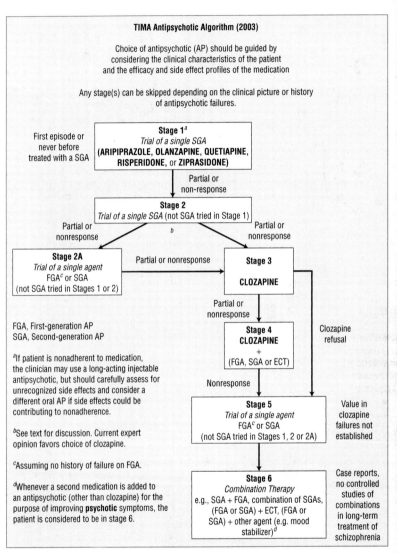

Figure 69–1. Patient entry into the algorithm is determined by individual patient history and by clinical presentation. Algorithm stages can be skipped if clinically appropriate, and one may go back stages if indicated. In general, inadequately responding patients should not remain in stages 1 through 3 longer than 12 weeks at therapeutic doses. Stage 3 may be up to 6 months. Algorithm updates may be obtained at http://www.dshs.state.tx.us/mhprograms/timasczman.pdf. This figure is in the public domain and may be reproduced, with appropriate citation to the authors and source (Miller et al. and Miller et al.) TIMA, Texas Implementation of Medication Algorithms; ECT, electroconvulsive therapy.

TABLE 69-1. Available Antipsychotics: Doses and Dosage Forms

Generic Name	Trade Name	Traditional Equivalent Dose (mg)[a]	Usual Dosage Range (mg/day)	Manufacturer's Maximum Dose (mg/day)	Dosage Forms[b]
Traditional antipsychotics (first-generation antipsychotics)					
Chlorpromazine	Thorazine	100	100–800	2000	T, L, LC, I, C-ER, SR
Fluphenazine	Prolixin	2	2–20	40	T, L, LC, I, LAI
Haloperidol	Haldol	2	2–20	100	T, LC, I, LAI
Loxapine	Loxitane	10	10–80	250	C, LC
Molindone	Moban	10	10–100	225	T, LC
Mesoridazine	Serentil	50	50–400	500	T, LC, I
Perphenazine	Trilafon	10	10–64	64	T, LC, I
Thioridazine	Mellaril	100	100–800	800	T, LC
Thiothixene	Navane	4	4–40	60	C, LC
Trifluoperazine	Stelazine	5	5–40	80	T, LC, I
Atypical antipsychotics (second-generation antipsychotics)					
Aripiprazole	Abilify	NA	15–30	30	T
Clozapine	Clozaril	NA	50–500	900	T
Olanzapine	Zyprexa	NA	10–20	20	T, I, O
Quetiapine	Seroquel	NA	250–500	800	T
Risperidone	Risperdal	NA	2–8	16	T, O, L
Risperidone	Risperdal Consta	NA	25–50 every 2 wk	50 every 2 wk	LAI
Ziprasidone	Geodon	NA	40–160	200	C, I

[a]NA, This parameter does not apply to atypical antipsychotics.
[b]T, tablet; C, capsule; ER or SR, extended- or sustained-release; I, injection; L, liquid solution, elixir, or suspension; LC, liquid concentrate; O, orally disintegrating tablets; LAI, long-acting injectable.

symptoms, family history of affective illness, compliance with the prescribed regimen, and good premorbid adjustment.
- Negative symptoms are generally less responsive to antipsychotic therapy.

MECHANISM OF ACTION

- Recent work has focused on the antipsychotics' relative affinities to block D_2 versus 5-HT_{2A} receptors.
- Antipsychotics can be classified into three categories:
  - High D_2 antagonism and low $5HT_{2A}$ antagonism (FGA-like)
  - Moderate to high D_2 antagonism and high 5-HT_{2A} antagonism (SGA-nonclozapine-like)
  - Low D_2 antagonism and high 5-HT_{2A} antagonism (SGA-clozapine-like)
- **Aripiprazole** is unusual in that it is a potent $5HT_{1A}$ agonist. It is a weak 5-HT_{2A} antagonist. It is a partial dopamine agonist in the hypodopaminergic state and a weak dopamine antagonist in the hyperdopaminergic state.
- **Ziprasidone** has the highest 5-HT_{2A}-to-D_2 affinity ratio of any of the antipsychotics. It is also a potent 5-HT_{1A} agonist and a modest inhibitor of presynaptic reuptake of norepinephrine and 5-HT.
- **Quetiapine** has the lowest D_2 binding.
- 60% to 65% occupation of D_2 receptors is thought to be necessary to decrease positive symptoms; 77% blockade of D_2 receptors is associated with EPS.
- The antipsychotic effects of the FGAs are proposed to occur in the limbic system, including the ventral striatum. The EPS results from DA blockade in the dorsal striatum.
- FGAs are dopaminergic antagonists with high affinity for D_2 receptors. Newer SGAs have variable D_2 binding.
- Transient blockade of dopamine receptors may be adequate to produce antipsychotic effect and transient rise in serum prolactin concentrations, but long-term D_2 blockade is required for production of EPSs and sustained hyperprolactinemia.
- FGAs, especially the low-potency antipsychotics (e.g., **chlorpromazine** and **thioridazine**), also block muscarinic, α_1-adrenergic, and histaminic receptors resulting in dry mouth, constipation, sinus tachycardia, and orthostatic hypotension. XIII

PHARMACOKINETICS

- Pharmacokinetic parameters and major metabolic pathways of antipsychotics are summarized in Table 69–2.
- Antipsychotics are highly lipophilic and highly bound to membranes and plasma proteins.
- They have large volumes of distribution and are largely metabolized through the cytochrome P450 pathways.
- **Risperidone** and its active metabolite 9-OH-resperidone are metabolized by CYP 2D6. Polymorphic metabolism should be considered in those with side effects at low doses (approximately 40% of African Americans and Asians).
- Most antipsychotics have half-lives of elimination in the range of 20 to 40 hours. After dosage stabilization, most antipsychotics (except **quetiapine** and **ziprasidone**) can be dosed once daily. It may be possible to dose SGAs less often than their plasma kinetics would suggest.
- A 12-hour postdose **clozapine** serum concentration of at least 250 ng/mL is recommended for patients taking divided doses of clozapine, or 350 ng/mL if the patient is taking once-daily dosing.

▶ XIII

TABLE 69–2. Pharmacokinetic Parameters of Selected Antipsychotics

Drug	Bioavailability (%)	Half-life (h)	Major Metabolic Pathways	Active Metabolites
Selected first-generation antipsychotics				
Chlorpromazine	10–30	8–35	FMO3, CYP 3A4	7-hydroxy, others
Fluphenazine	20–50	14–24	CYP 2D6	?
Fluphenazine decanoate		14.2 ± 2.2^a days		
Haloperidol	40–70	12–36	CYP 1A2, 2D6, 3A4	Reduced haloperidol
Haloperidol decanoate		21 days		
Second-generation antipsychotics				
Aripiprazole	87	48–68	CYP 3A4, 2D6	Dehydroaripiprazole
Clozapine	12–81	11–105	CYP 1A2, 3A4, 2C19	Desmethylclozapine
Olanzapine	80	20–70	CYP 1A2, 3A4, FMO3	N-glucuronide; 2-OH-methyl; 4-N-oxide
Quetiapine	9 ± 4	6.88	CYP 3A4	7-OH-quetiapine
Risperidone	68	3–24	CYP 2D6	9-OH-risperidone
Risperidone Consta		3–6 days	CYP 2D6	9-OH-risperidone
Ziprasidone	59	4–10	Aldehyde oxidase, CYP 3A4	None

^{a}Based on multiple-dose data. Single-dose data indicate a β half-life of 6–10 days.

- Serum concentration monitoring of clozapine should be done before exceeding 600 mg daily in patients who develop unusual or severe adverse side effects, in those taking concomitant medications that might cause drug interactions, in those with age or pathophysiologic changes suggesting altered kinetics, and in those suspected of being nonadherent to their regiments.
- **Risperidone Consta** is a suspension of drug in glycolic acid lactate copolymer microspheres. The polymer is slowly hydrolyzed after IM injection, and drug begins to be absorbed after about 3 weeks. Therapeutic concentrations are achieved after about 2 months with dosing every 2 weeks.
- The depot FGAs **fluphenazine decanoate** and **haloperidol decanoate** are esterified drugs formulated in sesame seed oil for deep intramuscular (IM) injection. Absorption from the muscle is the rate-limiting step.

INITIAL THERAPY

- The goals during the first 7 days are decreased agitation, hostility, anxiety, and aggression and normalization of sleep and eating patterns.
- After 1 week at a stable dose, a modest dosage increase may be considered. If there is no improvement within 3 to 4 weeks at therapeutic doses, then an alternative antipsychotic should be considered (i.e., move to the next treatment stage in the algorithm; see Figure 69–1).
- No data support giving larger daily doses to more severely symptomatic patients; however, in partial responders who are tolerating the antipsychotic well, it may be reasonable to titrate above the usual dose range.
- In general, rapid titration of antipsychotic dose is not recommended.
- IM antipsychotic administration (e.g., ziprasidone 10 to 20 mg, olanzapine 2.5 to 10 mg, or haloperidol 2 to 5 mg) can be used to calm agitated patients. However, this approach does not improve the extent of response, time to remission, or length of hospitalization.
- Intramuscular **lorazepam**, 2 mg, as needed in combination with the maintenance antipsychotic may actually be more effective in controlling agitation than using additional doses of the antipsychotic.

STABILIZATION THERAPY

XIII

- During weeks 2 and 3, the goals should be to improve socialization, self-care habits, and mood. Improvement in formal thought disorder may require an additional 6 to 8 weeks.
- Most patients require a dose of 300 to 1000 mg of chlorpromazine equivalents (of FGAs) daily or SGAs in usual labeled doses. Dose titration may continue every 1 to 2 weeks as long as the patient has no side effects.
- If symptom improvement is not satisfactory after 8 to 12 weeks, a different strategy (see Figure 69–1) should be tried.

MAINTENANCE THERAPY

- Medication should be continued for at least 12 months after remission of the first psychotic episode. Continuous treatment is necessary in most patients.
- Antipsychotics (especially FGAs and **clozapine**) should be tapered slowly before discontinuation to avoid rebound cholinergic withdrawal symptoms.
- In general, when switching from one antipsychotic to another, the first should be tapered and discontinued over 1 to 2 weeks after the second antipsychotic is initiated.

Depot Antipsychotic Medications

- The principle for conversion from oral antipsychotics to depot formulations is as follows:
  - Stabilize on an oral dosage form of the same agent (or at least a short trial of 3 to 7 days to be sure the medication is tolerated adequately).
- Risperidone is the first SGA to be available as a long-acting injectable. Usual dosing range is 25 to 50 mg IM every 2 weeks. It is a suspension of drug in glycolic acid-lactate copolymer microspheres. Significant risperidone serum concentrations are measurable about 3 weeks after single-dose administration. Thus oral medication must be administered for at least 3 weeks after beginning injections. Dose adjustments should be made no more often than every 4 weeks.
- For **fluphenazine decanoate**, the simplest conversion is the Stimmel method, which uses 1.2 times the oral daily dose for stabilized patients, rounding up to the nearest 12.5-mg interval, administered in weekly doses for the first 4 to 6 weeks (1.6 times the oral daily dose for patients who are more acutely ill). Subsequently, fluphenazine decanoate may be administered once every 2 to 3 weeks. Oral fluphenazine may be overlapped for 1 week.
- For **haloperidol decanoate**, a factor of 10 to 15 times the oral daily dose is commonly recommended, rounding up to the nearest 50-mg interval, administered in a once-monthly dose with oral haloperidol overlap for one month.
- Haloperidol and fluphenazine decanoate should be administered by a deep, "Z-track" IM method. Long-acting risperidone is injected by deep IM injection in the gluteus maximus, but Z-tracking is not necessary.
- In patients previously unexposed to the drug, an oral test dose of the medication is recommended before long-acting antipsychotics are given.

MANAGEMENT OF TREATMENT-RESISTANT SCHIZOPHRENIA

- Only **clozapine** has shown superiority in randomized clinical trials for the management of treatment-resistant schizophrenia.
- Symptomatic improvement with clozapine often occurs slowly in resistant patients, and as many as 60% of patients may improve if clozapine is used for up to 6 months.
- Because of the risk of orthostatic hypotension, clozapine is usually titrated more slowly than other antipsychotics. If a 12.5-mg test dose does not produce hypotension, then 25 mg of clozapine at bedtime is recommended, increased to 25 mg twice daily after 3 days, and then increased in 25- to 50-mg/day increments every 3 days until a dose of at least 300 mg/day is reached.
- Augmentation therapy involves the addition of a non-antipsychotic drug to an antipsychotic in a poorly responsive patient, while combination treatment involves using two antipsychotics simultaneously.
- Responders to augmentation therapy usually improve rapidly. If there is no improvement, the augmenting agent should be discontinued.
- Mood stabilizers (e.g., **lithium, valproic acid,** and **carbamazepine**) used as augmentation agents may improve labile affect and agitated behavior. A placebo-controlled trial supports fast symptom improvement when **divalproex** is combined with either **olanzapine** or **risperidone**.
- **Selective 5-HT reuptake inhibitors (SSRIs)** have been used with FGAs with improvement of negative symptoms. SSRIs have been used for obsessive-compulsive symptoms that worsen or arise during **clozapine** treatment.
- **Propranolol**, **pindolol**, and **nadolol** have been used for antiaggressive effects, especially in organic aggressive syndrome. If propranolol is used, a 20-mg test dose should be given to assess tolerability. If well tolerated, it can be initiated

XIII

at 20 mg three times daily. Increments can then be 60 mg/day every 3 days. Six to 8 weeks may be needed to evaluate response.

- Combining a FGA and a SGA and combining different SGAs have been suggested, but no data exist to support or refute these strategies. If a series of antipsychotic monotherapies fails, a time-limited combination trial may be attempted. If there is no improvement within 6 to 12 weeks, one of the drugs should be tapered and discontinued.

ADVERSE EFFECTS

Table 69–3 presents the relative incidence of common categories of antipsychotic side effects.

Autonomic Nervous System

- Anticholinergic (ACh) side effects include impaired memory, dry mouth, constipation, tachycardia, blurred vision, inhibition of ejaculation, and urinary retention. Elderly patients are especially sensitive to these side effects.
- Dry mouth can be managed with increased intake of fluids, oral lubricants (Xerolube), ice chips, or use of sugarless chewing gum or hard candy.
- Constipation can be treated with increases in exercise, fluid, and dietary fiber intake.

Central Nervous System
Extrapyramidal System
DYSTONIA

- Dystonias are prolonged tonic muscle contractions, with rapid onset (usually within 24 to 96 hours of dosage initiation or dosage increase); they may be life threatening (e.g., pharyngeal-laryngeal dystonias).
- Dystonic reactions occur primarily with FGAs.
- Treatment includes intramuscular or intravenous (IV) anticholinergics (Table 69–4) or **benzodiazepines**. **Benztropine mesylate**, 2 mg, or **diphenhydramine**, 50 mg, may be given IM or IV, or **diazepam,** 5 to 10 mg slow IV push, or **lorazepam**, 1 to 2 mg IM, may be given. Relief usually occurs within 15 to 20 minutes of IM injection or within 5 minutes of IV administration. The dose should be repeated if no response is seen within 15 minutes of XIII IV injection or 30 minutes of IM injection.
- Prophylactic ACh medications (e.g., the anticholinergics, not amantadine) are reasonable when using high-potency FGAs (e.g., **haloperidol, fluphenazine**), in young men, and in patients with a history of dystonia.

AKATHISIA

- Symptoms include subjective complaints (feelings of inner restlessness) and objective symptoms (pacing, shuffling, or tapping feet).
- Treatment with anticholinergics is disappointing, and reduction in antipsychotic dose may be the best intervention. Another alternative is to switch to a SGA, although akathisia occasionally occurs with the SGAs. **Quetiapine** and **clozapine** appear to have the lowest risk for causing akathisia.
- **Diazepam** (5 mg three times daily) is commonly used, but some researchers have failed to show efficacy.
- **Propranolol** (up to 160 mg/day), **nadolol** (up to 80 mg/day), and **metoprolol** (up to 100 mg/day) were reported to be effective.

PSEUDOPARKINSONISM

- Symptoms are (1) akinesia, bradykinesia, or decreased motor activity, including mask-like facial expression, micrographia, slowed speech, and decreased

TABLE 69–3. Relative Side-Effect Incidence of Commonly Used Antipsychotics

	Sedation	EPS	Anticholinergic	Orthostasis	Weight Gain	Prolactin
Aripiprazole	+	+	±	±	±	±
Chlorpromazine	++++	+++	+++	++++	++	+++
Clozapine	++++	±	++++	++++	++++	±
Fluphenazine	+	++++	+	+	+	++++
Haloperidol	+	++++	+	+	+	++++
Olanzapine	++	++	++	++	++++	+
Perphenazine	++	++++	++	++	+	++++
Quetiapine	++	±	+	++	++	±
Risperidone	+	++	+	++	++	++++
Thioridazine	++++	+++	++++	++++	+	+++
Thiothixene	+	++++	+	+	+	++++
Ziprasidone	++	++	±	+	±	+

Note: Side effects shown are relative risk based on doses within the recommended therapeutic range. Individual patient risk varies depending on patient-specific factors. Relative side-effect risk: ±, negligible; +, low; + +, moderate; + + +, moderately high; + + + +, high.
EPS, extrapyramidal side effects.

TABLE 69–4. Agents Used to Treat Extrapyramidal Side Effects

Generic Name	Equivalent Dose (mg)	Daily Dosage Range (mg)
Antimuscarinics		
Benztropine[a]	1	1–8[b]
Biperiden[a]	2	2–8
Trihexyphenidyl	2	2–15
Anithistaminic		
Diphenhydramine[a]	50	50–400
Dopamine agonist		
Amantadine	NA	100–400
Benzodiazepines		
Lorazepam[a]	NA	1–8
Diazepam	NA	2–20
Clonazepam	NA	2–8
β Blockers		
Propranolol	NA	20–160

[a]Injectable dosage form can be given intramuscularly for relief of acute dystonia.
[b]Dosage may be titrated to 12 mg/day with care; nonlinear pharmacokinetics have been demonstrated.

arm swing; (2) tremor (predominantly at rest and decreasing with movement); (3) rigidity, which may present as stiffness; cogwheel rigidity is seen as the patient's limbs yield in jerky, rachet-like fashion when moved passively by the examiner; and (4) stooped, unstable posture and slow, shuffling, or festinating gait.

- Accessory symptoms include seborrhea, sialorrhea, hyperhidrosis, fatigue, dysphagia, and dysarthria. A variant is rabbit syndrome, a perioral tremor.
- The onset of symptoms is usually 1 to 2 weeks after initiation of antipsychotic therapy or dose increase. The risk of pseudoparkinsonism with SGAs is low except in the case of **risperidone** in doses greater than 6 mg/day. XIII ◄
- Anticholinergics are an effective treatment. **Benztropine** has a longer half-life, which allows once- to twice-daily dosing. Dose increases above 6 mg/day must be slow because of nonlinear pharmacokinetics. **Trihexyphenidyl**, **diphenhydramine**, and **biperiden** usually require three-times-daily dosing.
- **Amantadine** is as efficacious as anticholinergics and has less effect on memory.
- An attempt should be made to taper and discontinue these agents 6 weeks to 3 months after symptoms resolve.

TARDIVE DYSKINESIA
- Tardive dyskinesia (TD) is sometimes irreversible and is characterized by abnormal involuntary movements (AIMs) occurring with chronic antipsychotic therapy.
- The classic presentation is buccolingual-masticatory (BLM) movements. Symptoms may become severe enough to interfere with chewing, speech, respiration, or swallowing. Facial movements include frequent blinking, brow arching, grimacing, upward deviation of the eyes, and lip smacking. Involvement of the extremities occurs in later stages (restless choreiform and athetotic movements of limbs). Truncal movements are classically reported in young adults. Movements may worsen with stress, decrease with sedation, and disappear with sleep.

- The Abnormal Involuntary Movement Scale (AIMS) and the Dyskinesia Identification System: Condensed User Scale (DISCUS) can be used to screen, but neither are diagnostic.
- Dosage reduction may have significant effect on outcome, with a complete disappearance of symptoms in some patients.
- Prevention of TD is best accomplished by (1) using antipsychotics only when there is a clear indication and at the lowest effective dose for the shortest duration possible; (2) using SGAs as first-line agents; (3) using the DISCUS or other scales to assess for early signs of TD at least quarterly; (4) discontinuing antipsychotics or switching to an SGAs (e.g., **risperidone** or **olanzapine**) at the earliest symptoms of TD, if possible; and (5) using antipsychotics only short term to abort aggressive behavior in nonpsychotic patients.
- α-**Tocopherol (vitamin E)**, 1200 to 1600 International Units, may prevent deterioration of TD, but it does not improve symptoms.

To date, there are no reports of TD with **clozapine** monotherapy, and it decreased AIMs in some trials.

- Limited evidence suggests that **olanzapine** may decrease TD symptoms. No data are available for other SGAs.

Sedation and Cognition
- Administration of most or all of the daily dose at bedtime can decrease daytime sedation and may eliminate the need for hypnotics.
- The SGAs as first-line treatment have been shown to improve cognition over a 9-month period.

Seizures
- There is an increased risk of drug-induced seizures in all patients treated with antipsychotics. The highest risk for antipsychotic-induced seizures is with the use of **chlorpromazine** or **clozapine**. **Olanzapine** may also be associated with greater risk. Seizures are more likely with initiation of treatment and with the use of higher doses and rapid dose increases.
- When an isolated seizure occurs, a dosage decrease is first recommended, and anticonvulsant therapy is usually not recommended.
- XIII If a change in antipsychotic therapy is required, **risperidone**, **molindone**, **thioridazine**, **haloperidol**, **pimozide**, **trifluoperazine**, and **fluphenazine** may be considered.

Thermoregulation
Hyperpyrexia can lead to heat stroke. Hypothermia is also a risk, particularly in elderly patients. These problems are more common with the use of low-potency FGAs and may also occur with **clozapine** and **olanzapine.**

Neuroleptic Malignant Syndrome (NMS)
- NMS occurs in 0.5% to 1% of patients taking FGAs. It may be more frequent with high-potency FGAs, injectable, or depot antipsychotics; in dehydrated patients; or in those with organic mental disorders. It has been reported with the SGAs, including **clozapine**, but is less frequent than with the FGAs.
- Symptoms develop rapidly over 24 to 72 hours and include body temperature exceeding 38°C (100.4°F), altered level of consciousness, autonomic dysfunction (tachycardia, labile blood pressure, diaphoresis, tachypnea, urinary or fecal incontinence), and rigidity.
- Laboratory evaluation frequently shows leukocytosis, increases in creatine kinase (CK), aspartate aminotransferase (AST), alanine aminotransferase (ALT), lactate dehydrogenase (LDH), and myoglobinuria.

- Treatment should begin with antipsychotic discontinuation and supportive care.
- **Bromocriptine**, used in theory to reverse DA blockade, reduces rigidity, fever, or CK in up to 94% of patients. **Amantadine** has been used successfully in up to 63% of patients. **Dantrolene** has been used as a skeletal muscle relaxant, with effects on temperature, respiratory rate, and CK in up to 81% of patients.
- Rechallenge with the lowest effective SGA dose may be considered only for patients in need of reinstitution of antipsychotics following observation for at least 2 weeks without antipsychotics. There must be careful monitoring and slow dose titration.

Endocrine System

- Galactorrhea and menstrual irregularities are common. These effects may be dose related and are more common with the use of FGAs and risperidone.
- Possible management strategies for galactorrhea include switching to an SGA (e.g., **olanzapine, quetiapine, aripiprazole**, or **ziprasidone**), adding **bromocriptine** (up to 15 mg daily), or adding **amantadine** (up to 300 mg daily).
- Weight gain is frequent with antipsychotic therapy including SGAs, especially **olanzapine** and **clozapine**. Weight gain may also occur with **risperidone** and **quetiapine**, but apparently **ziprasidone** and **aripiprazole** are least likely to have this effect.
- Schizophrenics have a higher prevalence of type 2 diabetes than non-schizophrenics. Antipsychotics may adversely affect glucose levels in diabetic patients. New onset diabetes has been reported with use of the SGAs, and the relative risk for the various SGAs is unknown.

Cardiovascular System

- Incidence of orthostatic hypotension (defined as a greater than 20-mm Hg drop in systolic pressure) is greatest with low-potency FGAs and SGAs, especially with IM or IV administration. Diabetics with cardiovascular disease and the elderly are predisposed.
- Tolerance to this effect usually occurs within 2 to 3 months. Reducing the dose or changing to an antipsychotic with less α-adrenergic blockade may also help.
- For severe hypotensive episodes, volume expansion (the use of IV fluids) should be tried before pressor agents. XIII
- Pure α-adrenergic pressor agents (e.g., **phenylephrine, metaraminol**) or **norepinephrine,** which has α agonist and β_1-adrenergic properties, can be used. **Epinephrine**, with α- and β-adrenergic effects, should not be used, and **isoproterenol** should also be avoided.
- Low-potency piperidine phenothiazines (e.g., **thioridazine**), **clozapine**, and **ziprasidone** are more likely to cause electrocardiogram (ECG) effects.
- ECG changes include increased heart rate, flattened T waves, ST-segment depression, prolongation of QT and PR intervals, and torsades de pointes. Torsades de pointes has been reported with **thioridazine** and **mesoridazine,** which may be a cause of cardiac sudden death.
- Ziprasidone prolonged the QTc interval about one-half as much as thioridazine. Ziprasidone's effect on the ECG are probably without clinical sequelea except in patients with baseline risk factors.
- In patients older than 50 years, pretreatment ECG and serum potassium and magnesium levels are recommended.

Lipid Effects

Some SGAs and phenothiazines cause elevations in serum triglycerides and cholesterol, and the extent to which this effect differs among antipsychotics is unclear. The risk for this effect may be less with risperidone, ziprasidone, or aripiprazole.

Ophthalmologic Effects

- Impairment in visual accommodation results from paresis of ciliary muscles. Photophobia may also result. If severe, **pilocarpine** ophthalmic solution may be necessary.
- Exacerbation of narrow-angle glaucoma can occur with use of antipsychotics or antiparkinson medication.
- Opaque deposits in the cornea and lens may occur with chronic phenothiazine treatment, especially with **chlorpromazine**. Although visual acuity is not usually affected, periodic slit-lamp examinations are recommended with long-term phenothiazines. Baseline and periodic slit-lamp examinations are also recommended for **quetiapine**-treated patients because of lenticular changes in animal studies.
- Retinitis pigmentosis can result from **thioridazine** doses greater than 800 mg daily (the recommended maximum dose) and can cause permanent visual impairment or blindness.

Hepatic System

- Liver function test abnormalities are common. If aminotransferases are greater than 3 times the upper limit of normal, the antipsychotic should be changed to a chemically unrelated antipsychotic. These changes are less common with the SGAs but are reported with **risperidone** and **clozapine**.
- Cholestatic hepatocanalicular jaundice can occur in up to 2% of patients receiving phenothiazines.

Genitourinary System

- Urinary hesitancy and retention are commonly reported, especially with low-potency FGAs and **clozapine**, and men with benign prostatic hypertrophy are especially prone.
- Urinary incontinence is especially problematic with **clozapine**.
- Risperidone produces at least as much sexual dysfunction as FGAs, but other SGAs are less like to have this effect.

XIII

Hematologic System

- Transient leukopenia may occur with antipsychotic therapy, but it typically does not progress to clinically significant parameters.
- If the white blood cell (WBC) count is less than 3000/mm^3 or the absolute neutrophil count (ANC) is less than 1000/mm^3, the antipsychotic should be discontinued, and the WBC count monitored closely until it returns to normal.
- Agranulocytosis reportedly occurs in 0.01% of patients receiving FGAs, and it may occur more frequently with **chlorpromazine** and **thioridazine**. The onset is usually within the first 8 weeks of therapy. It may initially manifest as a local infection (e.g., sore throat, leukoplakia, and erythema and ulcerations of the pharynx). These symptoms should trigger an immediate WBC.
- The 18-month treatment risk of developing agranulocytosis with **clozapine** is approximately 0.91%. Increasing age and female gender are associated with greater risk. The greatest risk appears to be between months 1 and 6 of treatment. Weekly WBC monitoring for the first 6 months (biweekly thereafter) is mandated in the product labeling. If the WBC drops to less than 2000/mm^3 or the ANC is less than 1000/mm^3, clozapine should be discontinued. In cases of mild to moderate neutropenia (granulocytes between 2000 and 3000/mm^3

or ANC between 1000 and 1500/mm^3), which occurs in up to 2% of patients, clozapine should be discontinued, with daily monitoring of complete blood counts until values return to normal.

Dermatologic System

- Allergic reactions are rare and usually occur within 8 weeks of initiating therapy. They manifest as maculopapular, erythematous, or pruritic rashes. Drug discontinuation and topical steroids are recommended when they occur.
- Contact dermatitis, including on the oral mucosa, may occur. Swallowing of the oral concentrate quickly may decrease problems.
- Both FGAs and SGAs can cause photosensitivity. Erythema and severe sunburns can occur. Patients should be educated to use maximal blocking sunscreens, hats, protective clothing, and sunglasses when in the sun.
- Blue-gray or purplish discoloration of skin exposed to sunlight may occur with higher doses of low-potency phenothiazines (especially **chlorpromazine**) long term.

USE IN PREGNANCY AND LACTATION

- There is a slightly increased risk of birth defects with low-potency FGAs.
- There is no relationship between **haloperidol** use and teratogenicity.
- Concern has been expressed over the use of SGAs in pregnancy because of the risk for weight gain, potential risk for gestational diabetes.
- Other potential, but largely unknown, risks of antipsychotic therapy include the possibility of behavioral teratogenicity on the neonate, receptor changes, and perinatal effects (e.g., tonicity, strength, and sucking), EPS, jaundice, respiratory depression, and intestinal obstruction.
- Antipsychotics appear in breast milk with milk-to-plasma ratios of 0.5 to 1.

DRUG INTERACTIONS

- Most antipsychotic drug interactions are relatively minor and often involve additive central nervous system (CNS), anticholinergic, or sedative effects.
- Antipsychotic pharmacokinetics can be significantly affected by concomitantly administered enzyme inducers or inhibitors. Smoking is a potent inducer of hepatic enzymes and may increase antipsychotic clearance by as much as 50%. The published literature may be consulted for a listing of antipsychotic drug interactions.
- Table 69–5 lists the major pathways thought to be involved in the metabolism of SGAs.

PHARMACOECONOMIC CONSIDERATIONS

- Although SGAs cost more than traditional agents, studies have fairly consistently shown total mental health care costs to be no higher or even lower when SGAs are used.
- Of greater controversy is whether differences in cost-effectiveness exist between the SGAs.

▶ EVALUATION OF THERAPEUTIC OUTCOMES

- Clinicians should use standardized psychiatric rating scales to rate response objectively. The four-item Positive Symptom Rating Scale and the Brief Negative Symptom Assessment are scales that are brief enough to be useful in the outpatient setting.

TABLE 69–5. Antidepressant/Antipsychotic P450 Inhibitor Drug Interactions

Inhibitor (Inhibits Substrate)	Substrate (Drug Metabolized By Pathway)		
	1A2	2D6	3A3/4
Bupropion (Wellbutrin) Citalopram (Celexa) Fluoxetine (Prozac)		**Phenothiazines (some)** Phenothiazines **PHENOTHIAZINES** **Risperidone,** Aripiprazole	**Clozapine, Quetiapine,** Ziprasidone[a] **Clozapine, Quetiapine,** Ziprasidone[a]
Fluvoxamine (Luvox)	**CLOZAPINE, THIORIDAZINE, HALOPERIDOL, OLANZAPINE, THIOTHIXENE**		
Nefazodone (Serzone)			**QUETIAPINE, Clozapine,** Ziprasidone[a]
Paroxetine (Paxil)		**PHENOTHIAZINES, Risperidone,** Aripiprazole	
Sertraline (Zoloft)		Phenothiazines	Clozapine, Quetiapine, Ziprasidone[a]

Note: The inhibitor drug inhibits the metabolism of the substrate drug; therefore increasing the amount of substrate drug in the body, and the potential for side effects from the substrate drug. Bold type and capital letters reflect the relative potential for the interaction to be clinically significant (i.e. **HIGH. Moderate.** Low).

[a]Indicates that this is a minor pathway for this substrate, and therefore the possibility of a clinically significant interaction through this pathway is decreased.

- Patient-rated self-assessments can also be useful, as they engage the patient in treatment and can open the door for patient education and addressing patient misconceptions.

See Chapter 68, Schizophrenia, authored by M. Lynn Crismon and Peter G. Dorson, for a more detailed discussion of this topic.

XIII ◄

Chapter 70

▶ SLEEP DISORDERS

▶ DEFINITION

The Diagnostic and Statistical Manual of Mental Disorders, 4th ed., text revision (DSM-IV-TR) classifies sleep disorders as shown in Table 70–1. One month of symptoms is required before a sleep disorder is diagnosed.

▶ SLEEP PHYSIOLOGY

- Humans typically have 4 to 6 cycles of non–rapid eye movement (NREM) and rapid eye movement (REM) sleep each night, each cycle lasting 70 to 120 minutes. Usually there is progression through four stages of NREM sleep before the first REM period.
- In stage 1 of NREM, alpha waves evolve into slower theta waves. Stage 2 is characterized by theta rhythms with sleep spindles and K complexes. Stage 3 and 4 sleep is called delta sleep.
- In REM sleep, there is a low-amplitude, mixed-frequency EEG, increased electric and metabolic activity, increased cerebral blood flow, muscle atonia, poikilothermia, vivid dreaming, and fluctuations in respiratory and cardiac rate.
- In the elderly, sleep is lighter and more fragmented with more arousals and a gradual disappearance of slow-wave sleep.
- Sleep is reduced when there is decreased serotonin activity or destruction of the dorsal raphe nucleus.
- REM sleep is turned on by cholinergic cells.

TABLE 70–1. DSM-IV-TR Classification of Sleep Disorders

Primary sleep disorders
Dyssomnias
    Primary insomnia
    Primary hypersomnia
    Narcolepsy
    Breathing-related sleep disorder
    Circadian rhythm sleep disorder
        Delayed sleep phase type
        Jet lag type
        Shift work type
        Unspecified type
    Dyssomnia not otherwise specified
Parasomnias
    Nightmare disorder
    Sleep terror disorder
    Sleepwalking disorder
    Parasomnia not otherwise specified
Sleep disorders related to another mental disorder
Insomnia related to another mental disorder
Hypersomnia related to another mental disorder
Other sleep disorders
Sleep disorder due to a general medical condition
Substance-induced sleep disorder

- Dopamine has an alerting effect. Neurochemicals involved in wakefulness include norepinephrine and acetylcholine in the cortex and histamine and neuropeptides (e.g., substance P and corticotropin-releasing factor) in the hypothalamus.
- Polysomnography (PSG) is a procedure that measures multiple electrophysiologic parameters simultaneously during sleep (e.g., electroencephalogram [EEG], electrooculogram [EOG], and electromyogram [EMG]). Two EOGs, one EEG, and one EMG are the minimal recordings used in scoring sleep stages.

▶ INSOMNIA

CLINICAL PRESENTATION

- Patients complain of difficulty falling asleep, maintaining sleep, or not feeling rested in spite of a sufficient opportunity to sleep.
- Transient (2 to 3 nights) and short-term (less than 3 weeks) insomnia are common and usually related to a precipitating factor. Chronic insomnia (greater than 1 month) may be related to medical or psychiatric disorders or medication, or it may be psychophysiologic.

DIAGNOSIS

Common causes of insomnia are shown in Table 70–2. In patients with chronic disturbances, a diagnostic evaluation includes physical and mental status examinations, routine laboratory tests, and medication and substance abuse histories.

TABLE 70–2. Common Etiologies of Insomnia

Situational
Work or financial stress
Interpersonal conflicts
Major life events
Jet lag or shift work
Medical
Cardiovascular (angina, arrhythmias, heart failure)
Respiratory (asthma, sleep apnea)
Chronic pain
Endocrine disorders (diabetes, hyperthyroidism)
Gastrointestinal (gastroesophageal reflux disease, ulcers)
Neurologic (delirium, epilepsy, Parkinson's disease)
Pregnancy
Psychiatric
Mood disorders (depression, mania)
Anxiety disorders (generalized anxiety disorder, obsessive-compulsive disorder, or panic disorder)
Substance abuse (alcohol or sedative-hypnotic withdrawal)
Pharmacologically induced
Anticonvulsants
Central adrenergic blockers
Diuretics
Selective serotonin reuptake inhibitors
Steroids
Stimulants

XIII

TREATMENT

- Management includes identifying the cause of insomnia, education on sleep hygiene, stress management, monitoring for mood symptoms, and elimination of unnecessary pharmacotherapy.
- Transient insomnia should be treated with good sleep hygiene and careful use of sedative-hypnotics.
- In short-term insomnia, nonpharmacologic treatment is important, but sedative-hypnotics can be used.
- Chronic insomnia calls for careful assessment for a medical cause, nonpharmacologic treatment, and careful and less frequent use of sedative-hypnotics to prevent tolerance and dependence.

Nonpharmacologic Therapy
Behavioral and educational interventions include short-term cognitive therapy, relaxation therapy, stimulus control therapy, light therapy, sleep restriction, and sleep hygiene education (see Table 70–3).

Pharmacologic Therapy
Nonbenzodiazepine Hypnotic Agents
- Antihistamines (e.g., **diphenhydramine**, **doxylamine**, and **pyrilamine**) are less effective than benzodiazepines, but side effects are minimal. Their anticholinergic side effects may be problematic, especially in the elderly.
- The antidepressants are good alternatives for patients with poor sleep who should not receive benzodiazepines, especially those with depression or a history of substance abuse.
- **Amitriptyline**, **doxepin**, and **nortriptyline** are effective, but side effects include anticholinergic effects, adrenergic blockade, and cardiac conduction prolongation.
- **Trazodone**, 25 to 75 mg, is often used for insomnia induced by selective serotonin reuptake inhibitors or bupropion. Side effects include serotonin syndrome

➤ XIII

TABLE 70–3. Nonpharmacologic Recommendations for Insomnia

Stimulus control procedures
1. Establish regular times to wake up and to go to sleep (including weekends).
2. Sleep only as much as necessary to feel rested.
3. Go to bed only when sleepy. Avoid long periods of wakefulness in bed. Use the bed only for sleep or intimacy; do not read or watch television in bed.
4. Avoid trying to force sleep; if you do not fall asleep within 20–30 min, leave the bed and perform a relaxing activity (e.g., read, listen to music, or watch television) until drowsy. Repeat this as often as necessary.
5. Avoid daytime naps.
6. Schedule worry time during the day. Do not take your troubles to bed.

Sleep hygiene recommendations
1. Exercise routinely (3–4 times weekly), but not close to bedtime because this may cause arousal.
2. Create a comfortable sleep environment by avoiding temperature extremes, loud noises, and illuminated clocks in the bedroom.
3. Discontinue or reduce the use of alcohol, caffeine, and nicotine.
4. Avoid drinking large quantities of liquids in the evening to prevent nighttime trips to the restroom.
5. Do something relaxing and enjoyable before bedtime.

(when used with other serotonergic drugs), oversedation, α-adrenergic block-ade, dizziness, and rarely priapism.

- **Zolpidem**, chemically unrelated to benzodiazepines or barbiturates, acts selectively at the benzodiazepine$_1$ receptor and has minimal anxiolytic and no muscle relaxant or anticonvulsant effects. It is comparable in effectiveness to benzodiazepine hypnotics, and it has little effect on sleep stages. Its half-life is approximately 6 to 8 hours, and it is metabolized to inactive metabolites. Common side effects are drowsiness, amnesia, dizziness, headache, and GI complaints. Rebound effects on discontinuation and tolerance with prolonged use are minimal, but theoretical concerns about abuse exist. It may have no significant effects on next-day psychomotor performance. The usual dose is 10 mg, which can be increased up to 20 mg nightly, but only 5 mg in elderly patients and those with hepatic impairment.
- **Zaleplon** also binds to the benzodiazepine$_1$ receptor. It has a rapid onset, a half-life of about 1 hour, and no active metabolites. It does not reduce night-time awakenings or increase the total sleep time. It may be best used for middle-of-the-night awakenings. It does not appear to cause significant rebound insomnia or next day psychomotor impairment. The most common side effects are dizziness, headache, and somnolence. The recommended dose is 10 mg for nonelderly adults and 5 mg in the elderly.
- **Valerian**, an herbal product, is also available without a prescription. Purity and potency concerns are an issue. It may cause daytime sedation.

Benzodiazepine Hypnotics

- The pharmacokinetic properties of benzodiazepine hypnotics are summarized in Table 70–4.
- Benzodiazines bind to γ-aminobutyric acid (GABA) receptors, and they have sedative, anxiolytic, muscle relaxant, and anticonvulsant properties. They increase stage 2 sleep and decrease REM and delta sleep.
- Overdose fatalities are rare unless benzodiazepines are taken with other central nervous system (CNS) depressants.
- **Triazolam** is distributed quickly because of its high lipophilicity, and thus it has a short duration of effect. **Erythromycin, nefazodone, fluvoxamine**, and **ketoconazole** reduce the clearance of triazolam and increase plasma concentrations.
- **Estazolam** and **temazepam** are intermediate in their duration of action.

TABLE 70–4. Pharmacokinetics of Benzodiazepine Hypnotic Agents

Generic Name	t_{max} (h)[a]	Parent $t_{1/2}$ (h)	Daily Dose Range (mg)	Metabolic Pathway	Clinically Significant Metabolities
Estazolam	2	12–15	1–2	Oxidation	
Flurazepam	1	8	15–30	Oxidation	Hydroxyethylflurazepam
					Flurazepam aldehyde
				N-dealkylation	N-DAF[b]
Quazepam	2	39	7.5–15	Oxidation	2-Oxo-quazepam
				N-dealkylation	N-DAF[b]
Temazepam	1.5	10–15	15–30	Conjugation	–
Triazolam	1	2	0.125–0.25	Oxidation	–

[a] Time to peak plasma concentration.

[b] N-desalkylflurazepam, mean half-life 47–100 h.

- The effects of **flurazepam** and **quazepam** are long because of active metabolites.
- With the exception of **temazepam**, which is eliminated by conjugation, all benzodiazepine hypnotics are metabolized by microsomal oxidation followed by glucuronide conjugation.
- *N*-desalkylflurazepam accounts for most of **flurazepam** pharmacologic effects. This metabolite may help when daytime anxiety or early morning awakening are present, but daytime sedation with impaired psychomotor performance may occur.

BENZODIAZEPINE ADVERSE EFFECTS

- Side effects include drowsiness, psychomotor incoordination, decreased concentration, and cognitive deficits.
- Tolerance to the daytime CNS effects (e.g., drowsiness, psychomotor impairment, decreased concentration) may develop in some individuals.
- Tolerance to hypnotic effects develops after 2 weeks of continuous use of **triazolam**. Efficacy of **flurazepam**, **quazepam**, and **temazepam** lasts for at least 1 month of continuous nightly use. **Estazolam** reportedly maintains efficacy at maximum dosage (2 mg nightly) for up to 12 weeks.
- Anterograde amnesia occurs more frequently with **triazolam** than **temazepam**; however, it has been reported with most benzodiazepines. Using the lowest dose possible minimizes amnesia.
- **Triazolam** is associated with a higher rate of confusion, bizarre behavior, agitation, and hallucinations than **temazepam**.
- Rebound insomnia occurs more frequently after high doses of **triazolam**, even when used intermittently.
- Rebound insomnia can be minimized by utilizing the lowest effective dose and tapering the dose upon discontinuation.
- There is an association between falls and hip fractures and the use of long-elimination half-life benzodiazepines; thus, **flurazepam** and **quazepam** should be avoided in the elderly.

XIII ▶ SLEEP APNEA

Apnea is the cessation of airflow at the nose and mouth lasting at least 10 seconds. The goals of therapy are to reduce apneic episodes and improve O_2 saturation.

OBSTRUCTIVE SLEEP APNEA

- Obstructive sleep apnea (OSA) is potentially life threatening and is characterized by repeated episodes of nocturnal breathing cessation with loud snoring and gasping. It is caused by an occlusion of the upper airway. Most individuals with OSA are overweight.
- In severe episodes there is heavy snoring, severe gas exchange disturbances, and respiratory failure causing gasping. This may occur up to 600 times/night.
- Episodes may be caused by obesity or fixed upper airway lesions, enlarged tonsils, amyloidosis, and hypothyroidism. Complications include arrhythmias, hypertension, cor pulmonale, and sudden death.
- The apneic episode is terminated by a reflex action to the fall in O_2 saturation that causes a brief arousal during which breathing resumes.
- OSA patients usually complain of excessive daytime sleepiness. Other symptoms are morning headache, poor memory, and irritability.

Treatment

- Patients with severe apnea (greater than 20 apneas per hour on polysomnography [PSG]) and moderate apnea (5 to 20 apneas per hour on PSG) have shown significant improvement and reduction in mortality with treatment.
- Nonpharmacologic approaches are the treatment of choice (e.g., weight loss, tonsillectomy, nasal septal repair, and nasal continuous positive airway pressure [CPAP]).
- The most important pharmacologic interventions are avoidance of all **CNS depressants**, but preliminary studies suggest that **zaleplon** does not interfere with respiratory function.
- Pharmacologic interventions should be reserved for patients with mild forms of OSA and in patients who have failed other treatments. **Protriptyline**, 10 to 30 mg/day, reduces the frequency of apneas and increases O_2 saturation. **Imipramine** may also be effective.
- **Fluoxetine** and **paroxetine** may be as effective as protriptyline, with fewer side effects.
- The only role for **medroxyprogesterone** is in patients with awake respiratory failure or noncompliance with CPAP.

CENTRAL SLEEP APNEA

- Central sleep apnea (CSA; less than 10% of all apneas) is characterized by repeated episodes of apnea caused by temporary loss of respiratory effort during sleep.
- Hypercapnic patients complain of morning headache and daytime sleepiness, while nonhypercapnic patients complain of insomnia and nocturnal awakenings with shortness of breath or gasping.

Treatment

- For hypercapnic patients, primary treatment is ventilatory support with O_2 and CPAP; **acetazolamide, theophylline,** and **medroxyprogesterone** have shown mixed results. Acetazolamide has caused a 70% reduction in CSA, but use is limited by side effects. Theophylline may be effective, but more study is needed.
- In nonhypercapnic patients, treatment may consist of benzodiazepines (**triazolam** or **temazepam**) and **acetazolamide**, CPAP, and oxygen to stabilize breathing patterns.

▶ NARCOLEPSY

- The essential features are sleep attacks, cataplexy, hypnagogic hallucinations, and sleep paralysis. Individuals with narcolepsy complain of excessive daytime sleepiness, sleep attacks that last up to 30 minutes, hypersomnia, fatigue, impaired performance, and disturbed nighttime sleep. They have multiple arousals during the night.
- Cataplexy is sudden bilateral loss of muscle tone with collapse, which is often precipitated by situations characterized by high emotion.
- It is accepted that narcolepsy results from defects in the hypocretin-orexin neurotransmitter system, perhaps as a result of an autoimmune process.

TREATMENT

- The goal of therapy is to maximize alertness during waking hours or at selected times.

XIII

TABLE 70–5. Drugs Used to Treat Narcolepsy

Generic Name	Trade Name (Manufacturer)	Daily Dosage Range (mg)
Excessive daytime somnolence		
Dextroamphetamine	Dexadrine (GlaxoSmithKline) generics (various)	5–60
Dextroamphetamine/amphetamine salts[a]	Adderall (Shire US)	5–60
Methamphetamine[b]	Desoxyn (Abbott)	5–15
Methylphenidate	Ritalin (Novartis), generics (various)	30–80
Modafinil	Provigil (Cephalon)	200–400
Pemoline	Cylert (Abbott)	37.5–112.5
Adjunct agents for cataplexy		
Fluoxetine	Prozac (Lilly), generics (various)	20–80
hydroxybutyrate	Xyrem (Orphan Medical)	60 mg/kg/night
Imipramine	Tofranil (Novartis), generics (various)	50–250
Nortriptyline	Aventyl (Lilly), Pamelor (Sandoz), generics (various)	50–200
Protriptyline	Vivactil (Merck), generics (various)	5–30
Selegiline	Eldepryl (Somerset)	20–40

[a] Dextroamphetamine sulfate, dextroamphetamine saccharate, amphetamine aspartate, and amphetamine sulfate.
[b] Not available in some states.

- Good sleep hygiene as well as two or more brief daytime naps daily (as little as 15 minutes) should be encouraged.
- Medications used to treat narcolepsy are shown in Table 70–5.
- **Modafinil** is considered the standard for treatment of excessive daytime sleepiness. Plasma concentrations peak in 2 to 4 hours, and the half-life is 15 hours. The dose is 200 to 400 mg/day. Preliminary evidence suggests no tolerance or withdrawal after abrupt discontinuation and no risk of abuse.
- Side effects of modafinil include headache, nausea, nervousness, and insomnia.
- **Amphetamines** and **methylphenidate** have a fast onset of effect and durations of 3 to 4 hours and 6 to 10 hours, respectively. Divided daily doses are recommended, but sustained-release formulations are available. Amphetamines are associated with more likelihood of abuse and tolerance. Side effects include insomnia, hypertension, palpitations, and irritability. Compliance with stimulants is usually poor.
- **Pemoline** has a delayed onset of effect, but its duration is 8 to 10 hours. Adherence is better than with the stimulants, but lethal liver toxicity and the need for liver function testing limit acceptance.
- The most effective treatment for cataplexy is the **tricyclic antidepressants** or **fluoxetine. Imipramine, protriptyline, clomipramine, fluoxetine,** and **nortriptyline** are effective in about 80% of patients.
- Of the new agents, **sodium oxybate** (γ-**hyroxybutyrate**) appears to be the most promising. It improves excessive daytime sleepiness and decreases episodes of sleep paralysis, cataplexy, and hypnogogic hallucinations.

XIII

▶ EVALUATION OF THERAPEUTIC OUTCOMES

- An algorithm for management of dyssomnias is shown in Figure 70–1. Patients with short-term or chronic insomnia should be evaluated after 1 week of

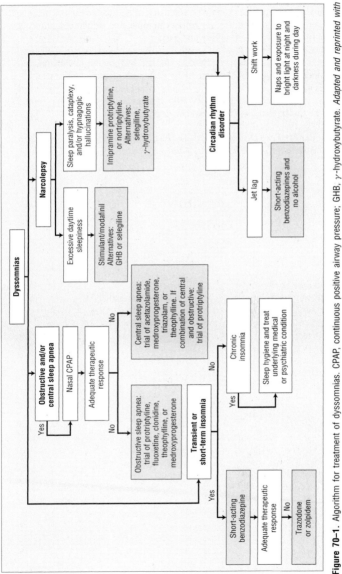

Figure 70–1. Algorithm for treatment of dyssomnias. CPAP, continuous positive airway pressure; GHB, γ-hydroxybutyrate. *Adapted and reprinted with permission from Jermain DM. Sleep disorders. In: Jann M, ed. Pharmacotherapy-Self-Assessment Program, 2nd ed: Kansas City, MO, American College of Clinical Pharmacy, 1995:139–154.*)

therapy to assess for drug effectiveness, adverse events, and compliance with nonpharmacologic recommendations. Patients should be instructed to maintain a sleep diary, including a daily recording of awakenings, medication ingestions, naps, and an index of sleep quality.

- Patients with sleep apnea should be evaluated after 2 to 4 weeks of treatment for improvement in alertness, daytime symptoms, and weight reduction. The bed partner can report on snoring and gasping.
- Monitoring parameters for pharmacotherapy of narcolepsy include reduction in daytime sleepiness, cataplexy, hypnagogic and hypnopompic hallucinations, and sleep paralysis. Patients should be evaluated monthly until an optimal dose is achieved, then every 6 to 12 months to assess adverse drug events (e.g., mood changes, sleep disturbances, cardiovascular abnormalities). If symptoms increase during therapy, PSG should be done.

See Chapter 71, Sleep Disorders, authored by Cherry Jackson and Judy L. Curtis, for a more detailed discussion of this topic.

XIII

Chapter 71

▶ SUBSTANCE-RELATED DISORDERS

▶ DEFINITION

The substance-related disorders include disorders related to the taking of drugs of abuse (including alcohol), to the side effects of a medication, and to toxin exposure. Substance dependence or addiction can be viewed as a chronic illness that can be successfully controlled with treatment, but cannot be cured, and is associated with a high relapse rate.

- *Addiction:* A primary chronic neurobiologic disease, with genetic, psychosocial, and environmental factors influencing its development and manifestations. It is characterized by behaviors that include one or more of the following 5Cs: chronicity, impaired control over drug use, compulsive use, continued use despite harm, and craving.
- *Intoxication:* Development of a substance-specific syndrome after recent ingestion and presence in the body of a substance, and it is associated with maladaptive behavior during the waking state caused by the effect of the substance on the central nervous system (CNS).
- *Physical dependence:* A state of adaptation that is manifested by a drug class–specific withdrawal syndrome that can be produced by abrupt cessation, rapid dose reduction, decreasing blood level of the drug, and/or administration of an antagonist.
- *Substance abuse:* The characteristic feature is a maladaptive pattern of substance use indicated by repeated adverse consequences related to the repeated use of the substance.
- *Substance dependence:* The essential feature is the continued use of the substance despite adverse substance-related problems.
- *Tolerance:* A state of adaptation in which exposure to a drug induces changes that result in a diminution of one or more of the drug's effects over time.
- *Withdrawal:* The appearance of the characteristic withdrawal syndrome or the use of the same or related drug to relieve or avoid withdrawal symptoms. Development of a substance-specific syndrome after cessation of or reduction in intake of a substance that was used regularly to induce a state of intoxication. It is usually associated with substance dependence and craving.

▶ CENTRAL NERVOUS SYSTEM DEPRESSANTS

ALCOHOL
- Table 71–1 relates the effects of **alcohol** to the blood alcohol concentration (BAC). Table 71–2 lists signs and symptoms of alcohol intoxication and withdrawal.
- There is 14 g of alcohol in 12 oz of beer, 4 oz of wine, or 1.5 oz (one shot) of 80-proof whiskey. This amount will increase the BAC by about 25 mg/dL in a healthy 70-kg male. Deaths generally occur when BACs are greater than 500 mg/dL.
- Absorption of alcohol begins in the stomach within 5 to 10 minutes of ingestion, but it is absorbed primarily from the duodenum. Peak concentrations are achieved 30 to 90 minutes after finishing the last drink.
- Alcohol is metabolized by alcohol dehydrogenase (a zero-order process except at very high and very low concentrations) to acetaldehyde, which is metabolized

TABLE 71–1. Specific Effects of Alcohol Related to the Blood Alcohol Concentration (BAC)

BAC (%)[a]	(Effect)
0.02–0.03	No loss of coordination, slight euphoria and loss of shyness. Depressant effects are not apparent.
0.04–0.06	Feeling of well-being, relaxation, lower inhibitions, sensation of warmth. Euphoria. Some minor impairment of reasoning and memory, lowering of caution.
0.07–0.09	Slight impairment of balance, speech, vision, reaction time, and hearing. Euphoria. Judgment and self-control are reduced, and caution, reason, and memory are impaired. It is illegal to operate a motor vehicle in some states at this level of intoxication.
0.10–0.125	Significant impairment of motor coordination and loss of good judgment. Speech may be slurred; balance, vision, reaction time, and hearing will be impaired. Euphoria. It is illegal to operate a motor vehicle at this level of intoxication.
0.13–0.15	Gross motor impairment and lack of physical control. Blurred vision and major loss of balance. Euphoria is reduced and dysphoria is beginning to appear.
0.16–0.20	Dysphoria (anxiety, restlessness) predominates, nausea may appear. The drinker has the appearance of a "sloppy drunk."
0.25	Needs assistance in walking; total mental confusion. Dysphoria with nausea and some vomiting.
0.30	Loss of consciousness.
≥0.40	Onset of coma, possible death due to respiratory arrest.

[a] Grams of ethyl alcohol per 100 mL of whole blood.

to carbon dioxide and water by aldehyde dehydrogenase. Catalase and the microsomal alcohol oxidase system are also involved.

- Most clinical labs report BAC in milligrams per deciliter. In legal cases, results are reported in percentage (grams of alcohol per 100 mL of whole blood). Thus, a BAC of 150 mg/dL = 0.15%.
- Alcohol withdrawal includes two main components: (1) history of cessation or reduction in heavy and prolonged alcohol use, and (2) presence of two or more of the symptoms of alcohol withdrawal (Table 71–2).

TABLE 71–2. Signs and Symptoms of Alcohol Intoxication and Withdrawal

Intoxication	Withdrawal
Slurred speech	Tremor
Ataxia	Tachycardia
Nystagmus	Diaphoresis
Sedation	Labile blood pressure
Flushed face	Anxiety
Mood change	Nausea and vomiting
Irritability	Hallucinations
Euphoria	Seizures
Loquacity	Hyperthermia
Impaired attention	Delirium

XIII

BENZODIAZEPINES (BZS) AND OTHER SEDATIVE–HYPNOTICS

- BZs with faster onset (e.g., **diazepam**) tend to be preferred by recreational users because they are reinforcing. They cause little respiratory depression.
- Adverse effects of BZs include decreased blood pressure, memory impairment, drowsiness, visual disturbances, confusion, gastrointestinal (GI) disturbances, and urinary retention.
- Intoxication is manifested as slurred speech, poor coordination, and swaying.
- Signs and symptoms of BZ withdrawal are similar to those of alcohol withdrawal, including muscle pain, anxiety, restlessness, confusion, irritability, hallucinations, delirium, seizures, and cardiovascular collapse. Withdrawal from short-acting BZs (e.g., **oxazepam, lorazepam, alprazolam**) has an onset within 12 to 24 hours of the last dose; other sedatives (e.g., **diazepam, chlordiazepoxide, clorazepate ,phenobarbital, amobarbital**) have elimination half-lives (or active metabolites with elimination half-lives) of 24 to greater than 100 hours. So, withdrawal may be delayed for several days after discontinuation.
- Sedative–hypnotic dependence is summarized in Table 71–3.
- Likelihood and severity of withdrawal are a function of dose and duration of exposure. Gradual tapering of dosage is associated with less withdrawal and rebound anxiety than abrupt discontinuation.
- **Flunitrazepam** (Rohypnol) is a BZ that is frequently taken with **alcohol, marijuana, cocaine,** or **heroin.** Onset of effects is within 30 minutes, and duration may be 8 hours or more. Sometimes called the "date-rape drug," it has been given to women in hope of lowering inhibitions.

γ-HYDROXYBUTYRATE (GHB)

- **GHB** is also called a "date-rape drug." It is sold as a liquid or powder, and effects include amnesia, hypotonia, abnormal sequence of rapid eye movement (REM) and non-REM sleep, and anesthesia.
- Toxic effects include decreased cardiac output, vomiting, respiratory depression, coma, and seizures.
- Withdrawal symptoms include mental status changes, elevated blood pressure, XIII tachycardia, diaphoresis, tremors, and severe agitation.

OPIATES

- Signs and symptoms of opioid intoxication and withdrawal are shown in Table 71–4. The onset of withdrawal ranges from a few hours after stopping heroin to 3 to 5 days after stopping methadone. Duration of withdrawal ranges from 3 to 24 days. Occurrence of delirium suggests withdrawal from another drug (e.g., **alcohol**).
- **Heroin** can be snorted, smoked, and given intravenously. Complications of heroin use include overdoses, anaphylactic reactions to impurities, nephrotic syndrome, septicemia, endocarditis, and acquired immunodeficiency syndrome (AIDS).
- **OxyContin** tablets, a controlled-release dosage form of oxycodone, are sometimes crushed by abusers to get the full 12-hour effect almost immediately. Snorting or injecting the crushed tablet can lead to overdose and death.
- **Hydromorphone** has a profile similar to heroin, but with the advantage of purity.
- **Opiates** are commonly combined with stimulants (e.g., cocaine [speedball]) or alcohol.

TABLE 71–3. Dependence on Sedative-Hypnotics

Generic Name	Common Trade Names (Manufacturer)	Oral Sedating (Dose (mg))	Physical Dependence Dose and Time Needed to Produce Dependence	Time Before Onset of Withdrawal (h)	Peak Withdrawal Symptoms (days)
Benzodiazepines					
Diazepam	Valium (Roche)	5–10	40–100 mg × 42–120 days	12–24	5–8
Chlordiazepoxide	Librium, Libritabs (Roche)	10–25	75–600 mg × 42–120 days	12–24	5–8
Clorazepate	Tranxene (Abbott)	7.5–15	45–180 mg × 42–120 days (est.)	12–24	5–8
Alprazolam	Xanax (Upjohn)	0.25–8	8–16 mg × 42 days (est.)	8–24	2–3
Flunitrazepam	Rohypnol (Roche)	1–2	8–10 mg × 42 days (est.)	24–36	2–3
Barbiturates					
Secobarbital	Seconal, Seco-8 (Lilly)	100	800–2200 mg × 35–37 days	6–12	2–3
Pentobarbital	Nembutal (Abbott)	100	Same	6–12	2–3
Equal parts of secobarbital and amobarbital	Tuinal (Lilly)	100	Same	6–12	2–3
Amobarbital	Amytal (Lilly)	65–100	Same	8–12	2–5
Nonbarbiturate sedative-hypnotics					
Ethchlorvynol	Placidyl (Abbott)	200	1–1.5 g × 30 days	6–12	2–3
Chloral hydrate	Noctec (various)	250	Exact dose unknown; 12 g/day chronically has led to delirium upon sudden withdrawal	6–12	2–3
Meprobamate	Equanil, Miltown, Meprotabs (various)	400	1.6–3.2 g × 270 days	8–12	3–8

Note: Withdrawal symptoms are tremor, tachycardia, diaphoresis, nausea, vomiting, elevated blood pressure, delirium, seizures, and hallucinations.

TABLE 71–4. Signs and Symptoms of Opioid Intoxication and Withdrawal

Intoxication	Withdrawal
Euphoria	Lacrimation
Dysphoria	Rhinorrhea
Apathy	Mydriasis
Motor retardation	Piloerection
Sedation	Diaphoresis
Slurred speech	Diarrhea
Attention impairment	Yawning
Miosis	Fever
	Insomnia
	Muscle aching

▶ CENTRAL NERVOUS SYSTEM STIMULANTS

CAFFEINE

- **Caffeine** is rapidly absorbed from the GI tract and reaches peak blood levels within 30 to 45 minutes. The half-life is 3.5 to 5 hours. It increases the heart rate and force of contraction and has a strong diuretic effect. Regular use is associated with tolerance.
- Signs and symptoms of excessive caffeine intake include anxiety, insomnia, flushed face, diuresis, GI disturbances, muscle twitching, rambling speech, tachycardia, arrhythmia, increased energy, and psychomotor agitation.
- The caffeine withdrawal syndrome begins within 18 to 24 hours of discontinuation and includes headache, drowsiness, and sometimes impaired psychomotor performance, difficulty concentrating, nausea, excessive yawning, and craving.

XIII ◀

COCAINE

- **Cocaine** may be the most behaviorally reinforcing of all drugs. Ten percent of people who begin to use the drug "recreationally" go on to heavy use.
- It blocks reuptake of catecholamine neurotransmitters and causes a depletion of brain dopamine.
- The hydrochloride salt is inhaled or injected. It can be converted to **cocaine base** (crack or rock) and smoked to achieve almost instant absorption and intense euphoria. Tolerance to the "high" develops quickly.
- In the presence of alcohol, cocaine is metabolized to cocaethylene, a longer-acting compound than cocaine with a greater risk for causing death.
- The elimination half-life of cocaine is 1 hour, and the duration of effect is very short.
- Adverse events include ulceration of nasal mucosa and nasal septal collapse, tachycardia, heart failure, hyperthermia, shock, seizures, psychosis, and sudden death.
- Signs and symptoms of cocaine intoxication and withdrawal are shown in Table 71–5.
- Withdrawal symptoms begin within hours of discontinuation and last up to several days.

TABLE 71–5. Signs and Symptoms of Cocaine Intoxication and Withdrawal

Intoxication	Withdrawal
Motor agitation	Fatigue
Elation/euphoria	Sleep disturbance
Grandiosity	Nightmares
Loquacity	Depression
Hypervigilance	Increased appetite
Tachycardia	
Mydriasis	
Elevated or lowered blood pressure	
Sweating or chills	
Nausea and vomiting	

METHAMPHETAMINE

- **Methamphetamine** (speed, meth, crank) can be taken orally, intranasally, by intravenous injection, and by smoking. The hydrochloride salt (ice, crystal, glass) is a clear crystal.
- Systemic effects of methamphetamine are similar to those of cocaine. Inhalation or intravenous injection results in an intense rush that lasts a few minutes. Methamphetamine has a longer duration of effect than cocaine. Pharmacologic effects include increased wakefulness, increased physical activity, decreased appetite, increased respiration, hyperthermia, euphoria, irritability, insomnia, confusion, tremors, anxiety, paranoia, aggressiveness, convulsions, increased heart rate and blood pressure, stroke, and death.
- Duration of withdrawal from methamphetamine ranges from 3 to 24 days. Occurrence of delirium suggests withdrawal from another drug (e.g., **alcohol**).
- **Ephedrine** and **pseudoephedrine** can be extracted from cold and allergy tablets and converted in illegal labs to methamphetamine.

XIII ▶ OTHER DRUGS OF ABUSE

NICOTINE

- More than 440,000 deaths annually, or 20% of the total deaths in the United States, are caused by smoking.
- **Nicotine** is a ganglionic cholinergic-receptor agonist with pharmacologic effects that are dose dependent. Effects include central and peripheral nervous system stimulation and depression; respiratory stimulation; skeletal muscle relaxation; catecholamine release by the adrenal medulla; peripheral vasoconstriction; and increased blood pressure, heart rate, cardiac output, and oxygen consumption. Low doses of nicotine produce increased alertness and improved cognitive functioning. Higher doses stimulate the "reward" center in the limbic system.

MARIJUANA

- **Marijuana** (reefer, pot, grass, weed) is the most commonly used illicit drug. The principal psychoactive component is Δ^9- **tetrahydrocannabinol (THC).** **Hashish**, the dried resin of the top of the plant, is more potent than the plant itself.

- Chronic exposure is not usually associated with a withdrawal syndrome, but sudden discontinuation by heavy users can cause a withdrawal syndrome.
- Initial effects of marijuana use include increased heart rate, dilated bronchial passages, and bloodshot eyes. Subsequent effects include euphoria, dry mouth, hunger, tremor, sleepiness, anxiety, fear, distrust, panic, incoordination, poor recall, and toxic psychosis. Other physiologic effects include sedation, difficulty in performing complex tasks, and disinhibition. Endocrine effects include amenorrhea, decreased testosterone production, and inhibition of spermatogenesis. Signs and symptoms of marijuana intoxication are tachycardia, conjunctival congestion, increased appetite, dry mouth, euphoria, apathy, and hallucinations.
- THC is detectable on toxicologic screening for up to 4 to 5 weeks in chronic users.
- Daily use of one to three joints appears to produce about the same lung damage and potential cancer risk as smoking five times as many tobacco cigarettes.

▶ OTHER DRUGS OF ABUSE

METHAMPHETAMINE ANALOGS

- The analogs of current concern include 3,4-methylenedioxy-amphetamine (**MDA**) and 3,4-methylenedioxy-methamphetamine (**MDMA**, ecstacy, Adam).
- MDMA is usually taken by mouth as a tablet, capsule, or powder, but it can also be smoked, snorted, or injected.
- MDMA stimulates the CNS, causes euphoria and relaxation, and produces a mild hallucinogenic effect. It can cause muscle tension, nausea, faintness, chills, sweating, panic, anxiety, depression, hallucinations, and paranoid thinking. It increases heart rate and blood pressure and destroys serotonin (5-HT)-producing neurons in animals.

PHENCYCLIDINE (PCP) AND KETAMINE

- **PCP** (angel dust, crystal) is often misrepresented as **lysergic acid diethy-lamide (LSD)** or THC. It is commonly smoked with marijuana but can be taken orally or IV. XIII
- Signs and symptoms of PCP intoxication include very unpredictable behavior, increased blood pressure, tachycardia, ataxia, slurred speech, euphoria, agitation, anxiety, hostility, and psychosis. At toxic doses, coma and seizures may occur.
- **Ketamine** (special K, jet, green), chemically related to PCP, is a veterinary anesthetic that can cause hallucinations, delirium, and vivid dreams.
- It is usually injected but can be evaporated to crystals, powdered, and smoked, snorted, or swallowed. Marijuana cigarettes can be soaked in ketamine solution.
- Side effects are increased blood pressure and heart rate, respiratory depression, apnea, muscular hypertonus, and dystonic reactions. In overdose, seizures, polyneuropathy, increased intracranial pressure, and respiratory and cardiac arrest may occur.

LYSERGIC ACID DIETHYLAMIDE

- Physical signs and symptoms of **LSD** intoxication include mydriasis, tachycardia, diaphoresis, palpitations, blurred vision, tremor, incoordination, dizziness, weakness, and drowsiness; psychiatric signs and symptoms include perceptual intensification, depersonalization, derealization, illusions, psychosis, and synesthesia. There is no withdrawal syndrome after discontinuation.

- LSD and similar drugs stimulate presynaptic 5-HT$_{1A}$ and 5-HT$_{1B}$, as well as postsynaptic 5-HT$_2$ receptors in the brain.
- Flashbacks may occur, especially in chronic users. It produces tolerance but is not addictive.
- LSD is sold as tablets, capsules, and a liquid. It is also added to absorbent paper and divided into small decorated squares, each square being one dose.

INHALANTS

- Organic solvents inhaled by abusers include **gasoline, glue, aerosols, amyl nitrite, typewriter correction fluid,** lighter fluid, cleaning fluids, paint products, nail polish remover, waxes, and varnishes. Chemicals in these products include **nitrous oxide, toluene, benzene, methanol, methylene chloride, acetone, methylethyl ketone, methylbutyl ketone, trichloroethylene,** and **trichorethane.** Other inhalants of abuse include **amyl nitrite** and **butyl nitrite.**
- Physiologic effects include CNS depression, headache, nausea, hallucinations, and delusions. With chronic use, the drugs are toxic to virtually all organ systems. Death may occur from arrhythmias or suffocation by plastic bags.

▶ DESIRED OUTCOME

The goals of treatment are cessation of use of the drug, termination of associated drug-seeking behaviors, and return to normal functioning. The goals of treatment of the withdrawal syndrome are prevention of progression of withdrawal to life-threatening severity, thus enabling the patient to be sufficiently comfortable and functional in order to participate in a treatment program.

▶ TREATMENT

XIII

INTOXICATION

- When possible, drug therapy should be avoided, but it may be indicated if patients are agitated, combative, or psychotic (Table 71–6).
- When toxicology screens are desired, blood or urine should be collected immediately when the patient presents for treatment.
- **Flumazenil** is not indicated in all cases of suspected BZ overdose, and it is contraindicated when cyclic antidepressant involvement is known or suspected because of the risk of seizures. It should be used with caution when BZ physical dependence is suspected, as it may precipitate BZ withdrawal.
- In opiate intoxication, **naloxone** may revive unconscious patients with respiratory depression. However, it may also precipitate physical withdrawal in dependent patients.
- **Cocaine** intoxication is treated pharmacologically (usually with lorazepam 2 to 4 mg intramuscularly every 30 minutes to 6 hours as needed) only if the patient is agitated and psychotic. Low-dose antipsychotics can be used short-term if necessary for psychotic symptoms.
- Many patients with **hallucinogen**, **marijuana**, or **inhalant** intoxication respond to reassurance, but short-term **antianxiety** and/or **antipsychotic** therapy can be used.

TABLE 71–6. Treatment of Substance Intoxication

Drug Class	Pharmacologic Therapy	Nonpharmacologic Therapy
Benzodiazepines	Flumazenil 0.2 mg/min IV initially, repeat up to 3 mg maximum	Support vital functions
Alcohol, barbiturates, and sedative-hypnotics (nonbenzodiazepines)	None	Support vital functions
Opiates	Naloxone 0.4–2.0 mg IV every 3 min	Support vital functions
Cocaine and other CNS stimulants	Lorazepam 2–4 mg IM every 30 min to 6 h as needed for agitation Haloperidol 2–5 mg (or other antipsychotic agent) every 30 min to 6 h as needed for psychotic behavior	Monitor cardiac function
Hallucinogens, marijuana, and inhalants	Lorazepam and/or haloperidol as above	Reassurance; "talk-down therapy"; support vital functions
Phencyclidine	Lorazepam and/or haloperidol as above	Minimize sensory input

- **PCP** intoxication is unpredictable, and "talk-down therapy" is not recommended. Sensory input should be minimized. Antianxiety and/or **antipsychotic** drug therapy may be necessary if behavior is uncontrollable.

WITHDRAWAL

Treatment of withdrawal from some common drugs of abuse is summarized in Table 71–7.

XIII

TABLE 71–7. Treatment of Withdrawal from Some Common Drugs of Abuse

Drug or Drug Class	Pharmacologic Therapy
Benzodiazepines	
Short- to intermediate-acting	Chlordiozepoxide 50 mg 3–4 times a day or lorazepam 2 mg 3–4 times a day; taper over 5–7 days
Long-acting	Chlordiazepoxide 50 mg 3–4 times a day or lorazepam 2 mg 3–4 times a day; taper over additional 5–7 days
Barbiturates	Pentobarbital tolerance test; initial detoxification at upper limit of tolerance test; decrease dosage by 100 mg every 2–3 days
Opiates	Methadone 20–80 mg orally daily; taper by 5–10 mg daily or clonidine 2 mcg/kg three times a day × 7 days; taper over additional 3 days
Mixed-substance withdrawal	
Drugs are cross-tolerant	Detoxify according to treatment for longer-acting drug used
Drugs are not cross-tolerant	Detoxify from one drug while maintaining second drug (cross-tolerant drugs), then detoxify from second drug
CNS stimulants	Supportive treatment only; pharmacotherapy often not used; bromocriptine 2.5 mg 3 times a day or higher may be used for severe craving associated with cocaine withdrawal

Alcohol

- Most clinicians agree that the **BZs** are the drugs of choice in treatment of **alcohol** withdrawal.
- The long-acting drugs (e.g., **chlordiazepoxide**, **diazepam**) control withdrawal effectively with few rebound effects. The long-acting drugs may be more effective in preventing seizures but may pose a risk of excess sedation, especially in the elderly and those with marked liver disease.
- A dosage regimen for alcohol detoxification with chlordiazepoxide is 50 to 100 mg orally every 6 hours for 1 day, then 25 to 50 mg every 6 hours for 2 days. Many clinicians, however, recommend individualizing the dosage, especially for patients with a history of seizures, acute medical or surgical illness, or delirium tremens.
- Some recommend front loading. For example, **diazepam** may be given in 20-mg doses every 2 hours until resolution of withdrawal symptoms. Typically, a total of 60 mg is required, and further doses are not needed.
- With symptom-triggered therapy, medication is given only if symptoms emerge. A typical regimen would include diazepam, 10 to 20 mg every hour, when a structured assessment scale indicates that symptoms are moderate to severe.
- Alcohol withdrawal seizures do not require anticonvulsant drug treatment unless they progress to status epilepticus. Patients with seizures should be treated supportively. An increase in the dosage and slowing of the tapering schedule of the **BZ** used for detoxification or a single injection of a BZ may be necessary to prevent further seizure activity.

Benzodiazepines

- For BZ withdrawal, the same drugs and dosages that are used for alcohol withdrawal are used (see Table 71–7).
- The onset of withdrawal from long-acting BZs may be up to 7 days after discontinuation of the drug. Detoxification is approached by initiating treatment at usual doses and maintaining this dose for 5 days. The dose is then tapered over 5 days. **Alprazolam** withdrawal may require a more gradual taper.

XIII

Opiates

- Unnecessary detoxification with drugs should be avoided if possible (e.g., if symptoms are tolerable). **Heroin** withdrawal reaches a peak within 36 to 72 hours, and **methadone** withdrawal peak is reached at 72 hours.
- Conventional drug therapy for opiate withdrawal has been **methadone**, a synthetic opiate. Usual starting doses have been 20 to 40 mg/day. The dosage can be tapered in decrements of 5 to 10 mg/day until discontinued. Some use discontinuation schedules over 30 days or over 180 days.
- **Buprenorphine** in two formulations (both assigned to schedule III) was recently made available for office-based management of opioid dependence by qualified physicians. Once-daily dosage is titrated to a target of 16 mg/day (range, 4 to 24 mg/day).

  - Subutex (buprenorphine) is used at the beginning of treatment for opiate abuse.
  - Suboxone, buprenorphine and naloxone, is used in maintenance treatment of opiate addiction.

- If **L-methadyl acetate hydrochloride (LAAM)** is used instead of methadone; dosing is 3 times weekly.

- **Clonidine** can attenuate the noradrenergic hyperactivity of opiate withdrawal without interfering significantly with activity at the opiate receptors. Monitoring should include blood pressure checks, supine and standing, at least daily.

Caffeine
- When **caffeine** is reintroduced, relief of withdrawal symptoms occurs within 30 to 60 minutes.
- Caffeinism is treated by reducing or discontinuing the drug. It may be necessary to taper the patient off the drug.

SUBSTANCE DEPENDENCE

The treatment of drug dependence or addiction is primarily behavioral. The goal of treatment is complete abstinence, and treatment is a lifelong process. Most drug-dependence treatment programs embrace a treatment approach based on Alcoholics Anonymous (AA).

Alcohol
- **Disulfiram** deters a patient from drinking by producing an aversive-reaction if the patient drinks. It inhibits aldehyde dehydrogenase in the pathway for alcohol metabolism, allowing acetaldehyde to accumulate, resulting in flushing, vomiting, headache, palpitations, tachycardia, fever, and hypotension. Severe reactions include respiratory depression, arrhythmias, myocardial infarction, seizures, and cardiovascular collapse. Inhibition of the enzyme continues for as long as 2 weeks after stopping disulfiram. Disulfiram reactions have occurred with the use of alcohol-containing mouthwashes and aftershaves. Usual dosage is 250 to 500 mg/day.
- Prior to starting disulfiram, baseline liver function tests (LFTs) should be obtained, and patients should be monitored for hepatotoxicity. LFTs should be repeated at 2 weeks, 3 months, and 6 months, then twice yearly. The prescriber should wait at least 24 hours after the last drink before starting disulfiram, usually at a dose of 250 mg/day.
- **Naltrexone**, 50 mg/day, has been associated with reduced craving and fewer drinking days. It should not be given to patients currently dependent on opiates as it can precipitate a severe withdrawal syndrome. XIII
- Naltrexone is hepatotoxic and contraindicated in patients with hepatitis or liver failure. LFTs should be monitored monthly for the first 3 months, then every 3 months. Side effects include nausea, headache, dizziness, nervousness, insomnia, and somnolence.

Nicotine
- Figure 1 is an algorithm for treating tobacco use.
- Every patient who uses tobacco should be offered at least brief treatment. All patients attempting tobacco cessation should be offered practical counseling (problem-solving/skills training), social support, stress management, and relapse prevention.
- First-line pharmacotherapies for smoking cessation are **bupropion sustained release**, **nicotine** gum, nicotine inhaler, nicotine nasal spray, and nicotine patch. Second-line pharmacotherapies include **clonidine** and **nortriptyline** and should be considered if first-line therapy fails.
- Interventions are more effective when they last greater than 10 minutes, involve contact with a professional, provide at least four to seven sessions, and provide **nicotine-replacement therapy (NRT)**.

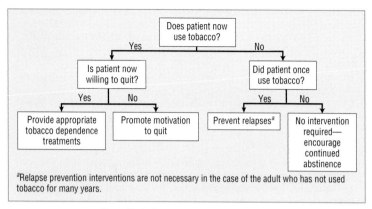

^aRelapse prevention interventions are not necessary in the case of the adult who has not used tobacco for many years.

Figure 71–1. Algorithm for treating tobacco use.

Nicotine-Replacement Therapy

- The role of pharmacotherapy is summarized in Tabl 71–8.
- NRTshould be used with caution in patients within 2 weeks post–myocardial infarction, those with serious arrhythmias, and those with serious or worsening angina.
- The **2-mg gum** is recommended for those smoking less than 25 cigarettes a day, and the **4-mg gum** for those smoking more than 25 cigarettes a day. Generally, the gum should be used for up to 12 weeks at doses of no more than 24 pieces per day. It should be chewed slowly until a peppery or minty taste emerges and then parked for about 30 minutes or until the taste dissipates. A fixed schedule may be more efficacious than as-needed use.
- The **patch** is available over-the-counter and as a prescription medication. Treatment of 8 weeks or less is as effective as longer treatments. The 16- and 24-hour patches have comparable efficacy. A new patch should be placed on a relatively hairless location each morning.
- **Nicotine nasal spray** requires a prescription. Recommended duration of therapy is 3 to 6 months at no more than 40 doses per day. A dose is one 0.5-mg delivery to each nostril (1 mg total). Initial doses are gradually increased as needed for symptom relief.
- NRT products have few side effects. Nausea and light-headedness may indicate nicotine overdose. The patch site may be rotated to minimize skin irritation, and over-the-counter **hydrocortisone** or **triamcinolone** cream may improve skin irritation. Sleep disturbances are reported in 23% of patients using the patch.

Bupropion

- **Bupropion sustained release (SR)** is an effective smoking-cessation treatment. It is contraindicated in patients with a seizure disorder, a current or prior diagnosis of bulimia or anorexia nervosa, and use of a **monoamine oxidase inhibitor** within the previous 14 days. It can be used in combination with NRT.
- Insomnia and dry mouth are the most frequent side effects.
- Bupropion SR should be dosed at 150 mg once daily for 3 days, then twice daily for 7 to 12 weeks or longer, with or without NRT. Patients should stop

XIII

TABLE 71–8. Summary of Clinical Guidelines for Prescribing Pharmacotherapy for Smoking Cessation

Who should receive pharmacotherapy for smoking cessation?	All smokers trying to quit, except in the presence of special circumstances. Special consideration should be given before using pharmacotherapy with selected populations: those with medical contraindications, those smoking fewer than 10 cigarettes/day, pregnant/breast-feeding women, and adolescent smokers.
What are the first-line pharmacotherapies recommended in this guideline?	All five of the FDA-approved pharmacotherapies for smoking cessation are recommended, including bupropion SR, nicotine gum, nicotine inhaler, nicotine nasal spray, and the nicotine patch.
What factors should a clinician consider when choosing among the five first-line pharmacotherapies?	Because of the lack of sufficient data to rank order these five medications, choice of a specific first-line pharmacotherapy must be guided by factors such as clinician familiarity with the medications, contraindications for selected patients, patient preference, previous patient experience with a specific pharmacotherapy (positive or negative), and patient characteristics (e.g., history of depression, concerns about weight gain).
Are pharmacotherapeutic treatments appropriate for lighter smokers (e.g., 10–15 cigarettes/day)?	If pharmacotherapy is used with lighter smokers, clinicians should consider reducing the dose of first-line nicotine replacement pharmacotherapies. No adjustments are necessary when using bupropion SR.
What second-line pharmacotherapies are recommended in this guideline?	Clonidine and nortriptyline.
When should second-line agents be used for treating tobacco dependence?	Consider prescribing second-line agents for patients unable to use first-line medications because of contraindications or for patients for whom first-line medications are not helpful. Monitor patients for the known side effects of second-line agents.
Which pharmacotherapies should be considered with patients particularly concerned about weight gain?	Bupropion SR and nicotine replacement therapies, in particular nicotine gum, have been shown to delay, but not prevent, weight gain.
Are there pharmacotherapies that should be especially considered in patients with a history of depression?	Bupropion SR and nortriptyline appear to be effective with this population.
Should nicotine replacement therapies be avoided in patients with a history of cardiovascular disease?	No. The nicotine patch in particular is safe and has been shown not to cause adverse cardiovascular effects.
May tobacco-dependence pharmacotherapies be used long term (e.g., 6 months or more)?	Yes. This approach may be helpful with smokers who report persistent withdrawal symptoms during the course of pharmacotherapy or who desire long-term therapy. A minority of individuals who successfully quit smoking use ad libitum nicotine replacement medications (gum, nasal spray, inhaler) long term. The use of these medications long term does not present a known health risk. Additionally, the FDA has approved the use of bupropion SR for long-term maintenance.
May pharmacotherapies ever be combined?	Yes. There is evidence that combining the nicotine patch with either nicotine gum or nicotine nasal spray increases long-term abstinence rates over those produced by a single form of nicotine replacement therapy.

XIII

smoking during the second week of treatment. For maintenance treatment, bupropion SR 150 mg twice daily for up to 6 months can be given.

Second-Line Medications
- **Clonidine**, delivered transdermally or orally, is an effective smoking-cessation treatment. It is given for 3 to 10 weeks and should not be discontinued abruptly. Abrupt discontinuation may cause nervousness, agitation, headache, tremor, and rapid rise in blood pressure.
- Dosing of clonidine initially is 0.1 mg orally twice daily or 0.1 mg/day transdermally, increasing by 0.1 mg/day each week if needed.
- The most common clonidine side effects are dry mouth, dizziness, sedation, and constipation. Blood pressure should be monitored.
- **Nortriptyline** is initiated 10 to 28 days before the quit date. The dose is initiated at 25 mg/day, gradually increasing to 75 to 100 mg/day. Treatment duration is commonly 12 weeks in trials, and common side effects were sedation, dry mouth, blurred vision, and light-headedness.

See Chapter 64, Substance-Related Disorders: Overview and Depressants, Stimulants, and Hallucinogens; and Chapter 65, Substance-Related Disorders: Alcohol, Nicotine, and Caffeine, authored by Paul L. Doering, for a more detailed discussion of the topic.

XIII

Chapter 72

▶ ACID-BASE DISORDERS

▶ DEFINITION

Acid-base disorders are caused by disturbances in hydrogen ion (H^+) homeostasis, which is ordinarily maintained by extracellular buffering, renal regulation of hydrogen ion and bicarbonate, and ventilatory regulation of carbon dioxide (CO_2) elimination.

▶ GENERAL PRINCIPLES

- General principles that are common to all types of acid-base disturbances are addressed first, followed by separate discussions of each type of acid-base disturbance.
- Buffering refers to the ability of a solution to resist change in pH after the addition of a strong acid or base. The body's principal buffer system is the carbonic acid/bicarbonate (H_2CO_3/HCO_3^-) system.
- Most of the body's acid production is in the form of CO_2 and is produced from metabolism of carbohydrates, proteins, and lipids.
- There are four primary types of acid-base disturbances, which can occur independently or together as a compensatory response.
  - Metabolic acidosis is characterized by decreased plasma bicarbonate concentrations (HCO_3^-), whereas metabolic alkalosis is characterized by increased HCO_3^-.
  - Respiratory acid-base disorders are caused by altered alveolar ventilation producing changes in arterial carbon dioxide tension ($Paco_2$). Respiratory acidosis is characterized by increased $Paco_2$, whereas respiratory alkalosis is characterized by decreased $Paco_2$.

DIAGNOSIS

- Blood gases (Table 72–1), serum electrolytes, medical history, and clinical condition are the primary tools for determining the cause of acid-base disorders and for designing therapy.
- Arterial blood gases are measured to determine oxygenation and acid-base status (Figure 72–1). Low pH values (less than 7.35) indicate acidemia, whereas high values (greater than 7.45) indicate alkalemia. The $Paco_2$ value helps to determine if there is a primary respiratory abnormality, whereas the HCO_3^- concentration helps to determine if there is a primary metabolic abnormality.
- The expected compensatory response can be calculated for each primary disturbance (Table 72–2). If the observed compensatory response is substantially different than that predicted by these empiric relationships, a mixed acid-base disturbance may be present.

DESIRED OUTCOME

Initial treatment is aimed at stabilizing the acute condition, followed by identifying and correcting the underlying cause(s) of the acid-base disturbance. Additional treatment may be needed depending on the severity of symptoms and likelihood of recurrence, especially in patients with ongoing initiating events.

Renal Disorders

TABLE 72–1. Normal Blood Gas Values

	Arterial Blood	Mixed Venous Blood
pH	7.40 (7.35–7.45)	7.38 (7.33–7.43)
P_{O_2}	80–100 mm Hg	35–40 mm Hg
Sa_{O_2}	95%	70–75%
P_{CO_2}	35–45 mm Hg	45–51 mm Hg
HCO_3^-	22–26 mEq/L	24–28 mEq/L

▶ METABOLIC ACIDOSIS

PATHOPHYSIOLOGY

- Metabolic acidosis is characterized by decreased pH and serum HCO_3^- concentrations, which can result from adding organic acid to extracellular fluid (e.g., lactic acid, ketoacids), loss of HCO_3^- stores (e.g., diarrhea), or accumulation of endogenous acids due to impaired renal function (e.g., phosphates, sulfates).
- The anion gap can be calculated to elucidate the cause of metabolic acidosis (Table 72–3). The anion gap is calculated as follows:

$$Anion\ gap = [Na^+] - [Cl^-] - [HCO_3^-]$$

The normal anion gap is approximately 9 mEq/L, with a range of 3 to 11 mEq/L.
- The primary compensatory mechanism is to decrease Pa_{CO_2} by increasing the respiratory rate.

CLINICAL PRESENTATION

- The major manifestation of chronic metabolic acidosis is bone demineralization with the development of rickets in children and osteomalacia and osteopenia in adults.
- The manifestations of acute severe metabolic acidosis (pH less than 7.15 to 7.20) involve the cardiovascular, respiratory, and central nervous systems. Hyperventilation is often the first sign of metabolic acidosis. Respiratory compensation may occur as Kussmaul's respirations (i.e., deep, rapid respirations characteristic of diabetic ketoacidosis).

TREATMENT

- The primary treatment of metabolic acidosis is to correct the underlying disorder. Additional treatment depends on the severity and onset of acidosis.
- Asymptomatic patients with mild to moderate acidemia (HCO_3^-, 12 to 20 mEq/L; pH, 7.2 to 7.4) can usually be managed with gradual correction of the acidemia over days to weeks using oral **sodium bicarbonate** or other alkali preparations (Table 72–4). The dose of bicarbonate can be calculated as follows:

$$Loading\ dose\ (mEq) = (Vd\ HCO_3^- \times body\ weight)$$

$$(desired\ [HCO_3^-] - current\ [HCO_3^-])$$

where Vd HCO_3^- is the volume of distribution of HCO_3^- (0.5 L/kg).

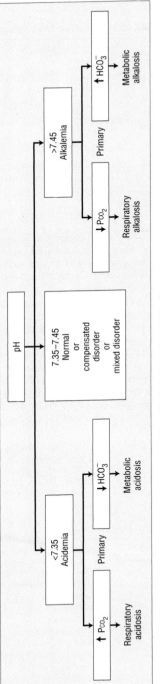

Figure 72–1. Analysis of arterial blood gases.

XIV

TABLE 72–2. Guidelines for Initial Interpretation of Acid-Base Disorders

Metabolic acidosis	$Paco_2$ (in mm Hg) should fall by 1.0–1.5 times the fall in plasma $[HCO_3^-]$ (in mEq/L)
Metabolic alkalosis	$Paco_2$ (in mm Hg) should increase by 0.25–1.0 times the rise in plasma $[HCO_3^-]$ (in mEq/L)
Acute respiratory acidosis	Plasma $[HCO_3^-]$ should rise by 0.1 times the increase in $Paco_2 \pm 3$
Acute respiratory alkalosis	Plasma $[HCO_3^-]$ should fall by 0.1–0.3 times the decrease in $Paco_2$ but usually not to less than 18 mEq/L
Chronic respiratory acidosis	Plasma $[HCO_3^-]$ should rise by 0.4 times the increase in $Paco_2 \pm 4$
Chronic respiratory alkalosis	Plasma $[HCO_3^-]$ should fall by 0.2–0.5 times the decrease in $Paco_2$ but usually not to less than 14 mEq/L

- Alkali therapy can be used to treat patients with acute severe metabolic acidosis due to hyperchloremic acidosis, but its role is controversial in patients with lactic acidosis. Therapeutic options include **sodium bicarbonate** and **tromethamine.** Two other options, **Carbicarb** and **dichloroacetate,** are investigational and not routinely available.
  - Sodium bicarbonate has been recommended to raise arterial pH to 7.15 to 7.20. However, no controlled clinical studies have demonstrated reduced morbidity and mortality compared with general supportive care. If intravenous (IV) sodium bicarbonate is administered, the goal is to increase, not normalize, pH to 7.20 and HCO_3^- to 8 to 10 mEq/L.
- Tromethamine, or THAM, a highly alkaline solution, is a sodium-free organic amine that acts as a proton acceptor to prevent or correct acidosis. However, no evidence exists that THAM is beneficial or more efficacious than sodium bicarbonate. The usual empiric dosage for THAM is 1 to 5 mmol/kg administered IV over 1 hour. An individualized THAM dose can be calculated as follows:

$$\text{Dose of THAM (in mL)} = 1.1 \times \text{body weight (in kg)}$$
$$\times (\text{normal } [HCO_3^-] - \text{current } [HCO_3^-])$$

XIV

TABLE 72–3. Common Causes of Metabolic Acidosis

Increased Anion Gap	Normal Anion Gap/Hyperchloremic States
Alcoholic ketoacidosis	Acid ingestion (hydrochloric acid or ammonium chloride)
Diabetic ketoacidosis	Carbonic anhydrase inhibitors
Lactic acidosis	Cholestyramine
Renal failure (acute or chronic)	Diarrhea
	Dilutional acidosis
Methanol ingestion	Gastrointestinal disorders
Ethylene glycol ingestion	Pancreatic fistula
Salicylate overdose	Potassium-sparing diuretic
Starvation	Renal tubular acidosis
	Ureterosigmoidostomy, ileostomy

TABLE 72–4. Therapeutic Alternatives for Oral Alkali Replacement

Generic Namic	Trade Name(s)	mEq Alkali	Dosage Form(s)
Shol's solution Sodium citrate/citric acid	Bicitra (Willen)	1 mEq Na/mL; equivalent to 1 mEq bicarbonate	Solution (500 mg Na citrate, 334 mg citric acid/ 5 mL)
Sodium bicarbonate	Various	3.9 mEq bicarbonate/tablet (325 mg)	325 mg tablet
		7.8 mEq bicarbonate/tablet (650 mg)	650 mg tablet
	Baking soda (various)	60 mEq bicarbonate/tsp (5 g/tsp)	Powder
Potassium citrate	Urocit-K (Mission)	5 mEq citrate/tablet	5 mEq tablet
Potassium bicarbonate/ potassium citrate	K-Lyte (Bristol) K-Lyte DS (Bristol)	25 mEq bicarbonate/tablet 50 mEq bicarbonate/tablet (DS)	25 mEq tablet (effervescent) 50 mEq tablet (effervescent)
Potassium citrate/ citric acid	Polycitra-K (Willen)	2 mEq K/mL; equivalent to 2 mEq bicarbonate 30 mEq bicarbonate/UD packet	Solution (1100 mg K citrate, 334 mg citric acid/5 mL) Crystals for reconstitution (3300 mg K citrate, 1002 mg citric acid/UD packet)
Sodium citrate/ potassium citrate/ citric acid	Polycitra (Willen) Polycitra-LC (Willen)	1 mEq K, 1 mEq Na/mL; equivalent to 2 mEq bicarbonate	Syrup (Polycitra) Solution (Polycitra-LC) (both contain 550 mg K citrate, 500 mg Na citrate, 334 mg citric acid/5 mL)

DS, double strength; UD, unit dose.

▶ METABOLIC ALKALOSIS

PATHOPHYSIOLOGY

XIV ◀

- Metabolic alkalosis is *initiated* by increased pH and HCO_3^-, which can result from loss of H^+ via the gastrointestinal tract (e.g., nasogastric suctioning, vomiting) or kidneys (e.g., diuretics, Cushing's syndrome), or from gain of bicarbonate (e.g., administration of bicarbonate, acetate, lactate, or citrate).
- Metabolic alkalosis is *maintained* by abnormal renal function that prevents the kidneys from excreting excess bicarbonate.
- The respiratory response to metabolic alkalosis is to increase $Paco_2$ by hypoventilation.

CLINICAL PRESENTATION

- No unique signs or symptoms are associated with mild to moderate metabolic alkalosis. Some patients complain of symptoms related to the underlying disorder (e.g., muscle weakness with hypokalemia or postural dizziness with volume depletion) or have a history of vomiting, gastric drainage, or diuretic use.
- Severe alkalemia (pH greater than 7.60) can be associated with cardiac arrhythmias and neuromuscular irritability.

TREATMENT

- Treatment of metabolic alkalosis should be aimed at correcting the factor(s) responsible for maintaining the alkalosis.
- Treatment depends on whether the disorder is sodium chloride responsive (urinary chloride concentration less than 10 mEq/L) or resistant (urinary chloride concentration greater than 20 mEq/L) (Figure 72–2).

▶ RESPIRATORY ALKALOSIS

PATHOPHYSIOLOGY

- Respiratory alkalosis is characterized by a decrease in $Paco_2$ and an increase in pH.
- $Paco_2$ decreases when ventilatory excretion exceeds metabolic production, usually because of hyperventilation.
- Causes of respiratory alkalosis include increases in neurochemical stimulation via central or peripheral mechanisms, or physical increases in ventilation via voluntary or artificial means (e.g., mechanical ventilation).
- The earliest compensatory response is to chemically buffer excess bicarbonate by releasing hydrogen ions from intracellular proteins, phosphates, and hemoglobin. If respiratory alkalosis is prolonged (more than 6 hours), the kidneys attempt to further compensate by increasing bicarbonate elimination.

CLINICAL PRESENTATION

- Although usually asymptomatic, respiratory alkalosis can cause adverse neuromuscular, cardiovascular, and gastrointestinal effects.
- Light-headedness, confusion, decreased intellectual functioning, syncope, and seizures can be caused by decreased cerebral blood flow.
- Nausea and vomiting can occur, probably as a result of cerebral hypoxia.
- Serum electrolytes can be altered secondary to respiratory alkalosis. Serum chloride is usually increased; serum potassium, phosphorus, and ionized calcium are usually decreased.

TREATMENT

- Treatment is often unnecessary because most patients have few symptoms and only mild pH alterations (i.e., pH less than 7.50).
- Direct measures (e.g., treatment of pain, hypovolemia, fever, infection, or salicylate overdose) can be effective. A rebreathing device (e.g., paper bag) can help control hyperventilation.
- Respiratory alkalosis associated with mechanical ventilation can often be corrected by decreasing the number of mechanical breaths per minute, using a capnograph and spirometer to adjust ventilator settings more precisely, or increasing dead space in the ventilator circuit.

▶ RESPIRATORY ACIDOSIS

PATHOPHYSIOLOGY

- Respiratory acidosis is characterized by an increase in $Paco_2$ and a decrease in pH.
- Respiratory acidosis results from disorders that restrict ventilation or increase CO_2 production, airway and pulmonary abnormalities, neuromuscular abnormalities, or mechanical ventilator problems.

XIV

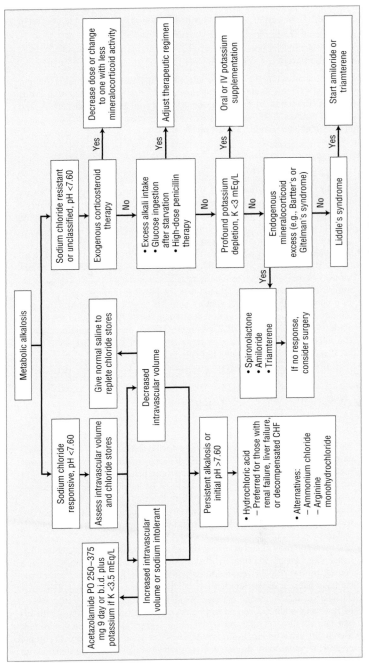

Figure 72–2. Treatment algorithm for patients with primary metabolic alkalosis.

- The early compensatory response to acute respiratory acidosis is chemical buffering. If respiratory acidosis is prolonged (more than 12 to 24 hours), renal excretion of H^+ increases, which generates new bicarbonate.

CLINICAL PRESENTATION

Neuromuscular symptoms include altered mental status, abnormal behavior, seizures, stupor, and coma. Hypercapnia can mimic a stroke or central nervous system (CNS) tumor by producing headache, papilledema, focal paresis, and abnormal reflexes. CNS symptoms are caused by increased cerebral blood flow and are variable, depending in part on the acuity of onset.

TREATMENT

- If carbon dioxide excretion is acutely and severely impaired ($Paco_2$ more than 80 mm Hg) or if life-threatening hypoxia is present (arterial oxygen tension [Pao_2] less than 40 mm Hg), adequate ventilation should be provided. Ventilation can include maintaining a patent airway (e.g., emergency tracheostomy, bronchoscopy, or intubation), clearing excessive secretions, administering oxygen, and providing mechanical ventilation.
- The underlying cause of acute acidosis should be treated aggressively (e.g., administration of bronchodilators for bronchospasm or discontinuation of respiratory depressants such as narcotics and benzodiazepines). Bicarbonate administration is rarely necessary and is potentially harmful.
- In a patient with chronic respiratory acidosis (e.g., chronic obstructive pulmonary disease), treatment is essentially similar to that for acute respiratory acidosis with a few important exceptions. Oxygen therapy should be initiated carefully and only if the Pao_2 is less than 50 mm Hg because the drive to breathe depends on hypoxemia rather than hypercarbia.
- For information on chronic respiratory acidosis, see Chapter 79.

▶ MIXED ACID-BASE DISORDERS

PATHOPHYSIOLOGY

XIV

- Failure of compensation is responsible for mixed acid-base disorders such as respiratory acidosis and metabolic acidosis, or respiratory alkalosis and metabolic alkalosis. In contrast, excess compensation is responsible for metabolic acidosis and respiratory alkalosis, or metabolic alkalosis and respiratory acidosis.
- Respiratory and metabolic acidosis can develop in patients with cardiorespiratory arrest, with chronic lung disease and shock, and with metabolic acidosis and respiratory failure.
- The most common mixed acid-base disorder is respiratory and metabolic alkalosis, which occurs in critically ill surgical patients with respiratory alkalosis caused by mechanical ventilation, hypoxia, sepsis, hypotension, neurologic damage, pain, or drugs; and with metabolic alkalosis caused by vomiting or nasogastric suctioning and massive blood transfusions.
- Mixed metabolic acidosis and respiratory alkalosis occur in patients with advanced liver disease, salicylate intoxication, and pulmonary-renal syndromes.
- Metabolic alkalosis and respiratory acidosis can occur in patients with chronic obstructive pulmonary disease and respiratory acidosis who are treated with salt restriction, diuretics, and possibly glucocorticoids.

TREATMENT

- Mixed respiratory and metabolic acidosis should be treated by responding to both the respiratory and metabolic acidosis. Improved oxygen delivery must be initiated to improve hypercarbia and hypoxia. Mechanical ventilation can be needed to reduce Paco$_2$. During initial therapy, appropriate amounts of alkali should be given to reverse the metabolic acidosis.
- The metabolic component of mixed respiratory and metabolic alkalosis should be corrected by administering **sodium** and **potassium chloride solutions**. The respiratory component should be treated by readjusting the ventilator or by treating the underlying disorder causing hyperventilation.
- Treatment of mixed metabolic acidosis and respiratory alkalosis should be directed at the underlying cause.
- In metabolic alkalosis and respiratory acidosis, pH does not usually deviate significantly from normal, but treatment can be required to maintain Pao$_2$ and Paco$_2$ at acceptable levels. Treatment should be aimed at decreasing plasma bicarbonate with **sodium** and **potassium chloride** therapy, allowing renal excretion of retained bicarbonate from diuretic-induced metabolic alkalosis.

▶ EVALUATION OF THERAPEUTIC OUTCOMES

- Patients should be monitored closely because acid-base disorders can be serious and even life threatening.
- Arterial blood gases are the primary tools for evaluation of therapeutic outcome. They should be monitored closely to ensure resolution of simple acid-base disorders without deterioration to mixed disorders due to compensatory mechanisms. For example, arterial blood gases should be obtained every 2 to 4 hours during the acute phase of respiratory acidosis and then every 12 to 24 hours as acidosis improves.

See Chapter 51, Acid-Base Disorders, authored by Gary R. Matzke and Paul M. Palevsky, for a more detailed discussion of this topic.

XIV

Chapter 73

▶ ACUTE RENAL FAILURE

▶ DEFINITIONS

- Acute renal failure (ARF) has no unifying definition. Most criteria include a combination of absolute serum creatinine (S_{cr}) value with change in either S_{cr} or daily urine output.
- A popular definition is an increase in S_{cr} of 0.5 mg/dL in patients with previously normal renal function or an increase of more than 1.0 mg/dL in patients with chronic renal disease. Unfortunately, S_{cr} is not a sensitive test; its use can delay recognition of ARF.

▶ PATHOPHYSIOLOGY

- Alterations to any of the basic kidney components (vasculature, glomeruli, tubules, and interstitium) can cause ARF. The manifestations of ARF depend on which components are involved.
- ARF can be categorized as prerenal (resulting from decreased renal perfusion), intrinsic (resulting from structural damage to the kidney), postrenal (resulting from obstruction of urine flow from the kidney out of the body), and functional (resulting from hemodynamic changes at the glomerular level) (Table 73–1).

▶ CLINICAL PRESENTATION

- The presentation can be subtle and depends on the setting. Outpatients often are not in acute distress; hospitalized patients may develop ARF after a catastrophic event.
- Symptoms in the outpatient setting include change in urinary habits, weight gain, or flank pain. Clinicians typically notice symptoms of ARF before they are detected by inpatients.
- Signs include edema, colored or foamy urine, and, in volume-depleted patients, orthostatic hypotension.

▶ DIAGNOSIS

- Rapid diagnosis of ARF is essential; delayed recognition can worsen nephrologic injury.
- Physical examination should include assessment of the patient's volume and hemodynamic status.
- Monitoring changes in urine output can help diagnose the type of ARF. Acute anuria (less than 50 mL urine/24 h) is secondary to complete urinary obstruction or a catastrophic event (e.g., shock). Oliguria (450 mL urine/24 h, or less) suggests prerenal azotemia, functional ARF, or acute intrinsic renal failure. Nonoliguric renal failure (more than 450 mL urine/24 h) usually results from acute intrinsic renal failure or incomplete urinary obstruction.
- Urinalysis can help clarify the cause of ARF. High urinary specific gravity, in the absence of glucosuria or mannitol administration, suggests prerenal azotemia or functional ARF. Proteinuria and hematuria suggest glomerular injury. Glucosuria, aminoaciduria, and phosphaturia suggest acute proximal tubular dysfunction. Benign urine sediment suggests prerenal azotemia, functional ARF, or urinary obstruction. Red blood cells and red blood cell casts

TABLE 73–1. Classification of Acute Renal Failure

Category	Classification of Acute Renal Failure	Differential Diagnosis
Prerenal renal failure	Systemic hypoperfusion	Intravascular volume depletion
		Dehydration
		Hemorrhage
		CHF
		Liver disease
		Nephrotic syndrome
		Overdiuresis
	Isolated renal hypoperfusion	Bilateral renal artery stenosis (unilateral renal artery stenosis in solitary kidney)
		Emboli
		Cholesterol
		Thrombotic
Functional acute renal failure		Medications
		Cyclosporine
		ACEIs
		NSAIDs
		Hypercalcemia
		Hepatorenal syndrome
Actute intrinsic renal failure	Vascular	Vasculitis
		Polyarteritis nodosa
		Thrombotic thrombocytopenic purpura
		Hemolytic uremic syndrome
		Emboli
		Cholesterol
		Thrombotic
	Glomerular	Systemic lupus erythematosus
		Poststreptococcal glomerulonephritis
		Antiglomerular basement membrane disease
	Acute tubular necrosis	Ischemic
		Hypotension
		Vasoconstriction
		Exogenous toxins
		Contrast dye
		Heavy metals
		Drugs (amphotericin B, aminoglycosides, etc.)
		Endogenous toxins
		Myoglobin
		Hemoglobin
	Acute interstitial nephritis	Drugs
		Pencillins
		Ciprofloxacin
		Sulfonamides
		Infection
		Streptococcal
Postrenal renal failure (obstruction)	Bladder outlet obstruction	Prostatic hypertrophy
		Improperly placed bladder catheter
	Ureteral (bilateral or unilateral with solitary functioning kidney)	Cervical cancer
	Renal pelvis or tubules	Retroperitoneal fibrosis
		Crystal deposition
		Oxalate
		Indinavir
		Sulfonamides
		Acyclovir
		Tumor lysis syndrome

XIV

TABLE 73–2. Diagnostic Parameters for Differentiating Causes of Acute Renal Failure

Laboratory Test	Prerenal Azotemia	Acute Intrinsic Renal Failure	Postrenal Obstruction
Urine sediment	Normal	Casts, cellular debris	Cellular debris
Urinary RBC	None	2 − 4+	Variable
Urinary WBC	None	2 − 4+	1+
Urine sodium	<20	>40	>40
FE_{Na} (%)	<1	>2	Variable
Urine/serum osmolality	>1.5	<1.3	<1.5
Urine/serum creatinine	>40:1	<20:1	<20:1
BUN/S_{Cr}	>20	15	15

Note: Common laboratory tests are used to classify the cause of acute renal failure. Functional acute renal failure, which is not included in this table, would have laboratory values similar to those seen in prerenal azotemia. However, the urine osmolality to plasma osmolality ratios may not exceed 1.5 depending on the circulating levels of antidiuretic hormone. The laboratory results listed under acute intrinsic renal failure are those seen in acute tubular necrosis, the most common cause of acute intrinsic renal failure.

BUN, blood urea nitrogen; FE_{Na}, fractional excretion of sodium; S_{Cr}, serum creatinine; RBC, red blood cell; WBC, white blood cell.

indicate glomerular injury. White blood cells and white blood cell casts result from interstitial inflammation (i.e., interstitial nephritis), secondary to an allergic, granulomatous, or infectious process.

- Simultaneous measurement of plasma and urinary chemistries and calculation of the fractional excretion of sodium (FE_{Na}) can help determine the etiology of ARF (Table 73–2). The FE_{Na} is calculated as

$$FE_{Na} = (U_{Na} \times P_{Cr} \times 100)/(U_{Cr} \times P_{Na})$$

where U_{Na} = urine sodium, P_{Cr} = plasma creatinine, U_{Cr} = urine creatinine, and P_{Na} = plasma sodium.
- Creatinine and blood urea nitrogen (BUN) are easy to measure, but they are insensitive to rapid changes in glomerular filtration rate (GFR).
- Diagnostic procedures include inserting a urinary catheter into the bladder (exclude postrenal obstruction); plain film radiograph (document the presence of two kidneys or renal stones); radioisotope scan, renal angiography, renal ultrasound, or cystoscopy with retrograde pyelography (document obstruction); and renal biopsy.

▶ DESIRED OUTCOME

The primary goal of therapy is to prevent ARF. If ARF develops, the goals are to avoid or minimize further renal insults that would delay recovery and to provide supportive measures until kidney function returns.

▶ TREATMENT

PREVENTION OF ACUTE RENAL FAILURE

- Nephrotoxin administration (e.g., radiocontrast dye) should be avoided whenever possible.
- When patients require contrast dye and are at risk of ARF because of diabetes mellitus, chronic kidney disease, or old age, renal perfusion should be

maximized. For example, hydration with normal saline can be started at 1 mL/kg on the morning of contrast dye administration. Additional preventive strategies include **oral acetylcysteine** 600 mg twice daily on the day before and the day of contrast dye administration in patients with chronic renal disease, glycemic control in diabetics, and **calcium channel blockers** in patients with kidney transplants.

- **Amphotericin B** nephrotoxicity can be reduced by slowing the infusion rate to 24 hours or, in at-risk patients, substituting **liposomal amphotericin B**.
- Many other strategies are popular but *lack* supportive evidence, including **mannitol**, **loop diuretics**, **dopamine**, and **fenoldopam**.

TREATMENT OF ESTABLISHED ACUTE RENAL FAILURE

No drugs have been found to accelerate ARF recovery. Therefore, patients with established ARF should be supported with nonpharmacologic and pharmacologic approaches through the period of ARF.

Nonpharmacologic Approaches

- Supportive care goals include aggressive fluid management to maintain euvolemia, tissue perfusion, and electrolyte balance.
- Avoidance of nephrotoxins is essential in the management of patients with ARF.
- Renal replacement therapy, the most popular nonpharmacologic therapy, is indicated for some patients with ARF (Table 73–3). Intermittent and continuous options have different advantages (and disadvantages) but, after correcting for severity of illness, have similar outcomes. Consequently, hybrid approaches (e.g., sustained low-efficiency dialysis and extended daily dialysis) are being developed to provide the advantages of both. The hybrid approach, however, makes drug dosing difficult to manage.
- Intermittent renal replacement therapy (e.g., hemodialysis) has the advantage of widespread availability and the convenience of lasting only 3 to 4 hours. Disadvantages include difficult venous dialysis access in hypotensive patients and hypotension due to rapid removal of large amounts of fluid.
- Of the continuous renal replacement therapies (CRRTs), peritoneal dialysis is usually not suitable except for children. CRRT, performed as continuous hemodialysis, continuous hemofiltration, or both, is becoming increasingly popular. CRRT gradually removes solute resulting in better tolerability by critically ill patients. Disadvantages include limited availability, need for 24-hour nursing care, high expense, and incomplete guidelines for drug dosing (see Chapter 75).

TABLE 73–3. The AEIOUs That Describe the Indications for Renal Replacement Therapy

Indication for Renal Replacement Therapy	Clinical Setting
A Acid-base abnormalities	Metabolic acidosis resulting from the accumulation of organic and inorganic acids
E Electrolyte imbalance	Hyperkalemia, hypermagnesemia
I Intoxications	Salicylates, lithium, methanol, ethylene glycol, theophylline, phenobarbital
O fluid Overload	Postoperative fluid gain
U Uremia	High catabolism of acute renal failure

Pharmacologic Approaches

- Loop diuretics have not been shown to accelerate ARF recovery or improve patient outcome; however, diuretics can facilitate management of fluid overload (Figure 73-1). The most effective diuretics are mannitol and loop diuretics.
- **Mannitol** 20% is typically started at a dose of 12.5 to 25 g intravenously (IV) over 3 to 5 minutes. Disadvantages include IV administration, hyperosmolality risk, and need for monitoring because mannitol can contribute to ARF.
- Equipotent doses of loop diuretics (**furosemide, bumetanide, torsemide, ethacrynic acid**) have similar efficacy. Ethacrynic acid is reserved for sulfa-allergic patients. Continuous infusions of loop diuretics appear to be more effective and to have fewer adverse effects than intermittent boluses. An initial

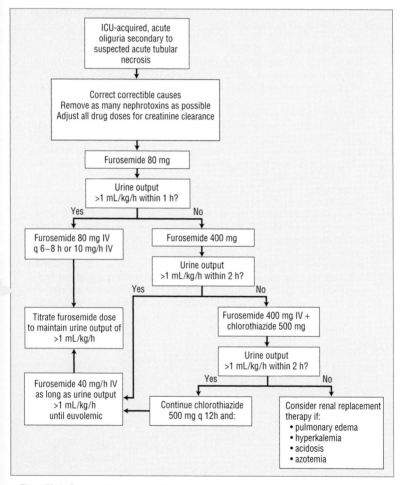

Figure 73–1. Suggested treatment algorithm for ICU-acquired oliguric acute renal failure resulting from acute tubular necrosis.

TABLE 73–4. Common Causes of Diuretic Resistance in Patients with Acute Renal Failure and Measures Used to Counteract Them

Classification of Diuretic Resistance	Potential Therapeutic Solution
Excessive sodium intake (sources may be dietary, IV fluids, and drugs)	Remove sodium from nutritional sources and medications
Inadequate diuretic dose or inappropriate regimen	Increase dose, use continuous infusion or combination therapy
Reduced oral bioavailability (usually furosemide)	Use parenteral therapy; switch to oral torsemide or bumetanide
Nephrotic syndrome (loop diuretic protein binding in tubule lumen)	Increase dose, switch diuretics, use combination therapy
Reduced renal blood flow	
Drugs (NSAIDs ACEIs, vasodilators)	Discontinue these drugs if possible
Hypotension	Intravascular volume expansion and/or vasopressors
Intravascular depletion	Intravascular volume expansion
Increased sodium resorption	
Nephron adaptation to chronic diuretic therapy	Combination diuretic therapy, sodium restriction
NSAID use	Discontinue NSAID
Congestive heart failure	Treat CHF, increase diuretic dose, switch to better absorbed loop diuretic
Cirrhosis	High-volume paracentesis
Acute tubular necrosis	Higher dose of diuretic, diuretic combination therapy, add low-dose dopamine

NSAID, nonsteroidal antinflammatory drug; ACEI, angiotensin-converting enzyme inhibitor; CHF, congestive heart failure.

IV loading dose (equivalent to furosemide 40 to 80 mg) should be administered before starting a continuous infusion (equivalent to furosemide 10 to 20 mg/h).

- Strategies are available to overcome diuretic resistance (Table 73–4), a common problem in patients with ARF. Agents from different pharmacologic classes, such as diuretics that work at the distal convoluted tubule (thiazides) or the collecting duct (**amiloride, triamterene, spironolactone**), may be synergistic when combined with loop diuretics. **Metolazone** is commonly used because, unlike other thiazides, it produces effective diuresis at GFR less than 20 mL/min.

NUTRITION THERAPY

- Enteral (see Chapter 56), but not parenteral, nutrition has been shown to improve patient outcomes.
- The most common interventions are management of fluid and electrolyte balance (see Chapter 76).
- Hyperkalemia is the most common and serious electrolyte abnormality in ARF. Typically, potassium must be restricted to less than 3 g/day and monitored daily.
- Additional electrolytes (and restrictions) that should be monitored include sodium (less than 3 g/day), magnesium, and phosphorus. The choice of treatment for hyperphosphatemia depends on whether the calcium-phosphate product is more than 55 (treat with **sevelamer** or oral aluminum-containing phosphate-binding antacids) or less than 55 (treat with calcium-containing antacids).

TABLE 73–5. Key Monitoring Parameters for Patients with Established Acute Renal Failure

Parameter	Frequency
Fluid ins/outs	Every shift
Patient weight	Daily
Vital signs	Every shift
Blood cultures and sensitivities	Check for results daily; obtain more when clinical signs of infection present
Blood chemistries	
Sodium, potassium, chloride, bicarbonate, calcium, phosphate, magnesium	Daily
BUN/S_{Cr}	Daily
Albumin	Once or twice weekly
Complete blood cell count with white cell differential	Daily
Drugs and their dosing regimens	Daily
Nutritional regimen	Daily
Blood glucose	Every shift for critically ill patients
Serum concentration data for drugs	After regimen changes and after RRT has been instituted
Times of administered doses	Daily
Doses relative to administration of RRT	Daily
Urinalysis	
Calculate measured creatinine clearance	Every time measured urine collection performed
Calculate fractional excretion of sodium	Every time measured urine collection performed
Plans for renal replacement	Daily
Invasive monitoring parameters	As indicated
Swan-Ganz readings	Every shift

BUN, blood urea nitrogen; S_{Cr}, serum creatinine; RRT, renal replacement therapy.

►XIV ► EVALUATION OF THERAPEUTIC OUTCOMES

- Close monitoring of patient status is essential (Table 73–5).
- Drug concentrations should be monitored frequently because of changing volume status, changing renal function, and renal replacement therapies in patients with ARF.

See Chapter 42, Acute Renal Failure, authored by Bruce A. Mueller, for a more detailed discussion of this topic.

Chapter 74

► CHRONIC KIDNEY DISEASE

► DEFINITION

- Chronic kidney disease (CKD) is a progressive loss of function over several months to years, characterized by gradual replacement of normal kidney architecture with interstitial fibrosis. Progressive kidney disease or nephropathy is generally synonymous with CKD.
- End-stage kidney disease (ESKD) occurs when the glomerular filtration rate (GFR) falls below 15 mL/min per 1.73 m^2 body surface area and requires dialysis or transplantation to remove uremic toxins and maintain hemodynamic stability.

► PATHOPHYSIOLOGY

- Susceptibility factors increase the risk for kidney disease but do not directly cause kidney damage. Susceptibility factors include advanced age, reduced kidney mass and low birth weight, racial or ethnic minority, family history, low income or education, systemic inflammation, and dyslipidemia.
- Initiation factors initiate kidney damage and can be modified by drug therapy. Initiation factors include diabetes mellitus, hypertension, autoimmune disease, polycystic kidney disease, and drug toxicity.
- Progression factors hasten decline in kidney function after initiation of kidney damage. Progression factors include glycemia in diabetics, hypertension, proteinuria, and smoking.
- Most progressive nephropathies share a final common pathway to irreversible renal parenchymal damage and ESKD. Key pathway elements are loss of nephron mass, glomerular capillary hypertension, and proteinuria.
- Many uremic toxins accumulate in patients with ESKD and alter organ, immune, and other bodily functions. Patients ultimately develop secondary complications such as anemia, hyperparathyroidism, renal osteodystrophy, and metabolic acidosis.

► CLINICAL PRESENTATION

- The clinical presentation of CKD depends on the patient's residual renal function and is initially silent (Figure 74–1).
- Every major organ system is affected by CKD. Classic signs and symptoms are asterixis, pruritus, dysgeusia, nausea, vomiting, anorexia, encephalopathy, and bleeding. Signs and symptoms are not useful for detecting CKD because they do not occur in early stages.

► DESIRED OUTCOME

- The primary goal is to identify at-risk patients and initiate appropriate interventions early, thereby slowing or halting progression of CKD to ESKD.
- Another goal is to manage and prevent progression of secondary complications.

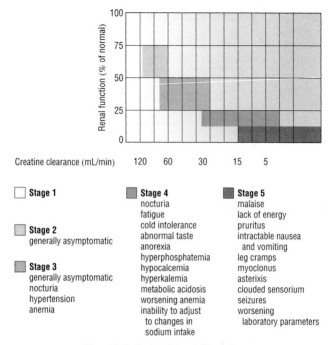

Figure 74–1. Staging of chronic kidney disease

Stage 1

Stage 2
generally asymptomatic

Stage 3
generally asymptomatic
nocturia
hypertension
anemia

Stage 4
nocturia
fatigue
cold intolerance
abnormal taste
anorexia
hyperphosphatemia
hypocalcemia
hyperkalemia
metabolic acidosis
worsening anemia
inability to adjust
   to changes in
   sodium intake

Stage 5
malaise
lack of energy
pruritus
intractable nausea
   and vomiting
leg cramps
myoclonus
asterixis
clouded sensorium
seizures
worsening
   laboratory parameters

▶ TREATMENT: PROGRESSIVE KIDNEY DISEASE

The treatment of progressive kidney disease includes nonpharmacologic and pharmacologic strategies. Strategies differ depending on the presence (Figure 74–2) or absence of diabetes (Figure 74–3).

NONPHARMACOLOGIC THERAPY

A low-protein diet (0.6 to 0.75 g/kg/day) can delay progression to ESKD in patients with or without diabetes, but compliance can be problematic.

PHARMACOLOGIC THERAPY

Hyperglycemia
• Intensive blood glucose control in patients with type 1 diabetes has been reported to reduce the frequency, decrease severity, and delay development or progression of diabetic complications, including nephropathy.
• For more information on diabetes, see Chapter 18.

Hypertension
• Adequate blood pressure control (Figures 74–2, 74–3, and 74–4) can reduce the rate of decline in GFR and albuminuria in patients with or without diabetes.

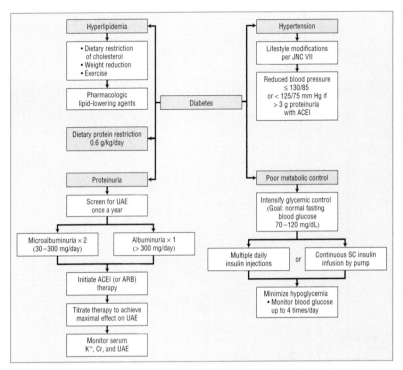

Figure 74–2. Therapeutic strategies to prevent progression of renal disease in diabetic individuals. UAE, urinary albumin excretion; SC, subcutaneous; JNC VII, the seventh report of the Joint National Committee on Prevention, Detection, Evaluation, and Treatment of High Blood Pressure.

- There is no consensus regarding the optimal antihypertensive agent, starting dosage, or maximum dosage. No class of antihypertensive agents reduces blood pressure better than the others. Angiotensin-converting enzyme inhibitors (ACEIs), followed by nondihydropyridine calcium channel blockers (CCBs) and angiotensin II receptor blockers (ARBs), have been the most thoroughly evaluated in diabetic and nondiabetic patients with CKD. XIV
- Treatment should begin with the lowest possible dose followed by gradual titration to achieve target blood pressure and, secondarily, to minimize proteinuria. Preliminary evidence suggests that combining an ACEI with a nondihydropyridine CCB or an ARB may yield further benefits.
- GFR typically decreases after starting ACEI therapy because this class reduces intraglomerular pressure. Serum creatinine (S_{Cr}) increases 25% to 30% within 3 to 7 days after starting therapy. S_{Cr} elevations of more than 0.5 mg/dL may signify drug-induced acute kidney failure and the need to stop ACEI therapy.
- For more information on hypertension, see Chapter 10.

Hyperlipidemia
- Lipid-lowering therapies decrease proteinuria and slow the rate of decline of GFR in nondiabetic patients with CKD.

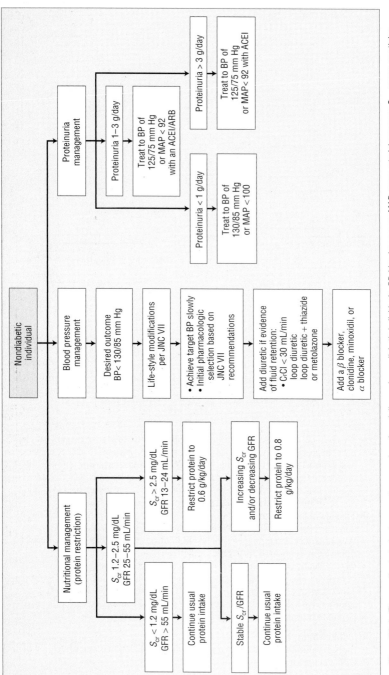

Figure 74–3. Therapeutic strategies to prevent progression of renal disease in nondiabetic individuals. BP, blood pressure; MAP, mean arterial pressure; S_{cr}, serum creatinine.

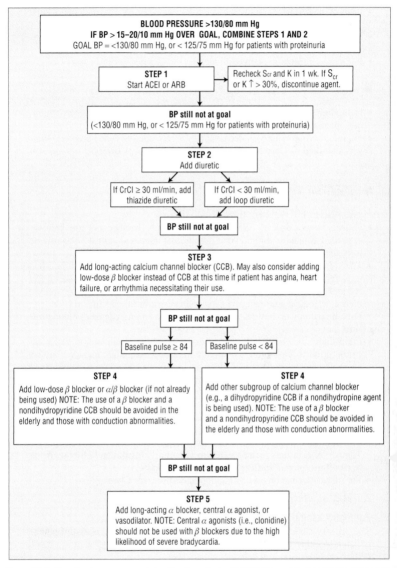

Figure 74–4. Hypertension management algorithm for patients with CKD. Dosage adjustments should be made every 2 to 4 weeks as needed. The dose of one agent should be maximized before another is added.

- Patients with CKD should be treated aggressively for dyslipidemia (Table 74–1).
- In addition to their lipid-lowering effects, statins (HMG-CoA reductase inhibitors) may have other effects that reduce progression of kidney disease.
- For more information on hyperlipidemia, see Chapter 9.

▶ TREATMENT: END-STAGE KIDNEY DISEASE

- Hemodialysis and peritoneal dialysis are the primary renal replacement therapies for patients with ESKD.
- For information on dialysis, see Chapter 45, Hemodialysis and Peritoneal Dialysis, authored by Gary Matzke, in *Pharmacotherapy: A Pathophysiologic Approach.*

▶ TREATMENT: SECONDARY COMPLICATIONS

FLUID AND ELECTROLYTE ABNORMALITIES

- Patients with CKD or ESKD maintain sodium balance but are volume-expanded. The most common manifestation of increased intravascular volume is systemic hypertension.
- The kidney's ability to adjust to abrupt changes in sodium intake is diminished in patients with ESKD. Sodium restriction beyond a no-added-salt diet is not recommended unless hypertension or edema is present. A negative sodium balance can decrease renal perfusion and cause a further decline in GFR.
- Diuretic therapy or dialysis may be necessary to control edema or blood pressure.
- Loop diuretics, particularly when administered by continuous infusion, increase urine volume and renal sodium excretion. Although thiazide diuretics are ineffective when creatinine clearance is less than 30 mL/min, adding them to loop diuretics can enhance excretion of sodium and water.

POTASSIUM HOMEOSTASIS

- Serum potassium concentration is usually maintained in the normal range until the onset of ESKD (GFR less than 15 mL/min).
- The definitive treatment of severe hyperkalemia in ESKD is hemodialysis. Temporary measures include **calcium gluconate**, **insulin** and **glucose,** nebulized **albuterol,** and **sodium polystyrene sulfonate.**
- For more information on potassium homeostasis, see Chapter 76.

ANEMIA

Pathophysiology

The primary cause of anemia in patients with CKD or ESKD is erythropoietin deficiency. Other contributing factors include decreased lifespan of red blood cells, blood loss, and iron deficiency.

▶ TREATMENT

- **Iron** supplementation is necessary to replete iron stores (Figure 74–5). Parenteral iron therapy improves response to erythropoietic therapy and reduces the dose required to achieve and maintain target indices. In contrast, oral therapy is often inadequate.
- Intravenous (IV) iron preparations have different pharmacokinetic profiles, which do not correlate with pharmacodynamic effect.

XIV

TABLE 74–1. Management of Dyslipidemia in Patients with CKD

Dyslipidemia	Goal	Initial Therapy	Modification in Therapy[a]	Alternative[a]
TG ≥500 mg/dL	TG <500 mg/dL	TLC	TLC + fibrate or niacin	Fibrate or niacin
LDL 100–129 mg/dL	LDL <100 mg/dL	TLC	TLC + low-dose statin	Bile acid sequestrant or niacin
LDL ≥130 mg/dL	LDL < 100 mg/dL	TLC + low-dose statin	TLC + max dose statin	Bile acid sequestrant or niacin
TG ≥200 mg/dL and non-HDL ≥130 mg/dL	Non-HDL <130 mg/dL	TLC + low-dose statin	TLC + max dose statin	Fibrate or niacin

[a]Dosing of selected agents by class: fibrate (gemfibrozil 600 mg twice a day); niacin (1.5–3 g/day of immediate-release product); statin (simvastatin 10–40 mg/day if glomerular filtration rate [GFR] <30 mL/min, 20–80 mg/day if GFR >30 mL/min); bile acid sequestrant (cholestyramine 4–16 g/day). HDL, high-density lipoprotein; LDL, low-density lipoprotein; Non-HDL, total cholesterol minus HDL cholesterol; TG, triglycerides; TLC, therapeutic lifestyle changes. See Chapter 9 for more complete dosing information.

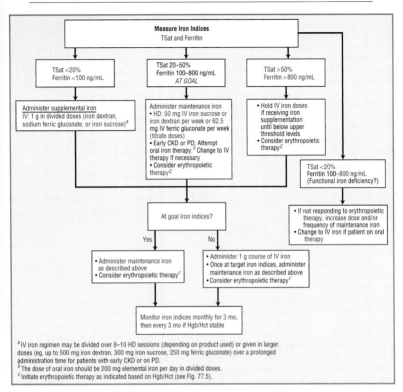

Figure 74–5. Guidelines for erythropoietic therapy in the management of the anemia of CKD.

- Adverse effects of IV iron include allergic reactions, hypotension, dizziness, dyspnea, headaches, lower back pain, arthralgia, syncope, and arthritis. Some of these reactions can be minimized by decreasing the dose or rate of infusion. Sodium ferric gluconate and iron sucrose have better safety records than iron dextran. Iron dextran requires a test dose to reduce the risk of anaphylactic reactions.
- Of the erythropoietic agents (Figure 74–6), **epoetin alfa** has been the mainstay of therapy for anemia. Subcutaneous (SC) administration is preferable because IV access is not required and because the SC dose that maintains target indices is 15% to 50% lower than the IV dose.
- **Darbepoetin alfa**, the newer erythropoietic agent, has a longer half-life and prolonged biologic activity. Therefore, doses are administered less frequently, starting at once a week or every other week when administered IV or SC.
- Erythropoietic agents are well tolerated. Hypertension is the most common adverse event.

Evaluation of Therapeutic Outcomes
- Iron indices (transferrin saturation [TSat]; ferritin) should be evaluated before initiating an erythropoietic agent (Figure 74–5). To avoid errors, clinicians should wait at least 2 weeks after a loading dose of IV iron to reassess iron indices.

XIV

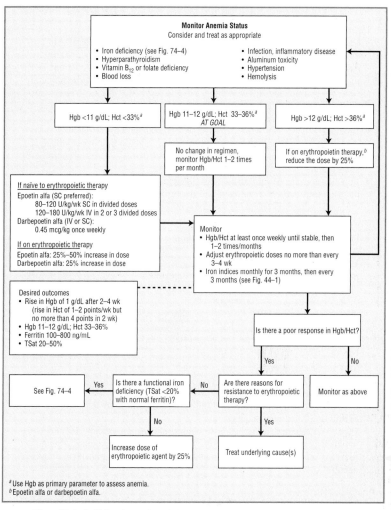

Figure 74–6. Guidelines for erythropoietic therapy in the management of the anemia of CKD.

- For monitoring purposes, hemoglobin is preferred to hematocrit because the latter fluctuates with volume status. The target hemoglobin is 11 to 12 g/dL (hematocrit 33% to 36%).
- After an erythropoietic agent is initiated, hemoglobin response is typically delayed. Steady-state hemoglobin levels do not occur until after the life span of a red blood cell (RBC) (mean 2 months; range 1 to 4 months). To avoid making premature dosing changes, clinicians should evaluate response over several weeks (Figure 74–6).
- Patients should be monitored for potential complications, such as hypertension, which should be treated before starting an erythropoietic agent.
- For more information on anemia, see Chapter 32.

SECONDARY HYPERPARATHYROIDISM AND RENAL OSTEODYSTROPHY

Pathophysiology and Clinical Presentation

- Calcium-phosphorus balance is mediated through a complex interplay of hormones and their effects on bone, gastrointestinal (GI) tract, kidney, and parathyroid gland. As kidney disease progresses, renal activation of vitamin D is impaired, which reduces gut absorption of calcium. Low blood calcium concentration stimulates secretion of parathyroid hormone (PTH). As renal function declines, serum calcium balance can be maintained only at the expense of increased bone resorption, ultimately resulting in renal osteodystrophy.
- Secondary hyperparathyroidism can cause skeletal complications such as osteitis fibrosa cystica (high bone-formation rate), altered lipid metabolism, altered insulin secretin, resistance to erythropoietic therapy, impaired neurologic and immune functions, and increased mortality.
- Renal osteodystrophy progresses insidiously for several years before the onset of symptoms such as bone pain and fractures. When symptoms appear, the disease is not easily amenable to treatment.

Treatment

- Preventive measures should be initiated in patients in early stages of CKD (GFR less than 60 mL/min).
- The new guidelines provide desired ranges of calcium, phosphorus, calcium-phosphorus product, and PTH for each stage of CKD (Table 74–2). Measurements should be repeated every 12 months for stage 3, every 3 months for stage 4, and more frequently for stage 5.
- Dietary phosphorus restriction (800 to 1000 mg/day) should be first-line intervention for stage 3 or higher CKD.
- By the time ESKD develops, most patients require a combination of phosphate-binding agents and Vitamin D therapy.

Phosphate-Binding Agents

- Phosphate-binding agents decrease phosphorus absorption from the gut and should be administered with meals to maximize this effect (Table 74–3).
- Oral calcium compounds are first-line agents for controlling both serum phosphorus and calcium concentrations.
- Elemental calcium from phosphate binders should not exceed 1500 mg/day, which may necessitate combination of calcium- and noncalcium-containing (magnesium, aluminum, or nonabsorbable hydrogel) phosphate-binding agents.

Vitamin D Therapy

- Calcium (less than 9.5 mg/dL) and phosphorus (less than 4.6 mg/dL) must be controlled before vitamin D therapy is initiated.

TABLE 74–2. K/DOQI Guidelines for Calcium, Phosphorus, Calcium Phosphorus Product, and Intact Parathyroid Hormone

Parameter	Stage 3 CKD	Stage 4 CKD	Stage 5 CKD
Corrected calcium (mg/dL)	"Normal"	"Normal"	8.4–9.5
Phosphorus (mg/dL)	2.7–4.6	2.7–4.6	3.5–5.5
Ca × P (mg^2/dL^2)	<55	<55	<55
Intact PTH (pg/mL)	35–70	70–110	150–300

K/DOQI, Kidney Disease Outcomes Qualitiy Initiative.

TABLE 74–3. Phosphate-Binding Agents Used in the Treatment of Hyperphosphatemia in CKD

Compound	Trade Name	Compound (Elemental Calcium Content)	Starting Doses	Comments
Calcium carbonate[a] (40%) elemental calcium)	Tums	500 (200), 1250 (500)	0.5–1 g (elemental calcium) t.i.d with meals	First-line agent; dissolution characteristics and phosphate-binding effect may vary from product to product; try to limit daily intake of elemental calcium to 1.5 g/day
	Oscal-500	1250 (500)		Approximately 39 mg phosphorus bound per 1 g calcium carbonate
	Catrate 600	1500 (600)		
	Nephro-Calci	1500 (600)		
	LiquiCal	1200 (480)		
	CalciChew	1250 (500)		
Calcium acetate (25% elemental calcium)	PhosLo	667 (167)	0.5–1 g (elemental calcium) t.i.d with meals	First-line agent; comparable efficacy to calcium carbonate with half the dose of elemental calcium; do not exceed 1.5 g/day
				Approximately 45 mg phosphorus bound per 1 g calcium acetate
				By prescription only
Sevelamer	Renagel	400, 800	800 mg t.i.d with meals	First-line agent; lowers LDL cholesterol
				More expensive than calcium products; preferred in patients at risk for extraskeletal calcification

Continued

TABLE 74-3. (Continued)

Compound	Trade Name	Compound (Elemental Calcium Content)	Starting Doses	Comments
Aluminum hydroxide	Alterna GEL Amphojel	600 mg/5 mL 300, 600 (tablet) 320 mg/ 5 mL (suspension)	300–600 mg t.i.d with meals	Third-line agents; do not use concurrently with citrate-containing products
	Alu-Cap	400		Reserve for short-term use (4 weeks) in patients with hyperphosphatemia not responding to other binders
Aluminum carbonate	Basaljel	500 (tablet, capsule) 400 mg/5 mL (suspension)	450–500 mg t.i.d with meals	Same as for aluminum hydroxide
Magnesium carbonate	Mag-Carb	70 mg capsule	70 mg t.i.d with meals	Third-line agent; diarrhea common; monitor serum magnesium
Magnesium hydroxide	Milk of magnesia	300, 600 (tablet) 400 mg/5 ml, 800 mg/5 mL (suspension)	300–400 mg t.i.d with meals	Same as for magnesium carbonate
Magnesium carbonate/calcium carbonate	MagneBind 200	200 (160)	200 mg t.i.d with meals (based on magnesium content)	Same as for calcium carbonate and magnesium carbonate

*a*Multiple preparations available, which are not listed.

LDL, low-density lipoprotein.

TABLE 74-4. Dosing Recommendations for Vitamin D in Patients with Stage 5 CKD on Hemodialysis (HD)[a]

PTH (pg/mL)	IV and PO Calcitriol Dose per HD	IV Paricalcitol Dose per HD	PO and IV Doxercalciferol Dose per HD
300–600[b]	0.5–1.5 mcg PO or IV	2.5–5.0 mcg	5 mcg PO 2 mcg IV
600–1000[b]	1–4 mcg PO 1–3 mcg IV	6.0–10 mcg	5–10 mcg PO 2–4 mcg IV
>1000[c]	3–7 mcg PO 3–5 mcg IV	10–15 mcg	10–20 mcg PO 4–8 mcg IV

[a]Peritoneal dialysis patients may be treated with PO doses of calcitriol (0.5–1.0 mcg) or doxercalciferol (2.5–5.0 mcg) two or three times weekly. May also use PO calcitriol at 0.25 mcg daily.
[b]If serum calcium <9.5 mg/dL, phosphorus >5.5 mg/dL, and Ca × P <55 mg^2/dL^2.
[c]If serum calcium <10 mg/dL, phosphorus <5.5 mg/dL, and Ca × P <55 mg^2/dL^2.
PTH, parathyroid hormone.

- **Calcitriol,** 1,25-dihydroxyvitamin D_3, has been used for the management of secondary hyperparathyroidism since the 1980s. Calcitriol directly suppresses PTH synthesis and secretion and appears to upregulate vitamin D receptors, which ultimately may reduce parathyroid hyperplasia. The dose depends on the stage of CKD and type of dialysis (Table 74–4).
- The newer vitamin D analogues **paricalcitol** and **doxercalciferol** may be associated with less hypercalcemia and, for paricalcitol, hyperphosphatemia.

Calcimimetics
- **Cinacalcet** reduces PTH secretion by increasing the sensitivity of the calcium-sensing receptor. The most common adverse events are nausea and vomiting.
- The most effective way to use cinacalcet with other therapies has not been decided. Cinacalcet should not be started if serum calcium is less than 8.4 mg/dL. The starting dose is 30 mg daily, which can be titrated to the desired PTH and calcium concentrations every 2 to 4 weeks and to a maximum of 180 mg daily.

METABOLIC ACIDOSIS

- A clinically significant metabolic acidosis is commonly seen when the GFR drops below 20 to 30 mL/min. ^{XIV}
- Consequences of metabolic acidosis include renal bone disease, fatigue, decreased exercise tolerance, reduced cardiac contractility, increased vascular irritability, and protein catabolism.
- Oral alkalinizing salts (e.g., **sodium bicarbonate**, **Shohl's solution**, and **Bicitra**) can be used in patients with stage 3 or higher CKD. **Polycitra**, which contains potassium citrate, should *not* be used in patients with severe renal insufficiency or ESKD because hyperkalemia may result.
- The replacement alkali dose can be approximated by multiplying bicarbonate's volume of distribution (0.5 L/kg) by the patient's weight (in kg) and by their deficit (24 mEq/L minus patient's serum bicarbonate value). The dose should be administered over several days. The daily maintenance dose is usually 12 to 20 mEq/mL and should be titrated as needed.
- Metabolic acidosis in patients undergoing dialysis can often be managed by using higher concentrations of bicarbonate or acetate in the dialysate.
- For more information on acid-base disorders, see Chapter 72.

HYPERTENSION

- The pathogenesis of hypertension in patients with CKD is multifactorial and includes fluid retention, increased sympathetic activity, an endogenous digitalis-like substance, elevated levels of endothelin-1, erythropoietin use, hyperparathyroidism, and structural arterial changes.
- The target blood pressure is controversial because of the greater potential for complications in patients with ESKD than in those with less advanced CKD. A higher target of more than 150/90 mm Hg has been proposed for patients with ESKD.
- Salt (2 to 3 g/day) and fluid intake should be restricted.
- Most patients with ESKD require three or more antihypertensive agents to achieve target blood pressure. As with less advanced CKD (see Figure 74–4), ACEIs, ARBs, and dihydropyridine CCBs are the preferred agents.
- Blood pressure should be monitored at each visit, and patients should perform home monitoring.
- For more information on hypertension, see Chapter 10.

HYPERLIPIDEMIA

- The prevalence of hyperlipidemia increases as renal function declines.
- Hyperlipidemia should be managed aggressively in patients with ESKD to an LDL-C goal of less than 100 mg/dL. Statins are the drugs of first choice. Although well tolerated by otherwise healthy patients, statins have the potential to cause myotoxic effects when administered in patients with hepatic disease or with interacting drugs such as azole antibiotics, cyclosporine, gemfibrozil, niacin.
- In patients with ESKD, lipid profile should be reassessed at least annually and 2 to 3 months after changing treatment.
- For more information on hyperlipidemia, see relevant section under progressive kidney disease in this chapter, Table 74–1, and Chapter 9.

MALNUTRITION

- Protein-energy malnutrition is common in patients with stage 4 or 5 CKD. Food intake is often inadequate because of anorexia, altered taste sensation, intercurrent illness, and unpalatability of prescribed diets.
- Daily protein intake should be 1.2 g/kg for patients undergoing hemodialysis and 1.2 to 1.3 g/kg for those undergoing peritoneal dialysis.
- Daily energy intake should be 35 kcal/kg for patients undergoing any type of dialysis. The intake should be lowered to 30 to 35 kcal/kg for patients older than 60 years.
- Water-soluble vitamins should be supplemented to replace dialysis-induced loss. L-carnitine is not recommended for patients with ESKD unless the disorders for which it has shown benefit (e.g., hypertriglyceridemia, hyper-cholesterolemia, and anemia) do not respond to standard therapies.
- For more information on nutrition requirements, see Chapter 55.

OTHER SECONDARY COMPLICATIONS

Uremic Bleeding

- The pathophysiology of uremic bleeding is multifactorial. The primary mechanisms are platelet biochemical abnormalities and alterations in platelet-vessel wall interactions.
- Dialysis shortens, but usually does not normalize, the bleeding time. The effect is short lived (1 to 2 days).

XIV

- Nondialytic therapies that may temporarily shorten increased bleeding time include **cryoprecipitate**, **desmopressin** (1-deamino-8-D-arginine vasopressin), and estrogens.

Pruritus

- Pruritus is a common problem in patients with ESKD. The pathogenesis is poorly understood but has been attributed to inadequate dialysis, skin dryness, secondary hyperparathyroidism, increased concentrations of vitamin A and histamine, and increased sensitivity to histamine.
- For more information on pruritus, see Chapter 45, Hemodialysis and Peritoneal Dialysis, authored by Gary Matzke, in *Pharmacotherapy: A Pathophysiologic Approach*.

See Chapter 43, Chronic Kidney Disease: Progression-Modifying Therapies, authored by Melanie S. Joy, Abhijit Kshirsagar, and James Paparello, and Chapter 45, Chronic Kidney Disease: Therapeutic Approach for the Management of Complications, authored by Joanna Q. Hudson and Kunal Chaudhary, for a more detailed discussion of this topic.

XIV

Chapter 75

▶ DRUG DOSING IN RENAL INSUFFICIENCY

▶ GENERAL PRINCIPLES

- The pathophysiology, clinical manifestations, diagnosis, and treatment of acute renal failure and chronic kidney disease (or end-stage kidney disease [ESKD]) are discussed in chapters 73 and 74, respectively.
- Drug therapy individualization for patients with renal insufficiency sometimes requires only a simple proportional dose adjustment based on creatinine clearance (CL_{cr}). Alternatively, complex adjustments are required for drugs that are extensively metabolized or undergo dramatic changes in protein binding and distribution.
- Patients can also have an altered pharmacodynamic response to a given drug because of the physiologic and biochemical changes associated with progressive renal insufficiency.

EFFECT ON DRUG ABSORPTION

- There is little quantitative information regarding influence of impaired renal function on drug absorption and bioavailability.
- Factors that theoretically affect bioavailability include alterations in gastrointestinal (GI) transit time, gastric pH, edema of the GI tract, vomiting and diarrhea, and concomitant drug therapy, especially antacid or H_2-antagonist administration.
- Increased bioavailability has been reported for **bufuralol, oxprenolol, propranolol, tolamolol, dextropropoxyphene,** and **dihydrocodeine** in patients with renal insufficiency. However, clinical consequences have been demonstrated only with dextropropoxyphene and dihydrocodeine.

EFFECT ON DRUG DISTRIBUTION

- The volume of distribution of many drugs is significantly increased or decreased in patients with ESKD. Changes result from altered protein or tissue binding, or pathophysiologic alterations in body composition (e.g., fractional contribution of total body water to total body weight).
- Generally, plasma protein binding of acidic drugs (e.g., **warfarin, phenytoin**) is decreased in ESKD, whereas binding of basic drugs (e.g., **quinidine, lidocaine**) is usually normal or slightly decreased or increased.
- Ideally, unbound (versus total) drug concentrations should be monitored, especially for drugs that have a narrow therapeutic range, are highly protein bound (free fraction less than 20%), and have marked variability in the free fraction (e.g., **phenytoin, disopyramide**).
- Methods for calculating volume of distribution (V_D) can be influenced by renal disease. Of the commonly used terms (i.e., volumes of central compartment [V_c], terminal phase [V_β, V_{area}], and distribution at steady state [V_{SS}]), V_{SS} is the most appropriate for comparing patients with renal insufficiency versus those with normal renal function because V_{SS} is independent of drug elimination.

EFFECT ON METABOLISM

- Chronic kidney disease affects metabolism of drugs by some cytochrome P450 (CYP450) enzymes in the liver and possibly in the intestines (e.g., CYP450 3A4 and 2C9). Prediction of the effect on the metabolism of a particular drug

TABLE 75–1. Effect of End-Stage Kidney Disease on Nonrenal Clearance

		Decreased	
Acyclovir	Aztreonam	Bufuralol	Captopril
Cefmenoxime	Cefmetazole	Cefonicid	Cefotaxime
Cefotiam	Cefsulodin	Ceftizoxime	Cilastatin
Cimetidine	Ciprofloxacin	Cortisol	Encainide
Erythromycin	Imipenem	Isoniazid	Methylprednisolone
Metoclopramide	Moxalactam	Nicardipine	Nimodipine
Nitrendipine	Procainamide	Quinapril	Repaglinide
Verapamil	Zidovudine		
		Unchanged	
Acetaminophen	Chloramphenicol	Clonidine	Codeine
Diflunisal	Indomethacin	Insulin[a]	Isradipine
Lidocaine	Morphine	Metoprolol	Nisoldipine
Nortriptyline	Pentobarbital	Propafenone	Quinidine
Theophylline	Tocainide	Tolbutamide	
		Increased	
Bumetanide	Cefpiramide	Fosinopril	Nifedipine
Phenytoin	Rosiglitazone	Sulfadimidine	

[a]May be unchanged or decreased.

is difficult, and a general quantitative strategy for adjusting treatment regimens is not available.
- Nonrenal clearance of a drug can be increased, decreased, or unaffected by renal failure (Table 75–1).
- Patients with severe renal insufficiency can experience accumulation of metabolite(s), which can contribute to pharmacologic activity or toxicity (Table 75–2).

EFFECT ON RENAL EXCRETION

- Altered renal filtration, secretion, and/or absorption can have dramatic effects on the pharmacokinetics of a drug. The impact depends on the fraction of drug normally eliminated unchanged by the kidney and on the degree of renal insufficiency.
- Quantitative investigation of renal handling of drugs is needed to elucidate the relative contribution of tubular and glomerular function to renal drug clearance. In the absence of clinically useful techniques to quantitate tubular function, clinical measurement or estimation of CL_{cr} remains the guiding factor for calculating drug dosage.

XIV

▶ DRUG-DOSAGE REGIMEN DESIGNS

- Most dosage adjustment guidelines use a fixed dose or interval for patients with broad ranges of renal function. However, these categories encompass up to a 10-fold range in renal function and are not optimal for all patients.
- The optimal dosage regimen for patients with renal insufficiency requires an individualized assessment. The optimal regimen depends on an accurate characterization of the relationship between the drug's pharmacokinetic parameters and renal function and on an accurate assessment of the patient's renal function.
- Consideration must be given to stability of renal function and type of dialysis.

TABLE 75–2. Pharmacologic Activity of Selected Drug Metabolites

Parent Drug	Metabolite	Pharmacologic Activity of Metabolites
Acetaminophen	N-acetyl-p-benzo-quinoneimine	Responsible for hepatotoxicity
Allopurinol	Oxypurinol	Metabolite primarily responsible for suppression of xanthine oxidase
Azathioprine	Mercaptopurine	All of the immunosuppressive activity resides in the metabolite
Cefotaxime	Desacetyl cefotaxime	Similar antimicrobial spectrum, but one-fourth to one-tenth as potent
Chlorpropamide	2-Hydroxychlorpropamide	Similar in vitro insulin-releasing activity
Clofibrate	Chlorophenoxyisobutyric acid	Primarily responsible for hypolipidemic effect and direct muscle toxicity
Codeine	Morphine-6-glucuronide	Possibly more active than parent compound; may contribute to prolonged narcotic effect in renal failure patients
Imipramine	Desmethylimipramine	Similar antidepressant activity
Ketoprofen	ketoprofen glucuronide	Accumulation of acyl glucuronide may worsen toxic effects (gastrointestinal disturbances and impairment of renal function)
Meperidine	Normeperidine	Less analgesic activity than parent, but more CNS-stimulatory effect
Morphine	Morphine-6-glucuronide	Possibly more active than parent compound; may contribute to prolonged narcotic effect in renal failure patients
Mycophenolic acid	Mycophenolic acid glucuronide	Lacks pharmacologic activity but may be associated with dose-limiting (gastrointestinal) side effects
Procainamide	N-acetyl procainamide	Distinct antiarrhythmic activity, the mechanism of which is different from that of the parent compound
Sulfonamides	Acetylated metabolites	Devoid of antibacterial activity, but elevated concentrations are associated with toxicity
Theophylline	1,3-Dimethyl uric acid	Cardiotoxicity has been demonstrated
Zidovudine	Zidovudine triphosphate	Primarily responsible for antiretroviral activity

▶ XIV

PATIENTS WITH RENAL INSUFFICIENCY

- If the relationship between CL_{cr} and the kinetic parameters of a drug (i.e., total body clearance [CL], elimination rate constant [k], and V_D) is known, these data should be used to individualize drug therapy (Table 75–3).
- If the relationship between CL_{cr} and the kinetic parameters is unknown, then the patient's kinetic parameters can be based on the fraction of drug eliminated renally unchanged (f_e) in subjects with normal renal function. This approach assumes that f_e is known, the decreases in CL and k are proportional to CL_{cr}, renal disease does not alter drug metabolism, any metabolites are inactive and nontoxic, the drug obeys first-order (linear) kinetic principles, and the drug is adequately described by a one-compartment model. The kinetic parameter/dosage

TABLE 75–3. Relationship between Renal Function and Pharmacokinetic Parameters of Selected Drugs

Drug	Total Body Clearance
Acyclovir	$CL = 3.37\,(CL_{cr}) + 0.41$
Amikacin	$CL = 0.6\,(CL_{cr}) + 9.6$
Cefmetazole	$CL = 1.18\,(CL_{cr}) - 0.29$
Ceftazidime	$CL = 1.15\,(CL_{cr}) + 10.6$
Ciprofloxacin	$CL = 2.83\,(CL_{cr}) + 363$
Digoxin	$CL = 0.88\,(CL_{cr}) + 23$
Gentamicin	$CL = 0.983\,(CL_{cr})$
Lithium	$CL = 0.235\,(CL_{cr})$
Netilmicin	$CL = 0.65\,(CL_{cr}) + 3.72$
Ofloxacin	$CL = 1.04\,(CL_{cr}) + 38.7$
Piperacillin	$CL = 1.36\,(CL_{cr}) + 1.50$
Teicoplanin	$CL = 7.09\,(CL_{cr}) - 16.2$
Tobramycin	$CL = 0.801\,(CL_{cr})$
Vancomycin	$CL = 0.69\,(CL_{cr}) + 3.7$

CL, total body clearance; CL_{cr}, creatinine clearance.

adjustment factor (Q) can be calculated as

$$Q = 1 - [f_e(1 - KF)]$$

where KF is the ratio of the patient's CL_{cr} to the assumed normal value of 120 mL/min per 1.73 m^2. The estimated total body clearance of the patient (CL_{PT}) can then be calculated as

$$CL_{PT} = CL_{norm} \times Q$$

where CL_{norm} is the mean total body clearance in patients with normal renal function.

- The best method for adjusting the dosage regimen depends on whether the goal is maintaining a similar peak, trough, or average steady-state drug concentration. The principal choices are to decrease the dose, prolong the dosing interval, or both. Prolonging the interval is generally preferred because it saves costs by reducing nursing and pharmacy time as well as associated supplies.
- The prolonged dosing interval (τ_f) or reduced maintenance dose (D_f) is calculated from the following relationships, where τ_n is the normal dosing interval and D_n is the normal dose:

$$\tau_f = \tau_n / Q$$
$$D_f = D_n \times Q$$

- If V_D is significantly altered or a specific concentration is desired, estimation of a dosage regimen becomes more complex. The dosing interval (τ_f) is calculated as

$$\tau_f = \{(-1/k_f)[\ln\,(C_{min}/C_{max})]\} + t_{peak}$$

where C_{min} and C_{max} are minimum and maximum concentrations, respectively, and t_{peak} is time of peak concentration. The dose is calculated as

$$D = [S \cdot F \cdot C_p^t \cdot V_D(k_a - k)]/\{k_a[e^{-kt}/(1 - e^{-k\tau})][e^{-k_a t}/(1 - e^{-k_a \tau})]\}$$

where S equals the salt fraction, F equals the bioavailability, C_p^t equals the desired plasma concentration at time t, and k_a is the absorption rate constant. If the drug is absorbed extremely rapidly, τ_f is calculated as

$$\tau_f = (-1/k_f)[\ln(C_{min}/C_{max})]$$

and dose as

$$D = V_D(C_{max} - C_{min})$$

PATIENTS RECEIVING CONTINUOUS RENAL REPLACEMENT THERAPY

- Drug therapy individualization for patients receiving continuous renal replacement therapy (CRRT) is complicated by higher residual nonrenal clearance of some drugs in patients with acute versus chronic renal insufficiency. Furthermore, there are marked differences in drug removal between intermittent hemodialysis and the three primary types of CRRT (i.e., continuous arteriovenous or venovenous hemofiltration [CAVH or CVVH], hemodialysis [CAVHD or CVVHD], and hemodiafiltration [CAVHDF or CVVHDF]). Additionally, there are differences in drug removal rates between the types of CRRT and within each type.
- During CAVH/CVVH, drug clearance is a function of membrane permeability for the drug, which is called the sieving coefficient (SC), and the rate of ultrafiltrate formation (*UFR*). The SC is often approximated by the unbound fraction (f_u) because this information is more readily available. Thus, clearance by CAVH/CVVH can be calculated as

$$CL = UFR \times f_u$$

- Clearance by CAVHDF/CVVHDF is calculated as the product of the combined ultrafiltrate and dialysate volume (V_{df}) and drug concentration in this fluid (C_{df}), divided by the plasma concentration going into the filter (C_p^{mid}) at the midpoint of the V_{df} collection period:

$$CL = (V_{df} \times C_{df})/C_p^{mid}$$

- Factors that influence drug clearance during CRRT include the filter membrane composition, ultrafiltration rate, blood flow rate, and dialysate flow rate.
- Initial dosing regimens for patients receiving CRRT can also be designed using published CRRT clearance values (Table 75–4).

PATIENTS RECEIVING CHRONIC AMBULATORY PERITONEAL DIALYSIS

- Peritoneal dialysis has the potential to affect drug disposition; however, drug therapy individualization is often less complicated because of the continuous nature of chronic ambulatory peritoneal dialysis (CAPD).
- Factors that influence drug dialyzability include drug-specific characteristics (e.g., molecular weight, solubility, degree of ionization, protein binding, and V_D) and intrinsic properties of the peritoneal membrane (e.g., blood flow, pore size, and peritoneal membrane surface area).
- In general, peritoneal dialysis is less effective in removing drugs than hemodialysis and, in fact, does not contribute substantially to total body clearance.

TABLE 75–4. Clearance of Selected Drugs by CAVH/CVVH and/or CAVHD/CVVHD

| | CAVH/CVVH | | CAVHD/CVVHD | | |
| | | | Clearance | | |
Drug	SC	Clearance	SC	DFR 1 L/h	DFR 2 L/h
Amikacin	0.93 ± 0.16	10.1			
Amrinone	$0.80–1.4$	$2.4–14.4$			
Cefuroxime		11.0 ± 5.2	0.90 ± 0.30	14.0 ± 2.2	16.2 ± 3.4
Ceftazidime			0.86 ± 0.07	13.1 ± 1.3	15.2 ± 1.3
Cilastatin	0.77	4.0 ± 2.3	0.68 ± 0.08	10.0 ± 3.0	18.0 ± 4.0
Ciprofloxacin				16.3	19.9
Digoxin				$6.4–10.0$	11
Gentamicin		3.5 ± 1.9		5.2 ± 1.8	
Imipenem	0.80	13.3	1.05 ± 0.19	16.0 ± 7.0	
Phenytoin	0.37 ± 0.08	1.0		6.5	
Theophylline				14.8	
Tobramycin		3.5 ± 1.9		$11.1–29$	14.9
Vancomycin	0.80	$6.7–13.3$	0.66 ± 0.08	121 ± 5.7	16.6 ± 5.7

Clearance is in mL/min. *SC*, sieving coefficient; DFR, dialysate flow rate; CAVH/CVVH, continuous arteriovenous or venovenous hemofiltration; CAVHD/CVVHD, continuous arteriovenous or venovenous hemodialysis.

PATIENTS RECEIVING CHRONIC HEMODIALYSIS

- The impact of hemodialysis on drug therapy depends on drug characteristics, dialysis prescription (e.g., dialysis membrane composition, filter surface area, blood and dialysate flow rates, and reuse of the dialysis filter), and clinical indication for dialysis.
- High-flux dialysis allows free passage of most solutes with molecular weights up to 20,000. Therefore, high-flux dialysis is more likely to remove high–molecular-weight drugs (e.g., **vancomycin**), and drugs with low- to mid-molecular weights (i.e., 100 to 1000), than conventional dialysis (Table 75–5).
- The dialysate recovery clearance approach has become the benchmark for determining dialyzer clearance. It can be calculated as

$$CL'_{D} = R/AUC_{0-t} \qquad \text{XIV}$$

where R is the total amount of drug recovered unchanged in dialysate and AUC_{0-t} is the area under the predialyzer plasma concentration-time curve during the time when the dialysate was collected. To determine AUC_{0-t}, at least two and preferably three to four plasma concentrations should be obtained during dialysis.

- Total clearance during dialysis can be calculated as the sum of the patient's residual clearance during the interdialytic period (CL_{RES}) and dialyzer clearance (CL_{D}):

$$CL_{T} \times CL_{RES} + CL_{D}$$

- Half-life between hemodialysis (HD) treatments and during dialysis can then be calculated from the following relationships using a published estimate of the drug's V_{D}:

$$t_{1/2, \text{offHD}} = 0.693\,[V_{D}/CL_{RES}] \qquad \text{and}$$

$$t_{1/2, \text{on HD}} = 0.693\,[V_{D}/(CL_{RES} + CL_{D})]$$

TABLE 75–5. Drug Disposition during Dialysis Depends on Filter Characteristics

Drug	Hemodialysis Clearance (mL/min)		Half-Life during Dialysis (h)	
	Conventional	*High-Flux*	*Conventional*	*High-Flux*
Ceftazidime	55–60	155[a]	3.3	1.2[a]
Cefuroxime	NR	103[b]	3.8	1.6[b]
Foscarnet	183	253[b]	NR	NR
Gentamicin	58.2	116[b]	3.0	4.3[b]
Netilmicin	46	87–109	5.0–5.2	2.9–3.4
Ranitidine	43.1	67.2[b]	5.1	2.9[b]
Vancomycin	9–21	31–60[c]	35–38	12.0[c]
		40–150[b]		4.5–11.8[b]
		72–116[d]		NR[d]

[a]Polyamide filter.
[b]Polysulfone filter.
[c]Polyacrylonitrile filter.
[d]Polymethylmethacrylate.
NR, not reported.

- Once key pharmacokinetic parameters are estimated (based on population data) or calculated, they can be used to simulate the plasma concentration-time profile of the drug for the patient and to ascertain how much drug to administer and when.
- Plasma concentrations of the drug over the interdialytic interval of 24 to 48 hours can be predicted. The concentration at the end of a 30-minute infusion (C_{max}) would be

$$C_{max} = [(D/t')(1 - e^{-kt'})]/CL_{RES}$$

The plasma concentration before the next dialysis session (C_{bD}) can be calculated as

$$C_{bD} \times C_{max} \times e^{-(Cl_{RES}/V_D) \times t}$$

- The hemodialysis clearance of most drugs is dialysis-filter dependent, and a value can be extrapolated from the literature. The concentration after dialysis can be calculated as

$$C_{aD} = C_{bD} \times e^{-[(CL_{RES}+CL_D)/V_D] \times t}$$

- The postdialysis dose can be calculated as follows if the elimination half-life is prolonged relative to the infusion time and thus minimal drug is eliminated during the infusion period:

$$D = V_D \times (C_{max} - C_{min})$$

See Chapter 48, Drug Therapy Individualization for Patients with Renal Insufficiency, authored by Reginald F. Frye and Gary R. Matzke, for a more detailed discussion of this topic.

Chapter 76

► ELECTROLYTE HOMEOSTASIS

► DEFINITION

Fluid and electrolyte homeostasis is maintained by feedback mechanisms, hormones, and many organ systems and is necessary for the body's normal physiologic functions. Disorders of sodium and water, calcium, phosphorus, potassium, and magnesium homeostasis are addressed separately in this chapter.

► DESIRED OUTCOME

The goals of therapy for disorders of electrolyte homeostasis are to promptly identify and correct reversible underlying causes, relieve symptoms, prevent complications, and normalize serum electrolyte concentrations.

► DISORDERS OF SODIUM AND WATER HOMEOSTASIS

- Two thirds of total body water is distributed intracelluarly, and one third is contained in the extracellular space. The effective arterial blood volume (EABV) is a component of the extracellular fluid (ECF) located in the vascular compartment and is responsible for organ perfusion.
- Adding an isotonic solution to the ECF does not change intracellular volume. Adding a hypertonic solution to the ECF decreases cell volume, whereas adding a hypotonic solution increases it (Table 76–1).
- Hypernatremia and hyponatremia can be associated with conditions of high, low, or normal ECF sodium and volume.

HYPONATREMIA (SERUM SODIUM LESS THAN 135 mEq/L)

Pathophysiology

- Hyponatremia predominantly results from an excess of extracellular water relative to sodium because of impaired water excretion.
- Causes of nonosmotic release of antidiuretic hormone (ADH) and hyponatremia include hypovolemia; decreased EABV, as seen in patients with congestive heart failure (CHF); nephrosis; cirrhosis; and syndrome of inappropriate ADH (SIADH) release.
- Depending on serum osmolality, hyponatremia is classified as isotonic, hypertonic, or hypotonic (Figure 76–1).

TABLE 76–1. Composition of Intravenous Replacement Solutions

| | | Distribution | | |
Solution	Tonicity	%ECF	%ICF	Free Water/L
5% Dextrose in water (D$_5$W)	Hypotonic	40	60	1000 mL
0.45% Saline ($^1/_2$ normal saline)	Hypotonic	73	37	500 mL
0.9% Saline (normal saline)	Isotonic	100	0	0 mL
3% Saline (hypertonic saline)	Hypertonic	100[a]	0	−2331 mL

[a] This solution will result in osmotic removal of water from the intracellular space.
ECF, extracellular fluid; *ICF*, intracellular fluid.

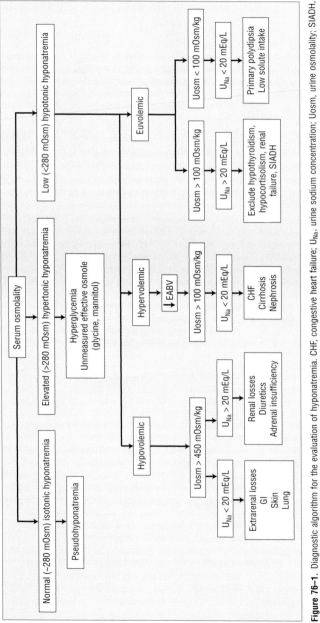

Figure 76–1. Diagnostic algorithm for the evaluation of hyponatremia. CHF, congestive heart failure; U$_{Na}$, urine sodium concentration; Uosm, urine osmolality; SIADH, syndrome of inappropriate antidiuretic hormone; EABV, effective arterial blood volume; GI, gastrointestinal.

- Hypotonic hyponatremia can be further classified as hypovolemic, euvolemic, or hypervolemic hyponatremia.
  - Hypovolemic hyponatremia is associated with a deficit of ECF volume and sodium, with a proportionally greater deficit of sodium than water.
  - Euvolemic hyponatremia is associated with a normal total body sodium content and small increases in ECF volume.
  - Hypervolemic hyponatremia (also referred to as dilutional hyponatremia) is associated with an elevated total body sodium content and an expanded ECF volume.

Clinical Presentation
- Most patients with hyponatremia are asymptomatic.
- Patients with hyponatremia and decreased ECF volume present with decreased skin turgor, orthostatic hypotension, and dry mucous membranes.
- Patients with serum sodium values more than 125 mEq/L are generally asymptomatic unless hyponatremia develops in less than 24 hours.
- Symptoms of acute hypotonic hyponatremia usually result from increased neuronal cell volume and consequent cerebral edema. Symptoms range from nausea, malaise, and headache in milder cases to coma and seizures in severe cases.

Treatment
Acute Symptomatic Hypotonic Hyponatremia
- Symptomatic patients, regardless of fluid status, should initially be treated with either a 0.9% or 3% concentrated saline solution. The serum sodium concentration should be titrated upward at a rate of 1.5 mEq/L for the first 2 to 4 hours in patients with severe symptoms. The total daily correction should not exceed 12 mEq.
- Patients with SIADH should be treated with 3% saline plus, if the urine osmolality exceeds 300 mOsm/kg, a loop diuretic (**furosemide**, 40 mg every 6 hours).
- Patients with hypovolemic hypotonic hyponatremia should be treated with 0.9% saline at 200 to 400 mL/h until hemodynamic stability is restored.
- Patients with hypervolemic hypotonic hyponatremia should be treated with 3% saline and prompt initiation of fluid restriction. Loop diuretic therapy will also likely be required to facilitate urinary excretion of free water.

Asymptomatic Hypotonic Hyponatremia
XIV
- Treatment of SIADH involves water restriction and correction of the underlying cause. Water should be restricted to approximately 1000 to 1200 mL/day. In some cases, administration of either sodium chloride or urea and a loop diuretic or of **demeclocycline** can be required.
- Treatment of asymptomatic hypervolemic hypotonic hyponatremia involves correction of the underlying cause and restriction of water intake to less than 1000 to 1200 mL/day. Dietary intake of sodium chloride should be restricted to 1000 to 2000 mg/day.

HYPERNATREMIA (SERUM SODIUM MORE THAN 145 mEq/L)
Pathophysiology and Clinical Presentation
- Hypernatremia can result from water loss (diabetes insipidus [DI]); hypotonic fluid loss; or, less commonly, hypertonic fluid administration or sodium ingestion.
- Symptoms of hypernatremia are primarily caused by decreased neuronal cell volume and can include weakness, restlessness, confusion, and coma.

TABLE 76–2. Drugs Used to Manage Central and Nephrogenic Diabetes Insipidus (DI)

Drug	Indication	Dose
Desmopressin acetate (DDAVP)	Central and nephrogenic DI	5–20 mcg intranasally q 12–24 h
Chlorpropamide	Central DI	125–250 mg PO daily
Carbamazepine	Central DI	100–300 mg PO b.i.d.
Clofibrate	Central DI	500 mg PO q.i.d.
Hydrochlorothiazide	Central and nephrogenic DI	25 mg PO q 12–24 h
Amiloride	Lithium-related nephrogenic DI	5–10 mg PO daily
Indomethacin	Central and nephrogenic DI	50 mg PO q 8–12 h

Treatment

- Treatment of hypovolemic hypernatremia should begin with 0.9% saline. After hemodynamic stability is restored and intravascular volume is replaced, free-water deficit can be replaced with 5% dextrose or 0.45% saline solution.
- The correction rate should be approximately 1 mEq/L/h for hypernatremia that developed over a few hours and 0.5 mEq/L/h for hypernatremia that developed more slowly.
- Patients with central DI are usually treated with intranasal **desmopressin**, beginning with 10 mcg/day and titrating as needed, usually to 10 mcg twice daily.
- Patients with nephrogenic DI should decrease their ECF volume with a thiazide diuretic and dietary sodium restriction (2000 mg/day), which often decreases urine volume by as much as 50%. Other treatment options include drugs with antidiuretic properties (Table 76–2).
- Patients with sodium overload should be treated with loop diuretics (furosemide, 20 to 40 mg intravenously [IV] every 6 hours) and 5% dextrose at a rate that decreases serum sodium by approximately 0.5 mEq/L/h or, if hypernatremia develops rapidly, 1 mEq/L/h.

EDEMA

Pathophysiology and Clinical Presentation

XIV

- Edema develops when excess sodium is retained either as a primary defect in renal sodium excretion or as a response to a decreased EABV despite an already expanded or normal ECF volume.
- Edema can occur in patients with decreased myocardial contractility, nephrotic syndrome, or cirrhosis.
- Edema is usually first detected in the feet or pretibial area in ambulatory patients and in the presacral area in bed-bound individuals. Edema is defined as pitting when the depression caused by briefly exerting pressure over a boney prominence does not rapidly refill.

Treatment

- Diuretics are the primary pharmacologic therapy for edema. Loop diuretics are the most potent, followed by thiazide diuretics and then potassium-sparing diuretics.
- Only pulmonary edema requires immediate pharmacologic treatment. Other forms of edema can be treated gradually with, in addition to diuretic therapy, sodium restriction and correction of underlying disease state.

▶ DISORDERS OF CALCIUM HOMEOSTASIS

- Extracellular fluid calcium is moderately bound to plasma proteins (46%), primarily albumin. Unbound or ionized calcium is the physiologically active form.
- Each 1 g/dL drop in serum albumin concentration below 4 g/dL decreases total serum calcium concentration by 0.8 mg/dL.

HYPERCALCEMIA (TOTAL SERUM CALCIUM MORE THAN 10.5 mg/dL)

Pathophysiology and Clinical Presentation

- The most common causes of hypercalcemia are cancer and hyperparathyroidism. The primary mechanisms are increased bone resorption, increased gastrointestinal (GI) absorption, and decreased renal elimination.
- The clinical presentation depends on the degree of hypercalcemia and rate of onset. Mild to moderate hypercalcemia (less than 13 mg/dL) can be asymptomatic.
- Hypercalcemia of malignancy develops quickly and is associated with anorexia, nausea and vomiting, constipation, polyuria, polydipsia, and nocturia. Hypercalcemic crisis is characterized by acute elevation of serum calcium to greater than 15 mg/dL, acute renal failure, and obtundation. Untreated hypercalcemic crisis can progress to oliguric renal failure, coma, malignant ventricular arrhythmias, and death.
- Chronic hypercalcemia (i.e., hyperparathyroidism) is associated with metastatic calcification, nephrolithiasis, and chronic renal insufficiency.
- Electrocardiogram (ECG) changes include shortening of the QT interval and coving of the ST-T wave. Very high serum calcium concentrations can cause T-wave widening.

Treatment

- The approach to hypercalcemia depends on the degree of hypercalcemia, acuity of onset, and presence of symptoms (Figure 76–2).
- Patients with hypercalcemic crisis or symptomatic hypercalcemia should be treated immediately and usually with hemodialysis, but it is not always readily available. In the interim, drug therapy (Table 76–3) and, if not contraindicated, volume expansion are usually initiated.
- Management of patients with asymptomatic, mild to moderate hypercalcemia XIV begins with attention to the underlying condition and correction of fluid and electrolyte abnormalities.
- Rehydration with saline and furosemide administration can decrease total serum calcium by 2 to 3 mg/dL within 24 to 48 hours.
- Bisphosphonates are indicated for hypercalcemia of malignancy. Newer bisphosphonates are preferred over **etidronate** because they are more potent and require only a single dose.

HYPOCALCEMIA (TOTAL SERUM CALCIUM LESS THAN 8.5 mg/dL)

Pathophysiology

- Hypocalcemia results from altered effects of parathyroid hormone and vitamin D on the bone, gut, and kidney. The primary causes are postoperative hypoparathyroidism and vitamin D deficiency.
- Symptomatic hypocalcemia commonly occurs because of parathyroid gland dysfunction secondary to surgical procedures involving the thyroid, parathyroid, and neck.

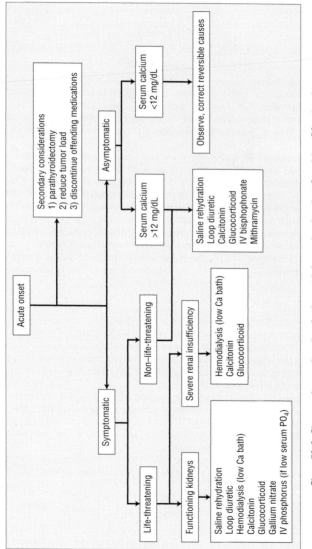

Figure 76–2. Pharmacotherapeutic options for the acutely hypercalcemic patient. Ca, calcium; PO₄, phosphorus.

TABLE 76–3. Drug Therapy Used to Treat Hypercalcemia

Drug	Starting Dosage	Time Frame to Initial Response (h)	Contraindications
0.9% saline ± electrolytes	200–300 mL/h	24–48	Renal insufficiency, congestive heart failure
Loop diuretics	40–80 mg IV every 1–4 h	N/A	Allergy to sulfas (use ethacrynic acid)
Calcitonin	4 U/kg q 12 h SC/IM 10–12 units/h IV	1–2	Allergy to calcitonin
Etidronate	7.5 mg/kg/day IV over 2 h	48	Renal insufficiency
Pamidronate	30–90 mg IV over 2–24 h	48	Renal insufficiency
Zoledronate	4–8 mg IV over 15 min	24–48	Renal insufficiency
Gallium nitrate	200 mg/m²/day	?	Severe renal insufficiency
Mithramycin	25 mcg/kg IV over 4–6 h	12	Decreased liver function; renal insufficiency; thrombocytopenia
Glucocorticoids	40–60 mg oral prednisone equivalents	?	Serious infections; hypersensitivity

- Hypoalbuminemia is a common cause of laboratory hypocalcemia. A corrected total serum calcium concentration can be calculated as follows:

$$\text{Corrected } S_{Ca} = \text{measured } S_{Ca} + [0.8 \times (4 \text{ g/dL} - \text{measured albumin})]$$

where S_{Ca} is serum calcium in mg/dL and measured albumin is serum albumin in g/dL.
- Hypomagnesemia can be associated with severe symptomatic hypocalcemia that is unresponsive to calcium replacement therapy.

Clinical Presentation
- Clinical manifestations are variable and depend on the onset of hypocalcemia.
- The hallmark sign of acute hypocalcemia is tetany, which manifests as paresthesias around the mouth and in the extremities; muscle spasms and cramps; carpopedal spasms; and, rarely, laryngospasm and bronchospasm.
- Cardiovascular manifestations result in ECG changes characterized by a prolonged QT interval and symptoms of decreased myocardial contractility often associated with heart failure.

XIV

Treatment
- Hypocalcemia associated with hypoalbuminemia requires no treatment because ionized plasma calcium concentrations are normal.
- Acute, symptomatic hypocalcemia requires IV administration of soluble calcium salts (Figure 76–3).
  - Initially, 100 to 300 mg of elemental calcium (e.g., 1 g **calcium chloride**, 2 to 3 g **calcium gluconate**) should be given IV over 5 to 10 minutes (60 mg or less of elemental calcium per minute).
  - The initial bolus is effective for only 1 to 2 hours and should be followed by a continuous infusion of elemental calcium (0.5 to 2.0 mg/kg/h) usually for 2 to 4 hours and then by a maintenance dose (0.3 to 0.5 mg/kg/h).
  - **Calcium gluconate** is preferred over **calcium chloride** for peripheral administration because the latter is more irritating to veins.

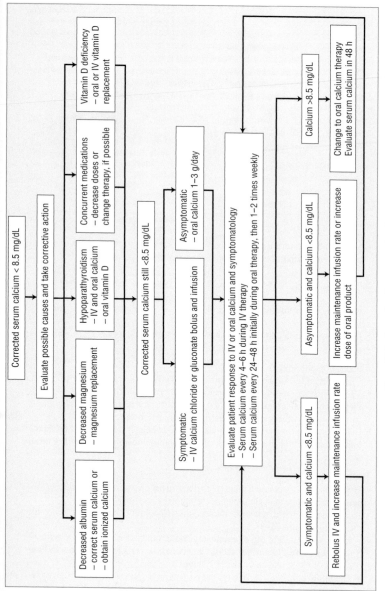

Figure 76-3. Hypocalcemia treatment algorithm.

- After acute hypocalcemia is corrected, the underlying cause and other electrolyte problems should be corrected.
  - Magnesium supplementation is indicated for hypomagnesemia.
  - Oral calcium supplementation (e.g., 1 to 3 g/day of elemental calcium) is indicated for chronic hypocalcemia due to hypoparathyroidism and vitamin D deficiency. If serum calcium does not normalize, a vitamin D preparation should be added (see Chapter 74).

▶ DISORDERS OF PHOSPHORUS HOMEOSTASIS

HYPERPHOSPHATEMIA (SERUM PHOSPHORUS MORE THAN 4.5 mg/dL)

Pathophysiology

- The most common cause of hyperphosphatemia is decreased phosphorus excretion, secondary to decreased glomerular filtration rate (GFR).
- Large amounts of phosphorus can be released from intracellular stores in patients who have rhabdomyolysis and in patients who receive chemotherapy for acute leukemia and lymphoma.

Clinical Presentation

- Some signs and symptoms of hyperphosphatemia are a result of the low solubility of the calcium-phosphate complexation product. Calcium-phosphate crystals are likely to form when the product of the serum calcium and phosphate concentrations exceeds 50 to 60 mg^2/dL^2.
- The major effect of hyperphosphatemia is related to the development of hypocalcemia and damage resulting from calcium phosphate deposits.
- For more information on hyperphosphatemia and renal failure, see Chapter 74.

Treatment

- The most effective way to treat hyperphosphatemia is to decrease phosphate absorption from the GI tract with phosphate binders (see Table 74–3).
- Severe symptomatic hyperphosphatemia manifesting as hypocalcemia and tetany is treated by the IV administration of calcium salts.

HYPOPHOSPHATEMIA (SERUM PHOSPHORUS LESS THAN 2.0 mg/dL)

Pathophysiology

XIV

- Hypophosphatemia can be the result of decreased GI absorption, increased urinary excretion, or extracellular to intracellular redistribution.
- Rapid refeeding of malnourished patients with high-carbohydrate, high-calorie nutritional diets with inadequate phosphorus can cause severe symptomatic hypophosphatemia.

Clinical Presentation

- Severe hypophosphatemia has diverse clinical manifestations that affect many organ systems.
- Neurologic manifestations include a progressive syndrome of irritability, apprehension, weakness, numbness, paresthesias, dysarthria, confusion, obtundation, seizures, and coma.
- Skeletal muscle dysfunction can cause myalgia, bone pain, weakness, and potentially fatal rhabdomyolysis. Respiratory muscle weakness and diaphragmatic contractile dysfunction can cause acute respiratory failure.
- Congestive cardiomyopathy, hemolysis, increased risk of infection, and platelet defects can also occur.

TABLE 76–4. Phosphorus Replacement Therapy

Product (Salt)	Phosphate Content
Oral Therapy	
Neutra-Phos (7 mEq/L each of Na and K)	250 mg/packet
Neutra-Phos K (14.25 mEq/mL K)	250 mg/capsule
K-Phos Neutral (13 mEq/tablet Na and 1.1 mEq/tablet K)	250 mg/tablet
Uro-KP Neutral (10.9 mEq/tablet Na and 1.27 mEq/tablet K)	250 mg/tablet
Intravenous Therapy	
Sodium PO_4 (4.0 mEq/mL Na)	3.0 mmol/mL
Potassium PO_4 (4.4 mEq/mL K)	3.0 mmol/mL

- Chronic hypophosphatemia can cause osteopenia and osteomalacia because of enhanced osteoclastic resorption of bone.

Treatment

- The route and dose of phosphorus replacement therapy are determined by the severity of hypophosphatemia (Table 76–4).
- Severe (less than 1 mg/dL) or symptomatic hypophosphatemia should be treated with IV phosphorus replacement. The recommended dosage of IV phosphorus is controversial and ranges from 5 to 45 mmol.
- Asymptomatic patients or those who exhibit mild to moderate hypophosphatemia can be treated with oral phosphorus supplementation.
- Patients should be closely monitored with frequent serum phosphorus and calcium determinations, especially if phosphorus is given IV or if renal dysfunction is present.
- Phosphorus, 12 to 15 mmol/L, should be routinely added to hyperalimentation solution to prevent hypophosphatemia.

▶ DISORDERS OF POTASSIUM HOMEOSTASIS

HYPOKALEMIA (SERUM POTASSIUM LESS THAN 3.5 mEq/L)

Pathophysiology

XIV
- Hypokalemia results from a total body potassium deficit or shifting of serum potassium into the intracellular compartment.
- Many drugs can cause hypokalemia (Table 74–5). Other causes of hypokalemia include diarrhea, vomiting, and hypomagnesemia.

Clinical Presentation

- Signs and symptoms are nonspecific and variable and depend on the degree of hypokalemia and rapidity of onset. Mild hypokalemia is often asymptomatic.
- Cardiovascular manifestations include hypertension and cardiac arrhythmias (e.g., heart block, atrial flutter, paroxysmal atrial tachycardia, ventricular fibrillation, and digitalis-induced arrhythmias). ECG effects include ST-segment depression or flattening, T-wave inversion, and U-wave elevation.
- Neuromuscular symptoms include muscle weakness, cramping, malaise, and myalgias.

Treatment

- In general, every 1-mEq/L fall of potassium below 3.5 mEq/L corresponds with a total body deficit of 100 to 150 mEq. To correct mild deficits, patients

TABLE 76–5. Drug-Induced Hypokalemia by Mechanism

Transcellular Shift	Enhanced Renal Excretion
β_2-Receptor Agonists	**Diuretics**
Epinephrine	Acetazolamide
Albuterol	Thiazides
Terbutaline	Indapamide
Pirbuterol	Metolazone
Salmeterol	Furosemide
Isoproterenol	Torsemide
Ephedrine	Bumetanide
Pseudoephedrine	Ethacrynic acid
Tocolytic Agents	**High-Dose Penicillins**
Ritodrine	Nafcillin
Nylidrin	Ampicillin
	Penicillin
Miscellaneous	**Mineralocorticoids**
Theophylline	**Miscellaneous**
Caffeine	Aminoglycosides
Insulin overdose	Amphotericin B
	Cisplatin

receiving loop or thiazide diuretics generally need 40 to 100 mEq of potassium.
- Whenever possible, potassium supplementation should be administered by mouth. Of the available salts, potassium chloride is most commonly used because it is the most effective for common causes of potassium depletion.
- IV use should be limited to patients who have severe hypokalemia (serum concentration less than 2.5 mEq/L), signs of hypokalemia, or inability to tolerate oral therapy. Potassium should be administered in saline because dextrose can stimulate insulin secretion and worsen intracellular shifting of potassium. Generally 10 to 20 mEq of potassium is diluted in 100 mL of 0.9% saline and administered through a peripheral vein over 1 hour. If infusion rates exceed 10 mEq/h, ECG should be monitored.

XIV

HYPERKALEMIA (SERUM POTASSIUM MORE THAN 5.5 mEq/L)

Pathophysiology
- Hyperkalemia develops when potassium intake exceeds excretion or when the transcellular distribution of potassium is disturbed.
- The primary causes of true hyperkalemia are increased potassium intake, decreased potassium excretion, tubular unresponsiveness to aldosterone, and redistribution of potassium to the extracellular space.

Clinical Presentation
- Hyperkalemia is frequently asymptomatic. Patients might complain of heart palpitations or skipped heartbeats.
- The earliest ECG change (serum potassium 5.5 to 6 mEq/L) is peaked T waves. The sequence of changes with further increases is widening of the PR interval, loss of the P wave, widening of the QRS complex, and merging of the QRS complex with the T wave resulting in a sine-wave pattern.

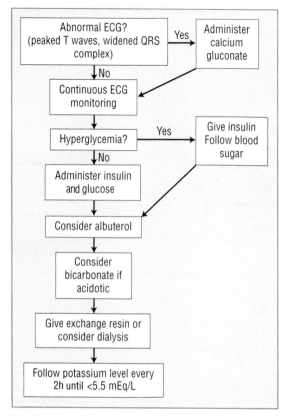

Figure 76–4. Treatment algorithm for hyperkalemia. ECG, electrocardiogram.

XIV

Treatment
- Treatment of hyperkalemia depends on the desired rapidity and degree of lowering (Figure 76–4; Table 76–6). Dialysis is the most rapid way to lower serum potassium concentration.
- Calcium administration rapidly reverses ECG manifestations and arrhythmias, but it does not lower serum potassium concentrations. Calcium is short acting and therefore must be repeated if signs or symptoms recur.
- Rapid correction of hyperkalemia requires administration of drugs that shift potassium intracellularly (e.g., insulin and dextrose, sodium bicarbonate, or β-adrenergic agonist).
- Sodium polystyrene sulfonate is a cation-exchange resin suitable for asymptomatic patients with mild to moderate hyperkalemia. Each gram of resin exchanges 1 mEq of sodium for 1 mEq of potassium. The sorbitol component promotes excretion of exchanged potassium by inducing diarrhea. The oral route is better tolerated and more effective than the rectal route.

TABLE 76–6. Therapeutic Alternatives for the Management of Hyperkalemia

Medication	Dose	Route of Administration	Onset/Duration of Action
Calcium	1 g (1 ampule)	IV over 5–10 min	1–2 min/10–30 min
Furosemide	20–40 mg	IV	5–15 min/4–6 h
Regular insulin	5–10 units	IV or SC	30 min/2–6 h
Dextrose 10%	1000 mL (100 g)	IV over 1–2 h	30 min/2–6 h
Dextrose 50%	50 mL (25 g)	IV over 5 min	30 min/2–6 h
Sodium bicarbonate	50–100 mEq	IV over 2–5 min	30 min/2–6 h
Albuterol	10–20 mg	Nebulized over 10 min	30 min/1–2 h
Hemodialysis	4 h	N/A	Immediate/variable
Sodium polystyrene sulfonate	15–60 g	Oral or rectal	1 h/variable

▶ DISORDERS OF MAGNESIUM HOMEOSTASIS

HYPOMAGNESEMIA (SERUM MAGNESIUM LESS THAN 1.4 mEq/L)

Pathophysiology

- Hypomagnesemia is usually associated with disorders of the intestinal tract or kidneys. Drugs (e.g., **aminoglycosides, amphotericin B, cyclosporine**, diuretics, **digitalis, cisplatin**) or conditions that interfere with intestinal absorption or increase renal excretion of magnesium can cause hypomagnesemia.
- Hypomagnesemia is commonly associated with alcoholism.

Clinical Presentation

- The dominant organ systems involved are the neuromuscular and cardiovascular systems. Typical signs include tetany, positive Chvostek's and Trousseau's signs, and generalized convulsions.
- Ventricular arrhythmias are the most important and potentially life-threatening cardiovascular effect.
- ECG changes include widened QRS complexes and peaked T waves in mild deficiency. Prolonged PR intervals, progressive widening of the QRS complexes, and flattening of T waves occur in moderate to severe deficiency.
- Many electrolyte disturbances occur with hypomagnesemia including hypokalemia and hypocalcemia.

XIV

Treatment

- The severity of magnesium depletion and presence of symptoms dictate the route of magnesium supplementation (Table 76–7). Intramuscular magnesium should be reserved for patients with severe hypomagnesemia and limited venous access. IV bolus injection is associated with flushing, sweating, and a sensation of warmth.
- Magnesium should be replaced over 3 to 5 days because 50% of the dose is excreted in the urine.

HYPERMAGNESEMIA (SERUM MAGNESIUM MORE THAN 2 mEq/L)

Pathophysiology

- Hypermagnesemia most commonly occurs in renal insufficiency when glomerular filtration is less than 30 mL/min.
- Other causes include magnesium-containing antacids in patients with renal insufficiency, enteral or parenteral nutrition in patients with multi-organ system

TABLE 76–7. Guidelines for Treatment of Magnesium Deficiency in Adults

1. **Serum Magnesium <1 mEq/L (1.2 mg/dL) with Life-Threatening Symptoms (seizure, arrhythmia)**
   Day 1
   2 g MgSO$_4$ (1 g MgSO$_4$ = 8.1 mEq Mg^{2+}) mixed with 6 mL 0.9% NaCl in 10-mL syringe and administer IV push over 1 min
   Follow with 0.5 mEq Mg^{2+}/kg lean body weight IV infusion over 5–6 h, then 0.5 mEq Mg^{2+}/kg lean body weight IV infusion over 17–18 h
   Days 2–5
   0.5 mEq Mg^{2+}/kg lean body weight per day divided in maintenance IV fluids

2. **Serum Magnesium <1 mEq/L (1.2 mg/dL) without Life-Threatening Symptoms**
   Day 1
   Total of 1 mEq Mg^{2+}/kg lean body weight per day as continuous IV infusion, or divided and given IM every 4 h for 5 doses
   Days 2–5
   Total of 0.5 mEq Mg^{2+}/kg lean body weight IV infusion per day as continuous IV infusion or divided and given IM every 6–8 h

3. **Serum Magnesium >1 mEq/L (1.2 mg/dL) and <1.5 mEq/L (1.8 mg/dL) without Symptoms**
   As in no. 2 above, *or*
   Milk of Magnesia 5 mL 4 times daily as tolerated, or
   Magnesium-containing antacid 15 mL 3 times daily as tolerated, or
   Magnesium oxide tablets 300 mg 4 times daily, increase to two tablets 4 times daily as tolerated

---

failure, magnesium for treatment of eclampsia, lithium therapy, hypothyroidism, and Addison's disease.

Clinical Presentation

- The sequence of neuromuscular signs as serum magnesium increases from 5 mEq/L to 12 mEq/L is sedation, hypotonia, hyporeflexia, somnolence, coma, muscular paralysis, and, ultimately, respiratory depression.
- The sequence of cardiovascular signs as serum magnesium increases from 3 mEq/L to 15 mEq/L is hypotension, cutaneous vasodilation, QT-interval prolongation, bradycardia, primary heart block, nodal rhythms, bundle branch block, QRS- and then PR-interval prolongation, complete heart block, and asystole.

Treatment

- IV calcium (100 to 200 mg of elemental calcium) is indicated to antagonize the neuromuscular and cardiovascular effects of magnesium. Doses should be repeated as often as hourly in life-threatening situations.
- Hemodialysis is the treatment of choice for patients with renal dysfunction. Forced diuresis with saline and loop diuretics is the treatment of choice for patients with adequate renal function.

▶ EVALUATION OF THERAPEUTIC OUTCOMES

- The primary endpoint for monitoring treatment fluid and electrolyte disorders is the abnormal serum electrolyte. The frequency depends on the presence of symptoms and degree of abnormality. In general, monitoring is initially performed at frequent intervals and, as homeostasis is restored, subsequently performed at less frequent intervals.

- Other electrolytes should also be monitored, especially if the electrolyte abnormality typically coexists with another abnormality (e.g., hypomagnesemia with hypokalemia and hypocalcemia, or hyperphosphatemia with hypocalcemia).
- Patients should be monitored for resolution of clinical manifestations of electrolyte disturbances and for treatment-related complications.

See Chapter 49, Disorders of Sodium, Water, Calcium, and Phosphorus Homeostasis, authored by Melanie S. Joy and Gerald A. Hladik, and Chapter 50, Disorders of Potassium and Magnesium Homeostasis, by Donald F. Brophy and Todd W. B. Gehr, for a more detailed discussion of this topic.

XIV

Chapter 77

▶ ALLERGIC RHINITIS

▶ DEFINITION

- Allergic rhinitis is inflammation of the nasal mucous membrane caused by exposure to inhaled allergenic materials that elicit a specific immunologic response mediated by immunoglobulin E (IgE). There are two types.
  - *Seasonal (hay fever):* occurs in response to specific allergens (pollen from trees, grasses, and weeds) present at predictable times of the year (spring and/or fall blooming seasons) and typically causes more acute symptoms.
  - *Perennial (intermittent or persistent):* occurs year round in response to non-seasonal allergens (e.g., dust mites, animal dander, molds) and usually causes more subtle, chronic symptoms.
- Some patients have both types, with symptoms year round and seasonal exacerbations.

▶ PATHOPHYSIOLOGY

- The initial reaction occurs when airborne allergens enter the nose during inhalation and are processed by lymphocytes, which produce antigen-specific IgE, thereby sensitizing genetically predisposed hosts to those agents. On nasal re-exposure, IgE bound to mast cells interacts with airborne allergens, triggering release of inflammatory mediators.
- An immediate reaction occurs within minutes, resulting in the rapid release of preformed mediators and newly generated mediators from the arachidonic acid cascade. Mediators of immediate hypersensitivity include histamine, leukotrienes, prostaglandin, tryptase, and kinins. These mediators cause vasodilation, increased vascular permeability, and production of nasal secretions. Histamine produces rhinorrhea, itching, sneezing, and nasal obstruction.
- From 4 to 8 hours after the initial exposure to an allergen, a late-phase reaction may occur, which is thought to be due to cytokines released primarily by mast cells and thymus-derived helper lymphocytes. This inflammatory response likely is responsible for persistent, chronic symptoms including nasal congestion.

▶ CLINICAL PRESENTATION

- Symptoms include clear rhinorrhea, sneezing, nasal congestion, postnasal drip, allergic conjunctivitis, and pruritic eyes, ears, or nose.
- Patients may complain of loss of smell or taste, with sinusitis or polyps the underlying cause in many cases. Postnasal drip with cough or hoarseness can also be bothersome.
- Untreated rhinitis symptoms may lead to insomnia, malaise, fatigue, and poor work or school efficiency.
- Allergic rhinitis is a risk factor for asthma; as many as 78% of asthma patients have nasal symptoms, and about 38% of allergic rhinitis patients have asthma.
- Recurrent and chronic sinusitis and epistaxis are complications of allergic rhinitis.

▶ DIAGNOSIS

- Physical examination may reveal dark circles under the eyes (allergic shiners), a transverse nasal crease caused by repeated rubbing of the nose, adenoidal breathing, edematous nasal turbinates coated with clear secretions, tearing, conjunctival injection and edema, and periorbital swelling.
- Microscopic examination of nasal scrapings typically reveals numerous eosinophils. The peripheral blood eosinophil count may be elevated, but it is nonspecific and has limited usefulness.
- Allergy testing can help determine whether rhinitis is caused by an immune response to allergens. Immediate-type hypersensitivity skin tests are commonly used. Percutaneous testing is safer and more generally accepted than intradermal testing, which is usually reserved for patients requiring confirmation. The radioallergosorbent test (RAST) can be used to detect IgE antibodies in the blood that are specific for a given antigen, but it is less sensitive than percutaneous tests.

▶ DESIRED OUTCOME

- The goal of treatment is to minimize or prevent symptoms with minimal or no side effects and reasonable medication expense.
- Patients should be able to maintain a normal lifestyle, including participation in outdoor activities and playing with pets as desired.

▶ TREATMENT

See Figure 77–1.

ALLERGEN AVOIDANCE

- Avoidance of offending allergens is difficult. Mold growth can be reduced by keeping household humidity below 50% and removing obvious growth with bleach or disinfectant.
- Patients sensitive to animals benefit most by removing pets from the home, if feasible. Exposure to dust mites can be reduced by encasing mattresses and pillows with impermeable covers and washing bed linens in hot water. Washable area rugs are preferable to wall-to-wall carpeting.
- High-efficiency particulate air (HEPA) filters can remove lightweight particles such as pollens, mold spores, and cat allergen, thereby reducing allergic respiratory symptoms.
- Patients with seasonal allergic rhinitis should keep windows closed and minimize time spent outdoors during pollen seasons. Filter masks can be worn while gardening or mowing the lawn.

PHARMACOLOGIC THERAPY

Antihistamines

- Histamine H_1-receptor antagonists bind to H_1 receptors without activating them, preventing histamine binding and action. They are more effective in preventing the histamine response than in reversing it.
- Oral antihistamines can be divided into two major categories: nonselective (first-generation or sedating antihistamines) and peripherally selective (second-generation or nonsedating antihistamines). However, individual agents should be judged on their specific sedating effects because variation exists among

XV ◀

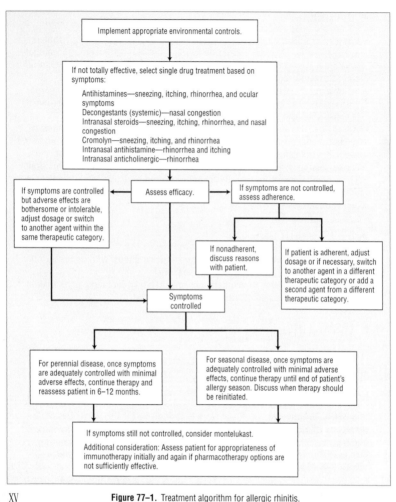

Figure 77–1. Treatment algorithm for allergic rhinitis.

XV

agents within these broad categories (Table 77–1). The central sedating effect may depend on the ability to cross the blood-brain barrier. Most older antihistamines are lipid soluble and cross this barrier easily. The peripherally selective agents have little or no central or autonomic nervous system effects.

- Symptom relief is caused in part by anticholinergic properties, which are responsible for the drying effect that reduces nasal, salivary, and lacrimal gland hypersecretion. Antihistamines antagonize capillary permeability, wheal-and-flare formation, and itching.

- Drowsiness is the most frequent side effect, and it can interfere with driving ability or adequate functioning at the workplace. Sedative effects can be beneficial in patients who have difficulty sleeping because of rhinitis symptoms.

TABLE 77–1. Relative Adverse-Effect Profiles of Antihistamines

Medication	Relative Sedative Effect	Relative Anticholinergic Effect
Alkylamine class, nonselective		
Brompheniramine maleate	Low	Moderate
Chlorpheniramine maleate	Low	Moderate
Dexchlorpheniramine maleate	Low	Moderate
Ethanolamine class, nonselective		
Carbinoxamine maleate	High	High
Clemastine fumarate	Moderate	High
Diphenhydramine hydrochloride	High	High
Ethylenediamine class, nonselective		
Pyrilamine maleate	Low	Low to none
Tripelennamine hydrochloride	Moderate	Low to none
Phenothiazine class, nonselective		
Promethazine hydrochloride	High	High
Piperidine class, nonselective		
Cyproheptadine hydrochloride	Low	Moderate
Phenindamine tartrate	Low to none	Moderate
Phthalazinone class, peripherally selective		
Azelastine (nasal only)	Low to none	Low to none
Piperazine class, peripherally selective		
Cetirizine	Low to moderate	Low to none
Piperidine class, peripherally selective		
Desloratadine	Low to none	Low to none
Fexofenadine	Low to none	Low to none
Loratadine	Low to none	Low to none

- Although anticholinergic (drying) effects contribute to efficacy, adverse effects such as dry mouth, difficulty in voiding urine, constipation, and potential cardiovascular effects may occur (Table 77–1). Antihistamines should be used with caution in patients predisposed to urinary retention and in those with increased intraocular pressure, hyperthyroidism, and cardiovascular disease.
- Other side effects include loss of appetite, nausea, vomiting, and epigastric distress. Taking medication with meals or a full glass of water may prevent gastrointestinal side effects.
- Antihistamines are more effective when taken approximately 1 to 2 hours before anticipated exposure to the offending allergen.
- Table 77–2 lists recommended doses of commonly used oral agents.
- **Azelastine** (Astelin) is an intranasal antihistamine that rapidly relieves symptoms of seasonal allergic rhinitis. However, patients should be cautioned about its potential for drowsiness because systemic availability is approximately 40%. Patients may also experience drying effects, headache, and diminished effectiveness over time.
- **Levocabastine** (Livostin) and **olopatadine** (Patanol) are ophthalmic antihistamines that can be used for allergic conjunctivitis that is often associated with allergic rhinitis. However, systemic antihistamines are usually effective for allergic conjunctivitis, making an ocular product unnecessary. They may be a logical addition to nasal glucocorticoids when ocular symptoms occur.

XV

TABLE 77–2. Oral Dosages of Commonly Used Antihistamines and Decongestants

Medication	Dosage and Interval[a]	
	Adults	*Children*
Nonselective (first-generation) anthihistamines		
Chlorpheniramine maleate, plain[b]	4 mg every 6 h	6–12 yr: 2 mg every 6 h
		2–5 yr: 1 mg every 6 h
Chlorpheniramine maleate, sustained-release	8–12 mg daily at bedtime or 8–12 mg every 8 h	6–12 yr: 8 mg at bedtime
		<6 yr: Not recommended
Clemastine fumarate[b]	1.34 mg every 8 h	6–12 yr: 0.67 mg every 12 h
Diphenhydramine hydrochloride[b]	25–50 mg every 8 h	5 mg/kg/day divided every 8 h (up to 25 mg per dose)
Peripherally selective (second-generation) antihistamines		
Loratadine[b]	10 mg once daily	6–12 yr: 10 mg once daily
		2–5 yr: 5 mg once daily
Fexofenadine	60 mg twice daily or 180 mg once daily	6–11 yr: 30 mg twice daily
Cetirizine[b]	5–10 mg once daily	>6 yr: 5 mg once daily
		infants 6–11 months[c]
Oral decongestants		
Pseudoephedrine, plain	60 mg every 4–6 h	6–12 yr: 30 mg every 4–6 h
		2–5 yr: 15 mg every 4–6 h
Pseudoephedrine, sustained-release[d]	120 mg every 12 h	Not recommended

Note: Fexofenadine and cetirizine are available by prescription only.
[a]Dosage adjustment may be needed in renal/hepatic dysfunction. Refer to manufacturers' prescribing information.
[b]Available in liquid form.
[c]0.25 mg/kg orally demonstrated to be safe.
[d]Controlled-release product available: 240 mg once daily (60–mg immediate-release with 180-mg controlled-release).

Decongestants

- Topical and systemic decongestants are sympathomimetic agents that act on adrenergic receptors in the nasal mucosa to produce vasoconstriction, shrink swollen mucosa, and improve ventilation. Decongestants work well in combination with antihistamines when nasal congestion is part of the clinical picture.
- Topical decongestants are applied directly to swollen nasal mucosa via drops or sprays (Table 77–3). They result in little or no systemic absorption.
- Prolonged use of topical agents (more than 3 to 5 days) can result in rhinitis medicamentosa, which is rebound vasodilation with associated congestion. Patients with this condition use more spray more often with less response. Abrupt cessation is an effective treatment, but rebound congestion may last for several days or weeks. Nasal steroids have been used successfully, but they take several days to work. Weaning the patient off the topical decongestant can be accomplished by decreasing the dosing frequency or concentration over several weeks. Combining the weaning process with nasal steroids may be helpful.
- Other adverse effects of topical decongestants include burning, stinging, sneezing, and dryness of the nasal mucosa.
- These products should be used only when absolutely necessary (e.g., at bedtime) and in doses that are as small and infrequent as possible. Duration of therapy should always be limited to 3 to 5 days.

XV

TABLE 77–3. Duration of Action of Topical Decongestants

Medication	Duration (h)
Short-acting	
Phenylephrine hydrochloride	Up to 4
Intermediate-acting	
Naphazoline hydrochloride	4–6
Tetrahydrozoline hydrochloride	
Long-acting	
Oxymetazoline hydrochloride	Up to 12
Xylometazoline hydrochloride	

- **Pseudoephedrine** (see Table 77–2) is an oral decongestant that has a slower onset of action than topical agents but may last longer and cause less local irritation. Also, rhinitis medicamentosa does not occur with an oral decongestant.
- Pseudoephedrine is the safest systemic decongestant; doses up to 180 mg produce no measurable change in blood pressure or heart rate. However, higher doses (210 to 240 mg) may raise both blood pressure and heart rate. Systemic decongestants should be avoided in hypertensive patients unless absolutely necessary. Severe hypertensive reactions can occur when pseudoephedrine is given concomitantly with monoamine oxidase inhibitors. Pseudoephedrine can cause mild central nervous system stimulation, even at therapeutic doses.
- Use of combination oral products containing a decongestant and antihistamine is rational because of the different mechanisms of action.

Nasal Corticosteroids
- Intranasal corticosteroids effectively relieve sneezing, rhinorrhea, pruritus, and nasal congestion with minimal side effects (Table 77–4). They reduce

TABLE 77–4. Dosage of Nasal Corticosteroids

Medication	Dosage and Interval
Beclomethasone dipropionate	>12 yr: 1 inhalation (42 mcg) per nostril 2–4 times a day (maximum, 336 mcg/day) 6–12 yr: 1 inhalation per nostril 3 times/day
Beclomethasone dipropionate, monohydrate	>12 yr: 1–2 inhalations once daily 6–12 yr: 1 inhalation per nostril (42 mcg) twice daily to start
Budesonide	>6 yr: 2 sprays (64 mcg) per nostril in AM and PM or 4 sprays per nostril in AM (maximum, 256 mcg)
Flunisolide	Adults: 2 sprays (50 mcg) per nostril twice daily (maximum, 400 mcg) Children: 1 spray per nostril 3 times a day
Fluticasone	Adults: 2 sprays (100 mcg) per nostril once daily; after a few days decrease to 1 spray per nostril Children > 4 yr and adolescents: 1 spray per nostril once daily (maximum, 200 mcg/day)
Mometasone furoate	>12 yr: 2 sprays (100 mcg) per nostril once daily
Triamcinolone acetonide	>12 yr: 2 sprays (110 mcg) per nostril once daily (maximum, 440 mcg/day)

XV

inflammation by blocking mediator release, suppressing neutrophil chemo-taxis, causing mild vasoconstriction, and inhibiting mast cell–mediated late-phase reactions.
- These agents are an excellent choice for perennial rhinitis and can be useful in seasonal rhinitis, especially if dosed in advance of symptoms. Some authorities recommend nasal steroids as initial therapy over antihistamines because of their high degree of efficacy when used properly along with allergen avoidance.
- Side effects include sneezing, stinging, headache, epistaxis, and rare infections with *Candida albicans.*
- Some patients improve within a few days, but peak response may require 2 to 3 weeks. The dosage may be reduced once a response is achieved.
- Blocked nasal passages should be cleared with a decongestant before admin-istration of glucocorticoids to ensure adequate penetration of the spray.

Cromolyn Sodium
- **Cromolyn sodium** (Nasalcrom), a mast cell stabilizer, is available as a non-prescription nasal spray for symptomatic prevention and treatment of allergic rhinitis.
- It prevents antigen-triggered mast cell degranulation and release of mediators, including histamine.
- The most common side effect is local irritation (sneezing and nasal stinging).
- The dosage for individuals at least 2 years of age is one spray in each nostril 3 to 4 times daily at regular intervals. Nasal passages should be cleared before administration, and inhaling through the nose during administration enhances distribution to the entire nasal lining.
- For seasonal rhinitis, initiate treatment just before the start of the allergens season and continue throughout the season.
- In perennial rhinitis, the effects may not be seen for 2 to 4 weeks; antihistamines or decongestants may be needed during this initial phase of therapy.

Ipratropium Bromide
- **Ipratropium bromide** (Atrovent) nasal spray is an anticholinergic agent useful in perennial allergic rhinitis.
- It exhibits antisecretory properties when applied locally and provides symp-tomatic relief of rhinorrhea associated with allergic and other forms of chronic rhinitis.
- The 0.03% solution is given as two sprays (42 mcg) 2 to 3 times daily. Adverse effects are mild and include headache, epistaxis, and nasal dryness.

Montelukast
- **Montelukast** (Singulair) is a leukotriene receptor antagonist approved for treatment of seasonal allergic rhinitis. It is effective alone or in combination with an antihistamine.
- The dosage for adults and adolescents older than 15 years is one 10-mg tablet daily. Children aged 6 to 14 years may receive one 5-mg chewable tablet daily. Children aged 2 to 5 may be given one 4-mg chewable tablet or oral granule packet daily. The timing of administration can be individualized. The dose should be given in the evening if the patient has combined asthma and seasonal allergic rhinitis.
- Although leukotriene antagonists represent a new therapeutic alternative, pub-lished studies to date have shown them to be no more effective than peripherally selective antihistamines and less effective than intranasal corticosteroids.

XV

IMMUNOTHERAPY

- Immunotherapy is the slow, gradual process of injecting increasing doses of antigens responsible for eliciting allergic symptoms in a patient with the intent of increasing tolerance to the allergen when natural exposure occurs.
- The effectiveness of immunotherapy probably results from diminished IgE production, increased IgG production, changes in T lymphocytes, reduced inflammatory mediator release from sensitized cells, and diminished tissue responsiveness.
- Because immunotherapy is expensive, has potential risks, and requires a major time commitment from patients, it should only be considered in selected patients. Good candidates include patients who have a strong history of severe symptoms unsuccessfully controlled by avoidance and pharmacotherapy and patients who have been unable to tolerate the adverse effects of drug therapy. Poor candidates include patients with medical conditions that would compromise the ability to tolerate an anaphylactic-type reaction, patients with impaired immune systems, and patients with a history of nonadherence to therapy.
- In general, very dilute solutions are given once or twice per week. The concentration is increased until the maximum tolerated dose is achieved. This maintenance dose is continued every 2 to 6 weeks, depending on clinical response. Better results are obtained with year-round rather than seasonal injections.
- Common mild local adverse reactions include induration and swelling at the injection site. More severe reactions (generalized urticaria, bronchospasm, laryngospasm, vascular collapse, and death from anaphylaxis) occur rarely. Severe reactions are treated with epinephrine, antihistamines, and systemic corticosteroids.

EVALUATION OF THERAPEUTIC OUTCOMES

- Patients should be monitored regularly for reduction in severity of identified target symptoms and the presence of side effects.
- Patients should be questioned about their satisfaction with the management of their allergic rhinitis. Management should result in minimal disruption to their life.
- The Medical Outcomes Study 36-Item Short Form Health Survey (SF-36) and the Rhinoconjunctivitis Quality of Life Questionnaire measure not only improvement in symptoms but also parameters such as sleep quality, nonallergic symptoms (e.g., fatigue, poor concentration), emotions, and participation in a variety of activities.

See Chapter 93, Allergic Rhinitis, authored by J. Russell May and Philip H. Smith, for a more detailed discussion of this topic.

XV

Chapter 78

▶ ASTHMA

▶ DEFINITION

The National Asthma Education and Prevention Program (NAEPP) has defined asthma as a chronic inflammatory disorder of the airways in which many cells and cellular elements play a role. In susceptible individuals, inflammation causes recurrent episodes of wheezing, breathlessness, chest tightness, and coughing. These episodes are usually associated with airflow obstruction that is often reversible either spontaneously or with treatment. The inflammation also causes an increase in bronchial hyperresponsiveness (BHR) to a variety of stimuli.

PATHOPHYSIOLOGY

- The major characteristics of asthma include a variable degree of airflow obstruction (related to bronchospasm, edema, and hypersecretion), BHR, and airway inflammation.
- Sudden asthma attacks are caused by both unknown and known factors such as exposure to allergens, viruses, or indoor and outdoor pollutants, and each may induce an acute inflammatory response.
- Inhaled allergens cause an early-phase allergic reaction characterized by activation of cells bearing allergen-specific IgE antibodies. There is rapid activation of airway mast cells and macrophages, which release proinflammatory mediators such as histamine and eicosanoids that induce contraction of airway smooth muscle, mucus secretion, vasodilation, and exudation of plasma in the airways. Plasma protein leakage induces a thickened, engorged, edematous airway wall and a narrowing of the airway lumen with reduced mucus clearance.
- The late-phase inflammatory reaction occurs 6 to 9 hours after allergen provocation and involves recruitment and activation of eosinophils, T lymphocytes, basophils, neutrophils, and macrophages.
- Eosinophils migrate to the airways and release inflammatory mediators (leukotrienes and granule proteins), cytotoxic mediators, and cytokines.
- T-lymphocyte activation leads to release of cytokines from type 2 (T_H2) T-helper cells that mediate allergic inflammation (interleukin [IL]-4, IL-5, IL-6, IL-9, and IL-13). Conversely, type 1 T-helper (T_H1) cells produce IL-2 and interferon γ that are essential for cellular defense mechanisms. Allergic asthmatic inflammation may result from an imbalance between T_H1 and T_H2 cells.
- Mast cell degranulation in response to allergens results in release of mediators such as histamine; eosinophil and neutrophil chemotactic factors; leukotrienes C_4, D_4, and E_4; prostaglandins; and platelet-activating factor (PAF). Histamine is capable of inducing smooth muscle constriction and bronchospasm and may play a role in mucosal edema and mucus secretion.
- Alveolar macrophages release a number of inflammatory mediators, including PAF and leukotrienes B_4, C_4, and D_4. Production of neutrophil chemotactic factor and eosinophil chemotactic factor furthers the inflammatory process.
- Neutrophils are also a source of mediators (PAFs, prostaglandins, thromboxanes, and leukotrienes) that contribute to BHR and airway inflammation.
- The 5-lipoxygenase pathway of arachidonic acid breakdown is responsible for production of leukotrienes. Leukotrienes C_4, D_4, and E_4 (cysteinyl leukotrienes) constitute the slow-reacting substance of anaphylaxis (SRS-A).

These leukotrienes are liberated during inflammatory processes in the lung and produce bronchoconstriction, mucus secretion, microvascular permeability, and airway edema.

- Bronchial epithelial cells also participate in inflammation by releasing eicosanoids, peptidases, matrix proteins, cytokines, and nitric oxide. Epithelial shedding results in heightened airway responsiveness, altered permeability of the airway mucosa, depletion of epithelial-derived relaxant factors, and loss of enzymes responsible for degrading inflammatory neuropeptides.
- The exudative inflammatory process and sloughing of epithelial cells into the airway lumen impair mucociliary transport. The bronchial glands are increased in size, and the goblet cells are increased in size and number, suggesting an increased production of mucus. Expectorated mucus from patients with asthma tends to have high viscosity.
- The airway is innervated by parasympathetic, sympathetic, and nonadrenergic inhibitory nerves. The normal resting tone of airway smooth muscle is maintained by vagal efferent activity, and bronchoconstriction can be mediated by vagal stimulation in the small bronchi. All airway smooth muscle contains noninnervated β_2-adrenergic receptors that produce bronchodilation. The importance of α-adrenergic receptors in asthma is unknown. The nonadrenergic, noncholinergic nervous system in the trachea and bronchi may amplify inflammation in asthma by releasing nitric oxide.

▶ CLINICAL PRESENTATION

CHRONIC ASTHMA

- Classic asthma is characterized by episodic dyspnea associated with wheezing, but the clinical presentation of asthma is diverse. Patients may also complain of chest tightness, coughing (particularly at night), or a whistling sound when breathing. These often occur with exercise but may occur spontaneously or in association with known allergens.
- Signs include expiratory wheezing on auscultation, dry hacking cough, or signs of atopy (e.g., allergic rhinitis or eczema).
- Asthma can vary from chronic daily symptoms to only intermittent symptoms. There are recurrent exacerbations and remissions, and the intervals between symptoms may be weeks, months, or years.
- The severity is determined by lung function and symptoms prior to therapy as well as by the number of medications required to control symptoms. Patients can present with mild intermittent symptoms that require no medications or only occasional use of short-acting inhaled β_2 agonists to severe chronic asthma symptoms despite receiving multiple medications.

XV

ACUTE SEVERE ASTHMA

- Uncontrolled asthma can progress to an acute state where inflammation, airway edema, excessive accumulation of mucus, and severe bronchospasm result in profound airway narrowing that is poorly responsive to usual bronchodilator therapy.
- Patients may be anxious in acute distress and complain of severe dyspnea, shortness of breath, chest tightness, or burning. They may be able to say only a few words with each breath. Symptoms are unresponsive to usual measures.
- Signs include expiratory and inspiratory wheezing on auscultation, dry hacking cough, tachypnea, tachycardia, pallor or cyanosis, and hyperinflated chest with

intercostal and supraclavicular retractions. Breath sounds may be diminished with very severe obstruction.

▶ DIAGNOSIS

CHRONIC ASTHMA

- The diagnosis of asthma is made primarily by a history of recurrent episodes of coughing, wheezing, or shortness of breath and confirmatory spirometry.
- The patient may have a family history of allergy or asthma or have symptoms of allergic rhinitis. A history of exercise or cold air precipitating dyspnea or increased symptoms during specific allergen seasons also suggest asthma.
- Spirometry demonstrates obstruction (FEV_1/FVC less than 80%) with reversibility after inhaled β_2-agonist administration (or at least a 12% improvement in FEV_1). Failure of pulmonary function to improve acutely does not necessarily rule out asthma. If baseline spirometry is normal, challenge testing with exercise, histamine, or methacholine can be used to elicit BHR.
- Studies for atopy such as serum IgE and sputum and blood eosinophils are not necessary to make the diagnosis of asthma, but they may help differentiate asthma from chronic bronchitis in adults.

ACUTE SEVERE ASTHMA

- Peak expiratory flow (PEF) and FEV_1 are less than 50% of normal predicted values. Pulse oximetry reveals decreased arterial oxygen and O_2 saturations. The best predictor of outcome is early response to treatment as measured by improvement in FEV_1 at 30 minutes after inhaled β_2 agonists.
- Arterial blood gases usually reveal mild metabolic acidosis (lactic acidosis from hypoxic metabolism in accessory respiratory muscles) and a low Pao_2.
- Criteria for impending respiratory failure and the need to intubate and mechanically ventilate a patient include (1) hypoxia unresponsive to O_2 (Pao_2 less than 60 mm Hg on Fio_2 greater than 60%), (2) $Paco_2$ greater than 65 mm Hg or increasing more than 5 mm Hg per hour despite adequate therapy, and (3) significant metabolic acidosis.
- A brief history and physical examination should be obtained while initial therapy is being provided. A history of previous asthma exacerbations (e.g., hospitalizations, intubations) and complicating illnesses (e.g., cardiac disease, diabetes) should be obtained. The patient should be examined to assess hydration status; use of accessory muscles of respiration; and the presence of cyanosis, pneumonia, pneumothorax, pneumomediastinum, and upper airway obstruction. A complete blood count may be appropriate for patients with fever or purulent sputum.

▶ DESIRED OUTCOME

CHRONIC ASTHMA

The NAEPP provides the following goals for chronic asthma management: (1) maintain normal activity levels (including exercise); (2) maintain (near) normal pulmonary function; (3) prevent chronic and troublesome symptoms (e.g., coughing or breathlessness in the night, in the early morning, or after exertion); (4) prevent recurrent exacerbations of asthma and minimize the need for emergency department visits or hospitalizations; (5) provide optimal pharmacotherapy with minimal or no adverse effects; and (6) meet patients' and families' expectations of care.

XV

ACUTE SEVERE ASTHMA

The goals of treatment are as follows: (1) correction of significant hypoxemia; (2) rapid reversal of airway obstruction (within minutes); (3) reduction of the likelihood of recurrence of severe airflow obstruction; and (4) development of a written action plan in case of a future exacerbation.

▶ TREATMENT

Figure 78–1 depicts current NAEPP recommendations for managing chronic asthma. Figure 78–2 illustrates the recommended therapies for treatment of acute asthma exacerbations in the home.

NONPHARMACOLOGIC THERAPY

- Patient education and the teaching of self-management skills should be the cornerstone of the treatment program. Self-management programs improve adherence to medication regimens, self-management skills, and use of health care services.
- Objective measurements of airflow obstruction with a home peak flow meter may not necessarily improve patient outcomes. The NAEPP advocates routine use of peak flow meters only for patients with moderate and severe persistent asthma.
- Avoidance of known allergenic triggers can improve symptoms, reduce medication use, and decrease BHR. Environmental triggers (e.g., animals) should be avoided in sensitive patients, and those who smoke should be encouraged to stop.
- Patients with acute severe asthma should receive supplemental oxygen therapy by mask or nasal cannulae titrated to maintain Sao_2 normal for altitude (greater than 95% at sea level). Significant dehydration should be corrected; urine specific gravity may help guide therapy in young children, in whom assessment of hydration status may be difficult.

PHARMACOLOGIC THERAPY

β_2 Agonists
See Table 78–1.

- The β_2 agonists are the most effective bronchodilators available. β_2-Adrenergic receptor stimulation activates adenyl cyclase, which produces an increase in intracellular cyclic AMP. This results in smooth muscle relaxation, mast cell membrane stabilization, and skeletal muscle stimulation.
- Aerosol administration enhances bronchoselectivity and provides a more rapid response and greater protection against provocations that induce bronchospasm (e.g., exercise, allergen challenges) than does systemic administration.
- **Albuterol** and other inhaled short-acting selective β_2 agonists are indicated for treatment of intermittent episodes of bronchospasm and are the first treatment of choice for acute severe asthma. Because short-acting inhaled β_2 agonists do not improve long-term control of symptoms, their use can be used to measure asthma control. They should be used only as needed for relief of symptoms.
- **Formoterol** and **salmeterol** are inhaled long-acting β_2 agonists indicated as adjunctive long-term control for patients with symptoms who are already on low to medium doses of inhaled corticosteroids prior to advancing to medium- or high-dose inhaled corticosteroids. Short-acting β_2 agonists should be continued for acute exacerbations. Long-acting agents are ineffective for acute

XV

Classify Severity: Clinical Features Before Treatment or Adequate Control			Medications Required to Maintain Long-Term Control
	Symptoms/Day Symptoms/Night	PEF or FEV$_1$ PEF Variability	Daily Medications
STEP 4 **Severe** **Persistent**	Continual Frequent	≤60% >30%	• **Preferred treatment:** – **High-dose inhaled corticosteroids** AND – **Long-acting inhaled β_2 agonists** AND, if needed, – Corticosteroid tablets or syrup long term (2 mg/kg/day, generally do not exceed 60mg/day). (Make repeat attempts to reduce systemic corticosteroids and maintain control with high-dose inhaled corticosteroids.)
STEP 3 **Moderate** **Persistent**	Daily >1 night/wk	>60% – <80% >30%	• **Preferred treatment:** – **Low-to-medium dose inhaled corticosteroids and long-acting inhaled β_2 agonists.** • Alternative treatment: – Increase inhaled corticosteroids within medium-dose range OR – Low- to medium-dose inhaled corticosteroids and either leukotriene modifier or theophylline. _ If needed (particularly in patients with recurring severe exacerbations): • **Preferred treatment :** – **Increase inhaled corticosteroids within medium-dose range and add long-acting inhaled β_2 agonists.** • Alternative treatment: – Increase inhaled corticosteroids within medium-dose range and add either leukotriene modifier or theophylline.
STEP 2 **Mild** **Persistent**	>2/week but < 1x/day >2 nights/month	≥80% 20-30%	• **Preferred treatment:** – **Low-dose inhaled corticosteroids.** • Alternative treatment (listed alphabetically): cromolyn, leukotriene modifier, nedocromil, OR sustained release theophylline to serum concentration of 5–15 mcg/mL.

STEP 1 Mild Intermittent	≤2days/wk ≤2 nights/month	≥80% <20%	• No daily medication needed. • Severe exacerbations may occur, separated by long periods of normal lung function and no symptoms. A course of systemic corticosteroids is recommended.

Quick Relief
All Patients

- Short-acting bronchodilator: 2–4 puffs short-acting inhaled β_2 agonists as needed for symptoms.
- Intensity of treatment will depend on severity of exacerbation; up to 3 treatments at 20-min intervals or a single nebulizer treatment as needed. Course of systemic corticosteroids may be needed.
- Use of short-acting β_2 agonists >2 times/wk in intermittent asthma (daily, or increasing use in persistent asthma) may indicate the need to initiate (increase) long term control therapy.

↓ **STEP DOWN**
Review treatment every 1–6 months;a gradual stepwise reduction in treatment may be possible.

↑ **STEP UP**
If control is not maintained, consider step up. First, review patient medication technique, adherence, and environmental control.

Goals of Therapy: Asthma Control

- Minimal or no chronic symptoms day or night
- Minimal or no exacerbations
- No limitations on activities; no school/work missed

- Maintain (near) normal pulmonary function
- Minimal use of short-acting inhaled β_2 agonist
- Minimal or no adverse effects from medications

Note

- The stepwise approach is meant to assist, not replace, the clinical decision making required to meet individual patient needs.
- Classify severity: assign patient to most severe step in which any feature occurs (PEF is % of personal best; FEV_1 is % predicted).
- Gain control as quickly as possible (consider a short course of systemic corticosteroids); then step down to the least medication necessary to maintain control.
- Minimize use of short-acting inhaled β_2 agonists. Over reliance on short-acting inhaled β_2 agonists (e.g., use of short-acting inhaled β_2 agonist every day, increasing use or lack of expected effect, or use of approximately one canister a month even if not using it every day) indicates inadequate control of asthma and the need to initiate or intensify long-term control therapy.
- Provide education on self-management and controlling environmental factors that make asthma worse (e.g., allergens and irritants).
- Refer to an asthma specialist if there are difficulties controlling asthma or if step 4 care is required. Referral may be considered if step 3 care is required.

Figure 78–1. Stepwise approach for managing asthma in adults and children older than 5 years.

TABLE 78–1. Relative Selectivity, Potency, and Duration of Action of the β-Adrenergic Agonists

Agent	Selectivity		Potency, $\beta_2{}^a$	Duration of Action[b]		Oral activity
	β_1	β_2		Bronchodilation (h)	Protection (h)[c]	
Isoproterenol	+ + + +	+ + + +	1	0.5–2	0.5–1	No
Metaproterenol	+ + +	+ + +	15	3–4	1–2	Yes
Isoetharine	+ +	+ + +	6	0.5–2	0.5–1	No
Albuterol	+	+ + + +	2	4–8	2–4	Yes
Bitolterol	+	+ + + +	5	4–8	2–4	No
Pirbuterol	+	+ + + +	5	4–8	2–4	Yes
Terbutaline	+	+ + + +	4	4–8	2–4	Yes
Formoterol	+	+ + + +	0.24	≥12	6–12	Yes
Salmeterol	+	+ + + +	0.5	≥12	6->12	No

[a] Relative molar potency to isoproterenol: 15, lowest potency.
[b] Median durations with the highest value after a single dose and lowest after chronic administration.
[c] Protection refers to the prevention of bronchoconstriction induced by exercise or nonspecific bronchial challenges.

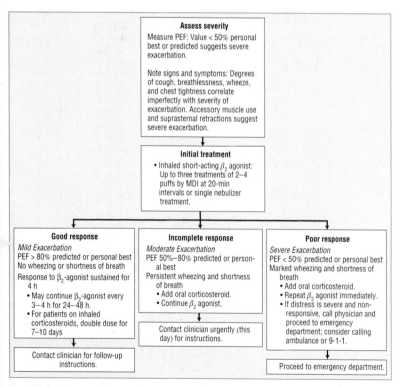

Figure 78–2. Home management of acute asthma exacerbation. Patients at risk of asthma-related death should receive immediate clinical attention after initial treatment. Additional therapy may be required. PEF, peak expiratory flow; MDI, metered dose inhaler.

severe asthma because it can take up to 20 minutes for onset and 1 to 4 hours for maximum bronchodilation after inhalation.

- In acute severe asthma, short-acting β_2 agonists (e.g., albuterol) should be given in high doses by nebulizer in frequent intervals or via metered dose inhaler (MDI); dosing guidelines are presented in Table 78–2.
- Inhaled β_2 agonists agents are the treatment of choice for exercise-induced bronchospasm (EIB). Short-acting agents provide complete protection for at least 2 hours after inhalation; long-acting agents provide significant protection for 8 to 12 hours initially, but the duration decreases with chronic regular use.
- In nocturnal asthma, long-acting inhaled β_2 agonists are preferred over oral sustained-release β_2 agonists or sustained-release theophylline. However, nocturnal asthma may be an indicator of inadequate anti-inflammatory treatment.

Corticosteroids

- **Corticosteroids** increase the number of β_2-adrenergic receptors and improve receptor responsiveness to β_2-adrenergic stimulation, thereby reducing mucus production and hypersecretion, reducing BHR, and preventing and reversing airway remodeling.
- Inhaled corticosteroids are the most effective long-term control therapy for persistent asthma, regardless of severity, and the only therapy shown to reduce the risk of death from asthma even in relatively low doses. Comparative doses are included in Table 78–3. Most patients with moderate disease can be controlled with twice-daily dosing; some products have once-daily dosing indications. Patients with more severe disease require multiple daily dosing. Because the inflammatory response of asthma inhibits steroid receptor binding, patients should be started on higher and more frequent doses and then tapered down once control has been achieved. The response to inhaled corticosteroids is delayed; symptoms improve in most patients within the first 1 to 2 weeks and reach maximum improvement in 4 to 8 weeks. Maximum improvement in FEV_1 and peak expiratory flow rates may require 3 to 6 weeks.
- Systemic toxicity is minimal with low to moderate inhaled doses, but the risk of systemic effects increases with high doses. Local adverse effects include dose-dependent oropharyngeal candidiasis and dysphonia, which can be reduced by the use of a spacer device. The ability of spacer devices to enhance lung delivery is inconsistent and should not be relied on.
- Systemic corticosteroids (Table 78–4) are indicated in all patients with acute severe asthma not responding completely to aggressive inhaled β_2 agonists (every 20 minutes for three to four doses). Intravenous therapy offers no advantage over oral administration. Multiple daily dosing appears warranted for initial therapy of acute exacerbations. It may take 6 to 8 hours for improvement in pulmonary function to occur after initiation of systemic therapy. Most patients achieve 70% of predicted FEV_1 within 48 hours and 80% by 6 days. Full doses should be continued until the patient's peak flow reaches 80% of predicted normal or personal best. Many patients require only 3- to 5-day courses of systemic corticosteroids. Tapering the steroid dosage after short courses is unnecessary.
- Systemic corticosteroids are also recommended for the treatment of impending episodes of severe asthma unresponsive to bronchodilator therapy. **Prednisone**, 1 to 2 mg/kg/day (up to 40 to 60 mg/day), is administered orally in two divided doses for 3 to 10 days. Because short-term (1 to 2 weeks) high-dose systemic steroids do not produce serious toxicities, the ideal method is to use a short burst and then maintain the patient on appropriate long-term control therapy with long periods between systemic corticosteroid treatments.

TABLE 78–2. Dosages of Drugs for Acute Severe Exacerbations of Asthma in the Emergency Department of Hospital

Medications	Dosages		Comments
	>6 yr old	<6 yr old	
Inhaled β-agonists			
Albuterol nebulizer soln. (5 mg/mL)	2.5–5 mg every 20 min for 3 doses, then 2.5–10 mg every 1–4 h as needed, or 10–15 mg/h continuously	0.15 mg/kg (minimum dose 2.5 mg) every 20 min for 3 doses, then 0.15–0.3 mg/kg up to 10 mg every 1–4 h as needed, or 0.5 mg/kg/h by continuous nebulization	Only selective β₂-agonists are recommended. For optimal delivery, dilute aerosols to minimum of 4 mL at gas flow of 6–8 L/min
Albuterol MDI (90 mcg/puff)	4–8 puffs every 30 min up to 4 h, then every 1–4 h as needed	4–8 puffs every 20 min for 3 doses, then every 1–4 h as needed	In patients in severe distress, nebulization is preferred; use holding-chamber–type spacer
Levalbuterol nebulizer soln.	Give at one-half the mg dose of albuterol above	Give at one-half the mg dose of albuterol above	The single isomer of albuterol is likely to be twice as potent
Bitolterol nebulizer soln. (2 mg/mL)	See albuterol dose	See albuterol dose; thought to be as potent to one-half as potent as albuterol on a microgram basis	Has not been studied in acute severe asthma; do not mix with other drugs
Pirbuterol MDI (200 mcg/puff)	See albuterol dose	See albuterol dose; one-half as potent as albuterol on a microgram basis	Has not been studied in acute severe asthma
Systemic β-agonists			
Epinephrine 1:1000 (1 mg/mL)	0.3–0.5 mg every 20 min for 3 doses SubQ	0.01 mg/kg up to 0.5 mg every 20 min for 3 doses SubQ	No proven advantage of systemic therapy over aerosol
Terbutaline (1 mg/mL)	0.25 mg every 20 min for 3 doses SubQ	0.01 mg/kg every 20 min for 3 doses, then every 2–6 h as needed SubQ	Not recommended
Anticholinergics			
Ipratropium Br. nebulizer soln. (0.25 mg/mL)	500 mcg every 30 min for 3 doses, then every 2–4 h as needed	250 mcg every 20 min for 3 doses, then 250 mcg every 2–4 h	May mix in same nebulizer with albuterol; do not use as first-line therapy; only add to β₂-agonist therapy
Ipratropium Br. MDI (18 mcg/puff)	4–8 puffs as needed every 2–4 h	4–8 puffs as needed every 2–4 h	Not recommended because dose in inhaler is low and has not been studied in acute asthma
Corticosteroids			
Prednisone, methylprednisolone, prednisolone	60–80 mg in 3 or 4 divided doses for 48 h, then 30–40 mg/day until PEF reaches 70% of personal best	1 mg/kg every 6 h for 48 h, then 1–2 mg/kg/day in 2 divided doses until PEF is 70% of normal predicted	For outpatient "burst" use 1–2 mg/kg/day, max. 60 mg, for 3–7 days; it is unnecessary to taper course

Note: No advantage has been found for very-high-dose corticosteroids in acute severe asthma, nor is there any advantage for intravenous administration over oral therapy. The usual regimen is to continue the frequent multiple daily dosing until the patient achieves an FEV₁ or PEF of 50% of personal best or normal predicted value and then lower the dose to twice-daily dosing. This usually occurs within 48 h. The final duration of therapy following a hospitalization or emergency department visit may be from 7 to 14 days. If patients are then started on inhaled corticosteroids, studies indicate there is no need to taper the systemic steroid dose. If the follow-up therapy is to be given once daily, studies indicate there may be an advantage to giving the single daily dose in the afternoon at around 3:00 PM.

TABLE 78–3. Available Inhaled Corticosteroid Products, Lung Delivery, and Comparative Doses

ICS	Product	Lung Delivery*a*
Beclomethasone dipropionate (BDP)	42 mcg/actuation CFC MDI, 200 actuations	4–10%
	40 and 80 mcg/actuation HFA MDI, 120 actuations	55–60%
Budesonide (BUD)	200 mcg/dose DPI, Turbuhaler, 200 doses	32% (16–59%)
	200 and 500-mcg ampules, 2 mL each	6%
Flunisolide (FLU)	250 mcg/actuation CFC MDI, 100 actuations	32%
Fluticasone propionate (FP)	44, 110, and 220 mcg/actuation CFC MDI, 120 actuations	26–30%
	50, 100, and 250 mcg/dose DPI, Rotadisk, 4 doses	15% (13–18%)
	50, 100, and 250 mcg/dose DPI, Diskus, 60 doses	15%
Mometasone furoate (MF)	200 and 400 mcg/dose DPI, Twisthaler, 14, 30, 60, and 120 doses	Unknown
Triamcinolone acetonide (TAA)	100 mcg/actuation CFC MDI, 240 actuations with spacer	22%

	Comparable Daily doses (mcg)		
	Low Dose, *Child/Adult*	*Medium Dose,* *Child/Adult*	*High Dose,* *Child/Adult*
BDP			
CFC MDI	84–336/168–504	336–672/504–840	>672/ >840
HFA MDI	40–160/80–240	160–320/240–400	>320/ >400
BUD			
DPI	100–200/200–400	200–400/400–800	>400/ >800
Nebules	250–500/UK	500–1000/UK	>1000/UK
FLU, CFC MDI	500–750/500–1000	750–1250/1000–2000	>1250/ >2000
FP			
CFC MDI	88–176/88–264	176–440/264–660	>440/ >660
DPIs	100–200/100–300	200–400/300–600	>400/ >600
MF, DPI	UK/200–400	UK/400–800	UK/ >800
TAA, CFC MDI	400–800/400–1000	800–1200/1000–2000	>1200/ >2000

a Lung delivery from in vivo radiolabel scintigraphy or pharmacokinetic studies
CFC, chlorofluorocarbon; HFA, hydrofluoroalkane; MDI, metered dose inhaler; UK, unknown; DPI, dry powder inhaler.

XV ◄

TABLE 78–4. Comparison of the Systemic Corticosteroids

Systemic	Anti-inflammatory Potency	Mineralocorticoid Potency	Duration of Biologic Activity (h)	Elimination Half-Life (h)
Hydrocortisone	1	1.0	8–12	1.5–2.0
Prednisone	4	0.8	12–36	2.5–3.5
Methylprednisolone	5	0.5	12–36	3.3
Dexamethasone	25	0	36–54	3.4–4.0

- In patients who require chronic systemic corticosteroids for asthma control, the lowest possible dose should be used. Toxicities may be decreased by alternate-day therapy or high-dose inhaled corticosteroids.

Methylxanthines

- **Theophylline** appears to produce bronchodilation by inhibiting phosphodiesterases (PDEs), which may also result in anti-inflammatory and other non-bronchodilator activity through decreased mast cell mediator release, decreased eosinophil basic protein release, decreased T-lymphocyte proliferation, decreased T-cell cytokine release, and decreased plasma exudation. Theophylline also inhibits vascular permeability, enhances mucociliary clearance, and strengthens contractions of a fatigued diaphragm.
- Methylxanthines are ineffective by aerosol and must be taken systemically (orally or IV). Sustained-release theophylline is the preferred oral preparation, whereas its complex with ethylenediamine (**aminophylline**) is the preferred parenteral product due to increased solubility. Intravenous theophylline is also available.
- Theophylline is eliminated primarily by metabolism via hepatic cytochrome P450 mixed-function oxidase microsomal enzymes (primarily CYP1A2 and CYP3A4) with 10% or less excreted unchanged in the kidney. The hepatic cytochrome P450 enzymes are susceptible to induction and inhibition by various environmental factors and drugs. Clinically significant reductions in clearance can result from cotherapy with cimetidine, erythromycin, clarithromycin, allopurinol, propranolol, ciprofloxacin, interferon, ticlopidine, zileuton, and other drugs. Some substances that enhance clearance include rifampin, carbamazepine, phenobarbital, phenytoin, charcoal-broiled meat, and cigarette smoking.
- Because of large interpatient variability in theophylline clearance, routine monitoring of serum theophylline concentrations is essential for safe and effective use. A steady-state range of 5 to 15 mcg/mL is effective and safe for most patients.
- Figure 78–3 gives recommended dosages, monitoring schedules, and dosage adjustments for theophylline.
- Sustained-release oral preparations are favored for outpatient therapy, but each product has different release characteristics and some products are susceptible to altered absorption from food or gastric pH changes. Preparations unaffected by food that can be administered a minimum of every 12 hours in most patients are preferable.
- Outpatient chronic theophylline administration can reduce asthma symptoms, reduce the amount of as-needed inhaled β_2 agonists used, and reduce oral corticosteroid requirements in steroid-dependent asthmatics. Sustained-release theophylline once nightly is effective for nocturnal asthma.
- In acute severe asthma exacerbations, addition of aminophylline to optimal inhaled β_2 agonists provides no further benefit and is not recommended.
- Significant disadvantages to chronic theophylline therapy are the dangers inherent in giving a drug that can produce severe cardiac arrhythmias, seizures, and death at serum concentrations only twofold greater than optimal therapeutic concentrations.
- Because of its high risk-benefit ratio, theophylline is considered a second- or third-line agent in the treatment of asthma.

Anticholinergics

- **Ipratropium bromide** and **tiotropium bromide** are competitive inhibitors of muscarinic receptors; they produce bronchodilation only in

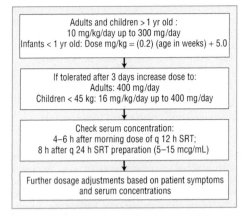

Figure 78–3. Algorithm for slow titration of theophylline dosage and guide for final dosage adjustment based on serum theophylline concentration measurement. For infants younger than 1 year, the initial daily dosage can be calculated by the following regression equation: Dose (mg/kg) = (0.2) (age in weeks) + 5. *Whenever side effects occur, dosage should be reduced to a previously tolerated lower dose.* SRT, sustained-release theophylline.

cholinergic-mediated bronchoconstriction. Anticholinergics are effective bronchodilators but are not as potent as β_2 agonists. They attenuate, but do not block, allergen- or exercise-induced asthma in a dose-dependent fashion.

- The time to reach maximum bronchodilation from aerosolized ipratropium is longer than from aerosolized short-acting β_2 agonists (2 hours vs. 30 minutes). This is of little clinical consequence because some bronchodilation is seen within 30 seconds, 50% of maximum response occurs within 3 minutes, and 80% of maximum is reached within 30 minutes. Ipratropium bromide has a duration of action of 4 to 8 hours.
- Inhaled ipratropium bromide is only indicated as adjunctive therapy in severe acute asthma not completely responsive to β_2 agonists alone. It generally produces a further improvement in lung function of 10% to 15%. Its addition to initial therapy may reduce the hospitalization rate in children and adults with severe exacerbations. It has not been shown to improve outcomes in chronic asthma.

XV

Cromolyn Sodium and Nedocromil Sodium

- **Cromolyn sodium** and **nedocromil sodium** have beneficial effects that are believed to result from stabilization of mast cell membranes. They inhibit the response to allergen challenge as well as EIB but do not cause bronchodilation.
- These agents are effective only by inhalation and are available as MDIs; cromolyn also comes as a nebulizer solution.
- Both drugs are remarkably nontoxic. Cough and wheezing have been reported after inhalation of each agent, and bad taste and headache after nedocromil.
- Cromolyn and nedocromil are indicated for the prophylaxis of mild persistent asthma in children and adults regardless of etiology. They may be particularly effective for allergic asthmatics on a seasonal basis or just prior to an acute exposure (i.e., animals or mowing the lawn). Nedocromil may allow some patients to decrease inhaled steroid dosage.

- Cromolyn is the second drug of choice for the prevention of EIB and may be used in conjunction with a β_2 agonist in more severe cases not completely responding to either agent alone.
- Most patients experience an improvement in 1 to 2 weeks, but it may take longer to achieve maximum benefit. Patients should initially receive cromolyn or nedocromil 4 times daily; after stabilization of symptoms the frequency may be reduced to 2 times daily for nedocromil and 3 times daily for cromolyn.

Leukotriene Modifiers

- **Zafirlukast** (Accolate) and **montelukast** (Singulair) are oral leukotriene receptor antagonists that reduce the proinflammatory (increased microvascular permeability and airway edema) and bronchoconstriction effects of leukotriene D_4. In adults and children with persistent asthma, they have been shown to improve pulmonary function tests, decrease nocturnal awakenings and β_2-agonist use, and improve asthma symptoms. However, they are less effective in asthma than low-dose inhaled corticosteroids. They are not used to treat acute exacerbations and must be taken on a regular basis, even during symptom-free periods. The adult dose of zafirlukast is 20 mg twice daily, taken at least 1 hour before or 2 hours after meals; the dose for children aged 5 through 11 years is 10 mg twice daily. For montelukast, the adult dose is 10 mg once daily, taken in the evening without regard to food; the dose for children aged 6 to 14 years is one 5-mg chewable tablet daily in the evening.
- Zafirlukast and montelukast are generally well tolerated. Rare elevations in serum aminotransferase concentrations and clinical hepatitis have been reported. An idiosyncratic syndrome similar to the Churg-Strauss syndrome, with marked circulating eosinophilia, heart failure, and associated eosinophilic vasculitis, has been reported in a small number of patients; a direct causal association has not been established.
- **Zileuton** (Zyflo) is an inhibitor of leukotriene synthesis. The dose is 600 mg four times daily with meals and at bedtime. Its use is limited due to the need for frequent dosing, the potential for elevated hepatic enzymes (especially in the first 3 months of therapy), and inhibition of the metabolism of some drugs metabolized by CYP3A4 (e.g., theophylline, warfarin). Serum alanine aminotransferase (ALT) should be monitored before treatment, once a month for the first 3 months, every 2 to 3 months for the remainder of the first year, and periodically thereafter.

Combination Controller Therapy

- The 2002 NAEPP guidelines recommend that the combination of inhaled corticosteroids and long-acting inhaled β_2 agonists is the preferred treatment for step 3 moderate persistent asthma. This combination is superior to doubling the dose of inhaled corticosteroids or adding leukotriene antagonists to inhaled corticosteroids.
- **Advair** is a combination product that treats both the inflammatory and bronchoconstrictive components of moderate to severe persistent asthma by delivering a dose of fluticasone (100, 250, or 500 mcg) with a fixed dose of salmeterol (50 mcg). It has a rapid onset (within 1 week), and the salmeterol component may allow reduction in inhaled corticosteroid dosage by 50% in patients with persistent asthma.

Omalizumab

Omalizumab (Xolair) is an anti-IgE antibody approved for the treatment of asthma not well controlled by high doses of inhaled corticosteroids. It is only indicated for corticosteroid-dependent atopic patients requiring oral corticosteroids

XV

or receiving high-dose inhaled corticosteroids with continued symptoms and high IgE levels. The dosage is determined by the patient's baseline total serum IgE (IU/mL) and body weight (kg). Doses range from 150 to 375 mg given subcutaneously at either 2- or 4-week intervals.

Methotrexate

Methotrexate in low doses (15 mg/wk) has been used to reduce the systemic corticosteroid dose in patients with severe steroid-dependent asthma. It results in a moderate reduction in systemic steroid dosage (approximately 23%) in some patients, but some studies have shown no beneficial effect. Methotrexate should be considered experimental and reserved for severe steroid-dependent asthmatics under the care of specialists, with careful monitoring of hepatic and pulmonary function.

▶ EVALUATION OF THERAPEUTIC OUTCOMES

CHRONIC ASTHMA

- Control of asthma is defined as achieving minimal need for rescue short-acting β_2 agonists (ideally none), no acute episodes, no limitation of activity, no emergency care visits, no nocturnal symptoms, normal pulmonary function, minimal or no medication side effects, and satisfaction of the patient and family with care.
- Monitoring consists of quantitating the use of inhaled short-acting inhaled β_2 agonists, days of limited activity, and number of symptoms (especially nocturnal).
- In moderate to severe persistent asthma, once-daily (on awakening) peak flow monitoring is recommended. The NAEPP recommends yearly spirometric studies.
- Patients should also be asked about exercise tolerance and nocturnal symptoms.
- All patients on inhaled drugs should have their inhalation technique evaluated monthly initially and then every 3 to 6 months.
- After initiation of anti-inflammatory therapy or an increase in dosage, most patients should begin experiencing a decrease in symptoms within 1 to 2 weeks and achieve maximum symptomatic improvement within 4 to 8 weeks. Improvement in baseline FEV_1 or peak expiratory flow (PEF) should follow a similar time frame, but a decrease in BHR as measured by morning PEF, PEF variability, and exercise tolerance may take longer and improve over 1 to 3 months.

ACUTE SEVERE ASTHMA

- Patients at risk for acute severe exacerbations should monitor morning peak flows at home.
- In young children, increased respiratory rate and heart rate and inability to speak more than one or two words between breaths are signs of severe obstruction.
- Lung function, either spirometry or peak flows, should be monitored 5 to 10 minutes after each treatment.
- Oxygen saturation by pulse oximetry and peak flows should be measured in all patients not completely responding to initial intensive inhaled β_2-agonist therapy.

See Chapter 26, Asthma, authored by H. William Kelly and Christine A. Sorkness, for a more detailed discussion of this topic.

XV

Chapter 79

▶ CHRONIC OBSTRUCTIVE PULMONARY DISEASE

▶ DEFINITION

- The National Heart, Lung, and Blood Institute (NHLBI) and World Health Organization (WHO) have proposed that chronic obstructive pulmonary disease (COPD) be defined as a disease characterized by progressive airflow limitation that is not fully reversible. The airflow limitation is usually both progressive and associated with an abnormal inflammatory response of the lungs to noxious particles or gases. The most common conditions comprising COPD are chronic bronchitis and emphysema.
  - Chronic bronchitis is associated with chronic or recurrent excess mucus secretion into the bronchial tree with cough that occurs on most days for at least 3 months of the year for at least 2 consecutive years when other causes of cough have been excluded.
  - Emphysema is defined as abnormal, permanent enlargement of the airspaces distal to the terminal bronchioles, accompanied by destruction of their walls, but without obvious fibrosis.

▶ PATHOPHYSIOLOGY

- The most common etiology is exposure to environmental tobacco smoke, but other chronic inhalational exposures can also lead to COPD. Inhalation of noxious particles and gases stimulates the activation of neutrophils, macrophages, and CD8+ lymphocytes, which release a variety of chemical mediators, including tumor necrosis factor α (TNFα), interleukin-8 (IL-8), and leukotriene B_4 (LTB$_4$). These inflammatory cells and mediators lead to widespread destructive changes in the airways, pulmonary vasculature, and lung parenchyma.
- Other pathophysiologic processes may include oxidative stress and an imbalance between aggressive and protective defense systems in the lungs (proteases and antiproteases). Increased oxidants generated by cigarette smoke react with and damage various proteins and lipids, leading to cell and tissue damage. Oxidants also promote inflammation directly and exacerbate the protease-antiprotease imbalance by inhibiting antiprotease activity.
- The protective antiprotease α_1-antitrypsin (AAT) inhibits several protease enzymes, including neutrophil elastase. In the presence of unopposed AAT activity, elastase attacks elastin, which is a major component of alveolar walls. A hereditary deficiency of AAT results in an increased risk for premature development of emphysema. In the inherited disease, there is an absolute deficiency of AAT. In emphysema resulting from cigarette-smoking, the imbalance is associated with increased protease activity or reduced activity of antiproteases. Activated inflammatory cells release several other proteases, including cathepsins and metalloproteinases (MMPs). In addition, oxidative stress reduces antiprotease (or protective) activity.
- An inflammatory exudate is often present in the airways that leads to an increased number and size of goblet cells and mucus glands. Mucus secretion increases, and ciliary motility is impaired. There is a thickening of the smooth muscle and connective tissue in the airways. Chronic inflammation leads to scarring and fibrosis. Diffuse airway narrowing occurs and is more prominent in small peripheral airways.

- Parenchymal changes affect the gas-exchanging units of the lungs (alveoli and pulmonary capillaries). Smoking-related disease most commonly results in centrilobular emphysema that primarily affects respiratory bronchioles. Panlobular emphysema is seen in AAT deficiency and extends to the alveolar ducts and sacs.
- Vascular changes include thickening of pulmonary vessels that may lead to endothelial dysfunction of the pulmonary arteries. Later, structural changes increase pulmonary pressures, especially during exercise. In severe COPD, secondary pulmonary hypertension leads to right-sided heart failure (cor pulmonale).

▶ CLINICAL PRESENTATION

- Initial symptoms of COPD include chronic cough and sputum production; patients may have these symptoms for several years before dyspnea develops.
- The physical examination is normal in most patients who present in the milder stages of COPD. When airflow limitation becomes severe, patients may have cyanosis of mucosal membranes, development of a "barrel chest" due to hyperinflation of the lungs, an increased resting respiratory rate, shallow breathing, pursing of the lips during expiration, and use of accessory respiratory muscles.
- Patients experiencing a COPD exacerbation may have worsening dyspnea, increase in sputum volume, or increase in sputum purulence. Other common features of an exacerbation include chest tightness, increased need for bronchodilators, malaise, fatigue, and decreased exercise tolerance.

▶ DIAGNOSIS

The diagnosis of COPD is based in part on the patient's symptoms and a history of exposure to risk factors such as tobacco smoke and occupational exposures.

PULMONARY FUNCTION TESTS

- Assessment of airflow limitation through spirometry is the standard for diagnosing and monitoring COPD. The forced expiratory volume after 1 second (FEV_1) is generally reduced except in very mild disease. The forced vital capacity (FVC) may also be decreased. The hallmark of COPD is a reduced FEV_1/FVC ratio to less than 70%.
- An improvement in FEV_1 of less than 12% after inhalation of a rapid-acting bronchodilator is considered to be evidence of irreversible airflow obstruction.
- Peak expiratory flow measurements are not adequate for diagnosis of COPD because of low specificity and a high degree of effort dependence. However, a low peak expiratory flow is consistent with COPD.

XV

ARTERIAL BLOOD GASES

- Significant changes in arterial blood gases are not usually present until the FEV_1 is less than 1 L. At this stage, hypoxemia and hypercapnia may become chronic problems. Hypoxemia usually occurs initially with exercise but develops at rest as the disease progresses.
- Patients with severe COPD can have a low arterial oxygen tension ($Pao_2 = 45$ to 60 mm Hg) and an elevated arterial carbon dioxide tension ($Paco_2 = 50$ to 60 mm Hg). Hypoxemia results from hypoventilation (V) of lung tissue relative to perfusion (Q) of the area. The low V/Q ratio progresses over several years, resulting in a consistent decline in the Pao_2.

- Some patients lose the ability to increase the rate or depth or respiration in response to persistent hypoxemia. This decreased ventilatory drive may be due to abnormal peripheral or central respiratory receptor responses. This relative hypoventilation leads to hypercapnia; in this situation the central respiratory response to a chronically increased $Paco_2$ can be blunted. Because these changes in Pao_2 and $Paco_2$ are subtle and progress over many years, the pH is usually near normal because the kidneys compensate by retaining bicarbonate.
- If acute respiratory distress develops (e.g., due to pneumonia or a COPD exacerbation) the $Paco_2$ may rise sharply resulting in an uncompensated respiratory acidosis.

DIAGNOSIS OF ACUTE RESPIRATORY FAILURE IN COPD

- The diagnosis of acute respiratory failure in COPD is made on the basis of an acute drop in Pao_2 of 10 to 15 mm Hg or any acute increase in $Paco_2$ that decreases the serum pH to 7.3 or less.
- Additional acute clinical manifestations include restlessness, confusion, tachycardia, diaphoresis, cyanosis, hypotension, irregular breathing, miosis, and unconsciousness.
- The most common cause of acute respiratory failure in COPD is acute exacerbation of bronchitis with an increase in the volume and viscosity of sputum. This serves to worsen obstruction and further impair alveolar ventilation, resulting in worsening hypoxemia and hypercapnia. Additional causes are pneumonia, pulmonary embolism, left ventricular failure, pneumothorax, and central nervous system depressants.

▶ DESIRED OUTCOME

The goals of therapy include smoking cessation; symptom improvement; reduction in the rate of FEV_1 decline; reduction in the number of acute exacerbations; improvement in physical and psychological well-being; and reduction in mortality, hospitalizations, and days lost from work.

▶ TREATMENT OF CHRONIC COPD

NONPHARMACOLOGIC THERAPY

- Smoking cessation is the most effective strategy to reduce the risk of developing COPD and the only intervention proven to affect the long-term decline in FEV_1 and slow the progression of COPD.
- Pulmonary rehabilitation programs include exercise training along with smoking cessation, breathing exercises, optimal medical treatment, psychosocial support, and health education. Supplemental oxygen, nutritional support, and psychoeducational care (e.g., relaxation) are important adjuncts in a pulmonary rehabilitation program.
- Annual vaccination with the inactivated intramuscular influenza vaccine is recommended. One dose of the polyvalent pneumococcal vaccine is indicated for patients at any age with COPD; revaccination is recommended for patients older than 65 years if the first vaccination was more than 5 years earlier and the patient was younger than 65 years.

PHARMACOLOGIC THERAPY

A stepwise approach to managing COPD is shown in Figure 79–1. Bronchodilators are used to control symptoms; no single pharmacologic class

XV

New	0: At risk	I: Mild	II: Moderate	III: Severe	IV: Very severe
Characteristics	• Chronic symptoms • Exposure to risk factors • Normal spirometry	• $FEV_1/FVC < 70\%$ • $FEV_1 \geq 80\%$ • With or without symptoms	• $FEV_1/FVC < 70\%$ • $50\% > FEV_1 < 80\%$ • With or without symptoms	• $FEV_1/FVC < 70\%$ • $30\% > FEV_1 < 50\%$ • With or without symptoms	• $FEV_1/FVC < 70\%$ • $FEV_1 < 30\%$ or presence of chronic respiratory failure or right heart failure

Avoidance of risk factor(s); influenza vaccination; pneumococcal vaccine

Add short-acting bronchodilator when needed

Add regular treatment with one or more long-acting bronchodilators
Add rehabilitation

Add inhaled glucocorticoids if repeated exacerbations

Add long-term oxygen if chronicrespiratory failure
Consider surgical treatments

Figure 79–1. Recommended therapy of stable COPD.

XV

has been proven to provide superior benefit over others, although inhaled therapy is generally preferred. Medication selection is based on likely patient adherence, individual response, and side effects. Medications can be used as needed or on a scheduled bases, and additional therapies should be added in a stepwise manner depending on response and disease severity. Clinical benefits of bronchodilators include increased exercise capacity, decreased air trapping, and relief of symptoms such as dyspnea. However, significant improvements in pulmonary function measurements such as FEV_1 may not be observed.

SYMPATHOMIMETICS

- β_2-Selective sympathomimetics cause relaxation of bronchial smooth muscle and bronchodilation by stimulating the enzyme adenyl cyclase to increase the formation of cyclic adenosine monophosphate (cAMP). They may also improve mucociliary clearance.
- Administration via metered-dose inhaler (MDI) or dry-powder inhaler (DPI) is at least as effective as nebulization therapy and is usually favored for reasons of cost and convenience. Refer to Table 78–1 in Chapter 78 for a comparison of the available agents.
- **Albuterol, levalbuterol, bitolterol, pirbuterol**, and **terbutaline** are the preferred short-acting agents because they have greater β_2 selectivity and longer duration of action than other short-acting agents (isoproterenol, metaproterenol, and isoetharine). The inhalation route is preferred to the oral and parenteral routes in terms of both efficacy and adverse effects. Short-acting agents can be used for acute relief of symptoms or on a scheduled basis to prevent or reduce symptoms. The duration of action of short-acting β_2 agonists is 4 to 6 hours.
- **Formoterol** and **salmeterol** are long-acting inhaled β_2 agonists that are dosed every 12 hours on a scheduled basis and provide bronchodilation throughout the dosing interval. Their use should be considered when patients demonstrate a frequent need for short-acting agents. Neither drug is indicated for acute relief of symptoms.

ANTICHOLINERGICS

- When given by inhalation, anticholinergic agents produce bronchodilation by competitively inhibiting cholinergic receptors in bronchial smooth muscle. This activity blocks acetylcholine, with the net effect being a reduction in cyclic guanosine monophosphate (cGMP), which normally acts to constrict bronchial smooth muscle.
- **Ipratropium bromide** has a slower onset of action than short-acting β_2 agonists (15 to 20 minutes vs. 5 minutes for albuterol). For this reason, it may be less suitable for as-needed use, but it is often prescribed in this manner. Ipratropium has a more prolonged bronchodilator effect than short-acting β_2 agonists. Its peak effect occurs in 1.5 to 2 hours and its duration is 4 to 6 hours. The recommended dose via MDI is 2 puffs four times a day with upward titration often to 24 puffs/day. It is also available as a solution for nebulization. The most frequent patient complaints are dry mouth, nausea, and, occasionally, metallic taste. Because it is poorly absorbed systemically, anticholinergic side effects are uncommon (e.g., blurred vision, urinary retention, nausea, and tachycardia).
- **Tiotropium bromide** is a long-acting agent that protects against cholinergic bronchoconstriction for more than 24 hours. Its onset of effect is within 30 minutes with a peak effect in 3 hours. It is delivered via the HandiHaler, a single-load, dry-powder, breath-actuated device. The recommended dose is

inhalation of the contents of one capsule once daily using the HandiHaler inhalation device. Because it acts locally, tiotropium is well tolerated; the most common complaint is dry mouth. Other anticholinergic effects have also been reported.

COMBINATION ANTICHOLINERGICS AND SYMPATHOMIMETICS

- The combination of an inhaled anticholinergic and β_2 agonist is often used, especially as the disease progresses and symptoms worsen over time. Combining bronchodilators with different mechanisms of action allows the lowest effective doses to be used and reduces adverse effects from individual agents. Combination of both short- and long-acting β_2 agonists with ipratropium has been shown to provide added symptomatic relief and improvements in pulmonary function.

- A combination product containing **albuterol** and **ipratropium** (**Combivent**) is available as an MDI for chronic maintenance therapy of COPD. Other similar combination products may become available in the future.

METHYLXANTHINES

- **Theophylline** and **aminophylline** may produce bronchodilation by inhibition of phosphodiesterase (thereby increasing cAMP levels), inhibition of calcium ion influx into smooth muscle, prostaglandin antagonism, stimulation of endogenous catecholamines, adenosine receptor antagonism, and inhibition of release of mediators from mast cells and leukocytes.

- Chronic theophylline use in COPD has been shown to produce improvements in lung function, including vital capacity and FEV_1. Subjectively, theophylline has been shown to reduce dyspnea, increase exercise tolerance, and improve respiratory drive. Nonpulmonary effects that may contribute to better functional capacity include improved cardiac function and decreased pulmonary artery pressure.

- Methylxanthines are no longer considered first-line therapy for COPD. Inhaled bronchodilator therapy is preferred over theophylline for COPD because of theophylline's risk for drug interactions and the interpatient variability in dosage requirements. Theophylline may be considered in patients who are intolerant or unable to use an inhaled bronchodilator. A methylxanthine may also be added to the regimen of patients who have not achieved an optimal clinical response to an inhaled anticholinergic and β_2 agonist.

- As with other bronchodilators in COPD, parameters other than objective measurements, such as FEV_1, should be monitored to assess efficacy. Subjective parameters, such as perceived improvements in dyspnea and exercise tolerance, are important in assessing the acceptability of methylxanthines for COPD patients.

- Sustained-release theophylline preparations improve patient compliance and achieve more consistent serum concentrations than rapid-release theophylline and aminophylline preparations. Caution should be used in switching from one sustained-release preparation to another because there are considerable variations in sustained-release characteristics.

- The role of theophylline in COPD is as maintenance therapy in non–acutely ill patients. Therapy can be initiated at 200 mg twice daily and titrated upward every 3 to 5 days to the target dose; most patients require daily doses of 400 to 900 mg.

- Dose adjustments should generally be made based on trough serum concentration results. A conservative therapeutic range of 8 to 15 mcg/mL is often preferable in the elderly to minimize the likelihood of toxicity. Once a dose is

XV

established, concentrations should be monitored once or twice a year unless the disease worsens, medications that interfere with theophylline metabolism are added, or toxicity is suspected.

- The most common side effects of theophylline include dyspepsia, nausea, vomiting, diarrhea, headache, dizziness, and tachycardia. Arrhythmias and seizures may occur, especially at toxic concentrations.
- Factors that may decrease theophylline clearance and lead to reduced dosage requirements include advanced age, bacterial or viral pneumonia, heart failure, liver dysfunction, hypoxemia from acute decompensation, and use of drugs such as cimetidine, macrolides, and fluoroquinolone antibiotics.
- Factors that may enhance theophylline clearance and result in the need for higher doses include tobacco and marijuana smoking, hyperthyroidism, and use of drugs such as phenytoin, phenobarbital, and rifampin.

CORTICOSTEROIDS

- The anti-inflammatory mechanisms whereby corticosteroids exert their beneficial effect in COPD include reduction in capillary permeability to decrease mucus, inhibition of release of proteolytic enzymes from leukocytes, and inhibition of prostaglandins.
- The clinical benefits of systemic corticosteroid therapy in the chronic management of COPD are often not evident, and there is a high risk of toxicity. Consequently, chronic, systemic corticosteroids should be avoided if possible.
- Appropriate situations to consider corticosteroids in COPD include (1) short-term systemic use for acute exacerbations and (2) inhalation therapy for chronic stable COPD.
- The role of inhaled corticosteroids in COPD is controversial. Major clinical trials have failed to demonstrate any benefit from chronic treatment in modifying long-term decline in lung function. However, other important benefits have been observed in some patients, including a decrease in exacerbation frequency and improvements in overall health status.
- Consensus guidelines indicate that inhaled corticosteroid therapy should be considered for symptomatic patients with stage III or IV disease (FEV_1 less than 50%) who experience repeated exacerbations.
- Side effects of inhaled corticosteroids are relatively mild and include hoarseness, sore throat, oral candidiasis, and skin bruising. Severe side effects such as adrenal suppression, osteoporosis, and cataract formation are reported less frequently than with systemic corticosteroids, but clinicians should monitor patients receiving high-dose chronic inhaled therapy.
- Several studies have shown an additive effect with the combination of inhaled corticosteroids and long-acting bronchodilators. Combination therapy with salmeterol plus fluticasone or formoterol plus budesonide was associated with greater improvements in FEV_1, health status, and exacerbation frequency than either agent alone. The availability of combination inhalers makes administration of both drugs convenient and decreases the total number of inhalations needed daily.

TREATMENT OF COPD EXACERBATION

DESIRED OUTCOMES

The goals of therapy for patients experiencing exacerbations of COPD are prevention of hospitalization or reduction in hospital stay, prevention of acute respiratory failure and death, and resolution of symptoms and a return to baseline clinical status and quality of life.

NONPHARMACOLOGIC THERAPY

- Oxygen therapy should be considered for any patient with hypoxemia during an exacerbation. Caution must be used because many COPD patients rely on mild hypoxemia to trigger their drive to breathe. Overly aggressive oxygen administration to patients with chronic hypercapnia may result in respiratory depression and respiratory failure. Oxygen therapy should be used to achieve a PaO_2 of greater than 60 mm Hg or oxygen saturation of greater than 90%. Arterial blood gases should be obtained after oxygen initiation to monitor carbon dioxide retention owing to hypoventilation.

- Noninvasive positive-pressure ventilation (NPPV) provides ventilatory support with oxygen and pressurized airflow using a face or nasal mask with a tight seal but without endotracheal intubation. In patients with acute respiratory failure due to COPD exacerbations, NPPV was associated with lower mortality, lower intubation rates, shorter hospital stays, and greater improvements in serum pH in 1 hour compared with usual care. Use of NPPV reduces the complications that often arise with invasive mechanical ventilation. NPPV is not appropriate for patients with altered mental status, severe acidosis, respiratory arrest, or cardiovascular instability.

- Intubation and mechanical ventilation may be considered in patients failing a trial of NPPV or those who are poor candidates for NPPV.

PHARMACOLOGIC THERAPY

Bronchodilators

- The dose and frequency of bronchodilators are increased during acute exacerbations to provide symptomatic relief. Short-acting β_2 agonists are preferred because of their rapid onset of action. Anticholinergic agents may be added if symptoms persist despite increased doses of β_2 agonists.

- Bronchodilators may be administered via MDIs or nebulization with equal efficacy. Nebulization may be considered for patients with severe dyspnea who are unable to hold their breath after actuation of an MDI.

- Clinical evidence supporting theophylline use during exacerbations is lacking, and thus theophylline should generally be avoided. It may be considered for patients not responding to other therapies.

Corticosteroids

- Results from clinical trials suggest that patients with acute COPD exacerbations should receive a short course of intravenous or oral corticosteroids. Because of the large variability in dose ranges used in those trials, the optimal dose and duration of treatment are unknown.

- It appears that short courses (9 to 14 days) are as effective as longer courses and have a lower risk of adverse effects. If treatment is continued for longer than 2 weeks, a tapering oral schedule should be employed to avoid hypothalamic-pituitary-adrenal (HPA) axis suppression.

XV

Antimicrobial Therapy

- Although most exacerbations of COPD are thought to be caused by viral or bacterial infections, as many as 30% of exacerbations are caused by unknown factors.

- Antibiotics are of most benefit and should be initiated if at least two of the following three symptoms are present: increased dyspnea, increased sputum volume, and increased sputum purulence. The utility of sputum Gram stain and culture is questionable because some patients have chronic bacterial colonization of the bronchial tree between exacerbations.

- Selection of empiric antimicrobial therapy should be based on the most likely organisms. The most common organisms for any acute exacerbation of COPD are *Haemophilus influenzae, Moraxella catarrhalis, Streptococcus pneumoniae,* and *Haemophilus parainfluenzae.*
- Therapy should be initiated within 24 hours of symptoms to prevent unnecessary hospitalization and generally continued for at least 7 to 10 days. Five-day courses with some agents may produce comparable efficacy.
- In uncomplicated exacerbations, recommended therapy includes a **macrolide (azithromycin, clarithromycin), second-** or **third-generation cephalosporin**, or **doxycycline**. Trimethoprim-sulfamethoxazole should not be used because of increasing pneumococcal resistance. Amoxicillin and first-generation cephalosporins are not recommended because of β-lactamase susceptibility. Erythromycin is not recommended because of insufficient activity against *H. influenzae.*
- In complicated exacerbations where drug-resistant pneumococci, β-lactamase-producing *H. influenzae* and *M. catarrhalis,* and some enteric gram-negative organisms may be present, recommended therapy includes **amoxicillin/clavulanate** or a fluoroquinolone with enhanced pneumococcal activity (**levofloxacin, gatifloxacin, moxifloxacin**).
- In complicated exacerbations with risk of *Pseudomonas aeruginosa,* recommended therapy includes a fluoroquinolone with enhanced pneumococcal and *P. aeruginosa* activity (**levofloxacin, gatifloxacin, moxifloxacin**).If intravenous therapy is required, a β-lactamase resistant penicillin with antipseudomonal activity or a third- or fourth-generation cephalosporin with antipseudomonal activity should be used.

▶ EVALUATION OF THERAPEUTIC OUTCOMES

- In chronic stable COPD, pulmonary function tests should be assessed with any therapy addition, change in dose, or deletion of therapy. Other outcomes measures include dyspnea score, quality-of-life assessments, and exacerbation rates (including emergency department visits and hospitalizations).
- In acute exacerbations of COPD, pulmonary function tests, white blood cell count, vital signs, chest x-ray, and changes in frequency of dyspnea, sputum volume, and sputum purulence should be assessed at the onset and throughout the exacerbation. In severe exacerbations, arterial blood gases and oxygen saturation should also be monitored.
- Patient adherence to therapeutic regimens, side effects, potential drug interactions, and subjective measures of quality of life must also be evaluated.

See Chapter 27, Chronic Obstructive Pulmonary Disease, authored by Sharya V. Bourdet and Dennis M. Williams, for a more detailed discussion of this topic.

XV

Urologic Disorders
Edited by Cindy W. Hamilton

Chapter 80

▶ BENIGN PROSTATIC HYPERPLASIA

▶ DEFINITION

Benign prostatic hyperplasia (BPH), a nearly ubiquitous condition, is the most common benign neoplasm of American men and occurs as a result of hormone-driven prostate growth.

▶ PATHOPHYSIOLOGY

- The prostate gland comprises three types of tissue: epithelial or glandular, stromal or smooth muscle, and capsule. Both stromal tissue and capsule are embedded with α_1-adrenergic receptors.
- The precise pathophysiologic mechanisms that cause BPH are not clear. However, both intraprostatic dihydrotestosterone (DHT) and type II 5 α-reductase are thought to be involved.
- BPH commonly results from both static (gradual enlargement of the prostate) and dynamic (agents or situations that increase α-adrenergic tone and constrict the gland's smooth muscle) factors. Examples of drugs that can exacerbate symptoms include testosterone, α-adrenergic agonists (e.g., decongestants), anticholinergics (e.g., antihistamines, phenothiazines, tricyclic antidepressants, anticholinergic antispasmodics, and anticholinergics for Parkinson's disease).

▶ CLINICAL PRESENTATION

- Patients with BPH can present with a variety of signs and symptoms. Symptoms vary over time and can improve, remain stable, or worsen spontaneously.
- Obstructive signs and symptoms result when dynamic and/or static factors reduce bladder emptying. Patients experience urinary hesitancy; urine dribbles out of the penis, and the bladder feels full even after voiding.
- Irritative signs and symptoms result from long-standing obstruction at the bladder neck. Patients experience frequency, urgency, and nocturia.
- Complications include chronic kidney disease, gross hematuria, urinary incontinence, recurrent urinary tract infection, bladder diverticula, and bladder stones.

▶ DIAGNOSIS

- Diagnosis of BPH requires a careful medical history, physical examination, objective measures of bladder emptying (e.g., peak and average urinary flow rate, postvoid residual urine volume), and laboratory tests (e.g., blood urea nitrogen [BUN] and prostate-specific antigen [PSA]).
- Medication history should include all prescription and nonprescription medications as well as dietary supplements.
- On digital rectal examination, the prostate is usually, but not always, enlarged (more than 20 g), soft, smooth, and symmetric.

TABLE 80–1. Categories of Benign Prostatic Hyperplasia Disease Severity Based on Symptoms and Signs

Disease Severity	Typical Symptoms and Signs
Mild	Asymptomatic
	Peak urinary flow rate <10 mL/s
	Postvoid residual urine volume >25–50 mL
	Increased BUN and serum creatinine
Moderate	All of the above signs plus obstructive voiding symptoms and irritative voiding symptoms (signs of detrusor instability)
Severe	All of the above plus one or more complications of BPH

BPH, benign prostatic hyperplasia; BUN, blood urea nitrogen.

▶ DESIRED OUTCOME

BPH treatment is aimed primarily at relieving manifestations of the disease that are bothersome for the patient. A secondary, but controversial, aim is to prevent serious complications in selected patients.

▶ TREATMENT

- Management options for BPH include watchful waiting, drug therapy, and surgical intervention.
- The choice depends on the severity of signs and symptoms (Table 80–1), with an emphasis on the patient's perception.

WATCHFUL WAITING

- Watchful waiting is appropriate for patients with mild disease, and for those with moderate disease with only mildly bothersome symptoms and without complications.
- Watchful waiting involves reassessment at regular 6- to 12-month intervals. Patients should be educated about behavior modification such as fluid restriction before bedtime, avoiding caffeine and alcohol, frequent emptying of the bladder, and avoiding drugs that exacerbate symptoms.

PHARMACOLOGIC THERAPY

- Pharmacologic therapy is appropriate for patients with moderately severe BPH and as an interim measure for patients with severe BPH.
- ▶ XVI Pharmacologic therapy interferes with the stimulatory effect of testosterone on prostate gland enlargement (reduces the static factor) or relaxes prostatic smooth muscle (reduces the dynamic factor) (Table 80–2).
- Two approaches are frequently used in the United States and merit separate consideration in this chapter. In general, 5α-reductase inhibitors have the advantage of decreasing prostate volume. α-Adrenergic antagonists have faster onset and are more likely to relieve symptoms. Combination therapy with both approaches is ideal for patients with severe symptoms and a prostate gland of 40 to 50 g or more.
- Agents that interfere with androgen stimulation of the prostate are not popular in the United States because of adverse effects. The luteinizing hormone-releasing hormone agonists **leuprolide** and **goserelin** cause decreased libido,

TABLE 80–2. Summary of Medical Treatment Options for Benign Prostatic Hypertrophy

Mechanism	Drug (Brand Name)	Daily Dose
Reduces static factor		
Blocks 5α-reductase enzyme	Finasteride (Proscar)	5 mg PO daily
	Dutasteride (Avodart)	0.5 mg PO daily
Blocks dihydrotestosterone at its intracellular receptor	Bicalutamide (Casodex)	50 mg PO daily
	Flutamide (Eulexin)	100–250 mg PO t.i.d.
Blocks pituitary release of luteinizing hormone	Leuprolide (Lupron)	7.5 mg IM monthly or 22.5 mg IM every 3 months
	Nafarelin	400 mcg SC daily
Blocks pituitary release of luteinizing hormone and blocks androgen receptor	Megestrol acetate	40–250 mg PO t.i.d.
Reduces dynamic factor		
Blocks α_1-adrenergic receptors in prostatic stromal tissue	Alfuzosin (UroXatral)	10 mg PO daily
	Terazosin (Hytrin)	1–10 mg PO daily
	Doxazosin (Cardura)	1–8 mg PO daily
Blocks α_{1A} receptors in the prostate	Tamsulosin (Flomax)	0.4–0.8 mg PO daily

erectile dysfunction, gynecomastia, and hot flashes. The antiandrogens **bicalutamide** and **flutamide** cause nausea, diarrhea, and hepatotoxicity.

5α-Reductase Inhibitors

- 5α-Reductase inhibitors are the only agents approved for BPH by the Food and Drug Administration (FDA) that interfere with the stimulatory effect of testosterone. These agents slow disease progression and decrease the risk of complications.
- Compared with α-adrenergic antagonists, 5α-reductase inhibitors have the disadvantages of requiring 6 months to maximally shrink an enlarged prostate, being less likely to induce objective improvement, and causing more sexual dysfunction.
- Whether the pharmacodynamic advantages of **dutasteride** confer clinical advantages over **finasteride** is unknown. Dutasteride inhibits types I and II 5 α-reductase, whereas finasteride inhibits only type II. Dutasteride more quickly and completely suppresses intraprostatic DHT (versus 80% to 90% for finasteride) and decreases serum DHT by 90% (versus 70%). XVI
- The ideal candidate has a prostate gland of 50 g or more. 5α-reductase inhibitors might also be preferred in patients with uncontrolled arrhythmias, poorly controlled angina, use of multiple antihypertensives, or inability to tolerate hypotensive effects of α-adrenergic antagonists.
- 5α-Reductase inhibitors reduce serum PSA levels by 50%. Therefore, PSA should be measured at baseline and, for monitoring purposes, subsequent measurements should be doubled.
- 5α-Reductase inhibitors are in FDA pregnancy category X and are therefore contraindicated in pregnant females. Pregnant and potentially pregnant women should not have contact with semen from men receiving 5α-reductase inhibitors.

α-Adrenergic Antagonists

- α-Adrenergic antagonists relax the smooth muscle in the prostate and bladder neck, thereby increasing urinary flow rates by 2 to 3 mL/s in 60% to 70% of patients and reducing postvoid residual urine volumes. **Terazosin** and **tamsulosin** produce durable responses for 3 to 4 years.
- α-Adrenergic antagonists do not decrease prostate volume or PSA levels.
- Terazosin, **doxazosin**, and **alfuzosin** are second-generation α-adrenergic antagonists. They antagonize peripheral vascular α_1-adrenergic receptors in addition to those in the prostate. Therefore, their adverse effects include first-dose syncope, orthostatic hypotension, and dizziness. Alfuzosin is less likely to cause cardiovascular adverse effects than other second-generation agents.
- To minimize orthostatic hypotension and first-dose syncope with terazosin and doxazosin, patients should be slowly titrated to a maintenance dose and should take these drugs at bedtime.

**Terazosin Slow
Titration Schedule**
Days 1–3: 1 mg at bedtime
Days 4–14: 2 mg at bedtime
Weeks 2–6: 5 mg at bedtime
Weeks 7 and on: 10 mg at bedtime

**Terazosin Quicker
Titration Schedule**
Days 1–3: 1 mg at bedtime
Days 4–14: 2 mg at bedtime
Weeks 2–3: 5 mg at bedtime
Weeks 4 and on: 10 mg at bedtime

- Tamsulosin, the only third-generation α-adrenergic antagonist, is selective for prostatic α_{1A} receptors. Therefore, tamsulosin does not cause peripheral vascular smooth muscle relaxation.
- Tamsulosin is a good choice for patients who cannot tolerate hypotension; have severe coronary artery disease, volume depletion, cardiac arrhythmias, severe orthostasis, or liver failure; or are taking multiple antihypertensives. Tamsulosin is also suitable for patients who want to avoid the delay of dose titration or to avoid dosing only at bedtime.
- Caution is needed to avoid potential drug interactions. Tamsulosin decreases metabolism of **cimetidine** and **diltiazem**. **Carbamazepine** and **phenytoin** increase catabolism of α-adrenergic antagonists.

SURGICAL INTERVENTION

- Prostatectomy, performed transurethrally or suprapubically, is the gold standard for treatment of patients with moderate or severe symptoms of BPH and for all patients with complications.
- Prostatectomy does not relieve irritative voiding symptoms of BPH. These patients may benefit from anticholinergic agents (see Chapter 82).

PHYTOTHERAPY

XVI

Although widely used in Europe for BPH, phytotherapy with products such as saw palmetto berry (*Serenoa repens*), stinging nettle (*Urtica dioica*), and African plum (*Pygeum africanum*) should be avoided. Studies of these herbal medicines are inconclusive, and the purity of available products is questionable.

▶ EVALUATION OF THERAPEUTIC OUTCOMES

- The primary therapeutic outcome of BPH therapy is restoring adequate urinary flow without causing adverse effects.
- Outcome depends on the patient's perception of effectiveness and acceptability of therapy. The American Urological Association Symptom Index and

International Prostate Symptom Score are validated standardized instruments that can be use to assess patient quality of life.

- Objective measures of bladder emptying (e.g., uroflowmeter and postvoid residual urine volumes) are also useful after 6 to 12 months of 5α-reductase inhibitor therapy or 3 to 4 weeks of α-adrenergic antagonist therapy.
- Laboratory tests (e.g., BUN, creatinine, PSA) and urinalysis should be monitored regularly. In addition, patients should have an annual digital rectal examination. If PSA does not decrease by 50% after 6 months of 5α-reductase inhibitor therapy, the patient should be evaluated for prostate cancer.

See Chapter 82, Management of Benign Prostatic Hyperplasia, authored by Mary Lee, for a more detailed discussion of this topic.

Chapter 81

▶ ERECTILE DYSFUNCTION

▶ DEFINITION

Erectile dysfunction (ED) is the failure to achieve a penile erection suitable for sexual intercourse. Patients often refer to it as impotence.

▶ PATHOPHYSIOLOGY

- ED can result from an abnormality in one of the four systems necessary for a normal penile erection or from a combination of abnormalities. Vascular, nervous, or hormonal etiologies of ED are referred to as organic ED. Abnormality of the fourth system (i.e., patient's psychological receptivity to sexual stimuli) is referred to as psychogenic ED.
- The penis has two corpora cavernosa, which have many interconnected sinuses that fill with blood to produce an erection. The penis also has one corpus spongiosum, which surrounds the urethra and forms the glans penis.
- Acetylcholine works with other neurotransmitters (i.e., cyclic guanylate monophosphate [cGMP], cyclic adenosine monophosphate [cAMP], vasoactive intestinal polypeptide) to produce penile arterial vasodilation and ultimately an erection.
- Causes of organic ED include diseases that compromise vascular flow to the corpora cavernosum (e.g., peripheral vascular disease, arteriosclerosis, essential hypertension), impair nerve conduction to the brain (e.g., spinal cord injury, stroke), and are associated with hypogonadism (e.g., prostate or testicular cancer, hypothalamic or pituitary disorders).
- Causes of psychogenic ED include malaise, reactive depression or performance anxiety, sedation, Alzheimer's disease, hypothyroidism, and mental disorders. Patients with psychogenic ED generally have a higher response rate to interventions than patients with organic ED.
- Social habits (e.g., cigarette smoking, excessive ethanol intake) and medications (Table 81–1) can also cause ED.

▶ CLINICAL PRESENTATION

- Signs and symptoms of ED can be difficult to detect. The patient's mate is often the first to report ED to the health care provider.
- Emotional manifestations include depression, performance anxiety, or embarrassment.
- Nonadherence to drugs thought to cause ED can be a sign of ED.

▶ DIAGNOSIS

- The diagnostic workup should be designed to identify underlying causes of ED.
- Key diagnostic assessments include ED severity, medical history, concurrent medications, physical examination, and laboratory tests (i.e., serum blood glucose, lipid profile, thyroxine level, testosterone level).
- A standardized questionnaire can be used to assess the severity of ED.

TABLE 81–1. Medication Classes That Can Cause Erectile Dysfunction

Drug Class	Proposed Mechanism of Erectile Dysfunction	Special Notes
Anticholinergic agents: antihistamines, anti-parkinsonian agents, tricyclic antidepressants, phenothiazines	Anticholinergic activity	Second-generation nonsedating antihistamines (e.g., loratadine) are not associated with erectile dysfunction. Selective serotonin reuptake inhibitor antidepressants can be substituted for tricyclic antidepressants if erectile dysfunction is a problem. Phenothiazines with fewer anticholinergic effects can be substituted in some patients it erectile dysfunction is a problem.
Dopamine agonists (e.g., metoclopramide, phenothiazines)	Inhibit prolactin inhibitory factor, thereby increasing prolactin levels	Increased prolactin levels are associated with blocking testosterone production from the testes. Depressed libido results.
Estrogens, antiandrogens (e.g., luteinizing hormone-releasing hormone superagonists, digoxin, spironolactone, ketoconazole, cimetidine)	Suppress testosterone stimulation of libido	In the face of a decreased libido, a secondary erectile dysfunction develops.
Central nervous system depressants (e.g. barbiturates, narcotics, benzodiazepines, short-term use of large doses of alcohol)	Suppress perception of psychogenic stimuli	
Agents that decrease penile blood flow (e.g., diuretics, β-adrenergic antagonists, or central sympatholytics [methyldopa, clonidine, guanethidine])	Reduce arteriolar flow to corpora	Any diuretic that produces a significant decrease in intravascular volume can decrease penile arteriolar flow. Safer antihypertensives include angiotensin-converting enzyme inhibitors, postsynaptic α_1-adrenergic antagonists (terazosin, doxazosin), calcium channel blockers, and angiotensin II antagonists.

▶ DESIRED OUTCOME

The goal of treatment is to improve the quantity and quality of penile erections suitable for intercourse.

▶ TREATMENT

- The first step in management of ED is to identify and, if possible, reverse underlying causes. Psychotherapy can be used as monotherapy for psychogenic ED or as an adjunct to specific treatments.
- Treatment options include medical devices, drugs (Table 81–2), and surgery. Although no option is ideal, the least invasive options are chosen first.

MEDICAL DEVICES

- Vacuum erection devices (VEDs) are first-line therapy for older patients. VEDs should be limited to patients who have stable sexual relations, because the onset of action is slow (i.e., approximately 30 minutes).
- To prolong the erection, the patient can also use constriction bands or tension rings, which are placed at the base of the penis to retain arteriolar blood and reduce venous outflow from the penis.
- VEDs can be used as second-line therapy after failure of oral or injectable drugs. Adding **alprostadil** to a VED improves the response rate.
- VEDs are contraindicated in patients with sickle cell disease. VEDs should be used cautiously in patients on **warfarin** because, through a poorly understood and idiosyncratic mechanism, it can cause priapism.

PHARMACOLOGIC TREATMENTS

Phosphodiesterase Inhibitors

- Phosphodiesterase decreases catabolism of cGMP, a vasodilatory neurotransmitter in the corporal tissue.
- Unless otherwise stated, general information applies to the entire class of phosphodiesterase inhibitors. **Sildenafil** is highlighted because it was the first to be marketed and is the most thoroughly studied. The newer agents **tadalafil** and **vardenafil** have different pharmacokinetic profiles (Table 81–3), drug-food interactions, and adverse effects.
- Phosphodiesterase inhibitors are selective for isoenzyme type 5 in genital tissue. Inhibition of this isoenzyme in nongenital tissues (e.g., peripheral vascular tissue, tracheal smooth muscle, and platelets) can produce adverse effects.
- Phosphodiesterase inhibitors are first-line therapy for younger patients. Sildenafil, 25–100 mg, induces satisfactory erections in 56% to 82% of patients. Approximately half of the remaining patients can have satisfactory responses after being instructed on proper use of phosphodiesterase inhibitors.
  - For the best response, patients must engage in sexual stimulation (foreplay).
  - For the fastest response, patients should take sildenafil on an empty stomach, at least 2 hours before meals. The other two agents can be taken without regard to meals.
  - For maximal absorption, patients should avoid taking sildenafil or vardenafil with a fatty meal. A fatty meal does not affect absorption of tadalafil.
  - If the first dose is not effective, patients should continue trying for 5 to 8 doses. Some patients benefit from titration up to 100 mg of sildenafil, 20 mg of vardenafil, or 20 mg of tadalafil.
- Sildenafil and vardenafil have similar pharmacokinetic profiles with a rapid onset of action and short duration. Tadalafil has a delayed onset of action and

TABLE 81-2. Dosing Regimens for Selected Drug Treatments for Erectile Dysfunction

Route of Administration	Generic Name (Brand Name)	Dosage Form	Common Dosing Regimen
Oral	Yohimbine (Aphrodyne, Yocon, Yohimex)	5.4-mg tablet or capsule	5.4 mg t.i.d
	Sildenafil (Viagra)	25-mg, 50-mg, 100-mg tablets	25–100 mg 1 hour before intercourse
	Apomorphine (Uprima)[a]	Sublingual tablets	
	Methyltestosterone (Oreton, Android)	10-mg, 25-m tablets and capsules	10–40 mg daily
	Fluoxymesterone (Halotestin)	2-mg, 5-mg, 10-mg tablets	5–20 mg daily
	Trazodone (Desyrel)[b]	50-mg, 100-mg, 150-mg, 300-mg tablets	50–150 mg daily
	Phentolamine (Spontane, Vasomax)[a]	Oral or buccal tablets	
	Vardenafil (Levitra)	2.5-mg, 5-mg, 10-mg, 20-mg tablets	5–10 mg 1 hour before intercourse
	Tadalafil (Cialis)	5-mg, 10-mg, 20-mg tablets	5–20 mg prior to intercourse
Topical	Testosterone patch (Testoderm)	4 mg/patch, 6 mg/patch	4–6 mg/day; apply to scrotum
	Testosterone patch (Testoderm TTS)	4 mg/patch, 6 mg/patch	4–6 mg/day; apply to arm, buttock, back
	Testosterone patch (Androderm)	2.5 mg/patch	2.5–5 mg/day; apply to arm, back, abdomen, thigh
	Testosterone gel (AndroGel 1%)	5 g/pkt, 10 g/pkt	5–10 g/day; apply to shoulders, upper arms, abdomen
Intramuscular	Testosterone cypionate (Depo-Testosterone)	100 mg/mL, 200 mg/mL	200–400 mg every 2–4 weeks
	Testosterone enanthate (Delatestryl)	100 mg/mL, 200 mg/mL	200–400 mg every 2–4 weeks
	Testosterone propionate	100 mg/mL	25–50 mg 2–3 times a week
Intraurethral	Alprostadil (MUSE)	125-mcg, 250-mcg, 500-mcg, 1000-mcg pellets	125–1000 mcg 5–10 minutes before intercourse
Intracavernosal	Alprostadil (Caverject)	5 mcg, 10 mcg, 20 mcg injection	2.5–60 mcg 5–10 minutes before intercourse
	Alprostadil (Edex)	5 mcg, 20 mcg, 20 mcg, 40 mcg injection	2.5–60 mcg 5–10 minutes before intercourse
	Papaverine[b]	30 mg/mL injection	Variable, usually used in combination
	Phentolamine[b]	2.5 mg/mL injection	Variable, usually used in combination

[a] Not yet commercially available in the United States at the time this chapter was written.
[b] Not FDA-approved for this use.

TABLE 81–3. Pharmacodynamics and Pharmacokinetics of Phosphodiesterase Inhibitors

	Sildenafil[a]	Vardenafil[a]	Tadalafil[a]
Trade name	Viagra	Levitra	Cialis
Inhibits PDE-5	Yes	Yes	Yes
Inhibits PDE-6	Yes	Minimally	No
Inhibits PDE-11	No	No	Yes
Time to peak plasma level (h)	0.5–1	0.7–0.9	2
Fatty meal decreases rate of oral absorption?	Yes	Yes	No
Mean plasma half-life (h)	3.7	4.4–4.8	18
Percentage of dose excreted in feces	80	91–95	61
Percentage of dose excreted in urine	13	2–6	36
Duration (h)	4	4	24–36
Usual daily dose (mg)	25–100	5–20	5–20
Daily dose in elderly patients (mg)	25	5	5–20
Daily dose in moderate renal impairment (mg)	25–100	5–20	5
Daily dose in severe renal impairment (mg)	25	5–20	5
Daily dose in mild hepatic impairment (mg)	25–100	5–20	10
Daily dose in moderate hepatic impairment (mg)	25–100	5–10	10
Daily dose in severe hepatic impairment (mg)	25	Not evaluated	Not recommended
Dose in patients taking cytochrome P450 3A4 inhibitors[a]	25 mg daily	2.5–5 mg every 24–72 hours	10 mg every 72 hours

[a]Sildenafil doses should be decreased when any potent cytochrome P450 3A4 inhibitor is used (e.g., cimetidine, erythromycin, clarithromycin, ketoconazole, itraconazole, ritonavir, and saquinavir). Vardenafil doses vary according to which agent is used (2.5 mg every 72 hours for ritonavir, 2.5 mg every 24 hours for indinavir, ketoconazole 400 mg daily, and itraconazole 400 mg daily; and 5 mg every 24 hours for ketoconazole 200 mg daily, itraconazole 200 mg daily, and erythromycin). Tadalafil doses are reduced only when it is used with the most potent cytochrome P450 3A4 inhibitors (e.g., ketoconazole or ritonavir).
PDE, phosphodiesterase.

prolonged duration. All three are metabolized by cytochrome P450 enzymes, primarily 3A4.

- Patients should avoid exceeding prescribed doses because higher doses do not improve response. Depending on the phosphodiesterase inhibitor, the dose should be reduced if the patient is elderly, has renal or hepatic impairment, or receives an inhibitor of cytochrome P450 3A4 (see Table 81–3).
- In usual doses, the most common adverse effects are headache, facial flushing, dyspepsia, nasal congestion, and dizziness.
- Sildenafil and vardenafil decrease systolic/diastolic blood pressure by 8-10/5-6 mm Hg for 1 to 4 hours after a dose. Although most patients are asymptomatic, multiple antihypertensives, **nitrates,** and baseline hypotension increase the risk of developing adverse effects. Although tadalafil does not decrease blood pressure, it should be used with caution in patients with cardiovascular disease because of the inherent risk associated with sexual activity.
- Guidelines are available for stratifying patients on the basis of their cardiovascular risk (Table 81–4).
- Sildenafil is contraindicated in patients at risk of ophthalmologic problems (e.g., retinitis pigmentosa) and should be used with caution by pilots who rely on blue and green lights to land airplanes. Sildenafil should be used cautiously

XVI

TABLE 81–4. Cardiovascular Risk Stratification of Patients Being Considered for Phosphodiesterase Inhibitors

Risk Category	Description of Patients' Conditions	Management Approach
Low	Asymptomatic cardiovascular disease Well-controlled hypertension Mild, stable angina Mild congestive heart failure (NYHA Class I)	Patient can be started on phosphodiesterase inhibitor.
Moderate	$\geq$3 risk factors for coronary artery disease Moderate, stable angina Myocardial infarction or stroke within 6 weeks Moderate congestive heart failure (NYHA Class 2)	Patient should undergo complete cardiovascular workup and treadmill stress testing to determine tolerance to increased myocardial energy consumption associated with increased sexual activity.
High	Unstable or symptomatic angina, despite treatment Poorly controlled hypertension Severe congestive heart failure (NYHA Class III or IV) Myocardial infarction or stroke within 2 weeks Moderate or severe valvular heart disease	Phosphodiesterase inhibitor is contraindicated.

NYHA = New York Heart Association.

in patients taking **aspirin** or other antiplatelet agents and in patients with bleeding tendencies.

• Tadalafil inhibits type 11 phosphodiesterase, which is thought to account for the dose-related back and muscle pain seen in 7% to 30% of patients.

• Phosphodiesterase inhibitors are contraindicated in patients taking nitrates. Phosphodiesterase inhibitors should not be administered within 4 hours of an α-adrenergic blocking agent.

Testosterone-Replacement Regimens

• **Testosterone**-replacement regimens restore serum testosterone levels to the normal range (300 to 1100 ng/dL). These regimens are indicated for symptomatic patients with hypogonadism as confirmed by low testosterone concentrations.

• Instead of directly correcting ED, testosterone-replacement regimens correct secondary ED by improving libido. Usually within days or weeks of starting therapy, they restore muscle strength and sexual drive and improve mood.

• Testosterone can be replaced orally, parenterally, or topically (see Table 81–2). Injectable regimens are preferred because they are effective, are inexpensive, and do not have the bioavailability problems or adverse hepatotoxic effects of oral regimens. Testosterone patches and gel are more expensive than other forms and should be reserved for patients who refuse injections.

• Before starting testosterone replacement, patients 40 years and older should be screened for benign prostatic hyperplasia (BPH) and prostate cancer. To ensure an adequate treatment trial, the patient should continue treatment for 2 to 3 months.

• Testosterone replacement can cause sodium retention, which can cause weight gain or exacerbate hypertension, congestive heart failure, and edema; gynecomastia; deleterious serum lipoprotein changes; and polycythemia. Exogenous testosterone can also exacerbate BPH and enhance prostate cancer growth.

XVI

- Oral testosterone-replacement regimens can cause hepatotoxicity, ranging from mildly elevated hepatic transaminases to serious liver diseases (e.g., peliosis hepatitis, hepatocellular and intrahepatic cholestasis, and benign or malignant tumors).

Alprostadil

- **Alprostadil**, or prostaglandin E_1, stimulates adenyl cyclase to increase production of cAMP, a neurotransmitter that ultimately enhances blood flow to and blood filling of the corpora.
- Alprostadil is approved as monotherapy for the management of ED. It is generally prescribed after failure of VEDs and phosphodiesterase inhibitors and for patients who cannot use these therapies. Of the available routes, the intracavernosal route is preferred over the intraurethral route because of better efficacy.

Intracavernosal Injection

- Intracavernosal alprostadil is effective in 70% to 90% of patients. However, a high proportion of patients discontinue its use because of perceived ineffectiveness; inconvenience of administration; unnatural, nonspontaneous erection; needle phobia; loss of interest; and cost of therapy.
- Intracavernosal alprostadil has been used successfully in combination with VEDs or vasoactive agents (e.g., papaverine, phentolamine, atropine) that act by different mechanisms. Phosphodiesterase inhibitors should not be added to intracavernosal alprostadil because the combination can cause prolonged erections and priapism.
- Intracavernosal alprostadil acts rapidly with an onset of 5 to 15 minutes. The duration of action is dose related and, within the usual dosage range, lasts less than 1 hour.
- The usual dose of intracavernosal alprostadil is 10 to 20 mcg up to a maximum of 60 mcg. Patients should start with 1.25 mcg, which should be increased by 1.25 to 2.50 mcg at 30-minute intervals to the lowest dose that produces a firm erection for 1 hour and does not produce adverse effects. In clinical practice, however, most patients start with 10 mcg and titrate quickly.
- To minimize the risk of complications, patients should use the lowest effective dose.
- Intracavernosal alprostadil should be injected 5 to 10 minutes before intercourse using a 0.5-inch, 27- or 30-gauge needle or an autoinjector. The maximum number of injections is one per day and three per week.
- Intracavernosal alprostadil is most commonly associated with local adverse effects, usually during the first year of therapy. Adverse events include cavernosal plaques or fibrosis at the injection site (2% to 12% of patients), penile pain (10% to 44%), and priapism (1% to 15%). Penile pain is usually mild and self-limiting, but priapism (i.e., painful, drug-induced erection lasting more than 1 hour) necessitates immediate medical attention.
- Intracavernosal injection therapy should be used cautiously in patients at risk of priapism (e.g., sickle cell disease or lymphoproliferative disorders) and bleeding complications secondary to injections.

Intraurethral Administration

- Intraurethral alprostadil, 125 to 1000 mcg, should be administered 5 to 10 minutes before intercourse. Before administration, the patient should empty his bladder and void completely. The maximum number of doses is one per day.

XVI

- Intraurethral administration is associated with pain in 24% to 32% of patients, which is usually mild and does not require discontinuation of treatment. Prolonged painful erections are rare.
- Female partners may experience vaginal burning, itching, or pain, which is probably related to transfer of alprostadil from the man's urethra to the women's vagina during intercourse.

Unapproved Agents
- Many other remedies are used, which may or may not be effective.
- Examples of other agents include **trazodone** (50 to 200 mg/day), **yohimbine** (5.4 mg three times daily), **papaverine** (7.5 to 60 mg [single agent therapy] or 0.5 to 20 mg [combination therapy] intracavernosal injection), and **phentolamine** (1 mg [combination therapy] intracavernosal injection).

SURGERY
- Surgical insertion of a penile prosthesis, the most invasive treatment for ED, is used after failure of less invasive treatments and for patients who are not candidates for other treatments.
- After a penile prosthesis is inserted, the corporal tissue is destroyed and the patient will no longer have a response to oral or intracavernosal vasoactive therapies or VEDs.

▶ EVALUATION OF THERAPEUTIC OUTCOMES

- The primary therapeutic outcomes for ED are improving the quantity and quality of penile erections suitable for intercourse and avoiding adverse drug reactions and drug interactions.
- To assess improvement, the physician should conduct specific assessments at baseline and after a trial period of 1 to 3 weeks.
- To avoid adverse effects due to excessive use, patients with unrealistic expectations should be identified and should be counseled accordingly.

See Chapter 81, Erectile Dysfunction, authored by Mary Lee, for a more detailed discussion of this topic.

XVI ◀

Chapter 82

▶ URINARY INCONTINENCE

▶ DEFINITION

Urinary incontinence (UI) is the complaint of involuntary loss of urine.

▶ PATHOPHYSIOLOGY

- The urethral sphincter, a combination of smooth and striated muscles within and external to the urethra, maintains adequate resistance to the flow of urine from the bladder until voluntary voiding is initiated. Normal bladder emptying occurs with a decrease in urethral resistance concomitant with a volitional contraction of the bladder or detrusor muscle.
- Acetylcholine is the neurotransmitter that mediates both volitional and involuntary contractions of the bladder. Bladder smooth muscle cholinergic receptors are mainly of the M_2 variety; however, M_3 receptors are responsible for both emptying contraction of normal micturition and involuntary bladder contractions, which can result in UI. Therefore, most pharmacologic antimuscarinic therapy is anti-M_3 based.
- UI occurs as a result of overfunctioning or underfunctioning of the urethra, bladder, or both.
  - Urethral underactivity is known as stress UI (SUI) and occurs during activities such as exercise, lifting, coughing, and sneezing. The urethral sphincter no longer resists the flow of urine from the bladder during periods of physical activity.
  - Bladder overactivity is known as urge UI (UUI) and is associated with increased urinary frequency, urgency, and urge incontinence. The detrusor muscle is overactive and contracts inappropriately during the filling phase.
  - Urethral overactivity and/or bladder underactivity is known as overflow incontinence. The bladder is filled to capacity but is unable to empty, causing urine to leak from a distended bladder past a normal outlet and sphincter. Common causes of urethral overactivity include benign prostatic hypertrophy (see Chapter 80); prostate cancer (see Chapter 63); and, in women, cystocele formation or surgical overcorrection after UI surgery.
  - Mixed incontinence includes the combination of bladder overactivity and urethral underactivity.
- Functional incontinence is not caused by bladder- or urethra-specific factors but rather occurs in patients with conditions such as cognitive or mobility deficits.
- Many medications can aggravate voiding dysfunction and UI (Table 83–1).

▶ CLINICAL PRESENTATION

- Signs and symptoms of UI depend on the underlying pathophysiology (Table 83–2). Patients with SUI generally complain of urinary leakage with physical activity, whereas those with UUI complain of nocturia and nocturnal incontinence.
- Urethral overactivity and/or bladder underactivity is a rare, but important, cause of UI. Patients complain of lower abdominal fullness, hesitancy, straining to void, decreased force of stream, interrupted stream, and sense of incomplete bladder emptying. Patients can also have urinary frequency, urgency, and abdominal pain.

TABLE 82–1. Medications Influencing Lower Urinary Tract Function

Medication	Effect
Diuretics	Polyuria, frequency, urgency
α-Receptor antagonists	Urethral relaxation and SUI in women
α-Receptor agonists	Urethral constriction and urinary retention in men
Calcium channel blockers	Urinary retention
Narcotic analgesics	Urinary retention from impaired contractility
Sedative hypnotics	Functional incontinence caused by delirium, immobility
Antipsychotics	Anticholinergic effects and urinary retention
Anticholinergics	Urinary retention
Antidepressants, tricyclic	Anticholinergic effects, α-agonist effects
Alcohol	Polyuria, frequency, urgency, sedation, delirium
Angiotensin-converting enzyme inhibitors (ACEIs)	Cough as a result of ACEI can aggravate SUI by increasing intra-abdominal pressure

SUI = stress urinary incontinence.

▶ DIAGNOSIS

- Patients should undergo complete medical history with assessment of symptoms, physical examination (i.e., abdominal examination to exclude distended bladder, pelvic examination in women looking for evidence of prolapse or hormonal deficiency, and genital and prostate examination in men), and brief neurologic assessment of the perineum and lower extremities.
- For SUI, the preferred diagnostic test is observation of urethral meatus while the patient coughs or strains.
- For UUI, the preferred diagnostic tests are urodynamic studies. Urinalysis and urine culture should be performed to rule out urinary tract infection.
- For urethral overactivity and/or bladder underactivity, digital rectal exam or transrectal ultrasound should be performed to rule out prostate enlargement. Renal function tests should be performed to rule out renal failure.

▶ DESIRED OUTCOME

The goal of therapy is to decrease the signs and symptoms of most distress to the patient.

TABLE 82–2. Differentiating Bladder Overactivity from Urethral Underactivity

Symptoms	Bladder Overactivity	Urethral Underactivity
Urgency	Yes	Sometimes
Frequency with urgency	Yes	Rarely
Leaking during physical activity	No	Yes
Amount of urinary leakage with *each episode* of incontinence	Large if present	Usually small
Ability to reach the toilet in time following an urge to void	No or just barely	Yes
Nocturnal incontinence	Yes	Rare
Nocturia	Usually	Seldom

XVI

▶ TREATMENT

NONPHARMACOLOGIC TREATMENT

- Nonpharmacologic treatment (e.g., life-style modifications, scheduling regimens, pelvic floor muscle rehabilitation) is the chief form of UI management at the primary care level.
- Surgery rarely plays a role in the initial management of UI but can be required for secondary complications (e.g., skin breakdown or infection). Otherwise, the decision to surgically treat symptomatic UI requires that lifestyle compromise warrants an elective operation and that nonoperative therapy be proven undesirable or ineffective.

PHARMACOLOGIC TREATMENT

- The choice of pharmacologic therapy (Table 82–3) depends on the type of UI.
- Pharmacologic therapies should be combined with nonpharmacologic therapies.

Stress Urinary Incontinence (SUI)

The goal of treatment of SUI is to improve urethral closure by stimulating α-adrenergic receptors in the smooth muscle of the bladder neck and proximal urethra, enhancing supportive structures underlying the urethral epithelium, or enhancing serotonin and norepinephrine effects in the micturition reflex pathways.

Estrogens

- Historically, local and systemic **estrogens** have been the mainstays of pharmacologic management of SUI.
- In open trials, estrogens were administered orally, intramuscularly, vaginally, or transdermally. Regardless of the route, estrogens exerted variable effects on urodynamic parameters, such as maximum urethral closure pressure, functional urethral length, and pressure transmission ratio.
- Results of four placebo-controlled comparative trials have not been as favorable, finding no significant clinical or urodynamic effect for oral estrogen compared with placebo.

α-Receptor Agonists

- Many open trials support the use of a variety of α-receptor agonists in SUI. Combining an α-receptor agonist with an estrogen yields somewhat superior clinical and urodynamic responses compared with monotherapy with either agent alone.
- Contraindications to α-receptor agonists include hypertension, tachyarrhythmias, coronary artery disease, myocardial infarction, cor pulmonale, hyperthyroidism, renal failure, and narrow-angle glaucoma.

Duloxetine

- **Duloxetine**, a dual inhibitor of serotonin and norepinephrine reuptake indicated for depression and painful diabetic neuropathy, is expected to become first-line therapy for SUI. Duloxetine is thought to facilitate the bladder-to-sympathetic reflex pathway, increasing urethral and external urethral sphincter muscle tone during the storage phase.
- Six placebo-controlled studies showed that duloxetine reduces incontinent episode frequency and the number of daily micturitions, increases micturition interval, and improves quality-of-life scores. These benefits were statistically significant but clinically modest.

TABLE 82–3. Pharmacotherapeutic Options in Patients with Urinary Incontinence

Drug Class	Drug Therapy (Usual Dose)	Comments
Overactive bladder		
Anticholinergic agents/antispasmodics	Oxybutynin IR (2.5–5 mg bid-qid), oxybutynin XL (5–30 mg daily), oxybutynin TDS (3.9 mg/day) (apply 1 patch twice weekly), tolterodine IR (1–2 mg twice a day), tolterodine LA (2–4 mg daily), trospium chloride 20 mg twice a day, solifenacin 5–10 mg daily, darifenacin 7.5–15 mg daily[a]	First-line drug therapy (oxybutynin or tolterodine are preferred).
Tricyclic antidepressants (TCAs)	Imipramine, doxepin, nortriptyline, or desipramine (25–100 mg at bedtime)	Generally reserved for patients with an additional indication (e.g., depression, neuralgia).
Topical estrogen (only in women with urethritis or vaginitis)	Conjugated estrogen 0.5 g vaginal cream three times per week for up to 8 months. Repeat course if symptom recurrence. Or use estradiol vaginal insert/ring [2 mg (1 ring)] and replace after 90 days if needed.	Marginally effective. Few adverse effects with cream and vaginal insert.
Stress		
α–Adrenergic agonists	Pseudoephedrine (15–60 mg tid) with food, water, or milk	First-line therapy for women with no contraindication (notably hypertension). (Second-line once duloxetine is approved). Somewhat less-effective alternative to pseudoephedrine.
Estrogen	See estrogens (above). Works best if urethritis or vaginitis are present.	Combined pseudoephedrine and estrogen somewhat more effective than pseudoephedrine alone in postmenopausal women.
Dual serotonin–norepinephrine reuptake inhibitors	Duloxetine[a] 40–80 mg/day (1 or 2 doses)	Once approved, will become first-line therapy. Most adverse events diminish with time, so support patient during initial use.
Overflow (atonic bladder)		
Cholinomimetics	Bethanechol (25–50 mg tid or qid) on empty stomach	Avoid use if patient has asthma or heart disease. Short-term use only. Never give IV or IM because of life-threatening cardiovascular and severe gastrointestinal reactions.

IR, immediate-release; LA, long-acting; XL, extended-release; TDS, transdermal system.
[a]Investigational. Doses provided are those best supported by clinical trials to date.

- To avoid drug interactions, clinicians should be careful when administering duloxetine with substrates or inhibitors of cytochrome P450 (CYP450) isoenzymes 2D6 and 1A2.
- The adverse-event profile might make adherence problematic. Adverse events include nausea, headache, insomnia, constipation, dry mouth, dizziness, fatigue, somnolence, vomiting, and diarrhea.

Urge Urinary Incontinence (UUI)

The pharmacotherapy of first choice for UUI is anticholinergic/antispasmodic drugs, which antagonize muscarinic cholinergic receptors.

Oxybutynin

- **Oxybutynin immediate-release** (IR) has been the drug of first choice for UUI and the "gold standard" against which other drugs are compared. Financial considerations favor generic oxybutynin IR.
- Approximately 25% of patients discontinue oxybutynin IR because of adverse effects due to antimuscarinic effects (e.g., dry mouth, constipation, vision impairment, confusion, cognitive dysfunction, and tachycardia), α-adrenergic inhibition (e.g., orthostatic hypotension), and histamine H_1 inhibition (e.g., sedation, and weight gain).
- Oxybutynin IR is best tolerated when the dose is gradually escalated from less than or equal to 2.5 mg twice daily to 2.5 mg three times daily after 1 month. Oxybutynin IR can be further increased in 2.5-mg/day increments every 1 to 2 months until the desired response, maximum recommended dose of 5 mg three times daily, or maximum tolerated dose is attained.
- **Oxybutynin extended-release** (XL) is better tolerated than oxybutynin IR and is as effective in reducing the number of UI episodes, restoring continence, decreasing the number of micturitions per day, and increasing urine volume voided per micturition. Oxybutynin XL has some efficacy and safety advantages over **tolterodine long-acting** (LA); however, these findings are based on open-label studies.
- The maximum benefit of oxybutynin XL is not realized for up to 4 weeks after starting therapy or escalating the dose.
- **Oxybutynin transdermal system** (TDS) is better tolerated than oxybutynin IR presumably because this route avoids first-pass metabolism in the liver, which generates the metabolite thought to cause adverse events, especially dry mouth.

Tolterodine

- Tolterodine, a competitive muscarinic receptor antagonist is considered first-line therapy in patients with urinary frequency, urgency, or urge incontinence.
- Controlled studies demonstrate that tolterodine is more effective than placebo and as effective as oxybutynin IR in decreasing the number of daily micturitions and increasing the volume voided per micturition. However, most studies have not shown a decrease in the number of daily UI episodes as compared with placebo.
- Tolterodine undergoes hepatic metabolism involving CYP450 2D6 and 3A4 isoenzymes. Therefore, elimination can be impaired by CYP450 3A4 inhibitors including **fluoxetine, sertraline, fluvoxamine**, macrolide antibiotics, imidazoles, and grapefruit juice.
- Tolterodine's most common adverse effects are dry mouth, dyspepsia, headache, constipation, and dry eyes. Tolterodine is better tolerated than oxybutynin IR, and dry mouth occurs less often with tolterodine LA than with tolterodine IR.

Other Pharmacologic Therapies for UUI

- **Trospium chloride**, a quaternary ammonium anticholinergic, is superior to placebo and is equivalent to oxybutynin IR and tolterodine IR. However, clinical studies are limited by their focus on cystometric rather than clinical endpoints, small absolute benefits compared with placebo, and lack of comparisons with LR formulations.

- Trospium chloride causes the expected anticholinergic adverse effects. The positive electrical charge could prevent trospium chloride from crossing the blood-brain barrier, but there are no data supporting the hypothesis that the drug is less neurotoxic than non-quaternary ammonium anticholinergics.

- **Solifenacin succinate** and **darifenacin** are antagonists of M_1, M_2, and M_3 muscarinic cholinergic receptors. These antagonists do not offer significant advances over other anticholinergics despite being "uroselective" in preclinical studies. Both behave like nonselective anticholinergic in humans, causing dry mouth and other anticholinergic effects.

- Drug interactions are possible if CYP450 inhibitors are given with solifenacin succinate (metabolized by 3A4 isoenzyme) or darifenacin (metabolized by 2D6 and 3A4 isoenzymes).

- Other agents including tricyclic antidepressants, **propantheline, flavoxate, hyoscyamine**, and **dicyclomine hydrochloride** are less effective, not safer, or have not been adequately studied.

- Patients with UUI and elevated postvoid residual urine volume should be treated by intermittent self-catheterization along with frequent voiding between catheterizations.

Overflow Incontinence

Overflow incontinence secondary to benign or malignant prostatic hyperplasia may be amenable to pharmacotherapy (see Chapters 63 and 80).

▶ EVALUATION OF THERAPEUTIC OUTCOMES

- Total elimination of UI signs and symptoms may not be possible. Therefore, realistic goals should be established for therapy.

- In the long-term management of UI, the clinical symptoms of most distress to the individual patient need to be monitored.

- Survey instruments used in UI research along with quantitating the use of ancillary supplies (e.g., pads) can be used in clinical monitoring.

- Therapies for UI frequently have nuisance adverse effects, which need to be carefully elicited. Adverse effects can necessitate drug dosage adjustments, use of alternative strategies (e.g., chewing sugarless gum, sucking on hard sugarless candy, or use of saliva substitutes for xerostomia), or even drug discontinuation.

See Chapter 83, Urinary Incontinence, authored by Eric S. Rovner, Jean Wyman, Thomas Lackner, and David Guay, for a more detailed discussion of this topic.

XVI ◀

Appendix 1

▶ ALLERGIC AND PSEUDOALLERGIC DRUG REACTIONS

TABLE A1–1. Classification of Allergic Drug Reactions

Type	Descriptor	Characteristics	Typical Onset	Drug Causes
I	Anaphylactic (IgE mediated)	Allergen binds to IgE on basophils or mast cells resulting in release of inflammatory medicators	Within 30 min	Penicillin immediate reaction Blood products Polypeptide hormones Vaccines Dextran
II	Cytotoxic	Cell destruction occurs because of cell-associated antigen that initiates cytolysis by antigen-specific antibody (IgG or IgM). Most often involves blood elements.	Typically 5–12 h	Penicillin, quinidine, phenylbutazone, thiouracils, sulfonamides, methyldopa
III	Immune complex	Antigen–antibody complexes form and deposit on blood vessel walls and activate complement. Result is a serum-sickness-like syndrome.	3–8 h	May be caused by penicillins, sulfonamides, radiocontrast agents, hydantoins
IV	Cell mediated (delayed)	Antigens cause activation of lymphocytes, which release inflammatory mediators.	24–48 h	Tuberculin reaction

TABLE A1–2. Top 10 Drugs or Agents Reported to Cause Skin Reactions

	Reactions per 1000 Recipients
Amoxicillin	51.4
Trimethoprim-sulfamethoxazole	33.8
Ampicillin	33.2
Iopodate	27.8
Blood	21.6
Cephalosporins	21.1
Erythromycin	20.4
Dihydralazine hydrochloride	19.1
Penicillin G	18.5
Cyanocobalamin	17.9

TABLE A1–3. Procedure for Performing Penicillin Skin Testing

A. Percutaneous (prick) skin testing

Materials	Volume
Pre-Pen 6 × 10⁶M	1 drop
Penicillin G 10,000 U/mL	1 drop
β-Lactam drug 3 mg/mL	1 drop
0.03% albumin-saline control	1 drop
Histamine control (1 mg/mL)	1 drop

1. Place a drop of each test material on the volar surface of the forearm.
2. Prick the skin with a sharp needle inserted through the drop at a 45° angle gently tenting the skin in an upward motion.
3. Interpret skin responses after 15 min.
4. A wheal at least 2 × 2 mm with erythema is considered positive.
5. If the prick test is nonreactive, proceed to the intradermal test.
6. If the histamine control is nonreactive, the test is considered uninterpretable.

B. Intradermal skin testing

Materials	Volume
Pre-Pen 6 × 10⁶M	0.02 mL
Penicillin G 10,000 U/mL	0.02 mL
β-Lactam drug 3 mg/mL	0.02 mL
0.03% albumin-saline control	0.02 mL
Histamine control (0.1 mg/mL)	0.02 mL

1. Inject 0.02–0.03 mL of each test material intradermally (amount sufficient to produce a small bleb).
2. Interpret skin responses after 15 min.
3. A wheal at least 6 × 6 mm with erythema and at least 3 mm greater than the negative control is considered positive.
4. If the histamine control is nonreactive, the test is considered uninterpretable.

Antihistamines may blunt the response and cause false-negative reactions.

From Sullivan TJ. Current Therapy in Allergy. St Louis, Mosby, 1985:57–61.

TABLE A1–4. Treatment of Anaphylaxis

1. Place patient in recumbent position and elevate extremities.
2. Monitor vital signs often (or continuously if possible).
3. Apply tourniquet proximal to site of antigen injection; remove every 10–15 min.
4. Administer epinephrine 1:1000 into nonoccluded site: 0.3–0.5 mL subcutaneously or intramuscularly in adults and 0.01 mL/kg subcutaneously or intramuscularly in children.
5. Administer aqueous epinephrine 1:1000 into site of antigen injection; 0.15–0.25 mL subcutaneously in adults and 0.005 mL/kg subcutaneously in children.
6. Establish and maintain airway with oropharyngeal airway device, endotracheal intubation, transtracheal catheterization, or cricothyrotomy.
7. Administer oxygen at 6–10 L/min.
8. Institute rapid fluid replacement with 0.9% sodium chloride, lactated Ringer's, or colloid solution (e.g., 5% albumin or 4% hetastarch).
9. For hypotension in adults, administer norepinephrine, 32 mcg/min (use 8 mg in 500 mL dextrose 5%) with the rate adjusted to maintain low-normal blood pressure. Alternatively, administer dopamine at 2–10 mcg/kg/min intravenously.
10. If refractory hypotension is present, administer cimetidine 300 mg or ranitidine 50 mg, intravenously over 3–5 min.
11. If bronchospasm is present, administer aminophylline 6 mg/kg intravenously over 20 min.
12. Administer hydrocortisone sodium succinate 100 mg intravenously (push) and 100 mg intravenously in saline every 2–4 h to block the late-phase reaction.
13. Administer diphenhydramine 1–2 mg/kg intravenously (push) (up to 50 mg) over 3 min to block histamine-1 receptors.
14. For adults taking a β-adrenergic blocker, administer atropine (0.5 mg intravenously) every 5 min until heart rate is greater than 60 beats/min, or isoproterenol 2–20 mcg/min intravenously titrated to heart rate of 60 beats/min, or glucagon 0.5 mg/kg intravenously (push) followed by 0.07 mg/kg/h continuously intravenously.

From Weiss ME, Adkinson NF, Clin Allergy 1988;18:515–540.

TABLE A1–5. Protocol for Oral Desensitization

Step[a]	Phenoxymethyl Penicillin			
	Concentration (units/mL)	Volume (mL)	Dose (units)	Cumulative Dose (units)
1	1000	0.1	100	100
2	1000	0.2	200	300
3	1000	0.4	400	700
4	1000	0.8	800	1500
5	1000	1.6	1600	3100
6	1000	3.2	3200	6300
7	1000	6.4	6400	12,700
8	10,000	1.2	12,000	24,700
9	10,000	2.4	24,000	48,700
10	10,000	4.8	48,000	96,700
11	80,000	1.0	80,000	176,700
12	80,000	2.0	160,000	336,700
13	80,000	4.0	320,000	656,700
14	80,000	8.0	640,000	1,296,700
Observe for 30 min				
15	500,000	0.25	125,000	
16	500,000	0.5	250,000	
17	500,000	1.0	500,000	
18	500,000	2.25	1,125,000	

[a]The interval between steps is 15 min.

Appendices

TABLE A1–6. Parenteral Desensitization Protocol

Injection No.	Benzylpenicillin Concentration (units)	Volume (mL)	(Route)
1[a,b]	100	0.1	ID
2	100	0.2	SC
3	100	0.4	SC
4	100	0.8	SC
5[b]	1000	0.1	ID
6	1000	0.3	SC
7	1000	0.6	SC
8[b]	10,000	0.1	ID
9	10,000	0.2	SC
10	10,000	0.4	SC
11	10,000	0.8	SC
12[b]	100,000	0.1	ID
13	100,000	0.3	SC
14	100,000	0.6	SC
15[b]	1,000,000	0.1	ID
16	1,000,000	0.2	SC
17	1,000,000	0.2	IM
18	1,000,000	0.4	IM
19	Continuous IV infusion at 1,000,000 units/h		

[a]Administer doses at intervals of not less than 20 min.
[b]Observe and record skin wheal-and-flare response.

See Chapter 86, Allergic and Pseudoallergic Drug Reactions, authored by Joseph T. Dipiro and Dennis R. Ownby, for a more detailed discussion of this topic.

Appendix 2

▶ DRUG-INDUCED HEMATOLOGIC DISORDERS

TABLE A2–1. Drugs Associated with Aplastic Anemia

Observational study evidence	Case report evidence ("probable" or "definite" causality rating)
Carbamazepine	Acetazolamide
Diclofenac	Aspirin
Furosemide	Captopril
Gold salts	Chloramphenicol
Indomethacin	Chloroquine
Methimazole	Chlorothiazide
Oxyphenbutazone	Chlorpromazine
Penicillamine	Dapsone
Phenobarbital	Felbamate
Phenothiazines	Interferon-alfa
Phenytoin	Lisinopril
Propylthiouracil	Lithium
Sulfonamides	Pentoxifylline
Tocainide	Quinidine
	Sulindac
	Ticlopidine

TABLE A2–2. Drugs Associated with Agranulocytosis

Observational study evidence	Case report evidence ("probable" or "definite" causality rating)
β-Lactam antibiotics	Acetaminophen
Carbamazepine	Acetazolamide
Carbimazole	Captopril
Clomipramine	Chloramphenicol
Digoxin	Chlorpropamide
Dipyridamole	Chlorpheniramine
Ganciclovir	Clindamycin
Glyburide	Clozapine
Gold salts	Colchicine
Imipenem-cilastatin	Dapsone
Indomethacin	Desipramine
Macrolide antibiotics	Ethacrynic acid
Methimazole	Ethosuximide
Mirtazapine	Gentamicin
Phenobarbital	Griseofulvin
Phenothiazines	Hydralazine
Phenytoin	Hydroxychloroquine
Prednisone	Imipramine
Procainamide	Levodopa
Propranolol	Meprobamate
Propylthiouracil	Methazolamide
Spironolactone	Methyldopa
Sulfonamides	Metronidazole
Sulfonylureas	NSAIDs
Ticlopidine	Olanzapine
Valproic acid	Penicillamine
Zidovudine	Pentazocine
	Primidone
	Pyrimethamine
	Quinine
	Rifampin
	Streptomycin
	Terbinafine
	Tocainide
	Tolbutamide
	Vancomycin

NSAID, nonsteroidal anti-inflammatory drug.

TABLE A2–3. Drugs Associated with Hemolytic Anemia

Observational study evidence	Levofloxacin
Phenobarbital	Methyldopa
Phenytoin	Minocycline
	NSAIDs
Case report evidence ("probable"	Omeprazole
or "definite" causality rating)	*p*-Aminosalicylic acid
Acetaminophen	Phenazopyridine
Angiotensin-coverting enzyme inhibitors	Probenecid
β-Lactam antibiotics	Procainamide
Cephalosporins	Quinidine
Ciprofloxacin	Rifabutin
Erythromycin	Rifampin
Hydrochlorothiazide	Streptomycin
Indinavir	Sulfonamides
Interferon-alfa	Sulfonylureas
Ketoconazole	Tacrolimus
Lansoprazole	Tolbutamide
Levodopa	Tolmetin
	Triamterene

NSAID, nonsteroidal anti-inflammatory drug.

TABLE A2–4. Drugs Associated with Oxidative Hemolytic Anemia

Observational study evidence
Dapsone
Case report evidence ("probable" or "definite" causality rating)
Ascorbic acid
Metformin
Methylene blue
Nalidixic acid
Nitrofurantoin
Phenazopyridine
Primaquine
Sulfacetamide
Sulfamethoxazole
Sulfanilamide

TABLE A2–5. Drugs Associated with Megaloblastic Anemia

Case report evidence ("probable" or	Methotrexate
"definite" causality rating)	Oral contraceptives
Azathioprine	*p*-Aminosalicylate
Chloramphenicol	Phenobarbital
Colchicine	Phenytoin
Cyclophosphamide	Primidone
Cytarabine	Pyrimethamine
5-Fluorodeoxyuridine	Sulfasalazine
5-Fluorouracil	Tetracycline
Hydroxyurea	Vinblastine
6-Mercaptopurine	

TABLE A2–6. Drugs Associated with Thrombocytopenia

Observational study evidence
Carbamazepine
Phenobarbital
Phenytoin
Valproic acid

Case report evidence ("probable" or "definite" causality rating)
Abciximab
Acetaminophen
Acyclovir
Albendazole
Aminoglutethimide
Aminosalicylic acid
Aminodarone
Amphotericin B
Ampicillin
Aspirin
Atorvastatin
Captopril
Chlorothiazide
Chlorpromazine
Chlorpropamide
Cimetidine
Clarithromycin
Clopidogrel
Danazol
Deferoxamine
Diazepam
Diazoxide
Diclofenac
Diethylstilbestrol
Digoxin
Ethambutol
Felbamate
Fluconazole
Gold salts
Haloperidol
Heparin
Hydrochlorothiazide
Ibuprofen
Inamrinone
Indinavir

Indomethacin
Interferon-alfa
Isoniazid
Isotretinoin
Itraconazole
Levamisole
Linezolid
Lithium
Low-molecular-weight heparins
Measles, mumps, and rubella vaccine
Meclofenamate
Mesalamine
Methyldopa
Minoxidil
Morphine
Nalidixic acid
Naphazoline
Naproxen
Nitroglycerin
Octreotide
Oxacillin
p-Aminosalicylic acid
Penicillamine
Pentoxifylline
Piperacillin
Primidone
Procainamide
Pyrazinamide
Quinidine
Quinine
Ranitidine
Recombinant hepatitis B vaccine
Rifampin
Simvastatin
Sirolimus
Sulfasalazine
Sulfonamide antibiotics
Sulindac
Tamoxifen
Tolmetin
Trimethoprim
Vancomycin

See Chapter 102, Drug-Induced Hematologic Disorders, authored by S. Jay Weaver and Thomas E. Johns, for a more detailed discussion of this topic.

Appendix 3

▶ DRUG-INDUCED LIVER DISEASE

TABLE A3–1. An Approach to Evaluating a Suspected Hepatotoxic Reaction Using a Clinical Diagnostic Scale

Patient presents with elevated liver enzymes	Score	Component subscore
Literature		
Literature supports this drug (drug combination) and pattern of liver enzyme elevation	+2	
No literature supports this, but the drug has been on the market for less than 5 yr	+0	———
No literature supports this and the drug has been on the market for 5 yr or more	−3	
Alternative causes		
Alternative causes (i.e., viral, alcohol, etc.) are completely ruled out	+3	
Alternative causes are partially ruled out	+0	———
Alternative causes cannot be ruled out and are possible or even probable	−1	
Presentation		
The presentation includes 4 or more extrahepatic (fever, malaise, etc.) symptoms	+3	
The presentation includes 2–3 extrahepatic symptoms	+2	
The presentation includes only 1 identifiable extrahepatic symptom	+1	———
The presentation is essentially a laboratory abnormality, with no extrahepatic symptoms	+0	
Temporality		
Initiation of drug therapy to onset is 4–56 days	+3	
Initiation of drug therapy to onset is <4 or >56 days	+1	
Discontinuance of therapy to onset is 0–7 days	+3	
Discontinuance of therapy to onset is 8–15 days	+0	———
Discontinuance of therapy to onset is > 15 days	−1	
Rechallenge		
Rechallenge was positive	+3	———
Rechallenge was negative or not attempted	+0	
Total Score		

Note: The likelihood that this presentation is an adverse reaction in the liver increases linearly with an increasing score. The maximum score is 14, and scores below 7 are associated with an ever-decreasing likelihood that the drug or drug combination in question caused the problem. This approach is not designed for the assessment of hepatic cancers or cirrhotic conditions.

TABLE A3–2. Environmental Hepatotoxins and Associated Occupations at Risk for Exposure

Hepatotoxin	Associated Occupations at Risk for Exposure
Arsenic	Chemical plant, construction, agricultural workers
Carbon tetrachloride	Chemical plant workers, laboratory technicians
Copper	Plumbers, outdoor sculpture artists, copper foundry workers
Dimethylforamide	Chemical plant workers, laboratory technicians
2,4-Dichlorophenoxyacetic acid	Horticulturists
Fluorine	Chemical plant workers, laboratory technicians
Toluene	Chemical plant, agricultural workers, laboratory technicians
Trichloroethylene	Printers, dye workers, cleaners, laboratory technicians
Vinyl chloride	Plastics plant workers, also found as a river pollutant

TABLE A3–3. Relative Patterns of Hepatic Enzyme Elevation versus Type of Hepatic Lesion

Enzyme	Abbreviations	Necrotic	Cholestatic	Chronic
Alkaline phosphatase	Alk Phos, AP	↑	↑↑↑	↑
5′-Nucleotidase	5-NC, 5NC	↑	↑↑↑	↑
γ-Glutamyltransferase	GGT, GGTP	↑	↑↑↑	↑↑
Aspartate aminotransferase	AST, SGOT	↑↑↑	↑	↑↑
Alanine aminotransferase	ALT, SGPT	↑↑↑	↑	↑↑
Lactate dehydrogenase	LDH	↑↑↑	↑	↑

↑, <100% of normal; ↑↑, >100% of normal; ↑↑↑, >200% of normal.

TABLE A3–4. An Approach to Determining a Drug Monitoring Plan to Detect Hepatotoxicity

The patient is to be started on a drug that may cause a hepatotoxic reaction
↓
Is the patient pregnant?
Is the patient more than 60 yr old?
Is the patient exposed to an environmental hepatotoxin at work or at home?
Is the patient drinking more than one alcoholic beverage per day or binging on weekends?
Is the patient using any injected recreational drug?
Is the patient using herbal remedies or tisanes that are associated with hepatic damage?
Is the patient's diet deficient in magnesium, vitamin E, vitamin C, or α- or β-carotenes?
Is the patient's diet excessive in vitamin A, iron, or selenium?
Does the patient have hypertriglyceridemia or type 2 diabetes mellitus?
Does the patient have juvenile arthritis or systemic lupus erythematosus?
Is the patient HIV-positive, have AIDS, or is on reverse transcriptase inhibitors?
Does the patient have chronic or chronic remitting viral hepatitis (hepatitis B or C)?
↓
Draw a baseline set of blood samples for liver enzymes, bilirubin, albumin, and transferrin before
beginning the drug
↓
Does the patient have more than two risk factors?
Is the drug identified as one that may cause a predictable hepatotoxic reaction?[a]

↓ Yes	↓ No
Redraw liver enzymes every 60–90 days depending on the drug for the first year	Redraw liver enzymes if other signs or symptoms manifest

If no toxicity is manifested during the first year of therapy, then redraw liver enzymes every 6–12 months;
assess liver for cirrhosis every 1–2 yr by ultrasound and every 4–6 yr by CT or MRI scan; biopsy as directed
by other findings

[a]A drug can become a predictable risk if it is administered concurrently with another drug or food that is known to induce or inhibit its metabolism.

See Chapter 38, Drug-Inuced Liver Disease, authored by William R. Kirchain and Mark A. Gil, for a more detailed discussion of this topic.

Appendix 4

▶ DRUG-INDUCED PULMONARY DISORDERS

TABLE A4–1. Drugs That Induce Apnea

Central Nervous System Depression	
Narcotic analgesics	F[a]
Barbiturates	F
Benzodiazepines	F
Other sedatives and hypnotics	I
Tricyclic antidepressants	R
Phenothiazines	R
Ketamine	R
Promazine	R
Anesthetics	R
Antihistamines	R
Alcohol	I
Fenfluramine	R
L-Dopa	R
Oxygen	R
Respiratory Muscle Dysfunction	
Aminoglycoside antibiotics	I
Polymyxin antibiotics	I
Neuromuscular blockers	I
Quinine	R
Digitalis	R
Myopathy	
Corticosteroids	F
Diuretics	I
Aminocaproic acid	R
Clofibrate	R

[a]Relative frequency of reactions: F, frequent; I, infrequent; R, rare.

Appendices

TABLE A4–2. Drugs That Induce Bronchospasm

Anaphylaxis (IgE-Mediated)		Anaphylactoid Mast-Cell Degranulation	
Penicillins	F[a]	Narcotic analgesics	I
Sulfonamides	F	Ethylenediamine	R
Serum	F	Iodinated-radiocontrast media	F
Cephalosporins	F	Platinum	R
Bromelin	R	Local anesthetics	I
Cimetidine	R	Steroidal anesthetics	I
Papain	F	Iron–dextran complex	I
Pancreatic extract	I	Pancuronium bromide	R
Psyllium	I	Benzalkonium chloride	I
Subtilase	I	**Pharmacologic Effects**	
Tetracyclines	I	β-Adrenergic receptor blockers	I–F
Allergen extracts	I	Cholinergic stimulants	I
L-Asparaginase	F	Anticholinesterases	R
Pyrazolone analgesics	I	α-Adrenergic agonists	R
Direct Airway Irritation		Ethylenediamine tetraacetic acid (EDTA)	R
Acetate	R	**Unknown Mechanisms**	
Bisulfite	F	ACE inhibitors	I
Cromolyn	R	Anticholinergics	R
Smoke	F	Hydrocortisone	R
N-Acetylcysteine	F	Isoproterenol	R
Inhaled steroids	I	Monosodium glutamate	I
Precipitating IgG Antibodies		Piperazine	R
α-Methyldopa	R	Tartrazine	R
Carbamazepine	R	Sulfinpyrazone	R
Spiramycin	R	Zinostatin	R
Cyclooxygenase Inhibition		Losartan	R
Aspirin/NSAIDs	F		
Phenylbutazone	I		
Acetaminophen	R		

[a]Relative frequency of reactions: F, frequent; I, infrequent; R, rare.

TABLE A4–3. Tolerance of Anti-inflammatory and Analgesic Drugs in Aspirin-Induced Asthma

Cross-Reactive Drugs	Drugs With No Cross-Reactivity
Diclofenac	Acetaminophen[a]
Diflunisal	Benzydamine
Fenoprofen	Chloroquine
Flufenamic acid	Choline salicylate
Flurbiprofen	Corticosteroids
Hydrocortisone hemisuccinate	Dextropropoxyphene
Ibuprofen	Phenacetin[a]
Indomethacin	Salicylamide
Ketoprofen	Sodium salicylate
Mefenamic acid	
Naproxen	
Noramidopyrine	
Oxyphenbutazone	
Phenylbutazone	
Piroxicam	
Sulindac	
Sulfinpyrazone	
Tartrazine	
Tolmetin	

[a]A very small percentage (5%) of aspirin-sensitive patients react to acetaminophen and phenacetin.

TABLE A4–4. Drugs That Induce Pulmonary Edema

Cardiogenic Pulmonary Edema

Excessive intravenous fluids	F[a]
Blood and plasma transfusions	F
Corticosteroids	F
Phenylbutazone	R
Sodium diatrizoate	R
Hypertonic intrathecal saline	R
β_2-Adrenergic agonists	I

Noncardiogenic Pulmonary Edema

Heroin	F
Methadone	I
Morphine	I
Oxygen	I
Propoxyphene	R
Ethchlorvynol	R
Chlordiazepoxide	R
Salicylate	R
Hydrochlorothiazide	R
Triamterene + hydrochlorothiazide	R
Leukoagglutinin reactions	R
Iron–dextran complex	R
Methotrexate	R
Cytosine arabinoside	R
Nitrofurantoin	R
Dextran 40	R
Fluorescein	R
Amitriptyline	R
Colchicine	R
Nitrogen mustard	R
Epinephrine	R
Metaraminol	R
Bleomycin	R
Iodide	R
Cyclophosphamide	R
VM-26	R

[a]Relative frequency of reactions: F, frequent; I, infrequent; R, rare.

TABLE A4–5. Drugs That Induce Pulmonary Infiltrates with Eosinophilia (Loeffler's Syndrome)

Nitrofurantoin	F[a]	Tetracycline	R
para-Aminosalicylic acid	F	Procarbazine	R
Sulfonamides	I	Cromolyn	R
Penicillins	I	Niridazole	R
Methotrexate	I	Gold salts	R
Imipramine	I	Chlorpromazine	R
Chlorpropamide	R	Naproxen	R
Carbamazepine	R	Sulindac	R
Phenytoin	R	Ibuprofen	R
Mephenesin	R		

[a]Relative frequency of reactions: F, frequent; I, infrequent; R, rare.

TABLE A4–6. Drugs That Induce Pneumonitis and/or Fibrosis

Oxygen	F[a]	Chlorambucil	R
Radiation	F	Melphalan	R
Bleomycin	F	Lomustine and semustine	R
Busulfan	F	Zinostatin	R
Carmustine	F	Procarbazine	R
Hexamethonium	F	Teniposide	R
Paraquat	F	Sulfasalazine	R
Amiodarone	F	Phenytoin	R
Mecamylamine	I	Gold salts	R
Pentolinium	I	Pindolol	R
Cyclophosphamide	I	Imipramine	R
Practolol	I	Penicillamine	R
Methotrexate	I	Phenylbutazone	R
Mitomycin	I	Chlorphentermine	R
Nitrofurantoin	I	Fenfluramine	R
Methysergide	I		
Azathioprine, 6-mercaptopurine	R		

[a]Relative frequency of reactions: F, frequent; I, infrequent; R, rare.

TABLE A4–7. Possible Causes of Pulmonary Fibrosis

Idiopathic pulmonary fibrosis (fibrosing alveolitis)
Pneumoconiosis (asbestosis, silicosis, coal dust, talc berylliosis)
Hypersensitivity pneumonitis (molds, bacteria, animal proteins, toluene diisocyanate, epoxy resins)
Smoking
Sarcoidosis
Tuberculosis
Lipoid pneumonia
Systemic lupus erythematosus
Rheumatoid arthritis
Systemic sclerosis
Polymyositis/dermatomyositis
Sjögren's syndrome
Polyarteritis nodosa
Wegener's granuloma
Byssinosis (cotton workers)
Siderosis (arc welders' lung)
Radiation
Oxygen
Chemicals (thioureas, trialkylphosphorothioates, furans)
Drugs (see Tables A4–5, A4–6, and A4–8)

TABLE A4–8. Drugs That May Induce Pleural Effusions and Fibrosis

Idiopathic	
Methysergide	F[a]
Practolol	F
Pindolol	R
Methotrexate	R
Nitrofurantoin	R
Owing to Drug-Induced Lupus Syndrome	
Procainamide	F
Hydralazine	F
Isoniazid	R
Phenytoin	R
Mephenytoin	R
Griseofulvin	R
Trimethadione	R
Sulfonamides	R
Phenylbutazone	R
Streptomycin	R
Ethosuximide	R
Tetracycline	R
Pseudolymphoma Syndrome	
Cyclosporine	R
Phenytoin	R

[a]Relative frequency of reactions: F, frequent; I, infrequent; R, rare.

See Chapter 29, Drug-Induced Pulmonary Diseases, authored by Hengameh H. Raissy, Michelle Harkins, and Patricia L. Marshik, for a more detailed discussion of this topic.

▶ DRUG-INDUCED RENAL DISEASE

TABLE A5–1. Drug-Induced Renal Structural–Functional Alterations and Examples

Tubular epithelial cell damage
Acute tubular necrosis
- Aminoglycoside antibiotics
- Radiographic contrast media
- Cisplatin/carboplatin
- Amphotericin B
Osmotic nephrosis
- Mannitol
- Dextran
- Intravenous immunoglobulin

Hemodynamically mediated renal failure
- Angiotensin-converting enzyme inhibitors
- Angiotensin II receptor antagonists
- Nonsteroidal anti-inflammatory drugs

Obstructive nephropathy
Intratubular obstruction
- Acyclovir
- Sulfadiazine
- Indinavir
- Foscarnet
- Methotrexate
Extrarenal obstruction
- Tricyclic antidepressants
- Indinavir
Nephrolithiasis
- Triamterene

Glomerular Disease
- Gold
- Nonsteroidal anti-inflammatory drugs
- Pamidronate

Tubulointerstitial disease
Acute allergic interstitial nephritis
- Penicillins
- Ciprofloxacin
- Nonsteroidal anti-inflammatory drugs
- Omeprazole
- Furosemide
Chronic interstitial nephritis
- Cyclosporine
- Lithium
- Aristolochic acid
Papillary necrosis
- Combined phenacetin, aspirin, and caffeine analgesics

Renal vasculitis, thrombosis, and cholesterol emboli
Vasculitis and thrombosis
- Hydralazine
- Propylthiouracil
- Allopurinol
- Penicillamine
- Gemcitabine
- Mitomycin
- Methamphetamines
Cholesterol emboli
- Warfarin
- Thrombolytic agents

Pseudo–renal failure
- Corticosteroids
- Trimethoprim
- Cimetidine

TABLE A5–2. Potential Risk Factors for Aminoglycoside Nephrotoxicity

A. Related to aminoglycoside dosing:
   Large total cumulative dose
   Prolonged therapy
   Trough concentration exceeding 2 mg/L
   Recent previous aminoglycoside therapy
B. Related to synergistic nephrotoxicity. Aminoglycosides in combination with:
   Cyclosporine
   Amphotericin B
   Vancomycin
   Diuretics
C. Related to predisposing conditions in the patient:
   Preexisting renal insufficiency
   Increased age
   Poor nutrition
   Shock
   Gram-negative bacteremia
   Liver disease
   Hypoalbuminemia
   Obstructive jaundice
   Dehydration
   Potassium or magnesium deficiencies

TABLE A5–3. Drugs Associated with Allergic Interstitial Nephritis

Antimicrobials	Nonsteroidal anti-inflammatory drugs
Acyclovir	Aspirin
Aminoglycosides	Indomethacin
Amphotericin B	Naproxen
Aztreonam	Ibuprofen
Cephalosporins	Diflunisal
Ciprofloxacin	Piroxicam
Erythromycin	Ketoprofen
Ethambutol	Phenylbutazone
Indinavir	Diclofenac
Penicillins	Zomepirac
Rifampin	**Miscellaneous**
Sulfonamides	Acetaminophen
Tetracyclines	Allopurinol
Trimethoprim-sulfamethoxazole	Interferon-alfa
Vancomycin	Aspirin
Diuretics	Azathioprine
Acetazolamide	Captopril
Amiloride	Cimetidine
Chlorthalidone	Clofibrate
Furosemide	Cyclosporine
Triamterene	Glyburide
Thiazides	Gold
Neuropsychiatric	Methyldopa
Carbamazepine	Omeprazole
Lithium	*para*-aminosalicylic acid
Phenobarbital	Phenylpropanolamine
Phenytoin	Propylthiouracil
Valproic acid	Radiographic contrast media
	Ranitidine
	Sulfinpyrazone
	Warfarin sodium

See Chapter 46, Drug-Induced Kidney Disease, authored by Thomas D. Nolin, Jonathan Himmelfarb, and Gary R. Matzke, for a more detailed discussion of this topic.

Note: Page numbers followed by *t* refer to tables; page numbers followed by *f* refer to figures.

Index

Index

Index

Index

Index

Index

Index

Ketoprofen (cont.)
  for OA, 11*t*
  pharmacokinetics of, 551*t*
  for rheumatoid arthritis, 33*t*
  side effects of, 553*t*
Ketorolac
  dosage of, 552*t*
  for migraine, 538
  for OA, 11*t*
  pharmacokinetics of, 551*t*
  side effects of, 553*t*
Kidney disease. *See also* Chronic kidney
      disease
  end-stage, 781
    effect on nonrenal clearance, 797
    treatment of, 785–787
  progressive
    treatment of, 782–783

L

LAAM. *See* L-methadyl acetate
      hydrochloride (LAAM)
Labetolol
  for hypertension, 104*t*, 114
  for hypertension in pregnancy, 315
Labor
  analgesia, 321
  and delivery, 319–321
  induction of, 320–321
  preterm, 319–320
    antenatal glucocorticoids for, 320
    betamethasone for, 320
    tocolytic therapy for, 319–320
Lactated Ringer's solution, 131
Lactation
  drugs used during, 321
  with haloperidol, 739
Lactobacillus
  for diarrhea, 226
Lactulose
  for constipation, 218, 219
  dosages of, 218*t*
  for hepatic encephalopathy, 214
Lamivudine
  pharmacologic parameters of, 398*t*
Lamotrigine
  adverse effects of, 523*t*, 524
  for bipolar disorder, 695*t*, 699*t*–700*t*,
      703*t*
  drug interactions with, 525*t*
  for epilepsy, 530
  for epilepsy with pregnancy, 519
  for posttraumatic stress disorder, 679*t*
  serum ranges, 529*t*
Lansoprazole
  for gastroesophageal reflux disease,
      231–234, 233*t*, 234, 235
  for peptic ulcer disease, 278*t*
Laparoscopic surgery
  infection, 480
Latanoprost
  for closed-angle glaucoma, 651
  for glaucoma, 653*t*
Latent syphilis, 452

Latent tuberculosis
  treatment of, 485*t*
Laxatives
  abusers, 217
  dosages of, 218*t*
  emollient
    for constipation, 219
    dosages of, 218*t*
LDL. *See* Low-density lipoprotein (LDL)
Lean body mass
  albumin, 585*t*
  visceral proteins assessing, 585*t*
Leflunomide
  for rheumatoid arthritis, 29, 31*t*, 32*t*
Left ventricular (LV) hypertrophy
  regression from hypertension, 115
Left ventricular (LV) reserve, 121
Lente
  for diabetes mellitus, 191
Lepirudin
  for venous thromboembolism, 151, 152
Leptin
  effect on food intake, 599*t*
Lesch-Nyhan syndrome, 1
Letrozole
  for breast cancer, 619, 619*t*
Leucovorin
  adjuvant
    for colon cancer, 626*t*
  for colorectal cancer, 624
Leukopenia
  transient, 738
Leukotriene modifiers
  for asthma, 838
Leuprolide
  for benign prostatic hyperplasia, 850
  for breast cancer, 618, 619*t*
  for prostate cancer, 646
Levalbuterol
  for acute severe exacerbations of asthma,
      834*t*
  for chronic obstructive pulmonary disease,
      844
Levamisole
  for colorectal cancer, 624–625
Levetiracetam
  adverse effects of, 523*t*
  for bipolar disorder, 703*t*
  drug interactions with, 525*t*, 526
  for epilepsy, 530–531
Levitra. *See* Vardenafil (Levitra)
Levobunolol
  for glaucoma, 652*t*
Levocabastine (Livostin), 821
Levodopa
  for Parkinson's disease, 565–566
Levofloxacin, 497*t*
  for acute bacterial sinusitis, 438*t*
  for acute uncomplicated cystitis, 495
  for bacterial pneumonia, 429*t*
  for chronic bronchitis, 422*t*
  for chronic obstructive pulmonary disease,
      848
  dosages of, 489*t*
  for lower urinary tract infection, 498*t*
  for prostatitis, 503

Index

Loxapine
  for schizophrenia
    dosage of, 728*t*
LSD. *See* Lysergic acid diethylamide (LSD)
Lubricants
  for constipation, 219
Lunelle, 287*t*, 301–302
Lung cancer, 630–634
  clinical presentation of, 630
  definition of, 630
  diagnosis of, 630–631
  non-small cell
    chemotherapy of, 631–633
    combination regimens for, 632*t*–632*t*
    treatment of, 631–633
  pathophysiology of, 630
  small cell
    chemotherapy of, 633–634
    radiation therapy of, 633
    surgery of, 633
    treatment of, 633–634
  staging of, 631
  treatment of, 631–633
LV hypertrophy. *See* Left ventricular (LV)
    hypertrophy
LV reserve. *See* Left ventricular (LV) reserve
Lymphocyte
  total count, 584
Lymphogranuloma venereum
  treatment of, 461*t*
Lymphoma, 635–642. *See also*
    Non-Hodgkin's lymphoma
  definition of, 635
  follicular
    treatment of, 640–641
Lysergic acid diethylamide (LSD), 757–758

M

Maalox
  for gastroesophageal reflux disease, 232*t*
Macrolide
  for acute otitis media, 432
  interacting with antimicrobials, 341*t*
  for pneumonia, 428*t*
  for sickle cell disease, 332
Magnesium
  with cardiopulmonary resuscitation, 68
  dosage of, 552*t*
Magnesium citrate
  for acute pancreatitis, 270
  dosages of, 218*t*
Magnesium homeostasis disorders, 815–816
Magnesium hydroxide
  dosages of, 218*t*
Magnesium salicylate
  pharmacokinetics of, 551*t*
  side effects of, 553*t*
Magnesium sulfate
  dosages of, 218*t*
  for hypertension in pregnancy, 315
  osmolarities of, 608*t*
  for preterm labor, 320
  for Torsades de pointes, 62
Major depression
  treatment of, 723*f*

Major depressive episode, 682
  DSM-IV-TR criteria for, 707*t*
Major histocompatibility complex (MHC), 27
Malnutrition
  with chronic kidney disease, 793
Mania
  secondary causes of, 681*t*
Manic-depressive illness. *See* Bipolar disorder
Manic episode, 682
Mannitol
  for acute renal failure, 777, 778
  for closed-angle glaucoma, 651
Manometry
  esophageal
    for gastroesophageal reflux disease, 229
MAP. *See* Mean arterial pressure (MAP)
Maprotiline
  adverse effects of, 712
  for depressive disorder, 712
    dosages for, 709*t*
  drug interactions with, 719*t*
  pharmacokinetics of, 715*t*
  side effects of, 710*t*
Marijuana, 756–757
  intoxication, 758
    treatment of, 759*t*
Mastitis
  postpartum, 321
Mazindol
  for obesity, 601
MDA. *See* Methylenedioxy-amphetamine
    (MDA)
Mean arterial pressure (MAP), 75, 114, 130*t*,
    137
Mean pulmonary artery pressure (MPAP),
    130*t*
Measles
  children immunization schedule, 505*t*–506*t*
  immunization schedule for, 507*t*–509*t*
  vaccine, 512
Mechlorethamine
  emetogenicity of, 259*t*
Mechlorethamine, vincristine (MOPP)
  for Hodgkin's disease, 637
  for non-Hodgkin's lymphoma, 638*t*
Meclizine
  during pregnancy, 265
Meclofenamate (Meclomen)
  for acute gouty arthritis, 4*t*
  dosage of, 552*t*
  for osteoarthritis, 11*t*
  pharmacokinetics of, 551*t*
  for rheumatoid arthritis, 33*t*
  side effects of, 553*t*
Meclomen. *See* Meclofenamate (Meclomen)
Medium-chain triglycerides, 96
Medroxyprogesterone acetate, 306, 307
  for breast cancer, 619*t*
  for central sleep apnea, 747
  for endometrial protection, 307*t*
  for obstructive sleep apnea, 747
Mefenamic acid
  dosage of, 552*t*
  for osteoarthritis, 11*t*
  pharmacokinetics of, 551*t*
  side effects of, 553*t*

Index

Methimazole
for thyroid disorders with pregnancy, 319
Methotrexate (MTX)
for asthma, 839
for Crohn's disease, 255
for diffuse large B-cell lymphoma, 641
for early breast cancer, 616
emetogenicity of, 259t
for inflammatory bowel disease, 251
during pregnancy, 313
for prostate cancer, 648
for psoriasis, 171t, 172
for rheumatoid arthritis, 29, 30, 31t, 32t
for small cell lung cancer, 634
Methsuximide
serum ranges, 529t
Methylbutyl ketone, 758
Methylcellulose
dosages of, 218t
Methyldopa
for hypertension, 104t, 109
for hypertension in pregnancy, 315
interactions with oral contraceptives, 299t
Methylene chloride, 758
Methylenedioxy-amphetamine (MDA), 757
Methylethyl ketone, 758
Methylphenidate
for narcolepsy, 748, 748t
Methylprednisolone, 835t
for diffuse large B-cell lymphoma, 642
Methylprednisolone acetate
for rheumatoid arthritis, 36
Methyltestosterone (Oreton, Android)
for erectile dysfunction, 857t
for osteoporosis, 25
Methylxanthines
for asthma, 836
for chronic obstructive pulmonary disease,
845–846
Methysergide
for migraine, 544t, 546
Metipranolol
for glaucoma, 652t
Metoclopramide
for acute migraine, 537, 541t
with enteral nutrition, 591
for gastroesophageal reflux disease, 235
for headache with pregnancy, 316
for nausea and vomiting, 263
during pregnancy, 265
for relactation, 321
Metolazone
for acute renal failure, 779
for heart failure, 79
Metoprolol
for acute coronary syndrome, 46
for dystonia, 733
for heart failure, 76
for hypertension, 103t, 107
for migraine, 544, 544t
Metronidazole
for cholangitis, 417t
for Crohn's disease, 254
for dermatologic conditions with
pregnancy, 317
for enterotoxigenic diarrhea, 386t

for *Helicobacter pylori*, 278t
for hepatic encephalopathy, 214
interacting with antimicrobials, 341t
for peptic ulcer disease, 276
for toxic megacolon, 256
for trichomoniasis, 460t, 462
Mexiletine
for arrhythmias, 54, 55t
side effects of, 57t
MHC. *See* Major histocompatibility complex
(MHC)
MI. *See* Myocardial infarction (MI)
Micronized estradiol, 305t
for menopause, 306t
Micronized progesterone, 306
for endometrial protection, 307t
Micronutrients
requirements, 588
Midazolam
for GCSE, 577t
for refractory GCSE, 579, 580t
for status epilepticus, 576
Midrin
for migraine, 539
Migraine
acetaminophen for, 538, 539
acute
pharmacologic treatment of, 537–538
treatment of, 540t
clinical presentation of, 535–536
definition of, 535
diagnostic tests, 536–537
laboratory tests, 536–537
nonpharmacologic treatment, 537
with oral contraceptives, 291
pathophysiology of, 535
pharmacologic prophylaxis of, 543–544
precipitating factors associated with, 539f
public health, 544t, 545f
signs of, 536
symptoms of, 535–536
treatment algorithm for, 538f
treatment of, 537–548
Milk of magnesia
for constipation, 218, 219, 220
Milrinone
for heart failure, 82–83
hemodynamic effects of, 82t
MINE. *See* Mesna, ifosfamide, mitoxantrone,
etoposide (MINE)
Mineral oil
for constipation, 219
dosages of, 218t
Minimally invasive surgery
infection, 480
Minipills
progestin-only, 290, 297
as emergency contraceptives, 300
Minocycline
for acne, 163–164
for chronic bronchitis, 422t
for rheumatoid arthritis, 30
for urinary tract infection, 496t
Mirapex. *See* Pramipexole (Mirapex)
Mirtazapine
adverse effects of, 713

Index

Index

Index

Index

Pyrazinamide (cont.)
  for reduced renal function or hemodialysis,
    491*t*
  for tuberculosis in pregnancy, 490
  for tuberculous meningitis, 490
Pyridoxine
  during pregnancy, 265
Pyridoxine hydrochloride
  for *Mycobacterium tuberculosis,* 353
Pyrilamine
  for insomnia, 744
Pyrimethamine
  for toxoplasmic encephalitis with HIV, 402*t*
Pyrimidine
  for metastatic colorectal cancer, 627*t*

Q

Quality of Life (QOL) questionnaire, 14
Quazepam
  adverse effects of, 746
  for insomnia, 746
  pharmacokinetics of, 745*t*
Questionnaire
  quality of Life (QOL), 14
Quetiapine (Seroquel)
  for Alzheimer's disease, 661
  for bipolar disorder, 689, 698*t*, 703*t*
  for dementia, 661*t*
  for dystonia, 733
  for galactorrhea, 737
  for Parkinson's disease, 568
  pharmacokinetics of, 730*t*
  for posttraumatic stress disorder, 680
  for schizophrenia, 729
    dosage of, 728*t*
Quinapril
  for heart failure, 75*t*
  for hypertension, 103*t*
Quinidine
  for arrhythmias, 54, 55*t*
  effect on renal insufficiency, 796
  side effects of, 57*t*
  for ventricular tachycardia, 61
Quinolone, 497*t*
  interacting with antimicrobials, 341*t*
  for sickle cell disease, 332
Quinupristin
  intraventricular and intrathecal dosage
    recommendation, 351*t*

R

RA. *See* Rheumatoid arthritis (RA)
Rabeprazole
  for gastroesophageal reflux disease,
    231–234, 233*t*, 234, 236
  for peptic ulcer disease, 278*t*
Radiation-induced nausea and vomiting
  (RINV), 264
Radioactive iodine
  for thyrotoxicosis, 201
Raloxifene, 308, 310
  for osteoporosis, 23
  risks of, 310
Ramipril
  for acute coronary syndrome, 50

  for heart failure, 75*t*
  for hypertension, 103*t*
Ranitidine
  disposition during dialysis, 802*t*
  for gastroesophageal reflux disease, 231,
    232*t*, 233*t*
  for peptic ulcer disease, 278*t*
RAS. *See* Renin-angiotensin-aldosterone
    system (RAS)
Rebleeding prevention
  with acute variceal hemorrhage, 211
Receptor activity of
  dobutamine, 444
  epinephrine, 444
Receptors
  effect on food intake, 599*t*
Recombinant human insulin
  for gestational diabetes mellitus, 315
Rectal cancer
  adjuvant therapy of, 626, 626*t*
  neoadjuvant therapy of, 626
Rectal exam
  digital
    for prostate cancer, 643
REE. *See* Resting energy expenditure (REE)
Refractory GCSE, 579
Refractory patients
  antidepressants, 722
Refractory PVT alternatives for
  CPR, 68
Refractory VF alternatives for
  CPR, 68
Regional anesthesia, 559
Rehydralyte, 226*t*
Rehydration therapy of
  gastrointestinal infection, 383
Relactation, 321
Reminyl. *See* Galantamine (Reminyl)
Renal diseases
  in diabetics
    prevention of, 783*f*
  drug-induced, 885*t*
  etiology of, 112
  preventing progression of, 784*f*
Renal failure. *See also* Acute renal failure;
    Chronic kidney disease
  with bipolar disorder, 693*t*
  with tuberculosis, 490, 491*t*
Renal function
  with drugs, 799*t*
Renal insufficiency
  dextropropoxyphene, 796
  dihydrocodeine, 796
  drug dosage regimen designs, 797
  drug dosing in, 796–802
  effect on drug absorption, 796
  effect on drug distribution, 796
  effect on renal excretion, 797
  metabolic effect, 796–797
Renal osteodystrophy, 789–790
Renal replacement therapy, 777
  continuous, 777, 800
RenAmine
  in parenteral nutrition, 608
Renin-angiotensin-aldosterone system (RAS),
    99

Index

Index

Index